PEDIATRIC NEUROLOGY

FOR THE CLINICIAN

PEDIATRIC NEUROLOGY

FOR THE CLINICIAN

EDITED BY

Ronald B. David, MD
Children's Neurological Services

Associate Clinical Professor of Pediatrics
Medical College of Virginia
Virginia Commonwealth University
Richmond, Virginia

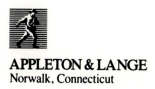

APPLETON & LANGE
Norwalk, Connecticut

Copyright ©1992 by Appleton & Lange
Simon & Schuster Business and Professional Group

92 93 94 95 96 / 10 9 8 7 6 5 4 3 2 1

Prentice Hall International (UK) Limited, *London*
Prentice Hall of Australia Pty. Limited, *Sydney*
Prentice Hall Canada Inc., *Toronto*
Prentice Hall Hispanoamericana, S.A., *Mexico*
Prentice Hall of India Private Limited, *New Delhi*
Prentice Hall of Japan, Inc., *Tokyo*
Simon & Schuster Asia Pte. Ltd., *Singapore*
Editora Prentice Hall do Brasil, Ltda., *Rio de Janeiro*
Prentice Hall, *Englewood Cliffs, New Jersey*

Library of Congress Cataloging-in-Publication Data

Pediatric neurology for the clinician / edited by Ronald B. David.
    p. cm.
  Includes bibliographical references.
  ISBN 0-8385-7905-1
  1. Pediatric neurology. I. David, Ronald B.
  [DNLM: 1. Nervous System Diseases—diagnosis. 2. Nervous System Diseases—in infancy & childhood. 3. Nervous System Diseases—therapy. WS 340 P3697]
  RJ486.P345 1992
  618.92'8—dc20
  DNLM/DLC
  for Library of Congress   91-17215

Designer: Michael J. Kelly

ISBN 0-8385-7905-1

PRINTED IN THE UNITED STATES OF AMERICA

To Candace,
to the children, Bryan, Susan, Elizabeth, Whitney, Thomas, and Jennifer,
and to all children who inspired and encouraged this effort.

Contributors

Richard J. Allen, MD
Professor
Director, Pediatric Neurology Metabolic Clinic
Section of Pediatric Neurology
Department of Pediatrics and Neurology
University of Michigan Medical School
Ann Arbor, Michigan

Russell A. Barkley, PhD
Professor
Psychiatry Department
University of Massachusetts Medical Center
Worcester, Massachusetts

Johan G. Blickman, MD, PhD
Assistant Professor
Department of Radiology
Harvard Medical School
Associate Radiologist
Acting Director, Division of Pediatric Radiology
Department of Radiology
Massachusetts General Hospital
Boston, Massachusetts

Warren T. Blume, MD, CM
Professor
Co-Director, Epilepsy Unit, University Hospital
Division of Neurology
Department of Clinical Neurological Sciences
University of Western Ontario
London, Ontario, Canada

John Bodensteiner, MD
Professor
Division of Pediatric Neurology
Departments of Neurology and Pediatrics
West Virginia University School of Medicine
Morgantown, West Virginia

Raymond W.M. Chun, MD
Professor
Division of Child Neurology
Department of Neurology
University of Wisconsin Hospitals
Madison, Wisconsin

Michael E. Cohen, MD
Professor and Chair
Department of Neurology
State University of New York at Buffalo
  School of Medicine
Buffalo, New York

Ronald B. David, MD
Children's Neurological Services
Associate Clinical Professor of Pediatrics
Medical College of Virginia
Virginia Commonwealth University
Richmond, Virginia

Ruthmary K. Deuel, MD
Professor
Departments of Pediatrics and Neurology
Washington University School of Medicine
St. Louis, Missouri

Patricia K. Duffner, MD
Professor and Associate Director
Division of Child Neurology
School of Medicine and Biomedical Sciences
State University of New York at Buffalo
Buffalo, New York

Paul R. Dyken, MD
Professor and Chairman
Pediatric Neurology
University of South Alabama
Mobile, Alabama

Patricia Ellison, MD
Professor
Department of Pediatrics
University of Colorado Health Sciences Center
Denver, Colorado

Pauline A. Filipek, MD
Instructor
Department of Neurology
Harvard Medical School
Assistant in Neurology
Division of Pediatric Neurology
Department of Neurology
Massachusetts General Hospital
Boston, Massachusetts

Marvin A. Fishman, MD
Professor
Division of Pediatric Neurology
Departments of Pediatrics and Neurology
Baylor College of Medicine
Chief, Neurology Service
Texas Children's Hospital
Houston, Texas

Richard H. Haas, MB, BChir
Associate Professor
Division of Pediatric Neurology
Department of Neurosciences
University of California, San Diego,
   School of Medicine
La Jolla, California

Jerome S. Haller, MD
Professor
Chief, Section of Pediatric Neurology
Department of Neurology
Albany Medical College
Albany, New York

Deborah G. Hirtz, MD
Medical Officer
Developmental Neurology Branch
National Institute of Neurological Disorders
   and Stroke
National Institutes of Health
Bethesda, Maryland

Gregory L. Holmes, MD
Director of Clinical Neurophysiology
Associate Professor of Neurology
Harvard Medical School
Children's Hospital
Boston, Massachusetts

H. Terry Hutchison, MD, PhD
Assistant Clinical Professor
Division of Pediatrics and Neurology
University of California, San Francisco,
   School of Medicine
San Francisco, California
Fresno-San Joaquin Teaching Program
Associate Medical Director
Rehabilitation Center
Valley Children's Hospital
Fresno, California

Diane Koch, PhD
Assistant Professor of Psychology in Pediatrics
University of South Florida School of Medicine
Tampa, Florida

Nancy L. Kuntz, MD
Assistant Professor
Division of Pediatric Neurology
Department of Pediatrics
John A. Burns School of Medicine
University of Hawaii
Honolulu, Hawaii

Diane Kurtzberg, PhD
Professor
Department of Neuroscience and Neurology
Rose F. Kennedy Center for Research in Mental
   Retardation and Human Development
Albert Einstein College of Medicine
Bronx, New York

Nicholas J. Lenn, MD, PhD
Professor
Division of Pediatric Neurology
Departments of Neurology and Pediatrics
State University of New York at Stony Brook
   Health Sciences Center
Stony Brook, New York

Paul Maertens, MD
Assistant Professor
Division of Child Neurology
Department of Neurology
University of South Alabama College of Medicine
Mobile, Alabama

Mary B. McMurray, MB, ChB
Associate Professor
Division of General Pediatrics
Department of Pediatrics
University of Massachusetts Medical Center
Worcester, Massachusetts

Ruth D. Nass, MD
Associate Professor of Neurology
New York University Medical Center
New York, New York

Karin B. Nelson, MD
Medical Officer
Neuroepidemiology Branch
National Institute of Neurological Disorders
    and Stroke
National Institutes of Health
Bethesda, Maryland

William L. Nyhan, MD, PhD
Professor
Division of Biochemical Genetics
Department of Pediatrics
University of California, San Diego,
    School of Medicine
La Jolla, California

Peter B. Rosenberger, MD
Assistant Professor
Department of Neurology
Harvard Medical School
Neurologist and Associate Pediatrician
Massachusetts General Hospital
Boston, Massachusetts

Barry S. Russman, MD
Professor
Division of Pediatric Neurology
Departments of Pediatrics and Neurology
University of Connecticut School of Medicine
Farmington, Connecticut
Chief, Pediatric Neurology
Division of Pediatric Neurology
Department of Pediatrics and Neurology
Newington Children's Hospital
Newington, Connecticut

Debora L. Scheffel, PhD
Assistant Professor
Special Education
Fort Hays State University
Hays, Kansas

Steven M. Shapiro, MD
Assistant Professor
Division of Child Neurology
Department of Neurology
Virginia Commonwealth University Medical College
    of Virginia School of Medicine
Richmond, Virginia

Shawke Soueidan, MD
Clinical Associate
Neuromuscular Division
National Institutes of Neurological Disorders
    and Stroke
National Institutes of Health
Bethesda, Maryland

Daniel W. Stowens, MD
Pediatric Neurologist
Children's Neurological Services
Richmond, Virginia

Doris A. Trauner, MD
Professor
Departments of Neurosciences and Pediatrics
University of California, San Diego,
    School of Medicine
La Jolla, California
Chief, Division of Pediatric Neurology
University of California, San Diego, Medical Center
San Diego, California

Contents

List of Pearls and Perils

List of Feature Tables

Introduction

Pediatric Neurology for the Clinician is for the physician, non-physician, student, resident, fellow, or professional of any discipline caring for a child with a neurologic disease or disorder. It is designed to be "user friendly" and "user helpful." It is divided into three sections: Pediatric Neurologic Evaluation, General Pediatric Neurologic Diseases and Disorders, and Common Pediatric Neurologic Problems: An Approach to Understanding, Diagnosis, and Treatment.

The first section provides the clinician with the tools for diagnosis. The second section is organized along the lines of a traditional disease and disorder textbook. It is designed principally to provide a rapid review of the subject matter to enable the clinician to answer quickly a parent's or professional colleague's question. The annotated bibliographies will enable the reader to access the best and most pertinent literature concerning a disorder or group of disorders, thereby extending the scope of the text. In combination with these selected citations, the text provides ample information for lectures, journal clubs, or an in-depth review of a disease or disorder. The additional, longer reference lists and bibliographies are designed to extend the text into a complete, although not thoroughly exhaustive, review of the subject matter.

The third section of the book provides a review of common pediatric neurologic disorders. These conditions may not generally be referred for subspecialty opinion. The section is therefore designed to round out and bolster the knowledge of the treating clinician.

The *Pearls and Perils* sections (see the list on p. xiii) throughout the book are a unique feature of this text. These collected bits of wisdom are presented to highlight the information provided and suggest appropriate cautions. They include not only diagnostic pearls and perils but also treatment pearls and perils.

The *Feature Tables* (see the list on p. xvii) are offered to make the text a diagnostic manual. Because of their importance they deserve further discussion. Classification science is important to medicine. Medical classification systems not only produce an orderliness in thinking, but also enhance one's ability to communicate effectively. A review of the medical classification systems of the last 2000 years, emphasizing those with the greatest utility and longevity, produced the following observations: the successful classification system should be simple, should group entities according to clearly discriminating features, and should be expandable and dynamic. Today's consistent feature may prove to be tomorrow's discriminating feature.

Classification domains in medicine usually are organized according to one of the following schema:

1. Anatomically, by the site of origin of the disorder.
2. Pathologically, by the gross or microscopic pathologic anatomy, revealed by either traditional pathologic study or imaging.
3. Pathophysiologically, by demonstrating altered chemical or electrophysiologic parameters.
4. Phenomenologically, by listing commonly agreed on observations and distinguishing between entities based on these observations (the best example of this would be the clinical classification of the epilepsies).
5. Etiologically, by cause.

It is this observer's belief that much of the confusion that arises in diagnosis is due to the clinician who crosses classification domains: for example, the frequent inclusion of anatomically oriented "temporal lobe seizures" in a phenomenologically based classification system that includes partial complex seizures.

Some conditions (e.g., pathologically classified brain tumors) lend themselves well to classification. Others (e.g., phenomenologically classified headaches and movement disorders) lend themselves much less well. Etiologic discriminators are the best and most powerful but are less commonly available. The goal, regardless of classification domain, is to seek the most powerful discriminating features that will produce the greatest diagnostic clarity. How well this is accomplished in this text reveals the state of the art in pediatric neurology. In some areas, it is easy to speak of a single discriminant. In other areas, several features, when clustered together, serve to discriminate. In still other areas, disriminators must include inclusionary as well as exclusionary features. Finally, at times we are left merely to design tables that compare features, for a discriminating feature should avoid crossing domains. Somewhat arbitrarily consistent features occur more than 75% of the time; variable, less than 75%. The feature tables should be viewed, therefore, only as a beginning in the extremely difficult effort to make diagnosis more precise.

There are other efforts made to facilitate the clinician's use of this text. These include lists of the *Feature Tables* and *Pearls and Perils* tables. A separate alphabetized listing of annotated references is also included. In the index an effort has been made to reduce the need for looking in several places for page citations. History and examination forms are available for clinical use and can be copied without the permission of the author or publisher.

It is my hope that this text will provoke new thinking, help solidify and enhance our decision-making, and perhaps even provoke new insights and questions on the part of those who will come after us. It is my fondest wish that, as you become closely acquainted with this text, it more often finds a place on your desk than on your bookshelf.

Ronald B. David
Richmond
March 1992

Acknowledgments

No singular effort can develop a text. No one contribution rises above another and the order of acknowledgment does not indicate the relative importance or contribution. Inevitably, it is principally and primarily the creative effort of the chapter authors. This text is the result of a truly cooperative effort. Without the knowledge and experience of these dedicated professionals, a portion of whose life's work is represented in the various chapters, we could not have developed this vehicle with which to sharpen and crystallize our search for knowledge in the diagnosis and treatment of neurologic diseases and disorders in children.

I would first like to acknowledge the valuable contribution of Mary Page, without whose editorial assistance this effort would not have been possible. My appreciation is extended to Dr. Peggy Ferry for her careful review of the manuscript, to the professional staff of Children's Neurological Services who taught me the meaning of interdisciplinary effort, and to the support staff at Children's Neurological Services, particularly Emma Bowery and Nancy Satterwhite, who always seemed to have the additional time and willingness to make this effort possible. Appreciation is extended to our interdisciplinary board and counsel including Drs. William Miller and John Nagle and M. Bruce Stokes, Esq.

A special acknowledgment is extended to Drs. Robin Morris, Jack Fletcher, Isabelle Rapin, Doris Allen, Dorothy Aram, Lynn Waterhouse, Deborah Fine, and Tera Yoder, who not only broadened my knowledge in the area of higher cortical function in children, but who developed and expanded my knowledge in classification science. The editor's collaboration with this group was only possible because of the support received from the Neurological Institute (N.I.N.D.S., Grant number [PO] NS20489–01A1). Acknowledgment is also extended to Drs. Sally and Bennett Shaywitz who sparked this effort and to the publishing team at Appleton & Lange, including Craig Percy, John Williams, and Edward Wickland, whose patient encouragement brought it to fulfillment.

Lastly, I would like to acknowledge the contribution of the pediatric and family practice communities of Richmond and Tidewater Virginia from whom I learned what is truly important to the clinician and how a text could speak to their needs. In this regard, I would particularly like to thank my close and trusted pediatrician friend, Dr. Grover Robinson, who, over a span of more than ten years, has served as a thoughtful and honest critic.

PEDIATRIC NEUROLOGY

FOR THE CLINICIAN

Section I

Pediatric Neurologic Evaluation

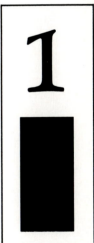

Chapter One

Neurologic History

Ronald B. David

Some clinicians have suggested that the taking of the neurologic history is as important as or potentially more important than the neurologic examination itself. Other clinicians have suggested that the neurologic history identifies the nature of the disorder or disease and the neurologic examination pinpoints its location. The history itself may be a narrative recapitulation of information provided by a child's primary caregiver(s) or it may be generated in response to a questionnaire or checklist. Experienced clinicians realize that the key to making a successful diagnosis often lies in asking the right questions and listening carefully to the answers. Responses to questionnaires or checklists can be used as part of a formal structured interview. They can be both reliable and valid diagnostically. For example, a patient may be queried with respect to headaches: (1) Are your head-

aches confined to one side of your head? (2) Are your headaches associated with vomiting or desire to sleep? (3) Do you have visual symptoms, such as dancing lights or other phenomena? A ''yes'' response to all three questions would permit accuracy of close to 100% for the diagnosis of migraine. No other questions or laboratory investigations may be necessary. Other questions provide clinical rather than diagnostic information, useful in practicing the art as well as the science of medicine. The questions that follow are those used by many clinicians to accomplish this end. Some are also valuable in answering research questions. They are all designed to be useful in the practice of pediatric neurology. *Note:* This form may be reproduced for clinical use without further permission from the author or publisher.

NEUROLOGIC HISTORY

A. Demographic and Family Data

1. Name _____

2. Date of birth: __ __ / __ __ / __ __

3. Age (years/months): __ __ / __ __

4. Sex:

   a. Male ___

   b. Female ___

5. Race:

   a. Caucasian ___

   b. Black ___

   c. Hispanic ___

   d. Oriental ___

   e. Other ___

Neurologic History Form from David RB: *Pediatric Neurology for the Clinician*. Norwalk, Conn: Appleton & Lange, 1992.

6. Birthplace: _____

7. Hospital name: _____

8. Siblings (*oldest first*):

Name	Age (*years, months*)	Sex (*M or F*)	Relation to child (*full, half, adopted, or step*)
_____	_____	_____	_____
_____	_____	_____	_____
_____	_____	_____	_____
_____	_____	_____	_____
_____	_____	_____	_____
_____			

9. Marital status of parents:
    a. Married   ____
    b. Single   ____
    c. Separated   ____
    d. Divorced   ____

10. Relationship of caregiver or individual accompanying child:
    a. Natural parent(s)   ____
    b. Adoptive parent(s)   ____
    c. Stepparent(s)   ____
    d. Foster parent(s)   ____
    e. Grandparent(s)   ____
    f. Aunt or uncle   ____
    g. Brother or sister   ____
    h. Other   _____

11. Parent's highest education experience:

	Father	Mother	Don't know
a. Eighth grade or less (*indicate level, if known*)	____	____	____
b. Attended high school	____	____	____
c. High school graduate	____	____	____
d. Attended college	____	____	____
e. Two-year degree	____	____	____
f. Four-year degree	____	____	____
g. Masters degree	____	____	____
h. Doctoral degree	____	____	____

12. Handedness of parents:

	Father	Mother	Don't know
a. Right	____	____	____
b. Left	____	____	____
c. Ambidexterous to some extent	____	____	____

13. Please check if a parent or blood relative has been
    or is considered to have any of following:

	Father	Mother	Relative
a. Mental retardation	_____	_____	_____
b. Mental illness or nervous breakdown	_____	_____	_____
c. Seizures or convulsions	_____	_____	_____
d. Difficulty walking	_____	_____	_____
e. Delayed or unintelligible speech	_____	_____	_____
f. Confusion of left and right hands	_____	_____	_____
g. Overactivity, restlessness, hyperactivity	_____	_____	_____
h. Being clumsy or awkward	_____	_____	_____
i. Difficulty with math	_____	_____	_____
j. Difficulty with spelling	_____	_____	_____
k. Difficulty with reading	_____	_____	_____
l. Impaired vision	_____	_____	_____
m. Impaired hearing	_____	_____	_____

B. Medical Information/History

1. Please check if your child has ever experienced or done
   any of the following:

	Yes	No	Don't know
a. Ear (myringotomy) tubes	_____	_____	_____
b. Visual difficulty	_____	_____	_____
c. Hearing difficulty	_____	_____	_____
d. Problems requiring the use of special shoes, splints, braces, or a wheelchair	_____	_____	_____
e. Encephalitis (brain fever) or meningitis	_____	_____	_____
f. Failure to thrive	_____	_____	_____
g. Poisoning or drug overdose	_____	_____	_____
h. Eating unusual substances (e.g., paint, plaster)	_____	_____	_____
i. Unconscious spells, fainting	_____	_____	_____
j. Convulsions, seizures, epilepsy	_____	_____	_____
k. Bedwetting beyond the age of 5 years	_____	_____	_____
l. Soiling beyond the age of 3 years	_____	_____	_____
m. Sleeping problems	_____	_____	_____
n. Poor growth or weight gain	_____	_____	_____
o. Unusual reactions to baby shots	_____	_____	_____
p. Toe walking	_____	_____	_____
q. Run or walk more awkwardly than other children	_____	_____	_____
r. Run or walk more slowly than other children	_____	_____	_____
s. Picked last or close to last in games where children pick sides	_____	_____	_____
t. Tics or unusual movements	_____	_____	_____

	Yes	No	Don't know
u. Headaches not relieved by nonprescription pain medicine	_____	_____	_____
v. Headaches not relieved by prescription pain medicine	_____	_____	_____
w. Headaches occurring in the middle of the night or upon awakening	_____	_____	_____
x. Production of unusual odors	_____	_____	_____
y. Unusual habits	_____	_____	_____
z. Difficulty swallowing	_____	_____	_____
aa. Excessive drooling	_____	_____	_____
bb. Poor sucking or feeding as an infant	_____	_____	_____
cc. Lost once-attained skills (speech/language or motor)	_____	_____	_____

2. Has your child ever been diagnosed with

	Yes	No	Don't know
a. Hyperactivity (hyperkinesis)	_____	_____	_____
b. Brain damage	_____	_____	_____
c. Retardation	_____	_____	_____
d. Developmental delay or disability	_____	_____	_____
e. Seizures or convulsions including febrile	_____	_____	_____
f. Motor delay	_____	_____	_____
g. Cerebral palsy	_____	_____	_____
h. Language/speech delay	_____	_____	_____
i. Immaturity	_____	_____	_____
j. Hearing impairment or deafness	_____	_____	_____
k. Blindness or partial sightedness	_____	_____	_____
l. Emotional or behavioral disturbance	_____	_____	_____
m. Hypotonia	_____	_____	_____
n. Spasticity	_____	_____	_____

3. Has your child ever

	Yes	No	Don't know
a. Had a special diet	_____	_____	_____
b. Received speech therapy	_____	_____	_____
c. Attended a preschool special education program	_____	_____	_____
d. Received counseling (family or individual)	_____	_____	_____
e. Been hospitalized overnight	_____	_____	_____
f. Been suspended or discharged or received detention from day care, kindergarten, or school	_____	_____	_____

4. Dates of interventions; speech, occupational, or physical therapy; or special education:

Type of service	Date begun	Date ended
_____	__ __ / __ __ / __ __	__ __ / __ __ / __ __
_____	__ __ / __ __ / __ __	__ __ / __ __ / __ __
_____	__ __ / __ __ / __ __	__ __ / __ __ / __ __

C. Treatment Information

1. Has your child ever been evaluated by a

	Yes	No	Don't know
a. Physician			
(1) Neurologist (child or general)	____	____	____
(2) Pediatrician	____	____	____
(3) Family doctor	____	____	____
(4) Psychiatrist	____	____	____
(5) Psychiatrist (physical medicine or rehabilitation specialist)	____	____	____
b. School psychologist	____	____	____
c. Teacher	____	____	____
d. Special education placement committee	____	____	____
e. Child development specialist	____	____	____
f. Physical or occupational therapist	____	____	____
g. Speech language pathologist	____	____	____

2. Has your child ever taken

	Yes	No	Don't know
a. Phenobarbital	____	____	____
b. Dilantin (phenytoin)	____	____	____
c. Mysoline (primidone)	____	____	____
d. Depakene, Depakote (valproate, valproic acid)	____	____	____
e. Tegretol (carbamazapine)	____	____	____
f. Zarontin (ethosuximide)	____	____	____
g. Valium (diazapam)	____	____	____
h. Haldol (haloperidol)	____	____	____
i. Klonopin or Clonopin (clonazepam)	____	____	____
j. Tofranil (imipramine)	____	____	____
k. Mephobarbital (mebaral)	____	____	____
l. Mellaril (thioridazine)	____	____	____
m. Dexedrine (dextroamphetamine)	____	____	____
n. Ritalin (methylphenidate)	____	____	____
o. Cylert (pemoline)	____	____	____
p. Asthma medication(s)	____	____	____
q. Antihistamine(s)	____	____	____

3. Has your child every had any unusual reactions to any medicine?

	Yes	No	Don't know
	____	____	____

4. Please list the drug and describe the reaction: _____

_____

_____

5. Describe each of your child's hospitalizations. Begin with the most recent.

Age (*years/months*)   Reason

__ __ / __ __   _____

__ __ / __ __   _____

__ __ / __ __   _____

__ __ / __ __   _____

__ __ / __ __   _____

__ __ / __ __   _____

6. Describe each of your child's emergency room visits. Begin with the most recent.

Age (*years/months*)   Reason

__ __ / __ __   _____

__ __ / __ __   _____

__ __ / __ __   _____

__ __ / __ __   _____

__ __ / __ __   _____

__ __ / __ __   _____

D. Pregnancy and Development

1. How many pregnancies has the child's mother had? _____   Don't know _____

2. Has she had any

	Yes	No	Don't know
a. Stillbirths	_____	_____	_____
b. Tubal pregnancies	_____	_____	_____
c. Miscarriages	_____	_____	_____
d. Abortions	_____	_____	_____

3. Were any medicines prescribed during pregnancy with this child, such as

	Yes	No	Don't know
a. Pills for nausea	_____	_____	_____
b. Antibiotics	_____	_____	_____
c. Water pills	_____	_____	_____
d. Pain pills	_____	_____	_____
e. Thyroid medicine	_____	_____	_____
f. Medicine to prevent miscarriage	_____	_____	_____
g. Medicine to suppress appetite	_____	_____	_____
h. Sedatives	_____	_____	_____
i. Tranquilizers	_____	_____	_____
j. Sleeping pills	_____	_____	_____
k. Blood pressure pills	_____	_____	_____
l. Other	_____	_____	_____

Name(s), if known _____

4. Were any of the following used during this
child's pregnancy?

	Yes	No	Don't know
a. Cigarettes	___	___	___
b. Alcohol (beer, wine, or hard liquor)	___	___	___
c. Coffee	___	___	___
d. Medicine that you bought at the drug store	___	___	___
e. Street drugs	___	___	___
(1) Marijuana	___	___	___
(2) Cocaine, crack	___	___	___
(3) Heroin	___	___	___
(4) LSD	___	___	___
(5) Amphetamines	___	___	___
(6) Methadone			

5. Were there any of the following complications during
the mother's pregnancy?

	Yes	No	Don't know
a. Significant abdominal injury	___	___	___
b. Any illness with fever and rashes	___	___	___
c. Diabetes	___	___	___
d. Operation	___	___	___
e. Emotional upset	___	___	___
f. Morning sickness	___	___	___
(1) Requiring special medicine	___	___	___
(2) Requiring hospitalization	___	___	___
g. Rh incompatibility	___	___	___
h. Bleeding from the vagina	___	___	___
i. Staining	___	___	___
j. Anemia	___	___	___
k. Swollen ankles	___	___	___
l. Heart disease	___	___	___
m. Toxemia, eclampsia, preeclampsia	___	___	___
n. High blood pressure	___	___	___
o. Kidney disease	___	___	___
p. German measles	___	___	___

		Don't know
6. How much weight was gained during pregnancy?	___ lb	___
7. How long was the total period of labor?	___ h	___
8. How long was the period of hard labor?	___ h	___
9. How long was it from the time water broke until the baby was delivered?	___ h	___

	Yes	No	Don't know
10. Was labor longer than 24 hours?	___	___	___

	Yes	No	Don't know
11. During pregnancy			
a. Was the mother confined to a bed for more than one day?	___	___	___
b. Was an ultrasound performed?	___	___	___
c. It so, were there any abnormalities on the ultrasound?	___	___	___
d. Were the baby's movements before birth			
(1) Normal	___	___	___
(2) Increased	___	___	___
(3) Decreased	___	___	___
e. Was amniocentesis performed?	___	___	___
f. If so, were there any abnormalities in the amniocentesis?	___	___	___
12. Was the baby considered premature?	___	___	___
13. Was the baby overdue by more than 2 weeks?	___	___	___
14. Was there internal manipulation of your baby?	___	___	___
15. Was a cesarean birth performed?	___	___	___
a. If performed, was the cesarean an emergency?	___	___	___
b. Was general anesthesia used?	___	___	___
16. Was the baby born head first?	___	___	___
17. Were forceps used?	___	___	___
18. Did the baby have any bruises?	___	___	___
19. Did the baby have any birthmarks?	___	___	___
20. Did the baby have breathing problems?	___	___	___
21. Was the cord wrapped around the baby's neck?	___	___	___
22. If so, was the cord wrapped more than once around the baby's neck?	___	___	___
23. Did the baby cry quickly?	___	___	___
24. Was the baby's color normal?	___	___	___
25. Was the baby blue?	___	___	___
26. Was the baby yellow (jaundiced)?	___	___	___
27. Did the baby require oxygen?	___	___	___
28. Did the baby require transfusions?	___	___	___
29. Did the baby require phototherapy (lights)?	___	___	___
30. Was the baby placed in an isolette, incubator, or intensive special care unit?	___	___	___
31. Did the baby have seizures or convulsions?	___	___	___
32. Was the baby placed on a respirator (breathing machine)?	___	___	___
33. Were there concerns about the baby's heart rate?	___	___	___
34. Was the fluid stained with the baby's meconium (bowel movement)?	___	___	___
35. Were there other complications before the baby was taken home?	___	___	___

List, if known _____

	Yes	No
36. Do you remember the baby's Apgar score?	_____	_____

a. Apgar score at 1 minute: _____

b. Apgar score at 3 minutes: _____

c. Apgar score at 5 minutes: _____

37. How long after birth did you take the baby home? _____ days   Don't know _____

38. What was baby's birth weight? _____ lb / _____ oz   Don't know _____

39. After the baby was brought home

	Yes	No	Don't know
a. Was the baby limp?	_____	_____	_____
b. Was the baby stiff?	_____	_____	_____
c. Did the baby have feeding or sucking problems?	_____	_____	_____

40. During the baby's first year of life, did the baby

	Yes	No	Don't know
a. Have difficulty sleeping?	_____	_____	_____
b. Fail to grow or gain weight?	_____	_____	_____
c. Show any unusual trembling or unusual movements of arms, legs, or head?	_____	_____	_____

41. How old was the child (your best guess, in months) when he or she first

	Under 6	6–12	12–18	18–24	24–36	36–48	48+	Don't know
a. Sat alone	_____	_____	_____	_____	_____	_____	_____	_____
b. Crawled	_____	_____	_____	_____	_____	_____	_____	_____
c. Stood alone	_____	_____	_____	_____	_____	_____	_____	_____
d. Walked with assistance	_____	_____	_____	_____	_____	_____	_____	_____
e. Walked without assistance	_____	_____	_____	_____	_____	_____	_____	_____
f. Showed hand preference	_____	_____	_____	_____	_____	_____	_____	_____
g. Was toilet-trained (urine)	_____	_____	_____	_____	_____	_____	_____	_____
h. Was toilet-trained (bowel)	_____	_____	_____	_____	_____	_____	_____	_____
i. Began to vocalize (babble)	_____	_____	_____	_____	_____	_____	_____	_____
j. Began to use words	_____	_____	_____	_____	_____	_____	_____	_____
k. Began to talk in sentences	_____	_____	_____	_____	_____	_____	_____	_____
l. Rode a tricycle	_____	_____	_____	_____	_____	_____	_____	_____
m. Rode a bicycle	_____	_____	_____	_____	_____	_____	_____	_____

	Left	Right	No preference
42. Which hand does your child prefer?	_____	_____	_____

43. Does the child

	Yes	No
a. Cry excessively	_____	_____
b. Rarely or never attempt to communicate	_____	_____
c. Use mainly gestures to communicate	_____	_____
d. Have a hearing problem	_____	_____
e. Turn head to distinguish from where a sound is coming	_____	_____

44. General language skills (see Table 3-5)

	Yes	No
Does your child		
a. Have difficulty learning new vocabulary words	_____	_____
b. Omit words from sentences (i.e., do his or her sentences sound telegraphic)	_____	_____
c. Speak in short, incomplete sentences	_____	_____
d. Have trouble with verbs, such as *is, am, are, was,* and *were*	_____	_____
e. Have difficulty following directions	_____	_____
f. Have difficulty understanding long sentences	_____	_____
g. Have difficulty responding appropriately to questions	_____	_____
h. Have problems asking questions beginning with *who, what, where,* and *why*	_____	_____
i. Have trouble using present and past tense verbs correctly	_____	_____
j. Show little or no progress in speech and language in the last 6 to 12 months	_____	_____
k. Omit sounds from words	_____	_____
l. Do you feel your child's speech is more difficult to understand than it should be in view of his or her age	_____	_____
m. Does it seem that your child uses *t, d, k,* or *g* in place of most other consonants when speaking	_____	_____

45. Receptive language skills (see Table 3-6)

	Yes	No
Does your child		
a. Understand "Where is mother?"	_____	_____
b. Point to one body part	_____	_____
c. Follow two-step commands two times out of three	_____	_____
d. Know six body parts	_____	_____
e. Understand the concept of "one"	_____	_____
f. Point to spoon, ball, and cup by use	_____	_____
g. Recognize day and night	_____	_____
h. Know three out of four prepositions (*on, under, in front, behind,* etc.)	_____	_____
i. Understand the concept of "three"	_____	_____
j. Identify right and left on self	_____	_____

46. Expressive language skills

Does your child   Yes   No

   a. Know two to four single words   _____   _____

   b. Use two-word sentences   _____   _____

   c. Refer to self by name   _____   _____

   d. Use plurals   _____   _____

   e. Converse in sentences   _____   _____

   f. Give full name   _____   _____

   g. Comprehend "tired," "old," and "hungry"   _____   _____

   h. Name opposite analogies two times out of three (up/down, mother/father, in/out)   _____   _____

   i. Comprehend senses (taste, feel, smell, see, hear)   _____   _____

   j. Define words correctly six out of nine times (ball, lake, desk, house, banana, curtain, ceiling, bush, sidewalk)   _____   _____

47. Other language skills

Does your child   Yes   No

   a. Have difficulty finding the correct words to use in conversation   _____   _____

   b. Have difficulty in getting the correct word out in conversation   _____   _____

   c. Put words in wrong order   _____   _____

   d. Confuse words that have similar sounds   _____   _____

   e. Have difficulty pronouncing words or sounds   _____   _____

   f. Hesitate or stop before he or she completes sentences   _____   _____

   g. Stutter or stammer   _____   _____

   h. Respond inconsistently to sound and speech   _____   _____

   i. Understand what is said to him or her   _____   _____

   j. Label objects (house, tree, car, ball)   _____   _____

   k. Label actions (walk, run, sleep, ride, jump, read, write)   _____   _____

   l. Understand stories read to him or her   _____   _____

   m. Tell about events happening during the day   _____   _____

   n. Comment on what he or she is doing   _____   _____

   o. Relay a short message   _____   _____

   p. Label his or her own emotions (happy, sad, fearful)   _____   _____

48. Is the child   Yes   No

   a. Understood by parents and family   _____   _____

   b. Understood by other adults   _____   _____

   c. Understood by other children   _____   _____

   d. Teased by children about his or her voice   _____   _____

   e. Teased by children about his or her speech   _____   _____

49. Does your child's voice sound different from those of other children the same age (too high/too low)?   Yes   No

                                                        _____   _____

50. Basic education skills

   a. Can the child   Yes   No

      (1) Count from 1 to 10

         Count from 10 to 20   _____   _____

	Yes	No
(2) Count 1 to 10 objects	_____	_____
Count 10 to 20 objects	_____	_____
(3) Identify the numbers 1 to 10	_____	_____
Identify the numbers 10 to 20	_____	_____
(4) Recognize his or her name in print	_____	_____
(5) Name letters in his or her name	_____	_____
(6) Identify other letters in the alphabet	_____	_____
(7) Print his or her first name correctly	_____	_____
(8) Point to primary colors (red, green, blue, yellow, black, white) when named	_____	_____
Name primary colors when pointed to	_____	_____
(9) Understand the concept of "money"	_____	_____
(10) Identify coins (penny, nickel, dime, quarter)	_____	_____
(11) Print the numbers 1 to 10	_____	_____
(12) Print all the letters of the alphabet	_____	_____
(13) Include at least six body parts (head, arms, body, legs, eye, ears, nose, fingers, hair) when drawing a person	_____	_____
(14) Understand concept of "same or different"	_____	_____
(15) Repeat a short sentence	_____	_____
(16) Recognize similar letters	_____	_____
Recognize similar words	_____	_____
Recognize similar numbers	_____	_____
b. Does your child have problems in	_____	_____
(1) Reading	_____	_____
Word identification	_____	_____
Comprehension	_____	_____
Phonics	_____	_____
(2) Spelling	_____	_____
Oral	_____	_____
Written	_____	_____
(3) Writing	_____	_____
Legibility	_____	_____
Slow speed	_____	_____
Sentence construction	_____	_____
Basic grammar	_____	_____
(4) Math	_____	_____
Memory of basic facts (addition, subtraction, multiplication, division)	_____	_____
Operations (addition, subtraction, multiplication, division)	_____	_____
Word problems	_____	_____
(5) Organization	_____	_____
Completing classroom assignments	_____	_____
Completing and turning in homework	_____	_____
Planning study time or morning routine	_____	_____

	Yes	No
(6) Reasoning and problem solving (personal or in school)	____	____
(7) Science, social studies, humanities, foreign languages	____	____

E. Attention/Activity/Behavior Habits

1. Does your child

	Yes	No
a. Sit still for a fascinating activity, such as television or being read to	____	____
(1) For under 5 minutes	____	____
(2) For 5–10 minutes	____	____
(3) For 10–15 minutes	____	____
(4) For greater than 15 minutes	____	____
b. Sit and listen to a story when being read to individually	____	____
c. Sit and listen to a story as a part of a group	____	____
d. Seem inattentive	____	____
e. Seem to daydream	____	____
f. Seem to be easily distracted	____	____
g. Go quickly from one task to another	____	____
h. Perform better in a calm, nondistracting setting	____	____
i. Hear, but not appear to listen	____	____
j. Appear overly frightened or anxious about new experiences	____	____
k. Avoid written work, such as printing or coloring	____	____
l. Produce poor schoolwork, even though he or she tries hard	____	____
m. Desire to make friends, but frequently make them angry	____	____
n. Insist on being in charge or he or she will not play	____	____
o. Have verbal fights with other children	____	____
p. Have physical fights with other children	____	____
q. Have a violent temper	____	____
r. Have temper tantrums	____	____
s. Steal	____	____
t. Swear or use vulgar language	____	____
u. Act verbally abusive to parents	____	____
v. Act verbally abusive to other adults	____	____
w. Act physically abusive to parents	____	____
x. Act physically abusive to other adults	____	____
y. Cheat in order to be the winner	____	____
z. Lose his or her temper quickly	____	____
aa. Allow his or her feelings to be quickly hurt	____	____
bb. Engage in		
(1) Head banging	____	____
(2) Bed rocking	____	____
(3) Hand flapping	____	____

cc. Frequently place his or her hands over ears   _____ _____

dd. Show a lack of interest in people   _____ _____

ee. Speak in a mechanical, machinelike voice   _____ _____

ff. Speak in a whisper   _____ _____

gg. Seem preoccupied with strange creatures or monsters   _____ _____

hh. Avoid affection from others   _____ _____

ii. Avoid eye contact with or looking at people   _____ _____

jj. Seem impulsive   _____ _____

kk. Seem explosive   _____ _____

ll. Change moods quickly   _____ _____

mm. Have difficulty in appreciating danger   _____ _____

nn. Seem easily frustrated   _____ _____

oo. Have trouble waiting his or her turn   _____ _____

pp. Seem extremely talkative   _____ _____

qq. Show shame or remorse   _____ _____

rr. Learn from his or her mistakes   _____ _____

ss. Accept discipline   _____ _____

2. What type of school does your child attend?   Public _____   Private _____

3. At what age did your child begin preschool or daycare? _____ years Don't know _____

4. At what age did your child begin kindergarten?   _____ years   Don't know _____

5. What grade does your child attend now?   _____

	Yes	No	Don't know
6. If in a regular grade (class), does your child receive special help?	_____	_____	_____
7. Has your child ever been absent from school for two weeks or longer?	_____	_____	_____
8. Has your child had frequent short absences from school resulting in absences for more than a total of 30 days during the school year?	_____	_____	_____
9. Has your child ever been suspended from school?	_____	_____	_____
10. Has your child ever been retained by either your decision or the school's?	_____	_____	_____

F. Skills or Abilities

	Yes	No	Don't know
1. Sports			
a. Baseball or softball	_____	_____	_____
b. Tennis	_____	_____	_____
c. Swimming	_____	_____	_____
d. Football	_____	_____	_____
e. Soccer	_____	_____	_____
f. Computer or video games	_____	_____	_____
g. Other	_____	_____	_____

2. Music

   a. Singing   _____ _____ _____

   b. Dancing (including ballet)   _____ _____ _____

   c. Instruments   _____ _____ _____

      Specify: _____ _____

                _____ _____

3. Art

   a. Drawing   _____ _____ _____

   b. Copying   _____ _____ _____

   c. Other   _____ _____ _____

4. Academic

   a. Reading   _____ _____ _____

   b. Creative writing   _____ _____ _____

   c. Math   _____ _____ _____

   d. Computer literate   _____ _____ _____

   e. Typing (keyboarding)   _____ _____ _____

5. Is your child a member of a

   a. Club   _____ _____ _____

   b. Other student organization _____ _____ _____

      Specify: _____ _____

                _____ _____

6. Has your child ever been elected to an office? _____ _____ _____

7. In what skill or ability area(s) does your child seem to excel over most children his or her age?

_____

_____

_____

The Neurologic Examination of the Newborn and Infant

Patricia Ellison

THE NEONATAL NEUROLOGIC EXAMINATION

Why perform a neurologic examination on a newborn? Perhaps the primary reason is reassurance of the parents. Parents have always wanted information about their newborns. There is an expectation that each baby must be normal—and preferably superior.

As physicians, we have never presumed to distinguish the normal from the superior in newborns. Indeed, we have barely managed to agree on the distinction between normal and abnormal. Much of our thinking about abnormality is based on neuropathology. Pathology of the neonatal brain, although long described, has only recently achieved the potential for on-the-spot diagnosis through modern imaging techniques. These methods identify hemorrhage, certain malformations, size of the ventricles, and certain evidence of ischemia (Rumack and Johnson, 1984). Function is variously affected even with the same pathology, but certain functions or, more properly, dysfunctions, have prognostic value; thus the utility of the neonatal neurologic examination.

History of the Neonatal Neurologic Examination

Two approaches have been taken to the development of the neonatal neurologic examination—neurologic and behavioral or "psychologic." The approaches were quite different and directed at answering different questions about the neonate. Yet both lines of inquiry were ultimately directed at answering these questions: How well will the baby/child learn? How well will the baby/child locomote? In other words, will the child be mentally retarded and will the child have cerebral palsy?

The major figures in the study of the neurologic approach were Peiper (1956) in Leipzig, Thomas and St. Anne Dargassies (1952) in Paris, and Prechtl (1977, 1980; Prechtl and Dijktstra, 1960) in Gronigen. Prechtl described the neurologic status of large samples of newborns. He then described the relationships between the neurologic abnormalities and conditions of pregnancy, labor, and delivery. He scored the neurologic items and performed data analyses, including factor analyses. He noted that the neurologic examination changed with the state of the baby; he described six states. He reported correlations of .53 between the neonatal and infancy neurologic evaluations (Prechtl, 1965, 1968), concluding that there were limitations in predicting later neurologic function from the neonatal examination. The French school emphasized assessment of active and passive tone. Both St. Anne Dargassies (1954, 1955, 1972, 1979) and Amiel-Tison (1976; Amiel-Tison and Grenier, 1986) followed samples of neonates into infancy and beyond. They described well how neurologic abnormality progresses and lessens. Scoring for items was not utilized until recently. Prechtl's use of scoring, which permitted description of the relationships between observations made at an earlier and a later time, had no parallel in the French work.

The psychologic approach first emphasized the acquisition of milestones and the responses to various test objects as indicators of neurologic integrity, as in the work of Gesell (1925). Major contributions to the neurologic examination of neonates were made by Graham (1956a,b; Graham et al., 1957) and Rosenblith (1961, 1968; Rosenblith and Anderson, 1968). Items were scored and included measures of alertness and apathy-irritability. Brazelton (1973) incorporated several of their items into his examination of the neonate, which combined neurologic and psychologic items. However, his neurologic items largely excluded the extensive work that had been done in Europe. Dubowitz and Dubowitz (1981) also included neurologic and psychologic items in their methods of examination of the neonate. They included neurologic items from both Prechtl and the French school.

Value of the Neonatal Neurologic Examination

The neonatal neurologic examination offers the following benefits:

1. The newborn with moderate to severe neurologic abnormality can be identified. The diagnosis is more accurate for newborns with acute injury than for those with chronic injuries. Of the available methods of assessment, a neonatal neurologic examination that includes sufficient behavioral items remains the best method for ascertaining chronic (or earlier) brain injury.
2. The at-risk newborn can be identified and followed further.
3. With serial evaluations, the neurologic evaluation is an indicator of both the *severity* and the *duration* of insult. For example, the asphyxiated or depressed neonate with clearing of abnormalities within 5 to 7 days has a better prognosis. Similarly, preterm neonates who demonstrate improvement to normal or near normal by 40 weeks gestation tend to do well.

Who Needs a Neonatal Neurologic Examination?

While it is accepted practice—indeed a standard of care—that all newborns receive a physical examination on admission to the nursery, the neurologic portion may be limited. The key questions are whether the baby focuses and follows and indicates other evidence of *"alertness"*, whether *limb tone* is normal, whether *head and neck* control is normal, whether *general body tone* is normal, and whether *patellar reflexes* are present.

Neonates in intensive care units should have neurologic examinations at least weekly, as soon as the neonates are able to tolerate them. Weekly reviews should also include assessment of head circumference, hematocrit, caloric intake, and weight gain. Neurologic examinations of near-term, term, and postterm neonates with acute illness are important indicators of their condition. For asphyxiated neonates, a daily neurologic examination is helpful for the first 7 days; then one should be performed weekly.

The neurologic findings are an important indicator of the *severity* and *duration* of neonatal illness. Serial examinations are rarely directed toward a medical diagnosis; rather, they are directed toward a different concept—that of diagnosing or predicting subsequent evidence of "brain damage." The neurologic examination is an *adjunct* in this regard to other modalities, which include electroencephalograph, measurement of evoked potentials, and imaging procedures.

Who Should Perform the Neonatal Neurologic Examination?

In many neonatal intensive care units, serial neurologic examination has been assigned to the physical or occupa-

tional therapists and, in some instances, to the nurses. There are advantages to this approach. Through experience and interest many professionals from these disciplines become skillful in these examinations. Ideally, the physicians, nurses, occupational therapists, and physical therapists should all perform the same neurologic examination. If the examination is worth doing, can be properly interpreted, and measures well, the credentials of the examiner become less important.

THE TRANSITIONAL PERIOD NEUROLOGIC EXAMINATION

The transitional period is defined as birth to 3 to 4 months corrected gestational age. The use of a single method of neurologic examination from birth through infancy has perhaps been best typefied by clinicians of the French school. However, Amiel-Tison (1976; Amiel-Tison and Grenier, 1986) has cautioned us about interpretation of findings during this period. The reliability of testing in this time period is not as high as that in older patients.

One way to increase the reliability of the assessment is to include items from the behavioral assessment. Amiel-Tison does this, although not in a precise fashion, when she comments on the importance of apathy or hyperirritability in this period. We recommend that an extended neonatal examination with both neurologic and behavioral items be used until age 3 to 4 months.

THE INFANT NEUROLOGIC EXAMINATION

Why perform a neurologic examination on an infant? As noted previously, perhaps the primary reason remains reassurance of the parents. Parents closely observe the developmental progress of their infant, often checking it against the development sections of various baby books. Neurologic assessment is sought when a delay in development is noted by either parent, a grandparent, or a physician, or there is another reason to be concerned, e.g., the infant was premature, was a sick neonate, or had had interim illnesses.

In infancy, separate assessments have been developed for neurologic examination and for development. In general, the premise of Gesell holds true: the infant who performs at age level is neurologically intact. This assumes that a sufficient number of items of development have been tested. Otherwise the reliability of the developmental examination is not sufficient to make judgments. To ask the mother such questions as "Does the baby smile?", "Does the baby sit?", and "Does the baby vocalize?" is not sufficient. Many clinicians now screen infant development formally with either the Denver Developmental Screening Test (Frankenbert et al., 1971) or the Gesell Screening Inventory (Knobloch et al., 1980). Infants who fail or who are borderline on two or more occasions merit two further assessments: a comprehensive neurologic examination and a more complete developmental evaluation.

History of the Infant Neurologic Examination

Brief descriptions follow for five methods of infant neurologic evaluation.

1. Milani-Comparetti and Gidoni (1967a,b). This method is richest in its assessment of the ability of the infant to determine position in space. Nine of the 27 items do this specifically: the four parachutes (forward, sideways, downward, and backward) and the five tiltboard items (prone, supine, sitting, all fours, and standing). Other items, often classified as "righting" items, must test a similar neurologic function. Delay in acquisition of these neurologic functions is highly correlated with delay in acquisition of motor skills such as sitting or standing; an infant could not be expected to move well if he or she cannot readily appreciate his or her position in space. We have described a scoring system for the Milani-Comparetti and Gidoni method (Ellison et al., 1983).

2. Vojta (1981). For most items the infant is suspended in space—horizontally, upside down, or vertically. This method is excellent for description of extensor posturing (Figure 2–1). The method is scored. It is however, limited by the small number of items.

3. French Method (St. Anne Dargassies, 1972; Amiel-Tison, 1976; Amiel-Tison and Grenier, 1986). This method has been used from the neonatal through infancy periods. It is one of the best ways to ascertain early hypertonia, particularly with the use of heel to ear and popliteal angle in early infancy (Ellison, 1984a). These mild changes are not well described by the suspensions of Vojta or the righting, parachute, and tiltboard items of Milani-Comparetti and Gidoni. Many pediatricians are already acquainted with the items as they are used to assess gestational age (scarf sign, heel-to-ear, popliteal angle, leg abduction). The addition of a chart for infancy is all that is necessary for proper interpretation.

4. Capute and associates (1984; Capute, 1979) This method incorporates testing of selected primitive reflexes: neurologic reflexes in the neonate that disappear in the course of infancy. Capute and associates (1984) have scored the reflexes and they have provided excel-

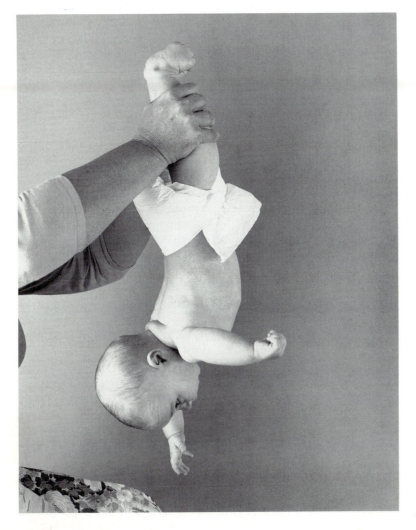

Figure 2–1. An infant in suspension, with extension of head, neck, and arms.

lent information on normal values (the ages at which normal infants lose each reflex). However, there are only a few such reflexes, a fact that will tend to decrease the internal consistency (reliability) of the test. For hypertonia (spasticity) of four limbs, this method is useful; for other abnormalities, the method is less useful.

5. *Paine and Oppe (Paine, 1960).* These clinicians provided the neurologic examinations for the National Collaborative Perinatal Project (Collaborative Study, 1966). The examinations in infancy were detailed in their attention to cranial nerves and selected reflexes, including some primitive reflexes. Items for tone and posture were less well represented.

Who Should Perform the Infant Neurologic Examination?

It would be preferable if every physician who cared for infants were comfortable in performing and interpreting the neurologic examination. However, because the majority of infants are neurologically normal, it is often difficult for a pediatrician or family practitioner to develop good criteria for neurologic abnormality. Assessment methods with scoring systems should help. These have been developed for full-term newborns (the Neo Neuro; Sheridan-Pereira et al., 1991) and for infants (the Infanib; Ellison et al., 1985a).

In many settings, including follow-up programs for neonatal intensive care units, the physical therapist performs the examination. In follow-up programs in rural areas and in some countries in Europe, the visiting nurse performs the neurologic examination. Each setting requires a method of examination with criteria for categorizing the infant without causing undue excitement about mild abnormalities (especially for the benefit of the parents).

REQUIREMENTS FOR NEUROLOGIC EXAMINATIONS OF NEONATES AND INFANTS

1. *The assessment should measure reasonably well whatever the examiner sets out to measure.* Physicians usually do not associate the concept of "measuring" with the neurologic examination. We consider ourselves diagnosticians, not measurers. However, many of us do not have the capacity to consider diagnoses because we cannot make sense out of that which we are measuring. This situation is not likely to improve in a setting in which the frequency of the condition is so low that the clinician cannot build a baseline for normality and abnormality *unless* the abnormality is extreme (and in that case the grandmother often also makes the proper identification). Surely skillful, experienced clinicians have engendered a system of measurement and a weighting of those measures through the intellectual process by which they declare the

neonate normal or abnormal, and more especially so when they pronounce finer gradations of normality/ abnormality. If the experienced clinician can do this, then this process can be "captured" in a form that can be utilized by the less experienced clinician. That is the premise on which our work on neonatal and infant neurologic examinations is based.

If any item is to be measured, it must be scored. The concept of scoring is certainly not new; Prechtl scored items in his work. Whenever possible, gradations of scoring should be made.

2. *It is important to understand how the items on the assessment interrelate* (see Tables 2–1 and 2–2). The best method for seeing this is the correlation (or covariance) matrix. Such a matrix cannot be formed without scoring the items.

Usually some items interrelate weakly and some strongly; that is, they have lower or higher correlation coefficients. Those items that have stronger relationships can then be grouped for subscores by a process of factor analysis or cluster analysis. It is generally considered that items that interrelate strongly are measuring similar qualities.

3. *Subscores should be formed on a mathematical/ statistical basis rather than on an a priori basis.* I make this statement strongly after years of data analysis with large sample sizes from some a priori scoring systems, e.g., the Denver Development Screening Test (Frankenberg et al., 1971) and the Dubowitz Neurological Examination (Dubowitz and Dubowitz, 1981). Many of the items simply do not group or cluster with the subscores designated by their creators. They make more sense in the groups or clusters achieved mathematically. The relationships between subscores can then be described, as shown in Tables 2–3 and 2–4 for the Neo Neuro and Infanib instruments.

4. *The first test of reliability for an assessment method should be a measure of internal consistency (Nunnally, 1978).* This criterion is foremost because it determines whether the assessment instrument has sufficient items that are strongly enough related to each other to measure that which the test purports to measure. Sometimes it is not possible to add more items to the test and increase the internal consistency. Either one is not clever enough to use the correct items or the dimension being measured cannot be measured well because of other limitations. In newborns and infants the limitation is stage of development. In such a case, one could conclude that a particular assessment instrument is about as reliable as one could expect, given the limitations of a cerain age. One might still use the test with full knowledge of the level of reliability. This observer considers this to be the situation with regard to the neonatal neurologic examination.

The reliability of the neurologic examinations as we have scored them increases from prematurity through infancy (Ellison et al., 1985a; Sheridan-Pereira et al., 1991).

TABLE 2–1. CORRELATION MATRIX OF ITEMS IN THE NEONEURO

	Heel-to-ear	Scarf sign	Posture	ATNR	Arm traction	Leg recoil	Popliteal angle	Head lag	Arm flexion	Held sit	Posterior neck	Anterior neck	Movement amount	Movement type	Tremor	Clenched hands	Abnormal posture	Persistent foot grasp	Knee reflexes	Ankle reflexes	Ankle clonus	Palmar grasp	Plantar grasp	Suck	Auditory orientation	Visual orientation	Alertness	Irritability	Consolability	Cry	Moro	Ventral suspension
Heel to ear	1.00																															
Scarf sign	.43	1.00																														
Posture	.13	.08	1.00																													
ATNR	.00	.04	.11	1.00																												
Arm traction	.22	.18	.08	.11	1.00																											
Leg recoil	.12	.01	.16	.11	.24	1.00																										
Popliteal angle	.43	.21	.15	.02	.21	.18	1.00																									
Head lag	.12	.15	.23	.15	.24	.12	.15	1.00																								
Arm flexion	.19	.27	.23	.11	.45	.12	.19	.35	1.00																							
Held sit	.19	.26	.17	.16	.33	.14	.09	.49	.34	1.00																						
Posterior neck	.03	.12	.03	.01	.12	.00	.07	.24	.14	.28	1.00																					
Anterior neck	.08	.23	.22	.09	.19	.00	.09	.53	.25	.59	.36	1.00																				
Movement amount	-.02	.06	.19	.13	.19	.14	.07	.12	.19	.18	.12	.19	1.00																			
Movement type	.11	.09	.21	.13	.17	.22	.19	.15	.20	.22	-.02	.17	.37	1.00																		
Tremor	.02	.05	.04	.00	.09	.05	.02	.10	.05	.14	.03	.08	.04	.22	1.00																	
Clenched hands	.01	-.03	.19	.26	.09	.25	.13	.16	.08	.06	-.02	.08	.19	.33	.17	1.00																
Abnormal posture	-.02	-.04	.19	.17	-.01	.12	.13	.15	.05	.06	.07	.17	.14	.16	.07	.37	1.00															
Persistent foot grasp	-.02	-.01	.10	.10	-.04	.08	.05	.14	-.01	.13	-.01	.12	.08	.23	.15	.36	.29	1.00														
Knee reflexes	-.06	-.01	.05	.09	.12	.09	.04	.08	.02	.14	.03	.10	.09	.01	.15	.10	.12	.05	1.00													
Ankle reflexes	.06	.06	.08	.13	.16	.13	.09	.09	.12	.08	.00	.07	.16	.16	.14	.12	.14	.02	.36	1.00												
Ankle clonus	.03	.04	.11	.08	.12	.18	.00	.11	.08	.12	.04	.05	.11	.17	.19	.15	.08	.08	.17	.19	1.00											
Palmar grasp	.03	.14	.15	.12	.11	.19	.02	.07	.22	.07	.11	.11	.18	.05	.07	.18	.08	.03	.06	.06	.11	1.00										
Plantar grasp	.08	.17	.08	.05	.16	.12	.11	.12	.19	.17	.10	.17	.22	.11	.04	.09	.03	.04	.12	.08	.11	.43	1.00									
Suck	.09	.11	.07	.10	.17	.11	-.05	.12	.16	.19	.12	.10	.21	.18	.08	.08	.04	-.01	.07	.03	.10	.14	.17	1.00								
Auditory orientation	.07	.11	.16	.02	.17	.14	.08	.15	.18	.11	.09	.16	.19	.19	.06	.11	.11	.05	.10	.12	.08	.05	.08	.13	1.00							
Visual orientation	.18	.18	.10	.11	.09	.14	.11	.10	.16	.16	.06	.08	.13	.21	.07	.13	.07	.06	-.04	.00	.10	.07	.05	.25	.17	1.00						
Alertness	.17	.14	.05	.00	.12	.14	.10	.10	.16	.18	.06	.14	.25	.23	.07	.13	.09	.00	-.01	.04	.09	.02	.05	.21	.24	.45	1.00					
Irritability	.06	.04	.13	.08	.14	.18	.13	.14	.14	.11	-.01	.08	.06	.15	.16	.24	.13	.06	.06	.13	.00	.07	.01	.05	.13	.10	.15	1.00				
Consolability	-.01	-.02	.03	.03	.07	.19	.05	.05	.02	-.01	-.05	-.05	-.03	.07	.11	.28	.08	.12	.05	.11	.05	.00	-.03	-.06	.12	.06	.11	.51	1.00			
Cry	-.00	.08	.04	.01	.12	.12	.05	.13	.12	.09	-.02	.09	.09	.19	.11	.18	.09	.19	.03	.09	.02	.01	.00	.02	.13	.05	.07	.36	.38	1.00		
Moro	.05	.23	.10	.17	.15	.09	.04	.14	.17	.26	.15	.21	.13	.03	.03	.04	.09	.06	.02	.02	.11	.27	.09	.12	.15	.12	.18	.07	.02	.05	1.00	
Ventral suspension	.04	.17	.17	.10	.19	.05	.16	.32	.25	.25	.11	.22	.12	.13	.06	.10	.12	.06	.09	.12	.07	.08	.06	.12	.10	.15	.10	.07	.02	.09	.09	1.00

TABLE 2-2. CORRELATION MATRIX OF ITEMS IN THE INFANIB

	ATNR	Pull to sitting	Sitting	Sideways parachute	Backward parachute	Standing	Foot grasp	Forward parachute	All fours	Body derotative	Body rotative	Scarf sign	Heel to ear	Popliteal angle	Leg abduction	Dorsiflexion of foot	Positive support reflex	Tonic labyrinthine supine	Tonic labyrinthine prone	Hands closed/open
ATNR	1.00																			
Pull to sitting	.50	1.00																		
Sitting	.45	.64	1.00																	
Sideways parachute	.51	.67	.81	1.00																
Backwards parachute	.03	.21	.23	.11	1.00															
Standing	.31	.50	.64	.60	.23	1.00														
Foot grasp	.30	.30	.40	.35	35	.55	1.00													
Forward parachute	.36	.47	.43	.54	.30	.36	.29	1.00												
All fours	.32	.53	.53	.60	.28	.54	.39	.29	1.00											
Body derotative	.51	.70	.70	.67	.15	.62	.43	.38	.61	1.00										
Body rotative	.10	.23	.25	.14	.80	.32	.41	.34	.40	.27	1.00									
Scarf sign	.53	.31	.34	.34	.18	.32	.37	.31	.22	.32	.23	1.00								
Heel to ear	.54	.40	.47	.45	.25	.42	.51	.41	.41	.49	.34	.58	1.00							
Popliteal angle	.56	.46	.48	.46	.24	.46	.48	.39	.40	.55	.33	.60	.81	1.00						
Leg abduction	.45	.34	.30	.28	.30	.31	.41	.27	.26	.32	.32	.59	.66	.77	1.00					
Dorsiflexion of foot	.20	.26	.28	.30	.14	.43	.56	.23	.28	.32	.19	.27	.46	.41	.36	1.00				
Positive support reflex	.33	.25	.25	.31	.13	.45	.49	.19	.23	.27	.19	.38	.43	.45	.38	.41	1.00			
Tonic labyrinthine supine	.76	.59	.59	.58	.12	.44	.38	.36	.39	.61	.19	.54	.57	.58	.47	.29	.36	1.00		
Tonic labyrinthine prone	.64	.54	.53	.53	.08	.41	.39	.31	.33	.55	.13	.43	.47	.47	.38	.35	.30	.80	1.00	
Hands closed/open	.69	.52	.54	.58	.17	.45	.52	.40	.39	.56	.20	.50	.58	.61	.48	.30	.43	.74	.60	1.00

In the neonatal period the reliability is .80. Under 7 months of age the reliability is .88; at 8 months or more it is .93 (Ellison et al., 1985). For either of these later ages the reliability is high enough for research purposes or for clinical work (separating one child from all others, placing the child in a category, and describing the implications for that category). More elaborate discussions of the reliability and validity of the infancy neurologic examination are provided elsewhere (Ellison, 1990).

5. *The scoring method should be computer compatible.* Larger sample sizes require the use of a computer.

6. *The examination must be capable of being administered in a reasonable period of time.*

THE NEUROLOGIC EXAMINATION DESCRIBED AND ILLUSTRATED

The examination has been divided into four subsections: (I) general description, (II) cranial nerves, (III) special situations: altered mental status and spinal cord lesions, and (IV) tone and posture (plus behavior for the neonate). The neonate and infant will be described together except for the separate examinations of tone and posture (and behavior), for which we would use, depending on the child's age, the Neo Neuro or the Infanib scoring sheet.

TABLE 2-3. CORRELATIONS OF NEONEURO FACTORS

	Head on neck	Irritability	Passive tone	Alertness	Reflex excitability	Extensor	Primitive reflexes
Head on neck	1.00						
Irritability	0.08	1.00					
Passive tone	0.20	0.07	1.00				
Alertness	0.22	0.09	0.16	1.00			
Reflex excitability	0.16	0.12	0.05	0.07	1.00		
Extensor	0.18	0.26	0.05	0.10	0.18	1.00	
Primitive reflexes	0.25	0.04	0.16	0.18	0.14	0.14	+1.00

TABLE 2-4. CORRELATIONS OF INFANIB FACTORS

	Extensor	Vestibular function	Head and trunk	French angles (passive tone)	Legs
Extensor	1.00				
Vestibular function	0.35	1.00			
Head and trunk	0.63	0.59	1.00		
French angles (passive tone)	0.57	0.19	0.49	1.00	
Legs	0.44	0.24	0.53	0.51	1.00

I. General Description

Most experienced examiners are continually assessing the baby from the initial encounter, constantly forming and reforming a "gestalt" of the neurologic condition.

Head. The *size* of the head is recorded, preferably at every evaluation. The initial newborn head circumference may be misleading because of molding during the birth process. In some instances this molding may be excessive with marked overlap of the sutures, which should be noted and recorded. The neonate may be mistakenly labeled as microcephalic on the basis of the initial head circumference. A definition of microcephaly should not be set at the tenth percentile. A more appropriate definition of microcephaly is one of greater than two standard deviations away from the mean (approximately the 2.5 percentile). Most of our head charts designate either a second or third percentile line. Even two standard deviations is not highly predictive of lesser mental function (mental retardation). Three standard deviations from the mean (the .6 percentile) is preferable for prediction of brain dysfunction.

Serial head circumferences are particularly useful in infancy as indicators of abnormal brain growth or ventricle size. A decrease of percentiles to the third percentile in the first 6 months or even somewhat later may indicate severe damage to the brain through a process such as hypoxia-ischemia. Excessively rapid growth may indicate hydrocephalus, subdural hematoma effusion, or rapid brain growth.

The *shape* of the skull is noted with particular attention to unusual configurations. Most of the craniosynostoses can be diagnosed by inspection. In infancy, the unusual head shapes that result from *constant assumption of the same position* (plagiocephaly) should be added to the differential diagnosis. Frequently overlooked is the rather remarkable skull configuration secondary to trauma and secondary fibrosis of the sternocleidomastoid muscle (torticollis).

The *size* of the anterior and posterior *fontanelles* is noted and recorded as is any bulging, fullness, or tension. The size of the anterior fontanelles for those infants with either larger or smaller head circumference should be recorded.

For newborns, the size and location of any *caputi* are recorded, either cephalohematoma (restricted to one section of the skull) or caput succudeum (crossing a suture line.

Eyes. Particularly in the newborn, the eyes may offer clues to abnormal brain processes, especially seizures. Conjugate deviation and repetitive nystagmus are especially good indicators. Wandering eye movements and sustained nystagmus may indicate any of several abnormalities: coma, malformation or decreased visual acuity. Other noteworthy findings may include abnormal pupil shape and various malformations of the anterior eye (e.g., coloboma, "setting sun" sign, and conjunctival hemorrhage).

By infancy, most congenital malformations of the brain have been noted. Sometimes sustained nystagmus is first observed in infancy, although there is no evidence that a new process has occurred. Nevertheless, special attention must be directed to acquired signs such as nystagmus (otherwise lesions such as optic glioma, hypothalamic tumors, or metabolic disorders will be missed).

The most common eye abnormality of infancy is strabismus. While strabismus per se does not equal brain dysfunction, those infants with a history of brain insults are at particular risk. These include those with a history of neonatal hypoxia-ischemia or intraventricular hemorrhage, infants who had prolonged use of the respirator as neonates, or those with delay in regaining birth weight.

Skin. Every inch of the skin is inspected for cafe au lait spots, depigmented spots, hemiangiomas, and nevi. Particularly for babies with seizures, neurophakomatoses are a consideration.

Both newborns and infants should be inspected for bruises or ecchymoses. The size and location of all must be recorded. For all ages, trauma is an important etiology; other important etiologies include bleeding disorders and meningococcemia.

Dysmorphologic Features. Most babies with obvious dysmorphologic features will eventually be formally evaluated. If, however, the primary care physician cannot recognize basic dysmorphologic features, the diagnosis may be delayed. Particular attention should be paid to distance between the eyes, ear shape and placement, hair whorls, hair texture, hair line, coarseness of facial features, shortness or webbing of neck, distance between nipples, presence of a gibbus formation, pectus excavatun, dermatoglyphics, number and placement of digits, webbing of fingers or toes, contracture of joints, and malformations of the limbs. These and other features should be noted and then be utilized to key the syndrome through one of the texts of dysmorphology (e.g., Smith, 1981; Goodman and Gorlin, 1977). Appropriate diagnostic tests can then be ordered. The expertise of a dysmorphologist may be needed for genetic counseling or for further diagnostic evaluation when a diagnosis has not been reached.

Organomegaly. The assessment of the size of the organs is usually accomplished quickly and may give an important clue to a neurologic diagnosis (e.g., hepatomegaly may suggest glycogen storage disease).

Seizures. Attention to seizures is of key importance in the neonatal period. In infancy, obvious seizures receive immediate attention by physicians. More subtle seizures—particularly the frequent, brief extension or flexion of infantile spasms—may be delayed in both diagnosis and treatment.

Apnea. The absence or presence and approximate frequency of apnea are noted.

Brachial Plexus Injury. This injury is usually noted in the hospital nursery, although this observer has examined neonates in whom the lesion was not noted during the initial examination. In general, the injury is easily distinguished from hemiparesis on the basis of different neurologic findings. Brachial plexus injuries are associated with depressed reflexes and hypotonia of the arm. Hemiparesis can be associated with facial weakness and increased tone and reflexes in both arms and legs. The timing is also different: brachial plexus injury is noted through early observation by the physician, nurse, or parents. Hemiparetic lesions tend to be noted later in the first year of life.

Hand Preference. Asymmetry of hand fisting, especially excessive clenching versus open position, is an important indicator of hemiparesis from the neonatal period through infancy. A second clue may be the early development of "handedness," suggesting weakness in or less use of the opposite hand.

II. Cranial Nerves

With an alert, conscious neonate or infant the following examinations should be carried out.

A. Vision and Hearing

Funduscopic Examination. For the neonate, the most important aspects are evaluation of cataracts, retinal hemorrhages, chorioretinitis, and anomalies such as optic nerve hypoplasia. For infants who are normal developmentally, the most one usually sees is a glimpse of the outline of the passing fundi. For at-risk or neurologically abnormal infants a more thorough examination is needed to find a "cherry-red spot," a phakoma or chorioretinitis. The extra patience needed to seek this information will often yield for the examiner these more obscure diagnoses.

Visual Acuity. Ordinarily we do not test visual acuity. However, we should be very careful to test whether the neonate or infant sees. (The use of a black-and-white bull's-eye is strongly recommended for testing, especially in neonates.) Testing of cranial nerves III, IV, and VI will help assess vision in infants. For infants who do not respond, further testing is often necessary to separate decreased visual function from limited cognitive function.

Assessment of a visual field cut, as in a hemiparetic infant, can be performed by having the child sit on the mother's lap. The infant's attention is first attracted by a small toy; then the examiner brings another object from the back of the head and observes the infant's head turning to that object. A dangling stethoscope or tape measure works well.

Often the determination of progressive loss of visual acuity is even more difficult. The mother may offer clues, e.g., the observation that her baby used to pick up small items (such as Cheerios) and no longer does.

Cranial Nerves III, IV, and VI. Although a human face or red yarn ball has been recommended as a stimulus for the neonate, a black-and-white bull's-eye is preferred, as indicated previously. Brazelton would consider following 30° through 60° a normal response. By 1 month of age, most neonates should track well if care is taken to test them while they are in an alert state. For older infants either a human face or a red yarn ball is a satisfactory stimulus. The yarn ball can also be used to check the infant's ability to focus while the examiner covers one eye for the cover test, then removes the cover to observe for eye movement as a test for strabismus.

Cranial Nerve VIII. For infants, hearing can be tested by response to crinkling paper at either ear, unobserved by the infant. Another person may speak in a low voice and call the infant's name. Or the examiner may ring a bell, again unobserved by the infant. Any neonate or infant for whom there is evidence of poor response to sound deserves further evaluation, including behavioral audiometry first and/or measurement of brainstem auditory evoked responses. As with vision, either decreased hearing or decreased mental function may contribute to the observed response. Fortunately, study of brainstem auditory evoked responses has considerably increased our ability to distinguish between the two and to provide amplification for hearing where indicated.

B. Facial

Cranial Nerve V. Respose to tactile or painful stimuli on the face may be used to assess the function of this nerve.

Cranial Nerve VII. Facial movement is generally best observed through spontaneous facial expression. The examiner may choose to test further for facial asymmetry by flicking the bottom of the foot to stimulate a cry, if the infant has not already done so spontaneously.

C. Bulbar Function

Cranial Nerves IX, X, and XI. Testing of the gag reflex is readily done with a wooden tongue blade. Ability to swallow is best evaluated by report of the mother or nurse.

Cranial Nerve XII. Fasciculations of the tongue have been observed, but may be difficult to distinguish from normal movements. Unusual tongue movements such as tongue thrusting and a large, obtrusive tongue should be noted.

III. Special Situations

A. Altered Mental Status

Special attention should be directed to the cranial nerves in all neonates or infants with altered mental states. This strategy can aid in localizing the site(s) of central nervous system injury. The degree of alteration should be noted.

Pupillary Responses to Light. Constricted pupils generally indicate brainstem dysfunction. Conversely, the dilated, poorly responsive pupil or pupils indicate impairment of brainstem function, often from increased intracranial pressure owing to third-nerve compression.

Corneal Reflexes. The examiner holds the lids apart and uses a small wisp of cotton to touch the cornea and elicit the reflex. Absence indicates brainstem dysfunction.

Doll's Eyes (Oculocephalic) Reflex. The so-called doll's eyes reflex is the most readily elicited response indicating brainstem dysfunction. The baby's head is turned from side to side. Failure of the eyes to move so as to main-

tain midposition indicates brainstem dysfunction. Note that this is true only in unresponsive or comatose older infants who, when alert, will focus or fix their gaze voluntarily.

Gag Reflex. In the comatose baby, the gag reflex, when absent, also reflects brainstem dysfunction.

Spontaneous Respirations. Clinicians have long used the presence and vigor of spontaneous respirations as an indicator of brainstem dysfunction.

B. Spinal Cord

For the neonate or infant with suspected or obvious spinal cord lesion, e.g., myelomeningocele, further testing is mandatory.

Sensation to Touch or Pinprick. When a sensory level is sought, pinprick testing is most effective. The skin of the neonate, and even of the infant, may be readily marred by pinprick. The testing should be done under optimal circumstances: the baby should be quiet; several examiners may wish to watch, rather than each performing separate trials; testing should begin distally and proceed proximally.

Sweating. The level of a cord lesion may also be detected by the observance of abnormal sweating, but this method is less precise for localization.

Stream of Urination. Observation of the stream is preferable. Percussion of the bladder outline may help confirm suspicions of a neurogenic bladder. Further information about infants may be gained from questioning the mother about the stream and the length of periods for which the diaper is dry. Constant dribbling also often indicates a neurogenic bladder.

Anal Wink. Testing for anal wink is done with a pin. In general, this is reserved for infants about whom there is concern about a cord lesion.

Colon Function. Decreased colon innervation generally results in constipation such that the bowel becomes distended and filled with feces. Then there may be recurrent diarrhea-like stools. The combination of a history of constipation and palpation of the abdomen for firm lumps of stool generally yields the correct interpretation. Many infants with abnormal neurologic function, particularly those with poor spontaneous movements, have constipation or less-frequent stools. They do not necessarily have poor innervation of the colon. As in most neurologic diagnoses, the constellation of findings yields the correct localization of the lesion.

IV. A. Tone, Posture, Behavior: Neonate (Neo Neuro Scoring Sheet)

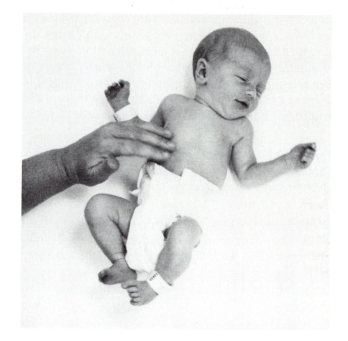

1. *Posture.* Observe the predominant posture at rest. Make separate note of extension, semiflexion, flexion, or strong flexion for arms and for legs. Also note recurrent asymmetry. The normal position for a full-term neonate is one of semiflexion or flexion of both arms and legs.

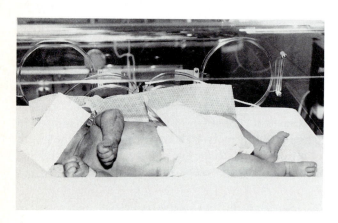

A

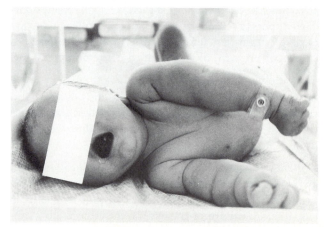

B

2. *Abnormal Posturing.* Observe throughout the examination for decorticate, decerebrate, or opisthotonic posturing. In **A**, there is flexion of the arms and extension of the legs (decorticate). There is also some neck retraction. In **B**, there is extension of the arms and extension of the legs (decerebrate). In **C**, the neonate assumes an opisthotonic posture. Note also extension of the arms and the clenched hands.

C

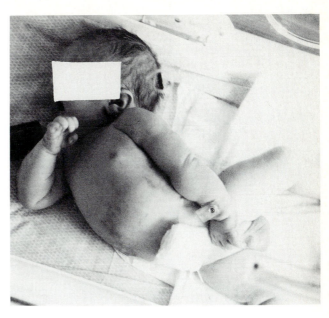

A

3. *Hand Clenching.* Observe whether the hands are never or rarely clenched, are intermittently clenched, or are persistently clenched. In **A**, the hands of a normal newborn are shown. In **B**, the hands are persistently clenched. Note also the opisthotonic posturing.

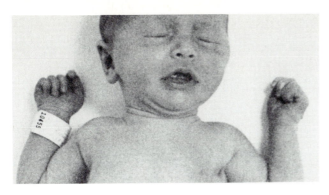

B

4. *Spontaneous Plantar Grasp.* Observe whether the toes curl persistently, intermittently, or only with stimulation (see item 5). In **B** in item 2, the toes curl persistently.

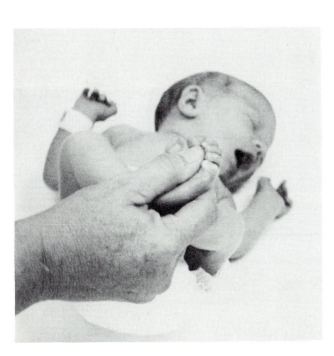

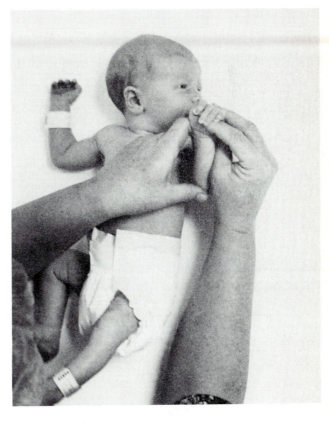

5. *Plantar Grasp.* Press a thumb or finger against the balls of the feet and observe the degree of plantar flexion of the toes. The normal degree of flexion is shown.

6. *Palmar Grasp.* Place a finger across the palm from the little finger side of the neonate's hand. Observe the degree of flexion of the fingers and arm. The normal degree of flexion is shown.

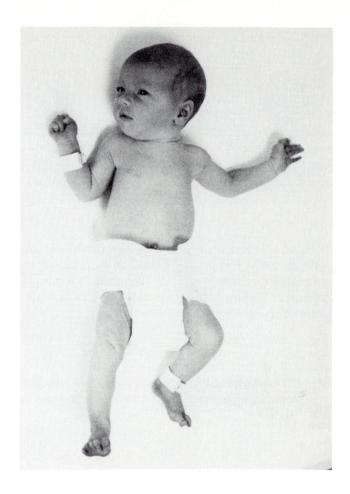

7. *Asymmetric Tonic Neck Reflex.* Turn the head slowly to one side and hold it. Observe for a fencing position: extension of the arm near the face and flexion of the opposite arm. Repeat on the other side. Observe whether this response is absent or present. If present, observe for ability of the neonate to overcome the position and for persistence of the position. The position for a normal newborn is shown.

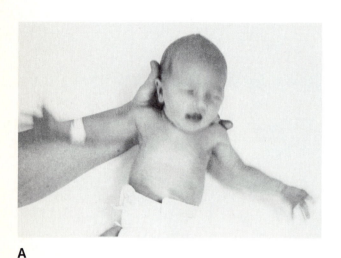

A

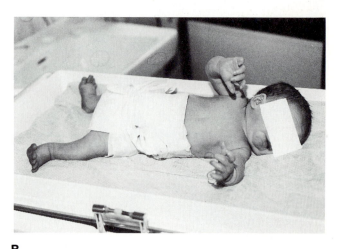

B

8. *Moro Reflex.* Support the neonate's head with one hand and the back in the midline with the other hand. Suddenly drop the neonate 10 to 20 cm and observe the response of the hands and arms. In **A**, the neonate demonstrates a normal response. In **B**, the neonate has a spontaneous exaggerated Moro reflex. Each time the neonate changes position, the Moro response is elicited.

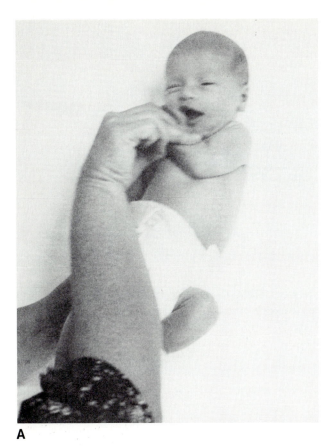

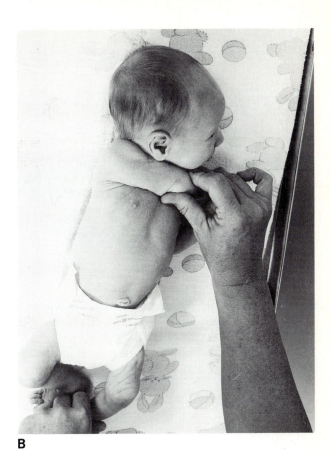

A   B

9. *Scarf Sign.* Grasp the upper arm near the elbow and move the arm across the chest. Observe the angle formed by the upper arm and a line parallel to the body. In **A,** the angle is shown for a normal neonate. In **B**, the infant demonstrates the excessive excursion of hypotonia.

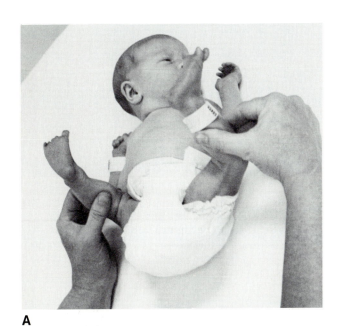

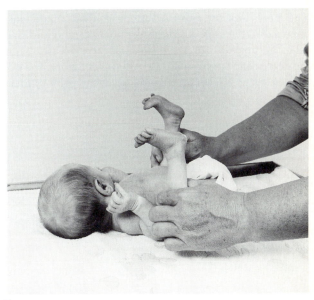

A   B

10. *Popliteal Angle.* Grasp the legs near the knee. Extend the lower leg by gentle pressure. Observe the angle formed by the neonate's upper leg and lower leg with the back of the knee as the fulcrum. In **A,** the normal popliteal angle is shown. In **B**, the excessively wide angle of hypotonia is demonstrated.

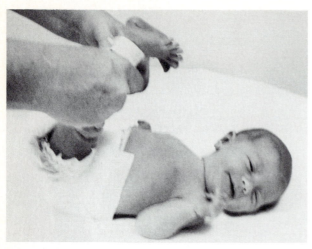

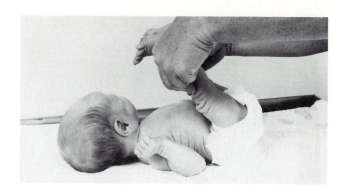

A   **B**

11. *Heel to Ear.* Grasp the legs near the ankles. Draw the feet as close to the head as they will go, keeping the buttocks on the table. Observe the angle between the neonate's trunk and legs with the hips as the fulcrum. In **A**, the normal angle is shown. In **B**, the neonate's toes may be brought near this nose more readily than is normal for age, again indicating hypotonia.

12. *Leg Recoil.* Flex both legs for 5 seconds. Then extend both legs by ankle traction with one hand and pressure on the kneecaps with the other hand. Hold this extended position for 2 seconds and then release. Note the degree and speed of hip flexion. In the figure, the examiner has positioned the legs in extension, prior to their release.

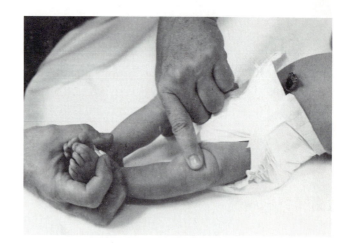

13. *Arm Traction.* With the neonate supine, grasp the wrists and slowly pull the arms to vertical. Score the angle of arm flexion at the moment the neonate is lifted from the surface. See item 17/18 for the maneuver; please note that in 17/18 the neonate has already been lifted from the surface.

14. *Held Sit.* Hold the neonate in an upright position with the examiner's hands used to support the neonate's shoulders. Observe the length of time the head is held in an upright position. See item 15 for support at the shoulders; please note that in 15 the head has been allowed to fall forward.

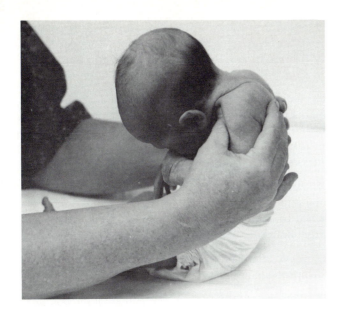

15. *Posterior Neck.* Support the neonate at the shoulders as in item 14. Allow the head to fall forward and wait 30 seconds. Note attempts to raise the head and ability to maintain the head in an upright position.

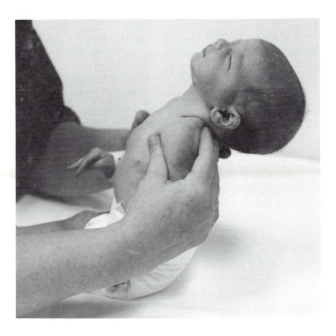

16. *Anterior Neck.* Support the neonate at the shoulders as in item 15. Allow the head to fall backward and wait 30 seconds. Note attempts to raise the head and maintain the head in an upright position.

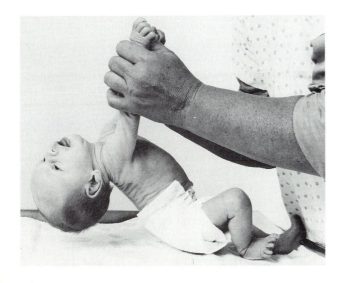

17/18. *Pull to Sit.* Use traction on both wrists to pull the neonate slowly to the sitting position. Score the *head lag* and *arm flexion* separately. In the figure, the delayed head lag and lack of arm flexion associated with hypotonia are demonstrated.

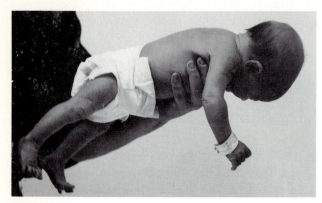

A

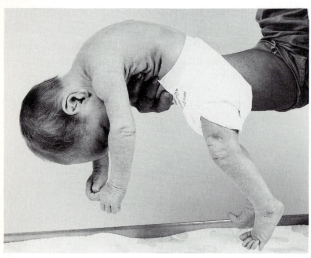

B

19. *Ventral Suspension.* Place one hand under the neonate's abdomen in the prone position and suspend the neonate horizontally. Observe the curvature of the back, the position of the head in relation to the trunk, and the flexion of the arms and legs. In **A**, normal ventral suspension is shown. In **B**, the drooping quality of neonatal hypotonia is demonstrated.

20. *Knee reflex.* Relax the leg by slight flexion at the knee. Tap the patellar area with a finger or with a small reflex hammer.

21. *Ankle reflex.* With the neonate in the prone position, flex the knee a little, then tap the ankle with two fingers horizontally or a small reflex hammer.

22. *Ankle Clonus.* Rapidly press the distal side of the foot while maintaining the leg slightly flexed. Observe for a response of quick, jerking movements of the foot.

23. *Tremor.* Observe the frequency of tremor throughout the examination. Observe also the state of the neonate at the time of tremor.

24. *Auditory Orientation* (to rattle). Support the neonate's head in the midline supine position, permitting the head to rotate. Present the auditory stimulus 6 to 10 in. from either ear in turn. Grade the response.

25. *Visual Orientation* (to black-and-white bull's-eye). Support the neonate's head in the midline supine position. Present the bull's-eye in the midline about 12 in. from the face. Move it laterally in either direction, then vertically, and finally in an arc.

26. *Alertness.* Observe the neonate throughout the examination but grade chiefly on the basis of responses obtained to auditory and visual stimuli. Note duration of attention.

27. *Suck.* Place index finger in the mouth with finger pad toward the palate. Assess strength and rhythm of suck.

28. *Movement Type.* Observe throughout the examination for sluggish, uncoordinated, jerky, athetoid, stretching, or smooth, alternating movements.

29. *Movement Amount.* Observe throughout for amount of movement.

30. *Consolability.* If the neonate does not console spontaneously, console first by talking, placing hand on belly, or wrapping. If the neonate still does not console, pick him or her up and place your finger in his or her mouth.

31. *Irritability.* Throughout the examination observe the number of stimuli required to elicit crying.

32. *Quality of Cry.* Note the absence or presence of the cry. If a cry is present, note the quality.

Using the Neonatal Neurologic (Neo Neuro) Scoring Sheet

(*Forms appear on the following pages.*) The Neo Neuro scoring sheet consists of two facing pages. The left-hand side of each page is used for the description of each item. The items are listed in an order that is logical from a clinical viewpoint. Each one should be evaluated and circled at the time of examination.

To the right of the description for each item lies the scoring for the neonatal period. The points for each item are then entered in the scoring columns at the far right. Each column is summed to yield a factor score. Factor scores are then summed to yield a total score. Two time periods are given: 0 through 48 hours and 72 hours through one week.

Scoring ranges for four categories of normality/abnormality are indicated for each of the two time periods. The categories are: normal, mildly abnormal, moderately abnormal, and severely abnormal.

The short form of the Neo Neuro consists of three items from each factor. The internal consistency for the short form is .73. It should be used only for newborns

Date of birth _____

Gestational age _____

Day of life _____

Name _____

Date _____

NEO NEURO

Item		Asymmetry	Scoring	Factors			
				1	2	3	4
1.	**POSTURE** Upper limbs a) extended b) semi-flexed or flexed c) strongly flexed lower limbs a) extended b) semi-flexed or flexed c) strongly flexed	d) = levels ≥ 2 d) = levels ≥ 2	arms a, d = 1 c = 3 b = 5 legs a, d = 1 c = 3 b = 5 sum, divide by 2				
2.	**POSTURING** a) decorticate b) decerebrate c) opisthotonic d) none of these		a, b, c = 1 d = 5				
3.	**HANDS CLENCHED** a) persistent b) intermittent c) rarely	R L d) = levels ≥ 2	a, d = 1 b = 3 c = 5				
4.	**SPONTANEOUS PLANTAR GRASP** a) persistent b) intermittent c) rarely		a = 1 b = 3 c = 5				
5.	**PALMAR GRASP** a) absent b) weak flexion c) medium flexion d) strong flexion spread to forearm e) very strong: lifts off bed	R L f) = levels ≥ 2	a, b, e, f = 1 c, d = 5				
6.	**PLANTAR GRASP** a) absent b) weak c) medium d) strong e) very strong	R L f) = levels ≥ 2	a, b, e, f = 1 c, d = 5				
7.	**ASYMMETRICAL TONIC NECK REFLEX** a) persistent b) present, not persistent c) absent		a = 1 b = 3 c = 5				
8.	**MORO** a) absent or minimal b) partial c) full d) exaggerated — immediate brisk response	R L e) = levels ≥ 2	a, d, e = 1 b = 3 c = 5				
9.	**SCARF SIGN** a) > 85° b) 60° to 85° c) 45° to 60° d) 15° to 45° e) 0° to 15°	R L f) = levels ≥ 2	a, b, c, f = 1 d = 3 e = 5				
10.	**POPLITEAL ANGLE** a) ≥ 180° b) 150° to 180° c) 130° to 150° d) 110° to 130° e) 90° to 110° f) < 90°	R L g) = levels ≥ 2	a, b, g = 1 c, f = 3 d, e = 5				
11.	**HEEL TO EAR** a) < 10° b) 10° to 40° c) 40° to 60° d) 60° to 90° e) 90° to 100° f) ≥ 100°	R L g) = levels ≥ 2	a, b, g = 1 c, d = 3 e, f = 5				
12.	**LEG RECOIL** a) no flexion by 5 sec. b) partial flexion by 5 sec. c) total flexion by 5 sec. d) immediate total flexion e) legs cannot be extended — flex strongly	R L f) = levels ≥ 2	a, e, f = 1 b = 3 c, d = 5				
13.	**ARM TRACTION** a) ≥ 180° b) 160° to 180° c) 120° to 160° d) 100° to 120° e) < 100°	R L f) = levels ≥ 2	a, b, f = 1 c, e = 3 d = 5				
14.	**HELD SIT** a) head stays forward or backward b) head up < 3 seconds c) head up 3-10 seconds d) head up > 10 seconds		a, d = 1 b = 3 c = 5				
15.	**POSTERIOR NECK** a) no attempt to raise head b) tries but cannot raise head c) head upright by 30 seconds, drops head d) head upright by 30 seconds, maintained e) examiner cannot extend head		a, e = 1 b = 3 c, d = 5				
16.	**ANTERIOR NECK** a) no attempt to raise head b) tries but cannot raise head c) head upright by 30 seconds, drops head d) head upright by 30 seconds, maintained e) examiner cannot flex head		a, e = 1 b = 3 c, d = 5				
17.	**PULL TO SIT** a. Head Lag a) 170° b) 140° to 170° c) 110° to 140° d) 70° to 110° e) > 70°		a, e = 1 b = 3 c, d = 5				
18.	b. Arm Flexion	R L f) = levels ≥ 2	a, b, e, f = 1 b = 3 c, d = 5				
19.	**VENTRAL SUSPENSION** a) b) c) d) e)		a, e = 1 b = 3 c, d = 5				

FACTOR SCORES

NEO NEURO, page 2

				5	6	7	
20.	**KNEE REFLEX** a) absent b) 1+-2+ c) brisk	d) $=\dfrac{\text{R} \quad \text{L}}{\text{levels}}$ ≥ 2	c, d = 1 a = 3 b = 5				
21.	**ANKLE REFLEX** a) absent b) 1+-2+ c) brisk	d) $=\dfrac{\text{R} \quad \text{L}}{\text{levels}}$ ≥ 2	c, d = 1 a = 3 b = 5				
22.	**ANKLE CLONUS** a) > 2 beats b) 1-2 beats c) absent		a = 1 b = 3 c = 5				
23.	**TREMOR** a) all states b) only in states 5, 6 c) also in state 4 d) only in sleep or after moro or startle e) none		a = 1 b, c = 3 d, e = 5				
24.	**AUDITORY** a) no reaction or startle b) brightens or stills c) turns to stimuli d) shifts eyes e) shifts and turns f) prolonged head turning		a = 1 b = 3 c-f = 5				
25.	**VISUAL** a) no focus or following b) focuses c) follows 30° horizontally jerkily d) follows 30° horizontally smoothly e) follows 30°-60° horizontally f) also follows vertically		a = 1 b, c = 3 d-f = 5				
26.	**ALERT** a) 0-4 sec. b) 5-10 sec. c) 11-30 sec. d) 31-60 sec. e) > 60 sec.		a = 1 b, e = 3 c, d = 5				
27.	**SUCK** a) no attempt b) weak c) strong irregular d) strong regular e) jaw clenched		a, e = 1 b, c = 3 d = 5				
28.	**MOVEMENT TYPE** a) mostly sluggish, incoordinated, jerky or athetoid b) mostly stretching or smooth alternating with random, athetoid or jerky c) smooth, alternating movements d) markedly asymmetric		a, d = 1 b = 3 c = 5				
29.	**MOVEMENT AMOUNT** a) induced b) none or minimal c) medium d) excessive		a, d = 1 b = 3 c = 5				
30.	**CONSOLABILITY** a) never cries b) consoles spontaneously c) consoles by talking, hand on belly or wrapping d) consoles by picking up or finger in mouth e) inconsolable		e = 1 d = 3 a-c = 5				
31.	**IRRITABILITY** a) no irritable crying b) cries to 1-2 stimuli c) cries to 3-4 stimuli d) cries to 5-6 stimuli e) cries consistently with stimuli f) cries without stimuli		f = 1 d, e = 3 a, b, c = 5				
32.	**QUALITY OF CRY** a) absent b) whimpering c) normal pitch and volume d) high-pitched e) hoarse		d, e = 1 a, b, c = 5				

FACTOR SCORES

TOTAL SCORE

0-48 Hrs.

Severely abnormal = < 100
Moderately abnormal = 100-119
Mildly abnormal = 120-134
Normal = 135 up

72 Hrs. - One Week

Severely abnormal = < 95
Moderately abnormal = 95-121
Mildly abnormal = 122-140
Normal = 141 up

considered to be healthy. The scoring is pass/fail; any newborn who fails the short form should be evaluated more thoroughly with the long form.

Considerable thought has been given to further description of neonatal abnormality, other than factor scores and levels of abnormality. Our data indicated that a variety of types of abnormal newborns were present in the moderately and severely abnormal ranges. These types are more numerous than the three types described by Prechtl: hemisyndrome, apathetic, and hyperexcitable. However, we believe that further categorization of these abnormalities is not indicated at this time. The implications for various combinations of abnormal factor scores must be studied in subsequent work.

Date of birth _____

Gestational age _____

Day of life _____

NEO NEURO
(Short)

Name _____

Date _____

Item		Asymmetry	Scoring	Factors							
				1	2	3	4	5	6	7	
2.	**POSTURING** a) decorticate b) decerebrate c) opisthotonic d) none of these		a, b, c = 1 d = 5								
3.	**HANDS CLENCHED** a) persistent b) intermittent c) rarely	R L d) = levels ≥ 2	a, d = 1 b = 3 c = 5								
4.	**SPONTANEOUS PLANTAR GRASP** a) persistent b) intermittent c) rarely		a = 1 b = 3 c = 5								
5.	**PALMAR GRASP** a) absent b) weak flexion c) medium flexion d) strong flexion spread to forearm e) very strong: lifts off bed f) = levels ≥ 2	R L	a, b, e, f = 1 c, d = 5								
6.	**PLANTAR GRASP** a) absent b) weak c) medium d) strong e) very strong f) = levels ≥ 2	R L	a, b, e, f = 1 c, d = 5								
8.	**MORO** a) absent or minimal b) partial c) full d) exaggerated — immediate brisk response e) = levels ≥ 2	R L	a, d, e = 1 b = 3 c = 5								
9.	**SCARF SIGN** a) > 85° b) 60° to 85° c) 45° to 60° d) 15° to 45° e) 0° to 15° f) = levels ≥ 2	R L	a, b, c, f = 1 d = 3 e = 5								
10.	**POPLITEAL ANGLE** b) 150° to 180° c) 130° to 150° d) 110° to 130° e) 90° to 110° f) under 90° g) = levels ≥ 2	R L	a, b, g = 1 c, f = 3 d, e = 5								
11.	**HEEL TO EAR** b) 10° to 40° c) 40° to 60° d) 60° to 90° e) 90° to 100° f) ≥ 100° a) < 10° g) = levels ≥ 2	R L	a, b, g = 1 c, d = 3 e, f = 5								
14.	**HELD SIT** a) head flops forward b) head up < 3 seconds c) head up 3-10 sec. d) head up > 10 sec.		a, d = 1 b = 3 c = 5								
16.	**ANTERIOR NECK** a) no attempt to raise head b) tries but cannot raise head c) head upright by 30 seconds, drops head d) head upright by 30 seconds, maintained e) examiner cannot flex head		a, e = 1 b = 3 c, d = 5								
17.	**PULL TO SIT — HEAD LAG ONLY** a) b) c) d) e)		a, e = 1 b = 3 c, d = 5								
20.	**KNEE REFLEX** a) absent b) 1+ -2+ c) brisk	d) = levels ≥ 2	c, d = 1 a = 3 b = 5								
21.	**ANKLE REFLEX** a) absent b) 1+ -2+ c) brisk	d) = levels ≥ 2	c, d = 1 a = 3 b = 5								
22.	**ANKLE CLONUS** a) ≥ 2 beats b) 1-2 beats c) absent		a = 1 b = 3 c = 5								
25.	**VISUAL** a) no focus or following b) focuses c) follows 30° horizontally jerkily d) follows 30° horizontally smoothly e) follows 30°-60° horizontally f) also follows vertically		a = 1 b, c = 3 d-f = 5								
26.	**ALERT** a) 0-4 sec. b) 5-10 sec. c) 11-30 sec. d) 31-60 sec. e) > 60 sec.		a = 1 b, e = 3 c, d = 5								
27.	**SUCK** a) no attempt b) weak c) strong irregular d) strong regular e) jaw clenched		a, e = 1 b, c = 3 d = 5								
30.	**CONSOLABILITY** a) never cries b) consoles spontaneously c) consoles by talking, hand on belly or wrapping d) consoles by picking up or finger in mouth e) inconsolable		e = 1 d = 3 a-c = 5								
31.	**IRRITABILITY** a) no irritable crying b) cries to 1-2 stimuli c) cries to 3-4 stimuli d) cries to 5-6 stimuli e) cries constantly f) cries without stimuli		f = 1 d, e = 3 a, b, c = 5								
32.	**QUALITY OF CRY** a) absent b) whimpering c) normal pitch and volume d) high-pitched e) hoarse		d, e = 1 a, b, c = 5								

FACTOR SCORES

TOTAL SCORES

0-48 Hrs.

Fail < 91
Pass ≥ 91
(Normal)

72 Hrs. - One Week

Fail < 95
Pass ≥ 95
(Normal)

All neonates with fail scores
should be assessed with the
32-item (full) Neoneuro.

4/87

IV. B. Tone and Posture: Infant (Infanib Scoring Sheet)

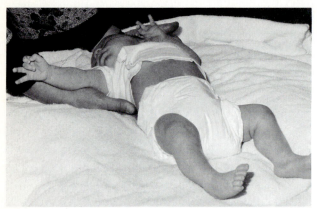

A

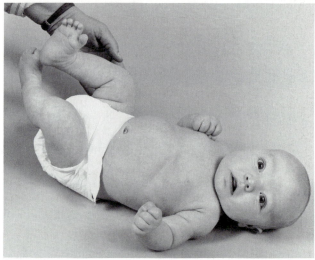

B

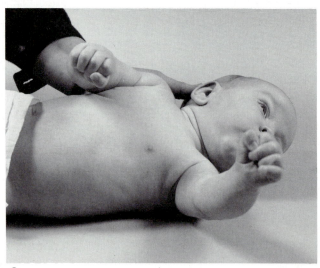

C

1. *Hands Open/Closed.* Observe the infant's hands. Constant return to a clenched hand or a tightly closed hand would be noted with any of the stress maneuvers. These may be induced by the examiner, as in the tonic labyrinthine supine maneuver, or induced spontaneously by the infant, as with even a slight turning of the head. At age 1 month, the normal infant in **A** holds his hands open even during an examiner-induced stress maneuver. At age 2 months, the infant with transient neuromotor abnormalities in **B** holds his hands clenched with even the slightest stimulation. At age 3½ months, the abnormal infant in **C** also clenches his hands with any stimulation, either examiner- or self-induced.

French Angles. The French angles form a part of the measure of gestational age by assessment when both physical and neurologic items are combined. The progressions are described from extreme immaturity to full term. Reversed progressions occur from full term to approximately 9 to 10 months in infancy. The scarf sign, heel to ear, popliteal angle, and leg abduction look similar in the preterm neonate who has a gestational age of 28 weeks and in the 9- to 10-month-old infant. Significant deviations are indicative of hypotonia or hypertonia.

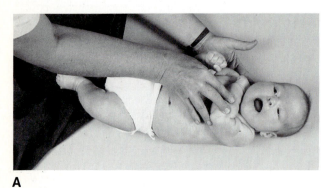

A   **B**

2. *Scarf Sign.* Hold the infant's arm near the elbow and move the arm across the infant's chest until resistance is met, as indicated in **C.** (In the other figures the maneuver is performed less well technically but the angle is seen more clearly.) Observe the angle between a vertical line dropped from the insertion of the arm and the upper arm.

A scarf sign with larger exertion than normal is an excellent indicator of hypotonia of the upper body,

Continued on next page.

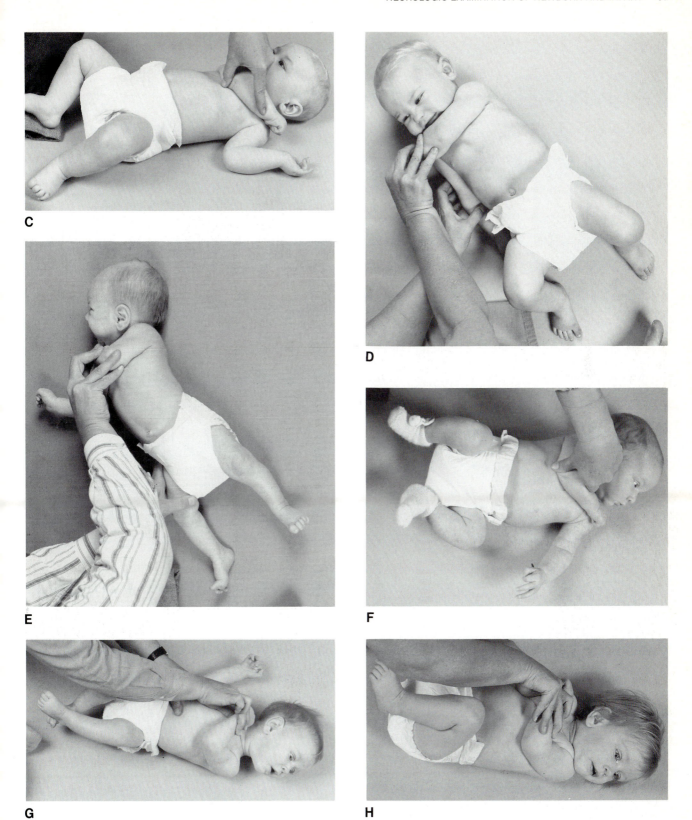

a very common finding in infants with other indicators of neurologic abnormality. Early hypertonia is uncommon. Progression from hypotonia to hypertonia in the upper body occurs in those infants with spastic tetraparesis/dyskinesia.

In the first series, the normal progression is shown from 0 to 3 **A,** to 4 to 6 **B,** to 7 to 9 **C,** to 10 to 12 months **D.** Note the increasing ease with which the shoulder (and trapezius muscle) extends and the arm is moved across the chest. In the second series (**E–H**), the progression is reversed. Initially (0 to 3 months), the arm is extended too easily, indicating hypotonia. At each subsequent step (4 to 6, 7 to 9, and 10 to 12 months), the shoulder extends less easily, indicating a progression from hypotonia to hypertonia.

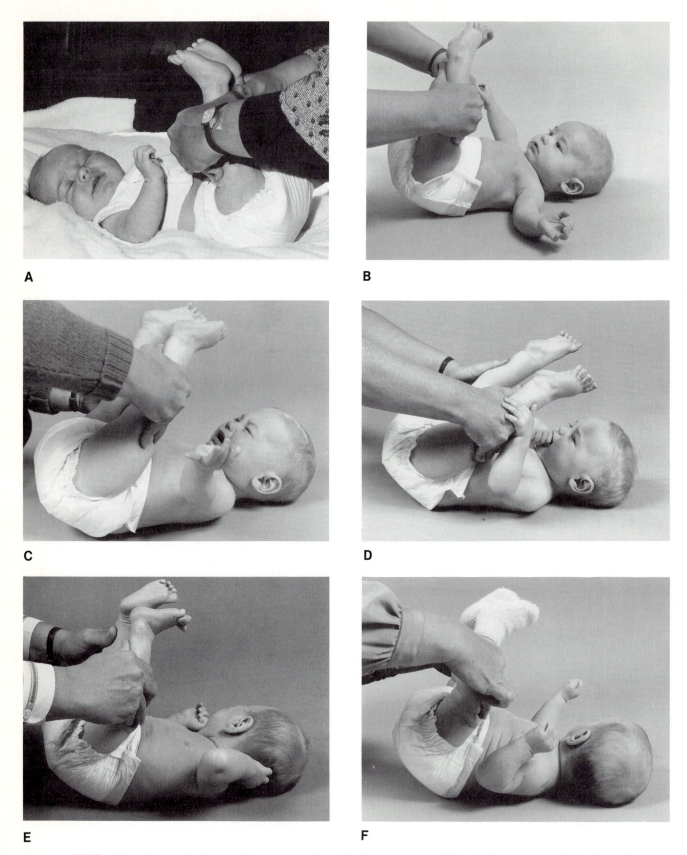

3. *Heel to Ear.* Grasp the legs at the knees so that the legs are extended and the position of the buttocks is well controlled. As much as possible, the buttocks should remain on or near the examining table (specifically this is not a measure of the flexibility of the spine; it is a measure of the flexibility of the hips). Measure the angle between the infant's trunk and legs.

Continued on next page.

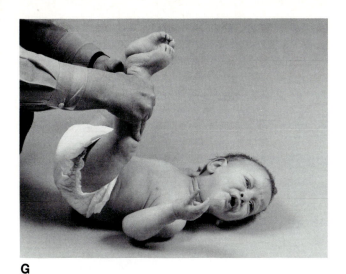

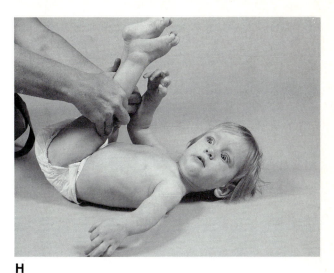

G

H

This is one of the best early indicators of hypertonia of the lower body. Infants with spastic diplegia or spastic tetraparesis/dyskinesia generally show change first in the flexibility of the hips or knees (see item 4). A developmental milestone that represents this progression is the item "plays with feet," used in the Gesell Screening Inventory at age 28 weeks.

In the first series (A–D), the normal infant shows the normal progression from 0 to 3, to 4 to 6, to 7 to 9, to 10 to 12 months. In the second series (E–H), the abnormal infant fails to decrease the heel-to-ear angle after 0 to 3 months. He departs increasingly from the normal progression as each interval passes (4 to 6 months, 7 to 9 months, 10 to 12 months). In addition, he assumes an asymmetric tonic neck posture and keeps his hands closed (H).

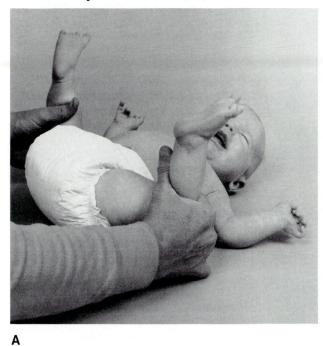

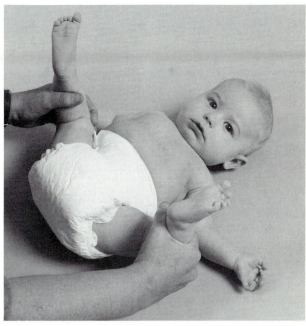

A

B

4. *Popliteal Angle.* Hold the legs near the knee, flex the leg at the hip, and abduct the legs, extending the lower leg until resistence is met. With the back of the knee as the fulcrum, measure the angle between the upper and lower parts of the leg. As indicated in item 3, popliteal angle is another excellent indicator of hypertonia in the lower body. Failure of the angle to increase throughout early and middle infancy often indicates spastic tetraparesis/dyskinesia, spastic diplegia, and, asymmetrically, spastic hemiparesis.

In the first series (A–D), the infant shows the normal progression from 0 to 3, to 4 to 6, to 7 to 9, to 10 to 12 months. In the second series (E–H), the popliteal angle is initially hypotonic, then becomes hypertonic.

Illustrations continued on next page.

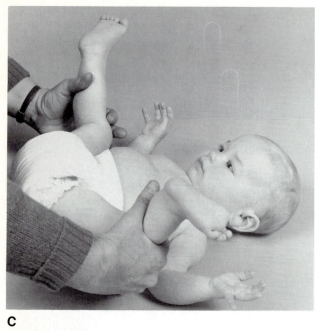

C

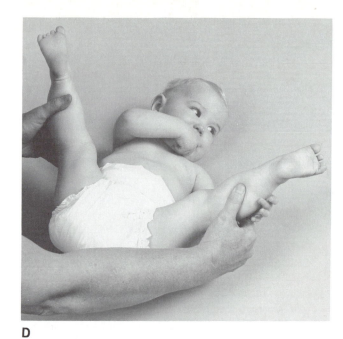

D

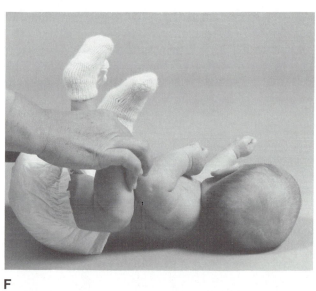

E

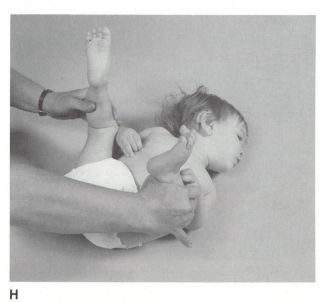

F

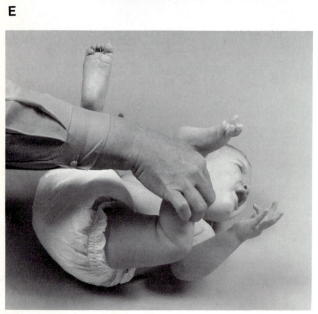

G

H

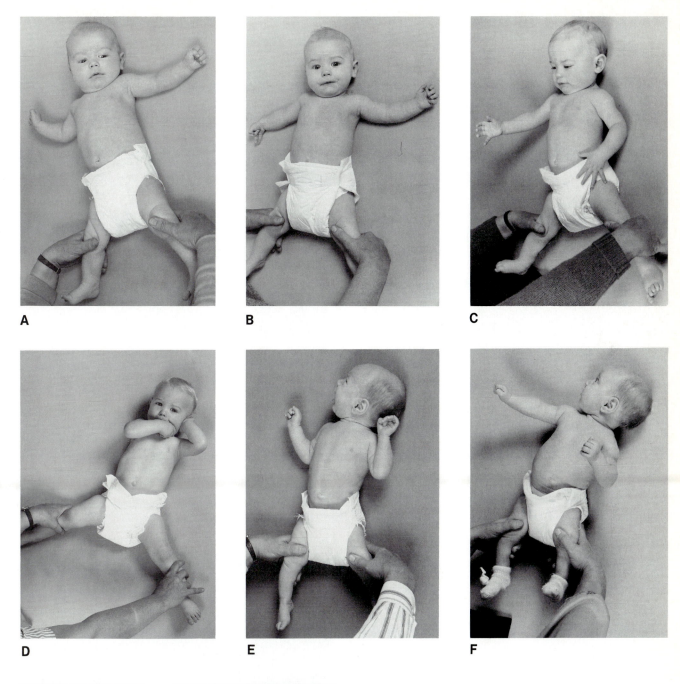

A

B

C

D

E

F

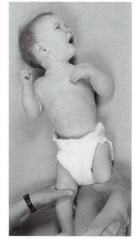

G

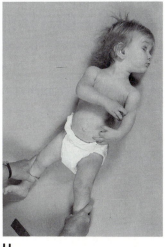

H

5. *Leg Abduction.* Hold the legs at the knee such that they are extended; abduct the legs. With the crotch as a fulcrum, measure the angle between the legs. This item is generally less sensitive than heel to ear or popliteal angle as an early indicator of hypertonia. It is an excellent indicator of hypotonia, but there are many other excellent indicators of hypotonia.

In the first series, the normal infant demonstrates the normal progression from 0 to 3 (**A**), to 4 to 6 (**B**), to 7 to 9 (**C**) to 10 to 12 months (**D**). In the second series, the abnormal infant has no increase in the angle at 4 to 6 months (**E**) or at any other age range.

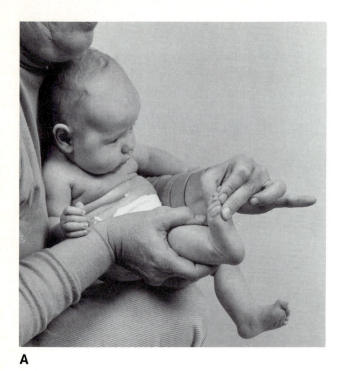

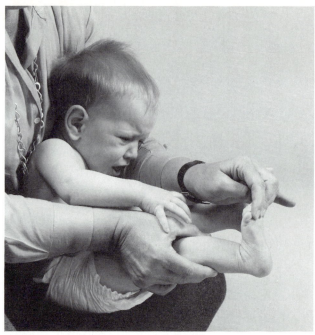

A   B

6. *Dorsiflexion of the Foot.* Flex the foot, pushing it against the leg until resistance is met. With the ankle as a fulcrum, measure the angle between the foot and the leg.

The feet are generally the last to show hypertonia, except in situations of very early severe hypertonicity, in which they may be in an extended position that is very difficult to change. More frequently, the feet are hypotonic until middle or late infancy, even in infants with spastic tetraparesis/dyskinesia.

At age 2 months, the normal infant (**A**) has a normal angle of dorsiflexion of the foot. At 4 months, the abnormal infant (**B**) has an increased angle of dorsiflexion of the foot.

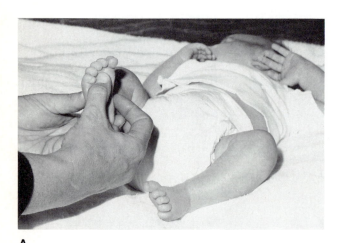

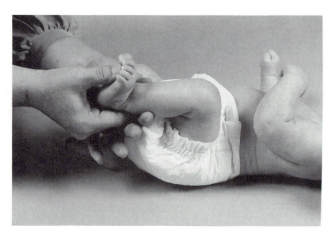

A   B

7. *Foot Grasp.* Place the thumb or finger firmly in the footpad and observe for curling of the infant's toes toward the bottom of the foot.

Foot grasp is a primitive reflex; specifically it is an item that is normal in the neonate but disappears in the course of infancy. For many of the primitive reflexes, the range of time that is considered normal for disappearance is quite long. It can also be exaggerated in its manifestation in early infancy; these exaggerations are abnormal. After the age at which the item should no longer be present, it can be graded to represent levels of normality/abnormality (no grasp, barely grasps, grasp).

At 1 month of age, the normal infant (**A**) has a prominent but not exaggerated foot grasp. At 3 months, the abnormal infant (**B**) has an exaggerated foot grasp.

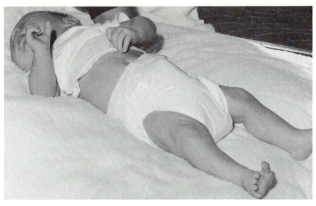

A

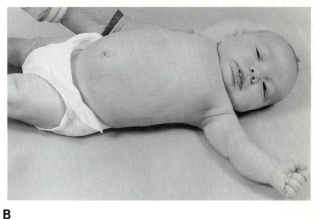

B

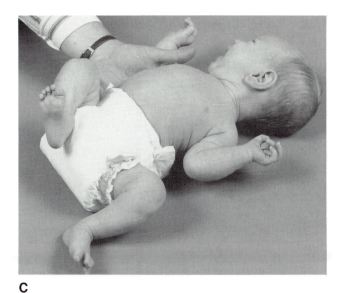

C

8. *Tonic Labyrinthine Supine.* Stimulate the intrascapular area with the hand. Observation is made of shoulder retraction and extension or flexion of arms, legs, or trunk. This item is also a primitive reflex.

At one month of age, the normal infant (**A**) demonstrates little response to this maneuver. The infant in (**B**) has a dramatic response with extension of both arms and legs; this response was graded as abnormal. The abnormal infant (**C**) has flexion of both arms and legs at 2 months; this response was also graded as abnormal.

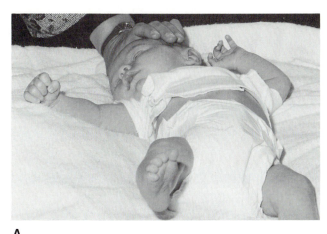

A

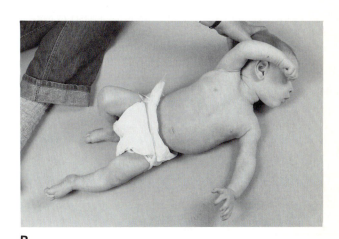

B

9. *Asymmetric Tonic Neck Reflex.* Turn the infant's head from side to side, observing the assumption of a fencing position, the extension of the arm faced, the flexion of the arm behind the head, and the extension of the leg faced. Also note the persistence of the posture: whether the infant assumes the posture and then moves out of it, in contrast to persisting in the posture. Persistence is abnormal at any age and is the manifestation of exaggeration of the reflex.

At age 1 month, the normal infant (**A**) manifests an asymmetric tonic neck reflex, which he then overcomes. The abnormal infant (**B**) at 5 months has a strong, persistent asymmetric tonic neck reflex. (It may be noted in many of the pictures of this infant that he goes into an asymmetric tonic neck reflex with many neurologic maneuvers, as well as spontaneously and repetitively when he is supine.)

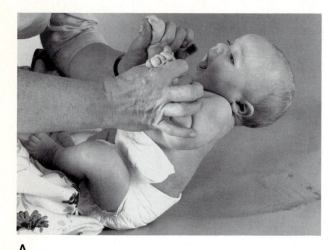

A

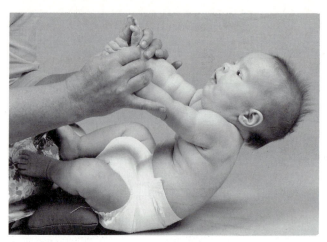

B

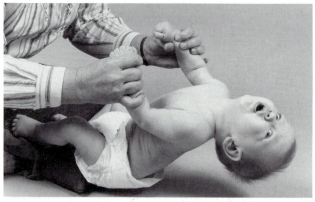

C

10. *Pull to Sitting.* Grasp the infant's hands and pull the infant to a sitting position. As seen in the figures, a small sandbag may be used as a weight to maintain the position of the buttocks. Observe first the position of the head: extended, straight up, or flexed. Second, observe the position of the arms: extended or flexed. If there is a discrepancy in the two observations, the scoring is based on the position of the head.

The most common abnormal finding is that of delay in head control or hypotonia of the neck and upper trunk. Hypertonia is noted much less frequently. The manifestation is precocious head control with extension of the head. This is demonstrated by the infant in (**A**) at age 2 months. His head control is "superior" to that expected for his age, an indication of the hypertonicity of his neck muscles. The normal infant (**B**) at 2 months has normal head control. The abnormal infant (**C**) at 7 months persists in poor head control, which he has had since his neonatal neurologic examination.

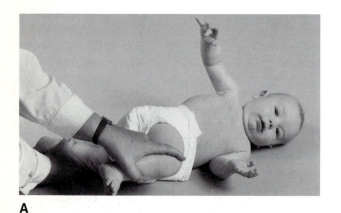

A

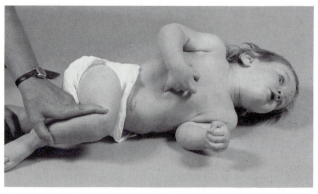

B

11. *Body Derotative.* Hold the infant by the lower legs, then rotate the legs to initiate rolling from supine to prone. Observe the infant's continuation of the maneuver. An infant with neurologic impairment may not be able to accomplish this or may do so slowly or awkwardly. To check for noncompliance, ask the parent if spontaneous rolling from supine to prone occurs at home. Full credit is given for a reported supine-to-prone roll.

At age 4 months, the normal infant readily raises the upper arm and participates in the maneuver. The abnormal infant flexes his arms, extends his trunk and head, and cannot complete the maneuver.

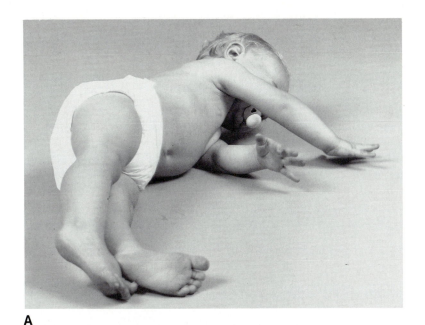

A

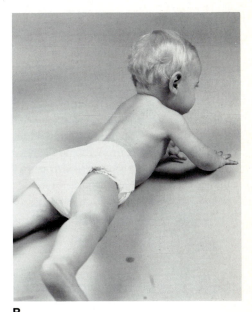

B

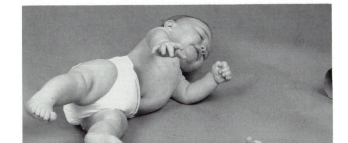

C

12. *Body Rotative.* The infant spontaneously rolls from supine to prone, then pulls to standing position. In normal infants the maneuver is often accomplished spontaneously in the course of the examination. The normal infant's ease with the maneuver is seen in (**A**) and (**B**). The abnormal infant accomplishes the maneuver, but he is slower and has a logrolling style: his upper and lower body are rolled as a unit.

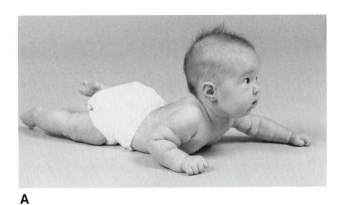

A

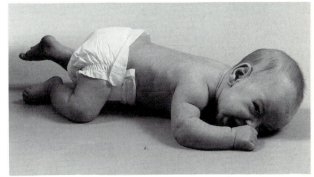

B

13. *All Fours.* Move the infant to the prone position. The rating of this item is based on observation of head position, arm position, and leg position. The major component is head position. The examiner is seeking optimal performance; encouragement of the infant is not only permitted but preferable.

The normal infant (**A**) at age 2 months holds her head up 90°; she extends the left arm and rests on the right forearm. The abnormal infant (**B**) at 4 months does not lift his head at all, even with much encouragement. His mother reported that he held his head up briefly at home.

14. *Tonic Labyrinthine Prone.* Move the infant to the prone position. Flex the infant's head and observe shoulder retraction and flexion of arms, hips, or legs under the trunk. The infant's body may be stabilized by placement of the examiner's hand under the abdomen. This is another primitive reflex, thus exaggeration is an abnormal response in early infancy. At 7 months, the abnormal infant has a prompt and vigorous response to head flexion.

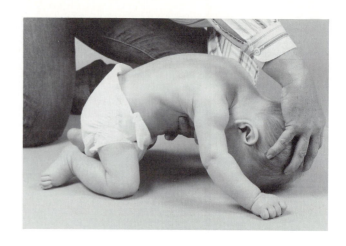

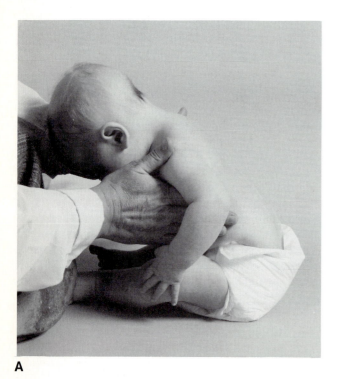

A

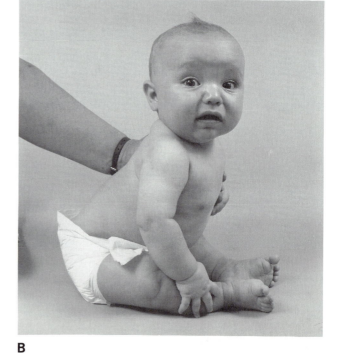

B

15. *Sitting.* The examiner holds or places the infant in a sitting position and notes the point at which bending occurs (L-3, L-5). It may not be possible to get the infant into a sitting position if there is repetitive extensor posturing. Other items (e.g., tonic labyrinthine prone, tonic labyrinthine supine, and asymmetric tonic neck reflex) should also be abnormal with extensor posturing of this degree. More frequently, abnormality is manifested by poor trunk control with a delay in the progression of sitting positions.

At age 4 months, the normal infant (**A**) bends forward from L-3. At the same age, the infant in (**B**) bends forward from L-5 and holds his head in an extended position. This precocious sitting position is abnormal, indicating excessive extension. At age 6 months, the abnormal infant (**C**) bends forward from L-3, indicating a delay in trunk control.

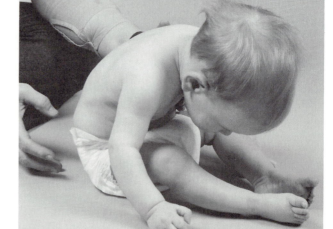

C

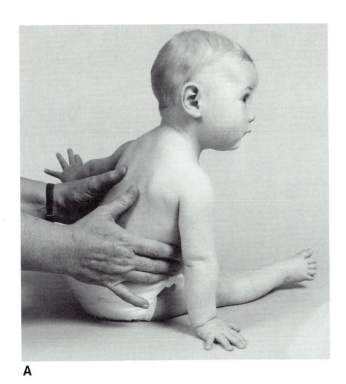

A

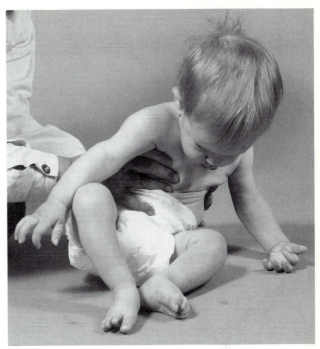

B

16. *Sideways Parachute.* Hold the infant in a sitting position, then tip the infant gently but firmly to each side and observe for the extension of the infant's hand to "prevent" falling or provide support. The parachute items, including sideways, forward, and backward parachutes, probably provide a measure of the maturation of vestibular function. Sideways and forward parachute maneuvers are also useful in the identification of hemiparesis. A hemiparetic infant demonstrates less thrust with the impaired arm.

At 8 months of age, the normal infant (**A**) readily thrusts his arm and head out in support. At the same age the abnormal infant (**B**) makes no effort to support himself with his arm and hand.

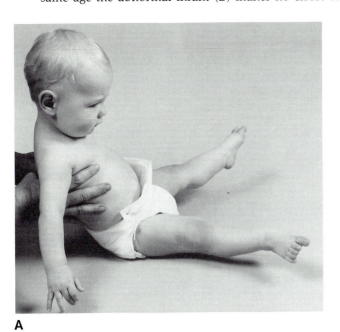

A

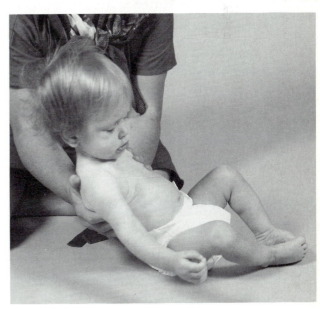

B

17. *Backward Parachute.* Gently but firmly thrust the infant backward, holding the infant at the trunk so that he or she will not lose balance and fall. Observe the posturing of the infant's arms. Some infants may turn to one side, appearing to use one arm more than the other. Because of this, the backward parachute maneuver is less useful in distinguishing asymmetry.

At 9 months of age, the normal infant (**A**) thrusts both arms toward the back. The abnormal infant (**B**) makes no effort to do so.

18. *Standing (Weight-Bearing).* Place the infant in a standing position and observe the position of the infant's body. Most newborns assume a standing position because of primitive reflexes. This tendency is lost variably but is almost always gone by age 2 months. Then the infant makes no attempt to weight-bear, or is at best unable to weight-bear.

Early weight-bearing, at approximately 2 to 5 months, should be associated with "buckling" at the knee. Specifically, the infant stands with legs straight, then bends or flexes the knees briefly and resumes a more straight-legged stance. Persistent standing without buckling often indicates hypertonia. Thus it is scored as abnormal. "Unequal" weight-bearing is less clear-cut; the infant may shift weight from one leg to another or stand such that the weight appears to be borne by one leg more than the other.

At 10 months, the normal infant (**A**) is sufficiently relaxed in a standing position that he appears casual and at ease. The abnormal infant (**B**) cannot maintain his trunk well and exhibits extensor posturing in a standing position (feet extended and head thrust back).

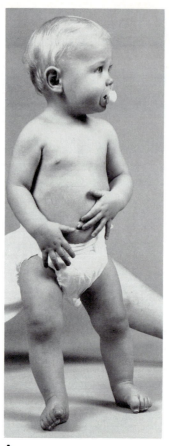

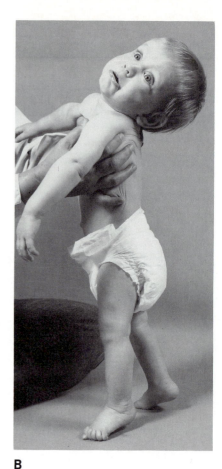

A

B

19. *Positive Support Reaction.* Observe the position of the infant's feet as the infant is placed in a standing position. The item is described and scored here a bit differently than usual, in order to focus attention on the feet. The item "belongs" with other items that describe the legs and feet: dorsiflexion of the foot, foot grasp, and weight-bearing. The abnormal infant fails to drop the heel flat to the floor.

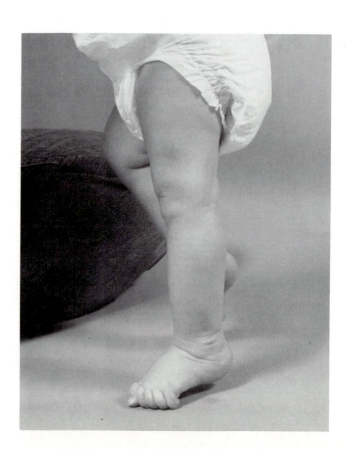

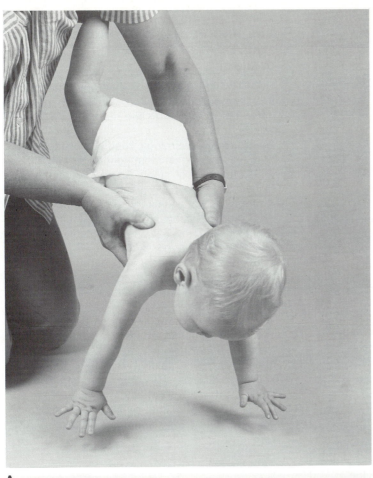

A

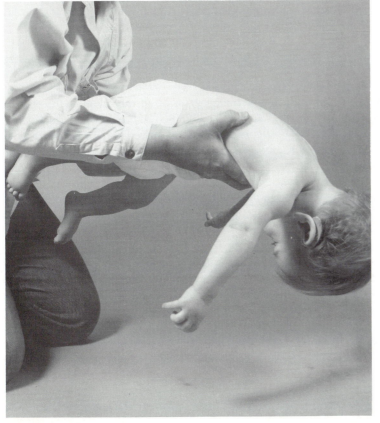

B

20. *Suspended Position: Forward Parachute.* Hold the infant at the trunk and propel the infant forward toward a surface, such as a table, thrusting the infant's head downward. Observe the infant's thrusting of arms forward for protection or support. As noted in item 16, this item is also an excellent indicator of asymmetry as manifested by unilateral arm thrust.

At age 7 months, the normal infant (**A**) thrusts his arms and hands forward. At the same age, the abnormal infant (**B**) makes no effort do do this.

Using the Infant Measure of Tone and Posture (Infanib) Scoring Sheet

(The Infanib appears on the following pages.) The items on the Infanib are listed in a logical order, progressing from supine to prone to sitting to standing to suspension. The age at which the item appears is listed at the far left. For each item, the examiner circles the description that most closely approximates the infant being examined. An item is not scored unless it is appropriate for the infant's corrected gestational age (thus 0 points are given for items below the infant's corrected gestational age). The age at which a major change occurs appears in the second column at the left.

The examiner uses the second page of the scoring sheet to ascertain the score per item. The age of the infant (corrected gestational age) is indicated at the top. Each item is scored by its relation to the infant's age. In general, items that are normal are scored 5, items that are mildly abnormal are scored 3, and items that are markedly abnormal are scored 1. For items that progress with age, a delay of one stage is scored 3 and a delay of two stages is scored 1. For the French angles items, the deviation may be in either direction, permitting a description of hypotonia (delay) or hypertonia (precocious). As noted previously, hands closed/open, foot grasp, tonic labyrinthine supine, asymmetric tonic neck reflex, and tonic labyrinthine prone are scored in the early months as abnormal only if the response is exaggerated. Early acquisition of a skill may be abnormal. For example, infants between 2½ and 5 months who do not "buckle" at the knee within 60 seconds receive a score of 1 (abnormal). Similarly young infants who bring their heads forward too well on pull to sit are scored as abnormal. All asymmetric positions are also given a score of 1. This approach assists in a diagnosis of hemiparesis.

The scores for each item should be placed in the allotted spaces on the first page of the scoring sheet. Each column is summed to obtain a factor score. This helps the examiner think about the items in groups. The factor scores are then summed to obtain a total score.

The degree of normality/abnormality based on the total score is ascertained from the chart on the second page of the scoring sheet for three age divisions: less than 4 months, 4 to 8 months, and eight months or more. For those infants whose scores fall in the range of abnormal, a category of abnormality is selected by the examiner.

In most of our work with infants, we have used a limited choice of categories for designation of neurologic abnormality: spastic tetraparesis/dyskinesia, spastic hemiparesis, spastic diplegia, and moderate to severe hypotonia. The mild hypotonias are included in transient neuromotor abnormalities. These categories evolved with experience and in working with other clinicians. When more categories of abnormality were utilized, we clinicians often disagreed. Thus the slightly broader categories were utilized when the research required that each category be graded for purposes of data analysis or for description of the progression of the category through infancy (Ellison et al., 1983). The types of abnormality and their outcome has been discussed in detail in other work (Ellison, 1984a,b). Any examiner who evaluates and scores an infant should have knowledge of these progressions before discussing the infant with the parents.

Summary. The Infanib provides a quantified, reliable measure of body tone and posture. It permits comparison of an infant between one visit and another; it permits comparison between one patient and another; it permits comparison between infants from one hospital and those from another. Three types of scores can be used for these comparisons: item scores, factor or dimension scores, and total scores. Serial examinations from larger numbers of infants can be readily stored in the computer for later data analysis.

For both clinical use and research purposes, the Infanib should help us in our quest for further knowledge about the neurology of infancy, its relationship to perinatal events, and its relationship to later function.

Pearls and Perils: Neurologic Examination of the Newborn and Infant

1. Do not wait for the developmentally delayed infant to "grow out of it." Perform or obtain careful developmental *and* neurologic evaluation.
2. Do not name a neurologic condition on the basis of one or two signs. Most conditions comprise a constellation of signs. Some exceptions include facial nerve palsy or brachial plexus injury.
3. Address parental anxiety. Parents are savvy. They read books on infant development. In the experiences of this examiner, their concerns are usually well founded.
4. Young (0 to 3 months) hypotonic infants may become spastic.
5. Older (6 to 12 months) hypotonic infants tend to become less hypotonic.
6. Monoparesis generally changes either by disappearing (most likely) or progressing to hemiplegia or diplegia.
7. Infants with early spasticity tend to appear more spastic as time passes—those with tetraparesis more so, those with diplegia less so.
8. Examination of the knee area with the popliteal angle measure is very helpful because both proximal and distal spasticity are thus identified.
9. As a constellation, delayed head control, hypotonia of arms, and limited popliteal angle or heel-to-ear angle are excellent early indicators of cerebral palsy.
10. Use of the reflex hammer is less reliable than evaluation of tone and posture.

INFANIB

CIRCLE ONE

Date of Exam _____

Corrected Gestational Age _____

ITEM	START SCORE	MAJOR CHANGE	NAME					
1	Birth		**SUPINE** Hands closed/open	Clenched	Clenched with stress maneuver	Closed	Sometimes closed	Open
2	Birth		Scarf sign	Less Than #1	0° to 15° (1)	15° to 45° (2)	45° to 60° (3)	60° to 85° (4) — Past #4
3	Birth		Heel to ear	Over 100°	90° to 100°	60° to 90°	40° to 60°	10° to 40° — Under 10°
4	Birth		Popliteal angle	Under 80°	80° to 90°	90° to 110°	110° to 150°	150° to 170° — Over 170°
5	Birth		Leg abduction	Under 40°	40° to 70°	70° to 100°	100° to 130°	130° to 150° — Over 150°
6	Birth		Dorsiflexion of foot	0° to 10°	10° to 40°	40° to 70°	70° to 80°	80° to 90°
7	Birth	9 mos.	Foot grasp		No Grasp	Barely Grasp	Average grasp	Excessive grasp or grasp with stress maneuver
8	Birth	6 mos.	Tonic labyrinthine supine		Absent	Some shoulder retraction or some extension of trunk or legs	Shoulder retraction and full leg extension or flexed arms and legs	
9	Birth	6 mos.	Asymmetric tonic neck reflex		Absent	Postures in, can move out	Persistent or spontaneous	
10	Birth		Pull to sitting		Head extended Arms extended	Head up Arms ext.	Head flexed Arms ext.	Head flexed Arms flexed
11	4 mos.		Body derotative		Present to both sides	Slow or mildly asymmetrical	Absent or markedly asymmetrical	
12	9 mos		Body rotative		Present to both sides	Slow or mildly asymmetrical	Absent or markedly asymmetrical	
13	Birth		**PRONE** All fours	Lifts Head	Head up 45°	Forearms only	Head up 90°	Bears weight on extended arms / Assumes all fours unsteadily / Assumes all fours well / Stands up through Plantigrade
14	Birth	9 mos.	Tonic labyrinthine prone		Absent	Some shoulder protraction or some flexion of legs	With Head Flexion — Shoulder protraction and arms, hips, or legs under trunk	
15	Birth		**SITTING** Sitting position			L3	L5	
16	6 mos.		Sideways parachute		Present in both arms	Slow or mildly asymmetrical	Absent or markedly asymmetrical	
17	9 mos.		Backwards parachute		Present in both arms	Slow or mildly asymmetrical	Absent or markedly asymmetrical	
18	Birth		**STANDING** Weight bearing	Primitive reflex	No weight bearing	Poor weight bearing Breaks at knees	Unequal weight bearing	
19	3 mos.		Positive support reaction		Feet flat	5 to 30 sec. on toes then drop to feet flat	>30 sec. on toes	
20	7 mos.		**SUSPENDED** Forward parachute		Present	Slow or mildly asymmetrical	Absent or markedly asymmetrical	

FACTOR SCORES

TOTAL SCORE

INFANIB, page 2

Overall: Normal = 5, Mildly abnormal = 3,
Markedly abnormal = 1

↓ Corrected gestational age
SCORING
Comments

ITEM	0-.9	1-1.9	2-2.9	3-3.9	4-4.9	5-5.9	6-6.9	7-7.9	8-8.9	9-18 months	matches age = 5
1.	Closed	Some times closed	Open				At any age, clenched or clenched with stress maneuver = 1				One stage delay = 3 Two stage delay = 1 One closed, one open = 1
2.	0 - 15°		15 - 45°			45 - 60°			60 - 85°		5 = Picture matches age 3 = One stage away ← or → 1 = Two stages away ← or →
3.	100 - 90°		90 - 60°			60 - 40°			40 - 10°		
4.	80 - 90°		90 - 110°			110 - 150°			150 - 170°		As above except definite asymmetry = 1
5.	40 - 70°		70 - 100°			100 - 130°			130 - 150°		As for # 2 & 3
6.	0-10° = 1 40-80° = 5 10-40° = 3 80-90° = 3		0-10° = 1 10 - 40° = 3			40 - 70° = 5		70 - 80° = 3		80 - 90° = 1	Definite asymmetry = 1
7.	Excessive grasp or grasp with stress maneuver = 1 , Other = 5							Absent = 5	Barely Grasp = 3	Grasp = 1	Definite asymmetry = 1
8.	Shoulder retraction and full leg extension or flexed arms and legs = 1, Other = 5							Absent = 5	Some = 3	Full = 1	
9.	Persistent or spontaneous = 1, Other = 5					Absent = 5	Postures in Can move out = 3			Persistent = 1	
10.						Full = 5 Partial head lag or not using arms = 3 Complete head lag and not using arms = 1					Picture matches age = 5 One stage delay = 3 Two stage delay = 1 0-4 months head flexion and arm flexion = 1
11.				Present to both sides = 5			Slow or mildly asymmetrical = 3		Absent or markedly asymmetrical = 1		
12.								Present = 5 Slow or mildly asymmetrical = 3 Absent or markedly asymmetrical = 1			
13.	Lifts Head	Head up 45°	Forearms only	Head up 90°	Bears weight on extended forearms	All fours unsteadily	All fours well	Plantigrade			Picture matches age = 5 One stage delay = 3 Two stage delay = 1
14.	Shoulder protraction , arms, hips or legs under trunk = 1, other = 5							Absent = 5	Some = 3	Full = 1	
15.				L3 →	L5 →						Picture matches age = 5 One stage delay = 3 Two stage delay = 1 0-5 months L5 break and head extension = 1
16.						Present in both arms = 5		Slow or mildly asymmetrical = 3	Absent or markedly asymmetrical = 1		
17.								As Above			
18.	Primitive Reflex	No Weight-bearing	Poor weight bearing Breaks at knee		Unequal weight bearing						Picture matches age = 5 One stage delay = 3 Two stage delay = 1
											Persistent weight-bearing (> 60 sec) at 2.5 - 5 months = 1
19.				Maintains weight feet flat = 5		5 - 30 sec. on toes then drop to feet flat = 3			> 30 sec on toes = 1		
20.							Present = 5	Slow or mildly asymmetrical = 3	Absent or markedly asym. = 1		

Degree of normality/abnormality based on total score

Less than 4 months	4 to 8 months	8 months or more
Abnormal ≤ 48	Abnormal ≤ 54	Abnormal ≤ 68
Transient 49 - 65	Transient 55-71	Transient 69-82
Normal ≥ 66	Normal ≥ 72	Normal ≥ 83

Category of abnormality

If abnormal, choose a category

☐ Spastic Tetraparesis/Dyskinesia   ☐ Spastic Hemiparesis   ☐ Spastic Diplegia   ☐ Hypotonia

WHAT IS THE PROGNOSIS FOR NEUROLOGIC ABNORMALITY?

Neonates

Newborns who are normal neurologically are, in general, normal at follow-up. This was noted in the studies of Prechtl, in which 8% of the normal neonates had neurologic aberrations at 2 to 4 years, (Prechtl and Dijkstra, 1960), and by Amiel-Tison (1976; Amiel-Tison and Grenier, 1986). Abnormal neonates, on the other hand, are much more difficult to classify in regard to prediction. Again, citing Prechtl, 68% of the abnormal neonates had neurologic aberrations at 2 to 4 years. (Prechtl's "neurologic abnormality of the neonate" and "neurologic aberrations at 2 to 4 years" are both broad-spectrum categories.)

One reason to group items in the neonatal neurologic examination and to give scores for these groups is that the groups (factors) may have very low relationships with each other (see Table 2–3). Even when the total neonatal scores were in the severely abnormal range, certain of the seven group scores were normal for some neonates in our original study. Neonates who scored in the moderately or severely abnormal categories had many different combinations of low group scores. For neonates with mildly abnormal total scores, the scores for irritability or the head-on-neck support dimensions were lower.

Theoretically, we should be able to determine through further research which combinations tend to improve and which do not. We should also be able to determine which combinations respond to which intervention therapies. In short, the use of the subscores should help us in untangling some of the unsolved problems.

Infants

Considerable information is already available about the progression of neurologic normality/abnormality from infancy through the early school years. Again, infants who are normal tend to remain so, unless there is an intervening event such as meningitis, seizures, or head injury.

Infants who are abnormal often look worse or score worse in the course of infancy. Many of them will improve in their neurologic function between infancy and early school years: they may even "outgrow" cerebral palsy. In the National Collaborative Perinatal Project, 16% of infants with a diagnosis of moderate or severe quadriplegia did not carry a diagnosis of cerebral palsy at age 7 years. In the same study, 72% of infants with mild spastic diplegia outgrew their cerebral palsy, and 50% percent of infants with moderate to severe spastic diplegia outgrew it. Only 48% of infants with mild hemiparesis and 13% of those with moderate to severe hemiparesis outgrew it by age 7 years (Nelson and Ellenberg, 1982).

Hypotonia, the most common category of abnormality for infants initially treated in the neonatal intensive care unit, tends to improve. We prefer to consider mild hypotonia as part of transient neuromotor abnormalities. In a series of 999 infants from the neonatal intensive care unit, 21% demonstrated transient neuromotor abnormalities in infancy (Ellison et al., 1982). Of these minor abnormalities, 79% had disappeared by 15 months. Infants with moderate to severe hypotonia also tend to outgrow it, more quickly if their other developmental skills (adaptive and personal-social) are normal.

Transient Neuromotor Abnormalities

This observer considers transient neuromotor abnormalities of infancy the most interesting category of neurologic abnormality. By infancy, much of the neurologic abnormality noted in the neonatal intensive care unit has disappeared, at varying ages in infancy depending on the assessment items utilized by the examiner. What remains is a reasonable marker that "something" happened to the brain. In follow-up in later years, this group has had an excess of abnormalities. In the National Collaborative Perinatal Project, children who were given a label of "suspected" cerebral palsy at 1 year and who did not have cerebral palsy at age 7 years had a significantly increased frequency of mental retardation, refractive errors, hyperactivity, and immature behavior (Nelson and Ellenberg, 1982). Drillien found significantly lower scores in reading and spelling achievement, speech, and motor tasks in those children from a sample of 261 low-birth-weight infants who had transient neurologic abnormalities (Drillien, 1972; Drillien et al., 1980). In our work, these children had an increased frequency of combinations of problems at age 7 years: cognitive deficits, motor dysfunction, learning disabilities, and behavioral problems (Ellison et al., 1985b).

In all of these studies, the majority of children with transient neurologic abnormalities were normal at preschool or early school years. The subscores on the Infanib should help us to separate better those infants who improve from those who do not improve. In addition, the range of neurologic sequelae is broad; we should be better able to predict the type of abnormal outcome (cognitive versus motor versus behavioral) and thus offer more specific and effective early intervention.

In other work, we have examined the relationship between early (neonatal) sicknesses and later neurologic function (Ellison, 1991). Several sicknesses or the processes that initiate them or occur during them have significant predictive value for later dysfunction.

Appendix I: The Courses of Three Typical Infants

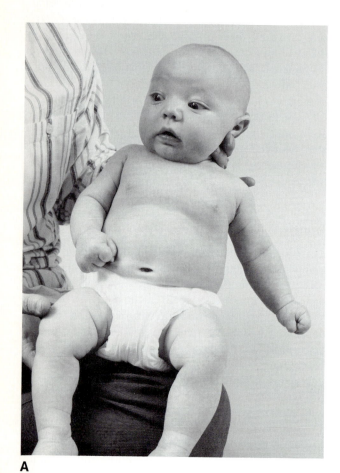

A

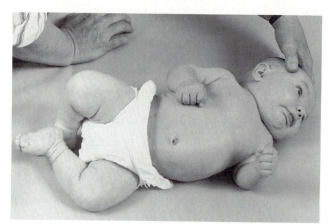

B

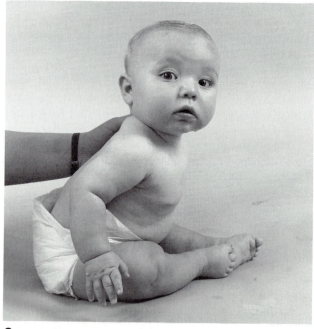

C

1. *Transient Neuromotor Abnormalities—Increased Early Extensor Tone (Hypertonia).* This infant was severely asphyxiated shortly after birth. In the early months of infancy, he exhibited a dull affect (**A**), interacting little with family members and responding poorly to stimuli. He exhibited clenched hands (**B**), especially with a stressed maneuver such as the asymmetric tonic neck reflex. He had "precocious" head control. He readily pulled his head up and flexed his arms on pull to sit (**C**) and he sat with a straight back, bending forward from L-5 and extending his head long before he should have.

   This infant had perhaps the most intensive physical therapy possible as well as directed visual and auditory stimulation. He learned to walk at 13 months of age. At 18 months of age his language and motor skills are average for age.

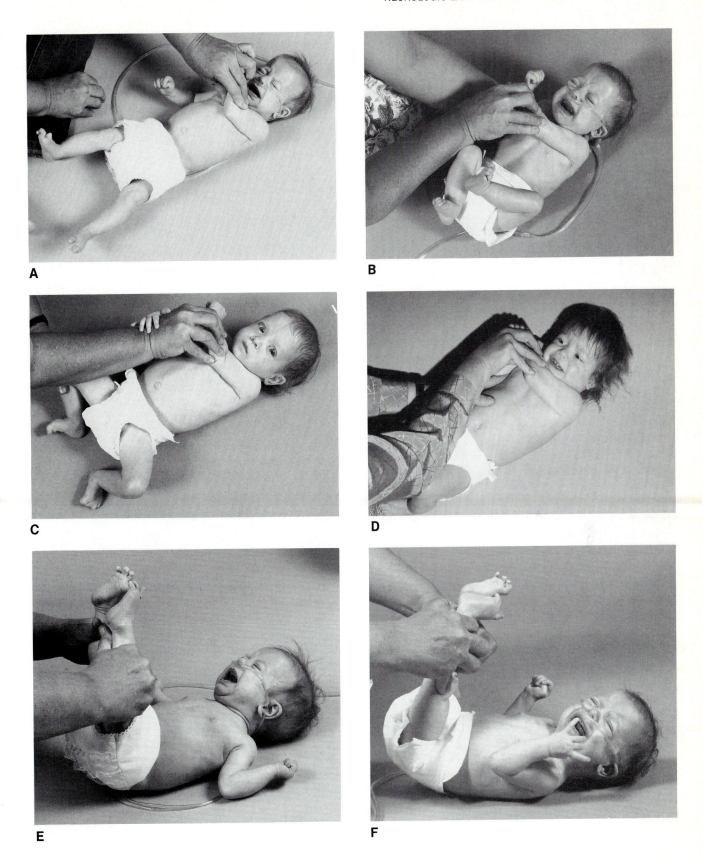

2. *Transient Neuromotor Abnormalities of the Premature.* This infant has a hypotonic scarf sign, which improves as she nears 1 year of age (**A-D**).

She has a mild increase in tone in her legs as indicated by the delayed progression in both heel to ear (**E-H**) and popliteal angle (**I-L**).

Text and illustrations continue on the next two pages.

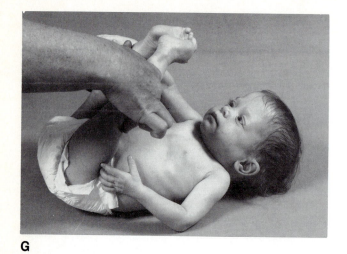

G

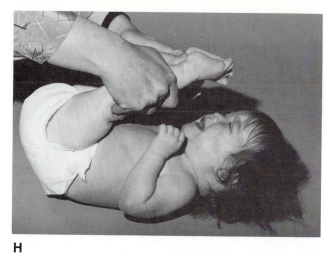

H

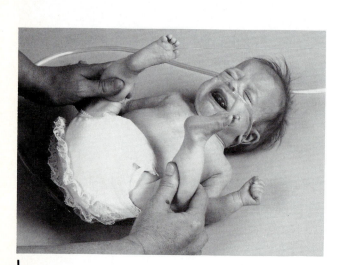

I

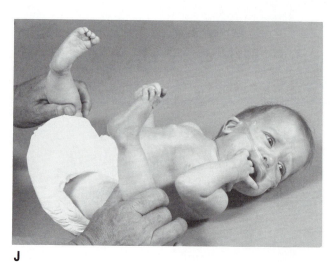

J

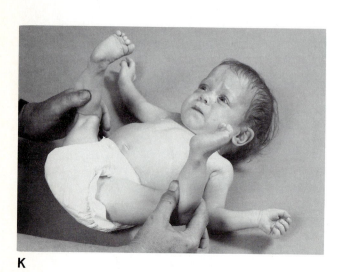

K

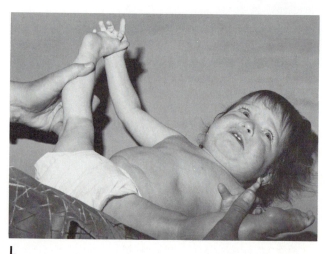

L

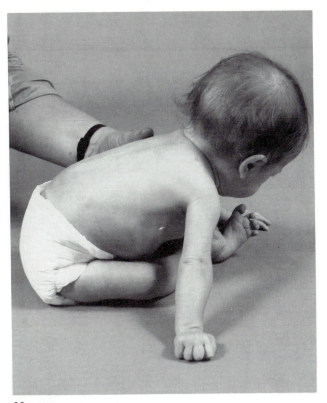

M

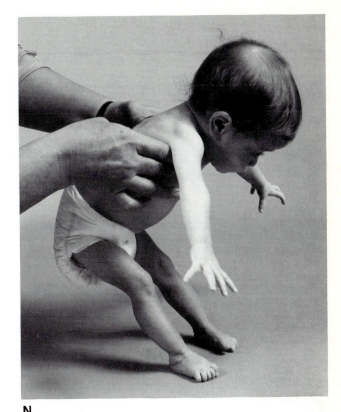

N

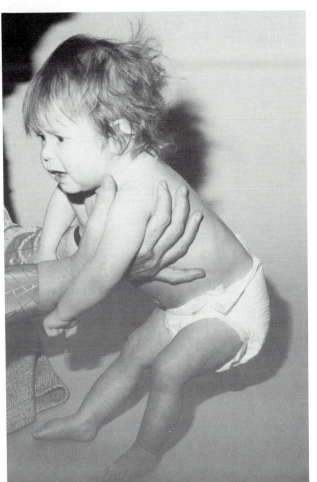

O

She had delay in truncal and leg control as well. Note the poor sit and the poor weight-bearing in the standing position (ages 7 and 11 months; M–O).

This infant learned to walk at 17 months of age. Her language at that age was within the range of normal for age. She had no evidence of spasticity.

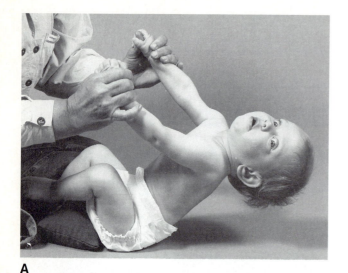

A

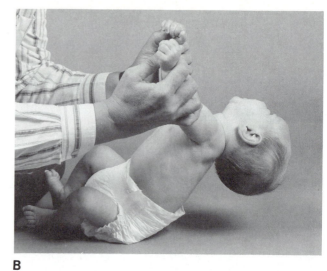

B

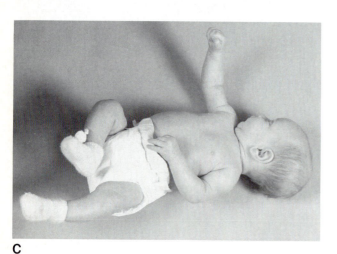

C

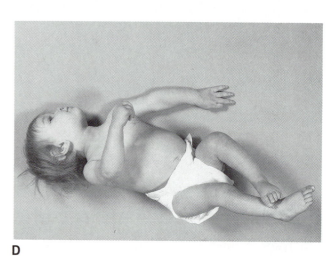

D

3. *Abnormality: Spastic Tetrapare-sis/Dyskinesia.* This infant had moderate to severe hypotonia as a neonate. His early head control was very poor (**A–B**).

In early infancy he began to assume the asymmetric tonic reflex position, particularly when placed supine on a firm surface (**C**). In later infancy, whenever he attempted to turn or roll, he adopted an asymmetric tonic neck reflex position (**D**). In midinfancy, he had difficulty weight-bearing (**E**). In late infancy, the standing position resulted in extensor posturing (**F**). He has not yet learned to walk.

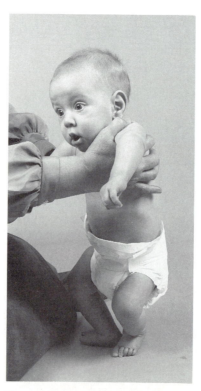

E

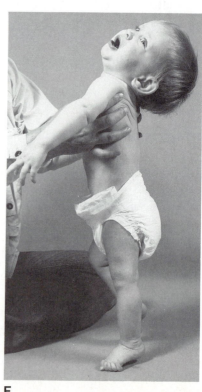

F

Appendix II: Neonatal and Infant Neurologic Exam

I. GENERAL DESCRIPTION

Head circumference
__ Centimeters
__ Percentile

__ Head configuration abnormalities
                          1 = No   2 = Yes
If yes, then check all that apply:
☐ Unilateral coronal suture
☐ Brachycephaly
☐ Dolichocephaly
☐ Oxycephaly
☐ Trigonencephaly
☐ Associated hand anomalies
    Describe: _____
☐ Other:_____

__ Anterior fontanelle abnormalities
                          1 = No   2 = Yes
If yes, then check all that apply:
☐ Bulging
☐ Concave
☐ Too large
☐ Too small

__ Size of fontanelle (centimeters)
☐ Other: _____

__ Other fontanelle abnormalities
                          1 = No   2 = Yes
If yes, then check all that apply:
☐ Open posterior fontanelle
☐ Third fontanelle
☐ Other: _____

__ Other skull abnormalities
                          1 = No   2 = Yes
    If yes, then check all that apply:
☐ Cephalohematoma
☐ Caput succudeum
☐ Molding
__   1 = Mild   2 = Moderate   3 = Severe
☐ Overlapping sutures
__   1 = Mild   2 = Moderate   3 = Severe
☐ Other: _____

__ Eye abnormalities   1 = No   2 = Yes
If yes, then check all that apply:
☐ "Setting sun"
☐ Wandering
☐ Conjugate deviation
☐ Nystagmus
☐ Strabismus
☐ Conjunctival hemorrhage
☐ Other: _____

__ Skin abnormalities   1 = No   2 = Yes
If yes, then check all that apply:
☐ Cafe au lait
☐ Depigmented spots
☐ Hemangiomas
☐ Nevi
☐ Ecchymoses
☐ Other: _____
and complete the following:
Size: _____
Location: _____

__ Dysmorphic features   1 = No   2 = Yes
If yes, then check all that apply:
☐ Eyes   ☐ Arms
☐ Hypertelorism   ☐ Legs
☐ Hypotelorism   ☐ Palmar creases
☐ Skull   ☐ Dermatoglyphics
☐ Neck   ☐ Digits
☐ Palate   ☐ Joints
☐ Chest   ☐ Genitalia
☐ Other: _____
and complete the following:
Describe:_____

__ Organomegaly   1 = No   2 = Yes
If yes, then check all that apply:
☐ Liver
☐ Kidney
☐ Spleen
☐ Heart
☐ Other: _____
and complete the following:
Describe:_____

__ Seizures
1 = No   2 = Infrequent
3 = Repetitive   4 = Status epilepticus
If yes, then check all that apply:
☐ Subtle
☐ Focal clonic
☐ Myofocal clonic
☐ Multifocal
☐ Tonic
☐ Myoclonic
☐ Other: _____

__ Apnea
1 = No   2 = Infrequent   3 = Recurrent

__ Brachial plexus injury   1 = No   2 = Yes
Describe: _____

__ Hand preference   1 = No   2 = Yes
If *yes,* check which applies:
☐ Right
☐ Left

II. CRANIAL NERVES

A. Vision and Hearing

__ Funduscopic examination abnormalities
                         1 = No   2 = Yes
If *yes,* then check all that apply:
☐ Retinal hemorrhage
☐ Chorioretinitis
☐ Optic nerve hypoplasia
☐ Cataract
☐ Cherry red spot
☐ *Other:* _____

__ Visual acuity abnormality
                         1 = No   2 = Yes
Describe: _____
_____

__ Cranial nerve III, IV, or VI abnormalities
                         1 = No   2 = Yes
If *yes,* then check all that apply:
☐ Paresis involving IV
☐ Paresis involving VI
☐ Strabismus
☐ *Other:* _____

__ Pupillary abnormalities   1 = No   2 = Yes
☐ Not round
☐ Unequal
☐ Unreactive to light
Describe: _____
_____

__ Hearing abnormalities   1 = No   2 = Yes
☐ Right
☐ Left
Indicate how this was determined:
☐ Clinical observation
☐ Brainstem auditory evoked response
☐ Behavioral audiometry
☐ *Other:* _____

B. Facial

__ Cranial nerve V abnormality
                         1 = No   2 = Yes
Describe finding: _____
_____

__ Cranial nerve VII abnormality
                         1 = No   2 = Yes
If yes, then check all that apply:
☐ Central paresis

☐ Peripheral paresis
☐ *Other:* _____

C. Bulbar function

__ Cranial nerve IX, X, or XI abnormalities
                         1 = No   2 = Yes
Describe finding: _____
_____

__ Sucking abnormality   1 = No   2 = Yes
Describe finding: _____
_____

__ Swallowing abnormality 1 = No   2 = Yes
Describe finding: _____
_____

__ Cranial nerve XII abnormalities
                         1 = No   2 = Yes
Describe finding: _____
_____

__ Tongue abnormality   1 = No   2 = Yes
If *yes,* then check all that apply:
☐ Large tongue
☐ Tongue atrophy
☐ Tongue fasciculation
☐ Tongue thrust
☐ *Other:* _____

III. SPECIAL SITUATIONS

A. Altered Mental Status

__ Impaired level of consciousness
                         1 = No   2 = Yes
☐ Hyperexitable
☐ Stuporous
☐ Comatose
__ Degree of coma   1 = Light   2 = Deep
If stupor or coma is present, then com-
complete the following:
__ Abnormal pupillary response to light
                         1 = No   2 = Yes
If *yes,* then check all that apply:
☐ Dilated
☐ Responsive
☐ Fixed
☐ Midpoint
☐ *Other:* _____

__ Other cranial nerve abnormalities
                         1 = No   2 = Yes
__ Corneal
   reflex   1 = *increased* 2 = *normal*
__ Doll's eyes   1 = *increased* 2 = *normal*
__ Gag reflex   1 = *increased* 2 = *normal*

__ Respiration	1 = *increased*	2 = *normal*
__ Heart rate	1 = *increased*	2 = *normal*
	3 = *decreased*	4 = *absent*
	3 = *decreased*	4 = *absent*
	3 = *decreased*	4 = *absent*
	3 = *decreased*	4 = *absent*
	3 = *decreased*	4 = *absent*

☐ *Other*: _____

B. Spinal Cord

__ Spinal cord abnormality   1 = *No*   2 = *Yes*
If yes, then check all that apply:
☐ Abnormal pinprick response
☐ Abnormal sweating
☐ Abnormal urination stream
☐ Neurogenic bladder
☐ Absent anal wink
☐ Constipation

☐ *Other*: _____
and complete the following:
__ Level of motor loss
__ Level of sensory loss
Describe: _____
_____

__ Dysraphism   1 = *No*   2 = *Yes*
If *yes*, then check all that apply:
☐ Open
☐ Closed
☐ Leaking cerebrospinal fluid
☐ Meningocele
☐ Encephalocele
☐ Myelomeningocele
___ Level of involvement
Describe: _____
_____

Acknowledgments

Mark Christensen (Denver, Colorado) took the photographs—a process that required the utmost patience and for which I am extremely grateful. Many thanks as well to the babies and their parents: Sammy Christensen, Andrew Flieder, Jeremy Pfauth, Kate, and Sarah.

ANNOTATED BIBLIOGRAPHY

Amiel-Tison C, Grenier A: *Neurological Assessment during the First Year of Life.* New York, Oxford University Press, 1986.
  This is a clear explanation of the French angles, plus additional items that two very experienced examiners have incorporated into their examinations over the years. For those with less experience, the assimilation of the many items for an overall "picture" of the infant may be less clear.
Ellison P: The infant neurological examination, *Adv Dev Behav Pediatr* 9:75–138, 1990.
  This article details the reasoning for recommending better measuring and more reliable, mathematically coherent neurologic assessments for infants.
Nelson K, Ellenberg J: Children who "outgrew" cerebral palsy. *Pediatrics* 69:529–536, 1982.
  This article provides basic information about changes in the neurologic examination during infancy and early childhood for a large sample, so that the examiner is less likely to make mistakes when discussing the future with parents.

REFERENCES

Amiel-Tison C: A method for neurologic evaluation within the first year of life. *Curr Probl Pediatr* 7:1–150, 1976.
Amiel-Tison C, and Grenier A: *Neurological Assessment during the First Year of Life.* New York, Oxford University Press, 1986.
Brazelton TB: Neonatal Behavioral Assessment Scale. *Clin Child Dev Med* 50, 1973.
Capute AJ: Identifying cerebral palsy in infancy through study of primitive reflex profiles. *Pediatr Ann* 8:34–42, 1979.
Capute AJ, Palmer FB, Shapiro BK, Wachtel RC, Ross A, Accardo PJ: Primitive reflex profile: A quantitation of primitive reflexes in infancy. *Dev Med Child Neurol* 26:375–383, 1984.
Collaborative Study on Cerebral Palsy, Mental Retardation and Other Neurological and Sensory Disorders of Infancy and Childhood. Part II: A forms. *Obstet Pediatr Neurol,* 1966.
Drillien CM: Abnormal neurologic signs in the first year of life in low birthweight infants: Possible prognostic significance. *Dev Med Child Neurol* 14:575–584, 1972.
Drillien CM, Thomson AJM, Burgoyne K: Low birth weight children at early school age: A longitudinal study. *Dev Med Child Neurol* 22:26–47, 1980.
Dubowitz L, Dubowitz V: *The Neurological Assessment of the Preterm and Full-term Newborn Infant.* Philadelphia, JB Lippincott, 1981.
Ellison P: Neurologic development of the high-risk infant. *Clin Perinatol* 11:41–57, 1984a.
Ellison P: Long-term follow-up studies: The prediction of the neurologic examination in infancy, in Moss AJ (ed): *Pediatrics Update.* New York, Elsevier Biomedical, 1984, p 187–200.
Ellison P: The neurological examination of infants. *Adv Dev Pediatr Behav* 9:75–138, 1990.
Ellison P: Neurological implications of perinatal complications, in Gray JW, Dean RS (eds): *Neuropsychology of Perinatal Complications,* New York, Springer, 1991, p 59–108.
Ellison P, Browning C, Trostmiller T: Evaluation of tone in infancy—Physical therapist versus pediatric neurologist. *J Calif Perinatal Assoc* 2:63–66, 1982.
Ellison P, Browning C, Larson B, Denny J: A scoring system for the Milani-Comparetti and Gidoni method of assessing neurologic abnormality in infancy. *Phys Ther* 63:1414–1423, 1983.

Ellison P, Horn JL, Browning C: The construction of an infant neurologic international battery (Infanib) for the assessment of neurologic integrity in infancy. *Phys Ther* 9:1326–1331, 1985.

Ellison P, Prasse D, Siewert J, Browning C: The outcome of neurological abnormality in infancy, in Harel S, Stern L (eds): *The At Risk Infant*. Baltimore, Md, Brookes, 1985, p 253–260.

Frankenberg W, Goldstein A, Camp B: The revised Denver Developmental Screening Test: Its accuracy as a screening instrument. *J Pediatr* 79:988–995. 1971.

Gesell A: *The Mental Growth of the Preschool Child*. New York, Macmillan, 1925.

Goodman RM, Gorlin RJ: *Atlas of the Face in Genetic Disorders*, 2nd ed. St. Louis, CV Mosby, 1977.

Graham FK: Behavioral differences between normal and traumatized newborns. I. The test procedures. *Psychol Monogr* 70 (427):1–16, 1956a.

Graham FK: Behavioral differences between normal and traumatized newborns. II. Standardization, reliability and validity. *Psychol Monogr* 70 (428):17–33, 1956b.

Graham FK, Pennoyer MM, Caldwell BM, Greenman M, Hartmann AF: Relationship between clinical status and behavior test performance in a newborn group with histories suggesting anoxia. *J Pediatr* 50:177–189, 1957.

Knobloch H, Stevens F, Malone A: *Manual of Developmental Diagnosis: The Administration and Interpretation of the Revised Gesell and Armatruda Developmental and Neurologic Examination*. Hagerstown, Md, Harper & Row, 1980.

Milani-Comparetti A, Gidoni EA: Pattern analysis of motor development and its disorders. *Dev Med Child Neurol* 9:625–630, 1967a.

Milani-Comparetti A, Gidoni EA: Routine developmental examination in normal and retarded children. *Dev Med Child Neurol* 9:631–638, 1967b.

Nelson K, Ellenberg J: Children who "outgrew" cerebral palsy. *Pediatrics* 69:529–536, 1982.

Nunnally JC: *Psychometric Theory*. San Francisco: McGraw-Hill, 1978.

Paine R: Neurologic examination of infants and children. *Pediatr Clin North Am* 7:471–510, 1960.

Peiper A: Die Eigenart der kindlichen Hirntätigkeit. Leipzig, Georg Thieme, 1956.

Prechtl HFR: Prognostic value of neurological signs in the newborn infant. *Proc R Soc Med* 58:3–4, 1965.

Prechtl HFR: Neurological findings in newborn infants after pre- and paranatal complications, in Jonxis JHP, Visser HKA, Troelstra JA (eds): *Aspects of Prematurity and Dysmaturity*. Leiden, HE Stenfert Kroese, 1968.

Prechtl HFR: The neurologic examination of the full-term newborn infant. *Clin Dev Med* 63:303–321, 1977.

Prechtl, HFR: Assessment methods of the newborn infant: A critical evaluation, in Stratton P (ed): *Psychobiology of the Human Newborn*. New York, Wiley, 1980, p 21–52.

Prechtl, HFR, Dijkstra J: *Prenatal Care*. Groningen, Noordhoff, 1960.

Rosenblith JF: The modified Graham behavior test for neonates. Test-retest reliability, normative data, and hypotheses for future work. *Biol Neonat* 3:174–192, 1961.

Rosenblith JF: Prognostic value of neonatal assessment. *Child Dev* 37:623–631, 1966.

Rosenblith JF, Anderson R: Prognostic significance of discrepancies in muscle tension between upper and lower limbs. *Dev Med Child Neurol* 10:322–330, 1968.

Rumack CM, Johnson ML: *Perinatal and Infant Brain Imaging*. Chicago, Yearbook, 1984.

Sheridan-Pereira M, Ellison P, Helgeson V: The construction of a scored form of the neonatal neurological examination. *J Dev Behav Pediatr* 12:25–30, 1991.

Smith DW: *Recognizable Patterns of Human Deformation*. Philadelphia, WB Saunders, 1981.

St. Anne Dargassies S: Neurodevelopmental symptoms during the first year of life. *Dev Med Child Neurol* 14:235–246, 1972.

St. Anne Dargassies S: La maturation neurologique des prématures. *Etudes Neonatales* 4:71–122, 1955.

St. Anne Dargassies S: Neurodevelopmental symptoms during the first year of life. *Dev Med Child Neurol* 14:235–246, 1972.

St. Anne Dargassies S: Normality and normalization as seen in a long-term neurological follow-up of 286 truly premature infants. *Neuropaediatrie* 10:226–244, 1979.

Thomas A, St. Anne Dargassies S: *Etudes Neurologiques sur le Nouveau né et le Jeune Nourisson*. Paris, Masson, 1952.

Vojta V: Die zerebralen Bewegungstorungen im Säulingsalter. Stuttgart, Ferdinand Enke, 1981.

The Neurologic Examination of the Young Child

Ruth D. Nass
Diane Koch

The goal of this chapter is to review comprehensively the neurologic and developmental/psychometric assessment of the toddler and preschool child. The reader is provided with an extensive prototype examination and the rationale behind it. Because no toddler or preschooler would cooperate for the entire exam, Table 3–2 provides a basic examination structure that, if completed, will provide sufficient information for most purposes.

Touwen and Prechtl's 1970 monograph *The Neurological Examination of the Child with Minor Central Nervous System Dysfunction* remains a classic. Some of the general suggestions made therein about the approach to the examination of the younger child deserve mention. As children generally dislike being undressed for examination, this should be done in stages and as necessary. Shoes and socks should be removed initially so that movements of the feet and legs can be monitored throughout. At some point the child must be completely undressed to look for skin markings suggestive of a neurocutaneous syndrome. Should the history be suggestive, a Woods lamp examination for previously unseen ash leaf spots should be undertaken. The child should be dressed again with some help by the examiner prior to the examination of the head, the final phase of the assessment. The inspection of the head, as well as that of the hands and feet, should also include assessment for the minor physical anomalies listed in Table 3–1. Waldrop and colleagues (1968) report that among 74 normal 2½-year-olds a highly anomaly score correlated with conduct problems in both boys and girls. Waldrup and Halverson (1971) documented the stability of the anomaly score and of hyperactivity from ages 2½ to 7½ years. Anomalies at 2½ years were predictive of hyperactivity at age 7½ years. Head circumference should also be measured because there is an increased incidence of head size two standard deviations above or below the mean in the learning-disabled population. Macrocephaly should be pursued, for potentially treatable causes like hydro-cephalus and for familial causes like fragile X chromosome and external hydrocephalus. Special attention should be paid to the motor function of the child with a large head, as such children are at increased risk for both gross and fine motor dysfunction (Lewis et al., 1983).

Touwen and Prechtl (1970) are very precise about the order of the neurologic examination. This concern with sequence is probably particularly relevant to the examination of the toddler, a process in which the maintenance of cooperation is crucial. Initially, while the history is being taken from the parent(s), the child should be observed as he or she acquaints himself or herself with the examining room environment. The sitting exam is performed first (with a young child often sitting in the parent's lap), followed in order by those parts of the exam that are performed in the standing position, those dealing wtih locomotion, any part of the exam requiring a prone or supine position, and finally the examination of the head. This is obviously quite different from the traditional approach to the neurologic examination suitable to the older child and adult. Listed by position of patient in Table 3–2 are aspects of the neurologic examination suitable for the child of under 6 years. The scoring form on page 86 may be used for the examination of the preschool child by omitting the items with an asterisk and using the suggested alternatives.

THE SITTING EXAMINATION

Spontaneous Mobility

Spontaneous mobility is assessed over a 3-minute period during the taking of the history from the parents. Both quantity and quality of movements are assessed, each on a scale of 0 to 3. With respect to quantity, both gross and fine motor movements are considered. Speed,

TABLE 3-1. MINOR ANOMALIES SEEN WITH ATTENTION DEFICIT HYPERACTIVITY DISORDER

Head

Electric hair
  Very fine hair that won't comb down
  Fine hair that is soon awry after combing
Two or more whorls

Eyes

Epicanthus
  Where upper and lower lids join nose point of union is
    Deeply covered
    Partly covered
Hypertelorism: Approximate distance between tear ducts:
  Greater than or equal to 1½ in.
  Between 1¼ and 1½ in.

Ears

Low-seated ears
  Bottom of ears in line with
    Mouth (or lower)
    Area between mouth and nose
Adherent lobes: Lower edges of ears extend
  Upward and back toward crown of head
  Straight back toward rear of neck
Malformed ears
Asymmetric ears
Soft and pliable ears

Mouth

High palate
  Roof of mouth
    Definitely steepled
    Flat and narrow at the top
  Furrowed tongue (one with deep ridges)
  Smooth or rough spots on tongue

Hands

Fifth finger
  Markedly curved inward toward other fingers
  Slightly curved inward toward other fingers
Single transverse palmar crease
Index finger longer than middle finger

Feet

Third toe
  Definitely longer than second toe
  Appears equal in length to second toe
Partial syndactylia of two middle toes
Gap between first and second toe (greater than or equal
    to ¼ inch)

From Waldrop et al. (1968) with permission.

smoothness, and adequacy are the qualitative parameters. High scores in the quantity domain suggest attentional difficulties, although the diagnosis of ADHD is based on classroom behavior, not office behavior.

Muscle Power

Muscle power, tone, and mass are assessed in the same fashion as in the older child. Often functional assessment of the distal lower extremity during gait maneuvers proves more useful than standard push-pull testing.

Reflex Assessment

The procedure for reflex assessment is standard. Younger children are more likely to show nonpathologic spread—for example, to the adductors when the knee is tapped. Sometimes a gendrasic maneuver is needed to bring out the reflexes. Touwen and Precthl suggest that the plantar reflex be elicted by stroking with a sharp object or a thumbnail from toe to heel. The reverse technique is suggested to avoid eliciting a grasp reflex as one approaches the toes in standard elicitation procedure.

TABLE 3-2. SOFT-SIGN NEUROLOGIC EXAMINATION OF THE CHILD UNDER 6 YEARS

Sitting assessment

Spontaneous motility (3-minute observation)
Muscle power, tone, mass
Reflexes
Sensory examination: Finger localization, double simul-
  taneous stimulation, graphesthesia, stereognosis

Standing assessment

Posture
Spontaneous motility (2-minute observation)
Posture with arms extended palms up and palms down
Assessment for involuntary movements (Prechtl's sign)
Mouth opening/finger spreading phenomenon
Diadochokinesis and associated movements
Finger nose test
Fingertip touching test
Finger opposition test
Standing with eyes closed

Assessment of gait and station

Gait
Walking a straight line
Walking on tiptoes
Walking on heels
One-foot stand
Hopping on one foot
Catch a ball
Truck

Prone or supine assessment

Examine spine
Knee-heel test
Sitting up without the use of the hands

Sitting assessment of the head

Musculature of face
Eyes
Ears
Mouth

Sensory Examination

Although Touwen and Prechtl (1970) do not discuss the sensory exam, some data on the sensory exam of the preschooler are available.

Finger Localization

Lefford et al. (1974) evaluated the development of finger localization skills in preschool children, ages 3 to 6 years. Many 3-year-olds (the percentage indicated in parentheses) and almost all 4- and 5-year-olds could oppose the thumb to the finger touched by the examiner (85%), find the fingers touched by the examiner with his contralateral hand (75%), oppose the thumb to the finger pointed to by the examiner (70%), find the fingers pointed to by the examiner with his contralateral hand (65%), and oppose the thumb to the finger indicated by the examiner while the subject's view was obstructed (50%). Levine and Schneider (1985) have normed a finger imitation task for the 4- to 6-year-old. Sitting opposite the child, the examiner opposes his or her thumb to another finger on the same hand, holding that position for 5 to 8 seconds while the child imitates it. There are five trials. Mirror movements should be noted, although they are probably fairly common in this age group. Dyskinesia, which Levine and Schneider (1985) designate as opposition movements that are slow to release, should be noted. Children who require excessive visual input of their own hand movements may have true finger agnosia. Most 4- to 6-year-olds will score correctly on three to four trials. Galin et al. (1977) found that most 5-year-olds could even oppose the thumb to the proximal, distal, or middle phalanx of each finger when it was touched by the examiner out of the child's view (uncrossed localization). However, it was not until age 8 or 9 that children were able to perform a crossed localization task—touch the homologous spot on the opposite hand with the opposite thumb. A discrepancy of the same type in ability to perform crossed versus uncrossed tasks is seem in disconnection syndromes induced by corpus callosum surgery. The question then is whether the young child is functionally acallosal. The more classic finger agnosia tasks of "How many fingers were touched, one or two?" and "How many between?" are too difficult for the preschooler. They are performed by only 30% and 15%, respectively, of 5-year-olds, 45% and 30% of 6-year-olds, and 85% and 65% of almost-7-year-olds (Kinsbourne and Warrington, 1963).

Lefford and colleagues (1974) attribute the developmental progress of digital competence during the preschool years to the development of different sensory modalities as guides for selective actions, then to the development of intersensory transfer, and finally to the ability to use representational information as a guide for behavior. Notably, Lindgren (1978) found that finger localization skill in kindergarten predicted reading and arithmetic achievement at the end of the first grade.

Maturing at the right pace plays a role in optimizing academic achievement. It is of particular interest that finger localization ability in the preschooler predicted arithmetic skill, because finger agnosia and dyscalculia are two of the deficits (right-left disorientation and agraphia are the other two) seen in Gerstmann's syndrome, which can occur on a developmental basis in the school-age child (J.E. Schwartz et al., 1981). Levine (1988) notes that children with finger localization problems may try to compensate by adopting an awkward pencil grip, resulting in dysgraphia.

Double Simultaneous Stimulation

Extinction to face on double simultaneous stimulation of hand and face is common in the child until about age 10 years, presumably because the face is more elaborately represented and because the facial sensory pathways mature earlier than those of the hand. In the preschool child there is also a right-left distinction, the testable child (sometimes as young as 2 years old) being more likely to extinguish the stimulus presented to the left hand, when right and left are touched simultaneously (Roeltgen et al., 1986; Kinsbourne and Hicks, 1978). Roeltgen et al. (1986) also found performance on a line bisection task consistent with a hemispatial neglect pattern. They suggest that asymmetric lateralization of attention mechanisms may be part of normal development and responsible for the right-left sensory phenomenon.

Graphesthesia

Levine and Schneider (1985) suggest a matching format wherein the child can pick among drawings of a circle, line, square, and cross which have been made on his or her preferred hand. Three of four correct is the norm for the 4- to 6-year-old.

Stereognosis

The Pediatric Examination of Educational Readiness (PEER; Levine and Schneider, 1985) provides a kit of five duplicate shapes for this purpose. One by one, four of these are placed in the child's fisted hand and he or she is asked to pick visually the matching form. Most 4- to 6-year-olds will identify three of the four.

THE STANDING EXAMINATION

Posture

The standing exam begins with an assessment of *posture*. The posture of the preschooler differs from that of the older child. The 3-year-old stands in a slightly broad-based position in a rather "plump" fashion. The 5-year-old can hold his or her body straight and the base has narrowed.

Spontaneous Motility

Spontaneous motility is assessed in the standing position similarly to the sitting position. The observation period is 2 minutes, while the child is "standing around waiting for things to happen." The limits of acceptable spontaneous motility are clearly age related.

Posture with Extended Arms

Posture is checked in both the palms-up and the palms-down position for 20 seconds. The preschooler's arms tend to drift in the direction of the palms and to be laterally displaced on both tasks 30° to 60°. Spooning of the wrist and hands is often present through age 5 years.

Assessment for Involuntary Movements

Assessment for involuntary movements, including Precthl's sign, is only accurate if the child can maintain a quiet general standing position for 2 minutes, i.e., passes the initial motility test. Thus, a reliable result is unlikely in the child under 4 years. To assess for choreiform movements the child stands with feet together and with the fingers of the pronated outstretched hands apart for 20 seconds. Below 6 years the eyes are open, above 6 the eyes are closed. Normed data are not available on the frequency of Precthl's sign in the preschooler, but it is probably very common.

Overflow Movements

Examination for overflow movements is an important part of the soft sign assessment. Overflow movements, associated movements, and synkinesis are defined as movements occurring in parts of the body other than the one attempting the task; they may be symmetric or asymmetric. Mirror movements occur symmetrically. Overflow is common in young children and disappears around age 10 (Connolly and Stratton, 1968), implying maturational changes in the organization of the motor system. For example, the crossed pyramid motor system, mediating rapid independent finger movements (Kuypers, 1981), matures later than the less specific medial motor system, which provides proximal limb and ipsilateral motor innervation (Geschwind, 1975). The uncrossed motor pathways may function tonically in childhood, resulting in mirror movements. With maturation, these noncrossing pathways come under the inhibitory control of the contralateral hemisphere (Dennis, 1976). Because myelination of the corpus callosum is completed at about the same time that mirror movements disappear around age 10 years (Yakovlev and LeCours, 1967), the corpus callosum is thought to transmit the interhemispheric inhibitory impulses (Dennis, 1976; Nass, 1985). Based on the finding that the degree of interference, for example, between a right hand tapping task and a verbal recitation task is greatest for young children (range 3 to 11 years), Kinsbourne and Hicks (1978) suggest that mirror movements reflect the greater proximity in neural space of the crossed and uncrossed motor systems in the immature nervous system.

Touwen and Prechtl (1970) suggest three tasks to assess for overflow and mirror movements: mouth opening/finger spreading, diadochokinesis, and the finger opposition test. The first task requires the child to open his or her mouth, close his eyes, and stick out his tongue while his extended arms, with hands and wrists relaxed, are supported by the examiner. The response of spreading the fingers is marked in the preschooler and muted by age 7 to 8 years. The second and third tasks are standard parts of the neurologic assessment of cerebellar and motor function, respectively.

On the *diadochokinesis task* the preschooler will often manifest marked mirroring in the opposite limb, even to the point of flexing the limb involuntarily. Associated movements are scored as follows: 0, none; 1, barely visible or slight elbow flexion; 2, mirror movements without elbow flexion; 3, mirror movements with elbow flexion. On Denckla's (1973, 1974) time-for-20 version of this task about 20% of 5-year-olds evidence mirroring (Wolff et al., 1983). The extent of associated movements may decrease at different rates on the two sides of the body as the child grows older. Touwen and Prechtl (1970) found that when dominance is not well established mirror movements may occur to a greater degree in the nondominant arm (when the dominant arm is voluntarily performing the task). Once dominance is well established mirror movements may be more prominant in the dominant arm. Njiokikjien et al. (1986) found more mirroring in the right (presumed dominant) arm at all ages (Table 3–3). Among all children tested half showed no difference between the arms. About one quarter of preschoolers evidence little to no mirroring of the left arm on this task.

TABLE 3–3. MIRROR MOVEMENTS DURING SUPINATION/PRONATION

Score		Age				
		4	4½	5	5½	6
0	L	20	19	29	55	52
	R	0	14	14	10	24
1	L	60	57	43	40	28
	R	40	24	24	65	32
2	L	5	19	14	5	12
	R	35	43	29	20	36
3	L	15	5	14	0	8
	R	25	19	33	5	8

The percentage of children scoring 0–3 for mirror movements on the supination/pronation task is shown vertically. The upper row (L) represents mirror movements on the left while the right arm voluntarily performs the task. The lower row (R) represents mirror movements on the right while the left arm voluntarily performs the task.
From Njiokikjien et al. (1986) with permission.

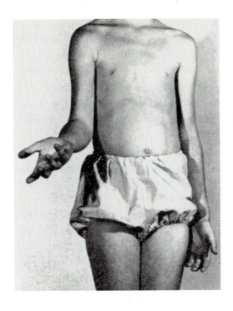
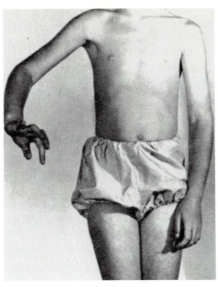

Figure 3-1. The diadochokinesis task. On the left, supination of the right hand provokes associated supination of the left hand. On the right, pronation of the right hand provokes associated pronation of the left hand. Movement of the right elbow during the diadochokinesis is clearly visible. (*From Touwen and Prechtl (1970), with permission.*)

The *finger opposition* test has been described by Touwen and Prechtl as five sequences to and fro of thumb to 2,3,4,5,4,3,2,3,4,5, and so on, and by Denckla (1973, 1974; Rudel et al., 1984) as time to do 20 movements, i.e., five sequences of thumb 2,3,4,5,2,3,4,5, and so on. Although excellent for bringing out associated movements (65% to 90% of 5-year-olds show mirroring; Wolff et al., 1983), these tests are often too difficult for children under 5 years. Denckla's time-for-20 finger tapping task, thumb to index finger, can be performed by many children 3 years old and up (Berger-Gross et al., 1984) and is, at least for the younger child, a good procedure for uncovering the overflow phenomenon (30% to 45% of 5-year-olds show mirroring; Wolff et al., 1983) as well as looking at fine motor function.

A number of other tasks have also been used to assess for associated movements, including clip pinching, finger spreading, and finger lifting (Wolff et al., 1983). Of these, only index finger lifting (passed by about 50% of 5-year-old boys and 70% of 5-year-old girls) would be a useful preschool measure. Interestingly, at all ages there is little difference between dominant- and nondominant-hand performance for clip pinching and finger spreading. Thus, an asymmetry here might be a useful marker of a hemisyndrome, unlike a number of other gross and fine motor skills, for which dominance effects are common until age 7 years.

Cerebellar Function

Tests of cerebellar function that Touwen and Prechtl (1970) perform in the standing position include *diadochokinesis, the finger/nose test* (the preschooler requires visual guidance and needs to hold his or her arm against his body for stabilization), the *fingertip touching test,* and *standing with eyes closed* for 15 seconds (the preschooler may move ankles and toes a bit to maintain balance, but this does not seem to be clinically significant). Obvious asymmetries of function are suggestive of ipsilateral cerebellar disease. On the diadochokinesis task the regularity of the movements and the presence of elbow movements are scored as follows (Touwen and Prechtl, 1970). 0, no movement; 1, irregular with elbow movements of more than 15 cm; 2, irregular with elbow movements of 5 to 15 cm; 3, correct with elbow movements of less than 5 cm (Figure 3-1). The percentage of children scoring 1 to 3 for quality of movement is shown in Table 3-4. It is the exception rather than the rule for the preschooler to perform this task with precision. Pronounced deviation of the elbow during rapid alternating movements suggests overuse of proximal musculature around the shoulder rather than maintaining the action at the wrist. In the majority of children the right arm performed better than the left throughout the age range tested (Njiokikjien et al., 1986). Denckla (1974) found little asymmetry on a time-for-20 pronation/supination task.

TABLE 3-4. QUALITY OF DIADOCHOKINESIS

Score		Age				
		4	4½	5	5½	6
1	L	60	29	14	5	12
	R	45	19	10	5	8
2	L	40	71	71	65	72
	R	50	76	71	55	64
3	L	0	0	14	30	16
	R	5	5	19	40	28

The percentage of children scoring 1–3 for quality of supination/pronation is shown vertically. The upper row (L) represents the left arm; the lower row (R) represents the right arm score.
From Njiokikjien et al. (1986) with permission.

Motor Coordination

The finger opposition tasks (Touwen and Precthl, 1970; Denckla, 1973, 1974) are more likely to be successful in the younger child. Timed finger tapping tasks can be used to assess fine motor coordination. A dominance effect is common in the young child.

ASSESSMENT OF GAIT AND STATION

The standing exam is followed by an examination of gait (Touwen and Prechtl, 1970). Children under 6 years generally show little arching of the foot when walking and little arm swing. The 2- to 4-year-old may show some minimal asymmetry of gait. The *normal gait* width after age 3 is 11 to 20 cm. Narrowing may result from hypertonia of the leg adductors and widening from hypotonia or sensory or cerebellar disease. Children under 5 years are not asked to *walk a straight line*, as even the 5- to 7-year-old is entitled to three deviations during the 20 paces forward and return walk. However, in the Collaborative Perinatal Study failure at age 4 on a very simple line walking task was a risk factor for both hyperactivity and the neurologic soft sign syndromes at age 7 (Nichols and Chen, 1981).

Children over 3 years should be able to walk on tiptoes. Any movements in upper extremities and face not present during the standard gait exam are considered associated movements. Diminishing degrees of extension of arms, ventroflexion of the hands, and lip and tongue movements are seen through age 7. Clenching of the fists is counted as an associated movement only if the arms are also extended. About 25% of 5-year-olds evidence overflow (Wolff et al., 1983).

Heel walking can be performed by children over 3 years. As with toe walking, any movements not seen during the normal walk are considered associated movements. They occur in about 50% to 80% of 5-year-olds (Wolff et al., 1983). Associated movements noted during heel walking persist longer, sometimes until 10 years, than do associated movements noted with toe walking. Arms are extended and wrists are dorsiflexed. Poor performance may also reflect hypotonia, paresis, or both. Touwen and Precthl (1970) note in particular that paresis of the peroneal muscles may occur without other muscles being impaired to the same degree. Such children will walk on the outer side of the foot rather than the heels. Children with even mild spastic diplegia will have trouble with heel walking.

The ability to *stand on one leg* develops suddenly and matures rapidly. At 3 years only a few children can stand on one leg for more than a few seconds. The one-foot stand can be sustained for 10 seconds by a 4-year-old given a couple of false starts (Levine and Schneider, 1985). By 5 years, most children can sustain the one-foot stand for about 10 seconds. There may be a marked difference between performance on the dominant and that on the nondominant leg between ages 4 and 5 years, a fact that does not necessarily indicate a hemiparesis.

Hopping on one foot is also abrupt in onset and rapid in progress. At 3 years only a few children are able to hop at all, and then only on the dominant foot. At age 4 5 to 8 times is normal and at age 5, 9 to 12 times. Prior to the age of 7 one leg is generally better than the other, although, as with the one-foot stand, the better leg may not be the one preferred for athletics. The possibility of a hemiparesis must be considered and the results here compared with other findings. Among a group of 150 5-year-olds 28% hopped more than 13 times on their left leg and 39% hopped more than 13 times on their right leg (Touwen and Prechtl, 1970). In the Collaborative Perinatal Study failure at age 4 on a hopping task was a risk factor for both hyperactivity and the neurologic soft sign syndromes at age 7 (Nichols and Chen, 1981).

Ability to *catch a ball* can be assessed in the toddler, Levine and Schneider (1985) use a 2-in. ball. The average 4- to 6-year-old will catch three to four of five tries. Associated movements of the face should be noted, since they are not present in most preschoolers. In the Collaborative Perinatal Study failure at age 4 on a ball catch task was a risk factor for the neurologic soft sign syndromes at age 7 (Nichols and Chen, 1981).

Touwen and Precthl (1970) suggest that *assessment of trunk* be performed while the child is standing. First the back is inspected and then the abdominal reflexes are elicited.

THE PRONE OR SUPINE EXAMINATION

Touwen and Precthl (1970) begin this phase of the assessment by inspecting the *spine*. This is followed by inspecting the posture of the *feet, legs, and hip joints*. The *knee-heel* test, although rarely within the capabilities of the child under 6 years, is of interest for dominance effects present through about age 7. The 5-year-old can perform the *sitting up without the use of the hands* task only by lifting his legs off the table, whereas by age 7 the legs stay in contact with the floor, another marker of diminishing overflow.

SITTING ASSESSMENT OF THE HEAD

Musculature of the Face

Assessment of the head begins with inspection of the musculature of the face for asymmetry at rest, during voluntary movement, and during emotional movement. Peripheral lesions, like those resulting from birth trauma or Bell's palsy, affect both the upper and lower face. After early injuries improvement is often accompanied by synkinesia like crocodile tears. Bilateral facial nerve palsies are often the most prominent finding in the Möbius sequence, which consists, in addition, of gaze palsies, esotropia, and sometimes abnormalities of cranial nerves IX through XII. Autopsy studies indicate four modes of developmental pathology: (1) nuclear absence, (2) destructive degeneration of nuclei, (3) peripheral nerve hypoplasia, and (4) myopathy. Generally, children present with feeding problems and lack of facial expression, as well as articulation difficulties. About one third have talipes equinovarus and about 15% are mentally retarded (Smith, 1982). Central upper motor neuron seventh-nerve deficits tend to involve primarily the lower face as the upper face is bilaterally innervated. The subcortically mediated emotional smile is relatively spared by supranuclear pathology, whereas with peripheral palsies the emotional smile is equally as impaired as the voluntary smile. Interestingly, congenital unilateral brain injuries tend to spare the face, possibly through sprouting of axons of normal ipsilateral corticobulbar innervation of rostral facial nerve nuclei (Lenn and Thurston, 1983). Congenital absence of the depressor obicularis oris muscle should not be confused with a facial palsy. In this disorder the abnormal side of the mouth is not pulled down when the child cries and the resting face is relatively normal. The side that droops during crying is the normal side and not the paralyzed one. The diagnosis is important, as the incidence of associated abnormalities, particularly cardiac, is high (Nelson and Eng, 1972).

EYES

The examination of the eyes includes an assessment for *strabismus*. About 5% of normal children and about 50% of children with brain damage have strabismus. Strabismus is classified in several ways. Heterophoria is a latent condition that is brought out only in certain circumstances like fatigue and testing. A heterotropia is constantly present and may be either exo- (outward) or eso- (inward) in the horizontal direction or hyper- or hypo- in the vertical direction. Strabismus may be alternating, with the fixating eye switching back and forth, or it may be monocular. In monocular strabismus the involved eye is at risk for a disuse amblyopia, since the immature organism can suppress fixation in order to prevent diplopia. Paralytic or noncomitant strabismus is due to paresis of one or more extraocular muscles. It is worst on gaze into the field of the affected muscle and diplopia may be a symptom. Acquired paralytic strabismus raises concern for intracranial pathology. The one exception is the benign sixth-nerve palsy, which sometimes is seen in children in a parainfectious setting. This is however, a diagnosis of exclusion. (Imaging should be performed to rule out intracranial pathology.) Congenital paralytic strabismus is usually caused by developmental defects of the extraocular system or birth trauma. Nonparalytic or

---

Pearls and Perils: Neurologic Examination of the Young Child

1. A position-oriented neurologic examination may be more useful in the preschooler than the classic systems-oriented exam.
2. A Babinski reflex elicited from toe to heel avoids a false negative—the masking of a true Babinski by the grasp reflex, which is often still apparent in the toddler.
3. Assessment for overflow movements can provide an index of neural maturation even in the preschooler, given the right elicitation procedures. Excess overflow may be a marker of later learning disabilities.
4. Gait and heel and toe walking are excellent sources of information about the neurologic status of the preschooler.
5. Preschoolers often show dominance effects in both gross and fine motor skills. Beware of overcalling a left hemisyndrome.

---

comitant strabismus is the more common type. Extraocular muscles function normally and the defect is equal in all directions of gaze. Sometimes nonparalytic strabismus is due to underlying ocular or visual pathology; mostly it is idiopathic. Pseudostrabismus must be differentiated from true strabismus. The former is a reflection of certain anatomic variations like prominent epicanthal folds, a broad and flat nasal bridge, and hypertelorism (Glazer, 1978).

Two simple tests can be used to identify strabismus. In the Hirschberg test the symmetry of the cornel reflex is documented. In the cover/uncover and cross/cover tests the eyes are observed for refixation movements. With the child fixing on a distant target alternately covering the two eyes elicits no movement. With esotropia the deviating eye will move outward as the fixating eye is occluded; with exotropia the deviating eye will move inward as the fixating eye is occluded. With a phoria the occluded eye tends to deviate, because binocular vision is temporarily disrupted, and refixation will be seen at the moment of uncovering (Glazer, 1978).

Extraocular motility is then assessed. Congenital anomalies of the oculomotor system consisting of omissions, substitutions, and duplications are often not brought to the attention of the physician until the preschool years. Distinguishing between congenital and acquired oculomotor problems has obvious therapeutic implications; old photographs are often very useful for this purpose (Glazer, 1978).

Duane's retraction syndrome is of three types, all involving retraction of the globe and narrowing of the lid fissure on attempted adduction: (1) palsy of adduction with retraction on adduction, (2) palsy of adduction with retraction and intact abduction, and (3) palsy of adduction and abduction with retraction on attempted adduction. Pfaffenbah et al. (1972) reviewed 186 cases and documented a female preponderance and a right eye preponderance (58% right eye compared with 20% left eye and 18% bilateral). Occasionally the Duane's retraction syndrome is mistaken for an acquired sixth-nerve palsy; however, diplopia is rare with congenital palsies (Glaser, 1978).

In Brown's tendon sheath syndrome, upgaze in the adducted position is restricted even during forced duction owing to the absence of the inferior oblique and thickening of the superior oblique tendon sheath. The deficit may be intermittent and even disappear during adulthood (Glaser, 1978).

A double elevator palsy has also been reported, involving both inferior oblique and superior rectus muscles. A homolateral ptosis is present but there is no diplopia and the pupil is spared. Preservation of Bell's phenomenon suggests that this is a supranuclear problem (Glaser, 1978).

The Marcus Gunn jaw winking phenomenon is a congenital trigeminal oculomotor synkinesis involving jaw and lid that is due to anomalous innervation. Generally the disorder presents in infancy as a (usually left) unilateral ptosis that jerks rhythmically upward during nursing. The jaw winking phenomenon is an exaggeration of a normally existing reflex. The phenomenon often disappears over time.

Congenital fourth-nerve palsies are not uncommon and are often discovered after minor head trauma. Review of old photographs will reveal the compensatory head tilt—head away from, chin toward the side of the paretic superior oblique muscle.

Examination of extraocular motility is concluded by assessment of the child's ability to *converge*. Accommodative esotropia tends to appear most commonly in the preschool years. This disorder is a reflection of excessive accommodation with overconvergence.

The *pupils* should then be examined. Anisocoria, which may actually have been congenital, is sometimes not noted until the toddler years. In general, anisocoria in which the difference is maintained in different illuminations is not pathologic; however, anisocoria that increases or diminishes when the light changes should be considered pathologic. If the pupillary difference is more pronounced in bright light, it is the larger pupil that is abnormal; if the anisocoria is worse in dim light, it is the smaller pupil that is abnormal. In Horner's syndrome, seen for example with traumatic brachial plexus palsy, anisocoria is more marked in dim light (which puts demands on the abnormal dilator mechanism) than in bright light (which puts demands on the intact constrictor mechanism) (Glaser, 1978). If Horner's syndrome occurs before age 2, the iris is often hypopigmented.

The examination of the pupils is followed by an assessment of *acuity* and of the *visual fields.* Acuity can be measured in the toddler using a finger mimicking game

with alternating eye occlusion. The acuity is recorded as finger counting at *X* feet (20 feet equals 20/200, 40 feet equals 20/100) and is limited only by the distance that the examiner can put between himself and the child (Glaser, 1978). Visual fields can be measured in the preschooler by finger mimicking of one, two, or five fingers flashed by the examiner. When fixation is a problem the face may be turned so that the abducted eye can be moved no further toward the right or left (Glaser, 1978).

Auditory acuity is then assessed with, for example, a ticking watch. The *tongue* and *pharyngeal arches* are inspected (cranial nerves IX through XII). Finally, the *funduscopic* examination is performed.

MENTAL STATUS

Much information about the child's cognitive functioning can be gleaned from observation during the neurologic exam. Attentional difficulties, for example, are seen as an inability to stay with such tasks as motor stance or heel or toe walking. An impression about the child's general language skills can be gleaned from his or her contribution to the history and ability to follow verbal commands during the examination. However, a formal assessment of higher cortical function should nonetheless be performed.

The asssessment of higher cortical function in the preschooler is limited not by the availability of appropriate measures, but by the cooperation of the child and the patience of the examiner. However, it is generally possible for the neurologist to get an impression of the child's functioning in the office and to obtain supporting and elaborating data from a psychometrician, neuropsychologist, and/or speech and language pathologist.

This section is divided into a presentation of useful office measures for assessing the preschooler and an introduction to the commonly used psychometric tests for this age group.

Office Measures

Historic
Although historic data are potentially biased by the historian, the advantages in the pre-school-age group are temporal closeness and the cooperative nature of the informant.

The *Anser system*, developed by Levine (1981), includes parent and teacher questionnaires for the 3- to 5-year-old. Although it is biased toward behavioral issues, a useful medical and developmental history can also be obtained using the parent questionnaire. The *Readiness for Kindergarten* workbook (Massey, 1975) also provides a history.

The *Denver Developmental Screening Test* (DDST, Frankenburg and Dodds, 1967) is a classic tool for assessing development in the personal-social, fine motor,

TABLE 3-5. PERTINENT QUESTIONS TO ASK PARENTS OF PRESCHOOL CHILDREN WITH SUSPECTED LANGUAGE DISORDERS

Key Quesions	Suspect Parent Responses
1. How old was your child when he began to speak his first words?	24 months or older
2. How old was your child when he began to put words into sentences?	36 months or older
3. Does your child have difficulty learning new vocabulary words?	Yes
4. Does your child omit words from sentences (i.e., do his sentences sound telegraphic)?	Yes
5. Does your child speak in short or incomplete sentences?	Yes
6. Does your child have trouble with verbs such as *is, am, are, was,* and *were*?	Yes
7. Does your child have difficulty following directions?	Yes
8. Does your child seem to have difficulty in understanding you if you use long sentences?	Yes
9. Does your child respond appropriately to questions?	No
10. Does your child ask questions beginning with *who, what, where,* and *why*?	No
11. Does your child use present and past tense verbs correctly?	No
12. Does it seem that your child has made little or no progress in speech and language in the last 6 to 12 months?	Yes
13. Does your child omit sounds from his words?	Yes
14. Do you feel your child's speech is more difficult to understand than it should be in view of his age?	Yes
15. Does it seem like your child uses *t, d, k,* or *g* in place of most other consonants when he speaks?	Yes

From A. Schwartz and Murphy (1975) with permission.

language, and gross motor domains. By and large, except for the personal-social domain, assessment beyond 2 years requires the cooperation of the child. However, a recently developed prescreening developmental questionnaire filled out by the parent identified 84% of nonnormal DDSTs (Frankenburg et al., 1987). An abnormal DDST predicts school problems at the end of the first grade with 84% accuracy (Sturner et al., 1985). The DDST is not as sensitive to speech and language problems, providing the equivalent of the Preschool Language Scale (Zimmerman et al., 1979) for receptive but not for expressive langage or articulation (Borowitz and Glascoe, 1986).

Table 3–5 lists pertinent questions to ask the parents of preschoolers suspected of experiencing language delay (A. Schwartz and Murphy, 1975).

Administerable in the Office

Language. Tables 3–6 and 3–7 list anticipated 50th-percentile receptive and expressive language milestones from ages 1 to 5. Assessment of language functioning using these milestones provides a general idea of language level. Additional information gleaned from observations of communicative language use (pragmatics); considering language in terms of its subcomponents of phonology, syntax, and semantics; and study of nonverbal cognitive capacities may provide the skilled clinician with enough information to make a subtype diagnosis from among the developmental language disorders (see Chapter 16). Finally, to obtain a measure of receptive vocabulary skills that correlates with overall language status, the *Peabody Picture Vocabulary Test* can be administered from 2½ years on by secretary, nurse, or physician. The *PEET* and *Peer*

TABLE 3-6. RECEPTIVE LANGUAGE SKILLS

Understands "Where is mother"?	12 months
Points to one body part	18
Follows two-step commands two times out of three (*me spoon/mom ball, me ball/ mom spoon, mom ball/cup me*)	18
Knows six body parts	2 years
Understands concept of "one"	2–2½
Points to spoon, ball, cup by use	2½
Recognizes day and night	3
Knows three out of four prepositions (*on, under, in front, behind*)	3½
Recognizes colors	4
Understands concept of "three"	4–4½
Identifies right and left on self	4½–5

TABLE 3-7. EXPRESSIVE LANGUAGE SKILLS

Knows two to four single words	12 months
Uses two-word sentences	18
Refers to self by name	2 years
Uses plurals, *I*	2–2½
Converses in sentences	2–2½
Gives full name	2½–3
Comprehends *old, tired, hungry*	3–3½
Can draw opposite analogies two times out of three (*fire/ice; mother/father; horse/mouse*)	3–3½
Comprehends senses	4
Defines words correctly six times out of nine (*ball, lake, desk, house, banana, curtain, ceiling, hedge, pavement*)	4½–5

(Levine and Schneider, 1985; Blackman et al., 1986) have language subtests—including spatial directions, complex sentences, categories, temporal directions, word span, and rote language skills (e.g., counting, days)—that can be used in isolation or in conjunction with the whole exam for the 3- to 6-year old.

Visual-Spatial and Motor. Table 3–8 lists anticipated 50th-percentile motor milestones from ages 1 to 5. Attention should be paid to crayon-holding posture. Sometime between the third and fifth years the pincer grasp established by 1 year gives way to the rigid tripod—thumb opposed to index finger supported by middle finger, but without flexion extension of the interphalangeal joints (the dynamic tripod, age 6 to 7 years). The *Beery Test of Visual Motor Integration* (1982) can be used in the office starting at age 2. Motor free tasks measuring perception (eliminating the possible confound of the motor component) are discussed subsequently. *Raven's Coloured Matrices* (Raven, 1962), a measure of nonverbal reasoning in which the child must complete a pattern in a six-choice format, can be administered to the 5-year-old. The *PEET* and *PEER* (Levine and Schneider, 1985; Blackman et al., 1986) have visuomotor subtests—including visual matching, copying figures, and drawing from memory—that can be used in isolation or in conjunction with the whole exam for ages 4 to 6 years.

Attention. Attentional deficit can be a problem in the preschool years (see Chapter 16) and is best assessed by observation. Unfortunately, Connors's questionnaire (1969) has not been validated for the preschooler. Levine's Anser questionnaires may prove useful here.

Dominance. Finally, dominance should be assessed by demonstration: show me which hand you use for writing. A dominance battery filled out by the parents is a useful way of assessing for mixed dominance. In general, it is atypical for the eventual right-hander to declare strongly prior to age 1 year or to have failed to declare by age 5 years. Although clear declaration of handedness does not generally take place until at least the end of the first year, numerous studies document a rightward bias, as evidenced by head turn preference in the neonatal period and grasping hand preferences in infancy (see Corballis, 1983, for review). Studies of handedness during the first year actually suggest a transient period during which there is a left hand bias, at least for reaching, in infants who ultimately are destined to be right-handed (Young et al., 1983).

Documentation of handedness declaration after age 1 has depended on both preference reports and performance skills. Gesell and Ames (1947) examined videotapes of situations contrived to secure handedness information on a variety of tasks. Other observation studies have used single tasks like writing or throwing. Examining both preference and ability in almost 300 2-year-olds, R. Schwartz (1988) found that 81% were right-handed. One year later, at age 3 years, 86% of the same cohort was right-handed. Assessing handedness by ball throwing in 2-year-olds, Churchill et al. (1962) found that 836/1102 were right-handed, 173 were ambidextrous, and 93 were left-handed. A number of dominance batteries designed to assess the spectrum of hand, foot, and eye preference on a variety of tasks are available (see Annett, 1985, for review). While there may be some minimal rightward evolution over the preschool years (Porac and Coren, 1981), the percentage of right-handers is in general already firmly fixed.

Relatively little information is available about the right versus left hand skill of right-handers during the preschool years. Annett (1985) found a stable right hand advantage on her peg moving task from ages 3½ to 15 years.

Berger-Gross et al. (1984) found a right hand advantage on finger tapping and sequencing tasks paralleling the right hand advantage to age 7 years found by Denckla (1973, 1974). Although left-handers are in general less strongly left-handed than right-handers are right-handed, the left hand of the young left-hander is the equal in terms of dextrous performance to the right hand of the young right-hander (Rudel et al., 1984).

Although in most instances sinistrality is genetically determined (Annett, 1985), some left-handedness is pathologically based. A disproportionately large number of left-handers may have presented at birth in the right occiput anterior position (Churchill et al., 1962). The investigators argued, however, that the left-handedness in these children was not due to brain damage during the birth process, as these children were otherwise normal. In addition, in separate studies of children with focal epilepsy and with hemiplegia, Churchill (1966, 1968) found no association between side of pathology and birth position. In contrast, others have argued that left-handedness occurs with increased birth stress and thereby have related it to brain damage during labor and delivery. Left-handedness is more common in the premature infant, again possibly owing to brain injury in the prenatal or perinatal period (Ross et al., 1987). The entity of pathologic left-handedness as described by Satz (1972) is a genetic right-hander who, because of perhaps more extreme perinatal injury to the left hemisphere, becomes a manifest left-hander, usually declaring excessively early. The pathologic right-hander probably

TABLE 3-8. VISUAL MOTOR SKILLS

Scribbles	1 year
Copies vertical line	2
Copies circle	2½
Copies + , draws circle	3½
Draws square	4½
Draws triangle	5–6

also exists, but may be more difficult to tease out. Bishop (1984) found an association between poor motor performance with the nonpreferred hand and left-handedness consistent with the view of shifted pathologic handedness. She also documented impaired cognitive performance relative to controls for a population selected on the basis of poor scores with the nonpreferred hand.

There is an increased incidence of left-handedness among the mentally retarded as well as among the learning disabled (Annett, 1985). Geschwind and Behan (1982) report ten times the incidence of dyslexia in the left-hander as compared to the right-hander and three times the incidence in the families of left-handers. Annett (1985) speculated that those not carrying her postulated right shift gene are at increased risk for learning problems, but that a variety of other factors, including gender, modify this risk. Certainly family history should include information about handedness and the presence of learning disabilities. Geschwind and Behan's (1982) finding of a high frequency of migraine and allergies in families with learning disabilities supports inquiry about these features as well. The recent suggestion that blonds are more likely to be learning disabled (Schacter el al., 1987) supports the inclusion of hair color in the general physical exam. The facts that more males are left handed and that the incidence of learning disabilities is higher among males than females led Geschwind (Geschwind and Behan, 1982), to postulate that androgens, perhaps by slowing maturation of the left hemisphere, play a causative role. Consistent with this hypothesis is the finding of a left hand bias among girls with congenital adrenal hyperplasia, who are exposed to excess androgens in utero, as compared to their unaffected female siblings (Nass et al., 1987).

Mixed dominance (hand, foot, eye, and sometimes ear preference) is also said to be associated with an increased risk for learning disabilities (Orton, 1937). As seen in Table 3–9 (Porac and Coren, 1981), showing dominance for hand, foot, eye and ear in adults, mixed dominance among the non-learning-disabled population also is inevitable. Mixed dominance is probably not a useful measure in the preschooler because of the relative paucity of data for this age group and the indication that dominance patterns may still be in transition (for review see Porac and Coren, 1981).

TABLE 3–9. PERCENTAGE OF ADULTS SHOWING CONSISTENT PREFERENCE

	Females (N = 2391)	Males (N = 2756)
Hand	80.6	74.0
Foot	57.7	42.2
Eye	72.4	65.4
Ear	53.7	46.4

From Porac and Coren (1981) with permission.

PRESCHOOL PSYCHOMETRIC ASSESSMENT INSTRUMENTS

Screening Tests

The *Goodenough-Harris Drawing Tests* (Goodenough and Harris, 1963) screen for intellectual maturity and are normed for children 3 through 15 years. The child is asked to draw a picture of a man, a woman, and him- or herself. Drawings are scored for the presence of 73 details. Raw scores are converted into standard scores distributed similarly to IQ scores. The numer of body part details expected increases with age. Two parts are expected at age 3½, six parts at 4½, and ten parts at 5½.

The *Boehm Test of Basic Concepts—Preschool Version* (Boehm, 1986) measures children's understanding of 26 basic relational concepts considered necessary for early school achievement. The test is appropriate for use with 3- to 5-year-old children or older children with identified language difficulties. The test presents a multiple-choice format wherein the child is asked to select the picture that best illustrates a concept. Relational concepts tested refer to characteristics of people and objects, such as size, direction, position in space, quantity, and time. Testing time is only 10 to 15 minutes.

The *Vineland Adaptive Behavior Scale* (Sparrow et al., 1985) assesses an individual's personal and social skills in daily activities. A survey form (297 items) and an expanded form (577 items) present questions in semi-structured format to parents or to teachers (the classroom form) concerning the adaptive behavior of the child in four domains: communication, daily living skills, socialization, and motor skills. The test is useful from birth through 18 years. It is especially useful in the evaluation of mental retardation and in preparing individual educational, habilitative, and treatment programs.

Intelligence Tests

The *Wechsler Preschool and Primary Scale of Intelligence—Revised* (WPPSI-R) (Wechsler, 1990) is a downward extension of the revised Wechsler Intelligence Scale for Children (WISC-R) designed to assess the intellectual abilities of the preschool child, age 3 to 6½ years. It is a well-standardized, reliable instrument used extensively by clinicians and school psychologists. Like the WISC-R, the WPPSI-R consists of subtests that measure diverse areas of ability. Most subtests provide the same measures as on the WISC-R and are seen as continuous with the WISC-R. The WPPSI-R therefore may be useful in providing baseline assessment for the young child who may be seen serially in follow-up evaluation during the school-age years. Separate verbal, performance, and full-scale IQs are obtained. The test is less useful for children at the upper and lower ends of IQ ranges than it is for children within the average ranges. Gifted children do not reach a ceiling and the test does not differentiate abilities at the lower levels. Up to four scale points are received for no correct responses on some subtests.

The *Stanford-Binet Intelligence Scale—Fourth Edition* (Thorndike et al., 1986) is a revision of the 1960 Stanford-Binet, Form L-M,, designed to eliminate culturally biased items in the earlier edition. This IQ test is based on a three-level hierarchical model of cognitive abilities, with a general reasoning factor as the highest level. Second-level abilities are divided among "crystallized," "fluid-analytic," and short-term memory. Specific verbal, quantitative, and abstract-visual reasoning factors make up the third level.

The *McCarthy Scales for Children's Abilities* (McCarthy, 1970) measure cognitive and motor skills in children 2½ to 8½ years of age through the use of game-like tasks. Scaled scores and percentiles are derived for six subscales: verbal, perceptual-performance, quantitative, general cognitive, memory, and motor. The General Cognitive Index is similar to an IQ, although the authors avoid the use of the term *IQ* because of the pitfalls of misinterpretation associated with it. Observations about laterality for hand and eye preference are included as part of the motor scale. Correlations with the Stanford-Binet and the WPPSI-R are moderately high.

The *Kaufman Assessment Battery for Children (K-ABC)* (Kaufman and Kaufman, 1983) measures intelligence and achievement in children aged 2½ to 12½ years. The K-ABC was designed to minimize the role of language skills in IQ assessment and was developed from research and theory in neuropsychology. It is based on the assumption that intelligence consists of two types of mental processing: sequential (reflected by subtests that present stimuli in serial or temporal order) and simultaneous (reflected by subtests that present gestalt-like, frequently spatial integration of information). Standard scores in five areas of functioning are obtained: Sequential Processing, Simultaneous Processing, Mental Processing Composite (Sequential and Simultaneous combined), Achievemnent, and Nonverbal (based on subtests that require no verbal response). The Nonverbal scale can be administered in pantomime and allows for the evaluation of hearing- and language-impaired and non–English-speaking children. Additional interpretation of the K-ABC for minority children is recognized by the inclusion of supplementary sociocultural norms.

The Achievement scale measures children's acquired knowledge, including reading, arithmetic, and general information, and provides a frame of comparison for evaluating the extent to which children apply their mental processing skills to learning situations. Clinical profiles for the learning-disabled, mentally retarded, and behaviorally disordered child are included in the interpretive testing manual. The test correlates well with other IQ tests. It is unique in its inclusion of neuropsychologic

tests appropriate for the preschooler, such as facial recognition, hand movements, and color interference.

The *Detroit Tests of Learning Aptitude—Primary* (Hammill, 1986) measures verbal, conceptual, attention, and motor domains in children 3 to 9 years. A general composite intelligence quotient is obtained. The test is particularly useful in assessing low-functioning children, providing a detailed profile of a child's abilities and deficiencies.

The *Hiskey-Nebraska Test of Learning Aptitude—Revised* (Hiskey, 1966) is a nonverbal intelligence test designed for deaf or hearing-impaired children aged 3 to 18½ years. Instructions for administration by gesture as well as verbal directions are provided. The test yields a "learning age" for deaf children and a "mental age" for hearing children. A Learning Quotient is derived by dividing the child's learning age by his or her chronologic age and is distributed similarly to an IQ score. Subtests are solely visual and include discrimination, memory, and constructional tasks.

The *Leiter International Performance Scale* (Leiter, 1979) is a nonverbal intelligence test designed to eliminate the language factor from IQ assessment. The test is appropriate for ages 2 to adult and yields a mental age and ratio IQ. Four subtests are presented at each age level. The child is presented with a series of visual sequences of increasing difficulty that he must match, continue in analogy, or construct associations with, using an array of appropriate blocks. A mental age and an IQ are derived.

The *Columbia Mental Maturity Scale* (Burgemeister et al., 1972) is a mental ability test requiring no verbal response and minimal motor response. It is particularly well suited for the young child, although it has norms from ages 3½ through 10 years, and for children who are physically or verbally impaired. Items are presented on cards at eight age levels, requiring the child to select from a series of drawings the one that does not belong.

Visuo-Spatial/Visual-Motor Tests

Raven's Coloured Progressive Matrices (Raven, 1962) is the children's version of the Standard Progressive Matrices Test, normed for children 5 through 11 years. It is a nonverbal test used to assess cognitive ability by presenting an incomplete visual design or a visual analogy of increasing abstraction. The child is asked to select from among six alternatives the design that best completes the initially presented design. Thirty-six test items are included to assess discrimination, problem solving, and logical analyses of visual-spatial information. Age norms and percentiles are derived.

The *Bender Visual-Motor Gestalt Test* (Bender, 1938) measures visual perception and motor behavior through the copying of geometric figures. The test is thought to be sensitive to brain injury and is appropriate for ages

4 through adult. It has been standardized by the Koppitz Scoring System for ages 5 through 10. The test presents a series of nine designs to be drawn on a single blank paper.

The *Beery Development Test of Visual-Motor Integration* (Beery, 1982) is a sequence of 24 geometric figures of increasing complexity to be copied into a test booklet. The test is normed for children 2 through 15 years and was designed as an educational assessment of visual-motor skills and remedial need. Information pertaining to remedial strategies is included as part of the test manual. The test includes items developmentally more appropriate for the preschooler than the Bender.

The *Motor Free Visual Perception Test (Colarusso and Hammill, 1972)* is a test of visual perception, including visual matching and discrimination, memory, figure-ground, and visual closure tasks. The test eliminates motor involvement from the performance assessment and thus allows for the measurement of perceptual skill without the confound of constructional ability. It is particularly useful for children who have motor impairments. Norms are available for children 4 through 8 years. Perceptual age and a perceptual quotient are derived.

Language Tests

The *Illinois Test of Psycholinguistic Abilities* measures the child's ability to understand and express verbal and nonverbal language for ages 2 to 10 years. Subtests include auditory reception, auditory-vocal association, auditory closure, and sequential memory, as well as visual reception, association, closure, memory, and gestural expression. The test is based on Osgood's model of communication. A psycholinguistic age and a psycholinguistic quotient are derived.

The *Test of Language Development—Primary* (Newcomer and Hammill, 1982) measures semantic and syntactic understanding and expression in children 4 through 8 years. Subtests include word articulation and discrimination, vocabulary, grammatic understanding and completion, and sentence imitation. Scores are converted to percentiles and age equivalents for each area.

The *Test of Early Language Development* (Hresko et al., 1981) is a measure of spoken language abilities for ages 3 through 7 years. Verbal and pictorial items are included, yielding information about receptive and expressive skills with respect to both the form and the content of language. A language quotient, percentile ranks, and age equivalents are derived.

The *Token Test for Children* (DiSimoni, 1978) assesses auditory comprehension of language through the presentation of directions of increasing length and complexity. The child responds to the directives by manipulating tokens of various sizes, shapes, and colors. The test assesses the child's ability to understand and follow instructions and yields information about attention, memory, and sequencing abilities as well as conceptual grouping. The test is appropriate for ages 1 through 15 years.

The *Goldman-Fristoe-Woodcock Auditory Skills Test Battery* (Goldman et al., 1976) assesses a broad range of auditory skills for ages 3 to adult, ranging from auditory attention and discrimination to complex association of sound-symbols in written language. The test provides detailed diagnostic information needed for instructional planning for the language pathologist or educator. Standardized scores on 12 subtests can be converted into age equivalents and percentile ranks.

ANNOTATED BIBLIOGRAPHY

Touwen BCL, Prechtl, HFR: *The Neurological Examination of the Child with Minor Central Nervous System Dysfunction.* London, Spastics International, 1970.
Levine M, Schneider E: *The Pediatric Examination of Educational Readiness.* Cambridge, Mass: Educators Publishing Service, 1985.
These are comprehensive references on the neurologic examination of the pre-school- and school-age child.
Nichols P, Chen T: *Minimal Brain Dysfunction.* Hillsdale, NJ, Lawrence Erlbaum, 1981.
This book presents the preschool neurologic examination and examines its predictive value.
Lefford A, Birch HG, Green G: The perceptual and cognitive basis for finger localization and selective finger movement in preschool children. *Child Dev* 45:335–343, 1974.
Kinsbourne M, Warrington EK: The development of finger differentiation. *J Exp Psychol* 15:132–137, 1963.
These articles provide a theoretic approach to the development of sensory skills and the understanding of body schema.
Nass R: Mirror movement asymmetries in congenital hemiparesis. *Neurology* 35:1059–1062, 1985.
This paper provides a good review of the theoretic basis for overflow in the child.
Wolff P, Gunnoe C, Cohen, C: Associated movements as a measure of developmental age. *Dev Med Child Neurol* 25:417–429, 1983.
This paper provides a good practical review of the extent of mirroring in the preschooler on common motor tasks.
Glaser JS: *Neuroophthalmology.* New York, Harper & Row, 1978.
This is a readable and, for its size, amazingly comprehensive neuroophthalmology text.
Levine MD: *The Anser System.* Cambridge, Mass. Educators Publishing Service, 1981.
This system, devised by a developmental pediatrician, provides parent and teacher history forms for the preschooler.
Frankenburg WK, Dodds JB: *The Denver Developmental Screening Test.* Denver, University of Colorado Press, 1969.
This remains the classic, easy-to-administer developmental screen.
Annett M: *Left, Right, Hand and Brain: The Right Shift Theory.* Hillsdale, NJ, Erlbaum Associates, 1985.
This is a comprehensive book on all aspects of dominance.

REFERENCES

Annett M: *Left, Right, Hand and Brain: The Right Shift Theory.* Hillsdale, NJ, Erlbaum Associates, 1985.

Beery KE: *Developmental Test of Visual-Motor Integration.* Chicago, Follett, 1982.

Bender L: *Bender Visual Motor Gestalt Test.* Los Angeles, Western Psychological Services, 1938.

Berger-Gross PM, Haggerty R, Rudel R, Kreiger J: Ontogenesis of Associated Movements: Is It a Cognitive Calendar? Presentation at American Psychological Association, Annual Meeting, 1984.

Bishop DVM: Using nonpreferred skill to investigate pathological left-handedness in an unselected population. *Dev Med Child Neurol* 26:214–226, 1984.

Blackman J, Levine M, Markowitz M: *Pediatric Extended Examination at Three.* Cambridge, Mass, Educators Publishing Service, 1986.

Boehm AE: *Boehm Test of Basic Concepts—Revised.* Cleveland, Psychological Corporation, 1986.

Borowitz KC, Glascoe FP; Sensitivity of the Denver Developmental Screening Test in speech and language screening. *Pediatrics* 78:1075–1078, 1986.

Burgemeister BB, Blum LH, Lorge I: *Columbia Mental Maturity Scale.* Cleveland, Psychological Corporation, 1972.

Churchill JA: On the origin of focal motor epilepsy. *Neurology* 16:49–58, 1966.

Churchill JA: A study of hemiplegic cerebral palsy. *Dev Med Child Neurol* 10:453–459, 1968.

Churchill JA, Igna E, Sent R: The association of position at birth and handedness. *Pediatrics* 29:307–309, 1962.

Colarusso RP, Hammill DD: *Motor Free Visual Perception Test.* Novato, Calif, Academic Therapy Publications, 1972.

Connolly K, Stratton P: Developmental changes in associated movements. *Dev Med Child Neurol* 10:49–56, 1968.

Connors KC: A teacher rating scale for use in drug studies with children. *Am J Psychiatry* 126:884–889, 1969.

Corballis MC: *Human Laterality.* New York, Academic Press, 1983.

Denckla MB: Development of speed in repetitive and successive finger movements in normal children. *Dev Med Child Neurol* 15:635–645, 1973.

Denckla MB: Development of motor coordination in normal children. *Dev Med Child Neurol* 16:729–741, 1974.

Dennis M: Impaired sensory and motor differentiation with callosal agenesis: A lack of callosal inhibition during ontogeny? *Neuropsychologia* 14:455–469, 1976.

DiSimoni F: *Token Test for Children.* Allen, Tex, DLM Teaching Resources, 1978.

Frankenburg WK, Dodds JB: The Denver Developmental Screening Test. *Pediatr* 71:181–186, 1967.

Frankenburg WK, Fandal AW, Thornton SM: Revision of Denver Prescreening Developmental Questionnaire. *J Pediatr* 110:653–658, 1987.

Galin D, Diamond R, Herron J: Development of crossed and uncrossed tactile localization of the fingers. *Brain and Language* 4:588–590, 1977.

Geschwind N: The apraxias: Neural mechanisms of disorders of learned movements. *Am Sci* 63:188–195, 1975.

Geschwind N, Behan P: Left handedness: Association with immune disease, migraine and developmental learning disorder. *Pro Nat Acad Sci* 79:5097–5100, 1982.

Gesell A, Ames LB: The development of handedness. *J Gen Psychol* 70:155–176, 1947.

Glaser JS: *Neuroophthalmology.* New York, Harper & Row, 1978.

Goldman R, Fristoe M, Woodcock RW: *Goldman-Fristoe-Woodcock Auditory Skills Test Battery.* Circle Pines, Minn, American Guidance Service, 1976.

Goodenough F, Harris D: *Goodenough-Harris Drawing Tests.* Los Angeles, Western Psychological Services, 1963.

Hammill P: *Detroit Test of Learning Aptitude—Primary.* Austin, Tex, Pro-Ed, 1986.

Hiskey M: *Hiskey-Nebraska Test of Learning Aptitude.* Lincoln, Neb, University of Nebraska Press, 1986.

Hresko WP, Reid DK, Hammill DD: *Test of Early Language Development.* Circle Pines, Minn, American Guidance Service, 1981.

Kaufman A, Kaufman A: *Kaufman Assessment Battery for Children.* Circle Pines, Minn, American Guidance Service, 1983.

Kinsbourne M, Hicks R: Functional cerebral space: A model for overflow, transfer and interference effects in human performance: A tutorial review, in Renquin J (ed): *Attention and Performance.* Hillsdale, NJ, Lawrence Erlbaum, 1978.

Kinsbourne M, Warrington EK: The development of finger differentiation. *J Exp Psychol* 15:132–137, 1963.

Kuypers H: Anatomy of the descending pathways in Brookhart J, Mountcastle V (eds): *Handbook of Physiology.* Baltimore, Md, American Physiological Society, 1981.

Lefford A, Birch HG, Green G: The perceptual and cognitive bases for finger localization and selective finger movement in preschool children. *Child Dev* 45:335–343, 1974.

Leiter RG: *Leiter International Performance Scale.* Los Angeles, Western Psychological Services, 1979.

Lenn N, Thurston S: Is facial sparing in children with prenatal hemiparesis evidence for neuronal plasticity? *Ann Neurol* 14:371, 1983.

Levine M: *The Anser System.* Cambridge, Mass, Educators Publishing Service, 1981.

Levine MD: *Developmental Variation and Learning Disorders.* Cambridge, Mass, Educators Publishing Service, 1988.

Levine M, Schneider E: *Pediatric Exam of Educational Readiness (PEER).* Cambridge, Mass, Educators Publishing Service, 1985.

Lewis B, Aram D, Horwitz S: Language and motor findings in benign megalencephaly. *Ann Neurol* 14:364, 1983.

Lindgren SD: Finger localization and the prediction of reading disability. *Cortex* 14:87–101, 1978.

McCarthy D: *McCarthy Scales of Children's Abilities.* Cleveland, Psychological Corporation, 1970.

Massey J: *Readiness for Kindergarten,* Palo Alto, Calif, Consulting Psychologists Press, 1975.

Nass R: Mirror movement asymmetries in congenital hemiparesis: The inhibition hypothesis revisited. *Neurology* 35:1059–1062, 1985.

Nass R, Baker S, Speiser P, et al: Hormonal effects on handedness: Left hand bias in females with congenital adrenal hyperplasia. *Neurology* 37:711–715, 1987.

Nelson K, Eng G: Congenital hypoplasia of the depressor anguli oris muscle: Differentiation from congenital facial palsy. *J Pediatr* 81:16–20, 1972.

Newcomer PL, Hammill DD: *The Test of Language*

Development—Primary. Circle Pines, Minn, American Guidance Service, 1982.

Nichols P, Chen T: *Minimal Brain Dysfunction: A Prospective Study*. Hillsdale, NJ, Lawrence Erlbaum, 1981.

Njiokikjien C, Driessen M, Habraken L: Development of supination-pronation movements in normal children. *Hum Neurobiol* 5:199–203, 1986.

Orton ST: *Reading, Writing and Speech Problems in Children*. London, Chapman and Hall, 1937.

Pfaffenbach DD, Cross HE, Kearns TP: Congential anomalies in Duane's retraction syndrome. *Arch Ophthamol* 88:635–641, 1972.

Porac C, Coren S: *Lateral Preferences and Human Behavior*. New York, Springer-Verlag, 1981.

Raven, JC: *Coloured Progressive Matrices*. London, ET Heron, 1962.

Roeltgen MG, Tucker DM, Roeltgen DP: Asymmetric lateralized attention in children. *Neurology* 20:413, 1986.

Ross G, Lipper E, Auld P: Hand preference in four-year-old children: Relation to prematurity. *Dev Med Child Neurol* 29:615–622, 1987.

Rudel RG, Healey J, Denckla MB: Development of motor coordination by normal left handed children. *Dev Med Child Neurol* 26:104–111, 1984.

Satz P: Pathological left handedness: An explanatory model. *Cortex* 8:121–135, 1972.

Schachter S, Ransil B, Geschwind N: Associations of handedness with hair color and learning disabilities. *Neuropsychologia* 25:269–276, 1987.

Schwartz A, Murphy M: Cues for screening language disorders in preschool children. *Pediatrics* 55:717–722, 1975.

Schwartz JE, Kaplan E, Schwartz AR: Childhood dyscalculia and Gerstmann syndrome: A clinical and statistical analysis. *Neurology* 31:81, 1981.

Schwartz R: Changing Patterns of Handedness with Age.

Presentation at International Neuropsychology Society Meeting, 1988.

Smith D: *Recognizable Patterns of Human Malformation*. Philadelphia, Saunders, 1982.

Sparrow S, Balla D, Cicchetti D: *Vineland Adaptive Behavior Scales*. Circle Pines, Minn, American Guidance Service, 1985.

Sturner RA, Green JA, Funk SG: Preschool Denver Developmental Screening Test as a predictor of later school problems. *J Pediatr* 107:615–621, 1985.

Thorndike RL, Hagen EP, Sattler JM: *Stanford-Binet Intelligence Scale—4th Edition*. Chicago, Riverside, 1986.

Touwen BCL, Prechtl HFR: *The Neurological Examination of the Child with Minor Central Nervous System Dysfunction*. London, Spastics International, 1970.

Waldrop M, Halverson CE: Minor physical anomalies and hyperactive behavior in young children, in Hellmuth J (ed): *The Exceptional Infant*. New York, Brunner/Mazel, 1971.

Waldrop M, Pedersen F, Bell RQ: Minor physical anomalies and behavior in preschool children. *Child Dev* 39:391–400, 1968.

Wechsler D: *Wechsler Preschool and Primary Scales of Intelligence—Revised*. Cleveland, Psychological Corporation, 1990.

Wolff P, Gunnoe C, Cohen C: Associated movements as a measure of developmental age. *Dev Med Child Neurol* 25:417–429, 1983.

Yakovlev PI, LeCours AR: The myelogenetic cycles of regional maturation of the brain, in Minkowski A (ed): *Regional Development of the Brain in Early Life*. Oxford, Blackwell Scientific, 1967.

Young G, Segalowitz S, Corter C, Trehub S: *Manual Specialization and the Developing Brain*. New York, Academic Press, 1983.

Zimmerman IL, Steiner VG, Pond RE: *Preschool Language Scale*. Toronto, CE Merrill, 1979.

The Neurologic Examination of the School-Age and Adolescent Child

Ruthmary K. Deuel

Virtually all items used in the neurologic examination of the adult may also be employed in the neurologic examination of the school-age child and adolescent. The items to be included must be chosen with care, commensurate with the information that is required from the examination.

Certain domains must always be evaluated in any neurologic examination. Thus, every neurologic exam should include an evaluation of the patient's mental status, cranial nerves, motor system, deep tendon reflexes, and responses to sensory stimulation. Depending on the presenting complaint and the general purposes of the examination, each of these domains may then be evaluated in greater or lesser detail.

Rapport with the child is a major factor in ensuring an efficient neurologic exam. The examiner should bear in mind that the child's best effort on each item is more informative than grudging or partial performance. In general, a cheerful, positive attitude toward the child and a stubborn insistence on repeated efforts if the first response to a command is insufficient are rewarded by a better exam. Just as developmental norms are important for the neurologic examination at younger ages, they are important in the school-age child, particularly on the mental status and motor performance items. To obtain as much information as possible with the least amount of effort, it is good to use certain items in the neurologic exam to define more than one factor. For instance, response to commands and negative or positive reinforcement on the part of the examiner give considerable information about the child's compliance. Hand preference and performance are other aspects of the exam that are readily examined concomitantly with the ongoing examination. If the child is instructed to use "your fastest hand first" or "your strongest hand first" on unimanual motor items, a measure of hand preference will be obtained

(Deuel and Moran, 1980). The historic information gathered before the examination concerning the child's behavior as well as physical aberrations should be supplemented by the physician's direct observations during the exam. In the course of the sections that follow, the individual items of the neurologic exam will not all be discussed in detail. An excellent standard text on the general subject is *The Neurologic Examination* (1979), edited by DeJong and Magee. The chapter by Dodge and Volpe in Farmer's textbook *Pediatric Neurology* (1983) gives a detailed overview of the more specialized pediatric neurologic exam.

The goal of conducting a neurologic examination in a school-age child is to arrive at the correct diagnosis. If one appropriately applies the examination to test hypotheses constructed from the chief complaint and history, at the end of 30 or so minutes sufficient information should be available to make a positive diagnosis of neurologic disease, mental retardation, or any of the several specific learning disabilities, as well as attention deficit disorder, developmental language disorder, or developmental apraxia. In addition, conduct disorder and childhood depression may generally be positively identified by a thorough neurologic examination.

ITEMS OF THE GENERAL PHYSICAL EXAMINATION

For a complete neurologic assessment, aspects of the general physical examination are pertinent and should always be evaluated. The number of the general exam items actually conducted is of course dependent on the question that the examination is attempting to resolve. In infants and children, height, weight, and head circumference should always be accurately measured and

be plotted according to the percentile for chronologic age. For school-age children, the Nellhaus Composite International and Interracial Graph for head circumference is most accurate (Nellhaus, 1968). Blood pressure and pulse rate are also part of the standard neurologic examination, as is evaluation of the head, eyes, ears, nose, throat, skin, skeleton, and thoracic and abdominal organs.

In observing the hair, texture and thickness are important. The skull should be palpated for bone defects and for unusual shape or contour, such as is seen in plagiocephaly or hydrocephalus. The facies should be described if any irregularities at all are observed. External examination of the eyes is important, including the anatomic structure of the lids, cornea, sclerae, conjunctivae, and irides. Interpupillary distance should be recorded. Hypertelorism or hypotelorism is an important stigma of some chromosomal disorders (Pryor, 1969). Excessive conjunctival vasculature is a subtle but important indicator of ataxia-telangiectasia (Taylor et al., 1975). The external examination of the ears likewise may yield information regarding branchial cleft and other less common anomalies. The otoscopic exam is best carried out after first testing for tympanic movement. A full examination of the mouth, lips, palate, and tongue structures pertinent to speech mechanisms and articulation should be carried out in any child with speech or language delay (Spriesterbach et al., 1978). Dentition may give a clue to skeletal abnormalities. In certain syndromes abnormal dentition is the rule (Beumer et al., 1973). Evaluation of the thyroid gland should be carried out by palpation and auscultation of the gland. The thorax should be examined, the heart and lungs auscultated, and pulses in the neck examined with auscultation of the head and neck after it is ascertained that the cardiac rhythm is regular and there are no intrinsic cardiac auscultatory findings. The radial, carotid, and femoral pulses also should be palpated. It is important to palpate the abdomen for enlarged organs. The genitalia should also be examined with a view to Tanner staging (Tanner, 1962). This is particularly important in suspected sex chromosome aneuploidies (Pennington et al., 1980; Ratcliffe, 1982; Waber, 1979). The spinal column should be examined with the patient prone, standing, and bending over to evaluate scoliosis and lordosis. The sacral region should be particularly carefully observed for dimples or bony defects, particularly if any lower extremity difficulties have been noted. Skin changes overlying the spine, such as hemangioma or hair tufts, are of importance as they may herald underlying bony and neural tube defects. Shagreen patches of tuberous sclerosis are also found in this location (Berg, 1985). The extremities should be carefully evaluated for structural abnormalities that may yield the clue to various heritable syndromes, such as homocysteinuria, the mucopolysaccharidoses, and pseudohypoparathyroidism (Grossman and Dorst, 1973; Steinback et al., 1965; Schimke, 1965).

During all phases of the exam, as the patient may remain passive, it is convenient to note whether the patient remains attentive to the examination, cooperative to commands, and responsive to positive and negative reinforcement. Because the physical exam is the primary observation being made, we have called this latter group of assessments concomitant observations (see the Appendix). It is usually easy to find at least two or three opportunities to use positive reinforcement. For example, when the child opens his mouth, one can say, "That's good" or when she relaxes her abdominal muscles, one can respond with, "You're doing a good job at that . . . would you keep it up?" Of course there are usually also opportunities for negative reinforcement, for example, "Don't breathe so fast" or "Don't put your shirt on yet." It is likewise valuable to consider the quality and quantity of the subject's distractability. Do external interruptions (e.g., comments from parents, knocks at the door) distract the child from following instructions for the exam? Does the child become distracted without any obvious external stimuli? Finally, as a concomitant observation, is the child impulsive, interrupting the exam with sudden self-initiated actions or talk? Structured conscious rating of these responses is valuable and necessary to the evaluation of the attentional cognitive and motivational abilities of the child. It is thus an integral part of the mental status examination. Although further testing may certainly be required to refine observations, a directed pediatric and neurologic exam should suffice for initial detection and designation of pervasive attentional, cognitive, and conduct disorders.

THE NEUROLOGIC EXAMINATION

The neurologic exam proper is a series of functional tests aimed at determining whether different segments and subsystems within the nervous system are normal. The functions to be assessed will vary, depending on what questions are asked. Thus the "standard" neurologic examination is perhaps more encompassing than some others, but it is designed to answer contemporary questions regarding motor and higher cortical function.

The subject of the examination cannot be passive during any of these tests, but must comply and attempt to carry out commands. For example, any detailed sensory examination is impossible without good patient compliance. In children the order of the neurologic exam items should be dictated by common sense and the need to maintain good compliance. It is more important to assess all the necessary items than to follow some set rule for their presentation. At the beginning of the exam of the school-age child it is often useful to introduce yourself by asking some of the "conversational items" in the mental status exam. For example, an assessment of orientation is often a good opener. This allows an evaluation

of the child's knowledge of where he or she is, who the doctor is, the day of the week, and, for older children, the date and year. Further items that can be used are the names of the child's school and school teacher. For junior-high-school-age children, the address and zip code of the child's school is a good item, as is the usual question about presidents of the United States.

Handedness may also be identified conversationally by inquiring about several everyday activities (Bryden, 1977) (and later checking the responses with performance during pantomime on command and use of actual objects; Provins and Cunliffe, 1972), such as "What hand do you use when you cut with a pair of scissors?", "What hand do you use when you eat with a fork?", or "Do you use the other hand better for doing something else?" The patient should be asked to identify his or her right hand, and then given a three-part command using left and right items (for example, put your left thumb on your right ear and close your eyes). If there is a question of left/right confusion, a test of finger identification with eyes closed and open then may be administered as well.

If the complaint is failure or poor performance in school, the mental status exam should definitely include grade- and age-appropriate testing of school skills: letter identification or reading, copying shapes, and writing spontaneously as well as to dictation and copying. The written output should be evaluated for speed and legibility. The child should be asked to count or work arithmetic problems, including word problems, as grade-appropriate. He or she should be asked to draw a picture of a person. Out of the corner of the eye, while ostensibly discussing historic information with the parent, the examiner should observe several facets of the patient's performance: (1) how the hands are used, (2) how attentive the child is to the task, and (3) how rapidly or painstakingly the task is accomplished. To present a certain distractor, the examiner may ask the parent a question about a subject emotionally charged for the child. The picture the child produces should be scored using the Goodenough criteria (Taylor, 1959, Rowe, 1987). Such a brief mental status screening allows the physician direct observational insight that may then be supplemented by formal individual psychometric and school achievement tests done at a school or other facility. The direct, firsthand testing of school skills by the neurologic examiner affords that examiner an opportunity to detect uneven development of different cognitive abilities. This portion of the exam should thus help evaluate the validity of any formal cognitive testing that may have been done, or point up areas where more detailed and quantitative testing should be requested. Without direct examination of these very important aspects of the child's development, the neurologic exam will not be helpful in solving diagnostic dilemmas concerning dyspraxia and several other specific learning and language disorders, or pinpointing these entities as a primary problem in a child

with secondary pervasive attention or conduct disorders. It is much less important in the evaluation of other common problems, such as seizures or neuropathy, and may be minimized if they are the primary concern.

Examination of the cranial nerves includes evaluation of the important special senses, vision and hearing. It is usually unnecessary to test smell. However, if there is a question of frontal lobe or anterior fossa pathology, this should be done. The use of commercially available scratch tablets allows one to present familiar fruit smells (orange and banana are most easily recognized by schoolchildren) to each nostril. Confrontation visual fields are usually easily undertaken with one eye covered with a 3 × 5 index card in the 10-year-old and over. The optimal object is a small white-headed pin. The tester should sight on the subject's pupil and use his or her own visual field as a measure of the subject's visual field, placing the pin equidistant between the tester and the subject. Using this technique, the blind spot that confirms accurate field mapping can usually be found in the alert cooperative school child (Traquiar, 1949; Thompson, 1979). In younger or less able children fingers may be presented spontaneously to both fields or to one for at least a gross estimate of field integrity. In any child who will fixate, optokinetic nystagmus can be used to estimate responses to visual stimuli (Dejong and Magee, 1979). Optokinetic nystagmus should definitely be tested when there is a question of subtle visual field defects in younger children, or with a question of cortical blindness in a child of any age (Brindley, 1969). Visual acuity can be tested using a standard Snellen chart at 20 feet.* Visual acuity testing should be performed with and without glasses. Eye position should be noted without glasses. A cover test—consisting of having the patient fixate with both eyes forward, then covering one eye and seeing if the position of the remaining uncovered eye changes—may be used if there is a question concerning extraocular muscle abormality (Cogan, 1956, Chapter 10). Versions of the eyes in conjugate following should also be tested. Pupillary symmetry and reactions to direct stimulation with light, and to light in the opposite eye, should be noted as should nystagmus. Spontaneous and reactive nystagmus may have various connotations, depending on the type and direction of the movements (Cogan, 1956, Chapter 5).

Funduscopy should be carried out so that both disks, both maculae, and the peripheral retina of each eye can be visualized. A short-acting pupillary dilator may be invaluable in achieving this end. Jaw movements should be assessed. The symmetry of both the upper and the lower face should be evaluated. To test hearing crudely, finger rustling or whispering in the right and left ear with the other ear occluded is a reasonable test of conversa-

---

*In first graders or older children, a Rosenbaum packet vision or screener may be used.

tion level. Deafness is still often undetected (Coplen, 1987); losses in selected frequences particularly may go unnoticed as a cause of "inattention." Taste is sometimes tested and children above age four usually readily respond to salt/sugar taste in the anterior two thirds for the seventh nerve or the posterior third for the ninth nerve of the tongue. Palate elevation must be tested, both voluntarily and as part of the gag reflex. The sterno-cleidomastoid muscle is tested by having the child turn his or her face away from the side of the muscle tested. Tilting the chin up toward the ear will make the contracting sternocleidomastoid more prominent for palpation. Shrugging of the shoulders also allows testing of the eleventh nerve. Tongue protrusion and lateral movements are evaluated to test the twelfth nerve. Repeated syllables such as *PA-TA-KA* (Spriesterbach et al., 1978) allow for evaluation of orobuccal agility. Obviously, it may be necessary to carry out further, more refined and quantitative tests of visual and auditory sensation, such as the measurement of visual evoked potentials or brainstem auditory evoked potentials (BAEP). It is well to bear in mind that measurement of BAEP to clicks (composed of multiple frequencies) is not designed for testing hearing threshholds.

Introducing the motor exam with gait testing allows the youngster a chance to stretch. Running should be tested with at least a 20-ft leeway; a hall is useful for this test. Children 8 years old or older should be able to skip or able to learn from a demonstration.* Tandem walking should be tested to evaluate lower extremity coordination. The Fog maneuver may be used, requiring the child to walk on the insides or the outside of the soles (Fog and Fog, 1963). This is useful in determining whether there are adventitious movements in the face and hands during this unpracticed and awkward gait. Toe and heel gait are also helpful to test active strength in the lower extremity muscle groups. The pronator drift test should be performed with the child standing, the arms extended, the palms up. The child should be asked to hold the posture for 20 seconds. To evaluate for chorea, the child should stand unsupported for 20 seconds with eyes closed, arms extended and hands pronated with wrists extended and fingers abducted and extended (Barlow, 1974). Resistive strength testing of the upper and lower extremities may be carried out in standard fashion in children 6 years old and older. For screening purposes, shoulder girdle, distal extremity, and hip girdle strength should be tested. Stair climbing or stepping up to the seat of a chair is an excellent test for the latter. If a musculo-skeletal or neuromuscular disorder is suspected, more thorough testing of each muscle group should be carried

out, with grading of muscle strength from 0 to 5. Of course, evaluation of sitting posture should be made during this portion of the exam.

Cerebellar coordination of the upper extremities is best tested with the finger-to-nose test. The elbow should come to full extension and the wrist to full pronation before the child's finger is allowed to touch the examiner's finger. It is best to require three positions—center, 30° to the left, and 30° to the right—with each hand, and to require two trials in each position for each hand. To evaluate coordination more proximally in the upper ex-

---

Pearls and Perils: Neurologic Examination of the School-Age Child

1. Turner's syndrome and its associated physical features are accompanied by a distinctive neuropsychologic profile of abnormal spatial understanding (Waber, 1979).
2. Williams's syndrome and its associated physical features are also accompanied by a distinctive neuropsychologic profile, including a fluent receptive language disorder and clumsiness (Pagon, 1987; Meyerson and Frank, 1987).
3. Hypertelorism may be a sign of congenital absence of the corpus callosum.
4. Mild degrees of hemiparesis may be markedly accentuated by the Fog maneuver with marked asymmetries of the upper extremities and assumption of a hemiparetic posture by the arm on the affected side.
5. The nondominant hand is often more accurate in stereognosis discrimination than the dominant one (Witelson, 1978).
6. There is no such thing as the standard neurologic exam. Rather, there are an infinite variety of neurologic exams, the items in which depend heavily on the individual performing them and the hypotheses being tested. Even when a standard protocol is recommended (as in the Collaborative Perinatal Project), different neurologic examiners will ascertain somewhat different incidences of disorders (Nichols and Chen, 1981).
7. Lack of direct testing of school skills may result in failure to diagnose specific cognitive deficits as the underlying cause of more pervasive, non-specific symptom complexes such as "attention deficit disorder" or "conduct disorder."
8. Most standardized psychometric tests—e.g., the WISC (Wechster, 1974), Stanford-Binet (Lewis and Merrill, 1973), and Slosson (Slosson, 1963)—depend heavily on verbal instructions. They cannot therefore differentiate between general decreased intellectual powers and a more specific deficit in language comprehension.

---

*Skipping requires a step on one foot, next a hop, landing on the first foot, then a step on the second foot, followed by a hop, landing on the second foot. If a child has no prior experience with skipping, he or she should be able to learn from one demonstration trial.

tremities, several tests are used. With all of them, observation of body parts not involved in the demanded action may yield information about synkinesis, particularly mirror movements. Resting tremor, intention tremor, titubation of the trunk or head, and other involuntary adventitious movements may also become apparent. To test the wrists, alternating taps of the palm and the dorsum of the hand on the knee should be done as rapidly as possible. Alternatively, the child may be given an object, such as a reflex hammer, to turn back and forth in a regular rhythmic fashion. The child may also be asked to pretend to screw a light bulb into a ceiling fixture. Movements are normally in rhythmic alternating fashion. With cerebellar disorders, however, they frequently assume an extremely erratic, nonrepetitive pattern. The heel-shin knee-ankle maneuver further tests coordination of the lower extremities.

The finger tapping task is often used as a measure of pyramidal tract function, and has the advantage of standardization as to rate expected at different ages and for both sexes (Denckla, 1973). During such unimanual distal movements it is valuable to have the other hand held in the air without support. One may then note whether associated mirror movements occur when the hand that is designated to be active is in fact carrying out the required action. Associated movements mirroring a variety of actions may occur in the hand not voluntarily engaged. Thus it is well to observe for them during the entire exam. Foot tapping can be done in the time-for-20 format described by Denckla (1974) and compared with standards. Hopping in place on either foot should be possible for any child over the age of 5 years.

Testing for developmental apraxia and clumsiness, a source of school and home failure that cannot be determined from paper and pencil tests, is very important in any child with school or attention difficulties. The tapping test just discussed is excellent to define clumsiness and accompanying adventitious movements, but does not suffice to demonstate apraxia. Apraxia (or dyspraxia) may be defined as the inability to carry out age-appropriate voluntary motor sequences in the absence of a primary motor or sensory deficit (David, 1981). It is only determined by direct testing during the neurologic exam. Copying hand postures (using for instance the Luria Fist Test), pantomiming acts (pouring milk into a glass), and using actual objects (putting a flashlight together and turning it on) are the three types of performance that should be covered in any complete examination for apraxia (Damasio et al., 1985). A standard manual apraxia battery is incorporated in the neurologic protocol in the appendix (items 115–148) (Deuel and Doar, 1990).

The upper extremity reflexes should be tested with the arms relaxed and in a symmetric position. Relaxation can sometimes be accomplished by asking complex questions of the patient as the respective tendons are tapped, or by reinforcement maneuvers. The Hoffman sign, otherwise called the Babinski of the upper extremity, should be attempted with a flick of the index fingernail. Examination of reflexes in the lower extremities may be done with the patient sitting and the legs in the symmetric dependent position, which is also advantageous for eliciting clonus. However, the deep tendon reflexes and clonus may also be checked in the supine position.

Sensation may be tested in 6- to 12-year-olds in the same manner as in adults. For a screening examination, light touch and position sense or light touch and vibration sense may be adequate. If there is any question of a spinal lesion, then examination of responses to thermal and pinprick stimuli becomes mandatory. Even in school-age children, it is wise to introduce the pin carefully before starting the exam, in which the entire dermatomal distribution should be tested, including the lower sacral segments. Stereognosis can be readily evaluated in this age group by using small common objects such as clips, safety pins, keys and coins. Graphesthesia (writing on the skin) may be evaluated. Normative data for graphesthesia of a relatively psychometric quality is given in the Halsted-Reitan battery (Russell et al., 1970, Chapter 2; Reitan, 1969), although the testing routine they recommend is quite lengthy. Bilateral simultaneous stimulation with fingers on the face, the hands, and the legs could be part of every screening examination. Finally, autonomic responses, vasomotor responses, and sweating should be noted.

In conclusion, the neurologic examination is a versatile diagnostic instrument. Using it, one should be reliably able to determine the maturational level of cognitive, emotional, and motor capacities as well as physical growth and development, and to detect localizing and lateralizing signs of nervous system abnormalities. Supplemented by a careful comprehensive history, the examination frequently yields all the basic information necessary to make a full diagnosis, not only of neurologic disease but also of neuropsychiatric and developmental disorders of higher cerebral function. To analyze quantitatively specific hearing and visual loss problems ascertained by the neurologic evaluation, or to evaluate nerve and muscle functions further, or developmental language disorders, dyslexia, dysgraphia, and dyscalculia, standardized tests may be helpful in amplifying the information yielded during the neurologic exam.

Appendix: Preschool and School-Age Pediatric and Neurologic Examination Scoring Form

This scoring form is useful as a reminder about the types of subtests entailed in an extensive physical and neurologic examination. Of course, as the neurologic exam is an "à la carte" rather than a "table d'hôte" menu, other individual items than those cataloged here may be substituted, and some listed items may be omitted. The suggested scoring is meant to facilitate computer entry. If an item is normal, the first box is checked. If an item is clearly abnormal, an 8 is circled, if it is not tested or questionable, a 9 is circled. Extra boxes are provided for concomitant observations on adventitious movements (AM,

see item P13), observed hand preference (first choice, see item N99; or hand used, see item N135), and quantitation (time in seconds, see item N101). For the dyspraxia items (N115–N149) there are three subscales, for use of actual objects (Object), imitation of nonsense gestures (Imitate), and pantomime (Pantomime). Of course, every time an abnormality is checked on the binary format, notes about its severity and quality should be made as usual. *Note:* This form may be reproduced for clinical use without further permission from the author or publisher.

PRESCHOOL AND SCHOOL-AGE PEDIATRIC AND NEUROLOGIC EXAM SCORING FORM

Items with an asterisk are inappropriate for the preschooler; items preceded with **PRE** are alternate versions for the preschooler.

S. Subject Identification

S1. Name _____ _____ _____
          Last   First   Middle

S2. Birthdate _____ _____ _____
              Month   Day   Year

S3. Age at examination _____

S4. Gender _____

S5. Handedness by subject report _____
                                          R-L-A

    a. Fork (R-L)
    b. Scissors (R-L)
    c. Other hand better at anything else? (Y-N)

E. Examiner Identification

E1. Examiner _____ _____ _____
              Last   First   Middle

E2. Title _____

E3. Place _____ _____
              Institution   Room Number

E4. Date _____ _____ _____
             Month   Day   Year

E5. Time exam started (0–24:0–60) _____

P. Pediatric Examination

P1. Weight _____ (kg) Percentile _____
P2. Height _____ (cm) Percentile _____
P3. OFC _____ (cm) Percentile _____
P4. Blood Pressure (right arm) ___ (S)/___ (D)

P5. Head shape and contour
    ☐ 8 9

P6. Hair
    ☐ 8 9

Preschool and School-age Pediatric and Neurologic Examination Scoring Form from David RB: *Pediatric Neurology for the Clinician.* Norwalk, Conn: Appleton & Lange, 1992.

SCHOOL-AGE SCORING FORM, page 2

P7. Facies
☐   8   9

P8. Eyes—structure (external exam): palpebral fissures, lids, cornea, sclera, conjunctiva, iris, pupils
☐   8   9

P9. Ears—size, shape, position
☐   8   9

P10. Ears—otoscopic exam
☐   8   9

P11. Nose: obstruction, mouth breathing
☐   8   9

P12. Lips—structure
Upper lip length
Lips meet when teeth in occlusion
☐   8   9

P13. Lips—function
Protrude (whistling position)
Retract ("Show me your teeth.")
☐   8   9   AM ☐

P14. Tongue—structure
Size in relation to dental arch
Fissures
Frenulum length
☐   8   9

P15. Tongue—function: curl up and down
☐   8   9   AM ☐

P16. Tongue—function: "Say *tsk tsk tsk tsk.*"
☐   8   9

P17. Hard palate: arch, width, integrity
☐   8   9

P18. Velopharyngeal port: soft palate and uvula structure
☐   8   9

P19. Dentition (include missing teeth in comments)
☐   8   9

P20. Articulator function: "Say *Pa-Ta-Ka.*"
☐   8   9
Time in seconds _____
PRE: "Say *Pa-Pa-Pa, Ta-Ta-Ta, Ka-Ka-Ka.*"

P21. Thyroid
☐   8   9

P22. Thoracic wall
☐   8   9

P23. Lungs
☐   8   9

P24. Heart size
☐   8   9

P25. Heart sounds
☐   8   9

P26. Heart rhythm
☐   8   9

P27. Heart rate
☐   8   9

P28. Radial, femoral and carotid pulses, bilaterally
☐   8   9

P29. Abdominal wall
☐   8   9

P30. Abdominal organs palpable
☐   8   9

P31. Abdominal masses
☐   8   9

P32. Genitalia
☐   8   9

P33. Tanner stage—pubic hair
☐   8   9
Stage number in arabic _____

P34. Tanner stage—breasts or penis
☐   8   9

P35. Lymph nodes
☐   8   9

P36. Skin vascular nevi
☐   8   9

P37. Skin pigmented or depigmented nevi
☐   8   9

P38. Skin—scars, eczema, vitigilous cyanosis
☐   8   9

P39. Spine and dimples, sinus, scoliosis, lordosis
☐   8   9

P40. Extremities—anatomy
☐   8   9

P41. Cooperation
☐   8   9

P42. Responsiveness to positive or negative reinforcement
☐   8   9

P43. Attention to commands
☐   8   9

P44. Attention shifts to external stimuli
☐   8   9

P45. Attention shifts or lapses without obvious external stimuli
☐   8   9

SCHOOL-AGE SCORING FORM, page 3

P46. Perseveration of attention in face of new command
☐   8   9

P47. Impulsiveness—sudden self-initiated talk or action
☐   8   9

P48. Impression of pediatric exam
☐   8   9

Neurologic Examination

N1. Alert—oriented (person and place)
☐   8   9

N2. Comprehends (number of fingers, age)
☐   8   9

*N3. Subject right hand identification ("Show me your right hand.")
☐   8   9

*N4. Subject left hand identification ("Show me your left hand.")
☐   8   9

*N5. One-part command ("Make a fist with your left hand.")
☐   8   9

*N6. Two-part command ("Cover your left eye with your right hand.")
☐   8   9

*N7. Three-part command ("Put your left thumb on your right ear and stick out your tongue.")
☐   8   9

*N8. Examiner left hand identification ("Point to my left hand.")
☐   8   9

N9. Finger identification—eyes open
☐   8   9

N10. Finger identification—eyes closed
☐   8   9

N11. Confrontation fields—right eye covered by card
☐   8   9

N12. Confrontation fields—left eye covered
☐   8   9

N13. Confrontation fields—bilateral simultaneous stimulation, upper and lower quadrants
☐   8   9

N14. Visual acuity—right eye without glasses to Snellen chart at 20 ft
☐   8   9

N15. Visual acuity—right eye with glasses to Snellen chart at 20 ft
☐   8   9

N16. Visual acuity—left eye without glasses to Snellen chart at 20 ft
☐   8   9

N17. Visual acuity—left eye with glasses to Snellen chart at 20 ft
☐   8   9

N18. Visual acuity—binocular vision to near card without glasses
☐   8   9

N19. Visual acuity—binocular vision to near card with glasses
☐   8   9

N20. Position of eyes in forward fixation (4 ft) without glasses
☐   8   9

N21. Cover test right eye (if *glasses*, use)
☐   8   9

N22. Cover test left eye (if *glasses*, use)
☐   8   9

N23. Extraocular muscles (right eye)
☐   8   9

Extraocular muscles (left eye)
☐   8   9

N24. Conjugate gaze—follow
☐   8   9

N25. Conjugate gaze—command
☐   8   9

N26. Pupils—symmetry
☐   8   9

N27. Pupil
Right eye react to direct light
Left eye consensual
☐   8   9

N28. Pupil
Left eye react to direct light
Right eye consensual
☐   8   9

N29. Conjugate gaze—converge
☐   8   9

N30. Pupils—accommodation
☐   8   9

SCHOOL-AGE SCORING FORM, page 4

N31. Nystagmus
☐   8   9

O **N32.** Funduscopy—right eye macula
☐   8   9

O **N33.** Funduscopy—right eye disk
☐   8   9

O **N34.** Funduscopy—right eye retina
☐   8   9

O **N35.** Funduscopy—left eye macula
☐   8   9

O **N36.** Funduscopy—left eye disk
☐   8   9

O **N37.** Funduscopy—left eye retina
☐   8   9

N38. Facial sensation (cotton swab)—right V
☐   8   9

N39. Facial sensation (cotton swab)—left V
☐   8   9

N40. Jaw open, close—right V
Versus resistance
☐   8   9

N41. Jaw open, close—left V
Versus resistance
☐   8   9

*****N42.** Jaw move left and right
☐   8   9

N43. Jaw jerk
☐   8   9

N44. Upper facial symmetry—VII
☐   8   9

N45. Lower facial symmetry—VII
☐   8   9

N46. "Open your eyes wide."
☐   8   9

N47. Finger rustle, right ear—VIII
☐   8   9

N48. Finger rustle, left ear—VIII
☐   8   9

N49. Palate elevation—IX, X (voluntary)
☐   8   9

N50. Gag reflex—right IX, X
☐   8   9

N51. Gag reflex—left IX, X
☐   8   9

N52. Sternocleidomastoid—right XI
☐   8   9

N53. Sternocleidomastoid—left XI
☐   8   9

N54. Tongue protrusion—XII
☐   8   9

N55. Tongue (left and right) lateral
movements—XII
☐   8   9

N56. Neck and trunk musculoskeletal anatomy
(scoliosis, torticollis)
☐   8   9

N57. Shoulder girdle musculoskeletal anatomy
A
☐   8   9

N58. Pelvic girdle musculoskeletal anatomy
A
☐   8   9

N59. Sitting posture
☐   8   9

N60. Muscle power neck flexion
☐ 0-5   8   9

N61. Muscle power neck exension
☐ 0-5   8   9

N62. Muscle power, deltoid—right
☐ 0-5   8   9

N63. Muscle power, deltoid—left
☐ 0-5   8   9

N64. Muscle power, biceps—right
☐ 0-5   8   9

N65. Muscle power, biceps—left
☐ 0-5   8   9

N66. Muscle power, wrist dorsi—right
☐ 0-5   8   9

N67. Muscle power, wrist dorsi—left
☐ 0-5   8   9

N68. Muscle power, finger extension—right
☐ 0-5   8   9

N69. Muscle power finger extension—left
☐ 0-5   8   9

N70. Muscle power, finger abduction—right
☐ 0-5   8   9

N71. Muscle power, finger abduction—left
☐ 0-5   8   9

N72. Muscle power, thumb-five oppose—right
☐ 0-5   8   9

N73. Muscle power, thumb-five oppose—left
☐ 0-5   8   9

SCHOOL-AGE SCORING FORM, page 5

N74. Muscle power, hip flexion—right
☐ 0–5   8   9

N75. Muscle power, hip flexion—left
☐ 0–5   8   9

N76. Muscle power, hip abduction—right
☐ 0–5   8   9

N77. Muscle power, hip abduction—left
☐ 0–5   8   9

N78. Muscle power, leg flexion—right
☐ 0–5   8   9

N79. Muscle power, leg flexion—left
☐ 0–5   8   9

N80. Muscle power, foot dorsiflexion—right
☐ 0–5   8   9

N81. Muscle power, foot dorsiflexion—left
☐ 0–5   8   9

N82. Muscle power, great toe dorsiflexion—right
☐ 0–5   8   9   AM ☐

N83. Muscle power, great toe dorsiflexion—left
☐ 0–5   8   9   AM ☐

N84. Muscle tone, upper extremities
☐ 0–5   8   9

N85. Muscle tone, lower extremities
☐ 0–5   8   9

N86. Gait (running in hall: 20 ft away, 20 ft toward)—speed, foot placement
☐ 0–5   8   9

N87. Gait (running in hall: 20 ft away, 20 ft toward)—hand and arm movement
☐   8   9

N88. Gait (walking in hall: 20 ft away, 20 ft toward)—foot placement, posture
☐   8   9

N89. Gait (walking in hall: 20 ft away, 20 ft toward)—hand and arm movement
☐   8   9

*N90. Skip eight paces in hall on command
☐   8   9

N91. Tandem ten paces—coordination (balance, foot placement)
☐   8   9
PRE: Tandem a few paces

N92. Tandem ten paces—adventitious movements (hand, arm, and face movement)
☐   8   9

*N93. Fog gait—feet *in*verted, five paces (adventitious hand, arm, and face movement)
☐   8   9

*N94. Fog gait—feet everted, five paces (adventitious hand, arm, and face movement)
☐   8   9

N95. Toe gait, five paces
☐   8   9   AM ☐

N96. Heel gait, five paces
☐   8   9   AM ☐

N97. Pronator drift (standing unsupported 20 seconds, eyes closed, arms extended, palms up)
☐   8   9

N98. Choreaform twitch (standing unsupported 20 seconds, eyes closed, arms extended, fingers extended and abducted, palms down)
☐   8   9

N99. Coordination (eyes open, standing unsupported)
Subject finger to examiner finger to subject nose—right hand
2 × 3 positions: left, center, right, arm full extension
☐   8   9   First choice _____

N100. Coordination (eyes open, standing unsupported)
Subject finger to examiner finger to subject nose—left hand
2 × 3 positions: left, center, right, arm full extension
☐   8   9   First choice _____

*N101. Coordination (sitting, alternating wrist supination, pronation): time for 20—right (reflex hammer in cross-palm grasp in tested hand, both arms adducted to waist, flexed at elbows)
☐   8   9   First choice _____ AM ☐
Time in seconds _____

*N102. Coordination (sitting, alternating wrist supination, pronation): time for 20—left (reflex hammer in cross-palm grasp in tested hand, both arms adducted to waist, flexed at elbows)
☐   8   9   First choice _____ AM ☐
Time in seconds _____

N103. Coordination (supination and pronation of wrist): time for 20—right
☐   8   9   First choice _____ AM ☐
Time in seconds _____

N104. Coordination (supination and pronation of wrist): time for 20—left
☐   8   9   First choice _____ AM ☐
Time in seconds _____

SCHOOL-AGE SCORING FORM, page 6

N105. Finger tap on thumb, time for 20—right (Denckla instructions)
☐ 8 9 First choice _____ AM ☐
Time in seconds _____

N106. Finger tap on thumb, time for 20—left (Denckla instructions)
☐ 8 9 First choice _____ AM ☐
Time in seconds _____

N107. Finger on successive fingers—left (Denckla instructions)
☐ 8 9 First choice _____ AM ☐
Time in seconds _____

N108. Thumb on successive fingers—left (Denckla instructions)
☐ 8 9 First choice _____ AM ☐
Time in seconds _____

N109. Hop in place, five times—right
☐ 8 9 First choice _____

N110. Hop in place, five times—left
☐ 8 9 First choice _____
Time in seconds _____

*N111. Foot tap—right (Denckla instructions)
☐ 8 9 First choice _____ AM ☐
Time in seconds _____

*N112. Foot tap—left (Denckla instructions)
☐ 8 9 First choice _____ AM ☐
Time in seconds _____

N113. Heel-shin, knee-ankle—right (subject lying down)
☐ 8 9

N114. Heel-shin, knee-ankle—left (subject lying down)
☐ 8 9

N115. Object—hand throw, Nerf ball, 3 ft—right
☐ 8 9 First choice _____

N116. Object—hand throw, Nerf ball, 3 ft—left
☐ 8 9 First choice _____

N117. Object—one-foot kick, Nerf ball, 3 ft—right
☐ 8 9 First choice _____

N118. Object—one-foot kick, Nerf ball, 3 ft—left
☐ 8 9 First choice _____

*N119. Object—"Erase this *E*."
☐ 8 9 Hand _____

*N120. Object—Wind the watch three times.
☐ 8 9 Hand that winds _____

N121. Imitate—two hands open, palms toward subject
☐ 8 9

PRE: Imitate—left, then right, hand up, fingers spread

N122. Imitate—left hand open, palm toward subject, right hand fisted
☐ 8 9

PRE: Imitate—left, then right, hand index finger up

*N123. Imitate—thumbs touch and index fingers touch (diamond shape)
☐ 8 9

*N124. Imitate—thumb touching index finger of other hand, palms toward subject
☐ 8 9

*N125. Imitate—thumbs and index fingers form interlocking circles
☐ 8 9

*N126. Imitate—right hand fisted, palm toward subject, with index and little fingers raised. Expect nonmirror response (child must use his or her right hand)
☐ 8 9

*N127. Imitate—begin in N113 position and climb up five times ("itsy-bitsy spider")
☐ 8 9

*N128. Imitate—Luria's fist test, one time quickly, right hand only ("Watch me. I'm going to show you what to do. I will do it only one time so look closely.")
1. Fist down on lap
2. Hand open, hit radial border of hand on lap
3. Fisted hand again, *palm side up* on lap
☐ 8 9

*N129. Imitate—Luria's fist test, one time quickly, left hand only ("Watch me. I'm going to show you what to do. I will do it only one time so look closely.")
1. Fist down on lap
2. Hand open, hit radial border of hand on lap
3. Fisted hand again, *palm side up* in lap
☐ 8 9

N130. Pantomime—"If this is a birthday cake, show me how to blow out the candles."
☐ 8 9

*N131. Pantomime—"Now, if this is a knife, show me how you would cut a piece of the cake."
☐ 8 9
Hand (if *single hand* used) _____

SCHOOL-AGE SCORING FORM, page 7

O **N132.** Pantomime—"Show me how you light a match."
☐   8   9
Hand that strikes _____

O **N133.** Pantomime—"Stand up and show me how you swing a baseball bat."
☐   8   9
Hand on top _____

N134. Pantomime—"Here is a book. Show me how you turn the pages."
☐   8   9
Hand that turns _____

N135. Pantomime—"If this is a comb, show me how you would use it to comb your hair."
☐   8   9
Hand used _____

N136. Pantomime—"Show me how you pour milk into a glass."
☐   8   9
Hand that pours _____

N137. Pantomime—"Show me how you would brush your teeth with a toothbrush."
☐   8   9
Hand holding toothbrush _____

*__N138.__ Pantomime—"Show me how you would open a locked door with a key."
☐   8   9
Hand holding key _____

N139. Object—Draw a square (8½ × 11 clean white paper, normal finish, #2 sharp pencil)
☐   8   9   Hand _____

N140. Object—Draw a triangle (8½ × 11 clean white paper, normal finish, #2 sharp pencil)
☐   8   9   Hand _____

N141. Object—Draw a rectangle (8½ × 11 clean white paper, normal finish, #2 sharp pencil)
☐   8   9   Hand _____
Pre: Object—draw a circle

*__N142.__ Object—"Please draw a clock with an hour hand and a minute hand." (8½ × 11 clean white paper, normal finish, #2 sharp pencil)
☐   8   9   Hand _____

*__N143.__ Copy the box
☐   8   9   Hand _____

N144. Object—Hand preference ("Write your first and last names.")
☐   8   9
Hand for pencil _____
PRE: "Write your first name."

*__N145.__ Object—"Now write it with the other hand."
☐   8   9

*__N146.__ Object—"Fold the paper neatly so it fits and put it into the envelope."
☐   8   9
Hand that puts paper in _____

*__N147.__ Object—"Put the batteries into the flashlight and turn it on."
☐   8   9
Hand that exerts torque _____

*__N148.__ Object—"Roll up the paper and then use it like a telescope to look at the doorknob."
☐   8   9   Eye _____

*__N149.__ Object—"Roll up the paper and then use it like a telescope to look at something in a different direction than the doorknob."
☐   8   9   Eye _____

N150. Romberg position, eyes open
☐   8   9

N151. Romberg position, eyes closed
☐   8   9

N152. Tremor, action—right hand
☐   8   9

N153. Tremor, action—left hand
☐   8   9

N154. Tremor, rest—right hand
☐   8   9

N155. Tremor, rest—left hand
☐   8   9

N156. Tremor, intention—right hand
☐   8   9

N157. Tremor, intention—left hand
☐   8   9

N158. Titubation
☐   8   9

N159. Reflex, biceps—right
☐   8   9

N160. Reflex, biceps—left
☐   8   9

N161. Reflex, triceps—right
☐   8   9

N162. Reflex, triceps—left
☐   8   9

SCHOOL-AGE SCORING FORM, page 8

N163. Reflex, knee—right
☐   8   9

N164. Reflex, knee—left
☐   8   9

N165. Reflex, ankle—right
☐   8   9

N166. Reflex, ankle—left
☐   8   9

N167. Reflex, clonus, sustained (6+ beats)—right ankle
☐   8   9

N168. Reflex, clonus, sustained (6+ beats)—left ankle
☐   8   9

N169. Reflex, plantar—right
☐   8   9

N170. Reflex, plantar—left
☐   8   9

N171. Sensation (touch recognition), C4—right (cotton swab, eyes closed)
☐   8   9

N172. Sensation (touch recognition), C4—left (cotton swab, eyes closed)
☐   8   9

N173. Sensation (touch recognition), C7—right (cotton swab, eyes closed)
☐   8   9

N174. Sensation (touch recognition), C7—left (cotton swab, eyes closed)
☐   8   9

N175. Sensation (touch recognition), T1—right (cotton swab, eyes closed)
☐   8   9

N176. Sensation (touch recognition), T1—left (cotton swab, eyes closed)
☐   8   9

N177. Sensation (touch recognition), L2—right (cotton swab, eyes closed)
☐   8   9

N178. Sensation (touch recognition), L2—left (cotton swab, eyes closed)
☐   8   9

N179. Sensation (touch recognition), L4—right (cotton swab, eyes closed)
☐   8   9

N180. Sensation (touch recognition), L4—left (cotton swab, eyes closed)
☐   8   9

N181. Sensation (touch recognition), S1—right (cotton swab, eyes closed)
☐   8   9

N182. Sensation (touch recognition), S1—left (cotton swab, eyes closed)
☐   8   9

N183. Sensation, position, right great toe (5+ trials)
☐   8   9

N184. Sensation, right index finger
☐   8   9

N185. Sensation, position, left great toe (5 trials)
☐   8   9

N186. Sensation, left index finger
☐   8   9

N187. Sensation, location of fingertip in space—right
☐   8   9

N188. Sensation, location of fingertip in space—left
☐   8   9

N189. Sensation, stereognosis (fine)—right (6 trials)
☐   8   9
PRE: Use 4 matching block shapes

N190. Sensation, stereognosis (fine)—left (6 trials)
☐   8   9
PRE: Use 4 matching block shapes

N191. Sensations graphesthesia (fingertip writing)—right
☐   8   9
PRE: Pick from drawn square, circle, cross

N192. Sensation, graphesthesia (fingertip writing)—left
☐   8   9
PRE: Pick from drawn square, circle, cross

N193. Autonomic—vasomotor
☐   8   9

N194. Autonomic—sweating
☐   8   9

N195. Time exam ended (0–24:0–60)

I. Impression

I1. Neurologic impression
☐   8   9

I2. Mental status—mood and affect throughout pediatric and neurologic exams
☐   8   9

I3. Estimated intellectual status
☐   8   9

ANNOTATED BIBLIOGRAPHY

Dodge PR, Volpe JJ: Neurologic history and examination, in Farmer TW (ed): *Pediatric Neurology*, 3rd ed. Philadelphia, Harper & Row, 1983, p 1–41.

This chapter is very succinctly written and very well illustrated. In addition, it explains how to take a good history and provides excellent advice on how to engage the patient's interest and cooperation. It contains good detail concerning examination of the cranial nerves and gives various "tricks of the trade" for eliciting valid sensory response.

Spriesterbach D, Morris HL, Darley FL: Examination of the speech mechanisms, in Darley FL, Spriesterbach D (eds): *Diagnostic Methods in Speech Pathology*, 2nd ed. New York, Harper & Row, 1978, p 215–231.

This chapter describes methods of examining speech mechanisms that are practical and often not covered by the medical school physical examination course. Examination of the speech mechanism is highly important in any school-age child suspected of having a language disorder, but is often omitted for lack of familiarity with the proper method.

Lewis TM, Merrill MA: *Stanford-Binet Intelligence Scale: Manual for the Third Revision, 1972 Norms Edition*. Boston, Houghton Mifflin, 1973.

The WISC-R is an individually administered, well-standardized test that breaks down cognitive function into "verbal" and "performance" scales. Although these scales (and the individual subtests that compose them) are useful, it is highly important to bear in mind that the WISC-R (as well as most other standard individual IQ tests) exclusively uses verbal communication for instruction and communication with the child. Thus, a child with a language disorder will likely have a depressed performance as well as verbal score. Recourse to nonverbal instruments may then be in order.

Slosson R: *Slosson Intelligence Test (SIT) for Children and Adults, 1963 Edition*. East Aurora, NY, Slosson Educational Publications, 1963.

The Slosson is a quick-screening IQ test that, with proper precautions against testing artifacts, can be very useful to the neurologic examiner. However, like all such screening tests, particularly if it provides an abormal estimate, it should be checked by the more reliable (and complex, requiring a person fully trained in its administration) WISC-R or Stanford-Binet.

REFERENCES

Barlow C: "Soft signs" in children with learning disorders. *Am J Dis Child* 128:605–606, 1974.

Berg B: Unusual neurocutaneous syndromes. *Neurol Clin North Am* 3:165–178, 1985.

Beumer J, Trowbridge HO, Silverman S Jr, Eisenberg EJ: Childhood hypophosphatasia and the premature loss of teeth: A clinical and laboratory study of seven cases. *Oral Med Oral Pathol* 35:631, 1973.

Brindley GS: Cortical blindness and the functions of non-geniculate fibers of the optic tracts. *J Neurol Neurosurg Psychiatr* 32:259–264, 1969.

Bryden M: Measuring handedness with questionnaires. *Neuropsychologia* 15:617–624, 1977.

Cogan DG: *Neurology of the Ocular Muscles*, 2nd ed, Springfield, Ill, Charles C Thomas, 1956.

Coplen J: Deafness: Ever heard of it? Delayed recognition of permanent hearing loss. *Pediatrics* 79:206–213, 1987.

Damasio A, Geschwind N, Klawans HL: Anatomic localization in clinical neuropsychology, in Vinken PU, Bruyn GW (eds): *Clinical Neuropsychology*. Handbook of Neurology, Vol 1(45). Amsterdam, Elsevier/North-Holland, 1985, p 7–22.

David R: *Nosology of Disorders of Higher Cerebral Function in Childhood*. Child Neurology Society, 1981.

DeJong R, Magee KR (eds): *The Neurologic Examination*, 4th ed. Hagerstown, Md, Harper & Row, 1979.

Denckla MB: Development of speed in repetitive and successive finger movements in normal children. *Dev Med Child Neurol* 15:635–645, 1973.

Denckla MB: Development of motor coordination in normal children. *Dev Med Child Neurol* 16:729–741, 1974.

Deuel RK, Doar BP: Testing manual praxis in school-aged children. *Ann Neurol* 28:425, 1990.

Deuel RK, Moran CC: Cerebral dominance and cerebral asymmetries on computed tomogram in childhood. *Neurology* 30:934–938, 1980.

Dodge PR, Volpe JJ: Neurologic history and examination, in Farmer TW (ed): *Pediatric Neurology*, 3rd ed. Philadelphia.

Fog E, Fog M: Cerebral inhibition examined by associated movements, in Bax M, MacKeith R (eds): *Clinics in Developmental Medicine*. London, Heineman, 1963, p 35–47.

Grossman H, Dorst J: The mucopolysaccharidoses, in Kaufman H (ed): *Progress in Pediatric Radiology*, Vol 4. Chicago, Year Book, 1973, p 495–544.

Lewis TM, Merrill MA: *Stanford-Binet Intelligence Scale: Manual for the Third Revision, 1972 Norms Edition*. Boston, Houghton Mifflin, 1973.

Meyerson M, Frank R: Language, speech and hearing in Williams syndrome. *Dev Med Child Neurol* 29:258–262, 1987.

Nellhaus G: Head circumference from birth to eighteen years. Practical composite international and interracial graphs. *Pediatrics* 41:106–114, 1968.

Nichols PL, Chen TC: *Minimal Brain Dysfunction: A Prospective Study*. Hillsdale, NJ, Lawrence Erlbaum, 1981.

Pagon R: Williams syndrome: Features in late childhood and adolescence. *Pediatrics* 80:85–91, 1987.

Pennington B, Puck M, Robinson A: Language and cognitive development in 47 XXX females followed since birth. *Behav Genet* 10:31, 1980.

Provins K, Cunliffe P: The reliability of some motor performance tests of handedness. *Neuropsychologia* 10:199–206, 1972.

Pryor HB: Objective measurement of interpupillary distance. *Pediatrics* 44:973–977, 1969.

Ratcliffe SG: Speech and learning disorders in children with sex chromosome abnormalities. *Dev Med Child Neurol* 24:80–84, 1982.

Reitan R: Manual for administration of Neuropsychological Test Batteries for Adults and Children. Tucson, Ariz, Neuropsychology Laboratory, 1969.

Rowe PC (ed): *The Harriet Lane Handbook*. Chicago, Year Book, 1987, p 109–110.

Russell E, Neuringer C, Goldstein K: *Assessment of Brain Damage.* John Wiley & Sons, New York, 1970.

Schimke R, McKusick VA, Huang T, Pollack AD: Homocysteinuria: Studies of 20 families with 38 affected members. *JAMA* 193:711–716, 1965.

Slosson R: *Slosson Intelligence Test (SIT) for Children and Adults, 1963 Edition.* East Aurora, NY, Slosson Educational Publications, 1963.

Spriesterbach DC, Morris HL, Darley FL: Examination of the speech mechanisms, in Darley FL, Spriesterbach DC (eds): *Diagnostic Methods in Speech Pathology,* 2nd ed. New York, Harper & Row, 1978, p 215–231.

Steinback H, Rudle U, Jonsson M, Young DA: Evaluation of skeletal lesions in pseudohypoparathyroidism. *Radiology* 85:670–677, 1965.

Tanner JM: *Growth at Adolescence,* 2nd ed. Oxford, Blackwell Scientific, 1962.

Taylor A, Handew DG, Arlett CF, et al: Ataxia telangectasia: A human mutation with abnormal radiation sensitivity. *Nature* 258:427–429, 1975.

Taylor E: Psychological Appraisal of Children with Cerebral Defects. Cambridge, Mass. Harvard University Press, 1959.

Thompson HS: Perimetry in neurophthalmology, in Frisen L (ed): *Topics in Neurophthalmology.* Baltimore, Md, Williams & Wilkins, 1979, p 3–90.

Traquiar, H: *An Introduction to Clinical Perimetry,* 6th ed. London, Kimpton, 1949.

Waber DP: Neuropsychological aspects of Turner's syndrome. *Dev Med Child Neurol* 21:58–70, 1979.

Weschsler D: *Weschsler Intelligence Scale for Children—Revised (WISC-R).* New York, Psychological Corporation, 1974.

Witelson S: Hemispheric specialization for linguistic and non-linguistic tactual perception using a dichotomous stimulation technique. *Cortex* 10:3–17, 1978.

Neurodiagnostic Laboratory Procedures

The Electroencephalogram
Warren T. Blume

THE NORMAL EEG

To read properly the electroencephalogam (EEG) of a child or adolescent, one must be aware of several aspects that distinguish it from that of an adult. Many of its features are age dependent and a brief review of these follows. Infants and young children often fall asleep during the recording and the consequent EEG changes are more marked than those found in older age groups. Maturational and state factors create a wider variety of waveforms than are usually found among adults; such multiple waveforms become superimposed to create sharply contoured waves that can be mistaken for spikes. These factors of maturation and state also create wider fluctuations of EEG among normal children, a factor that commonly leads to over-reading of the recording. Mild abnormalities therefore are often beyond the precision of this discipline. Finally, interhemispheric asymmetries of normally appearing features occur commonly in youth, including alpha activity, mu rhythm, and the so-called "posterior slow of youth."

The sometimes bewildering array of features can be simplified by asking four questions for each state of alertness in determining whether or not a recording is normal:

1. Is the background activity appropriate for age?
2. Are there any asymmetries, beyond those normally accepted for certain waveforms, that cannot be ascribed to artifact?
3. Are there any definite spikes?
4. Is there any focal or diffuse excessive delta activity?

Maturation Milestones

Wakefulness

The first discernible background frequency is 3 to 4 Hz, which appears at age 3 months. This increases to about 5 Hz at age 5 months, to 6 to 7 Hz at 12 months, and to 7 to 8 Hz at 2 years, and by 6 years stabilizes at about a 9-Hz rhythm (Figure 5-1). The mean frequency at 15 years is about 10 Hz. Alpha amplitude varies from 30 to 100 μV in the first year of life; it may increase to a maximum at 6 to 9 years and then decline. Passive eye closure can be helpful in eliciting background frequencies. An asymmetry of alpha is commonly seen in pediatric EEG; it is usually higher on the right, but a higher left amplitude is not clearly an abnormality. Asymmetries of amplitude are more accepted than asymmetries of frequency and a left-to-right frequency difference exceeding 1 Hz usually indicates an abnormality on the slower side.

The rhythmic background activity in youth is commonly interrupted by 250- to 500-ms waves occurring singly or repeating at 2 to 4 Hz and having an amplitude equal to or slightly greater than that of the background rhythms (Figure 5-2). Combination of such waveforms with alpha creates sharply contoured spike-like deflections in the occipital regions, which are not as sharp as occipital spikes. Such slow activity posteriorly blocks with eye opening and generally waxes and wanes with the alpha. The quantity and amplitude of such activity gradually increase in the first decade of life, reaching an apex in early adolescence. As with the background activity, the abundance of such "posterior slow of youth" can be considerably greater in the right hemisphere as compared to the left. Such activity can be rhythmic at about 3 to 4 Hz and may appear in prolonged runs. In

AWAKE   I yr

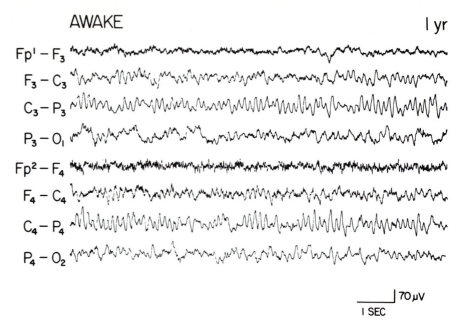

Figure 5-1. Rich mixture of waveforms in an alert infant. This tracing is dominated by 7- to 8-Hz central-parietal activity, but 1- to 2-Hz diffuse activity is also evident. The slightly greater quantity of delta on one side (*left*) is insignificant at this age. None of the apiculate waves is a spike. Normal recording.

addition to an intermittent and rhythmic form, a halving of the alpha frequency occurs on occasion in children, usually with drowsiness.

All such potentials are present with the eyes closed. In contrast, lambda waves may be particularly prominent as primarily electropositive, sharply contoured waves seen over the occipital head regions with the eyes open and particularly during scanning eye movements. Asymmetry of lambda waves is not an abnormality.

Theta (4 to 7 Hz) activity is present in varying amounts in the EEGs of pediatric patients. Its quantity relative to those of other waveforms increases considerably in the first years of life to reach a peak at age 5 to 6 years and then declines somewhat thereafter. Therefore, with the eyes closed or open, theta is the dominant dif-

fuse activity in recordings in the 2- to 5-year age group. With eyes closed, its quantity equals that of alpha activity at age 5 to 6 years, after which the alpha becomes the more prominent. As with adults, theta tends to predominate over the left hemisphere at most ages. It would be very difficult to interpret a pediatric recording as containing excess theta activity, given its normal predominance.

Delta (1 to 3 Hz) and theta are approximately equal in quantity during the first year of life. Although the absolute quantity of delta increases during the first year and continues to do so to the fifth year, proportionally it declines in relation to theta. However, low-voltage delta persists into adolescence in steadily declining quantities. Delta is never normally accentuated in drowsiness.

AWAKE   8 yrs

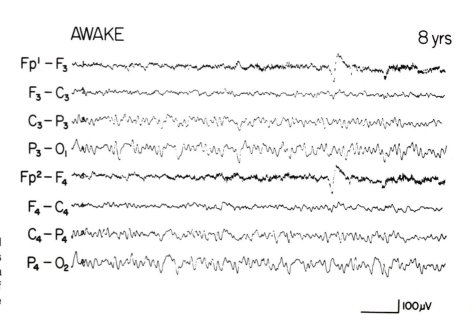

Figure 5-2. Electropositive occipital waves of 200 to 250 milliseconds separate the sharply contoured alpha to constitute the "posterior slow of youth," which can normally be quite abundant, as in this example.

Persistent background activity develops earlier in the central (Rolandic) head regions than in any other area. A 6- to 7-Hz rhythm may appear before 3 months of age and its frequency gradually increases to 8 to 10 Hz after 3 months. In the 1- to 5-year age group, the most prominent awake activity with eyes open resides in the central region. Asymmetries of such activity appear commonly and usually shift back and forth. A persistent central rhythm asymmetry usually suggests an abnormality on the lower side unless there is some defect in the skull. As such central rhythms combine with other rhythms, a sharply contoured appearance may result and this should be taken into account in identifying any central morphology as an epileptiform spike.

The main purpose of hyperventilation in children's recordings is to elicit spike wave discharges if they are not present during the resting recording. Regional spikes or excess slow waves are less commonly revealed than in adults. The accentuation of 2- to 3-Hz waves with hyperventilation is usually more marked in children than in adults, particularly around ages 10 to 12 years. Their location is often initially posterior in the early phases of hyperventilation, before becoming anterior.

Drowsiness

As the EEG signs of drowsiness appear commonly before the child looks drowsy, misinterpretations of excessive slow activity can be made. Sinusoidal theta is the most common drowsy pattern in children from ages 3 months to about 5 years. Its frequency is 3 to 5 Hz in the first year of life, increasing gradually to 4 to 6 Hz by age 4 years and then declining thereafter.

Prominent generalized bisynchronous bursts of 2- to 5-HZ rhythmic activity occasionally attaining 350 μV or more can be seen over the frontal and central regions in drowsiness from age 14 months to about 10 years (Figure 5–3). They are most common at ages 3 to 5 years. Such bursts are commonly mistaken for abnormalities and if there are sharply contoured waves intermingled they can be falsely identified as spike-waves. Such bursts disappear in moderate sleep, unlike spike-waves. From ages 6 to 16 years, rhythmic 5- to 7-Hz waves, maximum anteriorly, can accompany drowsiness. Beta activity at 20 to 25 Hz becomes more prominent in drowsiness and light sleep, and may be distributed diffusely with a maximum anteriorly.

Alpha activity classically disappears in moderate drowsiness, but the aforementioned phenomena may appear before alpha wanes.

In some children, the transition from wakefulness to sleep resembles an adult's pattern, without the aforementioned features.

Sleep

Rudimentary vertex (V) waves appear in light sleep as early as 3 to 4 months of age and become well developed by age 5 months. They achieve maximum expression as high-voltage sharply contoured monophasic or diphasic electronegative or electropositive waves at age 3 to 4 years and may be mistaken for Rolandic spikes (Figure 5–4). On bipolar montages, their amplitude may be quite asymmetrical, but such asymmetries should shift from side to side. When in doubt, use a referential montage to assess the symmetries of such V waves.

Spindles appear first at age 3 to 4 months and are almost invariably present during ages 3 to 9 months if adequate quantity and different levels of sleep are attained. Occasionally, a child of this age may descend too rapidly to very deep sleep and omit the spindle phase. Spindles may shift in prominence from side to side but the overall quantity should be approximately equal in the two hemispheres. Spindles are often at a maximum in the

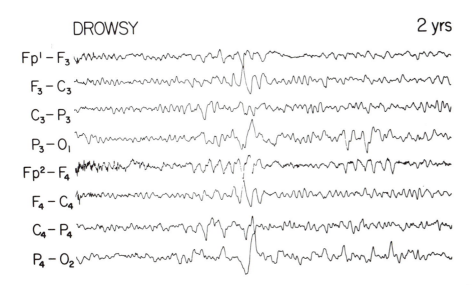

DROWSY   2 yrs

$Fp^1 - F_3$
$F_3 - C_3$
$C_3 - P_3$
$P_3 - O_1$
$Fp^2 - F_4$
$F_4 - C_4$
$C_4 - P_4$
$P_4 - O_2$

150 μV
1 SEC

Figure 5-3. Bursts of theta and delta in drowsiness, a normal phenomenon.

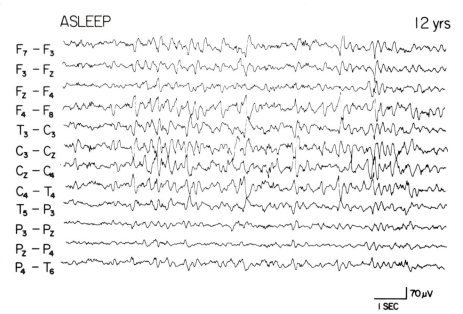

ASLEEP   12 yrs

$F_7 - F_3$
$F_3 - F_z$
$F_z - F_4$
$F_4 - F_8$
$T_3 - C_3$
$C_3 - C_z$
$C_z - C_4$
$C_4 - T_4$
$T_5 - P_3$
$P_3 - P_z$
$P_z - P_4$
$P_4 - T_6$

70 µV
1 SEC

Figure 5–4. Very apiculate V waves of varying morphology may appear in sequences, particularly in youth. Note their central-frontal (C_z-F_z) maxima.

central and parietal regions in youth. After infancy, almost all recorded sleep is non-REM. Therefore, the features previously discussed describe this phase.

Delta (1 to 3 Hz) activity is invariably present in non-REM sleep. In children it should be accentuated posteriorly, a feature best illustrated by bipolar anterior-posterior montages or ipsilateral ear references. Such posterior delta activity may be sharply contoured, and great caution should be exercised before identifying posteriorly situated waves as epileptiform sharp waves in sleep.

Arousal

In infants below 2 months of age, arousal consists of a decrease in the voltage of ongoing activity. At age 3 months, a diphasic slow wave may occur in response to

an afferent stimulus. This phenomenon, initially resembling a V wave, becomes better developed by 5 months, when it merges with a series of delta waves. If further arousal occurs, 4- to 8-Hz rhythmic theta lasting 1 to 5 seconds or longer may appear in children ages 7 months to 4 years. Following this theta with continuing arousal is, paradoxically, 1- to 3-Hz diffuse delta; this appears first at age 2 to 3 months, becomes maximally expressed at ages 12 to 18 months, and declines after age 5 years.

EEG AND EPILEPSY

Introduction

With access to a vast array of laboratory tests, the physician can easily forget that epilepsy is, and always will be, a clinical diagnosis—a differential diagnosis based on a painstaking history and physical examination. In many instances, these effective, safe, and relatively inexpensive diagnostic procedures (history and physical) will leave no unsolved questions. At other times, they will focus the attention on several questions to be addressed by the EEG, thus maximizing its clinical value: Is there a seizure disorder? Is it partial or generalized? If partial, is it unifocal (where?) or multifocal? How bad is the seizure disorder? Can one omit anticonvulsants after a seizure-free period?

To answer such questions with confidence, a recording of high technical quality is required. It must be interpreted by a physician knowledgeable in pediatric EEG.

Interictal EEG

Just as it is unusual for a patient to have an epileptic seizure in front of the physician, a clinical seizure occurs

---

Pearls and Perils: The Normal EEG

1. Maturation criteria must be considered when reading a child's EEG.
2. The modifications of the EEG with drowsiness are considerably greater for children than for adults and such modifications are age related.
3. Because of the rich mixture of waveforms in pediatric EEGs, sharply contoured waves appear commonly and these should not be interpreted as spikes.
4. A wide variety of normal findings exists in children's EEGs. Therefore, great caution should be exerted before stating that a mild abnormality exists.
5. When assessing the frequency of background activity, make sure the child is not drowsy, as this will slow the rate.

only rarely in routine EEG, with the exception of absence attacks with 3/s spike-waves. Therefore, interictal abnormalities, particularly spikes, are in practice the chief correlate of the epileptic condition that can help to answer the questions posed previously.

Of 242 children with spike foci, 82% were found by Trojaborg (1968) to have epilepsy, whereas Eeg-Olofsson et al. (1971) found epileptiform activity in only 1.9% of their 743 normal children. Thus, a reasonable correlation between epileptiform activity in the resting EEG and seizure disorders exists in children.

However, two cautionary notes should be added. The first concerns the normal sharply contoured waves that appear ubiquitously in the recordings of children, as mentioned earlier. In addition, several types of epileptiform waves, which can properly be called spikes, do not correlate with epileptic conditions (see Klass and Westmoreland, 1985, for review). These include small sharp spikes, 14/s and 6/s positive spikes, wicket spikes, 6/s spike-waves, and rhythmic midtemporal discharges. Definitions and descriptions of these phenomena are found in that article and in most EEG textbooks.

Generalized Epileptiform Abnormalities

Generalized Spike-Waves. The most classical of all EEG-clinical correlations is that observed between the bilaterally synchronous spike and the wave complex with absence attacks. Usually both the spike and the wave component emerge abruptly and distinctly from the background activity, but occasionally the spike discharge is obscure, leaving only a burst of rhythmic 3- to 4-Hz bilaterally synchronous waves. Descriptions of these phenomena appear in Blume (1982), Weir (1965), and Lemieux and Blume (1986). About 97% of patients with bilaterally synchronous spike-waves on the resting EEG or with hyperventilation have generalized seizure disorders (Blume, 1982). About 60% of these have absence attacks. The incidence of grand mal attacks varies considerably according to age at recording. A smaller number of patients with 3/s spike-waves, usually in the younger age groups, would have myoclonic seizures.

Because impairment of consciousness, as studied by reaction times, is most abnormal between 0.5 and 1.5 seconds after the onset of spike-wave complexes (Browne et al., 1974), some have considered that even a single spike-wave complex represents an absence attack! Although this may be theoretically true, an absence attack is unlikely to be clinically detectable unless sequential spike-wave complexes last more than 5 seconds (Niedermeyer, 1987).

Hyperventilation is the most effective means to elicit bisynchronous spike-wave discharges when they are not present in the resting recording. Hyperventilation was found to be more effective than a 6-hour recording in predicting clinical seizure frequency (Adams and Lueders, 1981). Photic stimulation may also elicit spike-waves, but these may appear in clinically normal subjects without a history of spontaneously appearing seizures.

Electrical status epilepticus during sleep (Patry et al., 1971; Tassinari et al., 1984) is a condition in which sequential bilaterally synchronous slow spike-waves are very abundant in non-REM sleep and therefore represent reiterative absence attacks. This condition is fortunately rare, as it impairs sleep, leading to episodes of diurnal microsleep. Varying quantities of 3/s spike-wave discharges may be seen during the awake recording.

Bilaterally synchronous myoclonic seizures are usually associated with bilateral spike-waves or poly–spike-waves. These may appear in an otherwise normal EEG, with slow spike-waves in the Lennox-Gastaut syndrome, or with excess delta in degenerative central nervous system disorders and metabolic encephalopathies. Although the spike-wave complexes accompany the myoclonus, the specific timing between the spike and the myoclonic jerk of the muscle varies (Gastaut et al., 1974). In some conditions, such as hereditary myoclonus epilepsy, the myoclonus may be present without any apparent EEG change.

The EEG in patients with grand mal seizures such as the grand mal seizure disorder of adolescence may be normal. In other cases it may show diffuse bursts of theta, or may contain sporadic spike-wave or poly–spike-wave complexes. During the rarely recorded grand mal attack, 20- to 40-Hz diffuse waves slowing to about 10 Hz appear during the tonic phase, followed by bilaterally synchronous and diffuse poly–spike-waves during the clonic phase. Unfortunately, muscle artifact rapidly obscures the tracing during grand mal attacks. Postictally, delta and theta predominate, with a return toward a normal recording within several minutes. No regional postictal abnormalities should occur if the attack was a primary generalized grand mal. In those patients with secondary generalized grand mal, the attack itself may predominate in one hemisphere and its postictal effects would reflect the side or area of most intense involvement.

Slow Spike and Wave. Gibbs et al. (1939) first distinguished slow spike and wave from the regular 3-Hz spike and wave, as the former repeats at 1.5 to 2 Hz. The epileptiform component may be either a spike or a sharp wave. These bilaterally synchronous discharges occupy a considerably greater quantity of the awake resting recording than do 3-Hz spike-waves (Figure 5–5). As compared to 3-Hz spike-waves, which appear principally in the 5- to 14-year age group, the maximum incidence of slow spike-waves is 1 to 5 years. In earlier years, this pattern may be intermixed with hypsarrhythmia; in later years, it may merge with 3-Hz spike-waves. The nonparoxysmal portion of the recording may be abnormally slow, in contrast to the traditionally normal findings with 3-Hz spike-waves. As with 3-Hz spike-waves, about 98% of patients with slow spike-waves have seizures. Tonic seizures are the most common, followed by

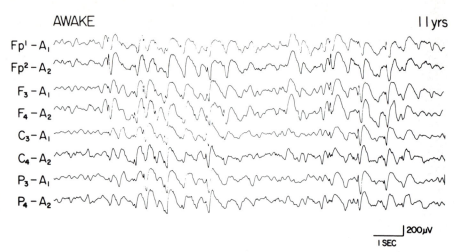

Figure 5-5. Abundant bisynchronous 1.5- to 2.5-Hz spike-waves are "slow spike-waves" seen with the Lennox-Gastaut syndrome or during absence status epilepticus.

atypical absence and myoclonic attacks. Intractable generalized seizures and bilaterally synchronous slow spike-waves on the EEG constitute the Lennox-Gastaut Syndrome. Most of these patients are mentally subnormal, but, when the syndrome appears in later ages, intelligence may be in the normal range. Hyperventilation less commonly elicits slow spike-waves and photic stimulation is not effective.

Sinusoidal-like waves at 10 to 20 Hz may appear diffusely in such recordings, accompanied by either tonic seizures or absence attacks.

Hypsarrhythmia. High-voltage 1- to 3-Hz waves with multifocal asynchronous spikes and sharp waves of varying morphology and amplitude constitute the pattern known as hypsarrhythmia (Figure 5–6). "Chaotic" is an appropriate description of the waveform in its full expression. Virtually continuous during wakefulness when fully present, hypsarrhythmia may become discontinuous in moderate and deep sleep, and this effect of state should be considered whenever sequential EEGs are compared.

Hrachovy et al. (1984) described dramatic changes in the character of hypsarrhythmia over the course of recordings from all of their 67 patients. In addition to the description already given, epochs of increased inter-

hemispheric synchronization were found that may be the forerunners of slow spike-waves. The pattern may predominate in one hemisphere or even be associated with a consistent focal spike discharge. Epochs of attenuation may interrupt the hypsarrhythmic pattern. Finally, asynchronous high-voltage delta activity with minimal epileptiform potentials can appear. The appearance of such EEG features depends on the duration of the recording, the clinical state of the patient, and the presence of structural abnormalities. For example, a large cystic defect in one hemisphere could impair the expression of hypsarrhythmia on that side, creating the asymmetrical form. Attenuation is most common in deep non-REM sleep, as already mentioned.

Despite the abundance of spikes and abnormal slow-waves, the hypsarrhythmic pattern is considered an interictal phenomenon, although one could consider the patient as being in an atypical absence during its presence. The most common clinical correlate of hypsarrhythmia is infantile spasms. During these the hypsarrhythmia pattern is abruptly and diffusely replaced by a single high-voltage wave with or without an accompanying spike. Immediately following this a diffuse or regional attenuation of electrical activity occurs, occasionally accompanied by low-voltage, high-frequency activity. Such

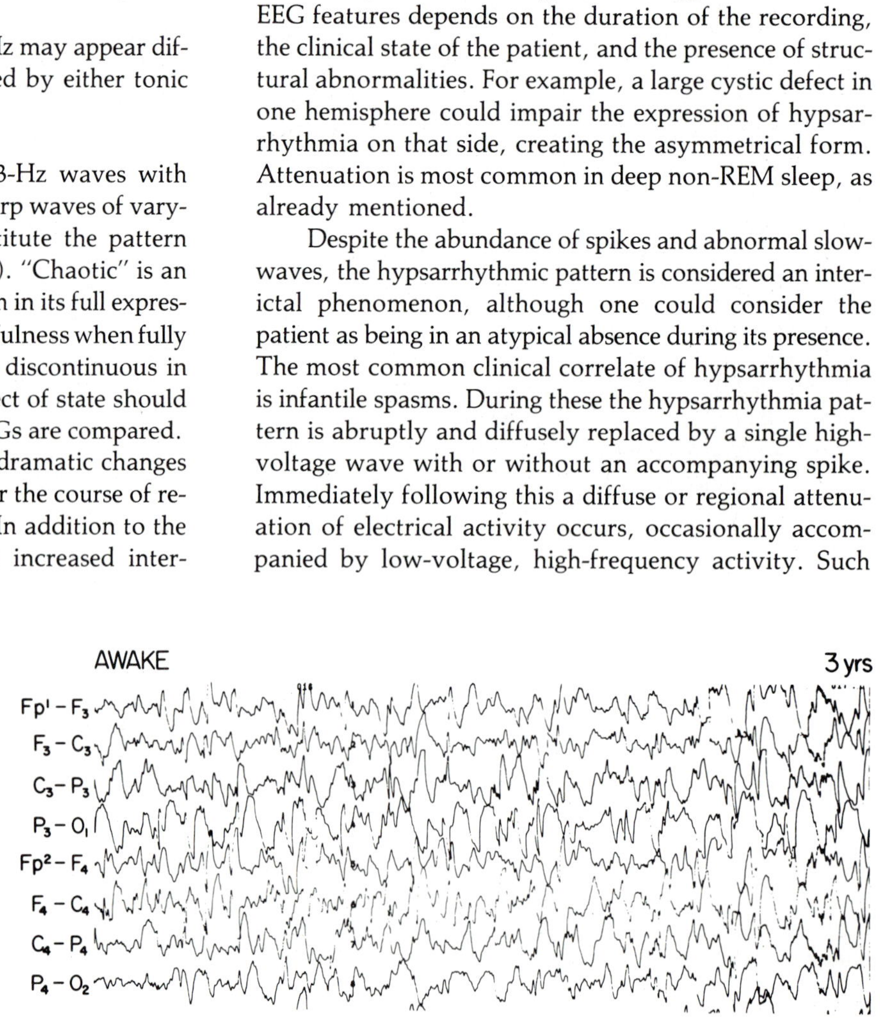

Figure 5-6. High-voltage diffuse delta with abundant multifocal spikes comprises the hypsarrhythmia pattern. These phenomena are at least moderately persistent in wakefulness but may appear in bursts in sleep.

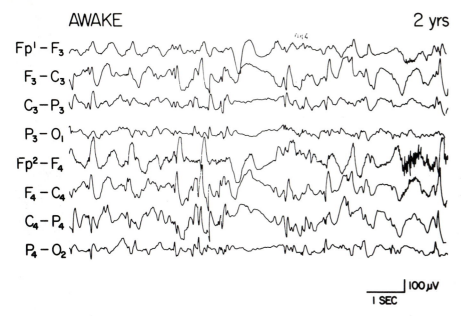

AWAKE   **2 yrs**

100 μV

1 SEC

Figure 5-7. An electrodecremental event. Sudden regional or diffuse (*center*) attenuation may interrupt the hypsarrhythmia or slow spike-wave pattern. Although no clinical change was evident on this occasion, such change may be associated with infantile spasms. Note chaotic hypsarrhythmia and bisynchronous slow spike-wave patterns here.

phenomena are termed electrodecremental events (EDEs) (Figure 5–7).

The hypsarrhythmia pattern is not always present when infantile spasms first occur but it ultimately appears. Therefore, the hypsarrhythmic pattern is helpful in differential diagnosis of epileptic and nonepileptic spasmodic conditions in infancy. Hypsarrhythmia is an age-related phenomenon, being confined usually to children aged 3 months to 5 years, approximately paralleling the time course of infantile spasms. At older ages, it may be replaced by slow spike-waves, focal or multifocal epileptiform abnormalities, or nonepileptiform abnormalities.

No aspect of the hypsarrhythmic pattern has been found to correlate reliably with the ultimate evolution of mental development. Etiology and clinical course are more likely to be of value in this respect.

Focal Epileptiform Potentials

Rolandic Spikes. Confined to children and adolescents, Rolandic spikes are frequent, stereotyped, and distinct discharges whose most prominent component is a downward deflection on anterior-posterior bipolar montages (Figure 5–8). This prominent downward deflection reflects the dipolarity of its field distribution, which can be proven by referential montages with positivity anteriorly and simultaneous negativity posteriorly (Blume, 1982). Although the negative component of the field is usually over the central-parietal regions with extension to the

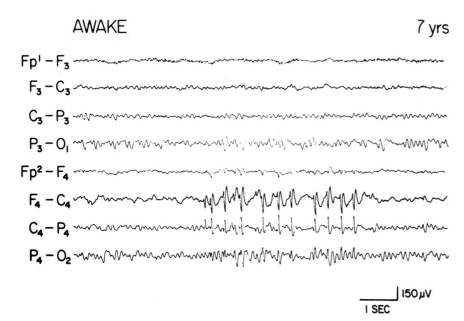

AWAKE   **7 yrs**

150 μV

1 SEC

Figure 5-8. Right Rolandic spikes. Their abundance is usually considerable, not in keeping with the infrequent associated seizures.

midtemporal areas, a sagittal or even parietal occipital location may be seen—all identified by the characteristic morphology and abundance. Such spikes may be virtually limited to one hemisphere in a recording but can be seen independently bilaterally and even synchronously bilaterally, in which case they resemble spike-waves. Distinction of these spikes from mu rhythm may be difficult. Their quantity would increase in non-REM sleep when the mu rhythm disappears.

When such spikes are abundant, they may be accompanied by slow waves in the same region. With this exception, the remainder of the EEG should be normal. In this case such focal spikes do not represent a structural lesion(s). However, when a persistent attenuation of background activity or focal delta appears, particularly if it is independent of the spikes, then a structural lesion might be present.

About 50% to 70% of patients with Rolandic spikes have seizures (Niedermeyer, 1987). Therefore, it is quite possible to find this pattern by accident in an EEG performed in the course of looking for another condition. For example, I have seen this pattern in patients with definite syncope.

The associated seizure disorder is benign Rolandic epilepsy of childhood, which most commonly occurs during non-REM sleep as grand mal or grand mal with unilateral predominance. During the daytime, partial sensory-motor attacks appearing principally in the face or arm may occur. Intellect and neurologic examinations are normal. Both the seizure tendency and the spikes tend to disappear by midadolescence, but the quantity of spikes bears no relationship to the quantity of epileptic seizures.

Occipital Spikes. Occipital spikes are well-defined electronegative spikes that appear unilaterally or bilaterally in synchronous or independent fashion over the occipital lobes and may spread to the posterior temporal or parietal regions. They are more abundant with eyes closed and therefore can be distinguished from lambda waves, which, in contrast, are normal electropositive potentials that occur when scanning a complex field.

Eeg-Olofsson et al. (1971) found occipital spikes in less than 1% of their normal children. Occipital spikes are the most common focal discharges in children less than 4 years of age and they appear most commonly at that time.

There are several types of occipital spikes. Children with epileptogenic lesions in the occipital lobe would have occipital spikes. Partial seizures with visual symptoms, complex partial attacks resembling temporal-lobe-originating seizures, and grand mal attacks all may occur in patients with unifocal or independent bi-occipital spikes. Spikes similar to Rolandic spikes in morphology and behavior may appear principally in the occipital lobe and they likely share clinical associations. Very brief occipital spikes may appear in congenitally blind children without any occipital lesion or seizure disorder (Lairy et al., 1964).

Smith and Kellaway (1964) found epilepsy in only 54% of their children with occipital spikes.

Photic stimulation may elicit occipital spikes in patients with both regional (D.C. Jones and W.T. Blume, unpublished results) and generalized encephalopathies, such as neuronal ceroid lipofuscinosis (Pampiglione and Harden, 1977).

Anterior Temporal Spikes. Although anterior temporal spikes are thought to be more common among adults, they do appear in childhood and have similar clinical correlates. This is not surprising, as complex partial seizures may begin as early as 3 to 4 years of age. Montages that distinguish these discharges from the temporal extension of Rolandic spikes are necessary; Rolandic spikes extend principally to the mid-temporal or posterior temporal region and are less prominent anteriorly and inferiorly.

Eeg-Olofsson et al. (1971) found temporal spikes in less than 1% of their series of normal children.

The etiology of such spikes includes any potential insult to the anterior temporal region. The classic antecedent would be febrile convulsions. If no plausible etiology exists for such anterior temporal spikes in young children with complex partial seizures of temporal lobe origin, a tumor or hamartoma may be lurking—even without CT evidence (Blume et al., 1982).

Ictal Epileptiform Potentials

In some instances, an electrographic seizure is manifested simply as sequential interictal potentials, such as a series of 3-Hz spike-wave discharges with absence attacks. Given the usual abundance of slow spike-wave discharges, it is at times difficult to determine if the patient is or is not in an atypical absence attack. Rhythmic waves of 10 to 20 Hz appearing diffusely may have absence or tonic seizures as the clinical correlate (Figure 5-9). Generalized myoclonic seizures have high-voltage diffuse and synchronous spikes with aftercoming slow waves as the clinical correlate even though the precise timing relationship between the EEG spike and the myoclonic jerk varies between patients and even in the same patient over time. Grand mal (tonic-clonic) seizures combine many of the aforementioned EEG features: very-low-voltage, high-frequency waves and/or 10- to 20-Hz rhythmic waves appear during the tonic phase. These are then interrupted by 300- to 400-millisecond bilaterally synchronous slow waves to constitute poly–spike-wave discharges during the clonic phase. The ictal phase of infantile spasms and hypsarrhythmia has been described. See Gastaut and Broughton (1972) for a full discussion of these ictal EEG–clinical relationships.

Focal seizures are characterized by the regional appearance of sequential waves that differ from background and whose morphology evolves over the course of the seizure (Blume et al., 1984). Such waves may resemble single or multiple sine wave sequences or a series of spikes or sharp waves.

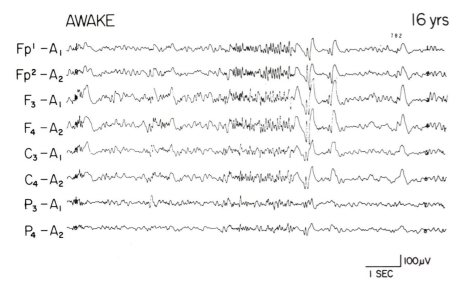

Figure 5-9. Fast rhythmic waves appear bilaterally in a 2-second burst (*center*) followed by bisynchronous slow spike-waves. Such fast waves may be associated with either absence or tonic seizures, but this burst ended before any clinical change could be discerned. The short (0.05) time constant of this segment abbreviated the slow waves of the slow spike-waves.

Activation Procedures

Any method that may elicit an EEG abnormality that has not occurred in a routine recording falls under the broad category of an activation procedure.

Hyperventilation

From age 4 years, children can cooperate with hyperventilation; their enthusiasm for the procedure is usually greater than that among adults. Consequently, and for reasons of brain immaturity, the effect of hyperventilation is more prominent in children than among adolescents and adults. Rythmic theta and delta activity appears initially posteriorly and then diffusely. It may not remit when the technologist asks the patient to stop hyperventilation as some patients may continue hyperventilating. Hypoglycemia may augment the response. Therefore, the degree of this response and its persistence are not criteria of abnormality.

The main purpose of hyperventilation is to elicit generalized spike-wave discharges when they are not present on the remainder of the recording. Focal spikes or other abnormalities may also appear, but such abnormalities must be convincingly focal and not simply transient hemispheric accentuation of the hyperventilation response.

Photic Stimulation

Photic stimulation can produce either no apparent response; a time-locked occipital response to the flash rate of varying morphology; myoclonus of the face and periocular and scalp musculature, also time-locked to the flash rate; and the photoconvulsive response. Full discussions of these phenomena can be found in EEG textbooks.

The most clinically significant response is the photoconvulsive response, a bilaterally synchronous polyspike or poly–spike-wave discharge that is not time-locked to the flash rate and that may continue beyond the cessation of the flash stimulus (Reilly and Peters, 1973) (Figure 5–10). This response is most readily elicited with flash

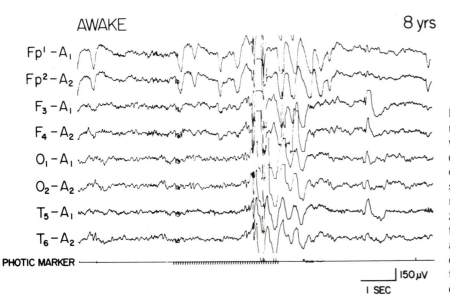

Figure 5-10. The photoconvulsive response, consisting of spike-waves whose repetition rate is wholly independent of flash rate and that outlast termination of the photic stimulation. Such spike-waves correlate better with a generalized seizure disorder than do spike-waves that are time-locked to the stimulus and do not outlast the flash. However, both types may be found in patients without a clinical seizure disorder.

rates of about 14 to 18 per second, particularly on eye closure. It is seen in about 3% of the laboratory population, in an approximately equal percentage of patients with partial seizure disorders, and in about 20% to 50% of patients with grand mal, myoclonic, or absence attacks (Takahashi, 1987). As the photoconvulsive response may be seen in normals and in patients with metabolic or drug withdrawal conditions, a diagnosis of a seizure disorder cannot conclusively be made on this basis. Moreover, relatives of patients with primary generalized seizures may demonstrate a photoconvulsive response without necessarily having a seizure disorder. On the other hand, such poly–spike-waves may confirm questionable spike-wave discharges on the resting recording and also establish the photosensitivity of patients with known primary generalized seizures. Spike-wave discharges to photic stimulation are uncommon under age 5 years and the incidence from 5 to 15 years is relatively stable. An exception would be those patients with myoclonic epilepsy of childhood, which may begin with a convulsion resembling a febrile convulsion; such patients were found by Dravet et al. (1985) and Dalla Bernardina et al. (1982) to exhibit the photoconvulsive response.

Ambulatory Electroencephalography

Techniques for prolonged ambulatory EEG monitoring have been developed using a wearable cassette-based, battery-powered EEG recording device permitting continuous 24-hour recording. Apparatuses with 4, 8, and 16 channels are available.

Ebersole's group (Leroy and Ebersole, 1983) devised montages to emphasize the anterior temporal and frontal regions, as most epileptiform discharges arise in these areas. With careful adherence to conservative standards of montage design and electrode application, about 80% of focal epileptiform abnormalities could be accurately identified and localized and 100% of seizures detected by ambulatory monitoring as compared to inpatient telemetry. Both systems were superior to routine EEG in this respect (Leroy and Ebersole, 1983; Bridgers and Ebersole, 1985). Routine EEG is probably superior for nonepileptiform abnormalities.

At this stage, the role of ambulatory EEG seems principally to support the diagnosis of an epileptic condition when there may have been some clinical doubt, to quantify epileptic seizures, and to lateralize and if possible localize the origin of some seizures. Technical limitations must be acknowledged, particularly when localization of seizure onset is the paramount goal. Epileptiform activity could arise from areas not covered by the limited montages and the design of such montages should be flexible.

Even ambulatory EEG samples only a limited duration of EEG, and many of the most difficult to diagnose epilepsy conditions occur in children or adults with infrequent attacks. Clues from seizure history and routine EEG suffice to categorize adequately most frequently occurring attack patterns.

Unfortunately, as with many medical innovations, economic factors have driven this technique to an accelerated popularity.

CERTAIN CENTRAL NERVOUS SYSTEM CONDITIONS WITH EPILEPSY

Febrile Convulsions

Three mechanisms may predispose to convulsions with a fever. The classic febrile convulsion is that representing a genetically determined susceptibility to generalized convulsions occurring only with fever. A second group of patients convulse with fever because of a thus far unrecognized brain insult occurring either prior to or during the febrile episode. A third group consists of children who have a chronic generalized epileptic condition that becomes evident first as convulsions during a febrile episode.

Complicated febrile convulsions are those that last for more than 15 minutes, are unilateral or focal, or are repeated within a single febrile episode. Such attacks tend to occur in patients whose neurologic development prior to the febrile attack was already abnormal and is usually associated with a higher risk of later epilepsy. Conversely, a single, brief, generalized febrile convulsion may have a relatively favorable prognosis. However, in practice, classifying each episode into either the simple or the complicated category may be clinically difficult, as may the determination of a prognosis. Therefore, EEG may help to categorize the mechanism of the febrile convulsion. EEGs carried out less than a week after a febrile convulsion may show various quantities of delta activity appearing either diffusely or posteriorly, the quantity depending on the duration of the febrile convulsion and the interval between its termination and the EEG recording. Such bilateral delta activity would fail to reveal the febrile convulsion mechanism. A postictal EEG with regionally accentuated delta or focal spikes would suggest that the seizure with a fever represented the second category outlined previously, i.e., a convulsion secondary to a previous or current central nervous system insult.

Pearls and Perils: EEG and Epilepsy

1. Slow spike-waves are characteristically more abundant than 3-Hz spike-waves.
2. Rolandic spikes are characteristically abundant, even though seizures are rare.
3. Distinction between sharply contoured mu rhythm and Rolandic spikes can occasionally be most difficult. When in doubt, consider it mu rhythm.

EEG could be valuable in the acute situation for any patient who fails to regain consciousness within a reasonable time after the apparent end of a febrile convulsion, to exclude the possibility of continuing seizure activity.

The presence of generalized spike-wave discharges on a routine EEG in a patient with febrile convulsions does not increase the incidence of nonfebrile generalized convulsions in later life. For example, about 20% of the patients of Frantzen et al. (1968) had sporadic generalized spike-waves that did not predict the recurrence of either febrile convulsions or the later development of nonfebrile seizures. Such spike-waves appear more commonly after age 4 years. On the other hand, abundant spike-waves suggest that the febrile convulsion is the first manifestation of a generalized nonfebrile seizure disorder.

An EEG is not mandatory in a patient with a simple febrile convulsion, and clinical judgment would be required as to whether an EEG could help unravel the mechanism of a more complicated attack.

Hemiconvulsion-Hemiplegia-Epilepsy

The hemiconvulsion-hemiplegia-epilepsy (HH&E) syndrome described by Gastaut et al. (1960) consists of a unilateral or predominantly unilateral prolonged convulsive seizure, a postictal hemiplegia that may or may not persist, and a partial epileptic seizure disorder, either as complex partial seizures from the implicated temporal lobe or focal motor and possible secondarily generalized seizures. As the young child is often febrile at the onset of the convulsive status epilepticus, a distinction from predominantly unilateral febrile convulsions is clinically and nosologically impossible. Postictally, high-voltage 1- to 2-Hz delta activity may be seen bilaterally with emphasis on the implicated hemisphere, and this EEG abnormality may persist in less prominent form for several years. Multifocal spikes chronically appear independently in either hemisphere but principally over the clinically implicated hemisphere. Secondarily generalized spike-waves are also a feature.

Acquired Epileptic Aphasia

Abundant spikes or spike-wave complexes appear bilaterally with predominance over the temporal and parietal regions in acquired epileptic aphasia, with the

emphasis shifting from side to side. Non-REM sleep may augment the spike quantity. Such EEG abnormalities become less prominent in adolescents, in rough parallel with the decline in the seizure disorder for most patients.

Rett's Syndrome

Reflecting the severe epilepsy that afflicts most girls with Rett's syndrome, epileptiform activity is prominent in the EEGs. Slow spike-waves are a major feature, and these usually achieve maximum expression posteriorly, as compared to the usual anterior field distribution of slow spike-waves in the Lennox-Gastaut syndrome (Niedermeyer and Naidu, 1987). Multifocal spikes may also appear. Trauner and Haas (1985) also found disorganized and slow background activity during wakefulness and quasi-periodic bursts of high-amplitude delta with interspersed epochs of attenuation lasting 3 to 4 seconds.

Epilepsy and Brain Tumors

The classic EEG sign of brain tumor is persistent regional delta activity with spike discharges in the same region if the tumor is slowly growing. Paroxysms of diffuse sinusoidal delta ("projected" activity) occur when intracranial pressure is raised. Thus we found persistent EEG delta activity in 10 of 16 patients whose tumors presented as chronic uncontrolled partial seizure disorders (Blume et al., 1982). However, multiple independent spike discharges occurred in a majority of epileptic patients with and without tumors; 4 of the 16 with tumors had generalized spike-wave discharges. Thus, the type and distribution of epileptiform discharges does not distinguish patients with tumors, but persistent delta activity over several recordings may suggest its presence. Of course, improved neuroimaging has lessened the EEG's value in tumor detection.

ACUTE CONDITIONS

Trauma

The magnitude of EEG changes following trauma is considerably greater in children than in adults with the same neurologic status. A mild head injury in a child may produce prominent EEG changes, and these therefore do not necessarily connote irreversible brain injury. Posteriorly accentuated excess delta activity is the most prominent single abnormality in the acute phase. The frequency of this delta activity is lower in the younger age groups. It declines rapidly after the second week postinjury (Silverman, 1962).

Because a head injury involves both direct and contre-coup effects, it is possible that the EEG would reveal effects that are not clinically apparent. For example, I have seen hemispheric arrhythmic delta activity ipsilateral to trauma-produced hemiplegia.

Pearls and Perils: CNS Conditions with Epilepsy

1. The patient with a simple febrile convulsion does not necessarily need an EEG.
2. Sporadic spike-wave discharges in a patient with febrile convulsions do not necessarily indicate that epilepsy will supervene.

When assessing the effects of head injury on EEG, the presence of preexisting EEG abnormalities must always be considered; for example, a 3-Hz bilaterally synchronous spike-wave pattern is most unlikely the result of trauma.

Epileptiform abnormalities are a not uncommon late consequence of trauma. To assure the relative or complete absence of these, one or more recordings including sleep may be required.

Encephalitis

Normal background rhythms are replaced by theta and rhythmic and arrhythmic excess delta activity. These slow waves are usually diffuse but may have regional accentuation. Although the abnormalities correlate reasonably well with the neurologic state of the patient, both the severity of the encephalitis and any associated systemic disease with metabolic derangements may contribute. Electrolytic derangements alter the EEG more prominently in children than in adults.

In the past, EEG was useful in localizing focal or multifocal abscesses, but advances in neuroimaging have largely supplanted this role.

Epileptic seizures may complicate encephalitis and their clinical manifestations may be unusual or subtle. The EEG, particularly if adequate recording time is allowed, can detect electrographic seizures or at least abundant epileptiform activity. In this manner it may also monitor the effectiveness of anticonvulsant therapy.

Periodic sharp waves are particularly characteristic of herpes simplex encephalitis; such sharp waves may be diffuse, temporal-frontal, unilateral, or bilateral in a shifting manner.

Meningitis

If the meningitis has a minimal encephalitic component, the associated EEG changes could be slight. Moreover, they could also represent any metabolic or electrolytic derangements attendant on the acute condition. Once again, focal delta activity should alert the clinician to the possibility of abscess as a complication.

Coma

Because the clinical examination of a patient with a subnormal level of consciousness, particularly coma, is primarily confined to assessment of brainstem function, the EEG provides a valuable adjunct by recording cortically originating activity.

Several phenomena can be seen in comatose conditions. The most common is diffuse persistent excess delta and theta activity. The reactivity to afferent stimuli of this activity correlates well with the depth of coma. Triphasic waves in association with a depressed level of consciousness indicate a metabolically induced comatose condition (Sundaram and Blume, 1987). Periodic lateralizing epileptiform discharges may be seen in patients with overriding regional abnormalities (Chatrian et al., 1964).

When recurrent seizures complicate the situation, the effectiveness of anticonvulsant treatment can be monitored by assessing the abundance of clinical and subclinical electrographic seizures and the quantity of spikes (Figure 5–11).

Burst suppression activity may appear in deep coma: bursts of brief runs of intermixed theta, delta, and spikes are separated by equal or longer periods of relative or complete inactivity, either diffusely or regionally. In other situations, diffuse, nonreactive sinusoidal patterns in the theta or alpha range have been described by several authors (see Bauer, 1987, for review).

The prognosis of any of these patterns depends on the etiology of the comatose condition, its duration, and the direction in which sequential EEG recordings are headed. Thus, if anesthetics or other central nervous system depressants have been used, the value of EEG patterns in prognosis is virtually nil. Metabolic and toxic

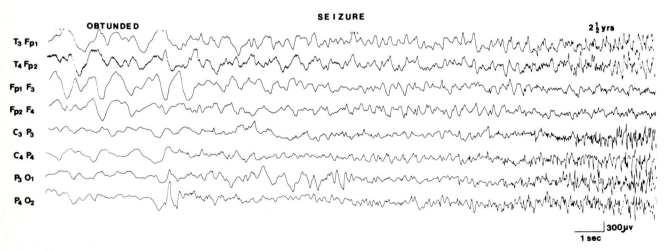

Figure 5–11. From an excessively slow, delta-dominated background, a gradually onsetting seizure occurs—first as theta (*center*), then as sequential polyspikes (*right*). Note the left-right alternating montage.

states usually have a better prognosis than structural or anoxic encephalopathies for a given EEG picture. Within this context, prognostically favorable signs are EEG reactions to exogenous stimuli, spontaneous variability, and normal sleep potentials. Lack of reactivity to deep painful afferent stimuli, the burst suppression pattern, monorhythmic alpha or theta frequencies, a very-low-voltage EEG, or electrocerebral silence all suggest an unfavorable outcome.

Pampiglione and Harden (1968) carried out EEGs within the first 12 hours of cardiac arrest in children aged 1 day to 10 years. Those children whose EEGs contained at least some normal features appropriate to age either on the initial recording or within a few hours recovered well. Patients with continuous delta that failed to resolve over several hours and those with burst suppression or electrocerebral inactivity died.

Focal or multifocal spikes or sharp waves appear to be present in the more deeply comatose states with Reye's syndrome and therefore may correlate with an unfavorable prognosis.

Reye's Syndrome
Aoki and Lombroso (1973) demonstrated a close relationship between the clinical staging of neurologic impairment with Reye's syndrome and EEG. Although the prognosis at each stage has likely improved since their original publication because of improvements in management, the close clinical-EEG relationship may be useful in monitoring patients who have been pharmacologically paralyzed as part of management.

As with any comatose condition, unfavorable EEG prognostic signs would include lack of reactivity to afferent stimuli, very-low-voltage activity or electrocerebral silence, and the burst suppression pattern.

The EEG in Determination of Irreversible Coma
It is to be hoped that the concept of irreversible coma will replace that of "brain death" in approaching this type of situation. Mohandas and Chou (1971) established criteria that would determine beyond reasonable doubt the state of irreversible damage to the brainstem: (1) a known, irreparable intracranial lesion, (2) no spontaneous movements, (3) apnea, (4) no brainstem reflexes, and (5) no change over 12 hours. No child or adult satisfying such criteria has ever survived (Pallis, 1983; Jorgenson, 1981; Tomlin et al., 1981; Rowland et al., 1983; Robinson, 1981; Moshe and Alvarez, 1986). It is therefore illogical to *require* that a physician verify the conclusions of one type of procedure for which no flaws have been shown (clinical evaluation) with one or more laboratory procedures for which many flaws have been uncovered (various laboratory procedures).

With respect to the EEG, even theoretic electrocerebral inactivity cannot be equated with total cessation of cortical function. A limiting factor is machine noise, from which cerebrally originating potentials of less than

<table>
<tr><td>

Pearls and Perils: Acute Conditions

1. EEG can help monitor the effectiveness of anticonvulsant medication in acutely ill patients whose epileptic seizures may have subtle or bizarre manifestations.
2. Sequential EEGs are often of greater prognostic value than a single EEG in assessing the prognosis of a comatose child.
3. EEG can be helpful in assessing whether coma is irreversible, but its value is considerably less than that of clinical data in this respect.

</td></tr>
</table>

2 μV cannot be distinguished. Neuronal discharges from the thalamus have been recorded in the presence of electrocerebral silence (Jonkman, 1969; Visser, 1969; Carbonell et al., 1963). Ashwal and Schneider (1979) showed the presence of EEG activity in patients up to 30 months of age who fulfilled other criteria for brain death; none of these five patients survived.

Instead of requiring physicians to utilize EEG in the determination of irreversible coma, it could be suggested as an ancillary test in situations during which full evaluation of brainstem function is not possible from a practical standpoint. This would occur when trauma to structures reflecting brainstem function had occurred. Even in this circumstance, EEG data would not necessarily assume primary importance, but would be considered along with other data in arriving at a clinical decision of irreversible coma.

If one accepts the concept of irreversible coma instead of brain death, demonstration of complete cortical electrical inactivity may not be required. Reactivity of any pattern to afferent stimuli would assume paramount importance. Technical requirements can be found in many publications, particularly that by Bauer (1987).

CHRONIC CONDITIONS

Syncope

Sequential EEG events occur in fortuitously recorded syncope: loss of alpha, a brief period of low-voltage beta, then rapidly augmenting diffuse theta, then delta activity followed by transient electrocerebral inactivity, then progressive recovery. Nonetheless, diagnosis of syncope does not depend on demonstration of this sequence, as was thought in the past.

The danger of performing an EEG in patients with syncope is that some irrelevant abnormality might be disclosed. Therefore, the purpose of the recording should be thoroughly established to the parents before the fact. When myoclonic or tonic movements are a prominent or prolonged feature of the syncopal attack (brief myoclonies are common), the clinician may be justified in wondering if a generalized epileptic condition is so represented. However, this is a rarity and an EEG is unnecessary in almost all cases of syncope.

Headache

Although a high percentage of nonspecific abnormalities may be seen in children and adults with migraine or other forms of headache, the value of such abnormalities in differential diagnosis has never been adequately established. Thus, an EEG would serve no better than clinical judgment in deciding whether a child's headache represented a brain tumor, arteriovenous malformation, or raised intracranial pressure.

Cerebral Palsy

Patients with hemiplegia have the highest incidence of EEG changes (90%), followed by quadriplegics (85%) (Gibbs and Gibbs, 1964). As the pathology is more deeply seated among patients with paraplegia and athetosis, EEG abnormalities are less common.

Asymmetries of awake and sleep potentials may appear among those with hemiplegia, the side of lower voltage corresponding to the clinically implicated hemisphere. Such abnormalities would be less common for patients with athetosis or diplegia.

Multiple independent spike foci are probably the most common single EEG abnormality. Usually these are more common over the implicated hemisphere, but, if both hemispheres are extensively involved, the spikes may be better expressed over the relatively healthy side.

Developmental Abnormalities of the Brain

Several EEG phenomena may be associated with congenital malformations of the brain, including a paucity of EEG activity either focally or diffusely, monorhythmic theta, or diffuse or focal delta activity. Encephalopathy caused by perinatal insults such as infection or trauma may have similar constellations of abnormalities, depending on the severity. In patients with relatively restricted abnormalities, such as porencephaly, most cerebral activity may be normal except in the implicated area, where paucity of activity, excessive slowing, or spike discharges may appear. Agenesis of the corpus callosum may be associated with a normal EEG or with hypsarrhythmia in infants with the Aicardi syndrome.

Degenerative Central Nervous System Disease

The EEG does not play a major role in the differential diagnosis of most degenerative diseases currently encountered; of greater significance are age, symptoms, neurologic examination, family history, and the course of the disease. However, EEG changes are often prominent and therefore their unexpected presence may signal the existence of a degenerative disorder.

Pearls and Perils:
Chronic Conditions

1. History and neurologic examinations are better than an EEG in diagnosing syncope and determining the cause of headache.

Slowing then disappearance of normal background rhythms combined with excess delta or theta activity is a common finding whether the gray or the white matter is primarily involved. Spike discharges are more common in primarily gray-matter disorders, whereas delta activity is relatively more prominent in white-matter disorders, but these distinctions are not absolute.

At younger ages, patients with neuronal ceroid lipofuscinosis may respond to low-frequency flash stimulation with large occipital spikes (Pampiglione and Harden, 1973). Early-onset degenerative conditions such as globoid leukodystrophy or phenylketonuria may be represented by the hypsarrhythmic pattern.

High-voltage posteriorly situated delta activity during both wakefulness and sleep may represent adrenoleukodystrophy in any patient without other likely causes, such as recent seizures or trauma.

The electroretinogram (ERG) may help in the differentiation of some degenerative conditions. For example, in GM_2 gangliosidosis (Tay-Sachs disease) the ERG remains normal, whereas it may be abolished with neuronal ceroid lipofuscinosis.

ANNOTATED BIBLIOGRAPHY

Niedermeyer E, Lopes da Silva F (eds): *Electroencephalography: Basic Principles, Clinical Applications and Related Fields,* 2nd ed. Baltimore, Md, Urban & Schwarzenberg, 1987.

Blume WT: *Atlas of Pediatric Electroencephalography.* New York, Raven Press, 1982.

These two textbooks, particularly that by Niedermeyer and Lopes da Silva, discuss the topics covered herein in greater detail. A more complete series of illustrations can be found in the atlas by Blume.

REFERENCES

Adams DJ, Lueders H: Hyperventilation and 6-hour EEG recording in evaluation of absence seizures. *Neurology* 31:1175–1177, 1981.

Aoki Y, Lombroso CT: Prognostic value of electroencephalography in Reye's syncrome. *Neurology* 23:333–343, 1973.

Ashwal S, Schneider S: Failure of electroencephalography to diagnose brain death in comatose children. *Ann Neurol* 6:512–517, 1979.

Bauer G: Coma and brain death, in Niedermeyer E, Lopes da Silva F (eds): *Electroencephalography: Basic Principles, Clin-*

ical Applications and Related Fields, 2nd ed. Baltimore, Md, Urban & Schwarzenberg, 1987, p 391–404.

Blume WT: Atlas of Pediatric Electroencephalography. New York, Raven Press, 1982, p 139.

Blume WT, Girvin JP, Kaufmann JCE: Childhood brain tumours presenting as chronic uncontrolled focal seizure disorders. Ann Neurol 12:538–541, 1982.

Blume WT, Young GB, Lemieux JF: EEG morphology of partial epileptic seizures. Electroencephalogr Clin Neurophysiol 57:295–302, 1984.

Bridgers SL, Ebersole JS: The clinical utility of ambulatory cassette EEG. Neurology 35:166–173, 1985.

Browne TR, Penry JK, Porter RJ, Dreifuss FE: Responsiveness before, during, and after spike-wave paroxysms. Neurology 24:659–665, 1974.

Carbonell J, Carrascosa G, Diersen S, et al: Some electrophysiological observations in a case of deep coma secondary to cardiac arrest. Electroencephalogr Clin Neurophysiol 15:520–525, 1963.

Chatrian GE, Shaw CM, Leffman, H: The significance of periodic lateralized epileptiform discharges in EEG: An electrographic, clinical and pathological study. Electroencephalogr Clin Neurophysiol 17:177–193, 1964.

Dalla Bernardina V, Capovilla G, Gattoni MV, Colamaria V, Bondavalli S, Bureau M: Epilepsie myoclonique grave de la première année. Rev Electroencephalogr Neurophysiol Clin 12:21–25, 1982.

Dravet C, Roger J, Bureau M: Severe myoclonic epilepsy of infants, in Roger J, Dravet C, Bureau M, Dreifuss FE, Wolf P (eds): Epilepsy Syndromes in Infancy, Childhood and Adolescence. London, John Libbey, 1985, p 58–67.

Eeg-Olofsson O, Petersen I, Sellden U: The development of the electroencephalogram in normal children from the age of 1 through 15 years. Paroxysmal activity. Neuropadiatrie 2:375–404, 1971.

Frantzen E, Lennox-Buchthal M, Nygaard A: Longitudinal EEG and clinical study of children with febrile convulsions. Electroencephalogr Clin Neurophysiol 24:197–212, 1968.

Gastaut H, Broughton R: Epileptic Seizures. Springfield, Ill, Charles C Thomas, 1972.

Gastaut H, Poirier F, Payan H, Salomon G, Toga M, Vigouroux M: HHE syndrome, hemiconvulsions-hemiplegia-epilepsy. Epilepsia 1:418–447, 1960.

Gastaut H, Broughton R, Roger J, Tassinari CA: Generalized convulsive seizures without local onset, in Vinken PJ, Bruyn GW (eds): Handbook of Clinical Neurology, Amsterdam, Elsevier, 1974, p 107–129.

Gibbs FA, Gibbs EL: Atlas of Electroencephalography, Vol 3: Neurological and Psychiatric Disorders. Reading, Mass, Addison-Wesley, 1964, p 185–198.

Gibbs FA, Gibbs EL, Lennox WG: Influence of the blood sugar level on the wave and spike formation in petit mal epilepsy. Arch Neurol Psychiatr 41:1111–1116, 1939.

Hrachovy RA, Frost JD Jr, Kellaway P: Hypsarrhythmia: Variations on the theme. Epilepsia 25:317–325, 1984.

Jonkman EJ: Cerebral death and the isoelectric EEG. Electroencephalogr Clin Neurophysiol 27:215, 1969.

Jorgenson EO: Brain death: Retrospective surveys. Lancet 1:378–379, 1981.

Klass DW, Westmoreland BF: Nonepileptogenic epileptiform electroencephalographic activity. Ann Neurol 18:627–635, 1985.

Lairy GC, Harrison A, Leger EM: Foyers EEG bi-occipitaux asynchrones de pointes chez l'enfant mal voyant et aveugle d'âge scolaire. Rev Neurol (Paris) 111:351–353, 1964.

Lemieux JF, Blume WT: Topographical evolution of spike-wave complexes. Brain Res 373:275–287, 1986.

Leroy RF, Ebersole JS: An evaluation of ambulatory cassette EEG monitoring: I. Montage design. Neurology 33:1–7, 1983.

Mohandas A, Chou SN: Brain death—A clinical and pathological study. J Neurosurg 35:211–218, 1971.

Moshe SL, Alvarez LA: Diagnosis of brain death in children. J Clin Neurophysiol 3:239–249, 1986.

Niedermeyer E: Epileptic seizure disorders, in Niedermeyer E, Lopes da Silva F (eds): Electroencephalography: Basic Principles, Clinical Applications and Related Fields, 2nd ed. Baltimore, Md, Urban & Schwarzenberg, 1987, p 415–416.

Niedermeyer E, Naidu S: Degenerative disorders of the central nervous system, in Niedermeyer E, Lopes da Silva F (eds): Electroencephalography: Basic Principles, Clinical Applications and Related Fields, 2nd ed. Baltimore, Md, Urban & Schwarzenberg, 1987, p 317–338.

Pallis C: ABC of brain death: The position in the USA and elsewhere. Br Med J 286:209–210, 1983.

Pampiglione G, Harden A: Resuscitation after cardiocirculatory arrest. Lancet 1:1261–1265, 1968.

Pampiglione G, Harden A: Neurophysiological identification of a late infantile form of "neuronal lipidosis." J Neurol Neurosurg Psychiatr 36:68–74, 1973.

Pampiglione G, Harden A: So-called neuronal ceroid lipofuscinosis. Neurophysiological studies in 60 children. J Neurol Neurosurg Psychiatr 40:323–330, 1977.

Patry G, Lyagoubi S, Tassinari CA: Subclinical "electrical status epilepticus" induced by sleep in children. Arch Neurol 24:242–252, 1971.

Reilly EL, Peters JF: Relationship of some varieties of electroencephalographic photosensitivity to clinical convulsive disorders. Neurology 23:1050–1057, 1973.

Robinson RO: Brain death in children. Arch Dis Child 56:657–658, 1981.

Rowland TW, Donnelly JH, Jackson AH, Jamroz SB: Brain death in the pediatric intensive care unit. Am J Dis Child 137:547–550, 1983.

Silverman D: Electroencephalographic study of acute head injury in children. Neurology 12:273–281, 1962.

Smith JMB, Kellaway P: The natural history and clinical correlates of occipital foci in children, in Kellaway P, Petersen I (eds): Neurological and Electroencephalographic Correlative Studies in Infancy. New York, Grune & Stratton, 1964, p 230–249.

Sundaram MBM, Blume WT: Triphasic waves: Clinical correlates and morphology. Cana J Neurol Sci 14:136–140, 1987.

Takahashi T: Activation methods, in Niedermeyer E, Lopes da Silva F (eds): Electroencephalography: Basic Principles, Clinical Applications and Related Fields, Baltimore, Md, Urban & Schwarzenberg, 1987, p 212.

Tassinari CA, Daniele O, Dravet C, et al: Sleep polygraphic studies in some epileptic encephalopathies from infancy to adolescence, in Degen R, Niedermeyer E (eds): Epilepsy, Sleep and Sleep Deprivation. Amsterdam. Elsevier, 1984, p 175–189.

Tomlin PJ, Martin JW, Honigsberger L: Brain death: Retrospective surveys. Lancet 1:378, 1981.

Trauner DA, Haas RH: Electroencephalographic abnormalities in Rett's syndrome. *Ann Neurol* 18:394, 1985.
Trojaborg W: Changes of spike foci in children, in Kellaway P, Petersen I (eds): *Clinical Electroencephalography of Children*. New York, Grune & Stratton, 1968, p 213–225.

Visser SL: Two cases of isoelectric EEGs (apparent exceptions proving the rule). *Electroencephalogr Clin Neurophysiol* 27:215, 1969.
Weir B: The morphology of the spike-wave complex. *Electroencephalogr Clin Neurophysiol* 19:284–290, 1965.

Electromyography
Nancy L. Kuntz

Electromyography (EMG) refers to a collection of diagnostic techniques, including nerve conduction studies and needle electromyography, that can be used selectively or in combination to obtain physiologic information about the motor unit. Limited information can be obtained regarding the central control over the motor unit. All of the techniques described in this chapter (and normative data for adults) have been established and diagnostically applied to adult medicine for several decades. However, only in the past 10 to 15 years have modifications of technique and equipment and careful study of the maturation of parameters allowed common application of these techniques to the pediatric population.

There is no "standard EMG" that will answer all questions about the motor unit—rather there exists a selection of different tests that complement each other to provide insight into most questions that can be posed about motor unit physiology. Many of the techniques are annoying to mildly painful for the subject. Therefore, infants and children will frequently not tolerate lengthy or prolonged examinations. These factors make it mandatory for the referring physician to have carefully worked out a clinical differential diagnosis and to establish, with the clinical electromyographer, a hierarchy of questions to be answered. In this way, the electromyographer approaches the study with a mental checklist of the data to be collected and a strict order of priority. Then, if the exam is prematurely terminated, the most valuable pieces of information have been obtained.

Practical problems exist that make EMG more difficult to perform in infants and children. Smaller extremity sizes make electrode separation and shock artifact more of a consideration. Additionally, shorter distances magnify the effect of small errors in measurement. The greater surface area in infants and children makes their extremities more susceptible to cooling, which changes nerve conduction parameters, neuromuscular transmission properties, and the appearance of motor units. Normal values for EMG studies for infants and children are very different than those for adults. Some of the techniques have well-described normal values, with the maturational changes worked out from extreme prematurity through adolescence—for example, ulnar motor nerve conduction studies. Normative data for other techniques—particularly sensory nerve conduction

studies and F-wave responses—are currently sparse, but data are currently being gathered in centers around the country.

Eliciting cooperation and comforting the infant or child through the procedure can be accomplished in many different ways. The referring physician has the opportunity to play an important role in this process by carefully preparing the patient and family. Graphic descriptions of "shocks" and "needles" provided for the sake of informed consent tend to become magnified into nightmares over the days or weeks between referral and testing. A simple explanation to the parent or older child is preferable: the testing consists of several different techniques and some portions may be annoying to mildly painful but should be brief. Assurance can be given that the electromyographer will carefully explain each technique prior to its being performed and that the parent or child will have control over terminating the examination, if necessary. The referring physician should also provide an estimate of the "mental age" of the patient. Most of the nerve conduction techniques can be slowly and patiently performed on a sleeping child or infant with a mental age of under 4 years without the child awakening or becoming frightened and uncooperative. Therefore, if there are no relative contraindications to sedation, many electromyographers (including this author) will sedate children functioning under this age level. Sedation can be accomplished through scheduling the testing at a normal nap time; considering sleep deprivation; using natural means such as a bottle and a favorite toy along with a quiet, darkened room; or by using chloral hydrate up to an oral dosage of 75 mg/kg 30 minutes prior to the scheduled time of the exam. Older children are most cooperative when they are well rested, awake, and feeling "in control."

NERVE CONDUCTION TECHNIQUES

Commonly used techniques include motor nerve conduction studies, sensory nerve conduction studies, F-wave latencies, H-reflex testing, blink reflex testing, and repetitive stimulation or paired stimuli to evaluate neuromuscular transmission. At times the testing of a single nerve or nerve/muscle combination provides adequate information. In other circumstances, multiple sites must be tested. For example, differentiation of acquired inflammatory peripheral nerve disease (e.g., Guillain-Barré syndrome) from genetically determined dysmyelinating peripheral neuropathies (e.g., Dejerine-Sottas disease or Refsum's disease) is facilitated by comparing involvement between multiple nerves in a single extremity or between nerves on opposite sides of the body. Other disorders, such as myasthenia gravis, can patchily affect different neuromuscular junctions, providing normal results when one nerve/muscle combination is tested and characteristically abnormal findings when another is tested.

All of these techniques involve the application of brief-duration, low-current electrical square wave pulses to peripheral sensory or mixed sensory-motor nerves with the use of various schemes to record the appropriate electrophysiologic response. The amount of current used is adequate to stimulate all of the nerve fibers of interest (usually large myelinated motor or sensory fibers) but is subthreshold for the unmyelinated "pain" fibers. The stimulus is therefore usually described as a tapping or a thumping, although some persons describe a stinging sensation that is mildly painful. If motor fibers are activated, an involuntary brief contraction of the muscles innervated by those fibers peripheral to the site of stimulation will occur. Occasionally subcutaneous needle electrodes must be employed to selectively stimulate or record from deeply placed nerves. Most commonly, tin disks can be taped or applied to the skin for both stimulation and recording. Surface electrodes are obviously better tolerated by infants and children.

Motor nerve conduction studies are performed by stimulating mixed nerves and recording over the endplate region of one of the muscles innervated by those fibers. The summated electrical response of all the muscle fibers appear as the M wave, or compound muscle action potential, whose onset latency, amplitude, and shape provide physiologic information. Stimulation at multiple points along the nerve along with a careful measurement of the distance between the points of stimulation provides an estimate of the maximal conduction velocity of the motor fibers (Figure 5–12). Any muscle/nerve combination that is anatomically suited to surface stimulation and re-

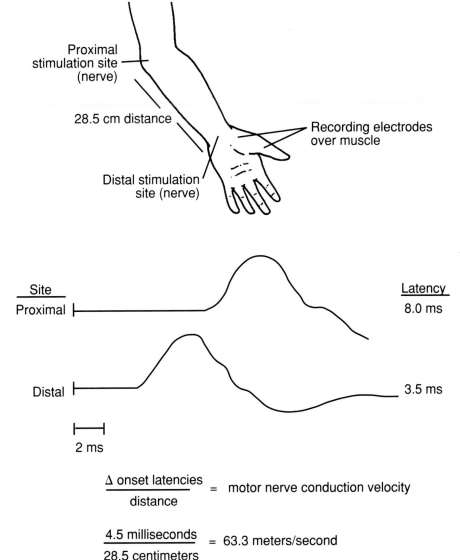

$$\frac{\Delta \text{ onset latencies}}{\text{distance}} = \text{motor nerve conduction velocity}$$

$$\frac{4.5 \text{ milliseconds}}{28.5 \text{ centimeters}} = 63.3 \text{ meters/second}$$

Figure 5–12. Technique for motor nerve conduction studies. Stimuli are applied to motor nerve fibers and the summated electrical response associated with the muscle contraction is recorded over the muscle.

cording can be tested. For example, in addition to the commonly tested nerves in the forearms and legs, the phrenic nerve can be stimulated in the neck and the response from the diaphragm recorded over the lower chest wall (Moosa, 1981). For most motor nerves, compound muscle action potential amplitudes are approximately one third of adult values in term infants, increase to approximately one half of adult values by 7 to 12 months of age, and increase proportionately thereafter. Motor nerve conduction velocities are approximately one half adult values in term infants, approach the lower limits of adult values between 7 months and 5 years of age, and approach mean adult normals by 5 to 10 years of age (Gamstorp, 1963; N.L. Kuntz, unpublished data) (Figure 5–13).

Sensory nerve conduction studies are performed by stimulating a mixed nerve and recording over a cutaneous sensory nerve or stimulating a cutaneous sensory nerve and recording over either a mixed nerve or the same cutaneous sensory nerve fibers at a distance (Figure 5–14) The amplitude of sensory nerve action potentials is much smaller than that of compound muscle action potentials (5 to 100 μV as compared to 2 to 20 mV), so these recordings are much more subject to technical problems. Sensory nerve action potential amplitudes are approximately one half of adult values in term infants. After 6 months of age, the range of amplitudes is roughly the came as that obtained in adults. Biphasic potentials are frequently recorded in infants and children, and the significance of this finding is controversial (Wagner and Buchthal, 1972; Kimura et al., 1977). The maturational changes in sensory nerve conduction velocities have not been as carefully established as those in motor nerve conduction velocities. However, they are approximately one

half of adult values in term infants and appear to reach adult mean values by 2 to 5 years of age. (Gamstorp, 1963; N.L. Kuntz, unpublished data) (Figure 5–15).

F-wave latencies are late responses, recorded over muscles after retrograde activation of motor axons, that activate a proportion of the anterior horn cells and induce an anterograde impulse. This latency includes conduction along the proximal portion of the motor axon that standard motor nerve conductions do not test. Because the response is measured as an absolute latency, this reflects both the conduction velocity as well as the distance traveled, which is proportional to the limb length. Normal values cannot, therefore, be directly extrapolated from motor nerve conduction velocities. Sparse normative data exist in infants and children (Miller and Kuntz, 1986; N.L. Kuntz, unpublished data) (Figure 5–16).

H reflexes (named after the initial recordings, which were made in hand muscles) are produced by activation of sensory fibers with a stimulation that is submaximal for activation of motor fibers. The motor response, elicited via activation of the same monosynaptic reflex arc responsible for clinical muscle stretch reflexes, is recorded. They are more easily elicited in infants than in older children and adults. Their main advantage lies in the low stimulation intensity required to elicit them and in their ability to evaluate the proximal sensory and motor pathways. Normal values exist for H reflexes recorded in hand and calf muscles (Mayer and Masser, 1969).

Blink reflexes consist of early and late electrical responses recorded over bilateral orbicularis oculi muscles after low-intensity electrical stimulation of the supraorbital branch of the trigeminal nerve. These responses

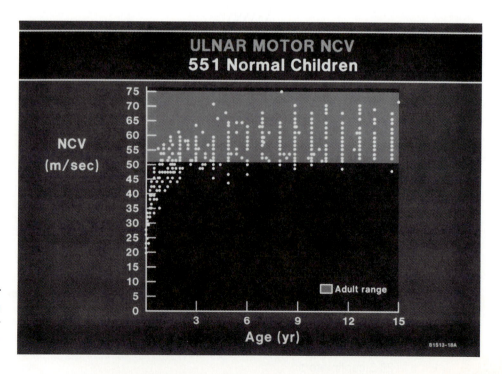

Figure 5–13. Normative data for ulnar motor nerve conduction velocity from 551 normal infants and children. (*N.L. Kuntz, unpublished data.*)

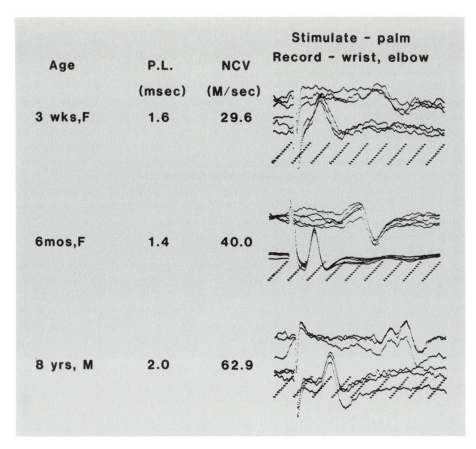

Age	P.L. (msec)	NCV (M/sec)	Stimulate – palm Record – wrist, elbow
3 wks,F	1.6	29.6	
6mos,F	1.4	40.0	
8 yrs, M	2.0	62.9	

Figure 5-14. Ulnar sensory nerve action potentials. Stimulation and recording are performed at different places along the same group of sensory nerve fibers. Age of subjects, peak latencies, and nerve conduction velocities are listed.

test polysynaptic pontine connections as well as the facial and trigeminal nerves. Responses in term infants are less consistent and occur with longer latencies than those in adults. Normative data have been obtained for infants and children (Kimura et al., 1977).

Neuromuscular transmission can be tested with pairs of stimuli or with trains of stimuli (repetitive stimulation), depending on the physiologic parameter to be assessed. Serial compound muscle action potential amplitudes and areas are compared. This technique can be difficult to use

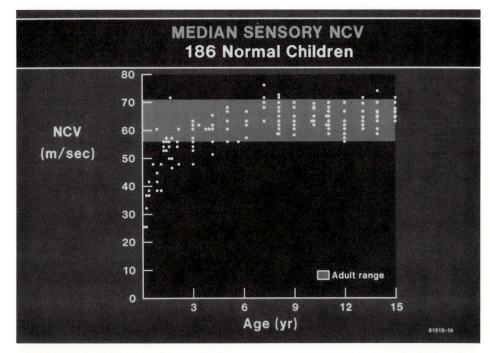

Figure 5-15. Normative data for median sensory nerve conduction velocity obtained from 186 normal infants and children. (*N.L. Kuntz, unpublished data.*)

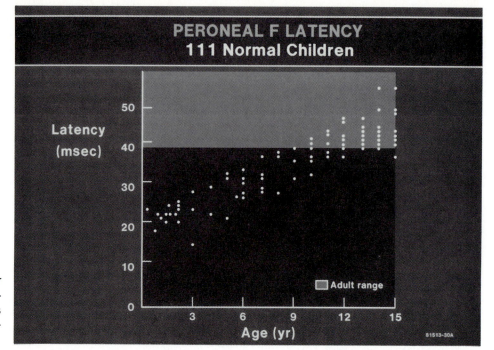

Figure 5–16. Normative data for peroneal F-wave latencies obtained from 111 normal infants and children. (*N.L. Kuntz, unpublished data.*)

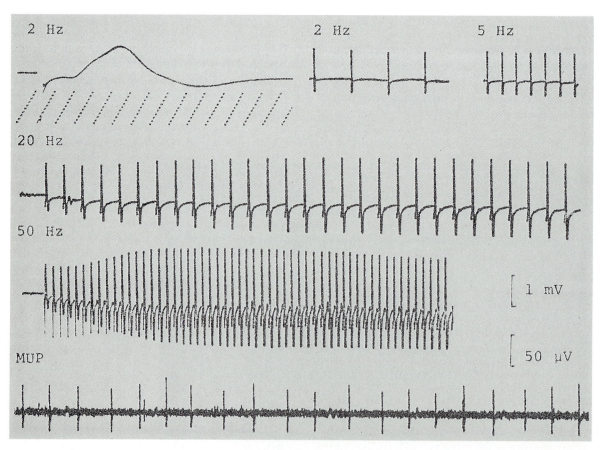

Figure 5–17. Repetitive stimulation of motor nerves to evaluate neuromuscular transmission. Responses from slow (2 Hz) and rapid (20 Hz, 50 Hz) repetitive stimulation are demonstrated from a 9-week-old infant with botulism.

in infants and children since voluntary movement of the extremity can produce artifacts. Repetitive stimulation at 2 to 3 Hz is used to evaluate most disorders of neuromuscular transmission. Neuromuscular transmission is mature enough in infants and children to respond to 2- to 3-Hz stimulation in a manner identical to that seen in adults. Rapid repetitive stimulation (20 to 50 Hz) is used to evaluate postsynaptic disorders of neuromuscular transmission (e.g., infantile botulism). Rapid repetitive stimulation is uncomfortable and can be technically difficult to perform in infants and children (Figure 5–17). The electromyographer must recognize that normal infants under 6 months of age can have decrements of up to 50% in amplitude in response to 20- to 50-Hz stimulation (Churchill-Davidson and Wise, 1963).

Nerve conduction studies can provide information about the type of nerve fibers involved (motor versus sensory), the pattern of involvement (uniform versus patchy, proximal versus distal), as well as the type of physiologic insult (conduction block versus axonal loss). Knowledge of whether the axons have been partially or totally severed can determine what the time course of recovery may be and whether surgical intervention should be con-

sidered. Conduction blocks lead to proportionately decreased amplitude of response when stimulation proximal to the site of the lesion is performed. When axons have been severed, they continue to function and to conduct stimuli applied *distal* to the site of the lesion for up to 5 to 7 days, until Wallerian degeneration disrupts their function. Therefore, nerve conduction studies performed a week after the lesion can differentiate axonal loss from conduction block. In the case of a complete brachial plexus lesion from birth, nerve conduction studies performed at 1 week of age will provide important physiologic and prognostic information. These principles are frequently used to determine the nature of peripheral nerve injury in adults but have been greatly underused in infants and children. Evidence of denervation does not appear on needle electromyography for up to 21 days after the injury.

NEEDLE EMG

Standard needle EMG is performed with a specialized recording electrode (equivalent to a 26-gauge needle with length adequate to reach the muscle), which is inserted into each muscle studied. Disposable electrodes are available to minimize the risk of transmissible diseases. For each needle placement, the electrical response to insertion, the resting muscle activity, an evaluation of any spontaneous electrical activity present, and an educated but nonetheless subjective assessment of the motor unit population are recorded.

Most infants and children experience some difficulty tolerating the needle examination owing to the discomfort involved. Even if they have slept through the nerve conduction studies with sedation, they usually wake up when the needle examination is started. Usually, the examination can be performed quickly and simultaneously tape-recorded for later detailed assessment or quantitation. In most cases, the support of a parent or a familiar adult, reassurance that the hurt will end quickly, and relaxation/distraction techniques will allow adequate information to be gathered in an awake child. If analgesia or a sedative or antianxiety medication is used, it must be tailored to allow the patient to be alert enough to follow requests to contract the muscle voluntarily. In most circumstances, the difficulty involved in attempting to premedicate the child for the needle exam portion of the test is greater than any comfort provided. Positioning and repositioning the extremity (particularly with the muscle at its shortest length) can aid in attaining a silent background for examination of spontaneous or insertional activity. In infants or children unable or unwilling to contract the muscle voluntarily, activation initiated by repeated passive movements, tactile stimulation, or infantile or protective reflexes can be used.

Most muscles in the body can be studied electromyographically. The muscles that are most superficial and distinct from vascular structures are the most easily studied. There is no standard set of muscles that are tested. The more complete and specific the differential diagnosis and physiologic questions to be answered are, the better able the electromyographer is to select and prioritize the muscles to be studied. If a muscle biopsy is planned, the electromyographer should be informed so that that particular muscle will not be tested, because such instrumentation can lead to artifacts difficult to differentiate from disease processes. Patients with bleeding tendencies are at some risk from needle electromyography; however, the process can usually still be safely performed under these circumstances.

The findings on needle examination are somewhat different in infants and children than in adults. Frequent motor endplate regions are encountered, especially in children under 1 year of age or with significant central nervous system immaturity. Initially positive, low-amplitude, short-duration "preinnervation infantile activity" has been described in premature infants and in developmental disorders such as myelomeningocele when innervation has not naturally occurred. There is no evidence that typical fibrillation potentials occur in full-term or older infants unless there is an abnormality in the peripheral nervous system. Motor unit potential recruitment does not differ significantly between children and adults. However, individual motor unit potential characteristics are different in infants than in adults. In infants, motor unit potentials are simpler in configura-

tion, shorter in duration (approximately one third the adult values), and lower in amplitude (approximately 20% to 50% of adult values) (Sacco and Buchthal, 1962). To obtain maximum information from needle electromyography, it is important to characterize motor unit potential recruitment separately from individual motor unit potential size. This is even more critical in infants and young children, in whom congenital malformations (such as hypoplasia of muscle) can produce findings not commonly seen in adults.

Disease processes that primarily involve abnormalities of the contractile mechanism of the muscle fiber tend to cause milder changes in the characteristics of the individual motor unit potentials: a tendency toward lower amplitude, briefer duration, and increased percentage of polyphasic motor unit potentials (Figure 5–18). There is a change in motor unit potential recruitment proportional to the degree of reduced strength: recruitment of greater numbers of motor unit potentials firing more rapidly and producing relatively less strength of contraction. Disease processes that involve loss of innervation to the muscle fibers are initially characterized by decreased numbers of motor unit potentials that can be voluntarily recruited. If the denervation persists, fibrillation potentials occur spontaneously that signal the presence of denervated muscle fibers (Figure 5–19). As reinnervation occurs, there are usually fewer but larger (higher amplitude, longer duration) motor unit potentials. Many disease states involve variable degrees of muscle fiber involvement and nerve fiber loss. In such cases, the concept of "myopathic" and "neurogenic" motor unit potentials being equivalent to clinical myopathy and neuropathy is too simplistic and can be misleading. Characterization of distinct motor unit populations is useful in understanding the pathophysiology of the disease process. For example, a population of low-amplitude, polyphasic, but varying motor unit potentials occurring along with enlarged motor unit potentials with decreased recruitment suggests a chronic neurogenic process with a component of ongoing reinnervation (Figure 5–20).

During routine needle EMG, judgments about motor unit potential characteristics are made by visual measurements of 20 to 40 individually isolated motor unit potentials during mild to moderate contractions. Quantitative methods increase the sensitivity to minor degrees of abnormality. These may vary from manual graphic measurements, to computer measurements on individual motor units, to theoretically derived computer programs for quantitating motor units or motor unit populations from partial interference patterns (a more moderate contraction with multiple motor units firing simultaneously). The latter methods are appealing for potential application to pediatric patients because they require less voluntary cooperation. However, they are still undergoing development and are not widely commercially available.

Pearls and Perils: Needle EMG

1. Standard needle EMG can reliably differentiate neurogenic processes from other motor problems in infants and children.
2. Needle EMG can provide important information about the pathophysiology of the disease process, e.g., the presence or absence of ongoing reinnervation.
3. Carrier states or subclinical phases of muscular dystrophies as well as congenital, structurally distinct myopathies can produce motor unit potentials with characteristics and recruitment patterns that are difficult to differentiate from normal values for age.
4. Muscles that are going to be biopsied should not be studied by needle EMG within several weeks prior to biopsy because the muscle trauma incurred can produce changes difficult to differentiate from disease states.
5. Serum muscle enzymes should be drawn prior to needle EMG, because the repeated needle insertions involved in most studies can produce a transient elevation of muscle enzymes that may confound the diagnostic effort.

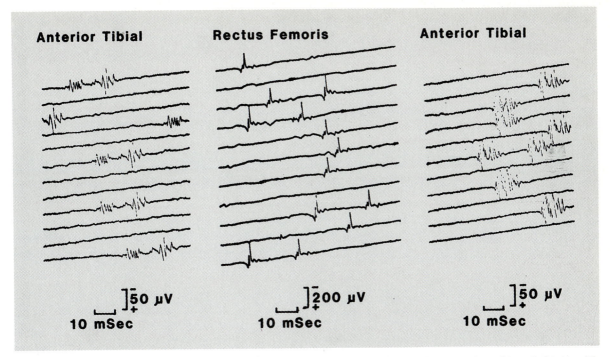

Figure 5–18. Individual motor unit potentials recorded from lower extremity muscles of two infants with congenital myotonic dystrophy.

The motor unit potentials recorded during routine needle EMG are a summation of the potentials from several dozen individual muscle fibers in proximity to the recording electrode that are innervated by a single anterior horn cell (the exact number of fibers that contribute depends on the characteristics of the recording electrode). Special techniques have been developed that can selectively record from a single or a pair of muscle fibers from a given motor unit (single-fiber EMG) or that can scan the muscle for a spatial map of contributing muscle fibers from a given motor unit (macroelectromyography). Both of these techniques are of limited

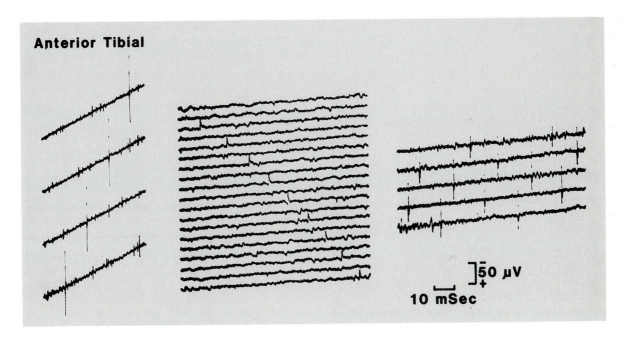

Figure 5–19. Fibrillation potentials recorded from the anterior tibial muscle of a 6-month-old infant with congenital myotonic dystrophy.

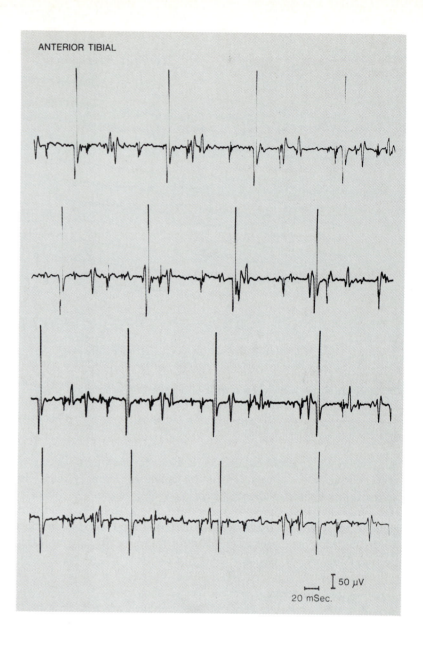

ANTERIOR TIBIAL

50 µV

20 mSec.

Figure 5–20. Motor unit potentials recorded from a 3-month-old infant with spinal muscular atrophy. Several distinct populations of motor unit potentials coexist, signifying denervation with ongoing reinnervation.

clinical usefulness in the pediatric population because of the increased cooperation required, the increased time required for the examination, and the limited experience to date to validate expected normal findings. Nevertheless, techniques have been developed that make voluntary cooperation less essential and the procedure more applicable to pediatric patients (Trontelj et al, 1986).

In summary, EMG refers to a collection of nerve conduction studies and techniques of needle EMG that can be used in various combinations to define disorders of the motor unit: anterior horn cell, peripheral nerve, nerve terminal, neuromuscular junction, and muscle. Increased technical problems relating to small size, decreased voluntary cooperation, the rapid change of normal values with maturation, and less well-defined normal values make the application of these techniques to infants and children

more challenging. Nevertheless, with close cooperation among the referring physician, parent, patient, and electromyographer, exacting pathophysiologic information can be obtained that may not be available by any other means. The potential exists to use these techniques not only for diagnostic purposes but also for prognostic purposes and for following the course of diseases during clinical treatment trials.

ANNOTATED BIBLIOGRAPHY

Nerve Conduction Studies

Miller RG, Kuntz NL: Nerve conduction studies in infants and children. *J Child Neurol* 1:19–26, 1986.

This reference provides a summary of technical issues unique to infants and young children as well as tables of normal values for the more commonly used nerve conduction techniques.

Electromyography and electric stimulation of peripheral nerves and muscle, in Aronson AE et al: *Clinical Examinations in Neurology*, 4th ed. Philadelphia, WB Saunders, 1976, p 320–329.

This reference contains a more complete description of the technical and theoretical aspects of nerve conduction studies. It does not contain any information specific to infants and children.

Needle Electromyography

Kimura J: *Electrodiagnosis in Diseases of Nerve and Muscle: Principles and Practice*. Philadelphia, FA Davis, p 235–258, 1983.

This reference contains an elegant discussion of needle EMG and will answer any questions left after the brief summary in this chapter. It does not contain any information specific to infants and children.

REFERENCES

Churchill-Davidson HC, Wise RP: Neuromuscular transmission in the newborn infant. *Anesthesiology* 24:271–278, 1963.

Gamstorp I: Normal conduction velocity of ulnar, median and peroneal nerves in infancy, childhood and adolescence. *Acta Paediatr Scand* 146:68–76, 1963.

Kimura J, et al: Electrically elicited blink reflex in normal neonates. *Arch Neurol* 34:246–249, 1977.

Mayer RF, Masser RS: Excitability of motoneurons in infants. *Neurology* 19:932–945, 1969.

Miller RG, Kuntz NL: Nerve conduction studies in infants and children. *J Child Neurol* 1:19–26, 1986.

Moosa A: Phrenic nerve conduction in children. *Dev Med Child Neurol* 23:434–448, 1981.

Sacco G, Buchthal F: Motor unit potentials at different ages. *Arch Neurol* 6:366–373, 1962.

Trontelj JV, Mihelin M, Fernandez JM, Stalberg E: Axonal stimulation for end-plate jitter studies. *J Neurol Neurosurg Psychiat* 49(6): 677–685, 1986.

Wagner AL, Buchthal F: Motor and sensory conduction in infants and childhood: Reappraisal. *Dev Med Child Neurol* 14:189–216, 1972.

Event-Related Potential Assessment of Sensory System Integrity

Diane Kurtzberg

The recording of event-related potentials (ERPs) in response to sensory stimulation in infants and children provides a noninvasive method for assessing the integrity of sensory systems (visual, auditory, somatosensory) from the periphery through the cerebral cortex. In the pediatric population, ERP recordings are particularly useful because we do not always have reliable behavioral measures of sensory function, especially in the very young infant and child. In addition to providing adequate indexes of sensory pathway abnormalities in patients with manifest neurologic disorders, they are important in the detection of sensory pathway abnormalities in babies and children who are known to be at high risk for sensory, cognitive, and language dysfunction, for example, very-low-birth-weight (VLBW) infants, babies experiencing perinatal asphyxia, or those with a family history of hearing impairment. In these cases, early detection of sensory dysfunction can lead to early intervention, which may ameliorate some of the long-term adverse effects of the deficit. This intervention is especially crucial in hearing and visual impairments.

SCALP-RECORDED EVENT-RELATED POTENTIALS

The electrical activity recorded from electrodes placed on the scalp includes the electroencephalogram (EEG) and the ERP. As described in the first section of this chapter, the EEG represents the spontaneous, ongoing electrical activity of the brain that is not related to specific sensory, motor, or cognitive processes. ERPs, by contrast, represent the neural activity that is specifically related or time-locked to sensory stimulation (evoked potentials, EP), motor acts (movement-related or motor potentials), or cognitive processes (cognitive ERP). Most clinical applications of ERPs currently use the obligatory brain responses to sensory stimuli, the EPs.

Because EPs are usually lower in voltage and embedded within the EEG, computers are needed to extract the ERP signal from the background EEG, which occurs randomly with respect to the stimulus. Averaged responses to repetitive presentations of the sensory stimulus are needed in order to obtain the ERP reliably. The number of presentations of the stimulus depends on the signal-to-noise ratio or the size of the ERP relative to the background EEG. In general, enhancement of the EP amplitude with respect to the random EEG is proportional to the square root of the number of stimuli used to compute the averaged EP. For example, the visual evoked potential (VEP) is larger in voltage ($<10\mu V$) than the auditory brainstem response (ABR) ($<1\mu V$). (The ABR is also called the brainstem auditory evoked potential or response.) Both are small relative to the background EEG. In order to extract the VEP from the background EEG it is necessary to have at least 50 to 100 repetitions of the visual stimulus, but the ABR requires as many as 2000 repetitions of the auditory stimulus. An inadequate number of stimuli will result in poorly defined and variable averaged EPs and preclude their use for reliable assessment of sensory pathway and cortical integrity.

EPs are often divided into near-field and far-field responses. Near-field responses are generated within cerebral cortex and recorded from scalp electrodes directly overlying the brain areas that are most likely to be active during sensory stimulation in a particular modality. For example, to record VEPs, electrodes are placed overlying primary visual cortex. Responses that differ in their waveshape and timing from those seen over primary sensory cortex can be recorded overlying secondary sensory cortical regions as well. In the presence of cortical pathology, the response recorded overlying primary sensory cortex may be within normal limits, with abnormalities occurring only in the processing of the sensory stimulation located in secondary cortical areas. These abnormalities may be indicative of dysfunction at higher levels of the processing of sensory information. Clinically important examples of this may be seen in cases of "cortical blindness" (Frank et al., 1988) or in cases of verbal auditory agnosia (Klein et al., 1988).

Far-field responses refer to EPs that are generated at a distance from the recording site, usually within the subcortical afferent pathways. The ABR is an example of a far-field response that is recorded from electrodes placed on the scalp; it reflects activity within the afferent auditory pathways from the eighth cranial nerve through the midbrain, occurring during the initial 15 milliseconds or so following a click or tone pip. It is important to point out that the cortical auditory EPs generated within primary auditory cortex are also far-field potentials because they are volume-conducted for several centimeters through the brain from the superior temporal plane to the central scalp, where they are recorded at their maximum amplitude. The short-latency somatosensory evoked potentials (SEPs) also reflect activity along the afferent pathway from the peripheral nerve to somatosensory cortex. Thus, the SEPs of subcortical origin (<20 milliseconds) are far-field responses when recorded from the scalp, whereas the cortical SEPs are near-field potentials.

The following sections will describe the procedures and clinical use of these sensory EPs (visual, auditory, and somatosensory) in the pediatric population.

VISUAL EVOKED POTENTIALS

The general question that the referring physician often asks when sending an infant or child for VEP testing is "What are his or her visual capabilities?" In some children, this information cannot always be obtained using

---

Pearls and Perils: Visual Evoked Potentials

1. The VEP is a noninvasive technique that can objectively assess visual pathway integrity in infants and children from whom it is not possible to obtain reliable behavioral measures of visual function.
2. The VEP to flash stimulation is useful in very young infants and children who are unable to maintain an awake and alert state and optimal fixation on a visual stimulator.
3. An objective estimate of visual acuity for each eye can be obtained using the VEP to pattern stimulation.
4. Owing to the rapid maturational changes in the waveshape, latency, and amplitude characteristics of flash and pattern VEPs recorded during infancy and childhood, an individual child's record must be compared against *age-matched* normative data. (Preterm infants must be corrected for gestational age.)
5. Before referring a child for VEP testing, a thorough ophthalmologic examination is necessary to identify ocular pathology (opacities, retinopathy) that can have an impact on the VEP.
6. Recording the pattern VEP requires an awake and alert infant or child who is able to maintain fixation on the visual stimulator during the entire testing session.
7. Owing to variability in the level of maturation of the visual system during the first 2 months of life, an absent or deviant pattern VEP does not necessarily imply visual pathway dysfunction. Repeat testing at 3 months of age or testing with larger checks or gratings is necessary.

---

standard behavioral and/or ophthalmologic techniques. VEPs have proven useful to assess visual pathway integrity in infants and children who show no signs of spontaneous or elicited visual behavior in the absence of ocular pathology; to assess amblyopia and monitor the treatment of strabismus; to evaluate the visual capabilities of children with ocular pathology, such as congenital cataracts or neuroophthalmologic conditions, such as nystagmus; and to assess the functional impact of lesions affecting the central visual pathways, such as optic nerve gliomas, pituitary tumors, or retrochiasmal lesions.

Two main EP procedures are available to assess the integrity of the visual pathways in infants and children. These are monitoring of the VEPs to light flash stimulation and to pattern reversal. Typically, electrodes are placed on the occipital region of the scalp overlying primary visual cortex (O_1 and O_2). Additional electrodes may be applied overlying secondary visual processing regions as well (parietal, temporal, central, and frontal areas of the scalp) when cortical pathology is suspected.

VEP to Flash Stimulation

The VEP to flash reflects the neural activity associated with diffuse light stimulation. Because flash VEPs are not very sensitive to sleep state, attention, and level of visual acuity in the young infant, they are useful in babies and some children who cannot maintain an alert state and fixate on patterned stimuli. Flash VEPs are also useful for assessing the integrity of the retro-cortical pathways in the presence of congenital cataract or corneal opacities.

The VEP to light flash undergoes striking maturational changes (as illustrated in Figure 5–21) during the preterm period (32 to 40 weeks postconception), and in full-term infants from birth to 6 months of age. The response recorded from primary visual cortex is sharply localized over the occipital scalp. Before 36 to 38 weeks postconceptional age it consists of a primarily surface negative component followed by a large positive wave. An early small positive component begins to emerge at 36 to 38 weeks postconceptional age and becomes very prominent by term. Responses, which differ in wave shape and timing from the occipital response, are recorded overlying parietal, temporal, central, and frontal regions of the scalp even in the youngest preterm infants, reflecting activation of secondary visual cortical centers. It is possible, therefore, to assess not only the integrity of primary visual cortical responsiveness, but also that of secondary cortical areas, even in preterm infants.

Because the flash VEP reflects the neural activity associated with diffuse light stimulation, it can tell us nothing about pattern processing, which is often the information that we hope to obtain. It is reasonable, therefore, to ask about the clinical utility of flash VEP recordings. We recorded flash VEPs in a group of 79 VLBW infants at 40 weeks postconceptional age and compared their occipital responses with those recorded from healthy full-term newborns (Kurtzberg, 1982). Fifty-one percent of the VLBW babies had normal VEPs to flash, whereas the remainder showed deviant responses. We re-

PRE TERM

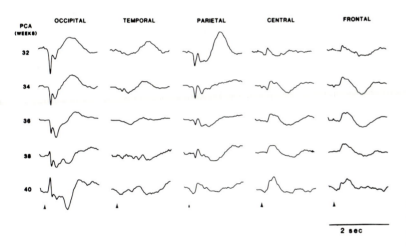

POSTTERM

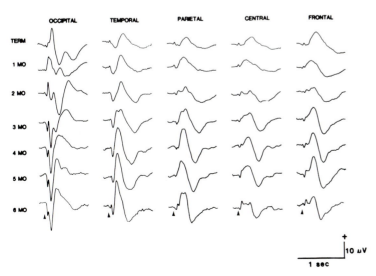

Figure 5–21. (*Top*) Grand mean VEPs to light flash recorded from 10 to 15 healthy preterm infants at 32 to 40 weeks postconceptional age. The occipital response consists of a negative deflection until about 38 weeks postconceptional age, when a positivity occurring at 200 milli-seconds after flash becomes prominent. Note the neural activity recorded over secondary visual processing areas (parietal, temporal, central, and frontal regions of the scalp). Arrow indicates onset of flash. (*Bottom*) Grand mean flash VEPs recorded from 15 to 20 healthy full-term infants during the first 6 months of life. The occipital VEP at term consists of a major positivity preceded by a small negative component and a positivity that appears as a shoulder on the larger component. This first positivity becomes more prominent during the first 6 months of life. The later large positive components become progressively shorter and more sharply defined, as do the components overlying secondary visual processing areas. Note the difference in time scale for preterm and postterm VEPs.

tested these infants at monthly intervals during the first 6 months of life and bimonthly to 1 year of age using pattern as well as flash stimulation. Ninety-two percent of the babies with normal flash VEP at 40 weeks postconceptional age had normal visual EPs during the first 6 months of life and 97% were normal at 1 year. Abnormalities persisted in greater than 50% of the infants who displayed abnormal VEPs at term. Thus, babies with normal flash VEPs at 40 weeks postconceptional age are likely to exhibit normal visual function as assessed by the pattern VEP at 1 year of age. Conversely, infants who have abnormal flash responses at term should be retested during the first year of life to evaluate further the nature and persistence of the apparent dysfunction.

VEP to Pattern Reversal

The VEP to reversal of checkerboard or grating patterns has several advantages in the assessment of visual function over the flash VEP. Because the total amount of luminance is held constant, the VEP to pattern reversal reflects the activity of neural mechanisms underlying pattern vision, not merely light sensitivity. In addition, objective measures of visual acuity for each eye can be obtained by systematically varying the element size within the pattern. Sokol and colleagues (e.g., Sokol, 1978;

Sokol et al., 1983) have developed a technique to obtain an estimate of visual acuity in young infants and children in which pattern VEPs are recorded to reversal of checks of different sizes and the amplitude of the response is measured and plotted against check size. A regression line is drawn and extrapolated to zero amplitude, which provides an estimate of visual acuity for each eye.

A major limitation of pattern VEP is the absolute requirement for an alert and attentive child who is able to maintain fixation on the pattern stimulator. This is often difficult to obtain in very young infants and the children who are in most need of this assessment. For example, when testing a child with amblyopia, patching the "good" eye will often cause the child to become fussy and avoid looking at the pattern with the eye that has diminished visual acuity. There are, however, measures that can be applied to maximize attentiveness and fixation on the pattern stimulator, such as careful questioning of the parents as to what time of the day the infant is most alert, having a cartoon superimposed on the reversing checks or grating pattern, or talking an older child through the procedure to engage attention and cooperation.

As with the flash VEP, the pattern VEP undergoes major maturational changes during childhood, with the most dramatic changes occurring during the first 3 months (Figure 5–22) (see also Moskowitz and Sokol,

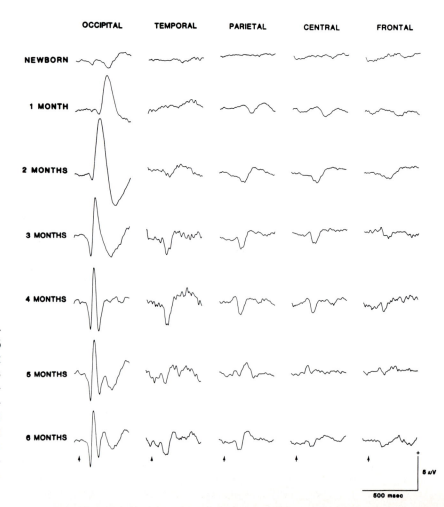

Figure 5–22. Grand mean pattern reversal VEPs recorded from 10 to 15 healthy full-term babies during the first 6 months of life. Stimuli were checks subtending 40' of visual angle. The occipital response at birth is not well defined, but becomes better formed and shorter in latency during the first 6 months of life. Responses overlying secondary visual processing areas begin to appear at 1 month of age. Arrow indicates pattern reversal.

1983). In the newborn infant, the pattern VEP recorded overlying the occipital region consists of a small negative-positive-negative complex followed by a larger positive wave. During the first few months of life, the pattern VEP becomes better defined and the most prominent peak of the response, the major positive component, decreases in latency. It is interesting to note that the responses recorded over secondary visual areas (parietal, temporal, and central regions) are not as prominent in the newborn period as is seen with the flash VEP (see Figure 5–21) and only begin to emerge during the first few months of life.

In using the pattern VEP to assess the visual system of the newborn infant, one must take into account the variability of the responses owing to differences in the level of maturation of the newborn's visual acuity. It is not uncommon to record very poorly formed responses

CHECK SIZE

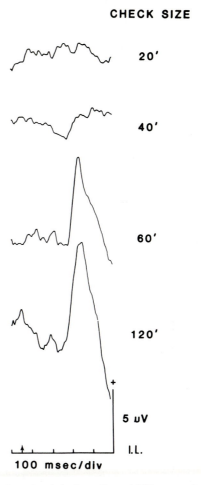

Figure 5–24. Occipital pattern VEP recorded from a healthy full-term infant to reversal of checks subtending 20′, 40′, 60′, and 120′ of visual angle. No identifiable response was recorded to 20′ checks; a low-voltage, poorly formed response is recorded to 40′ checks; and large well-formed VEPs are seen with larger checks. Arrow indicates pattern reversal.

in healthy full-term infants, and one must be cautious in interpreting these results as abnormal. Figure 5–23 illustrates pattern VEPs recorded from six healthy full-term infants shortly after birth and at 3 months to reversal of checks subtending 40′ of visual angle. Note the extreme variability in responsiveness among these children at term. By 3 months of age, however, this variability virtually disappears, signifying a more consistent maturational level of the visual system among infants at that age. It is always desirable, however, to increase check or grating size if no response is present to the smaller sizes (Figure 5–24).

Recording both flash and pattern VEP in high-risk infants at term, when the infant may be still hospitalized and accessible for testing, is not without its utility. As noted above, significant visual system impairment is unlikely in any infant who shows a response within normal limits at term. Occasionally, however, an infant with progressive visual impairment, such as retinopathy of prematurity, may not be picked up by the flash VEP at

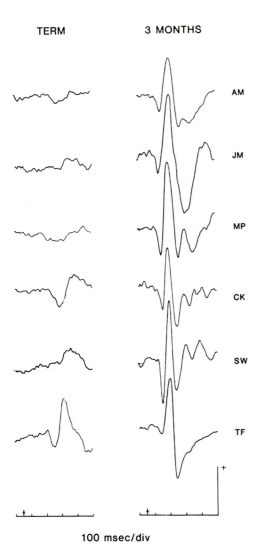

Figure 5–23. Pattern reversal VEPs recorded from six healthy full-term infants at birth and 3 months of age. Stimuli were checks subtending 40′ of visual angle. Note the variability in waveshape, latency, and amplitude at term, which is greatly reduced by 3 months of age. Calibration is 10 μV for all infants except AM and TF, for whom it was 20 μV. Arrow indicates pattern reversal.

term. The possibility of false negative VEPs cannot be entirely dismissed. Owing to the sensitivity of the pattern VEP to maturational factors, there may be a large number of deviant responses in the newborn period. Retesting at 3 months of age is recommended to determine if there are persistent visual pathway abnormalities. For efficient use of often limited resources, if the possibility of visual impairment is suspected, it is recommended that pattern VEP assessments be performed after 2 to 3 months of age.

In summary, the VEP procedure of choice for assessing visual pathway integrity in the pediatric population is the more sensitive pattern VEP, always keeping in mind the caveats described previously and listed in Pearls and Perils.

AUDITORY EVOKED POTENTIALS

The major purposes of recording auditory evoked potentials (AEPs) in infants and children are to measure objectively auditory system sensitivity or threshold and to assess the integrity of the central auditory pathways, from the cochlea through the cortex. The techniques available for this assessment are measurement of (1) the ABR for assessing peripheral and brainstem auditory pathways; (2) the middle latency response (MLR), reflecting the initial activation of primary auditory cortex; (3) the later occurring cortical auditory evoked potential (CAEP), reflecting activation of primary and secondary auditory cortexes; and (4) the discriminative response, which assesses the brain's ability to differentiate two auditory signals that vary acoustically. For clinical purposes, the most useful techniques at this time are the ABR and the CAEP; however, a brief discussion of the use of the MLR and discriminative response will also be included.

Auditory Brainstem Response

The ABR is a far-field response recorded from the scalp to rapid presentations of brief auditory stimuli, usually clicks or tone pips. In the adult (Figure 5–25, top left trace), the response, lasting less than 10 milliseconds, consists of a series of waves that reflects activation of the eighth cranial nerve (waves I and II) and brainstem auditory pathways through the thalamus (waves III to V). In the newborn infant, the ABR consists primarily of waves I, III, and V, although the other waves may be present (Figure 5–25, top right trace). The absolute latencies of these waves and their interpeak intervals are longer in the newborn response than in the adult response. The component latencies systematically decrease with maturation, with wave I reaching adult values by approximately 1 to 2 months of age and wave V decreasing rapidly in latency over the first 3 months and then slowly decreasing to reach adult latencies by 3 to 5 years of age (Eggermont, 1989; Salamy, 1984). Because of the differential maturation of these 2 waves, the interpeak interval

Pearls and Perils: Auditory Evoked Potentials

1. AEPs provide an objective assessment of auditory system threshold and the integrity of central auditory pathways from the ear through the cerebral cortex.
2. The ABR does not require an awake child, so threshold determination can be accomplished in infants and children who are behaviorally difficult to test.
3. Frequency-specific ABR assessment is an important supplement to the click-evoked ABR in determining threshold at audiometric frequencies.
4. CAEPs offer the possibility of assessing higher cortical auditory processing of more complex acoustic stimuli, such as speech sounds.
5. The combination of ABR and CAEP testing can indicate the specific level(s) at which damage to the auditory pathways is present.
6. The presence of an elevated auditory threshold as determined by the ABR does not preclude normal cortical responsivity at suprathreshold levels.
7. The auditory discriminative response offers the possibility of assessing higher levels of auditory processing, including mechanisms underlying the processing of language-related functions.
8. The responses recorded from infants and children must be compared against age-matched normative data.
9. In the presence of brainstem pathway abnormalities, assessment of peripheral threshold using the ABR is compromised and results must be interpreted with caution.
10. The ABR must be interpreted with the results of tests assessing middle ear status, such as tympanometry and otoscopy, because ABR abnormalities may be of conductive, rather than sensorineural, origin.
11. Because clicks contain a wide range of frequencies, ABR threshold elevations at specific frequencies may be missed.
12. Because the MLR is not reliably recorded in children, an absent response does not imply auditory pathway dysfunction.
13. Auditory system assessment using the ABR alone cannot detect pathology at higher levels. Dysfunction at levels above the auditory brainstem pathways must be assessed using CAEPs.

continues to shorten until early childhood, indicating that brainstem pathways continue to mature long after the cochlea has reached its mature state, as indexed by Wave I latency.

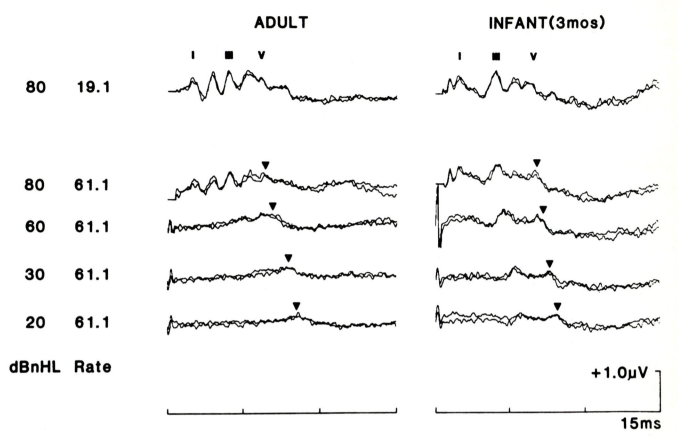

Figure 5–25. ABR to clicks recorded from a normal adult (*left*) and a preterm infant at 42 weeks postconceptional age (*right*). *Top traces:* Clicks were 80 dB nHL presented at 19.1/s, which elicit clear waves I through V in the adult and I, III, and V in the newborn. Latencies of the components are longer in the newborn compared with those in the adult. *Bottom set of traces:* Clicks were presented at 61.1/s at decreasing intensities (80, 60, 30, 20 dB nHL) to evaluate threshold. Note the presence of Wave V as indicated by the triangle in both the adult and newborn's records at 20 dB nHL, indicating normal thresholds. These data were collected by David Stapells.

Although the ABR cannot directly assess "hearing," which implies perception, it is sensitive to changes in stimulus intensity and end-organ impairment, and thus can be used to assess auditory system sensitivity, or response threshold.

Threshold Evaluation

The most frequent reason for referring a child for ABR testing is to assess auditory threshold. Detection of hearing impairment early in infancy can lead to timely therapeutic intervention, which can ameliorate the deleterious effects on the development of speech and language. The Joint Committee on Infant Hearing (1982) notes the following risk factors for hearing impairment: family history of childhood hearing impairment, congenital perinatal infection, anatomic malformations of the head and neck, very low birth weight ($\leq$ 1500 g), hyperbilirubinemia requiring exchange transfusions, bacterial meningitis, and severe neonatal asphyxia.

In applying the ABR for an assessment of auditory threshold, it is important to note that, in the presence of any brainstem pathway abnormalities, an accurate determination of threshold sensitivity is often problematic. In addition, normal "hearing" implies not only an intact peripheral and brainstem pathway, but a functional cortex as well. This can be evaluated by recording the CAEP and will be discussed in more detail shortly. The ABR must also be interpreted together with the results of tests assessing middle ear status, such as tympanometry and otoscopy, because abnormal thresholds obtained by ABR methods may be due to *conductive* rather than sensorineural dysfunction.

With these caveats kept in mind, the ABR has often proven to be an accurate reflection of auditory threshold (Finitzo-Hieber, 1982; Jerger et al., 1980). Thresholds are obtained by first rapidly presenting (11 to 19/s) the infant or child with high-intensity (60 to 80 dB nHL, i.e., above adult threshold) clicks. In the absence of pathology, this technique elicits clearly defined components of the ABR whose timing and amplitude characteristics can be compared against those in age-matched normal controls. The intensity of the click stimulation is then decreased, for example, to 60, 30, and 20 dB nHL.

To allow for more rapid data collection, the rate of stimulation is often increased, in our example from 19.1/s to 61.1/s, which does not degrade the response at high intensity (compare the responses for adult and newborn at 80 dB nHL at 19.1/s and 61.1/s). For this threshold evaluation, we are interested in the reliable presence or absence of wave V and its latency, because it is the wave most resistent to changes in stimulus characteristics. Normal threshold is defined as the presence of replicable wave Vs (within certain latency limits established with age-matched normal controls) to stimulation of clicks at ≤20 dB nHL. For neonates, normal ABR threshold is considered to be ≤30 dB nHL, but under proper testing conditions the vast majority of normal neonates have thresholds of ≤20 dB nHL.

Because the click contains a broad range of frequencies and therefore stimulates a large portion of the cochlea, it does not provide information concerning the sensitivity for *individual* frequencies. Thus, significant hearing losses (most importantly those within the frequencies present in speech sounds, which can substantially disrupt language acquisition) occasionally will be missed if only clicks are used to elicit the ABR. By recording the ABR to tones it is possible to provide the crucial information we need about sensitivity at individual frequencies (Stapells et al., 1985).

In the presence of a conductive involvement, such as otitis media or malformations of the ear such as atresia, ABR testing to *air-conducted* stimuli is often inaccurate. ABRs elicited by bone-conducted stimulation can circumvent this limitation and provide important information concerning cochlear sensitivity (Stapells and Ruben, 1989).

ABR testing for the detection or confirmation of neurologic dysfunction within the brainstem auditory pathways has also proven to be helpful in children with diverse neurologic impairments, such as leukoencephalopathies, brainstem gliomas, or hereditary degenerative disorders.

Thus, the ABR provides a useful tool for the identification of peripheral hearing impairment and auditory brainstem dysfunction. In order to assess auditory processing at levels higher than the brainstem, we must record cortical AEP.

Middle Latency Responses

The MLR, occurring between the ABR and the later CAEP, consists of a series of components that occur up to 50 to 100 milliseconds after stimulus onset. They are thought to reflect the initial activation of auditory cortex (Scherg and von Cramon, 1986). Up to six components (Na, Pa, Nb, Pb, Nc, and Pc) have been identified as part of the response, but only two of them, Na (occurring 15 milliseconds after stimulation) and Pa (occurring approximately 30 milliseconds after stimulation), are reliably recorded in normal adults (Figure 5–26, top

left). The clinical use of MLR recording in infants and young children is limited because the probability of reliably recording the responses is low in children under 5 years of age (see Figure 5–26), but increases with maturation (Kraus et al., 1985; Kurtzberg et al., 1988). If an MLR is reliably recorded in an individual child, it suggests that the pathway between the brainstem and cortical areas is intact. The absence of a response, however, cannot be taken as evidence of auditory pathway dysfunction (Stapells et al., 1988).

Cortical Auditory Evoked Potentials

Cortical auditory system processing at higher levels can be assessed by the later-occurring CAEP. Before the discovery of the ABR, attempts were made to use the CAEP as an objective measure of auditory system threshold (Barnet and Lodge, 1966; Rapin et al., 1970; Taguchi et al., 1969). Because the CAEPs are more variable than the ABR near threshold, their audiometric application was not successful and the recording of CAEPs for clinical purposes fell into disuse. CAEPs, however, offer the possibility of assessing higher levels of cortical processing of more complex suprathreshold auditory stimuli containing acoustic features that are essential for the normal acquisition of speech and language. Although click and tonal stimuli elicit CAEPs that can be used to assess cortical auditory responsiveness, more useful information can be obtained by using sounds with more complex acoustic features of linguistic stimuli. Stop-consonant vowel syllables (e.g., /da/, /ta/, /ba/, /pa/, /ga/, /ka/), which comprise the most salient characteristics of human speech, have been employed successfully in the evaluation of higher cortical auditory processing (e.g., Kurtzberg et al., 1988).

The CAEPs elicited by these speech sounds in the newborn infant recorded over the midline central region consist of a series of positive deflections followed by a negative wave (Figure 5–27). These potentials differ in timing and amplitude depending on the stimulus employed and the age of the child at recording. In the neonate, the largest positivity occurs at approximately 300 milliseconds and the later large negativity peaks at approximately 600 milliseconds after stimulus onset. On the basis of scalp topography and intracranial recordings of the same speech sounds in monkeys (Steinschneider et al., 1980, 1982), these potentials are believed to reflect neural activity generated in primary auditory cortex, located in the superior surface of the temporal lobe within the sylvian fissure.

A response with a different waveshape and maturational time course is recorded overlying the lateral temporal regions of the scalp (Figure 5–27). In the neonate, the most lateral response consists primarily of a negative wave peaking at approximately 275 milliseconds after the onset of the stimulus. This lateral temporal response, which is presumed to be generated in secondary auditory

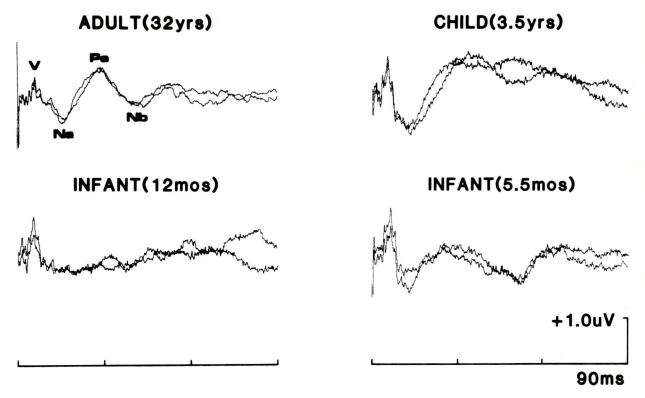

ADULT(32yrs)

CHILD(3.5yrs)

INFANT(12mos)

INFANT(5.5mos)

+1.0uV

90ms

Figure 5-26. MLRs recorded from a normal adult and three normal children at 3½ years, 12 months, and 5½ months. The adult record shows a clear ABR wave V and MLR waves Na, Pa, and Nb. The waveforms recorded from the children demonstrate three typical patterns seen in the pediatric population. The 5½-month-old infant's record is similar to that of the adult response. The 3½-year-old's MLR consists of an Na and a late, broad component, which may be Pa. The 12-month-old infant's recording shows only a wave V (ABR) and no MLR components. Stimuli were 70 dB nHL clicks delivered at 10.9/s with EEG amplifiers set at 10 to 1500 Hz. These data were collected by David Stapells.

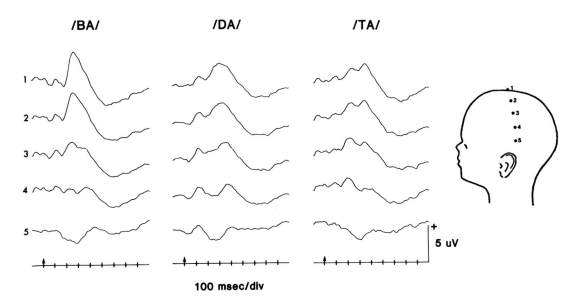

/BA/   /DA/   /TA/

5 uV

100 msec/div

Figure 5-27. Grand mean CAEPs recorded to the speech sounds /ba/, /da/, and /ta/ in a group of normal full-term infants. Note the series of positive deflections recorded overlying the midline central region of the scalp and the negative component overlying the lateral temporal area. These have a different maturational course, with the lateral temporal response lagging somewhat behind the CAEP recorded at the midline. The waveshape and amplitude of the responses differ as a function of the auditory stimulus. Arrow indicates stimulus onset.

cortex withing the superior temporal gyrus, shows a 2- to 3-month maturational sequence that lags behind the midline central response (Kurtzberg et al., 1984a).

There are progressive changes in waveshape, amplitude, and latency of these responses during the course of maturation, so, as with all EP studies, an individual patient's responses must be compared against age-matched normative data.

To assess the utility of early recordings of speech sound CAEPs in the assessment of auditory cortical processing integrity, we studied infants who were at high risk for subsequent speech and language dysfunction owing to extreme low birth weight (≤ 1500g), neonatal asphyxia, or both (Kurtzberg et al., 1988). CAEPs were recorded in these babies at 40 weeks postconceptional age and scored as being either normal or abnormal based on comparisons with the responses recorded from healthy full-term neonates. At 1 year corrected age, these children were tested at follow-up with the Sequenced Inventory of Communication Development, a standardized test of emerging receptive and expressive language function. The babies who showed normal CAEPs to speech sounds were significantly more likely to show normal receptive language function at 1 year of age than babies who had deviant CAEPs. Although still a research procedure, recording of CAEPs to speech sounds appears to be promising for predicting emerging language function in high-risk babies. In older children with possible developmental language dysfunction, the technique also provides a useful index of processing integrity at the cortical level.

Identification of Multilevel Involvement

Damage to the auditory system can occur at any level along the pathway, from the periphery through the cerebral cortex. The medical history of individual infants and children may place them at higher risk for selective and often diverse patterns of auditory system dysfunction. For example, premature infants are at risk for damage to the auditory system from the ear through the cerebral cortex. Middle-ear infections, ototoxicity owing to antibiotic therapy, and damage to brainstem pathways, subcortical white matter, and cortex associated with hypoxic-ischemic encephalopathy may produce quite varied patterns of dysfunction. Combined assessment using both ABR and CAEP can identify the level or levels of dysfunction. In our experience, using ABR and CAEP recordings, we have observed cortical auditory dysfunction without evidence of peripheral or brainstem dysfunction, and normal cortical functioning to complex speech signals is present despite evidence of peripheral or brainstem dysfunction (Cone-Wesson et al., 1987; Kurtzberg et al., 1988; Gravel et al., 1989).

The most important implication of these findings is that auditory system assessment using the ABR alone is incomplete and can fail to detect pathology at higher levels. Furthermore, the presence of an elevated auditory threshold as determined by the ABR does not necessarily preclude a normal cortical response at suprathreshold levels.

Discriminative Responses

Event-related potentials can be recorded in tasks that require discriminative stimulus processing. The best-known and most easily applied electrophysiologic technique for the pediatric population is provided by the "oddball" paradigm. One stimulus (e.g., the speech sound /da/) is presented repetitively and replaced on a small percentage of the trials by a second stimulus that varies along some acoustic dimension (e.g., /ta/). The ERP to the repetitively presented stimulus resembles the response to the same stimulus when presented alone. However, the response to the infrequent or "rare" stimulus differs. In addition to eliciting similar early components, additional longer-latency components appear; the most prominent one in the adult and older child is called P3 or P300. These potentials are seen not only when the subject actively responds to the oddball stimulus, but also when he or she is listening passively to the stimulus train. The latter circumstance, a cortical "orienting response," makes it possible to use the passive oddball paradigm in infants who cannot actively respond to the different stimulus. In the young infant, long-latency potentials are also elicited to the rare stimulus (Courchesne et al., 1981; Kurtzberg et al., 1988). These potentials are characterized by a large negative component overlying the frontal regions of the scalp. The occurrence of these potentials indicates that the infant's brain has processed the acoustic properties of the stimuli and has discriminated between them.

Although the discriminative potentials are not at present routinely used for clinical purposes, they offer the promise of evaluating higher cortical auditory processing, including more complex language-related functions, such as lexical and semantic abilities in young children.

SOMATOSENSORY EVOKED POTENTIALS

SEPs in young infants and children are used to evaluate the somatosensory pathways from the peripheral nerve through the cerebral cortex. As with EP measures of visual and auditory pathway integrity, the SEP is particularly useful in infants and children from whom it is impossible or difficult to obtain an accurate evaluation of sensory functioning using standard clinical procedures. Infants and children most often are referred for SEP testing when they present with possible spinal cord lesions, degenerative diseases, gait disturbances, and weakness (Fagan et al., 1987).

Although routine SEP recording can evaluate to a

limited degree the integrity of the peripheral nerve being stimulated, it is important to have a complete assessment of peripheral nerve function before the child is referred for SEP testing. Interpretation of central SEP abnormalities is not possible without complete information on the integrity of peripheral nerve function.

For SEP recording, stimulation usually consists of a brief shock to the skin overlying the peripheral nerve at an intensity sufficient to elicit a brief motor response (e.g., thumb twitch). Stimulation of the median nerve to assess the pathways of the upper extremities, and the peroneal or tibial for lower extremity evaluation, is most often used. Because recordings reflect afferent volleys of neural impulses within the peripheral nerve, dorsal columns, medial lemniscus, and thalamocortical radiations, as well as activity within somatosensory cortex (Arezzo et al., 1979, 1981; Desmedt and Cheron, 1982), localization of the specific level of dysfunction is possible. In addition, measures of peripheral nerve conduction velocity as well as central transmission times through the spinal cord, brainstem structures, and somatosensory cortex are obtainable.

For median nerve stimulation (Figure 5–28), the first response typically recorded overlies the brachial plexus (a negativity at 9 milliseconds after stimulation called N9, using the adult nomenclature for latency). The second component is called N11; it is recorded overlying the spinal cord at C7 and reflects activity within the cervical cord dorsal columns. The third component, N13, is recorded overlying the mid-inion region of the scalp and reflects the afferent volley of the brainstem lemniscal pathways. A component at a similar latency can be seen overlying the cervical cord and represents local synaptic activity within the dorsal horn. Two components reflect cortical activity: N20, representing the initial activation of somatosensory cortex within the banks of the central sulcus, and P23, reflecting neural activity within the crown of the post-central gyrus.

Lower-extremity SEPs most commonly are elicited by stimulation of the peroneal nerve at the knee or the posterior tibial nerve at the ankle. Responses are recorded from electrodes placed over the cauda equina, thoracic and lumbar spine, and contralateral somatosensory cortex, from which nerve conduction velocity, transmission time through the spinal cord, and thalamocortical pathways can be assessed.

In the pediatric population, it is important to remember that there are changes in the EPs with age as in the visual and auditory system. In the somatosensory system, however, it is crucial to remember that as the child grows there is an increase in the length of the somatosensory pathways, and, therefore, if conduction velocity remains constant, absolute conduction time will be increased. This increase is offset to various degrees, however, by the systematic decrease in conduction velocities that is presumably due to increased myelina-

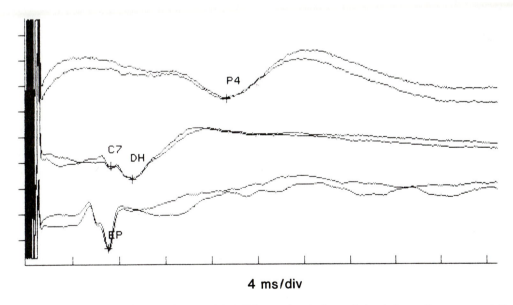

4 ms/div

Figure 5–28. SEPs recorded from a 2-year-old child to stimulation of the left median nerve at the wrist. Constant-current stimulation at a rate of 6.1/s was delivered at an intensity to elicit a motor response (thumb twitch). Each replicated trace consists of 1000 stimuli. *Bottom trace:* Erb's point potential (EP or N9) reflects the afferent volley from the median nerve to the brachial plexus and provides a measure of peripheral nerve conduction velocity. *Middle trace:* Responses recorded over C7 of the spinal cord indicating spinal root entry latency (N11) and response at dorsal horn (DH), which reflects synaptic activity within the spinal cord itself. *Upper trace:* SEP recorded over right parietal somatosensory cortex (at P4). Note the clearly formed negative component (N20), representing the initial activation of somatosensory cortex, followed by a large positive component (P23).

Pearls and Perils: Somatosensory Evoked Potentials

1. SEPs offer the possibility of objectively evaluating the integrity of peripheral and central somesthetic pathways in infants and children in whom standard clinical assessments are impossible or unreliable.
2. SEPs can determine the level of dysfunction along the somatosensory pathways from the peripheral nerve through somatosensory cortex.
3. SEPs are valuable when used intraoperatively to monitor spinal cord and brainstem structures during surgical procedures that might compromise their function.
4. Before referring a child for SEP testing, it is important to assess peripheral nerve function adequately, because interpretation of central somatosensory pathway abnormality is problematic in the presence of peripheral neuropathy.
5. Because the maturation of SEP components is rapid during childhood and the length of the pathway increases with the growth of the child, SEPs recorded from infants and children must be compared against age- and size-matched normative data.

tion within the nervous system. Thus, both age-specific and size-related normative data are mandatory (Taylor and Fagan, 1988).

Intraoperative recording of SEPs has also been used successfully to monitor the integrity of the spinal cord and brainstem during surgical procedures that might compromise these structures. This technique has been applied most commonly in the pediatric population during surgery for spinal cord lesions and scoliosis.

SEPs have not been as fully exploited in the pediatric as in the adult population, but their usefulness cannot be underestimated, especially for evaluating peripheral nerve and spinal cord dysfunction.

COGNITIVE EVENT-RELATED POTENTIALS

In the infant and the very young child, we are limited to recording ERPs to the passive presentation of stimuli. As noted in the preceding sections, much information about the integrity of sensory pathways and cortical responsiveness can be obtained by these methods. By the time a child is 4 to 5 years old, however, he or she is able to participate actively in studies that tap higher cognitive and language functions (Kurtzberg et al., 1979; Courchesne, 1983; Kurtzberg et al., 1984b). Although these techniques are largely in the "research and development" phase, a description of the clinical use of ERPs would be incomplete without mentioning the cognitive ERPs. In these studies, children are asked to evaluate and respond to the stimulation according to the demands of the task. For example, in the oddball paradigm, children would be asked to respond whenever the stimulus changes within a train of repeated stimuli. This behavioral response tells us that the child is successfully discriminating the stimuli. The timing and scalp configuration of the concurrently recorded cortical activity tell us about the neural mechanisms underlying this stimulus evaluation and decision-making process.

Complex tasks that assess specific functions, such as language processing are currently being used with children. These tasks engage specific aspects of the linguistic system, from simple phonemic discrimination to complex verbal and semantic processes, and have been successfully employed in the adult (e.g., Kutas and Hillyard, 1980; Novick et al., 1985). This work must first define the normal ERP patterns associated with various cognitive tasks, so that deviant patterns can be detected in children with possible linguistic or other cognitive dysfunction. In the near future, it is likely that the cognitive ERPs will provide clinically important tools for assessing disorders of higher cerebral function in children.

Acknowledgments

Preparation of this section and research reported herein were supported in part by grants from the USPHS (DC00224, HD01799, DC00223, and NS20489). I wish to thank Herbert G. Vaughan, Jr., and Judith A. Kreuzer for their valuable critique of the manuscript and David R. Stapells not only for his helpful suggestions, but also for providing Figures 5–25 and 5–26.

ANNOTATED BIBLIOGRAPHY

Kurtzberg D, Vaughan HG Jr: Electrophysiologic assessment of auditory and visual function in the newborn. *Clin Perinatol* 12:277–299, 1985.

  This paper is a review of the electrophysiologic techniques available to assess auditory and visual pathways in the newborn infant. It reviews not only the methodology but also research in the area.

Sokol S: Measurement of infant visual acuity from pattern reversal evoked potentials. *Vision Res* 18:33–39, 1978.

  This article provides a description of obtaining an objective estimate of visual acuity using the pattern reversal VEP.

Kurtzberg D, Stapells DR, Wallace IF: Event-related potential assessment of auditory system integrity: Implications for language development; in Vietze P, Vaughan HG Jr (eds): *Early Identification of Infants with Developmental Disabilities.* Philadelphia, Grune & Stratton, 1988, p 160–180.

  This chapter provides a comprehensive review of electrophysiologic techniques to evaluate sequential levels of the auditory system in infants and children and a discussion of how the results of these tests relate to early language outcome.

Fagan ER, Taylor MJ, Logan WJ: Somatosensory evoked potentials. Part I. A review of neural generators and special considerations in pediatrics. *Pediatr Neurol* 3:189–196, 1987.

Fagan ER, Taylor MJ, Logan WJ: Somatosensory evoked potentials. Part II. A review of the clinical applications in pediatric neurology. *Pediatr Neurol* 3:249–255, 1987.

These papers review the general methodology and usefulness of recording SEPs in infants and children based on over 900 studies performed in the authors' laboratories.

REFERENCES

Arezzo J, Legatt AD, Vaughan HG Jr: Topography and intracranial sources of somatosensory evoked potentials in the monkey. I. Early components. *Electroencephalogr Clin Neurophysiol* 46:155–172, 1979.

Arezzo J, Vaughan HG Jr, Legatt AD: Topography and intracranial sources of somatosensory evoked potentials in the monkey. II. Cortical components. *Electroencephalogr Clin Neurophysiol* 51:1–18, 1981.

Barnet AB, Lodge A: Diagnosis of deafness in infants with the use of computer averaged electroencephalographic responses to sound. *J Pediatr* 69:753–758, 1966.

Cone-Wesson B, Kurtzberg D, Vaughan HG Jr: Electrophysiologic assessment of auditory pathways in high risk infants. *Int J Ped Otorhinolaryngol* 14:203–214, 1987.

Courchesne E: Cognitive components of the event-related brain potential: Changes associated with development, in Gaillard AWK, Ritter W (eds): *Tutorials in Event Related Potentials Research: Endogenous Components.* Amsterdam, North-Holland, 1983, p 143–158.

Courchesne E, Ganz L, Norcia AM: Event-related brain potentials to human faces in infants. *Child Dev* 52:804–811, 1981.

Desmedt JE, Cheron G: Somatosensory evoked potentials in man: Subcortical and cortical components and their neural basis. *Ann NY Acad Sci* 388:388–411, 1982.

Eggermont JJ: The onset and development of auditory function: Contributions of evoked potential studies. *J Speech-Language Pathol Audiol* 13:5–16, 1989.

Fagan ER, Taylor MJ, Lorgan WJ: Somatosensory evoked potentials. Part I. A review of neural generators and special considerations in pediatrics. *Pediatr Neurol* 3:189–196, 1987.

Finitzo-Hieber T: Auditory brainstem response: Its place in infant audiologic evaluations. *Semin Speech Language Hearing* 3:76–87, 1982.

Frank Y, Kurtzberg D, Kreuzer JA, Vaughan HG Jr: Flash and pattern reversal visual evoked potential abnormalities in infants and children with "cerebral blindness." Poster presented at the Annual Meeting of the Child Neurology Society, Halifax, Nova Scotia, September 15–17, 1988.

Gravel JS, Kurtzberg D, Stapells DR, Wallace IF, Vaughan HG, Jr: Assessment of auditory system integrity in infants and young children. *Semin Hearing* 10, 1989.

Jerger J, Hayes D, Jordan C: Clinical experience with auditory brainstem response audiometry in pediatric assessment. *Ear and Hearing* 1:19–25, 1980.

Joint Committee on Infant Hearing. Position statement. *Pediatrics* 70:496–497, 1982.

Klein SK, Kurtzberg D, Rapin I: Auditory comprehension in children with verbal auditory agnosia. Poster presented at the Annual Meeting of the Child Neurology Society, Halifax, Nova Scotia, September 15–17, 1988.

Kraus N, Smith DI, Reed NL, Stein LK, Cartee C: Auditory middle latency responses in children: Effects of age and diagnostic category. *Electroencephalogr Clin Neurophysiol* 62:343–351, 1985.

Kurtzberg D: Event-related potentials in the evaluation of high-risk infants. *Ann NY Acad Sci* 388:557–571, 1982.

Kurtzberg D, Vaughan HG Jr, Kreuzer J: Task-related cortical potentials in children. *Progr Clin Neurophysiol* 6:216–223, 1979.

Kurtzberg D, Hilpert PL, Kreuzer JA, Vaughan HG Jr: Differential maturation of cortical auditory evoked potentials to speech sounds in normal full term and very low-birthweight infants. *Dev Med Child Neurol* 26:466–475, 1984a.

Kurtzberg D, Vaughan HG Jr, Courchesne E, Friedman D, Harter MR, Putnam LE: Developmental aspects of event related potentials. *Ann NY Acad Sci* 425:300–318, 1984b.

Kurtzberg D, Stapells DR, Wallace IF: Event-related potential assessment of auditory system integrity: Implications for language development, in Vietze P, Vaughan HG Jr (eds): *Early Identification of Infants with Developmental Disabilities.* Philadelphia, Grune & Stratton, 1988, p 160–180.

Kutas M, Hillyard SA: Reading senseless sentences: Brain potentials reflect semantic incongruity. *Science* 207:203–204, 1980.

Moskowitz A, Sokol S: Developmental changes in the human visual system as reflected by the latency of the pattern reversal VEP. *Electroencephalogr Clin Neurophysiol* 56:1–15, 1983.

Novick B, Lovrich D, Vaughan HG Jr: Event-related potentials associated with the discrimination of acoustic and semantic aspects of speech. *Neuropsychologia* 23:87–101, 1985.

Rapin I, Ruben RJ, Lyttle M: Diagnosis of hearing loss in infants using auditory evoked responses. *Laryngoscope* 80:712–722, 1970.

Salamy A: Maturation of the auditory brainstem response from birth through early childhood. *J Clin Neurophysiol* 1:293–329, 1984.

Scherg M, von Cramon D: Evoked dipole source potentials of the human auditory cortex. *Electroencephalogr Clin Neurophysiol* 65:344–360, 1986.

Sokol S: Measurement of infant visual acuity from pattern reversal evoked potentials. *Vision Res* 18:33–39, 1978.

Sokol S, Hansen VC, Moskowitz A, Greenfield P, Towle VL: Evoked potential and preferential looking estimates of visual acuity in pediatric patients. *Ophthalmologica* 90:552–562, 1983.

Stapells DR, Galambos R, Costello JA, Makeig S: Inconsistency of auditory middle latency and steady-state responses in infants. *Electroencephalogr Clin Neurophysiol* 71:289–295, 1988.

Stapells DR, Picton TW, Perez-Abalo M, Read D, Smith A: Frequency specificity in evoked potential audiometry, in Jacobson JT (ed): *The Auditory Brainstem Response.* San Diego, College Hill Press, 1985, p 147–177.

Stapells DR, Ruben RJ: Auditory brainstem responses to bone-conducted tones in infants. *Ann Otol Rhinol Laryngol* 98:941–949, 1989.

Steinschneider M, Arezzo JC, Vaughan HG Jr: Phase-locked cortical responses to a human speech sound and low-frequency tones in the monkey. *Brain Res* 198:75–84, 1980.

Steinschneider M, Arezzo JC, Vaughan HG Jr: Speech evoked activity in the auditory radiations and cortex of the awake monkey. *Brain Res* 252:353–365, 1982.

Taguchi K, Picton TW, Orpin JA, Goodman WS: Evoked response audiometry in newborn infants. *Acta Oto-Laryngol Suppl* 252:5–17, 1969.

Taylor MJ, Fagan ER: SEPs to median nerve stimulation: Normative data for pediatrics. *Electroencephalogr Clin Neurophysiol* 71:323–330, 1988.

Neuroimaging Techniques

Pauline A. Filipek and Johan G. Blickman

INDICATIONS FOR IMAGING STUDY

The relatively new ability to visualize brain tissue directly by means of cranial ultrasound (US), computed tomography (CT) and magnetic resonance imaging (MRI) has significantly enhanced the diagnostic capabilities of the pediatric neurologist. With the advent of each new technologic development, the information obtained has increased dramatically. It is therefore useful to review the capabilities, limitations, and indications of these new diagnostic modalities. The following guidelines are necessarily generalizations; each patient must always be considered individually in light of the need for, cost of, and diagnostic question(s) to be answered by an imaging study.

An imaging study is indicated in any child with evidence of increased intracranial pressure, enlarging head circumference, progressive focal neurologic signs, coma of uncertain etiology, suspected vascular malformation, hemorrhage, or mass lesion. With regard to chronic encephalopathy, an imaging study may not alter the treatment of the child, but, in specific situations, may be considered for the genetic, prognostic, and especially morphologic evaluation (Ferry, 1980). The prematurely born infant often routinely undergoes cranial US, as it has been well demonstrated that the sequelae of germinal matrix hemorrhage can be easily identified when screened for, while neurodevelopmental prognosis can be attempted (Blickman et al., 1991).

In most children with a normal neurologic examination, an imaging study is generally not necessary. This includes those children presenting with tension or migraine headaches (Ferry, 1980), and those who have had head trauma but either are asymptomatic or complain only of mild to moderate headache or dizziness, or have scalp hematoma or lacerations without loss of consciousness (Masters et al., 1987; Ferry, 1980).

CRANIAL ULTRASOUND

In the early 1970s, neonatal intensive care units were developed when it became obvious that very premature neonates of less than 32 weeks gestation could be kept alive (Volpe, 1987). There was, however, a high risk for intracranial hemorrhage and posthemorrhagic complications, for which cranial US became the screening method of choice. The procedure can be carried out in the neonatal intensive care unit as the machine is small, portable, and accurate.

Such real-time scanning through the anterior fontanelle can be performed by a sector scanhead or a linear array scanhead. These scanheads use either an isolating single oscillating crystal or an array of crystals with piezoelectric properties (a property of quartz and some ceramics that allows them to transform electrical impulses into sound waves and subsequently receive reflected sound waves and transform them back into electrical impulses). These electrical impulses are transformed into a gray scale that allows for structural differentiation based on how different tissue structures (such as cerebrospinal fluid (CSF), brain, or bone) reflect the ultrasonic beam.

Matrix cameras with six images per film are used to record these live images as hard-copy records. This procedure allows a standardized set of images in both the coronal and the sagittal scanning planes to be developed (Figure 5–29). However, the operator dependency of cranial ultrasonography needs to be kept in mind when interpreting these static images (Grant et al., 1988; Volpe, 1987; Blickman et al., 1991).

Doppler imaging allows the visualization of blood flow in the intracranial vessels, in particular the circle of Willis and the pericallosal arteries. This study has been shown to have predictive value, particularly when issues such as brain death and extracorporeal membrane oxygenation (ECMO) arise (McMenamin and Volpe, 1983; Taylor et al., 1987). Color flow Doppler imaging is a further refinement that will allow for more diagnostic information to be obtained in conjunction with clinical neurologic questions.

Indications for Cranial Ultrasound

Prematurity

It has been well demonstrated that US can identify and thus screen for ventricular dilatation and hemorrhage in the premature infant. Bleeding can occur intraparenchymally or intraventricularly, or be limited to the germinal matrix (Figure 5–30). Although many grading schemes for intracranial hemorrhage have been devised over the years, for practical purposes the following version (Blickman et al., 1991; Volpe, 1987) is most frequently used:

Grade I	Germinal matrix hemorrhage.
Grade II	Intraventricular hemorrhage with minimal dilatation of the ventricular system.
Grade III	Intraventricular hemorrhage with distended and/or blood-filled ventricular system.
Grade IV	Extension of the intraventricular hemorrhage into the brain parenchyma.

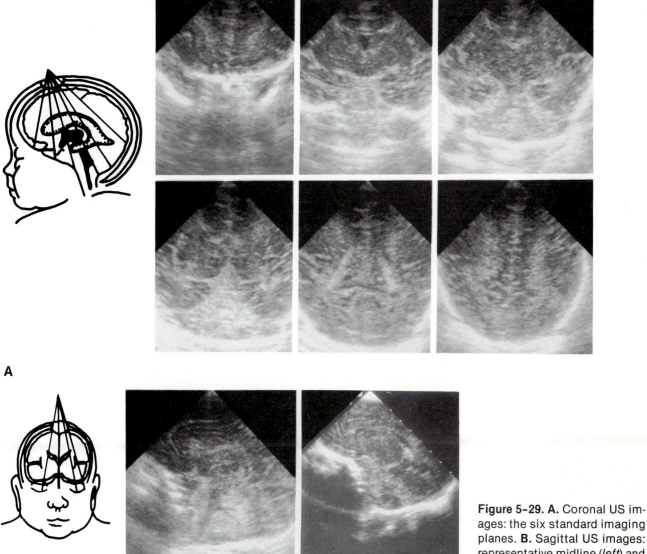

Figure 5–29. A. Coronal US images: the six standard imaging planes. **B.** Sagittal US images: representative midline (*left*) and off-center (*right*) planes.

Any grading system is only an attempt to arrive at a clinical prognosis from imaging information. As this is at best an imprecise process, rigid conclusions should not be inferred from it. In general, grades I and II have little, while grades III and IV have a significant impact on morbidity, mortality and neurodevelopmental outcome (Hayden and Swischuk, 1987).

The proper timing of cranial US in the premature neonate to follow intracranial hemorrhage and its sequelae is controversial. A consensus opinion states that infants of fewer than 32 weeks of gestation, or lower than 1500 g birth weight, should be screened within the first 7 days of life, as one third of premature infants with a normal study on day 1 may develop intracranial hemorrhage before 5 days of life (Pape and Wigglesworth, 1979). If major neurologic changes have occurred, or if there is a clinical change such as a significant drop in hematocrit or blood in the CSF, an immediate US evaluation is, of course, indicated. Subarachnoid or subdural hemorrhages are difficult to evaluate with cranial US as the convexities are difficult to image because of less than optimal lateral resolution.

If the findings are normal, no further examinations need be performed. If there is intracranial hemorrhage, weekly interval studies are recommended. Following discharge, a repeat study every 3 to 6 months for a year is sufficient.

A major screening role for US is found in patients undergoing ECMO, which may be instituted for extreme neonatal pulmonary insufficiency. ECMO will not be considered if intracranial hemorrhage or leukomalacia is identified by US.

Hemorrhage into the brain parenchyma can occur either as a sequela of germinal matrix hemorrhage, as

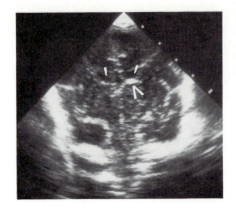

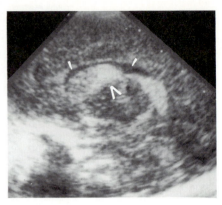

A   **B**

Figure 5-30. Coronal (**A**) and sagittal (**B**) cranial US images from a preterm infant with a grade I germinal matrix hemorrhage (*open arrowheads*), also showing the lateral ventricles (*solid arrowheads*).

mentioned previously, or as a sequela of birth trauma, Rh incompatibility, or other vascular insults. Cerebral infarctions, either iatrogenic as a consequence of intravascular catheters or idiopathic in etiology, can be diagnosed early by screening US.

Periventricular Leukomalacia

Periventricular infarction of the white matter is manifested by increased echogenicity projecting off the lateral ventricles, which, on sequential US examinations, may be seen to transform into cystic areas (Figure 5-31). It occurs in 5% to 10% of premature infants and is presumed to be due to hypoxemic damage to the white matter, causing necrosis. The commonly involved areas are the trigone of the lateral ventricles and at the level of the foramen of Monroe, corresponding to watershed areas of intracranial blood flow. These changes are characterized ultrasonographically by broad zones of increased periventricular echogenicity that can be symmetric but not necessarily homogeneous. The resulting "swiss cheese" appearance of the cystic transformation appears about 2 to 3 weeks after the appearance of the echodense areas (Grant et al., 1988; Creed and Haber, 1984; Volpe, 1987).

Hypoxic-Ischemic Encephalopathy

Anoxic states, either perinatal or secondary to brain edema, can also be diagnosed on US. Because these are insults primarily affecting the midline circle of Willis area, US is exquisitely suitable. It is characterized by hemorrhagic necrosis, primarily in the basal ganglia and thalamus. Intracranial edema is characterized by loss of normal sulcal marking the immature brain, but may be difficult to detect in the premature brain. Its sequelae, atrophy in virtually all cases, can be detected on coronal scans, particularly by detecting widening of the interhemispheric fissure (Volpe, 1987).

Developmental Malformations

Cranial US is a very sensitive and specific tool to evaluate congenital anomalies of the central nervous system. Congenital hydrocephalus, agenesis or lipoma of the corpus callosum, Dandy-Walker malformation (Figure 5-32), as well as arachnoid cysts, holoprosencephaly, and vein of Galen aneurysms, can be exquisitely delineated by US (Grant et al., 1988; Blickman et al., 1991). Any structural intracranial abnormality, however, can be better delineated by CT or MRI, which can define the anatomy in multiple planes. Conditions such as an encephalocele,

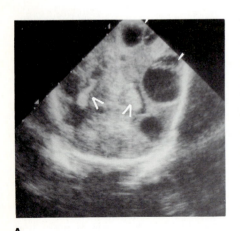

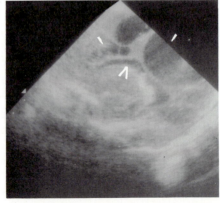

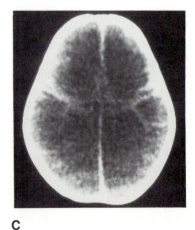

A   **B**   **C**

Figure 5-31. Coronal (**A**) and sagittal (**B**) US images from a preterm infant with periventricular leukomalacia. Note the large cystic regions (*solid arrowheads*) clearly defined on the US images, which are not visualized on the CT scan (**C**). Also note the lateral ventricles and choriod plexus (*open arrowheads*).

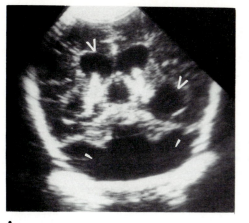
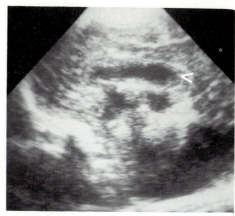
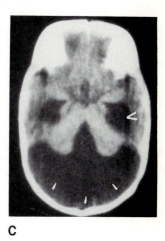

A   B   C

Figure 5–32. Coronal (**A**) and sagittal (**B**) US images next to a transaxial CT scan (**C**) of a Dandy-Walker cyst (*solid arrowheads*). Note also the enlarged frontal and temporal horns of the lateral ventricles (*open arrowheads*) as well as the clear definition of the cyst on the US images.

vein of Galen aneurysm, and malignancies—although are—necessarily benefit from a multimodal, imaging approach, especially from a clinical perspective.

Vascular Disease

Although ischemic or hemorrhagic insults in the parenchyma in infants are rare, cranial US will occasionally demonstrate them. Once again, however, owing to its limited definition of the convexities, CT or MRI will also be needed.

Techniques for Doppler evaluation, although still being developed, will no doubt further enhance the evaluation of intracranial vascular disease, in particular ischemic disease (Grant et al., 1988; Taylor et al., 1987).

Infection

The numerous sequelae of intracranial infection can be managed successfully by US. Meningitis is associated with echogenic sulci (seen in about 40% of patients), extra-axial fluid collections, and ventricular dilation. Abscess formation and cystic degeneration may also be identified. The most easily identifiable finding is ventriculitis, which occurs in up to 90% of cases of bacterial meningitis in infants. By the second or third week, debris may be seen within the ventricles. The TORCH infections, especially herpes simplex, are characterized by a particular pattern of periventricular and thalamic echogenic structures (Cleveland et al., 1987; Teele et al., 1988).

COMPUTED TOMOGRAPHY

During the past 15 years, CT scanning has revolutionized the diagnostic capabilities of clinicians by permitting direct radiologic visualization of brain parenchyma, its anatomic configuration, and any abnormalities resulting from disease states (Hershey and Zimmerman, 1985; Ferry, 1980). A CT scanner uses a narrow rotating x-ray beam and crystal detectors, which are located in a circle around the gantry of the scanner. The scanner itself is approximately 36 in. in diameter and 12 to 18 in. deep. During the acquisition of each tomographic slice, the x-ray tube and detectors rotate in a linear fashion around the head through 360°, thus obtaining x-ray absorption coefficient data for the entire field. The computer transforms this data by Fourier analysis into a gray scale to create the image, and the procedure is repeated for each slice (Gomez and Reese, 1976).

Indications for Contrast Agents

A cranial CT scan performed to diagnose intracranial hemorrhage or calcifications should be performed without

---

Pearls and Perils: Cranial Ultrasound

1. The portable sector scanner permits bedside evaluations in critically ill infants. Repeat examinations are performed with relative ease.
2. Because the transducer head is hand-held and easily maneuvered, patient sedation or positional manipulation is rarely necessary (Grant et al., 1988).
3. There are no known risks or deleterious effects associated with even repeated use of cranial US because it uses no ionizing radiation.
4. Only the central brain structures can be adequately imaged owing to limited peripheral resolution.
5. Cranial US is only useful up until about 12 months of age, when the anterior fontanelle closes.
6. The technique is extremely operator dependent, and its results are difficult to interpret for a clinician without imaging experience.

Pearls and Perils: CT Scanning

1. Relative to cranial US, CT can adequately visualize the entire brain parenchyma, including the convexities and peripheral regions of the hemispheres.
2. The requisite CT scanning time is relatively brief, approximately 20 minutes.
3. In trauma and other emergency settings, CT is the gold standard.
4. CT scans are usually obtained only in the transaxial plane, potentially limiting the visualization of anatomic structures or lesions. Direct coronal images can be obtained, but only as part of a procedure that involves uncomfortable patient positioning, thus decreasing the technique's effective use in the pediatric population.
5. A CT scan requires exposure to ionizing radiation to produce the images, although these measured doses are within accepted ranges (Ferry, 1980).
6. The use of intravenous contrast agents carries the risk of allergic reaction (Ferry, 1980). Nonionic contrast agents, although ten times as expensive, will reduce this risk by 40% to 60%.

the use of intravenous contrast agents, as either may be obscured by the vascular enhancement. The assessment of ventricular size alone does not require contrast enhancement.

Children with signs of increased intracranial pressure, enlarging head circumference, or focal neurologic dysfunction warrant a CT study with the use of intravenous contrast agents to delineate a possible mass lesion. About 80% of all cranial CT scans in children are performed without intravenous contrast administration.

At this time nonionic contrast media should be reserved for those children who have either a history of previous reaction to ionic agents, atopy, or difficult venous access.

MAGNETIC RESONANCE IMAGING

As a neuroimaging technique, MRI has provided an unprecedented method for radiologically visualizing the brain, producing anatomic definition of brain substructures and lesions at a level that was previously available only in postmortem anatomic studies. Although it is still considered a relatively "new" technologic advance, studies have shown MRI to be superior to CT in the visualization of the normal and diseased brain. In many situations, MRI may obviate the need for more invasive

imaging modalities, thus substantially reducing the risks inherent in a diagnostic evaluation. MRI has become a routine imaging modality—one that complements and, in many situations, supersedes the CT scan as the neuroimaging method of choice.

The conventional MR imaging system consists of a large magnet, with magnetic field strengths ranging up to 2.0 Tesla (T) (20 MG). The magnet is either of the permanent variety, up to 0.5 T, or a superconducting magnet, up to 2 T. The patient rests entirely within a tunnel (the gantry) during the imaging session, on an adjustable table that is 6 to 8 ft in length (Figure 5–33A). For brain imaging, a head coil is used, which resembles a helmet approximately 30 cm in diameter (Figure 5–33B), with an open window in front of the face. For spine imaging, the patient rests on a body coil, which resembles a firm flat cushion of variable size.

During the actual scan acquisition, a thumping or tapping noise is caused by the radiofrequency pulse crossing the magnetic field. It is occasionally loud enough to cause discomfort to the patient; ear plugs are usually available from the technicians. Currently, only proton (1H) imaging is clinically available, and this discussion will therefore be limited to proton MRI.

Sedation

The patient must be capable of remaining motionless for approximately 8 to 10 minutes for each of at least two acquisitions, plus the time necessary to tune the gradients. Because the MRI slices are obtained in a repetitive sequential fashion, isolated movements (even deep respirations) affect the entire acquisition; individual slices cannot be repeated, as with a CT scan. As a result, most young infants and developmentally impaired children will require sedation for a successful scanning procedure.

It has been the author's experience that many preschool and most early-school-age children will tolerate and cooperate fully with an MRI scan if they have been prepared prior to the actual appointment and are "talked through" the session with continuous encouragement by a parent or other individual who remains at the opening of the gantry during the procedure. The child must also be instructed not to speak to this individual, to avoid unnecessary motion. Informational brochures designed for this age group and their parents and given to them at the time of scheduling can eliminate the anxiety and fear of the unknown. Most children can readily imagine the MRI system to be a spaceship and do quite well if all their questions are answered prior to the session. The few extra moments required for this preparation can obviate the use of unnecessary sedation in most situations.

Basic Concepts of Nuclear Magnetic Resonance

Each individual hydrogen proton has a polar orientation, rotating around its own axis. These polar protons are randomly oriented in space throughout the brain (Figure

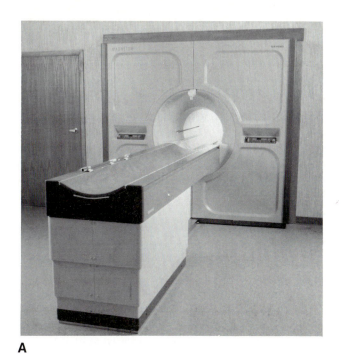

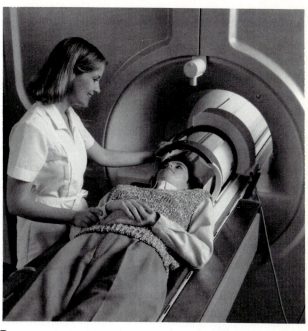

A   **B**

Figure 5–33. A. A conventional MRI system. **B.** Patient resting on the table, with the head coil being moved into position. Note the open "window" that will be positioned in front of the patient's face, and the deep narrow gantry. (*Both figures courtesy of Ann Deary, Siemens Medical Systems, Inc., Iselin, New Jersey*).

5–34A). When placed within a magnetic field, the protons align along the axis of the field (considered as the equilibrium state) (Figure 5–34B). When a radio-frequency pulse is applied to these aligned protons, this excitation causes the protons to deflect (or "flip") to a predetermined angle (Figure 5–34C).

After radio-frequency pulse excitation, the protons will return to the equilibrium state, precessing about the direction of the magnetic field in decreasing circles, much like a gyroscope rotates from the influence of gravity (Figure 5–34D). This precession or "wobbling" will decay, or relax, with time. The so-called relaxation parameters reflect the interaction of the precessing protons with the surrounding magnetic field and the neighboring protons. A gradient permits spatial localization; this creates each individual image slice in a scan series. Two measured time constants are used in MRI to characterize this relaxation: T_1 and T_2 (Pykett, 1982; Cohen, 1986). T_1 relaxation time represents the rate of return of the protons to the equilibrium state along the axis of the magnetic field. T_2 relaxation time represents the interactions of neighboring nuclei as the precession decays.

Abnormal shortening or prolongation of T_1 or T_2 is seen as a change in signal intensity (darker or lighter) relative to normal tissue (Table 5–1):

T_1 prolonged → decreased (darker) signal intensity
T_1 shortened → increased (brighter) signal intensity

T_2 prolonged → increased (brighter) signal intensity
T_2 shortened → decreased (darker) signal intensity

MRI Pulse Sequences

By adjusting the rate, duration, and intensity of the radio-frequency excitation pulses, various pulse sequences can be created to visualize different properties of the tissue in question. In routine clinical MRI, both T_1- and T_2-weighted sequences are obtained on each patient, with each complementary sequence averaging 10 minutes in duration.

T_1-weighted pulse sequences produce superior anatomic detail of the entire brain and spinal cord. The process of myelin development is readily visualized, as are any structural abnormalities. A T_1-weighted scan, such as an inversion recovery, can be considered as an in vivo neuroanatomic study (Cohen, 1986).

T_2-weighted pulse sequences are extremely sensitive to changes in tissue water content. These therefore produce visualization of most lesions, particularly those that disrupt the blood-brain barrier or myelin. A T_2-weighted scan, such as a spin echo, is very sensitive for identifying and characterizing the extent of lesions (Cohen, 1986).

Paramagnetic Contrast Agents

Several paramagnetic contrast agents have been recently approved by the Food and Drug Administration for use with MRI, in particular gadolinium-DTPA. This approval applies only for the neuroaxis and in patients over the age of 2 years. In areas with a disrupted blood-brain barrier, these paramagnetic agents indirectly affect MR image intensity by shortening relaxation times (primarily T_1), whereas iodinated CT contrast agents are

A. RANDOM ORIENTATION

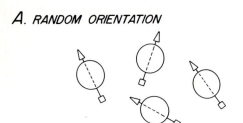

B. WITHIN MAGNETIC FIELD

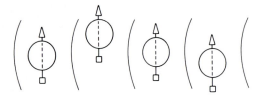

C. RADIO-FREQUENCY EXCITATION

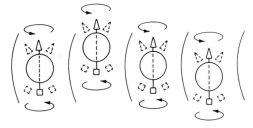

D. POST-RF-PULSE EXCITATION

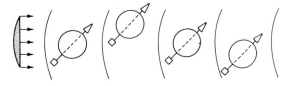

Figure 5–34. Basic concepts of nuclear magnetic resonance. *(Figure by Edith Tagrin, Massachusetts General Hospital.)*

directly imaged at these disrupted regions (Wolf et al., 1985; Cohen, 1986).

Risks of MRI

MRI is considered to be a safe procedure, essentially without risk in the routine clinical setting. No deleterious side effects have been reported as a consequence of the imaging procedure. However, there are potential hazards inherent in MRI. Strict guidelines govern the operation of conventional imaging systems, to assure that the thresholds for health effects are not exceeded (Cohen, 1986; Consensus, 1988).

Static magnetic fields at strengths of 2.0 T or less have not produced any harmful effects in studies of workers continuously exposed to high industrial magnetic fields. Changing magnetic fields (like those produced during the pulse sequences) induce electric currents, which are theoretically capable of interfering with nerve and cardiac conduction; however, the maximum threshold for the changing fields occurring in an MRI system is set at less than 1% of the electric current required to induce a nerve action potential. Radio-frequency-induced heating of tissue also occurs; but during an MRI scan it is limited to a level below the basal metabolic rate (Budinger, 1981; Cohen, 1986).

Further Considerations

The magnetic field gradients can potentially dislodge implanted metallic objects, such as surgical clips or cochlear

TABLE 5-1. APPEARANCE OF ABNORMALITIES ON MRI SCANS

	T_1-Weighted Sequence	T_2-Weighted Sequence
Hemorrhage		
Acute	Brighter	Brighter > Darker
Chronic		
Rim	Brighter	Brighter
Center	Darker	Brighter
Infarction		
Acute	Darker	Brighter
Chronic	Darkest	Brighter
Cerebral Edema	Darker	Brighter
Hydrocephalus—		
Periventricular Region	Darker	Brighter
Solid Tumor	Darker	Brighter
With Gadolinium-DTPA	Brighter	No change
Cystic Mass	Darkest	Brighter
Inflammation/Demyelination	Darker	Brighter
Vascular Malformations/Blood Vessel Lumen		
Patent	Darker	Darker
Thrombosed	Brighter	Brighter

Pearls and Perils: MRI

1. MRI can be performed in the coronal, sagittal, or transaxial plane, without repositioning the patient. This permits accurate visualization of substructures or lesions from multiple angles, expanding the clinical utility of the scan. The sagittal plane is particularly advantageous when abnormalities are suspected in the posterior fossa or brainstem (Cohen, 1986; Consensus, 1988).

2. In CT, severe osseous artifacts occur at cranial interfaces, particularly in the posterior fossa, and these obscure numerous critical areas; with MRI, the cerebral cortex, temporal lobes, posterior fossa, and brainstem are visualized with exquisite anatomic detail (Cohen, 1986; Consensus, 1988).

3. The overall sensitivity of MRI is greater than that of CT for lesions, particularly those disrupting the blood-brain barrier and those occurring in the white matter. This is particularly advantageous in the evaluation of disorders affecting myelin development or causing its disruption (Consensus, 1988).

4. MRI visualizes most abnormalities without the use of intravenous contrast agents. Paramagnetic contrast agents, primarily gadolinium-DTPA, are available when necessary to enhance the evaluation of blood-brain barrier integrity, the reticuloendothelial system, and the extracellular space (Consensus, 1988).

5. MRI can visualize the entire spinal cord in the sagittal plane, often eliminating the need for a more invasive myelogram (Cohen, 1986; Consensus, 1988).

6. There are no known risks incurred from a clinical MRI study.

7. Although MRI is a more sensitive indicator of many abnormalities, it is less specific in certain situations. For example, it is often difficult to differentiate tumor mass from surrounding edema, or tumor recurrence from the surrounding effects of radiation therapy, without the use of paramagnetic contrast agents (Cohen, 1986; Consensus, 1988).

8. MRI poorly differentiates calcifications or bony structures relative to CT. However, MRI is more sensitive for the detection of osteomyelitis, offering resolution equal to that of a radionuclide bone scan (Consensus, 1988).

9. Because the gantry is relatively narrow, many adult patients experience a claustrophobic reaction during the procedure. Children as a rule do not seem to mind the closeness, and often fall asleep. The long narrow gantry also makes it more difficult to reach a patient or to monitor cardiorespiratory function during procedures involving sedation (Cohen, 1986).

10. In small infants, anatomic discrimination is limited by the (normal) relative lack of myelin deposition (Cohen, 1986). Also, anatomic resolution is further diminished because of the relatively large head coil; infant-sized head coils are not as yet routinely available.

11. The thumping or tapping noise during scan acquisition may sometimes cause discomfort to the patient, although most children do not seem to mind it.

12. The longer scanning time may necessitate the use of sedation in younger children who might otherwise tolerate a CT scan.

---

implants. Most clips are situated in noncritical areas, and the magnetic effects would thus not be detrimental; within the imaged organ, artifacts from metallic clips may prevent adequate visualization.

Large metallic implants, such as orthopedic prostheses, may cause discomfort owing to local heating effects.

The magnetic field of an MRI system also affects metallic objects within the imaging room. Watches and credit or banking cards should not be brought into the scanner room. Modifications in anesthesia equipment, oxygen tanks (to avoid missile injuries), surgical instruments, cardiac monitors, intravenous poles, and stretchers have all become necessary to permit their safe use in the MRI environment (Consensus, 1988).

Two absolute contraindications exist for MRI: even slight movement of *surgical aneurysmal clips* could have catastrophic results; and *cardiac pacemakers* may revert from demand to fixed-rate output (Cohen, 1986).

CT OR MRI?

In summary, the advantages of MRI include multiplanar capability, superior contrast resolution, and the apparent absence of harmful effects on the patient. Its disadvantages include cost, long scanning times, sensitivity to motion, and limited availability for imaging critically ill patients. Although CT can approach the advantages and avoid some of the disadvantages, it must be considered that, particularly in the pediatric population, limited MRI/neuropathologic correlations have only recently become available. Extrapolation from the adult population, however, gives MRI a distinct advantage in the disease states affecting the pediatric neuroaxis.

The following section should be considered as offering guidelines. It reflects the current experience in both pediatric and adult populations, in unenhanced MRI scans, except where indicated.

Toxic/Metabolic Encephalopathies

Little is currently known about the utility of MRI in most acute encephalopathies, such as Reye's syndrome or severe anoxia, probably because the critical nature of the illness has precluded the use of a longer scanning procedure with difficult patient access.

Chemotherapy and cranial irradiation have been associated with various abnormalities by both CT and MRI. In general, MRI is more sensitive than CT in demonstrating treatment-related neurologic damage (Figure 5–35); these white matter abnormalities are often missed by CT. The changes seen on MRI have correlated well with the degree of neurologic dysfunction (Packer et al., 1986).

Rapid correction of hyponatremia resulting in central pontine myelinolysis may produce a brainstem lesion sufficiently small to be missed by CT. MRI has proved very useful in demonstrating brainstem signal abnormalities in many symptomatic patients with a negative CT scan (Rippe et al., 1987).

The contribution of MRI has not been well documented in other toxic-metabolic encephalopathies. Theoretically, MRI should prove more sensitive to any disturbance of water or myelin in any of these disorders.

Trauma

CT remains the first imaging modality of choice in acute head trauma for two reasons: the sensitivity of CT in demonstrating acute hemorrhage is superior to that of MRI, and the often critical nature of the clinical presentation again precludes the use of MRI, even if readily available. However, in the subacute phase, MRI can readily detect hematomas that become isodense with time

on CT (Figure 5–36). Also, nonhemorrhagic contusions or shearing injuries are more readily demonstrated by MRI than by CT. Therefore, MRI may play a more sensitive role in the subacute or chronic rehabilitation phase of head trauma (Consensus, 1988).

In spinal cord trauma, MRI can clearly identify the relationships of the cord to the surrounding vertebral elements and readily demonstrate cord compression (Cohen, 1986).

Seizures

CT can still be considered the first image modality of choice in the routine evaluation of generalized seizure disorders in children, if done both without and with intravenous contrast administration. MRI has been found to be far more sensitive than CT (which is usually negative) in identifying lesions in cases of both refractory and nonrefractory temporal lobe or partial epilepsy in the adult population, and should be included in the diagnostic evaluation of these conditions (Cohen, 1986; Schorner et al., 1987) as well as of any changing seizure disorder. The specific sensitivity of MRI in seizure disorders in children has not yet been well documented.

Movement Disorders

In general, MRI can be considered to be more sensitive to changes in the basal ganglia than is CT. In Huntington's disease, MRI is more sensitive to the morphologic changes, primarily subtle caudate atrophy, than is CT. In Wilson's disease, MRI demonstrates abnormalities in signal intensity occurring in the basal ganglia and thalamus, as well as within the subcortical white matter, presumably secondary to the paramagnetic effects of

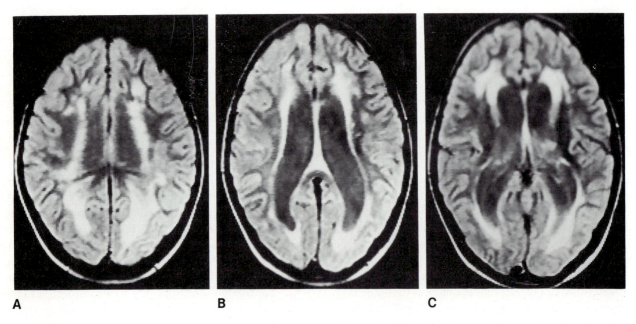

A   B   C

Figure 5–35. Spin echo MRI of methotrexate leukoencephalopathy. Note the abnormal high-intensity signal emanating from the periventricular white matter. (TR = 2000 ms, TE = 60 ms, slice = 7 mm.)

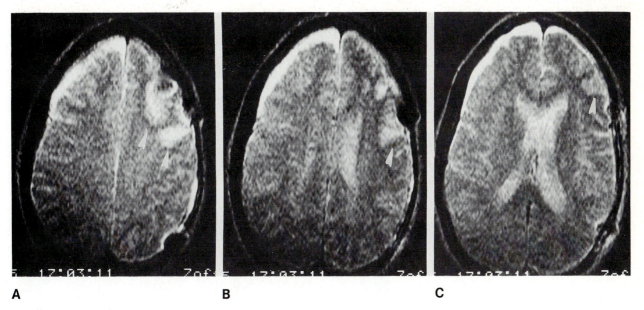

A B C

Figure 5–36. Chronic bilateral subdural hematomas (bright signal in frontal regions) 4 weeks after traumatic injury. Note also the large focal intraparenchymal region of high intensity in the left frontal area (*arrow*), anatomically corresponding to the patient's transcortical aphasia. The CT scan demonstrated only small subdural collections. (TR = 2000 ms, TE = 120 ms, slice = 7.5 mm.)

hemosiderin or copper deposition. In Hallervorden-Spatz disease, abnormal iron storage is readily visualized in the globus pallidus (Cohen, 1986; Rutledge et al, 1987). Lacunar infarcts or other small lesions have been recognized by MRI in the subthalamic nuclei in cases of hemiballismus; although no abnormalities have been described in cases of primary dystonias, neostriatal abnormalities have been seen in cases of secondary dystonias, including those caused by perinatal anoxia (Rutledge et al., 1987). In Gilles de la Tourette syndrome, no characteristic MRI abormalities have been identified to date.

Infectious Diseases

In uncomplicated acute meningitis, no abnormalities are usually noted by either CT or MRI. In severe pyogenic meningitis, diffuse enhancement over the surface of the brain may be seen with both contrast-enhanced CT and gadolinium-enhanced MRI. MRI is superior to CT in delineating any complicating infarctions or cortical venous/sinus thrombosis. MRI can also differentiate the relatively benign subdural effusion from the more insidious subdural empyema both of which appear equally hypodense on CT (Sze and Zimmerman, 1988).

In encephalitis, MRI is far more sensitive to both the early presence and the extent of abnormalities (Sze and Zimmerman, 1988) (Figure 5–37). This level of sensitivity may well prove to be diagnostically pathognomonic in fulminant cases in which prompt treatment is imperative, particularly in those etiologies with characteristic pathologic sites, such as the temporal lobes with herpes simplex.

Although MRI is more sensitive than CT in the detection of early cerebritis, patients usually present at the stage of late cerebritis or mature cerebral abscess, for the detection of which MRI and CT are essentially equivalent. MRI is better for determining the presence and extent of an extracerebral empyema, as well as any adjacent cortical ischemia, when compared with CT (Sze and Zimmerman, 1988).

Acute disseminated (postinfectious) encephalomyelitis, occurring subsequent to viral infection or immunization, has been increasingly detected by the use of MRI when the CT scan is often unremarkable (Sze and Zimmerman, 1988). In subacute sclerosing panencephalitis, MRI is again extremely sensitive to the extensive demyelination and cortical involvement (Figure 5–38).

The subacute encephalopathy in acquired immunodeficiency syndrome is usually associated with only diffuse cerebral atrophy by both CT scan and MRI; rare areas of signal abnormality have been reported by MRI. In cytomegalovirus encephalitis, the greater sensitivity of MRI is similar to that in the other encephalitides described previously. In cerebral toxoplasmosis, MRI can detect lesions at a far earlier stage than can CT, particularly small lesions in regions usually obscured by CT bony artifact (Sze and Zimmerman, 1988).

In progressive multifocal leukoencephalopathy, MRI has also proved to be far superior to CT for the early detection of the white matter lesions, as well as the recognition of cortical and deep gray nuclear involvement. An MRI is therefore the imaging modality of choice in immunocompromised patients with evidence of these disorders (Sze and Zimmerman, 1988).

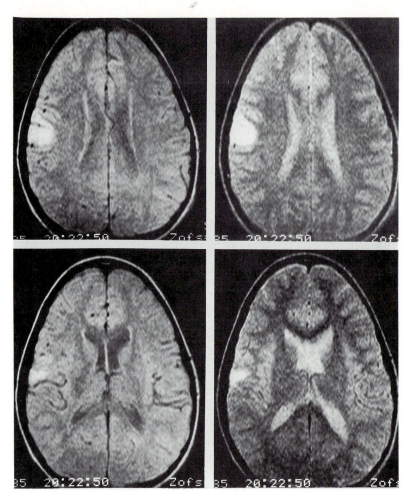

Figure 5-37. Spin echo MRI of focal Rasmussen's encephalitis. Note region of increased signal intensity in the right parietal lobe, corresponding to the EEG profile. The CT scan demonstrated only a much smaller, diffuse area of contrast enhancement. (TR = 2000 ms, TE = 60 ms (left) and 120 ms (right), slice = 7.5 mm.)

Immunologic Diseases

MRI has been found to be far superior to the CT scan in identifying plaques in multiple sclerosis (MS) (Consensus, 1988), demonstrating characteristic abnormalities in over 85% of adult MS patients (Ormerod et al., 1987; Sheldon et al., 1985) as compared to only 25% for CT (Sheldon et al., 1985); this level of sensitivity is vastly improved with the additional use of gadolinium-DTPA as a contrast agent. MRI is therefore the procedure of choice for the demonstration of disseminated lesions and for the prospective evaluation of disease evolution in MS (Haas et al., 1987) (Figure 5–39). In acute experimental allergic encephalomyelitis, the signal abnormalities seen on MRI have been shown to correlate with acute perivascular inflammatory changes and edema by histopathology, rather than with actual foci of demyelination (Grossman et al., 1987).

Although the current experience is limited, because most immunologic diseases affecting the central nervous system result in acute mononuclear perivascular changes, edema, and demyelination, one can postulate that MRI will be far more sensitive in the detection of parenchymal abnormalities in any of these disorders, particularly using gadolinium-DTPA.

Vascular Disease

Within hours after an acute ischemic event, MRI can detect and localize the arterial or venous infarction; a CT scan is often negative within the first 48 hours after the vascular occlusion, even with the use of intravenous contrast. In the subacute and chronic phases of infarction, both CT and MRI are essentially equivalent (Consensus, 1988), although MRI may readily detect smaller peripheral infarctions missed on CT.

In venous sinus thromboses, CT diagnosis relies on the appearance of the empty delta sign or cord sign. MRI appears to be more specific in the initial diagnosis of these disorders relative to CT, with increased sensitivity to the presence of the clot, the absence of flowing blood, and surrounding venous infarctions (Purvin et al., 1987). Comparison studies of the diagnostic usefulness of MRI relative to arteriography in these situations are not yet available.

As described previously, CT is indicated for evaluation of an acute hemorrhage, while MRI may be more sensitive in the subacute or chronic phases (Consensus, 1988). Vascular malformations and aneurysms are more readily detected and localized by MRI, which is particularly sensitive to following blood. Although MRI has

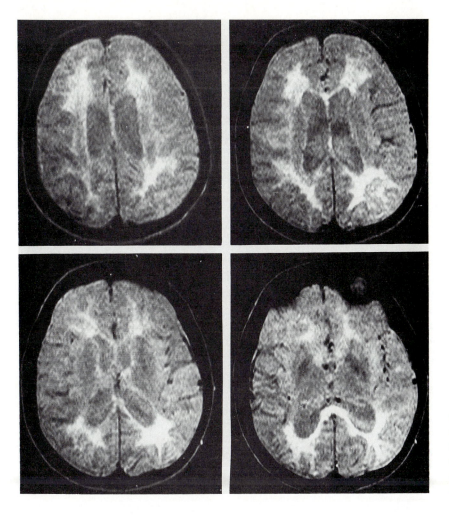

Figure 5–38. Spin echo MRI of subacute sclerosing panencephalitis. Note bilateral extensive abnormal signal from the subcortical and periventricular white matter. (TR = 2000 ms, TE = 60 ms, slice = 7.5 mm.)

demonstrated "cryptic" vascular malformations in patients with negative arteriograms, the two modalities should be considered complementary in these disorders (Consensus, 1988).

Neoplastic Disease

Unenhanced MRI and CT are essentially equivalent methods for the detection of most brain tumors (Consensus, 1988). CT can visualize calcifications, and, with

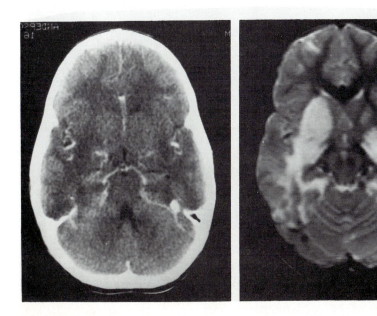

Figure 5–39. MRI slice (**B**) adjacent to the corresponding contrast-enhanced CT slice (**A**) in multiple sclerosis. Note extensive bilateral signal abnormalities predominantly in the white matter. (TR = 2000 ms, TE = 120 ms, slice = 7 mm.)

contrast enhancement, is better able than an unenhanced MRI to distinguish tumor margins from adjacent edema. MRI generally permits superior visualization at the vertex, in the posterior fossa and brainstem regions, and in any region adjacent to the cranium, such as at the base of the skull, in the suprasellar regions, or in the temporal lobes. Gadolinium-enhanced MRI is more sensitive in identifying small tumors, in defining the peritumor anatomy, and in delineating tumor margins from adjacent edema (Stack et al., 1988). Because of its multiplanar quality and superior anatomic discrimination, MRI can therefore provide more information pertaining to the precise location and extent of a lesion. Neither of these methods is superior in discriminating tissue diagnoses (Consensus, 1988).

In general, if there is suspicion of an intracranial mass lession and a negative CT scan, an MRI is indicated, particularly for evaluation of the temporal lobes, posterior fossa, and brainstem. An MRI would be the first modality of choice for the diagnostic evaluation of a spinal cord mass lesion, in lieu of a myelogram.

Neurocutaneous Disorders

In patients clinically diagnosed with tuberous sclerosis, CT scans usually demonstrate the characteristic subependymal nodules with or without calcifications, and occasionally visualize the subcortical hamartomas. In young children, however, there may not yet be sufficient

calcium deposition within these lesions to be visualized by CT. MRI demonstrates areas of prolonged T_2 signal abnormalities in the subcortical regions with greater sensitivity, which are consistent with the characteristic hamartomatous or gliotic tissue; a signal void results from the calcifications (Cohen, 1986).

Our experience suggests that MRI is the diagnostic modality of choice in both clinically diagnosed individuals with tuberous sclerosis and asymptomatic family members: MRI has detected the characteristic subcortical lesions in a previously undiagnosed parent with a normal CT scan and minimal clinical criteria (P. A. Filipek, P. Short, and J. Amos, unpublished results).

In bilateral acoustic neurofibromatosis, MRI is capable of detecting smaller intracanalicular acoustic neuromas when compared to the more invasive gas CT cisternography (Consensus, 1988), particularly with gadolinium enhancement (Stack et al., 1988). MRI is also more sensitive to neurofibromatous lesions of the optic pathway and spinal cord.

In von Hippel-Lindau disease, MRI is a noninvasive, sensitive method for the early presymptomatic detection and follow-up of both the central nervous system and abdominal visceral neoplasms, often before visualization is possible with other imaging modalities (Sato et al., 1988). It is the preferred imaging modality for the frequent multisystem radiologic evaluations necessary in the evaluation of patients with von Hippel-Lindau and those family members at risk.

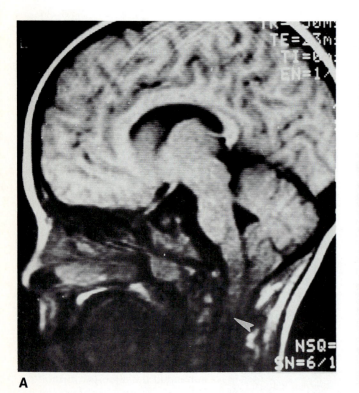

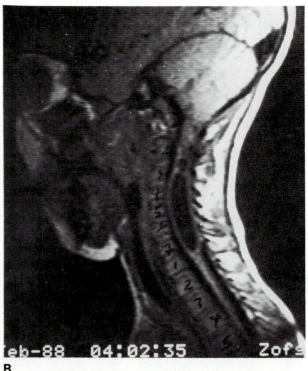

A

B

Figure 5-40. A. Sagittal T_1-weighted MRI demonstrating herniation of the cerebellar tonsils in Arnold-Chiari malformation. Note upper limits of cervical hydromyelia (*arrow*). (TR = 550 ms, TE = 23 ms, slice = 4 mm.) **B.** Sagittal cervical MRI on the same patient, demonstrating hydromyelia. This slice poorly represents the cerebellar herniation. (TR = 400 ms, TE = 23 ms, slice = 4 mm.)

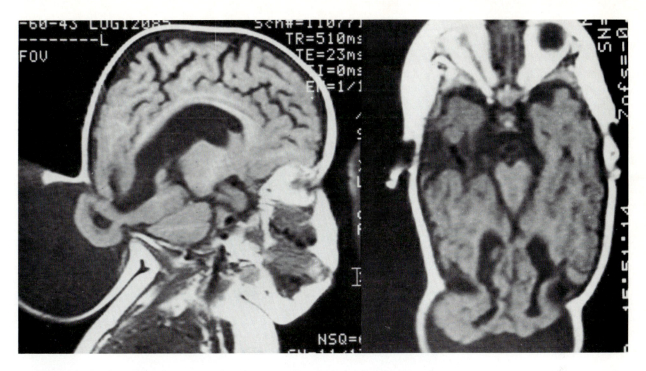

Figure 5–41. Preoperative sagittal and transaxial views of an occipital encephalocele. Note herniation of occipital lobe, including the occipital horns of the lateral ventricles, into the sac. (TR = 520 ms, TE = 23 ms, slice = 7 mm.)

Developmental Malformations

MRI is the imaging modality of choice for the evaluation of most potential malformations of the central nervous system. Its use in these evaluations, however, is limited in neonates and very young infants, because of the decreased anatomic resolution owing to the relative lack of myelin deposition (Cohen, 1986) and the unavailability of infant-sized head coils. Therefore, in this age group, other modalities may be preferable to MRI.

Neural tube defects are readily detected and localized by MRI. Arnold-Chiari malformations may not be apparent even on low CT slices through the foramen magnum, but are easily visualized on midsagittal MRI slices (Figure 5–40). Syringomyelia and diastematomyelia can be detected by MRI, eliminating the need for myelography with or without concomitant CT scanning (Cohen, 1986).

The use of MRI in the initial evaluation of myelomeningocele or encephalocele is obviously limited by the acute presentation of these malformations in a critically ill neonate. However, preoperatively, MRI can assist the neurosurgeon in anticipating the grossly altered neuroanatomy (Figure 5–41), and may be the imaging

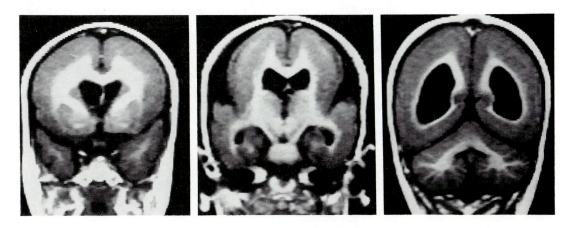

Figure 5–42. Coronal invesion-recovery MRI in lissencephaly. Note total absence of gyral formation and abnormal cortical thickness and configuration of the cerebral hemispheres. (TR = 1500 ms, TI = 450 ms, TE = 20 ms, slice = 7 mm.)

modality of choice for the long-term postsurgical follow-up of these infants (Cohen, 1986).

MRI is generally more sensitive for the detection of neuronal migration defects. Although many of these disorders, for instance lissencephaly (Figure 5–42), holoprosencephaly, or agenesis of the corpus callosum, can usually be diagnosed by CT scan, MRI permits the multiplanar visualization of the disrupted anatomic relationships as well as any associated abnormalities in myelin deposition. Since the advent of MRI, subtle cases of polymicrogyria and heterotopias (Figure 5–43) have been identified that were not recognized by CT.

Aquaductal stenosis can be directly visualized by MRI, and the periventricular extravasation of cere-

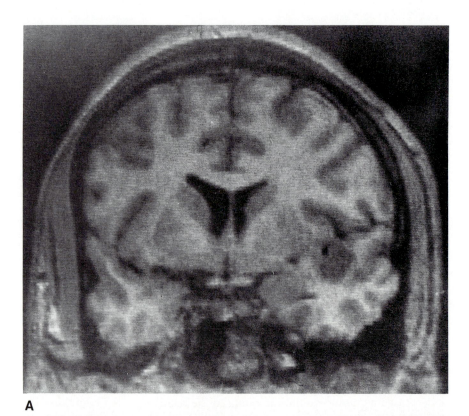

A

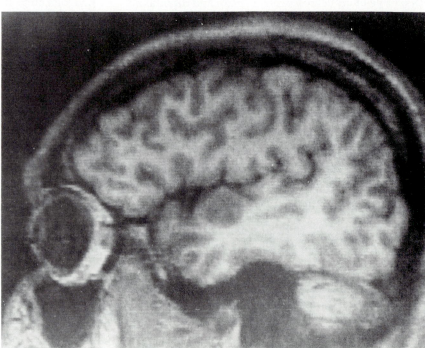

Figure 5–43. Coronal (**A**) and sagittal (**B**) MRI demonstrating left superior temporal heterotopia. CT scan (I – /I +) was unremarkable. (TR = 40 ms, TE = 15 ms, slice = 3.1 mm.)

B

brospinal fluid resulting from hydrocephalus is readily apparent (Cohen, 1986).

MRI is superior to CT for the determination of cerebellar or other posterior fossa malformations because of the lack of osseous artifact and the multiplanar capabilities of the scanner.

THE FUTURE OF MRI

The role of MRI in the future of pediatric neurology can only be anticipated from the explosive technologic evolution we have witnessed to date. The use of contrast agents promises to increase both the sensitivity and the specificity of the procedure, as well as to decrease imaging times substantially. New volumetric pulse sequences now permit thinner slices and allow one to image the entire brain without the interslice gap now seen in conventional CT or MRI scans. In addition, noninvasive angiographic studies may be permitted by the sensitivity of MRI to flowing blood.

Because of the exquisite anatomic detail afforded by MRI, in vivo volumetric studies are now possible, allowing the unprecedented opportunity to observe the brain in the course of normal development, to study it in those with developmental disabilities, or to chart the progression of disease (Fillipek et al., 1989). Current endeavors are also focused on human regional spectroscopy and spectroscopic imaging, virtually creating biochemic analyses and images of the brain and potentially providing in vivo characterization of neurotransmitter and peptide functions.

ANNOTATED BIBLIOGRAPHY

Cranial Ultrasound

Blickman JG, Jaramillo D, Cleveland RH: Neonatal cranial ultrasonography. *Curr Probl Diagn Radiol* 20(3), 1991.
    An updated review of practical cranial ultrasonography for the pediatric age group.

Computed Tomography

Hershey BL, Zimmerman RA: Pediatric brain computed tomography. *Pediatr Clin North Am* 32:1477–1508, 1985.
    This article reviews the findings of CT in a variety of pediatric neurologic disorders.

Magnetic Resonance Imaging

Cohen MD: *Pediatric Magnetic Resonance Imaging.* Philadelphia, WB Saunders, 1986.
    This monograph concisely covers pediatric MRI in an organized, informative fashion, including the basic physical properties of nuclear magnetic resonance, safety issues, spectroscopy, and MRI findings in the central nervous system, as well as the respiratory, cardiovascular, gastrointestinal, genitourinary, endocrine, and musculoskeletal systems.

Consensus Conference: Magnetic resonance imaging. *JAMA* 259:2132–2138, 1988.
    This report from NIH summarizes the findings of a multidisciplinary panel concerning the state-of-the art experience of the risks, advantages, and clinical indications for MRI in each organ system.
Pykett IL: NMR imaging in medicine. *Sci Am* 246:78–88, 1982.
    This article, written by one of the eminent researchers in the field, presents a clear description of the basic principles of nuclear magnetic resonance imaging for the nonphysicist.

REFERENCES

Blickman JG, Jaramillo D, Cleveland RH: Neonatal cranial ultrasonography. *Curr Probl Diagn Radiol* 20(3), 1991.
Budinger TF: Nuclear magnetic resonance (NMR) in vivo studies: Known thresholds for health effects. *J Comput Assist Tomogr* 5:800–811, 1981.
Cleveland RH, Herman TE, Oot RF, et al: The evolution of neonatal herpes encephalitis as demonstrated by cranial ultrasound with CT correlation. *Am J Perinatol* 4:215–219, 1987.
Cohen MD: *Pediatric Magnetic Resonance Imaging.* Philadelphia, WB Saunders, 1986.
Consensus Conference: Magnetic resonance imaging. *JAMA* 259:2132–2138, 1988.
Creed L, Haber K: Ultrasonic evaluation of the infant head. *CRC Crit Rev Diagn Imaging* 21:37–84, 1984.
Ferry PC: Computed cranial tomography in children. *J Pediatr* 96:961–967, 1980.
Filipek PA, Kennedy DN, Caviness VS, Rossnick SL, Spraggins TA, Starewicz PM: MRI-based brain morphometry: Development and application to normal subjects. *Ann Neurol* 25:61–67, 1989
Gomez MR, Reese DF: Computed tomography of the head in infants and children. *Pediatr Clin North Am* 23:473–498, 1976.
Grant EG, Tessler F, Perrella R: Infant cranial sonography. *Radiol Clin North Am* 26:1089–1110, 1988.
Grossman RI, Lisak RP, Macchi PJ, Joseph PM: MR of acute experimental allergic encephalomyelitis. *AJNR* 8:1045–1048, 1987.
Haas G, Schroth G, Krageloh-Mann I, Buchwald-Saal M: Magnetic resonance imaging of the brain of children with multiple sclerosis. *Dev Med Child Neurol* 29:586–591, 1987.
Hayden CK, Swischuk LE: *Pediatric Ultrasonography.* Baltimore, Md, Williams & Wilkins, 1987, p 1–8.
Hershey BL, Zimmerman RA: Pediatric brain computed tomography. *Pediatr Clin North Am* 32:1477–1508, 1985.
McMenamin JB, Volpe JJ: Doppler US in the determination of neonatal brain death. *Am Neurol* 14:302–307, 1983.
Masters SJ, McClean PM, Arcarese JS, et al: Skull x-ray examinations after head trauma. Recommendations by a multidisciplinary panel and validation study. *N Engl J Med* 316:84–91, 1987.
Ormerod IEC, Miller DH, McDonald WI, et al: The role of NMR imaging in the assessment of multiple sclerosis and isolated neurological lesions. *Brain* 110:1579–1616, 1987.
Packer RJ, Zimmerman RA, Bilaniuk LT: Magnetic resonance imaging in the evaluation of treatment-related central nervous system damage. *Cancer* 58:635–640, 1986.
Pape KF, Wigglesworth JJ: *Hemorrhage, Ischemia and the*

Perinatal Brain. Philadelphia, Lippincott, 1979.

Purvin V, Dunn DW, Edwards M: MRI and cerebral venous thrombosis. *Comput Radiol* 11:75–79, 1987.

Pykett IL: NMR imaging in medicine. *Sci Am* 246:78–88, 1982.

Rippe DJ, Edwards MK, D'Amour PG, Holden RW, Roos KL: MR imaging of central pontine myelinolysis. *J Comput Assist Tomogr* 11:724–726, 1987.

Rutledge JN, Hilal SK, Silver AJ, Defendini R, Fahn S: Study of movement disorders and brain iron by MR. *AJR* 149:365–379, 1987.

Sato Y, Waziri M, Smith W, et al: Hippel-Lindau disease: MR imaging. *Radiology* 166:241–246, 1988.

Schorner W. Meencke JH, Felix R: Temporal-lobe epilepsy: Comparison of CT and MR imaging. *AJR* 149:1231–1239, 1987.

Sheldon JJ, Siddharthan R, Tobias J, Sheremata WA, Soila K, Viamonte M: MR imaging of multiple sclerosis: Comparison with clinical and CT examinations in 74 patients. *AJR* 145:957–964, 1985.

Stack JP, Antoun NM, Jenkins JP, Metcalfe R, Isherwood I: Gadolinium-DTPA as a contrast agent in magnetic resonance imaging of the brain. *Neuroradiology* 30:145–154, 1988.

Sze G, Zimmerman RD: The magnetic resonance imaging of infections and inflammatory diseases. *Radiol Clin North Am* 26:839–859, 1988.

Taylor GA, Catena LM, Garin DB, et al: Intracranial flow patterns in infants undergoing ECMO: Preliminary observations with Doppler US. *Radiology* 165:671–674, 1987.

Teele RL, Hernanz-Schulman M, Sotrel A: Echogenic vasculature in the basal ganglia of neonates: A sonographic sign of vascularity. *Radiography* 169:423–427, 1988.

Volpe JJ: *Neurology of the Newborn.* Philadelphia, WB Saunders, 1987.

Wolf GL, Burnett KR, Goldstein EJ. Joseph PM: Contrast agents for magnetic resonance imaging, in Kressel HY (ed): *Magnetic Resonance Annual, 1985.* New York, Raven Press, 1985, p 231–266.

Section II

General Pediatric Neurologic Diseases and Disorders

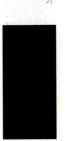

Toxic and Metabolic Encephalopathies

Doris A. Trauner

Any generalized disturbance in neuronal or glial metabolism can produce alterations in consciousness, or what is termed encephalopathy. This chapter will review common acquired metabolic and toxic disorders that disrupt normal brain metabolism and cause encephalopathic symptoms in children.

Regardless of the specific cause of the encephalopathy, symptoms that are typically present include confusion, hallucinations, indifference, and disorientation; alterations in level of consciousness, ranging from mild (lethargy) to severe (comatose); and seizures. The neurologic examination of the child with metabolic encephalopathy typically demonstrates (1) preserved cranial nerve function until the child is in deep coma; (2) intact pupillary responses to light, even in the presence of brainstem dysfunction, unless herniation of the brain has occurred; (3) diffuse hyperreflexia; (4) positive Babinski signs; (5) disturbances in respiratory pattern; and (6) often, generalized or multifocal seizures. Focal motor or sensory deficits are uncommon.

The electroencephalogram (EEG) in metabolic encephalopathies typically demonstrates diffuse slowing of background activity. At times, epileptiform activity may occur. Purely focal changes in the EEG are rare, but shifting or alternating asymmetries may be seen. Computed tomography (CT) scans or magnetic resonance imaging (MRI) of the brain are helpful in ruling out structural lesions; in metabolic disorders the CT scan or MRI is normal or shows evidence of cerebral edema with smaller than normal, even slit-like, ventricular size and obliteration of cisternal spaces.

HYPOXIC-ISCHEMIC ENCEPHALOPATHY

Insufficient oxygen supply to the brain leads rapidly to altered states of consciousness, extensor posturing, and seizures. Hypoxia, or lack of sufficient oxygen in the blood, can occur with severe pulmonary disease, cyanotic heart disease, and respiratory arrest. Ischemic conditions include hypertensive encephalopathy, systemic hypotension, and conditions in which cerebral blood flow is reduced, such as with generalized cerebral edema.

Signs and Symptoms. The progression of neurologic signs and symptoms with hypoxic/ischemic insults consists of early depression of the level of consciousness, with lethargy and obtundation followed by coma, and decorticate or decerebrate posturing. Progressive loss of cranial nerve function occurs in a rostral to caudal direction, and respiratory failure develops as a consequence of medullary damage. Generalized or multifocal seizures are frequently observed early in the course of a severe encephalopathy.

After a severe hypoxic insult, the patient may appear to be improving within 24 hours, only to deteriorate again as a consequence of cerebral edema on the second or third day, with deepening coma, recurrence of seizures, and evidence of brainstem dysfunction. Recovery from the hypoxic episode is gradual, and return of function occurs in a caudal to rostral progression.

Diagnosis. A history of respiratory compromise sufficient to impair brain oxygenation, or another event that could lead to reduced cerebral blood flow, will aid in the diagnosis of hypoxic-ischemic encephalopathy. Arterial blood gas determinations soon after the event may show decreased oxygen saturation, elevated carbon dioxide tension, and a respiratory acidosis.

Treatment. Intensive supportive therapy is necessary to minimize further complications of hypoxic insults. Maintenance of adequate oxygenation and systemic blood pressure and careful fluid and electrolyte balance are crucial. Prompt seizure control should be achieved with parenteral anticonvulsant medications. In severe cases, intracranial pressure should be monitored continuously because of the likelihood of cerebral edema. Elevated in-

Pearls and Perils: Metabolic Encephalopathy

1. Pupillary light reflexes are preserved until very late in the course of metabolic encephalopathies, and can be helpful in differentiating between metabolic and structural causes of coma.
2. It is uncommon for children with metabolic encephalopathies to have focal abnormalities on neurologic examination. They more typically have generalized or multifocal abnormalities.
3. The EEG in metabolic encephalopathy usually shows diffuse slowing of background activity without focality.
4. Focal findings on neurologic examination or focal seizures do not eliminate the possibility of a metabolic disorder.
5. It is easy to mistake lethargy or somnolence for "normal" in an infant or young child; parents are often the best judges of a child's altered mental status, especially in the early stages.

tracranial pressure should be treated with appropriate measures, such as controlled hyperventilation, osmotic diuretics, and neuromuscular blocking agents. If the child is iatrogenically paralyzed or sedated, continuous EEG monitoring is useful in detecting seizure activity.

DISORDERS OF FLUID AND ELECTROLYTE BALANCE

Although they are now less common, the importance of disorders of fluid and electrolyte balance worldwide in producing acquired brain damage still make this a subject worthy of discussion. Water and electrolytes are continually moving across capillary and cell membranes, maintaining an equilibrium among all organ components. Fluid volume is regulated by the interaction of several organs, including the kidney, skin, lung, adrenal glands, and brain. A malfunction of any one of these can result in problems with fluid and/or electrolyte balance. Excessive depletion of body water results in dehydration.

Dehydration in infants and children is usually caused by excessive loss of water and electrolytes from the gastrointestinal tract during vomiting or diarrhea. Other causes of excessive water loss include polyuria, diabetes insipidus, diabetes mellitus, and excessive sweating without adequate fluid replacement. Some sodium loss usually occurs with water loss. If more sodium than water is lost, hypotonic dehydration results; if more water than salt is excreted, a hypertonic state develops. Isotonic dehydration occurs when water and salt losses are balanced.

The central nervous system consequences of dehydration depend to some extent on the degree of salt loss. In hypertonic states, there may be shrinkage of cells and vascular stasis. Thrombosis of cerebral veins may occur. Rapid rehydration in this situation may result in tearing of cerebral veins and small hemorrhages. The hypotonic state may result in intracellular swelling and brain edema.

Symptoms and Signs. The clinical manifestations of dehydration depend on the rapidity of the fluid and electrolyte changes, and the degree of sodium imbalance. Rapid onset of isotonic dehydration is accompanied by lethargy and confusion; there is little other neurologic impairment until late in the course, when systemic hypotension develops and may lead to cerebral ischemia, obtundation, and coma. With hypotonic dehydration of acute onset, lethargy and confusion are also prominent, but the additional complication of seizures is present, particularly when serum sodium concentrations fall below 125. Chronic states of hypotonic dehydration are associated with more subtle changes, such as headache, vomiting, and abdominal pain, with little or no alteration in mental status.

Signs and symptoms of hypertonic dehydration include irritability, hypertonicity, hyperreflexia, lethargy or obtundation, and seizures. Occasionally opisthotonic posturing is seen. With too rapid rehydration and lowering of the serum sodium content, resulting hemorrhages into brain parenchyma may cause worsening of the neurologic condition, with deepening coma, focal or multifocal abnormalities on examination, and additional seizures.

FEATURE TABLE 6-1. METABOLIC ENCEPHALOPATHY

Discriminating Features	Consistent Feature	Variable Features
1. Diffuse neuronal dysfunction with altered mental state 2. Nonfocal abnormalities on neurologic exam 3. Laboratory evidence of metabolic derangement or organ dysfunction	1. Generalized slowing on EEG	1. Hyperreflexia 2. Altered muscle tone 3. Generalized or focal seizures

Pearls and Perils: Hypoxic-Ischemic Encephalopathy

1. Hypoxic-ischemic encephalopathy may occur as a complication of other disorders, such as severe Reye's syndrome, prolonged status epilepticus, or hypertensive encephalopathy; after trauma, as in near-drownings.
2. The appearance of improvement within 24 to 48 hours following a severe hypoxic insult is often more apparent than real, and may be followed by a second phase of more severe neurologic deterioration, as generalized cerebral edema evolves.

Diagnosis. The clinical diagnosis of dehydration states is usually apparent from a history of vomiting or diarrhea with poor oral intake of fluids, combined with a physical examination that discloses poor skin turgor, dried mucus membranes, sunken eyes, and little tear production. However, in hypertonic states, peripheral signs of dehydration may be less apparent, because extracellular fluid volume is relatively preserved owing to fluid shifts from intracellular to extracellular compartments. The history is extremely important in these instances. Inadvertent feeding by the mother of solutions that are too high or too low in salt, as a "home remedy" for diarrhea, may lead to altered electrolyte states much more rapidly than might otherwise be suspected from the history of the illness.

Other disorders that can present with features of dehydration should be considered. These include meningitis, encephalitis, and sepsis. Children with congenital heart disease, or hepatic or renal failure, may be taking diuretic medications or have a restricted salt intake; in certain situations, they may develop more chronic states of hypotonic imbalance. Laboratory tests to confirm the diagnosis of dehydration include blood urea nitrogen (BUN) determination, measurements of serum electrolytes and osmolality, and measurement of urine specific gravity and electrolyte content. With severe dehydration, the child may be acidotic, and serum bicarbonate and pH determinations will define the extent of acidosis.

Treatment. All forms of dehydration require fluid replacement, usually by the intravenous route if symptoms are severe or if the child is continuing to vomit. There are two steps to the treatment of dehydration. The first is rapid replacement of fluid and electrolytes in order to reestablish or maintain adequate cardiovascular and renal function. The second is slower administration of appropriate fluids to replace fully what has been lost and to maintain adequate fluid volume until the child is able to take in sufficient liquid by mouth to assure that normal hydration will be continued.

Bicarbonate solutions may be required if significant acidosis is present. In hypernatremic conditions, a hypotonic (but not sodium-free) salt solution may be used, although care should be exercised so that serum sodium concentration is reduced gradually, over a period of 72 hours, to minimize potential complications of rapid correction.

Specific decisions about fluid and electrolyte replacement must be made on a case-by-case basis, and frequent measurements of serum electrolytes and BUN are necessary to assess the effectiveness of treatment and to determine the course of further therapy.

If seizures occur as a result of the initial electrolyte imbalance, they usually respond to correction of the sodium abnormality and do not require specific anticonvulsant therapy. If the child has frequent or persistent seizures early in the course, phenobarbital may be given initally, but long-term treatment is generally not indicated.

Disorders of Calcium Homeostasis

Both hypocalcemia and hypercalcemia cause neurologic impairment. Calcium has a number of important functions in the nervous system: it is bound to cell membranes and it acts to stabilize the neuronal membrane, to modulate the excitable threshold of the cell, and to effect acetycholine release at the nerve terminals. In serum, calcium is present in three forms: about 33% is bound to protein and thus nondiffusible, 55% is ionized, and the remainder (about 12%) is diffusible but un-ionized. Deviations from normal values of ionized calcium concentrations lead to neurologic symptons such as seizures or tetany.

Regulation of calcium concentrations is the result of a number of factors, including the actions of parathyroid hormone, vitamin D, and thyrocalcitonin; renal function; and movement of calcium into and out of bone.

Hypocalcemia

Hypocalcemia occurs most commonly in the neonate, in particular in premature infants, infants of diabetic or toxemic mothers, and those who are small for gestational age or who have had severe hypoxic events. Symptoms usually begin in the second day of life. The etiology of hypocalcemia in these conditions is unclear. Elevated levels of parathyroid hormone have been documented in some patients, suggesting that immaturity of the parathyroid gland is not the explanation. In neonatal tetany, hypocalcemia develops late in the first week after birth. This condition is more often seen in infants fed cow's milk, which has a high phosphate content.

In older infants and children, hypocalcemia may develop as a consequence of vitamin D deficiency, hypoparathyroidism, pseudohypoparathyroidism, renal failure, acute pancreatitis, malabsorption syndromes, magnesium deficiency, treatment with phenytoin and

FEATURE TABLE 6-2. HYPOCALCEMIA

Discriminating Features	Consistent Features	Variable Features
1. Serum calcium < 7.0 mg/dL with normal serum protein 2. Positive Chvostek's and Trousseau's signs	1. Jitteriness 2. Seizures 3. Muscular irritability 4. Clonus	1. Muscle spasms 2. Focal seizures

other anticonvulsants, and infusion of large quantities of citrate with blood transfusions.

Signs and Symptoms. Infants may develop focal, multifocal, or generalized seizures as the first indication of hypocalcemia. Jitteriness, increased extensor tone, hyperreflexia, and clonus are common accompaniments. Older children may have classic signs and symptoms of tetany: muscle cramps, parasthesias, carpopedal spasms, and laryngospasm. Chvostek's sign may be elicited by tapping the lateral aspect of the face over the facial nerve; a positive response is indicated by a brief contraction of the facial muscles on the side percussed. Trousseau's sign may be elicited by applying pressure to the upper arm; a positive response consists of carpal spasm. Lethargy, hyperreflexia, and seizures are also prominent features of hypocalcemia in the older age group.

Diagnosis. Any infant who develops seizures or exhibits jitteriness or hypertonicity, in particular one who is at risk for developing hypocalcemia on the basis of the previously mentioned factors, should have measurements taken of serum calcium, phosphorus, and magnesium concentrations. Older infants and children who present with a first seizure should also have these tests as part of their initial evaluation. Symptoms are likely to occur with serum calcium concentrations below 7 mg/dL (if serum protein levels are normal). The electrocardiogram may show prolongation of the Q-T interval, and the EEG may exhibit diffuse slowing of background frequencies or dysrhythmias.

Serum phosphorus and alkaline phosphatase levels can help to discriminate among the various etiologies of hypocalcemia. In neonatal hypocalcemia, these are usually normal, with the exception of neonatal tetany, in which phosphorus levels are high. Hypoparathyroidism and pseudohypoparathyroidism are associated with high

phosphorus but normal alkaline phosphatase levels. In nutritional and vitamin-D-resistant rickets, phosphorus concentrations are decreased, whereas alkaline phosphatase is increased.

Treatment. Symptoms of hypocalcemia respond rapidly to intravenous infusion of calcium salt solutions. In most instances, this is sufficient to stop seizures and prevent recurrence. If magnesium concentrations are low as well, infusion of magnesium salts is also necessary. Seizures typically do not respond to administration of anticonvulsant medications, nor is there reason to place the child on long-term anticonvulsant therapy once a diagnosis of hypocalcemia has been established. If underlying disorders affecting calcium metabolism are found, these require treatment to prevent the hypocalcemia from recurring.

Hypercalcemia

Excessive calcium levels in children are found in association with vitamin D or A intoxication, thyrotoxicosis, hyperparathyroidism, bony metastases from malignant tumors, "idiopathic" hypercalcemia of infancy with failure to thrive, prolonged immobilization, hypophosphatasia, sarcoidosis, and Williams's elfin facies syndrome. High levels of calcium block synaptic transmission; many of the manifestations of this disorder are the result of neuromuscular blockade.

Signs and Symptoms. Infants with idiopathic hypercalcemia may fail to thrive in the first few months of life. Weakness and hypotonia are additional features. Infants with Williams's syndrome have characteristic "elfin" facial features and cardiac anomalies, in particular aortic stenosis. Older children with hypercalcemia from various causes may present with a constellation of symptoms, including headache, constipation, anorexia, vomiting, ir-

FEATURE TABLE 6-3. HYPERCALCEMIA

Discriminating Features	Consistent Features	Variable Feature
1. Serum calcium > 12 mg/dL 2. Muscle weakness 3. Irritability	1. Hypotonia 2. Hyporeflexia 3. Vomiting 4. Shortened Q-T interval	1. Dementia

ritability, lethargy, and weakness. Chronic hypercalcemia may result in formation of renal calculi and renal failure.

In hyperparathyroidism, serum phosphorus concentrations are decreased, wherease alkaline phosphatase levels may be normal or elevated. In most other causes, serum phosphorus is normal. Phosphorus and alkaline phosphatase values are both normal in infantile hypercalcemia. Vitamin intoxication and prolonged immobilization can be suspected from the history. Thyrotoxicosis should have associated clinical features, such as rapid heart rate, warm and dry skin, and exophthalmos.

Diagnosis. The differential diagnosis of hypercalcemic states includes primary myopathic disorders, because weakness and hypotonia are common to all of these. Serum calcium levels will readily differentiate myopathic from hypercalcemic disorders.

Treatment. Symptomatic treatment for hypercalcemia consists of administration of a chelating agent such as ethylenediamine tetraacetic acid (EDTA) to bind excess calcium. Infantile hypercalcemia responds to lowering of the vitamin D and calcium intake in the diet. The hypercalcemia associated with Williams's syndrome is usually transient, and may not require treatment. Hyperparathyroidism is corrected surgically.

Disorders of Magnesium Balance

Magnesium is an activator for numerous enzymatic reactions in the body. Regulation of magnesium balance is poorly understood. Parathyroid and adrenal hormones may play a role; transport across intestinal mucosa may also be a factor.

Hypomagnesemia is seen in neonates who are small for gestational age, in infants of diabetic or hypoparathyroid mothers, in the presence of liver disease, and after exchange transfusions. Rare instances of primary hypomagnesemia in male infants are thought to be due to defective intestinal transport. In such cases, hypocalcemia is present as well, but symptoms do not respond to calcium infusion unless magnesium supplementation is provided as well. Other causes of hypomagnesemia in older infants and children include prolonged vomiting or diarrhea, excessive use of diuretics, sprue, porphyria, hyperaldosteronism, malabsorption syndrome, rickets, diabetic ketoacidosis, acute pancreatitis, alcohol withdrawal, and hypoparathyroidism.

Excessive concentrations of magnesium are found after administration of magnesium salts, in uremia, and in adrenocortical insufficiency.

Signs and Symptoms. A deficiency of magnesium produces many symptoms similar to those of hypocalcemia. These include tetany, irritability, hypertonicity, hyperreflexia, seizures, carpopedal spasm, and positive Chvostek's and Trousseau's signs. Myoclonic jerks, mus-

---

Pearls and Perils: Disorders of Fluid and Electrolyte Balance

1. When seizures occur as a consequence of hyponatremic or hypernatremic dehydration, hypocalcemia, or hypoglycemia, long-term anticonvulsant therapy is not usually necessary unless evidence of permanent brain damage with a persistent epileptogenic focus on EEG is present.
2. Infants of diabetic mothers, premature infants, and those who are small for gestational age are most at risk for hypomagnesemia.
3. Hypomagnesemia is often found in combination with hypocalcemia, but may be present in isolation.
4. Muscle weakness, arreflexia, and hypotonia *in the presence of altered levels of consciousness* should suggest hypermagnesemia; patients with primary myopathic disorders do not have changes in mental status unless severe respiratory compromise has occurred.
5. Certain disorders, such as severe dehydration and hypernatremia, especially if the latter is reversed too rapidly, may cause tearing of superficial cortical veins and bleeding or thromboses, leading to focal neurologic deficits.
6. Infants with hypocalcemia and hypoglycemia may have focal motor seizures as a consequence of their metabolic disorder.

---

cle twitching, and tremors may be present. Changes in mental status include lethargy, confusion, agitation, hallucinations, and coma.

An excess of magnesium produces sedation, and very high levels may cause respiratory depression, hypotension, arreflexia, and flaccid paralysis.

Diagnosis. Normal magnesium concentrations are 1.5 to 2.5 mg/dL; symptoms develop at levels under 1.0 mg/dL and over 4 mg/dL.

Hypomagnesemic states must be differentiated from hypocalcemia by laboratory analysis of serum calcium, phosphorus, and magnesium levels. The differential diagnosis of hypermagnesemia includes neuromuscular disorders such as myasthenia gravis and infantile botulism, periodic paralysis, uremia, and toxin ingestions.

Treatment. The symptoms of hypomagnesemia respond rapidly to intravenous infusion of magnesium sulfate. Treatment of hypermagnesemic states includes liberal intravenous hydration, sometimes with diuretic therapy, and administration of calcium gluconate; in severe cases, hemodialysis may be necessary.

DISORDERS OF GLUCOSE HOMEOSTASIS

Hypoglycemia

Glucose is the primary energy substrate for the brain. A drop in serum glucose concentrations produces symptoms of neurologic dysfunction rapidly, within 30 to 45 minutes. Both the cerebral cortex and the reticular activating system are affected initially by hypoglycemia, so that alterations in consciousness occur early. If a normoglycemic state is not restored rapidly, permanent brain damage will result. Irreversible injury can take place within 90 minutes after the onset of severe hypoglycemia.

Causes of hypoglycemia in neonates include diabetic or toxemic mothers, intrauterine growth retardation, birth asphyxia, sepsis, Rh incompatibility, Beckwith's syndrome, and postmaturity. In infants and children, other etiologies include hereditary fructose intolerance, leucine sensitivity, insulinoma, galactosemia, panhypopituitarism, prediabetic state, malnutrition, malabsorption syndromes, liver disease, maple syrup urine disease, ketotic hypoglycemia, and glucose-6-phosphatase deficiency.

Signs and Symptoms. Because of its function as the primary energy substrate for the brain, deficiency of glucose produces rapid symptoms of altered mental status. Early changes consist of pallor, diaphoresis, confusion, syncope, tachycardia, and tremors. Apnea, jitteriness, hypotonia, poor suck, cyanosis, and tachypnea are particularly common in infants. Focal or generalized seizures may be the first sign of hypoglycemia. In severe instances, a comatose state evolves rapidly, accompanied by decerebrate posturing and hyperventilation, unlike the progression in most metabolic encephalopathies. Focal abnormalities, such as hemiparesis or aphasia, may be present.

Diagnosis. In the majority of instances, diagnosis is easily made on the basis of measurements of serum glucose concentrations. The level at which symptoms are likely to occur is partially determined by the age of the patient.

Pearls and Perils: Disorders of Glucose Homeostasis

1. Hypoglycemia may be present as one of the metabolic derangements in a number of acute encephalopathies, including Reye's syndrome, hepatitis, and salicylate intoxication.
2. Prolonged or recurrent attacks of hypoglycemia may lead to irreversible brain damage.
3. Chronic, low-grade hypoglycemia may cause insidious symptoms of confusion, cognitive impairment, and lethargy.

In neonates, a level of 30 mg/dL or below is considered abnormal; older infants and children become symptomatic at levels below 50 mg/dL.

Treatment. Prompt reversal of hypoglycemia with intravenous infusion of 25% glucose is imperative in order to prevent permanent neurologic sequelae.

Hyperglycemia

Abnormal elevations of serum glucose concentrations occur in diabetes mellitus and in certain iatrogenic situations. Hyperglycemia produces hyperosmolarity and intracellular dehydration. Central nervous system manifestations of neuronal dehydration include hallucinations, tremors, coma, and focal or generalized seizures. Management of such patients consists of reducing serum glucose concentrations with insulin, and cautious hydration. Rapid rehydration may worsen the neurologic condition by producing excessive movement of fluid into brain cells, resulting in cerebral edema.

NUTRITIONAL DISORDERS

Vitamins are necessary cofactors for many enzymatic reactions within the body. A well-balanced diet normally provides the necessary amounts of vitamins for metabolic needs. Neurologic disorders develop in the presence of vitamin deficiency, excess, or dependency states. In the latter case, the body requires more than the normal amount of a particular vitamin in order to carry out enzymatic functions.

Vitamin A

Vitamin A deficiency or intoxication may cause increased intracranial pressure (pseudotumor cerebri). Symptoms and signs are those found with any form of pseudotumor: headache, visual impairment, and papilledema are most common. Treatment of the deficiency state with vitamin A replacement usually reverses the problem. With vitamin excess, reducing intake to that required for metabolic needs may correct the intracranial pressure problem, but other modes of treatment such as repeated lumbar punctures or acetazolamide may be necessary for several days or weeks to reduce pressure in order to prevent permanent visual impairment.

Vitamin D

Vitamin D is a fat-soluble vitamin responsible for maintenance of normal calcium and phosphorus metabolism. Deficiency of vitamin D is associated with signs and symptoms of hypocalcemia, while excessive quantities can produce a clinical picture of hypercalcemia. Pseudotumor cerebri may also occur with vitamin D toxicity.

Vitamin B Complex

Vitamins of the B complex are directly involved in brain enzymatic reactions. These are water-soluble vitamins present in many dietary components. B vitamins of neurologic significance include thiamine, pyridoxine, B_{12}, and niacin.

Thiamine

Thiamine, or vitamin B_1, is a necessary cofactor in the intermediary metabolism of carbohydrates. Thiamine deficiency is caused by inadequate dietary intake, in particular when polished rice is a dietary staple. It also occurs with starvation, malnutrition states, hyperemesis gravidarum, gastrointestinal and liver disease, prolonged parenteral alimentation with inadequate vitamin replacement, and alcoholism.

Two clinical syndromes appear in the presence of thiamine deficiency, beriberi and Wernicke's encephalopathy. In the first case, a mixed motor and sensory peripheral neuropathy predominates, with weakness, absent deep tendon reflexes, paresthesias, sensory loss, and ataxia. Increased intracranial pressure and meningismus are additional features, and altered levels of consciousness appear in severe deficiency states. The syndrome of Wernicke's encephalopathy is rare in children. The classic clinical presentation of this disorder is the triad of ophthalmoplegia, ataxia, and mental changes (usually dementia, somnolence, or inattentiveness). Peripheral neuropathies are present as well. Prolonged thiamine deficiency may result in permanent neurologic disability. Severe cases may be fatal.

The presence of peripheral neuropathy and other typical features, as well as a history of malnutrition, inadequate diet, or other predisposing factors, should suggest the diagnosis of thiamine deficiency.

Treatment of severe forms of thiamine deficiency is best undertaken with intravenous thiamine replacement. Prompt treatment is necessary to prevent permanent neurologic disability or death.

Pyridoxine

Pyridoxine, or vitamin B_6, is an essential cofactor in numerous metabolic reactions in the nervous system, including the decarboxylation of several amino acids. Deficiency of this vitamin is rare. Cases occur on a genetic basis, during parenteral alimentation with inadequate replacement, in infants fed commercial formulas deficient in pyridoxine, in infants fed powdered goat's milk, after jejunal-ileal bypass, and in patients taking isoniazid or penicillamine, which are B_6 antagonists.

Symptoms of pyridoxine deficiency consist of hyperirritability and intractible seizures. In older children and adults, a peripheral neuropathy may be found. The diagnosis of both the deficiency and dependency states should be suspected in any infant with seizures of unknown etiology, especially if they do not respond to routine anticonvulsant medications. Treatment with intravenous doses of pyridoxine results in prompt cessation of seizures. Permanent neurologic impairment in the form of mental retardation and spasticity may occur after prolonged deficiency states.

A familial pyridoxine-dependency state has been documented, and causes intractible seizures in neonates and infants. The seizures are refractory to anticonvulsant medications, but respond promptly to intravenous administration of high doses of pyridoxine (25 to 100 mg). Occasional case reports have documented the need for even higher doses (200 to 400 mg).

An excess of pyridoxine may also result in neurologic impairment, in the form of a primarily sensory polyneuropathy.

Vitamin B₁₂

Deficiency of Vitamin B_{12} occurs with congenital pernicious anemia, with regional ileitis, with operative resection of the terminal ileum, in blind-loop syndrome, and with infestation with the tapeworm *Diphyllobothrium latum*. Symptoms and signs are those of subacute combined degeneration, and include ataxia, weakness of the lower extremities, and impairment of vibratory sensation. Vitamin replacement therapy will prevent the progression of symptoms, and may provide partial improvement, but some permanent disability is common.

Niacin

Niacin deficiency (pellagra) is found in children whose diet consists of corn as a staple food, with little intake of meat. The classic clinical triad consists of diarrhea, dermatitis, and dementia. Neurologic abnormalities include irritability, delirium or obtundation, coarse tremors, spasticity, polyneuropathy, and optic atrophy. Diagnosis is based on the dietary history and the characteristic triad of symptoms. There is usually a prompt response to administration of niacin.

Certain inherited metabolic disorders may respond to vitamin therapy, at least partially. These are listed in Table 6–1. The primary features of these disorders are

TABLE 6-1. VITAMIN-RESPONSIVE INBORN ERRORS OF METABOLISM

Disorder	Vitamin
Methylmalonic acidemia	B_{12}
Leigh's syndrome	Thiamine
Homocystinuria	Pyridoxine
Hartnup's disease	Niacin
Multiple carboxylase deficiency	Biotin
3-Methylcrotonyl-glycinuria	Biotin

varying degrees and types of neurologic impairment. They can be differentiated from primary vitamin deficiency states by their neurologic symptomatology, and by assays of serum lactate and pyruvate, urine and plasma amino acids, and urine organic acids.

ENCEPHALOPATHIES ASSOCIATED WITH SYSTEMIC DISEASE

Hepatic Encephalopathy and Reye's Syndrome

Damage to the liver produces a number of metabolic derangements, regardless of the etiology. These include hyperammonemia, impairment of carbohydrate metabolism, excessive fatty acidemia, hyperaminoacidemia, hyperbilirubinemia, abnormalities in neurotransmitter balance within the brain, and increased brain concentrations of octopamine, a putative neurotransmitter that may act as an inhibitor to normal neurotransmission. Treatment of any one of these metabolic abnormalities does not necessarily reverse the neurologic disorder, and it is likely that multiple factors are involved in producing hepatic encephalopathy.

Causes of liver disease include viral and parasitic infections, toxins such as carbon tetrachloride, ingestion of poisonous mushrooms (such as *Amanita phalloides*), primary and metastatic liver tumors, excessive alcohol use, inborn errors of metabolism (such as systemic carnitine deficiency and Wilson's disease), and medications (such as valproic acid).

Pathologic changes in liver are to some extent dependent on the etiology. Inflammatory changes are common with infectious causes; cellular necrosis is seen with toxins, infections, and medications; cirrhosis occurs with the use of some medications, Wilson's disease, and alcoholism. Fatty changes in liver are sometimes found with toxin exposure, in certain inborn errors of metabolism, and with valproic acid hepatotoxicity.

Reye's syndrome is an acute metabolic encephalopathy of childhood associated with hepatic dysfunction. The cause is unknown, although a virus-toxin interaction has been proposed as the most likely mechanism. It differs from other causes of liver disease in that serum bilirubin concentrations are normal; there is no cellular necrosis or fibrosis histologically; the primary pathologic changes in liver consist of diffuse microvesicular accumulation of fat, and swelling and pleiomorphism of mitochondria. Reye's syndrome appears to be primarily a disease of mitochondria, and all of the metabolic derangements found can be explained by failure of mitochondrial function.

Diffuse cerebral edema is a common complication of hepatic encephalopathy and Reye's syndrome.

Signs and Symptoms. Early manifestations of hepatic encephalopathy consist of lethargy and indifference; as the disease progresses, obtundation and coma ensue. The neurologic examination demonstrates no focal abnormalities; the alteration in consciousness and diffuse hyperreflexia are typically the only findings. In the early stages, asterixis may be elicited by having the patient extend the arms and hyperextend the wrists. An intermittent loss of tone in the outstretched wrists produces a flapping motion. As level of consciousness deteriorates, asterixis disappears. Respiratory changes, in particular hyperventilation, are prominent. Chronic hepatic encephalopathy causes a clinical picture of dementia, at times accompanied by a movement disorder, such as choreoathetosis or dystonia.

The presentation of Reye's syndrome in the child over 1 year of age is quite stereotyped in most cases. The child is recovering from a viral illness, most often influenza or varicella, and then begins vomiting repeatedly. Within 24 to 48 hours after the onset of vomiting, mental status changes are observed. Initially the child may be hyperexcitable and combative, with intermittent lethargy. There may be rapid progression of stupor and coma. Seizures sometimes accompany the other signs. Infants with Reye's syndrome have a more insidious presentation. There may be little or no vomiting. The first

FEATURE TABLE 6-4. HEPATIC ENCEPHALOPATHY

Discriminating Features	Consistent Features	Variable Features
1. Infectious, toxic, or neoplastic liver damage 2. Elevated serum NH_3 concentration 3. Abnormal liver function tests	1. Asterixis (in early stages) 2. Elevated serum short-chain fatty acids	1. Vomiting 2. Seizures

FEATURE TABLE 6-5. REYE'S SYNDROME

Discriminating Features	Consistent Features	Variable Features
1. Noninflammatory liver dysfunction with normal bilirubin 2. Biphasic illness 3. Persistent vomiting 4. Elevated serum ammonia 5. Histochemical evidence of decreased succinic dehydrogenase activity in liver	1. Metabolic acidosis 2. Respiratory alkalosis 3. Cerebral edema 4. Hyperventilation 5. High serum creatine phosphokinase 6. Fatty infiltration in liver 7. Mitochondrial swelling and pleiomorphism	1. Seizures 2. Hypoglycemia

indication of neurologic dysfunction may be seizure activity. Respiratory abnormalities are prominent early, and in fact the first sign of illness may be apnea.

Diagnosis. Tests of liver function should be performed in any child with unexplained encephalopathy. Elevation of serum transaminases and prolongation of prothrombin time suggest liver disease. Hypoglycemia may be present, and bilirubin concentrations are often abnormal (except in Reye's syndrome). Hyperammonemia accompanies most cases of hepatic encephalopathy. If there is evidence of liver dysfunction, a toxicology screen should be performed to look for toxic causes, a hepatitis A and B virus panel should be obtained, and a search for other viral agents such as cytomegalovirus may be warranted. Serum lactate and creatine phosphokinase concentrations are elevated in Reye's syndrome.

Examination of the cerebrospinal fluid is usually normal, with the exception of hypoglycorrhacia and elevated cerebrospinal fluid pressure. The EEG demonstrates diffuse slowing of background activity. In some cases of hepatic encephalopathy, bilaterally synchronous triphasic delta waves are found.

In recent years, several inborn errors of metabolism have been found to mimic Reye's syndrome in that the first manifestation may be an acute encephalopathy with liver dysfunction. These disorders must be considered in all cases of suspected Reye's syndrome, and ruled out using appropriate tests. The disorders include medium- and long-chain acyl CoA-dehydrogenase deficiency, systemic carnitine deficiency, urea cycle defects, and organic acidemias.

Treatment. The management of the child with hepatic encephalopathy is complicated because of the multiple metabolic derangements, excessive bleeding tendencies, and cerebral edema. In the early stages, careful control of fluid and electrolyte balance and correction of hypoglycemia are important. Reduction of serum ammonia concentrations can be accomplished using neomycin by oral or nasogastric tube administration or

enema, or lactulose orally. A low-protein diet will help to prevent further ammonia accumulation. In more advanced stages of encephalopathy, hypertonic glucose administration may help, in addition to the above measures. Administration of fresh frozen plasma, or whole blood in an exchange transfusion, will help to correct the clotting abnormalities. In cases of severe, fulminant hepatic necrosis, a liver transplant may be the only means of reversing the disease process.

Treatment of cerebral edema should be considered as part of the regimen for any child in a coma. When necessary, an intracranial pressure (ICP) monitoring device can be inserted for continuous recording of ICP. However, if clotting parameters are severely abnormal, this may not be possible. In either event, evidence of increased ICP, either by recording device or changes in clinical status, may be treated with osmotic diuretics such as mannitol, with intubation and controlled hyperventilation, and with neuromuscular blockade using an agent such as pancuronium bromide.

There is evidence that treatment of children with Reye's syndrome in the early stages with intravenous hypertonic (10% to 15%) glucose solutions may prevent

---

Pearls and Perils:
Hepatic Encephalopathy and
Reye's Syndrome

1. Correction of clotting disorders in patients with hepatic encephalopathy is difficult, and may require exchange transfusion or plasmapheresis.
2. Treatment of Reye's syndrome with intravenous hypertonic glucose solutions in the early stages may prevent progression of the disease.
3. Cerebral edema and increased intracranial pressure are major complications of hepatic encephalopathy and a frequent cause of death.
4. Bleeding tendencies are increased in patients with hepatic injury, and may lead to additional neurologic complications.

the progression of the disease. Thus, even if a child with suspected Reye's syndrome is awake and only minimally sleepy, it is best to administer this treatment as soon as the diagnosis is considered.

Renal Failure

Disease of the kidney produces a number of metabolic changes in the body, including uremia, hypocalcemia, hyperphosphatemia, acidosis, and hyperkalemia. Systemic hypertension is also a complication. The encephalopathy of renal disease is most often caused by uremia, but severe hypertension may also produce an acute encephalopathy.

Symptoms and Signs. With acute elevations of blood urea, patients become lethargic, restless, and agitated. They may complain of dysarthria and dysphagia. Generalized muscle weakness, fasciculations, tremors, and asterixis may be present. Deterioration in mental status to delirium, stupor, or coma accompanies disease progression. Focal or generalized seizures are common. Diffuse hyperreflexia, positive Babinski signs, and muscle rigidity are found on examination.

Chronic renal failure in children may produce growth failure, mental retardation, microcephaly, sensorimotor neuropathies, and seizure disorders.

Hypertensive encephalopathy has an abrupt onset, with generalized or focal seizures, and coma.

Diagnosis. Elevations of BUN (usually above 90 mg%); raised serum creatinine, potassium, and phosphorus concentrations; and hypocalcemia are typical laboratory findings. In addition to diffuse, high-amplitude slowing, triphasic waves may be seen on the EEG.

Treatment. Acute uremia is treated with hemo- or peritoneal dialysis. The neurologic manifestations of chronic renal failure in children do not respond well to dialysis. Long-term anticonvulsant therapy may be required for seizure management. Early renal transplantation appears to modify the course of the neurologic symptoms.

Dialysis Encephalopathy

A progressive neurologic syndrome has been described in children and adults undergoing chronic hemo- or peritoneal dialysis. Symptoms consist of progressive loss of speech, dysarthria, dementia, seizures, and myoclonus. The disorder initially may have intermittent symptoms, but eventually the deficits become fixed. The EEG is diffusely slow, with multifocal spike discharges showing

---

Pearls and Perils: Renal Failure

1. Asymptomatic peripheral neuropathy is found in most children with chronic uremia.
2. Children with chronic renal failure may decompensate and develop encephalopathic symptoms in the presence of acute infection or electrolyte imbalance, even when BUN concentrations are below 90 mg/dL.
3. Insidious onset of dementia and seizures may be a result of chronic renal failure, but may also be caused by dialysis encephalopathy.
4. Long-term treatment of renal failure with aluminum-containing antacids may produce a progressive clinical syndrome of dementia, speech arrest, and seizures.

---

frontal predominance. Elevated blood and tissue aluminum concentrations have been found in many patients with this disorder. However, the use of binding agents to clear aluminum from the body has not led to uniform improvement in symptomatology. Seizures and myoclonus may respond to benzodiazepine treatment.

Thyroid Dysfunction

Hypothyroidism may occur as a congenital abnormality owing to aplasia of the thyroid gland or deficiency of one of the thyroid enzymes, or may appear later in childhood, for example, as a consequence of Hashimoto's thyroiditis. When thyroid deficiency is present in utero, it results in severe neurologic deficits in the form of hypotonia, weakness, hoarse cry, and severe mental retardation. Other clinical features include macrocephaly with persistent patent posterior fontanelle; abdominal distention; umbilical hernia; coarse, dry skin; and large, protruding tongue. In some infants, diffuse muscular hypertrophy is prominent, leading to an erroneous consideration of muscular dystrophy. Older children with acquired hypothyroidism become sluggish and apathetic, with impaired memory and school performance. These children may also have generalized muscle weakness and hypertrophy.

Diagnosis of hypothyroidism is made by measuring serum levels of T_4, T_3, and thyroid-stimulating hormone (the latter is elevated in the presence of hypothyroidism). Thyroid insufficiency should be considered in any infant with developmental delay, in particular if the typical morphologic features are present, and in children with generalized muscle weakness and hypertrophy.

Treatment with synthetic thyroxine replacement will

FEATURE TABLE 6–6. RENAL FAILURE

Discriminating Feature	Consistent Features	Variable Features
1. Elevated BUN	1. Neuropathy	1. Seizures
	2. Altered mental state	2. Asterixis

reverse the symptoms in older children. Infants treated after 6 months of age continue to exhibit severe psychomotor retardation. Even if treatment is initiated within the first 6 months, residual neurologic deficits in the form of ataxia and speech and learning delays may persist.

Hyperthyroidism in children may be insidious, with hyperactivity and short attention span as the only manifestations. Other features include irritability, personality changes, inattentiveness, tremors, hyperreflexia, choreiform movements, and seizures. Exophthalmos and lid lag are characteristic features, but are not uniformly present in children. Neuromuscular symptoms, such as ophthalmoplegia and generalized weakness, are common in adults but are rarely found in children.

The diagnosis should be considered in any child with recent onset of hyperactive behavior or chorea. Palpation of the thyroid gland may demonstrate enlargement. Elevation of serum T_4 and/or T_3 concentrations confirms the diagnosis. Treatment with thyroid-blocking agents such as propylthiouracil restores euthyroid function and reverses the neurologic deficits.

NEUROLOGIC EFFECTS OF SYSTEMIC MALIGNANCY

In both children and adults, malignant tumors outside the nervous system can produce neurologic symptoms. The cause of these "remote" effects is not known. Possible etiologies include elaboration of autoimmune antibodies by the tumor, or a slow virus infection. The tumor most often associated with such an indirect effect in children is neuroblastoma. A characteristic syndrome of myoclonus and chaotic eye movements, or opsoclonus, is produced in the presence of neuroblastoma. This neurologic picture may be the initial presentation of the tumor, and may predate the ability to detect tumor presence by routine diagnostic tests.

Other causes of opsoclonus-myoclonus syndrome include viral infections, toxic exposure to the insecticide DDT, and other tumors. The diagnosis of neuroblastoma rests on detection of a mass by chest or abdominal radiographic examination, or by the presence of elevated levels of homovanillic and vanyllylmandelic acid in the urine.

Removal of the tumor does not uniformly improve the neurologic symptoms. About 40% of children have permanent neurologic deficits in the form of ataxia or other movement disorders, psychomotor retardation, and speech delays, and opsoclonus and myoclonus may persist as well.

TOXIC ENCEPHALOPATHIES

Heavy Metals: Lead

Lead poisoning continues to be a significant health risk. Approximately 4% of children under the age of 5 years have toxic blood lead levels of greater than 25 mcg/dL. There is evidence that even lower levels of exposure are associated with cognitive deficits in children. Studies of hyperactive children demonstrated blood lead levels of 25 mcg/dL or greater in over 50% of the children. Elevated dentine lead concentrations were associated with lower than expected IQ scores in another study. Chronic, low-level lead exposure may contribute to the etiology of mental retardation.

Sources of exposure to lead include paint in older buildings, improperly glazed pottery, contamination of drinking water by lead pipes or from industrial plants, leaded jewelry, industrial crayons, leaded toy soldiers, sniffing of leaded gasoline, and inhalation of fumes from burned storage batteries. Children at highest risk for lead exposure are poor, and often from inner-city areas. Black children have a higher incidence of lead exposure than do children from other ethnic groups. Children who are anemic or malnourished are also at higher risk.

FEATURE TABLE 6-7. LEAD TOXICITY

Discriminating Features	Consistent Features	Variable Features
1. Blood lead level > 25 mcg/dL 2. Elevated FEP	1. Irritability 2. Hyperactivity 3. Neuropathy 4. Dementia 5. Learning disabilities	1. Seizures 2. Basophilic stippling 3. Lead lines on gums, nails 4. Coma

---

Pearls and Perils: Lead Exposure

1. Lead exposure is not limited to poor children; exposure to lead may occur from jewelry, improperly glazed pottery, and other sources.
2. *No* level of lead exposure is safe; even low levels over a long period of time may produce subtle cognitive and behavioral deficits.

Signs and Symptoms. Both acute and chronic encephalopathies may result from lead exposure. Acute lead intoxication is often associated with vomiting, ataxia, seizures, and mental status changes with obtundation or coma. Increased intracranial pressure is a common and serious complication. In the chronic form, symptoms are nonspecific, and include irritability, anorexia, intermittent vomiting, abdominal pain, constipation, behavior problems, and hyperactivity. Lead exposure can produce a peripheral neuropathy, but this is more common in adults than children. The general physical examination provides few clues to the presence of lead poisoning, although gray lead lines may be present in the gingival margins in some chronic cases.

Diagnosis. Laboratory tests that are useful in supporting a diagnosis of lead poisoning include a hemogram and examination of the peripheral blood smear, looking for evidence of anemia and basophilic stippling. Concentrations of free erythrocyte porphyrin are elevated, because lead inhibits the enzyme heme synthetase, preventing the incorporation of iron into protoporphyrin III. Blood lead levels may also be measured directly.

Treatment. Treatment of acute and severe lead poisoning must be prompt and aggressive, in particular if coma and signs of increased intracranial pressure are evident. Intensive respiratory and cardiovascular support may be required, as well as the use of continuous ICP monitoring devices and management of intracranial hypertension. Chelating therapy with British anti-lewisite (BAL) and EDTA should be initiated immediately. Anticonvulsant therapy may be necessary if clinical or electrographic seizures are present.

Treatment of chronic lead exposure depends on the severity. For children with blood lead levels greater than 25 μcg/dL, inpatient or outpatient chelation therapy with EDTA may need to be initiated. The guidelines from the Centers for Disease Control may be used to determine which children require chelation therapy.

All children who are at risk for lead exposure, or who have documented lead exposure, should be followed with serial lead levels and free erythrocyte porphyrin (FEP) determinations for at least 6 months, and perhaps longer, to ensure that exposure is not continuing. Efforts should be made at the time of the initial visit or hospitalization to identify the sources of lead exposure and to make sure that steps are taken to eliminate them.

Pertinent information on other heavy metals is listed in Table 6–2.

Salicylism

Because of the presence of salicylates in a number of frequently used over-the-counter medicinal preparations, salicylate ingestion is a potential cause of accidental fatal poisoning in children under the age of 5 years. Toxic levels of salicylates produce a number of metabolic derangements, including metabolic acidosis, respiratory alkalosis, hypoprothrombinemia, hypoglycemia, hyperammonemia, hypokalemia, lactic acidosis, and accumulation of organic acids. Even in therapeutic concentrations, salicylates may produce hepatic injury, and this is common with toxic amounts. Histologic changes in the liver consist of focal necrosis, nonspecific inflammatory changes (usually of the mononuclear cell type and predominantly in the periportal areas), ballooning, and eosinophilic degeneration of hepatocytes. Occasionally, microvesicular fatty infiltration of liver parenchyma,

TABLE 6-2. HEAVY METAL TOXICITY

Element	Exposure	Nervous System Symptoms	Systemic Symptoms	Diagnosis	Treatment
Thallium	Insecticides Rodenticides	Headaches Ataxia Seizures Somnolence Cranial nerve palsies	Abdominal pain Diarrhea Hair loss Renal and cardiac failure	Urine thallium level	Bithizone KCl and charcoal Hemodialysis
Arsenic	Insecticides Herbicides	Headaches Irritability Seizures Sensory neuropathy	Anemia Vomiting Bloody diarrhea	Urine, hair arsenic levels	BAL, penicillamine
Organic mercury	Fungicides	Ataxia Choreoathetosis Tremor Blindness	Anemia Colitis Stomatitis Gingivitis	Red blood cell mercury level	Supportive care, ?thiol resins

FEATURE TABLE 6-8. SALICYLISM

Discriminating Features	Consistent Features	Variable Features
1. Serum salicylate level > 25 mg/dL	1. Hypoglycemia	1. Hyperammonemia (mild)
2. Hyperventilation	2. Lactic acidosis	2. Hyperglycemia
3. Lethargy, obtundation, coma		3. Hypoprothrombinemia
4. Metabolic acidosis/respiratory alkalosis		

reminiscent of that found in Reye's syndrome, has been reported following acute salicylate ingestion.

Cerebral edema with brain swelling is also a consequence of salicylate intoxication. No specific histologic changes have been reported in brain.

Signs and Symptoms. Symptoms of salicylate intoxication include repetitive vomiting, dizziness, tinnitus, and diaphoresis. These progress to dehydration, delirium, and coma. Hyperventilation is a prominent feature. Excess bleeding, from the gastrointestinal tract and elsewhere, may be noted. Clinical manifestations of salicylism are similar to those of Reye's syndrome, and both disorders must be considered in the infant or young child who presents with this clinical picture.

Diagnosis. Laboratory abnormalities reflect the underlying metabolic derangements. Disturbances of glucose and electrolyte balance are common. Arterial blood gas determinations typically demonstrate a mixed metabolic acidosis and respiratory alkalosis. Tests of liver function may be abnormal, and prothrombin time prolonged. Ketosis and lactic acidosis are present. A serum salicylate level of 25 mg/dL or greater is indicative of intoxication.

Differential diagnosis of salicylism includes Reye's syndrome, diabetic ketoacidosis, encephalitis, and meningitis.

Treatment. Treatment of mild forms of intoxication includes gastric lavage and generous intravenous fluid therapy. In the more severe cases, intensive respiratory and cardiovascular support may be necessary. Metabolic and electrolyte derangements should be corrected with appropriate intravenous solutions. The most advanced cases may require hemo- or peritoneal dialysis. Vitamin K may help to alleviate bleeding problems.

Barbiturate Poisoning

Signs and Symptoms. Accidental or deliberate ingestion of barbiturates may produce symptoms such as lethargy, ataxia, slurred speech, and nystagmus in mild cases, but massive overdoses cause coma, hyporeflexia, cardiorespiratory depression, and shock. The rapidity of onset and duration of symptoms depend on the amount and type of barbiturate ingested. Exposure to short-acting barbiturates leads to rapid onset of symptoms, but in mild cases these clear within a few hours. Phenobarbital in-

---

Pearls and Perils: Salicylism

1. Differentiation between salicylism and Reye's syndrome is difficult. Salicylism is more likely to be associated with a serum pH in the acidotic range. Marked hyperammonemia is more often seen in Reye's syndrome.
2. A serum salicylate level should be obtained in any child with acute onset of unexplained encephalopathy. Prompt treatment results in reversal of the neurologic and metabolic derangements.
3. Hyperbilirubinemia and clinical jaundice are not typical of salicylate-induced liver injury.
4. Massive hepatic necrosis has been reported in children on chronic salicylate therapy, even in the absence of toxic blood levels.

Pearls and Perils: Barbiturate Poisoning

1. In most metabolic encephalopathies, hyperreflexia is present on examination, and brainstem reflexes are preserved until late in the course; in contrast, barbiturates depress the reflexes and evidence of brainstem dysfunction is common.
2. Acute barbiturate intoxication can cause areflexia, absence of brainstem reflexes, and a flat EEG—all of which symptoms are reversible when the drug clears from the system. Thus, a diagnosis of brain death cannot be made on the basis of clinical and EEG findings in the presence of barbiturate intoxication.

TABLE 6-3. PLANT TOXINS

Plant or Toxin	Symptoms
Aflatoxin B₁ (cereal grains, peanut butter)	Reye's syndrome–like illness with vomiting, encephalopathy, and hypoglycemia
Mushrooms	
Amanita phalloides	Hepatic necrosis, encephalopathy
Amanita muscaria	Hepatic and renal damage; miosis, dizziness, ataxia, delirium, hallucinations, coma, seizures
Nutmeg	Delirium, excitability, drowsiness, hallucinations
Wolfsbane and larkspur	Tingling in mouth, stomach, and skin; weakness, impaired speech, coma; seizures
Mountain laurel	Salivation, lacrimation, vomiting; seizures
Nicotine	Nausea, vomiting, diarrhea; headache; dizziness, confusion, tremors
Jimsonweed	Mydriasis, bizarre behavior, visual hallucinations
Pokeweed	Vomiting, cramps, dizziness, lethargy, seizures

gestion results in a much longer duration of symptoms, and may take several days to clear.

Diagnosis. Diagnosis rests on the detection of barbiturates in blood or urine specimens. The EEG in mild cases shows low-voltage fast activity, but activity becomes progressively slower as symptoms progress, and in severe poisoning the EEG may be flat. This is completely reversible as the patient recovers.

Treatment. Treatment consists of gastric lavage to remove any remaining drugs from the stomach. Intensive cardiovascular and respiratory support is necessary in severe cases, and hypotension may necessitate the use of pressor agents. Forced alkaline diuresis is helpful, but hemodialysis may be necessary if the patient continues to deteriorate.

Plant Toxins

A number of plants commonly found in the environment contain substances that are toxic when ingested. A partial list of these is given in Table 6-3.

ANNOTATED BIBLIOGRAPHY

Agus ZS, Wasserstein A, Goldfarb S: Disorders of calcium and magnesium homeostasis. *Am J Med* 72:473, 1982.
  A summary of calcium and magnesium imbalance.
Bondy PK, Rosenberg LE (eds): *Metabolic Control and Disease*, 8th ed. Philadelphia, WB Saunders, 1980.
  A good overview of metabolic disorders.
Bresnan MJ, Hicks EM: Nutritional, vitamin, and endocrine disorders, in Farmer TW (ed): *Pediatric Neurology*, 3rd ed. Philadelphia, Harper & Row, 1983.
  A comprehensive review of disorders that can result in encephalopathy.
Forbes GB, McCormick KL: Disturbances of water and electrolytes, in Farmer TW (ed): *Pediatric Neurology*, 3rd ed. Philadelphia, Harper & Row, 1983.

A readable summary of fluid and electrolyte problems.
Plum F, Posner JB: *Disorders of Stupor and Coma*, 3rd ed. Philadelphia, FA Davis, 1980.
  An excellent overview of the encephalopathies.
Siesjo BK, Plum F: Pathophysiology of anoxic brain damage, in Gaull GE (ed): *Biology of Brain Dysfunction*. Vol 1. New York, Plenum Press, 1973.
  A good review of the basic mechanisms of anoxic encephalopathy.
Spencer PS, Schaumburg HH (eds): *Experimental and Clinical Neurotoxicology*, Baltimore, Md, Williams & Wilkins, 1980.
  Thorough coverage of toxins affecting the central nervous system.

BIBLIOGRAPHY

Fluids and Electrolytes

Book LS: Vomiting and diarrhea. *Pediatrics* 74(pt 2):950, 1984.
Cockburn F, Brown JK, Belton NR, Fortar JO: Neonatal convulsions associated with primary disturbance of calcium, phosphorus and magnesium. *Arch Dis Child* 48:99, 1973.
Fishman RA: Neurological manifestations of hyponatremia, in Vinken PJ, Bruhn GW (eds): *Handbook of Clinical Neurology*, Vol 28. Amsterdam, North-Holland, 1977.
Laureno R: Central pontine myelinolysis following rapid correction of hyponatremia. *Ann Neurol* 13:232, 1983.
Massry SG, Seelig MS: Hypomagnesemia and hypermagnesemia. *Clin Nephrol* 7:147, 1977.
Morris-Jones PH, Houston IB, Evans RC: Prognosis of the neurologic complications of acute hypernatremia. *Lancet* 2:1385, 1967.
Pizarro D, Posada G, Villavicencio N, Mohs E, Levine MM: Oral rehydration in hypernatremic and hyponatremic diarrhea dehydration. *Am J Dis Child* 137:730, 1983.
Rasch DK, Huber PA, Richardson CJ, L'Hommedieu CS, Nelson TE, Reddi R: Neurobehavioral effects of neonatal hypermagnesemia. *J Pediatr* 100:272, 1981.
Swanson PD: Neurological manifestations of hypernatremia, in Vinken PJ, Bruhn GW (eds): *Handbook of Clinical Neurology*, Vol 28. Amsterdam, North-Holland, 1977.

Glucose

Arieff AI, Doerner T, Zelig H, Massry SG: Mechanisms of seizures and coma in hypoglycemia. *J Clin Invest* 54:654, 1974.

Guisado R, Arieff AI: Neurologic manifestations of diabetic coma: Correlation with biochemical alterations in the brain. *Metabolism* 24:665, 1975.

Koivisto M, Blanco-Sequeiros M, Krause U: Neonatal symptomatic and asymptomatic hypoglycemia: A follow-up study of 151 children. *Dev Med Child Neurol* 14:603, 1972.

Rosenbloom AL, Riley WJ, Weber FT, Malone JI, Donnelly, WH: Cerebral edema complicating diabetic ketoacidosis in childhood. *J Pediatr* 96:357, 1980.

Nutritional Disorders

Bankier A, Turner M, Hopkins IJ: Pyridoxine dependent seizures, a wider clinical spectrum. *Arch Dis Child* 58:415, 1983.

Davis RA, Wolf A: Infantile beriberi associated with Wernicke's encephalopathy. *Pediatrics* 21:409, 1958.

Donaldson JO: Pathogenesis of pseudotumor cerebri syndromes. *Neurology* 31:877, 1981.

Evans D, Hansen JD, Moodie AD, van der Spuy HI: Intellectual development and nutrition. *J Pediatr* 97:358, 1980.

Goutieres F, Aicardi J: Atypical presentations of pyridoxine-dependent seizures: A treatable cause of intractable epilepsy in infants. *Ann Neurol* 17:117, 1985.

Hakim AM, Carpenter S, Pappius GM: Metabolic and histologic reversibility of thiamine deficiency. *J Cereb Blood Flow Metab* 3:468, 1983.

Pearson HA, Vinson R, Smith RT: Pernicious anemia with neurologic involvement in childhood. *J Pediatr* 65:334, 1964.

Still CN: Nicotinic acid and nicotinamide deficiency: Pellagra and related disorders of the nervous system, in Vinken PJ, Bruhn GW (eds): *Handbook of Clinical Neurology*, Vol. 28. Amsterdam, North-Holland, 1977.

Wilson JD, Madison LL: Deficiency of thiamine (beri beri), pyridoxine and riboflavin, in Isselbacher KJ, Adams RD, Braunwald E, et al (eds): *Harrison's Principles of Internal Medicine*, 9th ed. New York, McGraw-Hill, 1980.

Winick M: Malnutrition and brain development. *J Pediatr* 74:667, 1969.

Wyatt DT, Noetzel MJ, Hillman RE: Infantile beriberi presenting as subacute necrotizing encephalomyelopathy. *J Pediatr* 110:888, 1987.

Hepatic Encephalopathy

Cooper AJL, Ehrlich ME, Plum F: Hepatic encephalopathy: GABA or ammonia? *Lancet* 2:158, 1984.

Sherlock S: Hepatic encephalopathy. *Br J Hosp Med* 17:144, 1977.

Reye's Syndrome

Barrett MJ, Hurwitz ES, Schonberger LB, Rogers MF: Changing epidemiology of Reye syndrome in the United States. *Pediatrics* 77:598, 1986.

DeVivo DC: Reye syndrome. *Neurol Clin North Am* 3(1):95, 1985.

Hurwitz ES, Barrett MJ, Gregman D, et al: Public Health Service study on Reye's syndrome and medications: Report of the pilot phase. *N Engl J Med* 313:849, 1985.

Lichtenstein PK, Heubi JE, Daugherty CC, et al: Grade I Reye's syndrome. A frequent cause of vomiting and liver dysfunction after varicella and upper respiratory infection. *N Engl J Med* 309:133, 1983.

Trauner DA: Treatment of Reye syndrome. *Ann Neurol* 7:204, 1980.

Renal Failure

Mahoney CA, Arieff AI: Uremic encephalopathies: Clinical, biochemical and experimental features. *Am J Kidney Dis* 11:324, 1982.

Rasbury WC, Fennell RS, Morris MK: Cognitive functioning of children with end-stage renal disease before and after successful transplantation. *J Pediatr* 102:589, 1983.

Raskin HN, Fishman RA: Neurologic disorders in renal failure. N Engl J Med 294:143, 204, 1976.

Dialysis Encephalopathy

Alfrey AC, LeGendre GR, Kaehny WD: The dialysis encephalopathy syndrome: Possible aluminum intoxication. *N Engl J Med* 294:184, 1976.

Geary DF, Fennell RS, Andriola M, Gudat J, Rodgers BM, Richard GA: Encephalopathy in children with chronic renal failure. *J Pediatr* 97:41, 1980.

Pillion G, Loirat C, Blum C, et al: Aluminum encephalopathy: A potential risk of aluminum gels in children with chronic renal failure. *Int J Pediatr Nephrol* 2:29, 1981.

Thyroid Dysfunction

Mosier HD: Hyperthyroidism, in Gardner LI (ed): *Endocrine and Genetic Diseases of Childhood*, 2nd ed. Philadelphia, WB Saunders, 1975.

Murphy G, Hulse JA, Jackson D, et al: Early treated hypothyroidism: Development at 3 years. *Arch Dis Child* 61:761, 1986.

New England Congenital Hypothyroidism Collaborative. Neonatal hypothyroidism screening: Status of patients at 6 years. *J Pediatr* 107:915, 1986.

Price JF, Ehrlich RM, Walfish PG: Congenital hypothyroidism: Clinical and laboratory characteristics of infants detected by neonatal screening. *Arch Dis Child* 56:845, 1981.

Rovet J, Ehrlich R, Sorbara D: Intellectual outcome in children with fetal hypothyroidism. *J Pediatr* 110:700, 1987.

Toxins

Bismuth C: The principles of management of acute poisoning, in Tinker J, Rapin M (eds): *Care of the Critically Ill Patient*. Berlin, Springer-Verlag, 1983.

Robinson RR, Gunnells JC, Clapp JR: Treatment of acute barbiturate intoxication. *Mod Treat* 8:561, 1971.

Seidel J: Acute mercury poisoning after polyvinyl alcohol preservatives. *Pediatrics* 107:337, 180.

Snyder RD: The involuntary movements of chronic mercury poisoning. *Arch Neurol* 26:379, 1972.

Lead Poisoning

Bellinger DC, Needleman HL: Lead and the relationship between maternal and child intelligence. *J Pediatr* 102:523, 1983.

Chisolm JJ, Barltrop D: Recognition and management of children with increased lead absorption. *Arch Dis Child* 54:249, 1979.

Landrigan PJ, et al: Statement on childhood lead poisoning. *Pediatrics* 79:457, 1987.

Preventing lead poisoning in young children: A statement by the Centers for Disease Control, January 1985. Atlanta, US Department of Health, Education and Welfare, 1985.

Salicylism

Bray PF, Gardiner AY: Salicylism and severe brain edema. *N Engl J Med* 297:1235, 1977.

Kerzner B: Salicylate intoxication. *Drug Ther Bull* 6:94, 1976.

Pierce AW: Salicylate poisoning. *Pediatrics* 54:342, 1974.

Zimmerman HJ: Effects of aspirin and acetaminophen on the liver. *Arch Intern Med* 141:333, 1981.

Traumatic Encephalopathies

H. Terry Hutchison

ACUTE DIFFUSE TRAUMATIC BRAIN INJURY

Head injury is the leading cause of death and morbidity in children as well as in young adults. Nearly half of all head injuries result from motor vehicle accidents. The death rate from auto accidents increases nearly tenfold for young men after the driving age. A similar increase is *not* seen for young women. A large portion of the remainder of head injuries result from falls or child abuse. The overall incidence of head injury is 200 to 300 new cases per year per 100,000 population. In the United States, about one million children each year suffer a head injury. Of these about 165,000 visit a hospital. About 1 in 10 falls into the category of moderately to severely head injured. Most of these children will have some disability lasting months or years. Those with a minor head injury, defined as no loss of consciousness or at most a brief loss of consciousness, may have some neurologic deficits that will interfere with their lives for up to several months.

Acute injury to the brain may result from causes other than a blow to the head. Anoxic injury from near-drowning accounts for nearly half as many deaths in children as does trumatic injury from motor vehicle accidents. Cardiorespiratory arrest from a variety of causes, status epilepticus and various metabolic encephalopathies account for most of the remainder.

Pathology

Several mechanisms of injury occur simultaneously in severe traumatic brain injury. Direct contusion of the gray matter of the brain may occur at the site of impact. Laceration of the brain occurs with penetrating trauma. Contusion of the side of the brain opposite the point of impact is called contre-coup injury. More commonly the brain is contused on the undersurface of the temporal and frontal lobes, and on the anterior poles of the temporal lobes, regardless of the site of impact. This pattern results from the brain striking against the bony prominences at the base of the cranial vault. Shearing forces are thought to be involved in the pathogenesis of these contusions. Rotational acceleration appears to exaggerate their likelihood of occurrence. Contusions may be extensive without loss of consciousness. Their significance lies in their part in the genesis of the secondary events of edema, hemorrhage, and swelling.

Loss of consciousness occurs immediately in severe head trauma. Animal studies have suggested that injuries of increasing severity involve first the cerebral hemispheres and then the diencephalon. Only the most severe injuries involve dysfunction of the mesencephalon directly. Direct brainstem contusion without concomitant injury to the cerebral hemispheres is rarely seen pathologically. However, several lines of evidence suggest that transient functional changes in the reticular activating system without gross structural changes in the brainstem may be involved in the initial loss of consciousness in traumatic brain injury.

Diffuse white matter degeneration occurs directly as a result of shearing forces in head trauma. Extensive white matter destruction from any cause is associated with poor outcome.

Anoxic-ischemic injury complicates the majority of traumatic brain injuries. Hypoventilation and hypotension, as well as unequal distribution of blood flow, are present to some degree with most head injuries. Multiple trauma increases the risk of anoxic-ischemic injury. The neurons of gray matter are particularly sensitive to anoxia. The hippocampus and basal ganglia are the most easily damaged, and the cerebral cortex and cerebellum are also quite sensitive to anoxic injury. In the most severe anoxic injuries the white matter is also damaged and the outcome is poor.

Secondary brain damage occurring after the initial injury may be due to anoxic-ischemic events, or to transtentorial herniation. Herniation, in turn, may be due to diffuse brain swelling or to expanding intracranial masses. These secondary brain injuries may be more signficant than the primary injury and are discussed in more detail later in this chapter.

FEATURE TABLE 7-1. ACUTE DIFFUSE TRAUMATIC BRAIN INJURY

Discriminating Features	Consistent Features	Variable Features
1. Loss of consciousness is noted in all severe traumatic brain injuries, except for purely focal injuries. 2. Deepening coma following a rostral-caudal progression from hemispheric dysfunction through diencephalic, midbrain, pontine, and medullary stages from traumatic brain injury identifies acute diffuse traumatic brain injury. 3. A history of trauma sufficient to produce the injury in the absence of other causes of encephalopathy is a further discriminating feature.	1. Contusion of the undersurfaces of the temporal and frontal lobes, and of the anterior poles of the temporal lobes, are consistent features of nearly all traumatic brain injuries, regardless of the site of impact. 2. Brainstem dysfunction is invariably associated with hemispheric dysfunction. 3. Deepening coma is associated with the progressive appearance of flexor posturing, extensor posturing, and finally flaccidity. 4. Hypoventilation, or apnea, accompanies deeper levels of coma. 5. Some degree of anoxic-ischemic brain injury accompanies nearly all of the more severe traumatic head injuries.	1. Contusion of the brain sometimes occurs on the side opposite the point of impact. Such lesions are called contre-coup injuries. 2. Secondary injury often accompanies brain trauma. The major causes of secondary brain injury are anoxia-ischemia and transtentorial herniation. 3. In an individual child, the depth of coma is only roughly correlated with the severity of injury. Focal traumatic injury and anoxia account for some of this variability. 4. Mild or minor head injury, or concussion, are terms referring to those head injuries with brief or no loss of consciousness. Such injuries are sometimes associated with acute deterioration or lasting sequelae.

Signs and Symptoms

Loss of consciousness is characteristic of severe diffuse traumatic brain injury. The extent and duration of the loss of consciousness correlate well with outcome. However, in an individual child, it is not possible to predict outcome reliably from length of coma. A few children present an alarming but short-lived picture of deep coma with unreactive pupils, followed by rapid recovery. Others may have a relatively brief loss of consciousness followed by deterioration and a poor outcome. The presence of anoxic injury, or focal traumatic brain injury, may account for some of this individual variability.

The severity of loss of consciousness (or of coma) correlates with the severity of injury. Deeper levels of unconsciousness imply more severe injury. Plum and Posner have defined levels of consciousness corresponding to dysfunction of progressively more caudal structures in the brain. As discussed previously, this rostral-caudal progression reflects the observation that caudal structures are rarely damaged without there first having been damage to the more rostral brain structures. A rostral-caudal progression of symptoms also occurs in compromise owing to increasing brain swelling and transtentorial herniation. Recovery from loss of consciousness often follows this progression in reverse order.

The first of Plum and Posner's stages is the early diencephalic stage. At this level consciousness is altered, but not necessarily lost. Some children are agitated or combative. Others are somnolent, but may become agitated transiently with stimulation. Appropriate motor responses to noxious stimulation are present. Except for babies in the newborn period, children can usually move their limbs toward the source of noxious stimulation. Children of all ages withdraw from pain. Oculocephalic and pupillary reflexes are intact.

The second, or late diencephalic, stage is marked by loss of consciousness and flexor (decorticate) posturing. The posturing occurs in response to stimulation, or sometimes at rest. Oculocephalic and pupillary reflexes remain intact. Hypoventilation may occur and respirations are irregular.

The third stage correlates with dysfunction of the midbrain and upper pons. Extensor rigidity (decerebrate posturing) is the maximum motor response. Oculocephalic and pupillary reflexes are impaired because the brainstem nuclei controlling these reflexes are located in the damaged midbrain. Responsiveness, other than increasing rigidity, is deeply impaired. Respiration is usually irregular, with hyper- or hypoventilation.

The final stage corresponds to dysfunction of the lower pons and upper medulla. The limbs are motionless and flaccid except possibly for some leg flexion to stimulation above the neck. Spontaneous breathing is present, but hypoventilation is the rule.

Some period of apnea occurs commonly in more severely head-injured children. This, in part, accounts for the high incidence of anoxic damage complicating traumatic brain injury. On the whole, anoxic injury carries a worse prognosis than does purely traumatic injury producing the same level of coma.

In some cases symptoms are observed that do not fit a pattern of rostral-caudal progression. For example, a child may exhibit extensor rigidity with the eyes open and with conjugate eye movements. This suggests patchy brainstem compromise, and is often due to anoxic-ischemic injury to the brainstem. Careful examination may reveal other focal neurologic deficits even in a comatose patient. Such deficits are more likely to occur with more severe injury, but are easily overlooked because of the motor signs and lack of responsiveness associated with coma. These signs are important because they may indicate severe focal brain injuries that are not reflected in the level of consciousness.

At the other end of the spectrum of loss of consciousness are those children who have suffered no loss, or no more than a brief loss, of consciousness, and who have no focal neurologic deficits. These children are said to have suffered a minor, or mild, head injury. Concussion is another term with similar meaning. Injuries of this kind are not necessarily minor or mild. Some children with such an injury have persistent, subtle, but disabling symptoms of brain dysfunction lasting hours to months. Others, about 5%, may show marked deterioration owing to brain swelling or, less often, to an expanding intracranial hematoma.

Diagnostic Studies

Computer tomography (CT) has greatly aided the diagnosis and management of traumatic brain injury. This technique allows direct visualization of the brain and is particularly sensitive to the presence of intracranial bleeding. Skull fractures may also be seen on CT, although conventional plane skull films are often necessary to delineate the bony abnormalities. The value of routine skull films is debated, but it is clear that CT provides most of the information available from skull films, as well as additional information that cannot be obtained in any other way. Angiography has largely been supplanted by CT for routine evaluation.

Magnetic resonance imaging (MRI) may be superior to CT in some ways, but the problem of gaining access to a patient in a strong magnetic field precludes its routine use in head trauma, although this is changing. For example, MRI is particularly superior in the diagnosis of acute spinal chord injuries.

Radiographic examination of other body areas, including the cervical spine, is usually indicated. A long bone series should be obtained in cases of suspected child abuse.

Electroencephalography (EEG) is of little use in acute trauma. EEG is not a reliable indicator of brain death in children, and other criteria should be used in this situation. Continuous EEG and compressed EEG spectral array monitoring and evoked potential monitoring are of great interest, but their usefulness in the care of individual patients is still being studied.

Pearls and Perils: Acute Diffuse Traumatic Brain Injury

1. Worsening (blood pressure may be increased) vital signs owing to brain injury almost always occur after a decrease in the level of consciousness. Therefore, level of consciousness is the most sensitive indicator of neurologic deterioration. The Glasgow Coma Scale is widely used to monitor level of consciousness.
2. Coma is defined as being present in those children who do not open their eyes, speak, or obey commands. Coma is present in babies who do not open their eyes or cry.
3. People with GCS scores of less than 8 account for 30% of all head injury admissions, but more than 95% of deaths.
4. CT demonstrates most of the lesions identifiable on plane skull films, but the latter may be more valuable in the elucidation of fractures.
5. Maintenance of airway, breathing, and circulation are of the highest priority for the treatment of brain-injured children.
6. Some severe or fatal brain injuries occur without external evidence of trauma.
7. The presence of retinal hemorrhages in an infant suggests child abuse.
8. Secondary brain damage may be preventable. The major causes of secondary brain damage are anoxia-ischemia and transtentorial herniation.
9. In an individual child, it is not possible to predict outcome reliably from the length or severity of coma.
10. Severe focal brain injuries and cervical spinal cord injury may be overlooked in comatose children because of the lack of responsiveness and motor signs associated with coma.
11. The tendency to ascribe warning signs of other injury to brain dysfunction should be avoided. Hypotension rarely occurs as a result of acute brain injury. Hypertension is the usual response. Fever over 102°F is rarely due to brain dysfunction.
12. A long bone series should be done in cases of suspected child abuse.
13. The most common conditions resulting from inadequate treatment include hypoxia, hypotension, sepsis, and seizures.
14. Comatose children with traumatic brain injury usually require intubation, intravenous lines, and transfer to an appropriate intensive care unit.

Treatment

The importance of adequate management of traumatically brain-injured children cannot be overemphasized. It has been estimated that, in as many as 70% or 80% of acutely comatose children and adults, gross errors in management are made when they are first seen. Errors in management occur in urban as well as in rural hospitals, and in teaching as well as private hospitals. The most common conditions resulting from inadequate treatment include hypoxia, hypotension, sepsis, and seizures. Iatrogenic complications include misplacement of endotracheal tubes, pneumothorax following subclavian puncture, and fractured ribs from overzealous resuscitation. The excess morbidity and mortality from these errors cannot be estimated. There are a few basic principles in the management of acute brain injury that every physician should know and that could prevent more severe neurologic deficits and loss of life owing to inadequate management. A more complete discussion of brain damage secondary to events occurring after the initial injury is found in the following section.

Maintenance of airway, breathing, and circulation are the principles of basic life support and are of first priority.

The taking of a history and examination for other injuries are essential. Life-threatening injuries of the chest, abdomen, spine, and limbs are easily overlooked in children with impaired consciousness. This is particularly true of abdominal injuries, in which tenderness, guarding, and rigidity may be absent despite severe bleeding or peritonitis. Stabilization of the neck and subsequent imaging studies of the spine, the chest, and, if indicated, the limbs are the next important steps. A history is often difficult to obtain but may be of critical importance. The details of the injury as well as information regarding the onset of symptoms, prodromal illness or the ingestion of poisons, and the use of drugs or alcohol must be sought. Scalp injuries or other signs of trauma are important in the assessment of brain injury. But some severe or fatal traumatic brain injuries occur with no external evidence of trauma. Retinal hemorrhages accompany severe deceleration or shaking injuries, but also occur with asphyxia.

The tendency to ascribe warning signs of other injury or illness to brain dysfunction should be avoided. A few principles are important to remember and are listed in Pearls and Perils.

Assessment of the level of consciousness should be carried out accurately. The Glasgow Coma Scale (GCS) is widely used for this purpose and is described in Table 7–1. One great advantage of this scale is that it may be applied quickly, repeatedly, and accurately by professionals with all levels of training. The scale records responses in terms of eye opening, movements, and vocalization. This information can be quickly and unambiguously transmitted to others involved in the care of the patient. It is by no means necessary to use, or remember, the numbers of the scale; *words* are sufficient and communicate more information.

According to the GCS, a child is in coma who fails to open his or her eyes, to speak, and to obey commands. Coma in babies is less well characterized but may be defined as existing in those babies who fail to open their

TABLE 7-1. GLASGOW COMA SCALE

Response	Value	Explanation
Eye Opening		
Spontaneous	4	Eyes are open without stimulation
To speech	3	Eyes open to speech or sound. This does not imply obeying commands
To pain	2	Eyes open only to noxious stimuli
None	1	Do not score if eyes are swollen shut
Motor Response		
Obeys commands	6	Follows commands like "stick out your tongue"
Localizes pain	5	Limb moves toward source of pain
Withdrawal	4	Normal response with abduction of the shoulder (this is the maximum response babies can generate)
Flexion	3	"Decorticate" posturing with adduction of the shoulder, elbows flexed, legs extended, rigid
Extension	2	"Decerebrate" posturing with elbows and legs extended, rigid
No response	1	Tone is flaccid
Verbal Response		
Oriented	5	Knows time, place, person
Confused	4	Conversational speech but confused
Inappropriate	3	Words but no coherent speech—often swearing and combativeness
Incomprehensible	2	No recognizable words—moans and groans or crying in babies (this is the maximum response babies can generate)
No response	1	Makes no sounds—a score of 1 is given for intubated patients

The maximum score generated with maximum stimulation is added in each section. Maximum possible is 15 (10 in babies). Remember that *words* are a perfectly adequate form of communication, and that description of what happens in each area is more useful than numbers alone.
After Teasdale G, Jennett B: The Glasgow Coma Scale. Lancet 2:81, 1974.

eyes or to cry, or who have abnormal motor responses. All children whose GCS is 7 or below are in coma by these definitions. Furthermore, many children with a GCS score of 8 will also be in coma. This is of great predictive importance. Patients with GCS scores of greater than 8 account for 70% of all head injury admissions but less than 5% of deaths. Conversely, those with GCS scores of less than 8 account for only 30% of admissions but more than 95% of deaths. A similar dichotomy exists for other causes of acute brain injury, including drowning and metabolic encephalopathy.

Once the initial assessment and stabilization have been accomplished, ongoing careful observation and management are essential to prevent secondary brain injury, as well as to treat injuries not involving the brain directly. This is often best accomplished in an intensive care unit. This further management will be discussed in the following section.

Support of the family and friends of the acutely brain-injured child is mandatory. A wealth of printed material is available that is designed to answer some of their questions. This information can increase communication between families and health care personnel. It must be pointed out, however, that no booklet can replace the warmth of human compassion, which can be provided only by personal contact.

ANNOTATED BIBLIOGRAPHY

Bruce DA, Raphaely RC, Goldberg AI, et al: Pathophysiology, treatment and outcome following severe head injury in children. *Child's Brain* 5:174–191, 1979.

An excellent discussion of the acute management of traumatically brain-injured children, with particular reference to brain edema.

Clifton GL, Grossman RG, Makela ME, Miner ME, Handel S, Sadhu V: Neurological course and correlated computerized tomography findings after severe closed head injury. *J Neurosurg* 52:611, 1980.

A good discussion of the role of CT scanning in the management of head trauma.

Hutchison R, Hutchison HT: Head Injury: A Booklet for Families. Houston, Texas Head Injury Foundation, 1983. 21 p.

A compendium of answers to questions frequently asked by families of acutely head-injured persons. This booklet is written for families. It explains some of the equipment and terminology of the intensive care unit.

Jennett B, Teasdale G: *Management of Head Injuries.* Philadelphia, FA Davis, 1981.

An excellent monograph on acute management and outcome of head injury. It includes an excellent discussion of the pathology of head injury.

Levin HS, Benton AL, Grossman RG: *Neurobehavioral Consequences of Closed Head Injury.* New York, Oxford University Press, 1982.

An authoritative look at the outcome of head trauma. This book also includes a summary of the pathophysiology of head trauma.

Miner ME, Wagner KA (eds): *Neurotrauma: Treatment,* *Rehabilitation and Related Issues.* Boston, Butterworths, 1986.

An up-to-date summary of approaches to the acute management of head trauma. Issues of outcome are also discussed.

Plum F, Posner JB: *Diagnosis of Stupor and Coma,* 3rd ed. Philadelphia, FA Davis, 1981.

The standard monograph describing the pathophysiology of coma in eminently understandable terms.

DETERIORATION FOLLOWING ACUTE BRAIN INJURY

Neurologic deterioration following acute traumatic brain injury often warns of life-threatening complications. Many of these complications are treatable and most are preventable. The most sensitive indicator of neurologic deterioration is a progressive decrease in the level of consciousness. Brain damage secondary to events occurring after the initial injury is often more severe than the primary traumatic damage. Three mechanisms underlie these secondary injuries. First, there is a high risk of ongoing anoxic-ischemic injury in severely injured children. Other metabolic derangements, such as electrolyte imbalance, hypoglycemia, and hyperosmolar states, are also common. Second, diffuse brain swelling, an increase in the volume of the brain, may lead to herniation of the brain through the tentorium, or to global ischemic injury through lack of perfusion of the brain. Infection and fever may aggravate diffuse swelling. Finally, expanding intracranial mass lesions may damage the brain by exerting local pressure on it, or by transtentorial herniation.

SUBACUTE DIFFUSE BRAIN SWELLING

Subacute diffuse brain swelling is more likely to cause secondary neurologic deterioration in children than in adults. In young children this swelling is sometimes so dramatic that it has been called the syndrome of "malignant brain edema." This condition is often treatable with good outcome if herniation and brain ischemia are prevented. On the other hand, diffuse brain swelling may cause death owing to increased intracranial pressure or subsequent transtentorial herniation. The pressure in the head may become so high that the arterial pressure generated by the heart is not capable of perfusing the brain. This leads to ischemic death. Once blood flow to the whole brain, or to portions of the brain, has been interrupted, it is usually impossible to force blood back into the damaged vessels, even if the perfusion pressure is returned to normal. This accounts in part for the irreversibility of severe ischemic brain injury.

Pathology

Traumatic brain injury is often associated with disruption of the blood-brain barrier. This barrier is formed by tight junctions between the endothelial cells of brain

FEATURE TABLE 7–2. SUBACUTE DIFFUSE BRAIN SWELLING

Discriminating Features	Consistent Features	Variable Features
1. Subacute decreased level of consciousness is the most sensitive indicator of progressive brain and brainstem compromise. 2. Increased brain volume is due to greater quantities of extracellular fluid (vasogenic edema), intracellular fluid (cytotoxic edema), or blood (hyperemia).	1. Increased intracranial pressure is consistent with clinically significant diffuse brain swelling. 2. The clinical signs associated with diffuse brain swelling follow an orderly rostral-to-caudal progression, leading ultimately to death. 3. The CT picture of small ventricles and relatively lucent brain with blurring of the gray-white borders is consistent with diffuse brain swelling.	1. Increased intracranial pressure may not accompany brain swelling unless the compliance of the intradural space is exceeded. 2. Obliteration of the perimesencephalic cisterns may be seen in incipient or actual herniation. 3. Cerebral blood flow in head-injured children may be increased, normal, or decreased. 4. Seizures worsen brain swelling, but may not occur unless there is some focal injury to the brain as well. 5. Electrolyte abnormalities may be due to diabetes insipidus or to the syndrome of inappropriate antidiuretic hormone secretion. 6. A hypermetabolic state with arterial hypertension and tachycardia may accompany subacute diffuse brain swelling.

capillaries and prevents passage of larger molecules out of the capillaries. The capillary barrier is susceptible to traumatic damage which permits a transudate to fill the extracellular spaces in the brain. This vascular compromise involves biochemic mediators and is not due to direct mechanical disruption of the vessels. This process has been termed vasogenic edema. It affects the white matter preferentially. Cytotoxic edema, on the other hand, affects all parts of the brain and involves swelling of the neuronal and glial cells without an increase in extracellular fluid. Anoxic-ischemic injury and injury resulting from most metabolic causes are the major contributors to cytotoxic edema. Hyperemia also increases the volume of the brain and is often the major initial contributor to brain swelling in children. The cerebrospinal fluid is still another intracranial compartment that may contribute to increased intracranial pressure. Cerebrospinal fluid may be trapped within the ventricles, or it may fail to be absorbed into the venous system.

Signs and Symptoms

Brain swelling causes clinically significant signs and symptoms by two mechanisms: increased intracranial pressure and transtentorial herniation. The most sensitive indicator of progressive compromise owing to brain swelling is a decreasing level of consciousness. The GCS monitors the rostral-caudal progression of symptoms caused by downward herniation of the brain and brainstem. The GCS score reflects the sequential compromise of the diencephalon, midbrain, pons, and medulla, and the symptoms associated wtih compromise at each of these levels were discussed previously.

Inadequate ventilation with hypoxia and hypercarbia is the most common condition aggravating brain swelling and leading to neurologic compromise following head trauma. Hypoventilation sometimes occurs in association with acute brain injury, with its attendant deleterious effects, before medical assistance arrives. Further hypoventilation is then often preventable. Primary pulmonary complications cause hypoventilation and may include pneumonia or pneumonitis from aspiration of gastric contents, or of water in the case of drowning. Intubation, or sometimes tracheostomy, is often necessary to maintain an open airway. Almost every head-injured child has difficulty swallowing and handling secretions, a problem that may lead to airway obstruction or pneumonia. Infection and fever from any source may aggravate brain swelling.

The adult respiratory distress syndrome occurs in children and may make ventilation difficult. Pulmonary edema caused by injudicious fluid management, including giving hyperosmolar agents, is a preventable complication. On the other hand hypotension owing to inadequate fluid administration may further damage the brain as well as other organs. Good hemodynamic balance is essential.

Seizures complicate the hospital course of more than 5% of children with traumatic brain injury. Roughly 50% of children with penetrating injury or intracranial hematoma have seizures. The majority of seizures occur within the first 1 or 2 hours after injury. Seizures further aggravate the effects of brain injury by increasing brain metabolism and producing acidosis. Hypoxia, systemic acidosis, increased intracranial pressure, and fever may accompany the muscle contractions of seizures. These movements may worsen other injuries. Paralyzing the child does not reverse the central effects of seizures. Local brain hypoxia and acidosis may continue to damage the brain even though the clinical signs of seizure are masked with paralyzing drugs.

Late posttraumatic epilepsy (seizures occurring more than 1 week after the injury) is more likely to occur if there is penetrating brain injury or hematoma, or if early seizures have occurred. Early posttraumatic seizures occur more often, and late seizures less often, in children than in adults.

Electrolyte abnormalities are common following severe head trauma. Inattention to electrolyte balance may add to the problems caused by diabetes insipidus or inappropriate antidiuretic hormone secretion. These latter abnormalities may occur at different times in the same patient. Poor temperature regulation accompanies severe brain injury. However, as already noted, hypothermia rather than fever is the rule.

A hypermetabolic state occurs in many children with traumatic or metabolic brain injury. This condition seems to be mediated by increased catecholamine secretion by the injured brain and is characterized by arterial hypertension and tachycardia. Direct cardiac injury and cerebral perfusion disturbances may result when this condition is severe. Although the arterial blood pressure is high, the intracranial pressure may also be high and the cerebral blood flow compromised. This condition is to be distinguished from the Cushing reflex, consisting of arterial hypertension and bradycardia rather than tachycardia. The Cushing reflex occurs in response to intracranial hypertension. The hypermetabolic state caused by excess catecholamine secretion may be treated with β-adrenergic blockade. As the arterial blood pressure is reduced the intracranial pressure often follows, without further compromise of the cerebral perfusion pressure.

Nutrition is compromised by the need for fluid restriction and the relative inability to provide oral feedings. Hypermetabolism complicates this nutritional deficiency. Some children lose 20% of their body weight in the first 2 weeks in the hospital. This condition can be alleviated somewhat by early institution of nasogastric feedings or parenteral hyperalimentation.

Penetrating head trauma is a special problem because of the need for surgical intervention to debride the wound and because of the risks of infection. If the penetration is by a low-velocity object, the signs and symptoms are

---

Pearls and Perils: Subacute Diffuse Brain Swelling

1. Early posttraumatic seizures occur more often, and late seizures less often, in children than in adults.
2. The perfusion pressure (intracranial pressure minus mean arterial pressure) is an important determinant of brain perfusion and should generally be above 50 mm Hg.
3. Fever of any source aggravates brain swelling.
4. Nutrition is critically important in head-injured children. Orogastric feeding or parenteral nutrition should begin early.
5. With increasing intradural volume there is decreasing compliance, so that small additional increases in volume may be associated with large increases in intracranial pressure.
6. The Cushing reflex associated with intracranial hypertension involves arterial hypertension and bradycardia. Arterial hypertension and tachycardia are also often seen together, but this combination of symptoms is due to catecholamine release rather than intracranial hypertension.
7. Lumbar puncture is relatively contraindicated in the presence of diffuse brain swelling because of the risk of herniation.
8. Paralyzing drugs mask the clinical signs of seizure, but the brain hypoxia and acidosis caused by seizures may continue.

---

of purely focal brain injury. Unless there is involvement of both hemispheres, or the brainstem, there is no, or only brief, loss of consciousness. The sequelae are related to the injured portion of the brain.

Diagnostic Studies

CT is the major diagnostic tool for the evaluation of brain swelling, but it is limited because it cannot measure intracranial pressure. Thus clinically significant swelling may be accompanied by a normal CT, and marked swelling on CT may be accompanied by normal intracranial pressure. CT in acute head injury may often show small ventricles. The parenchyma may be lucent with blurring of the border between the gray matter and the white matter. In children these changes may be difficult to distinguish from normal. Acute or incipient herniation of the brainstem may be suspected if there is obliteration of the perimesencephalic cistern at the level of the quadrigeminal plate. The lateral recesses of this cistern separate the midbrain from the unci of the temporal lobes. MRI is considered useful in detecting early edema.

The ability to measure cerebral blood flow is rarely available, but may show increased blood flow in the case of hyperemia, or decreased flow in the case of ischemia.

Lumbar puncture is relatively contraindicated in the

presence of increased intracranial pressure because of the risk of herniation. (It is also probably unnecessary in most cases.)

Treatment

Intubation and hyperventilation are the most rapid and effective ways of treating progressive brain and brain-stem compromise owing to increased intracranial pressure. This procedure is not without risk because hyperventilation may, in some cases, exacerbate cerebral ischemia. It is often necessary to paralyze the patient to prevent "fighting" of the ventilator and to reduce intrathoracic pressure, which is transmitted to the brain. Hyperosmolar agents, such as mannitol, may be helpful to reduce brain water. However, early in the course in children, brain swelling may result from hyperemia with little increase in brain water. Hence mannitol may actually worsen the problem initially by increasing blood volume. Mannitol may also contribute to hyperosmolar damage and electrolyte imbalance. Thus mannitol should be used only in an intensive care unit and by medical and nursing personnel who are familiar with its effects.

Monitoring of intracranial pressure may aid in the management of brain swelling. Unfortunately, monitoring alone may not suggest a successful treatment modality. Ventricular catherterization is the most invasive of the monitoring procedures. Furthermore, the catheter cannot always successfully be placed because of small ventricular size, resulting from swelling. On the other hand ventricular catheterization allows for the most direct measurement of intracranial pressure and, in some instances, permits treatment of intracranial hypertension by venting cerebrospinal fluid. Other monitoring devices include the subarachnoid screw and a variety of epidural catheters.

There is little evidence that intracranial hypertension per se causes secondary brain injury. Rather the increased pressure is transmitted to the intracranial vascular tree and may compromise cerebral blood flow. The cerebral perfusion pressure (mean arterial pressure minus intracranial pressure) is a more direct, but still approximate, measure of brain perfusion. A potentially more useful, but rather invasive, means of measuring brain perfusion is by sampling the internal jugular venous blood. The arterial-venous oxygen difference is then a measure of oxygen extraction and brain perfusion. Low oxygen extraction suggests excess blood flow (hyperemia) or decreased brain metabolism (as occurs in brain death). High extraction suggests ischemia. Thus measurement of the arterial-venous oxygen difference may permit more rational treatment of intracranial hypertension with hyperventilation and other means of manipulating the cerebral circulation.

Children who are comatose, or whose deteriorating level of consciousness suggests they may become comatose, should be treated in an appropriate intensive care unit. The presence of other injuries, or systemic illness, increases the risk of deterioration and complicates the management of brain injury. As a rule of thumb all children whose GCS score is 8 or below should be treated in an intensive care unit.

The most important feature of an appropriate intensive care unit is nurses who are familiar and comfortable with the management of acutely brain-injured children. Round-the-clock availability of neurosurgeons who are committed to the management of traumatic brain injury is also important. CT capability should be immediately available.

Transport to an appropriate facility should involve initial stabilization, which usually includes intubation. Many units now have transport teams to ensure against secondary brain damage in transit.

ANNOTATED BIBLIOGRAPHY

Bruce DA, Alavi A, Bilaniuk L, Dolinskas C, Obrist W, Uzzel B: Diffuse cerebral swelling following head injuries in children: The syndrome of "malignant brain edema." *J Neurosurg* 54:170–178, 1981.

This article discusses deterioration caused by brain swelling in children with and without a "lucid period." The usefulness of CT in brain-injured children is illustrated. The role of hyperemia in acute brain swelling in children is presented.

Jennett B, Teasdale G: Management of head injuries. Philadelphia, FA Davis, 1981, p 19–75, 211–252.

A clear presentation of the pathophysiology of diffuse brain swelling and its management.

Miner ME, Wagner KA (eds): *Neurotrauma: Treatment, Rehabilitation and Related Issues.* Boston, Butterworths, 1986, p 27–88.

An up-to-date discussion of the management of head injuries. These sections are particularly useful for understanding the physiologic changes accompanying brain injury. Intensive monitoring devices are discussed.

Obrist WD, Langfitt TW, Jaggi JL, Cruz J, Gennarelli TA: Cerebral blood flow and metabolism in comatose patients with acute head injury. *J Neurosurg* 61:241–253, 1984.

This paper presents measurements of cerebral blood flow showing that hyperemia is common in the early course of head injury in younger patients.

Snoek JW, Minderhoud JM, Wilmink JT: Delayed deterioration following mild head injury in children. *Brain* 107:15–36, 1984.

A detailed look at causes of deterioration and outcome in children with mild head trauma. Brain swelling, seizures, and hematomas are discussed.

INTRACRANIAL HEMATOMAS

Intracranial hematomas occur in a minority of children with deteriorating neurologic signs. Focal deficits, such as hemiparesis or eye deviation, may warn of bleeding in the head. This is especially so when these signs appear gradually after an injury. Similarly, a gradual deterioration of consciousness may warn of bleeding, causing increasing intracranial pressure or pressure on the brainstem. Seizures are commonly associated with hematomas and may contribute to clinical deterioration in children with hematomas. If the child survives the initial deterioration, the outcome often has more to do with the underlying brain injury than with the presence of intracranial blood.

Pathology

Intracranial hematomas may arise from bleeding in the epidural space, in the subdural space, or within the parenchyma of the brain. The clinical and pathologic findings and the mechanisms of injury differ among these sites of bleeding.

Epidural hematomas are often associated with a fracture of the skull and the subsequent rupture of an artery lying next to the skull. The middle meningeal artery is often injured, leading to a temporal fossa clot. However, epidural hematomas may occur in the posterior fossa as well. The bleeding may be brisk, accounting for rapid neurologic deterioration. The clot often forms a lens-shaped mass as it dissects the dura away from the skull. This mass then deforms the underlying brain, which, if the bleeding continues, may herniate. Except for this mass effect, the underlying brain may be relatively uninjured.

Subdural hematomas, on the other hand, are more often associated with underlying brain injury. They appear to result from tearing of the veins bridging the subdural space. The bleeding is venous and therefore often slower and less forceful than epidural arterial bleeding. Strong shearing forces appear to mediate the formation of subdural hematomas. These shearing forces are particularly disruptive to cortical nerve fibers. Microscopic evidence of axonal disruption is frequently found in the brain underlying a subdural hematoma. This underlying brain may become quite edematous.

Intracerebral blood is often associated with focal

FEATURE TABLE 7-3. INTRACRANIAL HEMATOMAS

Discriminating Features	Consistent Features	Variable Features
1. The hallmark of intracranial bleeding is gradual neurologic deterioration with the appearance of focal neurologic deficits and a decreasing level of consciousness. However, in only a minority of children are these symptoms attributable to intracranial bleeding. 2. Collections of free blood may be found in the epidural space, in the subdural space, or within the brain parenchyma. These collections may be detected by CT scanning, or directly during surgery or at autopsy.	1. A gradually decreasing level of consciousness accompanies most symptomatic intracranial hematomas. 2. Focal neurologic signs are consistent with intracranial hematomas. 3. A hemiparesis is often seen with a supratentorial hematoma. 4. Pupillary and eye movement abnormalities and motor signs suggest a posterior fossa hematoma. 5. Headache, papilledema, nystagmus, and ataxia are consistent with less severe posterior fossa hematomas. 6. Seizures are frequently associated with intracranial hematomas. 7. A gradually developing third-nerve palsy suggests an intracerebral hematoma and may herald impending uncal herniation.	1. Epidural hematomas are often associated with fracture of the skull and rupture of an artery lying near the skull. 2. The brain underlying an epidural hematoma may be relatively uninjured. 3. Subdural hematomas are often associated with marked underlying brain injury owing to the shearing forces involved in the formation of the hematoma. 4. The damaged brain under a subdural hematoma may become quite edematous. 5. Intracerebral bleeding often complicates focal contusions and lacerations, and is found in more severely injured children. 6. Intracerebral bleeding is often delayed by hours or days following the injury. 7. Clotting abnormalities are often found in children with delayed posttraumatic intracerebral bleeding. 8. Retinal and preretinal hemorrhages may accompany intracerebral hematomas, especially those involving acceleration/deceleration injuries.

contusions or lacerations of the brain. Contusions, though they may be extensive, are rarely large enough to account for loss of consciousness in and of themselves. However, they are frequently accompanied by focal or diffuse brain edema, which accentuates their clinical importance.

Occasionally intraparenchymal bleeding is delayed by hours or days following the injury. The mechanism of this curious circumstance is unknown but may be related to local or diffuse clotting abnormalities induced by the trauma. Evidence of intravascular fibrinolysis is obtained in a majority of cases. The tendency to form delayed hematomas may be related to the severity of the underlying brain injury.

Signs and Symptoms

The hallmark of clinically significant intracranial bleeding is gradual neurologic deterioration with the appearance of focal neurologic signs and a decreasing level of consciousness. Seizures are frequently associated with hematomas, and may suggest their presence. While these signs and symptoms are consistent with an expanding intracranial mass, only a minority of children with these symptoms actually have clinically significant intracranial bleeding. Similarly, not all intracranial hematomas are symptomatic. Furthermore, the symptoms of the various kinds of intracranial bleeding often overlap. Thus the clinical evaluation of intracranial hematomas is not entirely reliable. CT scanning adds greatly to the clinical characterization of intracranial bleeding and is of obvious therapeutic importance.

A hemiparesis is sometimes associated with an intracranial hematoma. This condition may be difficult to evaluate in a comatose child, but careful observation of spontaneous movements and movements in response to stimulation may reveal the deficit. Reflex asymmetry, or the Babinski sign, is sometimes helpful. Conjugate eye deviation, or a gaze preference, sometimes correlates with a hemisphereic hematoma. The eyes usually, but not always, look toward the side of the lesion.

Unilateral pupil dilation, with ptosis and failure of adduction of the affected eye, suggests a third-nerve palsy. When this sign appears after an injury, it suggests an expanding intracranial mass and incipient uncal herniation. The affected eye is usually on the same side as the mass. This third-nerve sign is not usually seen in the central herniation syndrome discussed previously. Unfortunately, this clinical sign occurs late in the course and is more important as a herald of impending herniation than as an early sign of intracranial bleeding. Furthermore, traumatic third-nerve palsy is not entirely specific as it occurs commonly without intracranial bleeding.

Retinal and preretinal hemorrhages are often associated with traumatic hematomas, especially those involving acceleration/deceleration injury. Retinal hemorrhages may result from direct acceleration injury, from sudden increased intracranial pressure, from ob-

struction of venous drainage, and from hypoxic injury. Contrary to popular opinion, retinal hemorrhages occur in a variety of injuries and are not pathognomonic of child abuse. But their presence in a small infant with seizures should raise the possibility of abuse.

Hematomas may occur in the posterior fossa after mild or severe head injuries. Rapid deterioration accompanying larger hematomas may produce apnea and deep coma. Brainstem compression may be quickly fatal. Pupillary movement, eye movement, and motor signs often, but not always, accompany larger posterior fossa hematomas. Small hematomas in the parenchyma of the brainstem may produce devastating symptoms that belie their size. Headache, papilledema, nystagmus, and ataxia may be signs of less severe hematomas.

Epidural bleeding is often brisk. Neurologic deterioration may occur from a matter of minutes to several hours after the injury. Untreated, the deterioration associated with epidural hematomas may be profound. However, because the underlying brain may be relatively uninjured, prompt evacuation of the blood is often associated with a good outcome.

Subdural bleeding is usually less brisk than epidural

**Pearls and Perils:
Intracranial Hematomas**

1. The outcome in patients with intracranial hematomas has more to do with the underlying brain injury than with the presence of blood.
2. Most children with gradually deteriorating consciousness do not have an intracerebral hematoma.
3. CT scanning has become an essential part of the diagnosis of intracerebral hematomas.
4. Prompt drainage (within 4 hours) may yield dramatic improvement with subdural hematomas.
5. Prompt drainage of epidural hematomas may be lifesaving.
6. The appearance of a third-nerve palsy is often more useful as a sign of impending herniation than as an early sign of an intracranial hematoma.
7. Life-threatening intracranial hematomas may follow relatively mild head trauma.
8. New bleeding may occur for a week or more after head trauma.
9. Blindly placed burr holes are dangerous and frequently miss significant hematomas easily seen on CT.
10. Brain edema associated with a hematoma may be more dangerous to the child than the bleeding itself.
11. Retinal and preretinal hemorrhages in infants strongly suggest but are not pathognomonic of child abuse.

bleeding. Nonetheless, the accumulation of subdural blood may be equally life threatening. Furthermore, subdural hematomas are often associated with severe underlying brain injury. Thus the child may not respond as well as hoped to the evacuation of the clot. Brain edema associated with a subdural hematoma may produce more mass effect than does the accumulation of blood itself. This edema may be so severe as to cause herniation even if the hematoma is removed. In spite of these caveats, prompt drainage of subdural hematomas sometimes yields dramatic improvement.

Intracerebral hematomas often occur in more severely injured children. However, many children with intracerebral hematomas are able to respond to commands on admission to the hospital. The appearance of focal neurologic deficits, or of deteriorating consciousness, should prompt an investigation for intracranial bleeding. Seizures often occur with intracerebral hematomas. The onset of seizures in a child who had appeared stable may mark the onset of delayed intracerebral bleeding. New bleeding, or enlargement of an existing hematoma, may occur for a week or more following trauma to the brain. Brain edema surrounding the clot may pose additional danger for the child. Because intracerebral hematomas are associated with abnormalities of the brain substance, residual focal neurologic deficits are common.

Diagnostic Studies

CT scanning provides a rapid and reliable, and relatively noninvasive, means of diagnosing and following intracranial bleeding. A CT scanner is thus mandatory for any center treating head injuries. CT frequently allows the diagnosis of intracranial bleeding before symptoms associated with the hematoma appear or are recognized. This allows the physician to follow the course of the hematoma and be forewarned of possible problems relating to acute management and to rehabilitation.

MRI may detect some hematomas not seen on CT. However, the small increase in yield rarely justifies the expense and risk of placing an acutely ill patient in a device with which monitoring is difficult and all magnetic materials must be removed from the room.

Since the advent of CT, angiography is rarely used to identify hematomas. However, this procedure may be of value to the surgeon in defining vascular supply. Blindly placed skull trephine or burr holes are dangerous and frequently miss significant hematomas easily identified by CT. Subdural taps in an infant with an open fontanelle are less dangerous, but still much less sensitive than CT.

Plane skull X rays may be helpful in identifying fractures associated with epidural or subdural hematomas. These fractures are usually, but not always, visible on CT images as well.

Treatment

Prompt evacuation of larger extra-axial hematomas is often lifesaving. In spite of the underlying brain injury

associated with subdural hematomas, evacuation within 4 hours has been shown to improve chances for survival greatly. Survival rates with large epidural hematomas are dramatically better with prompt drainage. Thus the early diagnosis of intracranial hematomas is essential. CT scans should be obtained initially in all children with severe traumatic brain injuries, and should be done whenever evidence of neurologic deterioration appears.

Smaller clots that do not produce clinically significant mass effects need not be evacuated acutely. Debridement of contused and lacerated brain may be necessary because of increasing intracranial pressure and local mass effect. Delayed intraparenchymal hematomas usually do not require drainage. Furthermore, the location of these hematomas within the brain parenchyma, and the coagulopathy often associated with them, make surgical removal more difficult.

The brain edema associated especially with subdural and intracerebral hematomas may pose important therapeutic problems. Treatment of this edema is essentially similar to the treatment of diffuse brain edema discussed earlier. Craniectomy, or removal of portions of the damaged brain, may be of benefit in the treatment of expanding masses aggravated by focal brain edema. These modalities offer little to the treatment of diffuse edema.

ANNOTATED BIBLIOGRAPHY

Aoki N, Masuzawa H: Infantile acute subdural hematoma: Clinical analysis of 26 cases. *J Neurosurg* 61:273–280, 1984.
  A discussion of infantile subdural hematomas associated with minor trauma. Mechanism of injury is discussed with particular reference to the battered child syndrome.
Atluru V, Epstein LG, Zilka A: Delayed traumatic intracerebral hemorrhage in children. *Pediatr Neuro* 2:297–301, 1986.
  A discussion of delayed traumatic hematomas with particular reference to CT diagnosis.
Dhellemmes P, Lejeune JP, Christiaens JL, Combelles G: Traumatic extradural hematomas in infancy and childhood: Experience with 144 cases. *J Neurosurg* 62:861–864, 1985.
  This paper discusses the incidence and clinical course of extradural (epidural) hematomas in children.
Miner ME, Kaufman HH, Graham SH, Haar FH, Gildenberry PL: Disseminated intravascular coagulation fibrinolytic syndrome following head injury in children: Frequency and prognostic implications. *J Pediatr* 100:687–691, 1982.
  This article discusses clotting abnormalities in head-injured children with and without delayed intracerebral bleeding.

RECOVERY FROM TRAUMATIC BRAIN INJURY

Some children may die following traumatic brain injury, whereas others may remain in a coma or in a persistent vegetative state. Those who recover usually show some neurologic deficits, which may be transient or permanent. The rate and extent of recovery from various degrees of traumatic brain injury follow a course that is characteristic when one looks at a large number of patients. Except for those with mild head injury, few children exhibit only one pattern of impairment. Yet the similarities in the behavior patterns of many children tend to outweigh the individual differences. Early in the course, it is by no means possible to predict reliably the outcome of any particular patient. It is clear, however, that significant recovery can continue for several years following a traumatic brain injury.

At first glance one might expect that the prognosis for recovery from traumatic brain injury in children would be better than that for adults. This seems to be true for older children and adolescents. In contrast, the immature brains of young children seem to be particularly vulnerable to diffuse damage, and they are therefore more likely to demonstrate residual neuropsychologic deficits.

Injuries in primary cortical areas, such as visual field deficits, motor paralysis, and tactile deficits, usually show rapid initial recovery, which is often complete. However, recovery from problems persisting for more than a few months is likely to be incomplete.

Lesions in the posterior cortical association areas often involve more complex functions, such as constructional abilities, visual-motor coordination, and speech and language. The problems may demonstrate more gradual improvement that continues beyond the first year after injury.

Patterns of behavior involving the prefrontal and anterior temporal cortical areas, or that are symptomatic of more diffuse injury, may signify prolonged impairment. Even though a brain-injured child returns to fully independent and functional living, some subtle deficits may be apparent to the experienced eye that reflect the child's previous injury. Such children may demonstrate problems in organization, affective control, motivation, judgment, speed of thinking, and memory, as well as irritability and distractibility. These are the hallmarks of sequelae of traumatic brain injury in children.

Children with mild head trauma, involving brief or no loss of consciousness, transiently demonstrate some of these hallmarks of brain injury. These deficits may disappear completely within hours after the injury, or may persist for several months.

Pathology

Injury to the brain resulting in focal neurologic deficits may occur by direct contusion at the point of impact. Contre-coup injury may produce more or less severe focal deficits on the side opposite the blow. Injuries involving more force, or those characterized by significant rotational acceleration, produce direct contusion of the brain against the bony prominences of the calvarium. This pattern accounts for the most universal signs and symptoms of frontal and anterior temporal lobe dysfunction seen in traumatic brain injury.

Intracerebral hematomas account for a major por-

tion of focal symptoms. Encephalomalacia often persists in the area of the hematoma. Penetrating trauma produces similar focal injuries. Lesions of this kind are more frequently associated with posttraumatic epilepsy.

More diffusely distributed but multifocal gray matter contusions and lacerations may be present and may be reflected in more global symptoms in the areas of reasoning and judgment. Diffuse white matter injury often results in prolonged coma or in a persistent vegetative state. White matter injury may contribute to the marked slowing of motor and cognitive processes encountered in severe injury.

Some degree of anoxia or ischemia accompanies the majority of traumatic brain injuries. Anoxia affects the gray matter preferentially; the hippocampus and basal ganglia are the most sensitive areas. More severe anoxic-ischemic injury affects the gray matter globally, usually with severe sequelae. Diffuse white matter destruction follows some very severe anoxic-ischemic injuries.

Short-term memory is subserved by the limbic system and thalamus. The hippocampus, in particular, is exquisitely susceptible to anoxic injury, and to direct injury by contusion of the temporal poles.

Signs and Symptons

Receptive deficits following traumatic brain injury may include signs and symptoms related to primary cortical sensory areas. Visual field cuts often accompany severe hemispheric injury. Tactile sensory deficits are easily overlooked in children, for pain and touch are rarely lost completely because they are subserved by redundant systems. Discriminatory touch including stereognosis is more susceptible to injury, but may be quite difficult to test in children. Hearing loss is more easily tested and may account for delay in the acquisition or reacquisition of language.

More complex receptive deficits may appear in the perception of language from auditory or visual material or both. Reading and repetition involve the posterior association cortex. Deficits in visual-spatial perceptions may be more subtle, but still quite debilitating. Constructional abilities also reflect posterior association cortical functions.

Motor signs and symptoms involve more anterior cortical areas. Spastic paralysis may involve lesions anywhere along the length of the pyramidal tracts. The extrapyramidal system is often injured, and such injuries may be associated with abnormalities of tone and posture as well as tremors, adventitious movement disorders such as choreoathetosis and ballism, and inaccuracy and poor coordination of movements. Children with excellent functional recovery may have persistent, slow, irregular, robot-like movements and gait. These deficits may interfere with normal psychosocial development and preclude recreational activities requiring grace of movement.

Focal motor and sensory signs may reflect cir-

FEATURE TABLE 7-4. RECOVERY FROM TRAUMATIC BRAIN INJURY

Discriminating Features	Consistent Features	Variable Features
1. The hallmarks of sequelae of traumatic brain injury in children include problems in organization, affective control, motivation, judgment, speed of thinking, and memory, as well as irritability and distractibility. These deficits reflect global brain injury as well as injury to the prefrontal and anterior temporal areas of the brain.	1. The child has attention and concentration problems. Impulsivity, distractibility, and motor hyperactivity may be present.	1. Focal neurologic deficits often correlate with the site of a hematoma, penetrating trauma, or severe contusion.
2. To establish that a specific event caused the signs and symptoms of traumatic encephalopathy, it is necessary to document that the signs and symptoms appeared following the specific injury.	2. Difficulties with reasoning and tracking complex concepts exist.	2. Visual field deficits usually reflect severe hemispheric injury.
	3. There is a slow rate of cognitive processing.	3. Problems with discriminatory touch and stereognosis are more common than insensitivity to touch or pain, but are easily overlooked.
3. Memory of the events of the accident and immediately after is lost in all but the most trivial of injuries.	4. The child has memory difficulties, especially with short-term memory.	4. Hearing loss may account for delay in acquisition or reacquisition of language.
	5. Naming and word-finding difficulties are present.	5. Visual-spatial and constructional deficits may interfere with learning even when reading, repetition, and computation are intact.
	6. There are behavior changes, which may include explosive behavior, catastrophic anxiety, or intractable indifference.	6. Motor deficits may include spasticity, disorders of tone and posture, movement disorders, and ataxia, as well as deficits in the planning and execution of complex coordinated movements.
		7. Language problems may include comprehensional, visual perceptual, naming, and expressive difficulties. Nonaphasic speech disturbances may also occur. More complex problems with understanding and relating stories and humorous material are often present.
		8. Short-term memory problems are almost universally present. Memory retrieval difficulties and shrinking retrograde amnesia are also commonly encountered.

cumscribed injury anywhere in the brain or brainstem. The localization of these lesions benefits from the rich heritage of the study of vascular lesions in neurology. Brainstem signs, particularly gaze palsies, are common following severe head trauma and are often transient. Visual tracking problems owing to frontal lobe dysfunction are also quite common and often resolve. Transient blindness is occasionally seen and does not necessarily imply a severe injury.

More anteriorly placed motor deficits involve problems in the planning and execution of complex coordinated movements. Some motor aphasic symptoms are

in this category. The understanding and use of complex sentences, stories, and humorous material suffer from frontal damage, and this undoubtedly accounts for some of the peculiarities of language seen in head-injured children.

More global deficits affect attention, concentration, and the ability to track complex concepts and reasoning. Cognitive processing is often slow. These deficits may preclude normal school and social functioning even when primary cognitive skills such as reading and computation are intact. Impulsivity, distractibility, and motor hyperactivity are frequently seen in brain-injured children. Apathy and inactivity may be even more difficult to rehabilitate. Erratic carelessness in dress and hygiene is seen in children who are fastidious in other ways. Impaired ability to start and stop activities, or to shift activities, may make children rigid and apparently uncooperative. Explosive behavior, catastrophic anxiety, or intractable indifference are often exasperating to parents, teachers, and peers. These problems may seriously hamper goal-directed behavior in children who have shown excellent cognitive recovery.

The opportunity for the development of the secondary emotional problems is obvious. Unfortunately, the prejudices and emotional problems of parents and siblings, as well as of teachers and peers, may have forceful negative impact on the brain-injured child. There is no substitute for an appropriately supportive and structured home environment in the rehabilitation of a child with head injuries.

Memory is a highly complex brain function that depends on a number of structures. Thus it is not surprising that memory difficulties are virtually universal in severe and mild traumatic brain injuries. Immediate memory recovers quickly in patients who regain consciousness. Thus they have the ability to grasp and remember the events around them for some seconds. However, the next process, short-term memory, is highly susceptible to traumatic and anoxic brain injury. Conscious children with short-term memory deficits are unable to lay down any lasting new memories. They remain confused and disoriented even though they may be able to recognize faces, speak, and converse on a perfunctory level. After further recovery, children may have no memory of this period of disorientation following their injury, a phenomenon called posttraumatic amnesia. The length of posttraumatic amnesia statistically correlates well with recovery.

Retrograde amnesia—loss of memory of events preceding the trauma—also commonly occurs with any degree of traumatic brain injury. An injury sufficient to produce posttraumatic amnesia also disrupts those memories that, at the time of the accident, had not yet been consolidated into long-term memory. This period rarely exceeds 30 minutes before the injury. However, in another phenomenon, called shrinking retrograde amnesia, memories of events several months before the accident are lost. These memories gradually return with recovery and their loss reflects abnormalities in memory retrieval. Older and often-rehearsed memories are the most easily retrieved, but these represent only a small part of the stored experiences of a normal child.

Naming errors and word-finding difficulties frequently persist in brain-injured children. These deficits contribute to the use of inappropriate words and verbal approximations. While naming certainly involves memory, the language association areas of the posterior cortex are clearly involved. Word-finding disturbances, anomia, agrammatism, and impaired comprehension are termed aphasias. These problems often continue to show improvement for years after a severe head injury. Nonaphasic speech disturbances—including dysarthria, mutism, echolalia, palilalia, stuttering, and nonaphasic misnaming—also occur in brain-injured children. In contrast to speech disorders in head-injured adults, an extended period of mutism lasting a few days to several months is common in children. The overall recovery of speech and language in children is often more impressive than that seen in adults.

Younger children with focal left brain injuries may show excellent recovery of the language with time. This is apparently because there is bihemispheric language potential, particularly in younger children. This recovery of language is in contrast to the greater susceptibility of the immature brain to the effects of diffuse injury.

Diagnostic Studies

Assessment of the extent of injury and prediction of the course of recovery from traumatic brain injury in children are hampered by the relative paucity of studies in this

---

Pearls and Perils: Recovery from Traumatic Brain Injury

1. Transient blindness following a mild head injury often resolves without sequelae.
2. A few children will have an alarming but transient picture of deep coma with unreactive pupils. Recovery is rapid and complete.
3. An extended period of mutism following severe brain injury is common in children. Many of these children have impressive recovery of language skills once they start talking.
4. Gaze palsies and visual tracking problems are common in brain-injured children and often resolve completely.
5. The brains of young children appear to be more vulnerable to lasting damage than those of older children and adolescents.
6. It is not possible to predict reliably, for most individual children, the rate and extent of recovery.
7. Children with severe cognitive disability owing to traumatic brain injury do not necessarily score in the abnormal range on standardized tests.
8. The normal emergence of continuing developmental skills may limit the recognition of residual deficits of traumatic brain injury until the deficient skill would be expected to appear.
9. Mild head injury, minor head injury, or concussion is not necessarily minor. Some children are quite disabled by such seemingly trivial injuries, and the organic deficits may persist for months.

area. Furthermore, deficits from brain injury are superimposed on normally emerging and continuing developmental skills. Younger children have a limited ability to cooperate with testing, and many of the skills one would like to assess have not appeared yet, even in normal children. Thus different test instruments, each with age-adjusted norms, must be used. Even so, discovery of motor, cognitive, and behavior deficits resulting from brain injury may not be possible for years after the injury. By then the results of testing are often confused by the myriad factors influencing normal pathologic development.

Detailed assessment of a head-injured child is a complex process. The major purpose of such an assessment is to enable rational therapy in an inpatient or outpatient rehabilitation setting, or in school. Sometimes an assessment is done for legal reasons, or to better inform the parents about the child's condition. There is no simple test battery that will reliably identify all the areas of residual injury. In fact, many head-injured children are severely debilitated by their injuries and yet score within the normal range on standardized tests. This is particularly true in school settings, where only simple reading, word recognition, and computational skills are tested. The test situation is often designed to remove distraction and provide as much structure as possible. Thus the organic deficits preventing the child's success in the classroom are ascribed to "behavioral problems" and the child may be denied appropriate special education services. Furthermore, the standard categories of special education—"learning disabled," "emotionally disabled," "educably mentally retarded," and so on—do not address the patterns of deficits seen in traumatically brain-injured children.

In the acute period following a traumatic brain injury, the child's abilities may change daily. Thus the assessment of the child's deficits is best done on an ongoing basis by the team involved in his or her treatment. The team is often directed by a physiatrist, neuropsychologist, or neurologist and includes therapists from several disciplines. Individuals involved in assessments should be trained and skilled in working with often hard-to-test children.

The neuropsychologic assessment is the most comprehensive. This testing is often done when the child is relatively stable and at infrequent intervals to reduce practice effects. Neuropsychologic testing is often capable of documenting unmistakable signs of traumatic encephalopathy in the presence of cognitive and emotional dysfunction of other origins. The other team members supply additional information, which is essential to a full assessment and appropriate therapeutic approach.

CT, MRI, EEG, and evoked response testing provide important information about the structure and function of the brain. However, these tests do not measure performance directly, and therefore they are of limited usefulness in planning appropriate rehabilitation therapy.

Treatment

The more severely brain-injured children require acute inpatient rehabilitation, which should begin even while the child is in coma. A team approach to rehabilitation is essential because several overlapping areas of expertise are needed to address a child with multiple problems. Furthermore, a structured and supportive environment is essential for children with impaired executive functions and whose performance deteriorates with extraneous stimulation. The family is an essential part of the rehabilitation team, and appropriate social and family interactions are fostered by the team approach. The rehabilitation nurse often spends the most time with the child and may act as liaison between the team and the family. The speech and language pathologist assesses and treats language problems and also deficits in perceptual and visual-spatial skills. Learning styles and behavior responses to the therapy situation are assessed. The occupational therapist is concerned with the functional use of limbs as well as motor planning and activities of daily living. A feeding team is often assembled for children who are not able to take adequate nutrition by mouth. The physical therapist is concerned with tone and posture, seating and positioning, and ambulation. The psychologist addresses organic deficits in the control of emotions, anxiety, and aggressiveness. Secondary emotional problems of the hcild and the family are also addressed. Formal psychologic and neuropsychologic testing is done when appropriate. The child life specialist acts as an advocate for the child as a whole person. Patient education and play activities are designed to reduce stress and foster the integration of the child with family and community. The schoolteacher begins to involve the child in appropriate educational activities and begins the reintegration of the child into an appropriate school on discharge. The social worker is involved in maintaining and supporting the family as well as coordinating community resources for the child's benefit. The discharge planner provides a smooth and timely transition to home and community and also secures needed equipment to continue the child's rehabilitation outside the hospital.

Some children may benefit from a postacute rehabilitation setting, which may involve residential care. These are children who have recovered some measure of independent mobility and cognition and need additional intensive help in achieving successful reintegration into home and community.

Less severely injured children may not require a full team approach to rehabilitation. But an awareness of the problems unique to traumatic brain-injured children is essential to assess and treat them adequately.

School is the major occupational activity of children beyond 5 or 6 years of age. Reintegration into an appropriate school situation is essential for children with injuries of all degrees.

ANNOTATED BIBLIOGRAPHY

Jaffe KM (ed): Pediatric Head Injury. *J Head Trauma Rehabil* 1(4), 1986.

This entire issue is devoted to papers discussing outcomes in and rehabilitation of traumatically brain-injured children.

Jennett B, Teasdale G: *Management of Head Injuries.* Philadelphia, FA Davis, 1981, p 19–75.

A concise discussion of pathologic changes and pathophysiologic mechanisms underlying traumatic brain injury.

Levin HS, Benton AL, Grossman RG: *Neurobehavioral Consequences of Closed Head Injury.* New York, Oxford University Press, 1982, p 189–207.

A well-written discussion of outcome issues, including assessment, pathophysiology, and rehabilitation. Chapter 10, in particular, is devoted to children.

Lezak MD: *Neuropsychological assessment,* 2nd ed. New York, Oxford University Press, 1983, p 18–84, 165–175.

A discussion of the brain-behavior relationships underlying neuropsychologic assessment. This book also contains a detailed compendium of testing instruments.

Ylvisaker M (ed): *Head Injury Rehabilitation: Children and Adolescents.* San Diego, College Hill Press, 1985.

A compendium of papers dealing with a wide range of pediatric rehabilitation issues.

The Epilepsies
Gregory L. Holmes

Seizures are one of the most common of the neurologic disorders that occur in children. Fortunately, if the seizure disorder is correctly diagnosed medical therapy may greatly improve the child's life. This chapter will review current standards of care in the diagnosis and treatment of epilepsy in childhood.

A *seizure* may be defined as a sudden, involuntary, time-limited alteration in neurologic function secondary to an abnormal discharge of neurons in the central nervous system. *Epilepsy* refers to a chronic condition in which a patient experiences recurrent seizures. Epilepsy is a sign of underlying brain dysfunction rather than a single disease.

Seizures secondary to a provoked insult (e.g., fever, hypoglycemia, or acute head trauma) do not fall under the definition of epilepsy since they are secondary to a short-lived condition rather than a chronic condition. Although epilepsy is a chronic condition, it is not necessarily a lifelong disorder, because remissions frequently occur in children.

Epilepsy is common, with an incidence (number of new cases per year per unit of population) of approximately 50/100,000. The highest incidence occurs in childhood. Approximately 75% of patients who develop epilepsy will do so before age 20 years.

CLASSIFICATION OF EPILEPTIC SEIZURES

The most widely accepted classification of epileptic seizures is the International Classification of Epileptic Seizures. This classification, given in Table 8–1 will be used throughout the chapter.

The International Classification of Epileptic Seizures is based on three factors: (1) clinical seizure manifestations, (2) ictal (during seizure) electroencephalographic (EEG) patterns, and (3) interictal (between seizures) EEG patterns.

The classification is subdivided into two broad categories: (1) partial seizures (seizures that begin focally) and (2) generalized seizures (seizures that are bilateral-ly symmetric and without local onset). Seizures are then further classified by their clinical and EEG manifestations.

This classification system emphasizes clinical and EEG features, details readily available to the physician taking care of the patient. Based on a reliable history and interictal EEG, the physician can generally classify the seizure. Once the seizure is classified the type of workup and appropriate antiepileptic medication can be determined.

Whereas the International Classification of Epileptic Seizures adequately describes individual epileptic seizures, it does not describe the many clinical syndromes that are important in dealing with children with epilepsy. For that reason, in 1985 the International Classification of Epilepsies and Epileptic Syndromes was proposed. An epileptic syndrome is defined as an epileptic disorder characterized by a cluster of signs and symptoms customarily occurring together. The factors used to define the syndrome may be clinical (such as case history, seizure type, modes of seizure recurrence, and neurologic and psychologic findings) or findings detected by ancillary studies (such as EEG or computed tomography [CT] scan). A syndrome does not necessarily have a common etiology and prognosis. Common epileptic syndromes will be discussed in this chapter.

EVALUATION

The *history* and *neurologic examination* remain the cornerstone of neurologic diagnosis. It is important to determine by history whether the patient had a seizure, and, if so, what type. Generally speaking, if there is uncertainty about the diagnosis it is usually better to withhold treatment and wait for another attack before embarking on an extensive workup and initiation of antiepileptic drugs (AEDs).

Diagnostic Studies

Following the diagnosis of a seizure the clinician must determine the underlying or precipitating cause of the

TABLE 8-1. CLASSIFICATION OF EPILEPTIC SEIZURES

Clinical Seizure Type	Ictal EEG	Interictal EEG
I. Partial seizures		
A. Simple partial seizures (consciousness not impaired) 1. With motor symptoms 2. With somatosensory or special sensory symptoms 3. With autonomic symptoms or signs 4. With psychic symptoms	Local contralateral discharge starting over the corresponding area of cortical representation.	Local contralateral discharge.
B. Complex partial seizures (with impairment of consciousness; may sometimes begin with simple symptomatology) 1. Simple partial onset followed by improved consciousness 2. With impairment of consciousness only	Unilateral or bilateral discharges, diffuse or focal in temporal or frontotemporal regions.	Unilateral or bilateral generally asynchronous focus; usually in the temporal or frontal region.
C. Complex partial seizures evolving to secondary generalized seizures		
II. Generalized seizures		
A. Absence seizures 1. Impairment of consciousness only 2. With mild clonic components 3. With atonic components 4. With tonic components 5. With automatisms 6. With autonomic components	Usually regular and symmetrical 3 Hz but may be 2- to 4-Hz spike-wave complexes or multiple spike-wave complexes. Abnormalities are bilateral.	Background activity usually normal.
B. Atypical absence seizures	EEG more heterogeneous than typical absences; may include irregular spike-wave complexes, fast activity, or other paroxysmal activity. Abnormalities are bilateral but often irregular and asymmetrical.	Background activity usually abnormal.
C. Myoclonic seizures	Multiple spike-wave, or sometimes spike-wave or sharp-slow waves.	Same as ictal.
D. Clonic seizures	Fast activity (10 Hz or more) and slow waves; occasional spike-wave pattern.	Spike-wave or multiple spike-wave discharges.
E. Tonic seizures	Low-voltage fast activity, or a fast rhythm of 9 to 10 Hz or more decreasing in frequency and increasing in amplitude.	Background usually abnormal. Sharp-slow wave complexes.
F. Tonic-clonic seizures	Rhythm at 10 or more Hz decreasing in frequency and increasing in amplitude during tonic phase, interrupted by slow waves during clonic phase.	Multiple spikes, spike-wave, or sharp waves.
G. Atonic seizures	Multiple spikes-waves or flattening or low-voltage fast activity.	Multiple spikes-and-slow waves.

Adapted from Dreifuss (1981) with permission of the publisher.

seizure. The nature of the initial workup is partly determined by how the patient presents. Clearly the patient who arrives at the emergency room in status epilepticus or is comatose or febrile is approached differently than the patient who has totally recovered from the seizure by the time he or she presents to the clinician. Only the latter condition will be discussed in this section. The management of status epilepticus is discussed later in this chapter, and febrile seizures are discussed in Chapter 25.

Electroencephalography

Because EEGs are noninvasive, benign, and relatively inexpensive, it is reasonable to obtain at least one EEG on any patient with seizures or suspected seizures. The making of both an awake and an asleep recording is desirable. Epileptiform activity may occur only during the sleep state. If natural sleep cannot be obtained, a hypnotic agent such as chloral hydrate may be useful.

A question that frequently arises is when, following a seizure, an EEG should be obtained. Although spikes may be suppressed and postictal slowing may be seen on the EEG for up to a week following a seizure, this may be an important finding if the slowing is focal. Focal slowing may be indicative of focal pathology. Therefore, it is recommended that the EEG be obtained as soon as is practically possible. If the record is abnormally slow, it may have to be repeated after several weeks to determine if the slowing was a postictal phenomenon.

Table 8–2 lists the typical EEG findings in the various seizure types. It should be remembered that the EEG is only suggestive of epilepsy and rarely diagnostic of the disorder. The primary exception to this rule is absence seizures, since it is quite likely that in untreated patients hyperventilation, photic stimulation, or sleep will result in generalized spike-wave activity on the EEG. For practical purposes generalized spike-wave activity lasting longer than 3 seconds can be considered a seizure. EEGs are not infrequently normal in patients with generalized tonic-clonic or partial seizures. The diagnosis of epilepsy is based on clinical, not EEG, data.

Neuroimaging

The CT and magnetic resonance imaging (MRI) scans have now clearly been shown to be superior to the clinical examination, the EEG, and routine skull radiographs in the diagnosis of structural lesions of the central nervous system. The MRI is technically superior to the CT scan. There is, however, considerable debate in the literature as to whether all patients with seizures require MRI or CT scans. A significant number of CT scans are abnormal, in both children and adults with epilepsy. In series of CT scans in children with epilepsy, abnormal scans are seen in approximately one third of cases. Abnormal CT scans are most frequent in patients who have partial seizures, abnormal neurologic findings, focal paroxysmal discharges, or slowing on the EEG.

CT abnormalities may also be detected in children with normal neurologic examinations and EEGs. In a study by McAbee and colleagues (1989) of 101 pediatric patients presenting with their first seizure (febrile or afebrile), 7% had abnormal CT scans. The highest risk of having an abnormality (13%) was in children with afebrile focal seizures. Although an abnormal CT scan was more likely to be associated with an abnormal EEG, a normal result did not eliminate the possibility of an abnormal CT.

Although abnormal CT scans occur frequently in children with epilepsy, the abnormalities frequently do not alter the clinical management of the patient. In a study of CT scans in 309 pediatric patients with seizures, Lagenstein et al. (1980) found that 46% of the children had pathologic findings on the scan. Although 13 children had severe pathologic findings, in no cases were surgically correctable lesions found. Likewise, Yang et al. (1979) found that in only 7 of 256 children (3%) with seizures were abnormalities of therapeutic significance found on CT scan.

The MRI is more sensitive than the CT scan and is now the preferred test in the evaluation of a patient with seizures. Heinz and colleagues (1989) compared the "yield" of the CT to that of the MRI in patients with epilepsy. The MRI detected an abnormality in five patients (8%) in whom the CT was negative. The MRI was recommended to be the imaging procedure of choice for detection on an epileptogenic focus in seizure patients. Convers and colleagues (1990) performed MRI scans on 100 patients with intractable partial seizures, normal CT scans, and focal EEG abnormalities. The MRI was abnormal in 31 patients and was consistent with EEG data in 22 patients, of whom 20 had temporal lobe epilepsy. This study, in adult patients, demonstrated that the MRI was more often abnormal in temporal lobe epilepsy than in frontal lobe epilepsy.

TABLE 8–2. CHARACTERISTIC EEG FEATURES IN THE VARIOUS SEIZURE TYPES

Seizure Type	Interictal EEG Abnormalities
Partial Seizures	
Simple partial	Variable, spikes over involved area of cortex may be normal
Complex partial	Variable, frontal/temporal lobe spikes
Generalized Seizures	
Absence	Generalized spike-wave, often activated by sleep, hyperventilation, or photic stimulation
Generalized tonic-clonic	Variable, frequently normal
Myoclonic	Usually abnormal, generalized spike-wave, multiple spikes
Tonic/atonic	Usually abnormal, generalized abnormalities, spikes, multiple spike-waves

In summary, CT and MRI scans are frequently abnormal in children with partial seizures. Although the majority of the abnormalities will not alter management of the child, in a small but significant percentage an unexpected neoplasm or other treatable lesion will be discovered. In addition, even when the CT or MRI scan does not alter therapeutic management, it may offer the clinician valuable information regarding the etiology of the seizures. A normal CT or MRI scan also serves to comfort both the physician and the parents by assuring them that "nothing is being missed." However, even with a normal CT or MRI scan, it behooves the physician to follow the patient closely, because a change in neurologic examination or development of focal slowing on the EEG would indicate the necessity for a repeat study.

Treatment

The decision to treat a patient with seizures with AED therapy should never be taken lightly. All AEDs are associated with side effects, both dose-related and idiosyncratic. The frequency of unacceptable side effects requiring discontinuation of initial AED therapy in newly treated seizure patients was over 30% in the Veterans Administration Cooperative Trial (Smith et al., 1987), which was undertaken to determine the optimal drug for initial treatment of epilepsy. Neuropsychologic studies have found that AEDs, even when tolerated, are associated with a high frequency of cognitive difficulties.

In the not too distant past it was not unusual for children or adults to be placed on both phenytoin and phenobarbital for their first generalized tonic-clonic seizure or partial seizure. Now an increasing number of physicians decide not to treat the first seizure with AEDs at all. This trend will be reinforced by the recent paper by Shinnar and colleagues (1991). In a prospective study, 283 children in the Bronx with a first unprovoked seizure were closely followed for a mean of 30 months. The vast majority of the children were not treated with AEDs. Subsequent seizures occurred in only 36% of the cases. The cumulative risk for recurrence was 60% at 36 months in children with a history of a static neurologic insult (termed "remote symptomatic" by the authors), versus 36% in children with an idiopathic seizure. The EEG was the most important predictor of recurrence in children with idiopathic seizures. Children with an idiopathic seizure and a normal EEG had a cumulative recurrence risk of 26% at 36 months. Age of time of first seizure and duration of seizure did not affect recurrence risk.

This study of largely untreated children demonstrated that the recurrence risk following a first unprovoked seizure is low. Interestingly, the rate of seizure recurrence in children was similar to that reported in a study by Hauser and colleagues (1990) using similar methods in adults. Many factors must be considered when deciding whether to start AED therapy and each child must be evaluated as an individual. However, in view of the not insignificant risk encountered with AEDs, in most children it appears reasonable to wait for a second seizure before subjecting the child to years of drug therapy.

PHARMACOLOGY OF ANTIEPILEPTIC DRUGS

The principal means of therapy in children with seizures is AEDs. The pharmacologic management of epilepsy has changed decisively over the past decade in regard to the introduction of new drugs, improved methods of administration, and the development of AED serum levels. The goal in the treatment of epilepsy is to reduce or eliminate seizures while minimizing the adverse effects of the treatment. It should be recognized that drug management of children with epilepsy is only one component of the overall management strategy. Recognition of the psychologic, educational, and social complications in epilepsy is as critical as treating the seizures. Failure to address these problems will result in a treatment program failure, regardless of whether or not seizures are eliminated.

Pearls and Perils: Pharmacology of Antiepileptic Drugs

1. Published therapeutic levels of AEDs should be used only as a guide. It is likely that each patient has his or her own therapeutic level.
2. In some patients with severe seizures the goal should not be to stop all seizures regardless of drug toxicity but rather to allow the child to function well at home and school even though some seizures may occur.
3. Carbamazepine, phenobarbital, primidone, ethosuximide, and phenytoin serum levels correlate fairly well with seizure control and toxicity while VPA and clonazepam levels are less valuable.
4. The use of a single AED usually results in higher serum levels, less toxicity, and better seizure control than when polypharmacy is employed.
5. When using AEDs with short half-lives the time that the level is obtained is important. When using AEDs with long half-lives the time the level is obtained is not important.
6. Failure to heed parents' complaints about behavioral changes following introduction of barbiturates and benzodiazepines is a mistake. These drugs often lead to behavioral or cognitive impairment in children and should be avoided when possible.
7. Obtaining blood levels before a steady state is reached will give erroneous results. When obtaining AED levels it is essential to wait at least five half-lives following starting or adding a new drug or changing the dosage.

TABLE 8-3. EFFICACY OF ANTIEPILEPTIC DRUGS USED IN VARIOUS SEIZURE TYPES

Drug	Absence	Generalized Tonic-Clonic	Myoclonic	Simple Partial	Complex Partial
Carbamazepine	0	+	0	+	+
Clonazepam	+	+	+	±	±
Ethosuximide	+	0	±	0	0
Phenobarbital	0	+	±	+	+
Phenytoin	0	+	0	+	+
Primidone	0	+	±	+	+
Valproate	+	+	+	+	+

Adapted from Holmes (1987) with permission of the publisher.
0 = Rarely effective; ± = sometimes effective; + = frequently effective.

Following the establishment of the diagnosis the physician should determine the type of seizure. Although there is no "drug of choice" in the treatment of epilepsy, clinical trials have established that some drugs are more useful in reducing certain seizure types than others. Some AEDs, such as ethosuximide, are highly effective in controlling only one type of seizure (absence), whereas others, such as valproic acid, are useful in a broad spectrum of seizure types. Table 8–3 lists the AEDs found to be most useful in some of the seizure types. The treatment of individual seizure types is reviewed later in the chapter.

Medical treatment should always begin with a single AED. Even in patients with mixed seizure disorders a single drug is started and increased to therapeutic serum levels or until drug toxicity occurs. If at that time seizures are not eliminated or substantially reduced, a second drug can be started while the original AED is tapered and discontinued. If more than one AED is started initially, the physician is never certain which one is controlling the seizures or causing toxicity. There is little evidence that AEDs when used in combination have a synergistic effect. Conversely, numerous studies have demonstrated that polytherapy is unnecessary in *most* patients. The clinician should always strive for monotherapy.

The treatment of epilepsy has been significantly improved by the development of techniques allowing measurement of serum levels of AEDs. Therapeutic ranges, the plasma concentrations for which optimal seizure control is likely to occur without significant side effects, have now been established for most AEDs. It must be recognized that the therapeutic range serves only as a guide and that any given patient may respond to levels outside the therapeutic range. Individual patients may have complete seizure control with levels below those considered therapeutic while other patients may tolerate and require levels above those listed. Conversely some patients have intolerable side effects at levels within the therapeutic levels. Signs of clinical toxicity, in spite of the maintenance of "therapeutic" levels, are particularly common in patients on multiple AEDs. Despite these caveats, clinical responses and toxicity correlate much better with serum levels than dosage.

In most instances AEDs are administered orally on a long-term basis. Following initiation of therapy, the drug will accumulate in the body until such time as the rate of elimination equals the rate of administration. Over this period of time, body and plasma concentrations increase exponentially until they reach a steady state or plateau. Steady state, a balance between accumulation and elimination of the AED, results in a stable level below which the concentration in the serum will not fall. The time to reach a steady state is approximately five half-lives (Figure 8–1).

In the steady state the range of fluctuation of plasma concentrations remains relatively constant. The minimum concentration occurs prior to a dose whereas the maximum level is dependent primarily on absorption rate. Because bioavailability varies considerably among the AEDs, it is usually preferable to obtain "routine" levels at trough, immediately prior to the next dose. AEDs with a long half-life, such as phenobarbital, have small daily fluctuations and timing of serum sampling is not important. However, when using a drug with a short half-life,

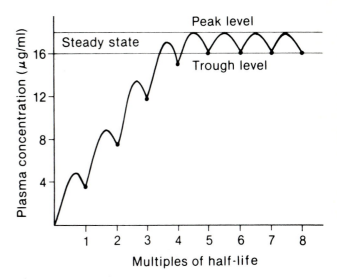

Figure 8-1. Plasma concentration of a drug (ordinate) following repeated oral drug administration. Interval of administration is a function of half-life of the drug. *(From Holmes, 1987, with permission of the publisher.)*

such as carbamazepine, the serum level will vary significantly depending on when the blood is sampled. If the physician is primarily concerned about toxicity, a level at peak, usually one to several hours after dosing, would be most valuable. Transient toxic effects of carbamazepine, such as diplopia, lethargy, and nausea, occur when the plasma carbamazepine is at peak concentration and dissipate when the level decreases. Fluctuations between minimum and maximum plasma levels of AEDs are more pronounced when children are on polytherapy. If a patient complains about the side effects of an AED at the time of peak serum concentration, the frequency of administration may be increased without changing the total daily dose. For example, if a child is taking carbamazepine, 400 mg tid, and has diplopia 2 hours after taking the drug, a trial of 300 mg qid may be helpful.

One common mistake in obtaining serum AED levels is to obtain them prior to development of the steady state. Obtaining the level before the steady state is reached will be misleading and the level measured will be lower than the eventual steady state. Because of the numerous drug interactions, it is very important to obtain serum levels of all AEDs when patients are receiving multiple AEDs. Measurements of AED levels are expensive and should always be used judiciously. Indications for monitoring plasma drug levels are given in Table 8–4. Summaries of some of the important pharmacokinetic properties of the AEDs are listed in Table 8–5.

Space limitations prohibit an extensive discussion of AEDs. The reader is referred to the textbook by Holmes (1987) for detailed discussions of the commonly used AEDs. The reader is encouraged to review the side effects of these drugs before prescribing the medications.

Phenobarbital

Phenobarbital remains one of the most widely used AEDs in pediatrics. Phenobarbital is effective in a variety of seizure types, is inexpensive, and is one of the safest AEDs available. However, non–life-threatening side effects such as behavioral changes and learning difficulties have limited the usefulness of the drug.

Phenobarbital is a broad-spectrum AED that is effective in the treatment of generalized tonic-clonic and partial seizures. The drug may also be helpful in almost all other seizure types. In addition, phenobarbital is effective in preventing recurrences of febrile seizures and is one of the primary drugs used in the treatment of status epilepticus.

Phenobarbital is likely the safest AED available, causing few serious side effects. While rashes are not infrequent with phenobarbital, discontinuation of the drug may not be required unless the rash is severe or persistent. The major side effects with phenobarbital consist of lethargy, learning difficulties, and behavioral changes. Hyperactivity is a common problem in children, as are mood changes, irritability or fussiness, and sleep disturbances. Sleep disturbances consist of difficulty falling asleep or early morning awakening with associated daytime irritability. There is now evidence in both children and adults that phenobarbital can affect cognitive abilities, such as short-term memory and perceptual-motor tasks.

Primidone

Primidone (Mysoline), a congener of phenobarbital, is useful in the treatment of generalized tonic-clonic and partial seizures. The drug is unique among AEDs because both the parent compound and its metabolites have antiepileptic properties. Primidone is metabolized through oxidation to phenobarbital and splitting of the ring to form phenylethylmalonamide (PEMA). Primidone, phenobarbital, and PEMA all have antiepileptic properties. Because of the antiepileptic properties of the three components, primidone may be effective in controlling seizures that do not respond to phenobarbital. Like phenobarbital, primidone is most effective in generalized tonic-clonic and partial seizures. Unfortunately, the drug has many of the side effects of phenobarbital.

Phenytoin

Phenytoin (Dilantin) is one of the most highly prescribed, inexpensive, and effective medications at the physician's disposal. Although there are numerous side effects, some of which are serious, it is considered to be a safe medication.

Phenytoin is a broad-spectrum AED that is effective in the treatment of generalized tonic-clonic, partial, and tonic seizures. The drug may be helpful in almost all other seizure types.

The metabolism of phenytoin differs from that of other AEDs because its biotransformation follows zero-order kinetics. Enzymes responsible for degradation of phenytoin become saturated at serum concentrations of phenytoin that fall within the serum therapeutic range. Once the hepatic enzymes are saturated the metabolic rate

TABLE 8–4. INDICATIONS FOR MONITORING PLASMA AED LEVELS

To determine serum level at steady state following initiation of therapy.

Following addition of another AED.

When interaction with a non-antiepileptic drug is suspected.

When drug biotransformation or elimination is altered as a consequence of a secondary disease.

When therapeutic effect is not achieved or symptoms of toxicity are observed.

When noncompliance is suspected.

When suspected maturational changes in absorption, biotransformation, or elimination occur.

When significant weight gain or loss occurs.

From Holmes (1987) with permission of the publisher.

TABLE 8-5. SUMMARY OF PHARMACOKINETIC DATA OF FREQUENTLY USED DRUGS

Drug	Absorption (%)	Peak Time of Effect (h)	Plasma Protein Binding (%)	Relative Volume of Distribution (L/kg)	Plasma Half-Life (h) Adults	Plasma Half-Life (h) Children	Dosage in Children (mg/kg)	Preferred Dosage Interval	Time to Steady State (days)	Therapeutic Plasma Concentration (μg/ml)
Phenobarbital	80–90	5–15	40–60	0.7–1.0	46–136	37–73 45–173 (neonate)	2–4	qd	14–21	15–40
Primidone	90–100	1–3	19	0.59	6–18	5–18	12–25	tid, qid	1–4	4–12
Phenytoin	85–95	4–8	69–96	0.6–0.7	10–34	5–18 10–60 (neonate) 10–140 (premature)	4–8	bid children qd adults	7–10	10–20
Ethotoin	—	2–4	46	—	5	5	20–50	4–6 times daily	1	15–50
Carbamazepine	70–80	3–6	70–80	0.8–1.9	14–27	8–25	10–30	tid, qid	3–4	6–12
Ethosuximide	100	1–7	0	0.62–0.72	50–60	24–36	15–40	tid, qid	7–10	40–100
Methsuximide	80–100	1–4	0	—	34–80	34–48	10–40	tid, qid	7–10	N-desmethyl-methsuximide (metabolite): 10–40
Valproic acid	100	1–4	80–95	0.2	6–18	4–14	30–60	qid (enteric coated, BID)	1–2	40–150
Clonazepam	98	1–4	47–80	3.2	20–40	20–40	0.1–0.2	tid	4–8	0.02–0.08 μg/ml (20–80 ng/ml)
Acetazolamide	100	2–4	90–95	1.8	10–15	10–15	10–20	tid	2–3	10–14

is no longer dependent on substrate load but proceeds at a constant pace (zero-order or nonlinear kinetics). Therefore, once hepatic saturation occurs half-life increases with increasing serum levels. Small increases in dosage will therefore result in a large increase in serum level and subsequent clinical toxicity (see Figure 8–2). Once the patient has levels in the lower therapeutic range it is necessary to increase the phenytoin dose by small amounts. A general rule is not to increase the dose by more than 25 mg/day once the patient has a serum phenytoin level above 10 μg/mL. Owing to the complex metabolism of phenytoin, monitoring of serum phenytoin levels is very important. Because intramuscular phenytoin crystallizes and is subsequently absorbed slowly and erratically the drug should *not* be given by this route.

Reported adverse effects of phenytoin include both dose-dependent and idiosyncratic reactions. Monitoring of serum phenytoin levels can eliminate many of the dose-related side effects. Common dose-related side effects of phenytoin include lethargy, gastrointestinal distress, dizziness, ataxia, tremors, and nystagmus. There is a correlation between serum levels and clinical signs of toxicity. Nystagmus appears at around 20 μg/ml, ataxia at 30 μg/ml, and drowsiness at levels greater than 40 μg/ml.

One of the most frequent yet serious idiosyncratic reactions is a skin rash. The clinical spectrum of skin rashes ranges from a common morbilliform rash occur-

ring 1 to 14 days after the onset of therapy to toxic epidermal necrosis, exfoliative dermatitis, and Stevens-Johnson syndrome. Though the morbilliform rash may be benign and self-limited, disappearing spontaneously, it is recommended that the drug be discontinued. If the rash is mild (measles-like or scarlatiniform), therapy may be resumed after the rash clears. If the rash recurs on reinstitution of therapy, further phenytoin usage is contraindicated.

Hepatic dysfunction is a rare but serious complication that usually occurs during the first 6 weeks of therapy. Lymphadenopathy is also a rare complication of phenytoin treatment, requiring that the drug be discontinued. Cosmetic side effects seen with chronic phenytoin use include gingival hypertrophy, hirsutism, coarsening of facial features, and increase in acne. Phenytoin has been associated with impairments in attention, memory, and speed of information processing, and with subjective feelings of fatigue, especially in association with high concentrations of the drug.

Carbamazepine

Carbamazepine (Tegretol), introduced in 1962, has emerged as one of the most valuable and widely used AEDs. It is now used in seizure types that had been treated in the past primarily with phenobarbital and phenytoin. Unlike those drugs, however, carbamazepine has no cosmetic side effects nor does it alter behavior, mood, or cognitive function. Unfortunately, an overemphasized fear about rare idiosyncratic hematologic side effects has prevented even wider use of this drug.

Carbamazepine is an effective treatment for partial seizures and generalized tonic-clonic seizures. It may also occasionally be helpful in other seizure types, such as tonic and myoclonic seizures. Absence seizures do not typically respond to carbamazepine. As discussed later in this section, atypical absence seizures may even be exacerbated by carbamazepine.

Carbamazepine has been associated with both dose-related and idiosyncratic reactions. The dose-related side effects are common and non–life-threatening while the idiosyncratic reactions are rare but serious. Common dose-related side effects include drowsiness, ataxia, gastrointestinal disturbances, diplopia, headache, irritability, clumsiness, and dizziness. These symptoms usually occur at peak concentrations and can often be relieved by increasing the dosing frequency without changing the total daily dose.

Idiosyncratic reactions of most concern are those involving the bone marrow. Fortunately, recent reviews of the subject have indicated that the hematopoietic toxicity of carbamazepine is much less than originally feared. It is estimated that the prevalence of carbamazepine hematologic toxicity is 0.002% for aplastic anemia, 10% for transient leukopenia, 2% for persistent leukopenia, 2% for thrombocytopenia, and less than 5% for anemia. As with other side effects, hematopoietic toxicity appears

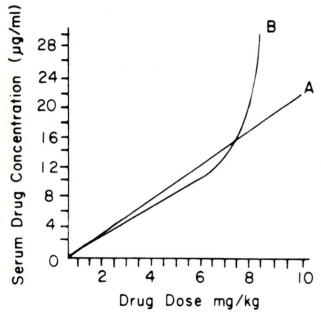

Figure 8–2. Relationship between serum drug concentration (ordinate) and drug concentration (abscissa) for a drug observing (A) first-order kinetics (linear) and (B) zero-order kinetics. Most antiepileptic drugs follow first-order kinetics whereas phenytoin follows zero-order kinetics. *(From Holmes, 1987, with permission of the publisher.)*

to be more frequent when the patient is on multiple AEDs. Pancreatitis has also been reported with carbamazepine.

Carbamazepine has been reported by Snead and Hosey (1985) to exacerbate seizures in some children. The most common seizure type that was exacerbated was atypical absence. These authors found that patients with bilaterally synchronous spike-wave discharges of 2.5 to 3 Hz on their EEGs were particularly susceptible to worsening of their seizures with carbamazepine administration. Numerous other authors have reported an exacerbation of some seizures with carbamazepine.

A major advantage of carbamazepine over phenobarbital and primidone is that carbamazepine usually results in no cognitive or behavioral changes. Children taking carbamazepine remain alert and do not demonstrate learning difficulties or personality changes.

It is recommended that a complete blood count (CBC) be obtained prior to initiation of therapy and at 2 weeks, 1 month, and 2 months, and then every 4 to 6 months. It is likely that these guidelines are too stringent and future recommendations will suggest less frequent CBCs. Unless there is clinical evidence of hepatic disease routine monitoring of liver function tests is not necessary. A mild leukopenia occurs in a significant number of patients and does not usually require discontinuation of the drug. Unfortunately, there are no well-established guidelines regarding the management of leukopenia. In some patients the white blood cell count (WBC) will increase once the dose is increased. I would recommend that the daily dose of carbamazepine be reduced if the total neutrophil count falls below 1000 mm^3. In addition, parents should be advised to notify their physician if easy bruising, petechial or purpuric hemorrhage, or other signs of hematologic toxicity appear in their child.

Ethosuximide

Ethosuximide (Zarontin) is an excellent first-line AED for the treatment of seizures. It is highly efficacious in this seizure type and has relatively few adverse side effects. It is rarely used for other seizure types.

Side effects occur in approximately one third of patients treated with ethosuximide. Many of the side effects are mild and include gastrointestinal distress, such as nausea, vomiting, anorexia, and discomfort; dizziness; headaches; hiccups; and drowsiness. Serious side effects with ethosuximide are quite rare. Ethosuximide has been associated with hematologic disorders such as leukopenia and pancytopenia. It is recommended that a CBC be obtained monthly for 2 months, then every 4 to 6 months.

Valproic Acid

Valproic acid (VPA, sodium valproate, Depakene, Depakote) is one of the most valuable AEDs to be released in the past decade. However, physicians prescribing the drug must be very familiar with the side effects, some of which are life threatening.

VPA is a broad-spectrum AED that has been successfully used in multiple seizure types. The drug has been primarily used in the treatment of absence, generalized tonic-clonic, tonic, atonic, and myoclonic seizures. In addition, it may be effective in other seizure types, including infantile spasms and partial simple and complex seizures. Although it has been shown to be an effective prophylactic drug for febrile seizures, VPA is not routinely recommended for this disorder.

Mild but annoying side effects are common in children started on VPA. Nausea and vomiting are two of the most common complaints following initiation of VPA therapy. These are usually a transient problem, although they persist in some children, even after they have been on the drug for weeks. Nausea and vomiting may result from a direct effect of VPA on the stomach shortly after ingesting the drug or a central effect occurring several hours after ingestion. These side effects can usually be eliminated or lessened by reducing the dosage, consuming the drug with food, or using the enteric-coated preparation (Depakote). Sedation occurs in a significant number of patients following initiation of VPA, especially when VPA is administered with other AEDs. This side effect usually disappears with continued usage. Tremors are common with VPA and may correlate with serum level. Transient hair loss, weight gain or loss, stomatitis, and skin rashes occasionally occur in some patients. Unlike many other AEDs, VPA has relatively few adverse effects on psychosocial development. Patients taking the drug rarely have a change in behavior, mood, learning abilities, or personality.

Pancreatitis is a rare, but serious, side effect reported in association with VPA. Thrombocytopenia or platelet dysfunction had been reported with VPA. Except in patients who are undergoing surgery, these findings usually have little clinical importance. Red cell aplasia, neutropenia, and bone marrow suppression have also been reported with VPA.

Cases of stupor and coma associated with nontoxic serum levels of VPA have been described. The symptoms may occur when VPA is used alone or in combination with other drugs and in most cases appear to be secondary to hyperammonemia. Although there is a poor correlation between clinical symptoms and serum ammonia levels, reductions of VPA dosage in symptomatic patients may result in clinical improvement. The most serious side effect associated with VPA is liver toxicity. Two types have been reported: a common, transient, dose-dependent, asymptomatic rise in serum transaminase (SGOT and SGPT) and a rare, idiosyncratic, severe, non-dose-related, symptomatic hepatitis that may be fatal. The first type usually occurs during the first 3 months of therapy and is very common. Usually SGOT and SGPT levels fall with a reduction of the VPA dosage; at other times the enzyme levels decrease spontaneously despite continuation of treatment.

Recently Dreifuss and colleagues (1989) reviewed the

cases of fatal hepatotoxicity associated with VPA in the United States. No hepatic fatalities were found in patients above the age of 10 years receiving VPA as monotherapy. The rate of hepatic fatalities was 0.08 in 10,000 in patients on monotherapy versus a rate of 0.38 in 10,000 in patients on polytherapy. The highest-risk group consisted of children below the age of 2 years treated with polytherapy (12.62 in 10,000). The initial signs and symptoms of hepatic dysfunction include vomiting, lethargy, jaundice, weakness, drowsiness, and an increase in seizure frequency. Although routine laboratory studies are warranted, parents must be warned that they do not guarantee safety because the onset of the hepatic dysfunction may be very rapid and fulminating.

All patients on VPA require monitoring of liver function and hematologic studies. It is recommended that baseline studies (CBC with platelet estimation, SGOT or SGPT) be obtained prior to administration of the drug. Repeat studies should then to be done at 2 weeks and then monthly until the child has been on the drug 6 months. At that time, repeat studies can be performed every 3 to 6 months. These studies should be repeated immediately if there is any clinical indication of liver disease. In addition, amylase levels may be helpful if the patient has abdominal pain. Easy bruising or bleeding should be pursued with a CBC, platelet count, and clotting studies. In patients with lethargy or other mental symptoms, a measurement of serum ammonia level may be helpful. It is also important to obtain the AED level of both VPA and other AEDs if used concurrently, because drug interactions are quite common.

Other AEDs

There are many other AEDs that may be occasionally useful in children. Clonazepam (Klonopin), a benzodiazepine, is useful in a variety of seizures, including absence, generalized tonic-clonic, and myoclonic. Acetazolamide (Diamox) is sometimes useful as an adjunctive agent in children with absence and generalized tonic-clonic seizures. Methsuximide (Celontin), like ethosuximide, is useful in absence seizures as well as partial complex seizures.

ANNOTATED BIBLIOGRAPHY

Mikati M: The newer antiepileptic drugs: Carbamazepine and valproic acid. *Pediatr Ann* 20:34–40, 1991.

This is a recent, comprehensive review of the use of the two newer AEDs, carbamazepine and valproic acid, in the treatment of childhood epilepsy.

Farwell JR, Lee YJ, Hirtz DG, Sulzbacher SI, Ellenberg JH, Nelson KB: Phenobarbital for febrile seizures—Effects on intelligence and on seizure recurrence. *N Engl J Med* 322:364–369, 1990.

In this study a total of 217 children with febrile seizures were randomized to prophylactic treatment with phenobarbital or a placebo. There was a small but significant difference in IQ between the phenobarbital and placebo-treated groups, which decreased but was still present at 6 months after medication withdrawal. However, until further follow-up IQ measurements are obtained, it will be uncertain as to whether phenobarbital causes permanent deficits in intelligence.

Camfield P, Camfield C, Dooley J, Smith E, Garner B: A randomized study of carbamazepine versus no medication after a first unprovoked seizure in childhood. *Neurology* 39:851–852, 1989.

The authors randomized 31 children with a first partial or generalized tonic-clonic afebrile seizure to either carbamazepine treatment or no treatment and found that carbamazepine reduced the recurrence risk of afebrile seizures. However, four patients discontinued carbamazepine because of side effects.

Ramsay RE: Use of phenytoin and carbamazepine in treatment of epilepsy. *Neurol Clin North Am* 4:585–600, 1986.

A review of the clinical indications, pharmacokinetics, and side effects of two drugs used for partial and generalized tonic-clonic seizures.

Holmes GL: *Diagnosis and Management of Seizures in Children.* Philadelphia, WB Saunders, 1987.

All of the AEDs commonly used in children are reviewed in this textbook.

SIMPLE PARTIAL SEIZURES

Classification

Partial seizures are those in which the first clinical and EEG changes indicate activation of a system of neurons

FEATURE TABLE 8-1. SIMPLE PARTIAL SEIZURES

Discriminating Features	Consistent Feature	Variable Features
1. Unlike partial complex seizures there is not an impairment of consciousness with simple partial seizures. 2. Seizures are usually brief and stereotyped. 3. Seizures frequently respond to carbamazepine, phenytoin, primidone, or phenobarbital.	1. No impairment of consciousness.	1. Motor symptoms. 2. Somatosensory symptoms. 3. Psychic symptoms. 4. Autonomic symptoms. 5. Postictal symptoms. 6. Association with structural lesions of the brain. 7. Interictal EEG abnormalities.

limited to part of one cerebral hemisphere. Partial seizures are further classified primarily on the basis of whether or not consciousness is impaired during the attack. When consciousness is not impaired, the seizure is classified as a simple partial seizure. When consciousness is impaired, that is, the patient is unable to respond normally to exogenous stimuli by virtue of altered awareness and/or responsiveness, the seizure is classified as a complex partial seizure.

The clinical manifestations of partial seizures are determined by the cortical area involved. For example, seizures arising from the occipital region present with visual phenomena, those from the precentral gyrus with motor phenomena, and those from the postcentral gyrus with sensory symptoms. Seizures arising from the temporal lobe are usually associated with an altered state of consciousness and therefore are classified as complex partial seizures.

Simple partial seizures may be further classified into those with motor signs, somatosensory or special sensory symptoms, autonomic symptoms, or psychic symptoms.

Clinical Characteristics

Partial seizures with motor symptoms are the most common type of simple partial seizures. Depending on the site or origin of the attack in the motor strip, any portion of the body may be involved in focal seizure activity. The type of seizures may vary from those involving only small groups of muscles, such as rhythmic twitching of a single finger or part of the tongue, to those involving multiple muscles, such as seen in clonic activity of the arm or leg. Partial seizures may remain strictly focal or may spread to adjoining cortical areas, producing a sequential involvement of body parts, formerly known as a "Jacksonian march." Following partial motor seizures, there may be paralysis of the muscle groups involved in the seizure. This weakness, termed Todd's paralysis, lasts from minutes to hours and is helpful in determining the focus of the seizure. One of the most common types of simple partial seizures with motor phenomena, benign Rolandic epilepsy, is described in more detail subsequently.

Autonomic symptoms consist of a variety of complaints, including abdominal pain, tachycardia, diaphoresis, pupillary dilatation, flushing, and piloerection. Abdominal pain as a manifestation of a seizure disorder is rare and has been termed abdominal epilepsy. Because the abdominal pain usually occurs during a complex partial seizure, it is discussed in the next section.

Somatosensory seizures arise from those areas of the cortex serving sensory functions. Like those of simple partial seizures, the clinical symptoms vary depending on the area of sensory cortex involved. Although any type of sensation may occur, typically the patient reports a feeling of "pins and needles" or numbness. Like seizures

Pearls and Perils: Simple Partial Seizures

1. Simple partial seizures are usually short, lasting less than a minute.
2. Structural brain lesions must be considered in children with simple partial seizures.
3. The lack of an EEG abnormality during a seizure does not rule out the possibility of a simple partial seizure.

with motor symptoms, somatosensory seizures also may spread to neighboring areas of the cortex. Olfactory sensations, usually in the form of unpleasant odors, may occur. Gustatory sensations are usually unpleasant and unrefined (salty, sour, sweet, bitter) rather than specific. Patients commonly describe the sensations as "metallic." Vertiginous symptoms include the sensations of falling or floating in space as well as vertigo. Special sensory seizures are accompanied by illusions, delusions, or hallucinations, which vary considerably in complexity from patient to patient.

Disturbances of higher cerebral function (psychic symptoms) are usually components of complex partial seizures and will be discussed in the section on complex partial seizures. Only rarely is this group of symptoms a manifestation of simple partial seizures.

All of the foregoing symptoms—motor, somatosensory, special sensory, autonomic, and psychic—may precede either a complex partial seizure or a generalized tonic-clonic seizure. The partial seizure is often referred to as an *aura*, because it may be the only part of the seizure recalled by the patient and serves to warn him or her that a tonic-clonic or complex partial seizure is pending.

Differential Diagnosis

It is usually not difficult to diagnose partial simple seizures correctly. Occasionally seizures with somatosensory, psychic, or special sensory symptoms may be confused with migraine. This differential diagnosis is discussed under Complex Partial Seizures. In addition, movement disorders such as ticks and chorea may be confused with partial motor seizures. This differential is further discussed under Myoclonic Seizures.

Electroencephalography

The EEG is frequently but not always abnormal in patients with partial simple seizures. Focal spikes or sharp waves are seen in 40% to 85% of patients and frequently correspond to the areas of focal cortical epileptogenic activity. Frequently the epileptogenic area is so limited that epileptiform activity is not seen even during a clinical seizure.

Etiology

Etiologic factors associated with simple partial seizures may be static, such as those following neonatal trauma or subarachnoid hemorrhage, or progressive, such as lesions associated with tumors or chronic encephalitis. The etiologic agents of both complex partial and simple partial seizures are similar and will be discussed in the section on complex partial seizures.

ANNOTATED BIBLIOGRAPHY

Holmes GL: Partial seizures in children. *Pediatrics* 77:725–731, 1986.

  This is a study of the clinical and EEG manifestations of 56 children with simple or complex partial seizures evaluated using EEG and videotape monitoring.

BENIGN ROLANDIC EPILEPSY

Benign Rolandic epilepsy is an important, distinct epileptic syndrome occurring in childhood that is characterized by nocturnal generalized seizures of focal onset and daytime partial seizures arising from the lower Rolandic area of the cortex, and by an EEG pattern consisting of a midtemporal-central spike foci. It is important for the clinician to be aware of this *syndrome* because its evaluation and prognosis differ considerably from those for other focal seizure disorders.

Clinical Characteristics

The disorder is limited to the pediatric age group. Seizures begin between the ages of 2 and 12 years although more typically the child is between 5 and 10 years of age. They remit spontaneously and rarely recur after 16 years of age. The developmental and neurologic examination is usually normal in these children. A single nocturnal seizure is the most common mode of presentation although diurnal seizures may also occur. In nocturnal seizures the initial event is frequently clonic movements of the mouth with salivation and gurgling sounds from the throat. Secondary generalization of the seizure occurs frequently and may be the only portion of the seizure witnessed by the parents. The initial focal component of the seizure may be quite brief and therefore may be missed by parents. Motor phenomena during the daytime attacks are usually restricted to one side of the body. These attacks frequently involve the face, although the arm and leg may also be involved. Arrest of speech may occur at the onset of the attack or be present during its course. The patient may describe stiffness or spasms of the tongue or jaw or a choking sensation. Salivation and guttural utterance often occur. Consciousness is rarely impaired during the daytime attacks, and postictal confusion and amnesia are unusual. It is extremely unusual for a patient to have a diurnal generalized tonic-clonic seizure. Status epilepticus does not occur in this syndrome. The seizures are clearly distinguishable from complex partial seizures because they lack automatisms; olfactory, gustatory, or epigastric auras; illusions; hallucinations; or affective symptomatology.

Electroencephalography

The disorder is characterized by a very distinctive, dramatic EEG pattern. The characteristic interictal EEG correlate is distinct high-amplitude spikes with a prominent following slow wave appearing singly or in groups at the midtemporal and central (Rolandic) region (C_3, C_4, T_3, T_4). As with other spikes, Rolandic spikes are not diagnostic of epilepsy and many occur in children without a history of seizures.

FEATURE TABLE 8-2. BENIGN ROLANDIC EPILEPSY

Discriminating Features	Consistent Features	Variable Features
1. Usually no difficulty in making diagnosis when consistent features are present. It is imperative to obtain sleep EEG if benign Rolandic epilepsy is suspected and patient has normal awake EEG. 2. Seizures respond to most AEDs.	1. Childhood seizure disorder: begins before age 13, not seen after second decade. 2. Associated with temporal-central spike focus. 3. Nocturnal generalized tonic-clonic seizures and/or diurnal seizures referable to the lower Rolandic area of the brain. 4. Normal neurologic examination and intellectual function. 5. Benign prognosis.	1. Seizures may occur during day, night, or both. 2. EEG abnormality may be seen during wakefulness and/or sleep.

Pearls and Perils: Benign Rolandic Epilepsy

1. Patients with benign Rolandic epilepsy and normal neurologic examination do not require CT scans. However, if the seizures do not respond to AEDs, focal slowing develops on the EEG, or the neurologic examination changes, a CT scan should be ordered.
2. Benign Rolandic epilepsy, unlike most partial seizure disorders, has a strong familial disposition.

Genetics

Benign Rolandic epilepsy is usually familial. The disorder is inherited via a single, autosomal dominant gene, with a low, age-dependent penetrance. Of close relatives (siblings, children, and parents of the proband), 50% demonstrate the EEG abnormality between the ages of 5 and 15 years. Before 5 and after 15 years of age there is a low penetrance, with few patients demonstrating the abnormality. Only 12% of patients that inherit the EEG abnormality have clinical seizures.

Evaluation and Treatment

If the patient has a clinical history and EEG characteristics of this disorder and a normal neurologic examination a further workup is not warranted. If the neurologic examination is abnormal or EEG demonstrates abnormalities other than the typical epileptiform discharge further evaluation with a CT or magnetic resonance imaging scan is necessry.

Because the seizures are benign and usually infrequent, most physicians do not treat the first or even the second seizure. When treated, the seizures are usually controlled with a single AED. AEDs used for partial simple and partial complex seizures, i.e., phenobarbital, phenytoin, and carbamazepine, are usually effective. Response is usually so dramatic that failure to respond should raise questions regarding compliance.

ANNOTATED BIBLIOGRAPHY

Lombroso C: Sylvian seizures and midtemporal spike foci in children. *Arch Neurol* 17:52–59, 1967.
This article was one of the first to call attention to this unique seizure type and remains one of the best descriptions of both the EEG and clinical manifestations of this disorder.
Beaussart M: Benign epilepsy of children with rolandic (centrotemporal) paroxysmal foci. A clinical entity. Study of 221 cases. *Epilepsia* 13:795–811, 1972.
In this, the largest study to date of this disorder, the benign prognosis is emphasized.

COMPLEX PARTIAL SEIZURES

Complex partial seizures (CPSs) are one of the most common seizure types to occur both in children and adults. Because the focus of CPSs often arises in the temporal lobe, an area concerned with memory and emotion, clinical symptoms may be quite complex and variable, encompassing the entire range of neuropsychiatric symptoms. The overlap of psychogenic behavioral manifestations and clinical phenomena associated with CPSs makes the differential diagnosis and management both difficult and challenging.

Clinical Characteristics

Although extremely variable, CPSs usually last from 30 seconds to several minutes. CPSs can occur during both the awake and sleeping states. When CPSs occur in sleep, they are most likely to appear shortly after the child falls asleep or during the early morning hours when the patient cycles frequently through stage 2 of sleep. When occurring at night, the seizures may be very difficult to differentiate from the parasomnias. This will be further discussed in Chapter 27.

Aura
A CPS may start as a simple partial seizure followed by impairment of consciousness or begin with impairment of consciousness. In patients with a simple partial onset to the seizure the initial phase of the seizure is often termed an aura. The aura is therefore defined as the portion of the seizure that occurs before consciousness is lost. The aura may consist of any of the manifestations of a simple partial seizure depending on the area of cortex involved. The aura varies considerably from patient to patient and includes somatosensory, auditory, visual, olfactory, and gustatory symptoms; hallucinations; vixceral sensations, such as oropharyngeal, epigastric, abdominal, genital, or retrosternal, sensations; and complex subjective experiences, such as fear, strangeness, embarrassment, dizziness, vertigo, deja vu, or jamais vu.

Automatisms
Automatisms consisting of involuntary motor activity occurring during the period of impaired consciousness either during the ictus or in the postictal period, are common in CPSs. The patient is partially or totally amnesic for the behavior. Examples of automatic behavior include chewing, tongue movements, lip smacking and swallowing, hand gestures, scratching, crying, laughing, and repeating a word or phrase. The activity may be complex and quasipurposeful, such as playing cards, drawing, or playing music. Automatisms can be seen in other seizure types, including absences and the postictal phase of a generalized tonic-clonic seizure.

FEATURE TABLE 8-3. COMPLEX PARTIAL SEIZURES

Discriminating Features	Consistent Features	Variable Features
1. There is always impairment of consciousness during CPSs. 2. CPSs usually are longer than absence seizures (average duration over 1 minute). Unlike absence seizures, CPSs may be associated with an aura. Whereas absence seizures have a sudden onset and ending, in CPSs there is usually not an abrupt onset and ending. 3. Usually respond to carbamazepine, phenytoin, primidone, or phenobarbital.	1. Altered state of consciousness.	1. Automatisms. 2. Affective symptoms. 3. Psychic symptoms. 4. Somatosensory symptoms. 5. Aura. 6. Postictal impairment. 7. Duration. 8. Association with structural brain lesions. 9. Interictal EEG findings.

Autonomic Symptoms

Like simple partial seizures, CPSs may be associated with a variety of autonomic symptoms. Partial seizures in which abdominal pain and vomiting are components have been termed abdominal epilepsy. This form of epilepsy, a seizure disorder occurring principally in children, usually occurs as a complex partial seizure with impairment of consciousness. The pain of abdominal epilepsy is often colic-like, severe, and periumbilical in location. The pain is brief in duration and occurs at unpredictable intervals. The attacks may be accompanied by other autonomic phenomena, such as borborygmi, sweating, salivation, and flatus.

Psychic Symptoms

Although psychic symptoms occur commonly in CPSs, they frequently precede the alteration of consciousness and serve as the aura to the patient. Psychic symptoms, defined as disturbances of higher cerebral function, include dysphasia, cognitive disturbances, affective symptoms, dysmnesic symptoms, illusions, and hallucinations.

Affective Symptoms. Emotional changes have been well recognized as ictal events in CPSs and consist of fear and sadness, depression, embarrassment, joy, or ecstasy. Any emotion may constitute the ictal experience, although some emotions occur more commonly than others. Because children often have difficulty verbalizing their experiences, their emotions may be evident only by their facial expressions. Fear—a common ictal emotion in both children and adults—may be evidenced by the child's facial expression or the need to run or be held by the parents.

Dysmnesic Symptoms. Dysmnesic symptoms consist of a distortion of memory and may consist of the sensation that an experience had occurred before (deja vu if visual,

deja entendu if auditory). Vivid "flashbacks" to specific events in the past may be reported by patients. Because the dysmnesic symptoms occur before the period of impaired consciousness, the symptoms serve as an aura to the patient. Some patients may have frequent, annoying episodes of deja vu or deja entendu as partial simple seizures, without impairment of consciousness. In my experience dysmnesic symptoms are unusual in young children.

Special Sensory Symptoms

Alterations of perception may occur during CPSs. These may consist of unusual clearness of vision or more commonly take the form of illusions or hallucinations. Illusions, defined as distortions of perception, may consist of macropsia (objects or people appearing larger than normal), micropsia (objects or people appearing smaller than normal), or similar distortions of sounds. The patient may experience altered perception of the body, depersonalization, a feeling that the patient is outside the body, or dissociative states. Hallucinations, perceptions with corresponding external stimuli, may occasionally occur in CPSs.

Seizures in which the patient has olfactory or gustatory hallucinations have been termed uncinate fits or seizures. The olfactory and gustatory sensations are typically of a disagreeable quality and accompanied by movements of the lips and tongue.

Postictal Symptoms

Postictal confusion and tiredness are typical for CPSs. It is often difficult to differentiate the ictal from the postictal events, since there is rarely an abrupt transition between the two phases. Although fatigue frequently follows CPSs, unlike the symptomatology of generalized tonic-clonic seizures, deep sleep is unusual. The most common postictal finding is confusion.

Differential Diagnosis

Because CPSs may consist of simple staring, with or without automatisms, the seizures may sometimes be confused with absence seizures. Helpful distinguishing features of typical absence seizures include a sudden onset, lack of an aura, brief duration (less than 30 seconds), and sudden cessation with immediate resumption of preictal activity and clarity of mind. CPSs usually last longer than absence seizures. CPSs are frequently followed by confusion and fatigue, which never occur with absence seizures. Another key differentiating point is that hyperventilation easily induces absence seizures in the untreated patient, whereas CPSs are much less likely to be induced by hyperventilation. The EEG is also very helpful in differentiating the two seizure types. The clinical and EEG features that differentiate CPSs from absence seizures are listed in Table 8–6.

A common diagnostic problem is differentiating between nonepileptic episodic rage or dyscontrol attacks and CPSs. Rage attacks occur with some type of provocation, albeit often minimal, and are completely out of character for the patient. Adding to the problems in differentiating these attacks from CPSs is the fact that the majority of patients with episodic dyscontrol have organic cerebral defects and some have documented epilepsy. Both CPSs and nonepileptic rage attacks may be of similar duration, lasting several minutes, and are frequently followed by fatigue, confusion, and amnesia for the event (see Table 8–7). Unlike rage attacks, CPSs are rarely, if ever, associated with person-directed violence. Whereas patients during CPSs have reactive automatic behavior and may become agitated and combative when restrained, directed violence does not occur. Conversely, in rage attacks, violence directed against individuals commonly occurs. Another differentiating point is that CPSs are usually stereotyped compared with the variable features of rage attacks. The most helpful differentiating point is that rage attacks are usually precipitated by some event, however trivial, that is disturbing to the patient. Although CPSs on occasion may be precipitated by stress, the consistent relationship seen in rage attacks is usually lacking.

On occasion migraines may be confused with CPSs with autonomic or sensory symptoms. The differentiation of migraine from abdominal epilepsy is one of the most difficult diagnoses to make. Like abdominal epilepsy, migraines may result in episodic abdominal pain. In children with migraine, the abdominal symptoms may not be associated with the headache. In addition, interictal EEGs may be abnormal in both abdominal epilepsy and childhood migraine. Because abdominal epilepsy usually occurs as a CPS, there is impairment of consciousness during the attack, whereas abdominal pain with migraine is rarely associated with impaired consciousness. A family history of migraines may be an important clue to the diagnosis. Migraines are discussed further in Chapter 24.

Electroencephalography

The interictal EEG findings in patients are variable. Abnormalities that occur on interictal EEGs in patients with CPSs include spikes, sharp waves, spike-wave discharges, or focal slowing activity. Although CPSs are frequently associated with focal interictal epileptiform activity, some patients will show generalized or diffuse abnormalities. When focal spikes are present they most frequently occur in the anterior temporal lobe. However, interictal discharges may be located outside the temporal region, most frequently in the frontal lobe. Bilateral temporal lobe spikes occurring either independently or synchronously are seen in approximately one third to one fourth of patients with CPSs.

The likelihood of detecting epileptiform activity can be increased by recording the EEG during drowsiness and

TABLE 8–6. DIFFERENTIAL DIAGNOSIS OF TYPICAL ABSENCE SEIZURES AND COMPLEX PARTIAL SEIZURES

Clinical Data	Absence Seizures	Complex Partial Seizures
Frequency per day	Multiple	Rarely more than 1 or 2
Duration	Frequently less than 10 s; rarely greater than 30 s	Average duration over 1 min; rarely less than 10 s
Aura	Never	Frequently
Eye blinking	Common	Occasionally
Automatisms	Common	Frequently
Postictal impairment	None	Frequently
Seizures activated by:		
Hyperventilation	Very frequently	Occasionally
Photic stimulation	Frequently	Rarely
EEG		
Ictal	Generalized spike-wave	Usually unilateral or bilateral temporal or frontal discharges
Interictal	Usually normal	Variable; may be spikes or sharp waves in frontal or temporal lobes

From Holmes (1987) with permission of the publisher.

TABLE 8-7. DIFFERENTIATION OF RAGE ATTACKS FROM COMPLEX PARTIAL SEIZURES

Clinical Data	Complex Partial Seizures	Rage Attacks
Duration	Seconds to minutes	Minutes
Stereotype of attacks	May vary but usually have consistent patterns	Patterns occasionally widely divergent
Aura	Frequent	Rare
Violence	Unusual, rarely directed	Frequent, may be directed
Precipitating event	No	Usually
Amnesia for event	Partial or total	None to total
Postictal confusion, lethargy, sleepiness	Common	Sometimes
Nocturnal occurrence	May occur	No
Interictal behavioral abnormalities	Sometimes	Usually
Responds to antiepileptic medication	Usually	Occasionally
EEG		
Ictal	Variable, temporal or frontal lobe spikes	Normal or nonspecific abnormalities
Interictal	Unilateral or bilateral frontal or temporal lobe discharges	No change

From Holmes (1987) with permission of the publisher.

sleep. Sleep deprivation may be a powerful activator of epileptiform activity. If an abnormality is not detected on the initial EEG, repeating the study following sleep deprivation may be useful. Finally the addition of supplementary electrodes, such as sphenoidal electrodes, may also increase the yield of the EEG. Hyperventilation and photic stimulation usually do not activate seizures in children with CPSs.

The diagnosis of CPSs, is always made on the basis of clinical criteria and a normal EEG should never be used to rule out CPSs. Conversely, the clinician must be aware that epileptiform EEG patterns may occur in children who do not, and never will, have seizures. An abnormal EEG should never be construed as definite evidence of CPSs in the absence of a convincing clinical history.

Etiology

In a classic study of CPSs of temporal lobe origin in 100 children, Ounsted and colleagues found that 35% of the patients had a major cerebral insult before the seizures began. Associated etiologic factors included birth asphyxia, head injury, infections, and tumors. In another 32% status epilepticus began before the seizures, and in 33% no etiology could be determined for the seizures.

The pathologic examination of tissue obtained at the time of total or partial temporal lobectomies for intractable seizures has greatly enhanced our knowledge about the etiologic factors associated with CPSs. Falconer and associates examined temporal lobes from 100 patients, primarily adults, with CPSs of temporal lobe origin. The authors found that mesial temporal lobe sclerosis was present in 47 cases, small cryptic tumors in 24 cases, miscellaneous focal lesions such as scars or infarcts in 13 cases, and equivocal lesions such as subpial and white

matter gliosis in 22 cases. Although it is beyond the scope of this chapter to discuss the etiologies of CPS in detail, a few comments about tumors are warranted.

Although brain tumors are a rare cause of seizures in children, accounting for only approximately 1% to 2% of cases, 25% to 40% of children with supratentorial brain tumors have seizures. However, the probability of a tumor is not the same in all seizure types. Partial seizures are more frequently associated with tumors than other seizure types. In large series of patients with CPSs, tumors have comprised a significant percentage of the etiologies.

Evaluation

Unlike absence seizures, which usually occur multiple times daily, CPSs rarely occur more than once or twice daily. Only rarely will the physician have an opportunity to actually observe a seizure. For that reason the history is critically important. Altered consciousness is the sine qua non of CPSs, and if the child is totally alert and responsive during the attack the diagnosis of CPSs cannot be made. The physician should evaluate the history for factors that may have precipitated the seizure. For example, sleep, fatigue, stress, and hypoglycemia may play a role in inducing seizures.

The past medical history may offer clues to the etiology of the seizures. As noted earlier, frequent causes of CPSs include birth asphyxia or trauma, head injuries, severe febrile seizures, and meningitis or encephalitis. The review of symptoms from patients with CPSs is essential and a careful history of other neurologic symptoms must be obtained. A recent history of headaches or vomiting, especially if the symptoms occur at night, should raise the possibility of a structural lesion as the etiology of the seizures.

Pearls and Perils:
Complex Partial Seizures

1. The patient with epileptic "staring spells," especially if they occur less than once daily, is more likely to have PCSs than absence seizures.
2. Children with CPSs, who do not respond to phenytoin, carbamazepine, VPA, primidone, and phenobarbital are unlikely to achieve seizure control and should be considered for possible surgery.
3. It is an error to attribute violence to an epileptic seizure. Although patients may become agitated during a seizure or postictal period, especially when restrained, directed violence is extremely rare.
4. Patients with abdominal pain rarely have seizures as an etiology of the pain. Abdominal epilepsy, a very rare disorder, is usually partial complex in type and is associated with impairment of consciousness.

It is important for the physician to do a careful neurologic examination on a child with CPSs. Any abnormal neurologic finding on physical examination in a child without prior documented neurologic impairment requires further evaluation.

Although the interictal EEG is never diagnostic of CPSs, it can be helpful in supporting the diagnosis. An EEG should be obtained when the diagnosis is first suspected clinically and preferably prior to initiation of AEDs. Routine EEGs are not indicated in CPSs and should be obtained only if there is a change in the neurologic examination, character of the seizures, or seizure frequency. The EEG may also be of value in deciding when to withdraw AEDs.

It is recommended that all children with CPSs have a CT or MRI scan. CT scans are frequently abnormal in children with partial seizures. Although the majority of the abnormalities will not alter management of the child, in a small but significant percentage an unexpected neoplasm or other treatable lesion will be discovered. In addition, even when the CT or MRI scan does not alter therapeutic management, it may offer the clinician valuable information regarding the etiology of the seizures. A normal CT or MRI scan also serves to comfort both the physician and parents that "nothing is being missed." However, even with a normal CT or MRI scan, it behooves the physician to follow the patient closely, because a change in neurologic examination or development of focal slowing on the EEG would indicate the necessity for a repeat study.

Treatment

Carbamazepine, phenytoin, phenobarbital, and primidone are the primary AEDs used in the treatment of CPSs. As previously discussed, frequent behavioral changes and cognitive impairment are seen with the barbiturates and this group of drugs is generally avoided. CPSs are frequently refractory to pharmacologic therapy. Only 25% to 60% of patients will have a good to excellent response, that is, either complete or almost complete cessation of seizure activity. The remainder will continue with slight or no reduction in seizure frequency. Because some patients, even with optimal pharmacologic management, continue to have CPSs, they may be candidates for surgical treatment.

There are no firm guidelines as to when AEDs should be withdrawn in patients who are seizure free. Recurrence risk is related to a number of factors including age of onset, seizure frequency and duration, and neurologic examination. All of these factors must be considered in each patient. A general recommendation is that, once a child is seizure free for 2 years, slow AED withdrawal should be initiated.

ANNOTATED BIBLIOGRAPHY

Ounsted C, Lindsay J, Norman R: Biological factors in temporal lobe epilepsy. *Clin Dev Med* 22, 1966.
   This monograph is an excellent longitudinal study of temporal lobe seizures in children.
Falconer MA, Serafetinides EA, Corsellis JA: Etiology and pathogenesis of temporal lobe epilepsy. *Arch Neurol* 10:233–248, 1964.
Mathieson G: Pathology of temporal lobe foci, in Penry JK, Daly DD (eds): *Advances in Neurology*, Vol II: *Complex Partial Seizures and Their Treatment.* New York, Raven Press, 1975, p 163–185.
   Both articles deal with the pathologic findings at surgery in patients undergoing temporal lobectomies for CPSs. Although the series are composed primarily of adults who had seizures refractory to medical treatment, the results are likely to be applicable to the pediatric population.
Holmes GL: Partial seizures in children. *Pediatrics* 77:725–731, 1986.
   This is a study of the clinical and EEG manifestations of 56 children with simple or complex partial seizures evaluated using EEG and videotape monitoring.

GENERALIZED TONIC-CLONIC SEIZURES

Generalized tonic-clonic (GTC) seizures, previously termed grand mal seizures, are the most dramatic and frightening seizures the clinician will encounter. There is rarely any difficulty in making the diagnosis.

Classification

There are two basic types of GTC seizures: primary GTC seizures, which are bilaterally symmetric and without focal features at onset, and secondary GTC seizures, which begin focally and then become generalized.

FEATURE TABLE 8-4. GENERALIZED TONIC-CLONIC SEIZURES

Discriminating Features	Consistent Features	Variable Features
1. Rarely confused with other disorders except pseudoseizures. Unlike pseudoseizures epileptic GTC seizures are rarely associated with vulgarity, writhing or thrashing movements, or asymmetric movements. 2. Prolactin levels usually elevated following GTC seizure; normal following pseudoseizures. 3. Usually respond to carbamazepine, phenytoin, primidone, phenobarbital, or VPA.	1. Loss of consciousness. 2. Tonic-clonic movements of all four extremities. 3. Postictal period.	1. Aura. 2. Urinary incontinence. 3. Self-injury, i.e., tongue biting. 4. Duration.

Clinical Characteristics

Some children with GTC seizures or their parents are aware of the impending seizure days or hours before it occurs. Headaches, insomnia, changes in mood, irritability, and changes in appetite may occur before the seizure. These prodromal symptoms are to be distinguished from the aura, which generally precedes the GTC by seconds or minutes.

The aura is a partial seizure, reflecting an abnormal focal electrical discharge from the brain, while the prodrome is not associated with epileptiform discharges. The physiologic basis of the prodrome has not been established.

The aura is useful in distinguishing between primary and secondary GTC seizures because it indicates that the seizure began focally and becomes secondarily generalized. Auras vary considerably from patient to patient and may encompass any of the manifestations of simple partial seizures, including focal motor, sensory, autonomic, or psychic symptoms.

The stereotyped nature of the motor activity in GTC seizures is dramatic and easily recognized. The most dramatic manifestations consist of the extension or tonic phase, which is characterized by sudden rigid extension of the arms and legs. As the thoracic and abdominal muscles contract, air is forced over the vocal cords, and this phenomenon may result in a cry. Apnea is possible at this time and may persist through the clonic phase. During the clonic phase, muscle relaxation is interspersed with tonic contractions. The alternating increase and decrease in muscle tone result in rhythmic jerks, which decrease in frequency as the seizure continues. Following the last clonic jerk, the bladder sphincter relaxes and incontinence may occur. The combination of a rigidly closed jaw and increased secretions during the seizure can lead to partial airway obstruction and results in noisy, labored respirations.

The duration and extent of the postictal impairment are related to the duration of the GTC seizure. The postictal sleep after GTC seizures is much more intense than that following CPSs.

Differential Diagnosis

GTC seizures are readily diagnosed and only rarely present the clinician with a difficult differential diagnosis. Pseudoseizures may resemble GTC seizures, although there are usually clinical features that may help the physician differentiate the two (Table 8–8). GTC seizures may also occur following breath-holding attacks. Long or complicated syncopal attacks may also occasionally resemble GTC seizures.

Electroencephalography

The interictal manifestations of GTC seizures are quite varied. The EEGs may be normal during both the awake and sleep states. Focal or multifocal paroxysmal activity is seen in the interictal EEG of 20% to 40% of patients with GTC seizures. This focal or multifocal paroxysmal activity may consist of spikes, sharp waves, or theta activity.

Etiology

GTC seizures may be secondary to acquired lesions (symptomatic) or may be idiopathic. Primary GTC seizures are usually idiopathic and have a strong genetic influence, whereas secondary GTC seizures usually have an acquired etiology. Primary GTC seizures are rare and it is likely that, with improving neurodiagnostic and neuropathologic capabilities, more patients will be demonstrated to have focal lesions.

TABLE 8-8. CRITERIA USEFUL FOR DIFFERENTIATING EPILEPTIC SEIZURES FROM PSEUDOSEIZURES

Clinical Data	Pseudoseizures	Generalized Tonic-Clonic Seizures
Changes in seizure frequency with medication change	Rare	Usual
Increased seizure frequency with stress	Frequently	Occasionally
Combativeness	Common	Rare
Vulgar language	Frequent	Rare
Self-injury	Rare	Common
Incontinence	Rare	Common
Tongue biting	Rare	Common
Nocturnal occurrence	Rare	Common
Stereotype of attacks	Often variable	Little variation
Postictal confusion, lethargy, or sleepiness	Rarely	Always
EEG		
Interictal	Often normal	Frequently abnormal
During attack	Normal	Always abormal

From Holmes (1987) with permission of the publisher.

Toxins, environmental stresses, or systemic diseases may result in primary GTC seizures. The most common identifiable stress in children is fever (Chapter 25). Systemic disorders such as hypoglycemia, uremia, hepatic failure, and hypoxia may result in primary GTC seizures.

Evaluation

The nature and extent of the evaluation of a patient with GTC seizures is dependent to a great extent on whether the GTC seizures are primary or secondary in type. It is therefore important for the physician to obtain a careful description of the seizures. An aura or focal onset indicates that the patient has secondary GTC seizures. A history of absence or myoclonic seizures is frequently obtained in primary GTC seizures, whereas partial seizures may occur in patients with secondary GTC seizures. Patients with primary GTC seizures often have a family history positive for absence or GTC seizures. Primary GTC seizures usually are associated with normal neurologic and developmental examinations, whereas patients with secondary GTC seizures are more likely to have abnormal neurologic examinations and intelligence.

If the patient is seen immediately following a GTC seizure, laboratory studies should include measurement of glucose, calcium, blood urea nitrogen, and electrolytes; liver function tests; CBC; and a toxin screen. If there is a possibility of meningitis or encephalitis a spinal tap is indicated. Patients with evidence of increased intracranial pressure should have an immediate CT scan.

Because primary GTC seizures are not associated with intracranial pathology, a CT scan is theoretically not necessary. However, the clinician can never be entirely certain that the seizure is generalized from onset rather than partial with secondary generalization. It is therefore recommended that all patients with unexplained GTC seizures receive a CT scan as part of their evaluation.

Treatment

The drugs of first choice in the treatment of GTC seizures are phenobarbital, primidone, phenytoin, carbamazepine, and valproic acid. The drugs have similar efficacy although carbamazepine is usually better tolerated than the other AEDs.

Patients with partial seizures that secondarily generalize and do not respond to AEDs may benefit from focal resections. If the patient has multifocal disease or has seizures in which a focal onset cannot be detected, a corpus callosotomy may offer some benefit.

No firm guidelines are available as to when to withdraw AEDs in patients with GTC seizures. As a general rule, I recommended that consideration be given to withdrawing antiepileptic drugs after the patient has been seizure free for 2 to 3 years.

ANNOTATED BIBLIOGRAPHY

Mattson RH, Cramer JA, Collins JF: Comparison of carbamazepine, phenobarbital, phenytoin, and primidone in partial and secondarily generalized tonic-clonic seizures. *N Engl J Med* 313:145–151, 1985.

Pearls and Perils: Generalized Tonic-Clonic Seizures

1. Most patients with GTC seizures have secondary generalized seizures, that is, the seizures have a partial onset and then become generalized.
2. Seizures in a given patient are generally stereotyped. In patients who are having a variety of symptoms with their attacks, pseudoseizures should be considered.

Forsythe WI, Sills MA: One drug for childhood grand mal: Medical audit for three-year remissions. *Dev Med Child Neurol* 26:742–748, 1984.

These two studies compared the effectiveness of the commonly used AEDs in the treatment of GTC seizures. That by Mattson and associates involved only adults.

ABSENCE SEIZURES

Absence seizures are probably the most frequently missed seizure disorders. Although absence seizures are not life threatening, it is still very important that the physician be able to detect these seizures, because, if they go undetected, the child may suffer a decline in school performance and possible self-injury. Fortunately, these seizures usually respond quite well to AEDs.

Classification

The term *petit mal* has been replaced in the classification of seizures by the term *absence seizures. Petit mal* is still used, however, by a large number of health workers and the lay public. Most physicians use *petit mal* to describe what are now considered typical absence seizures.

Clinical Characteristics

Absence seizures rarely begin before the age of 2 years or after the teenage years. The hallmark of the typical absence is the abrupt suppression of mental functions, usually to the point of complete abolition of awareness, responsiveness, and memory. The seizures are never preceded by an aura. Typical absences last from a few seconds to half a minute, although at times the seizures may last over a minute. Ongoing activity is interrupted; the patient changes facial expression and becomes transfixed like a statue. In a simple absence, the child has statue-like facies with a dull, motionless, distant appearance to the face. The child frequently returns to the gesture, sentence, or other interrupted activity at the end of the seizure. Postictal fatigue never occurs, although the chlid may be momentarily confused and disoriented owing to the "time loss." This time loss may serve as a clue to the child that a seizure occurred, even though there may be complete amnesia for events during the seizure.

At times, the suspension of mental function is less complete. This is particularly true for brief attacks (those lasting less than 5 seconds) and occasionally for longer attacks, which may consist of mild confusion without complete loss of contact. The child may be able to continue simple and automatic behavior during some seizures. At times, the impairment of consciousness is so slight that it is not perceptible by observers and may be detected only during refined psychologic tests of higher cortical functioning during EEG monitoring.

Although it is often assumed that simple absence seizures are common, in fact this is a rare seizure type. Penry and colleagues reviewed 374 recorded absence seizures from 48 patients and found simple absences, characterized by staring and cessation of activities, to constitute only 9.4% of the seizures. The absence seizures of the majority of patients had complex features, consisting of clonic or myoclonic activity, automatisms, and changes in postural tone.

Automatisms occur frequently in absence seizures. The automatic behavior is similar to that which occurs in CPSs, and may consist of licking the lips, chewing, grimacing, scratching, or fumbling with the clothes. However, much more complex activity may also occur, such as dealing playing cards, moving pieces in a game, and even playing patty-cake. There is almost always a slowing of the activity, although this may not be discernible to the casual observer. Speech may occur during absence seizures although it may slow or be slurred.

The frequency of absence seizures varies considerably from day to day and even hour to hour. In some patients the variable frequency appears to be related to stress and fatigue. Most untreated children with absence seizures have over 10 seizures a day and may have several hundred.

FEATURE TABLE 8–5. ABSENCE SEIZURES

Discriminating Features	Consistent Features	Variable Features
1. Unlike partial complex seizures, absence seizures are usually brief (under 10 seconds), have a clear onset and cessation, and have no aura or postictal period.	1. Impairment of consciousness.	1. Duration.
	2. Clear onset and cessation.	2. Automatisms.
	3. No aura or postictal period.	3. Changes in body tone.
2. When absence seizures are recorded during an EEG there is a generalized spike-wave discharge.		4. Autonomic dysfunction.
3. Absence seizures usually respond to ethosuximide or VPA.		

The majority of children with typical absence seizures have normal neurologic examinations and intelligence, although school performance may be impaired owing to the frequent seizures. GTC seizures occur in 40% to 60% of patients with typical absence seizures. Occasional children will also have myoclonic seizures. Typical absences are rarely associated with other seizure types except for GTC seizures.

Electroencephalography

In absence seizures, the EEG shows the sudden onset of either generalized symmetric spike or multiple spike–slow-wave complexes. In typical absence seizures, the spike-wave complexes usually occur at a frequency of 2.5 to 3.5 Hz while in atypical absences the frequency is usually less than 2.5 Hz.

Hyperventilation is a potent activator of typical absence seizures. Failure to induce an absence seizure with several trials of hyperventilation of 3 to 5 minutes' duration in an untreated patient would make the diagnosis of absence seizures unlikely. Photic stimulation may also induce absence seizures, although the likelihood of producing a seizure is not as high as with hyperventilation.

Atypical Absences

Atypical absences are those seizures in which the onset or cessation is not as abrupt as in typical absences and in which changes in tone are more pronounced than in typical absences. Atypical absences, like typical absences, may be associated with automatisms, clonic components, and autonomic components as well as changes in tone. However, automatisms are not as frequently seen in atypical absences as in typical absences. Atypical absence seizures frequently have a longer duration than typical absences, sometimes lasting several minutes.

Unlike the usual 3-Hz spike-wave discharges that occur in typical absence seizures, a slow spike-wave discharge occurring at a frequency of around 1.5 to 2.5 Hz is characteristic of atypical absence seizures. The interictal EEG is usually abnormal in patients with atypical absences. Many patients with atypical absences have the Lennox-Gastaut syndrome, which is discussed next.

Differential Diagnosis

Diagnosing absence seizures is relatively easy for the alert clinician. The differential diagnosis of staring attacks includes CPSs and daydreaming as well as absence seizures. Table 8–6 summarizes factors that can be used to differentiate the three disorders. Absence seizures can be confirmed by having the patient hyperventilate for 3 to 5 minutes. In the untreated child, failure to induce an absence seizure with hyperventilation should serve to alert the physician that the patient is unlikely to have absence seizures. The routine EEG obtained during hyperventilation, photic stimulation, and sleep is useful in substantiating the diagnosis. Although a normal EEG

does not rule out the possibility that the child has absence seizures, the likelihood that frequent absence seizures are occurring is slim. If a clinical suspicion remains, the child may require repeated EEGs or prolonged EEG monitoring.

Etiology

A diverse group of etiologic factors has been associated with absence seizures. Although there has been a long-standing debate about whether absence seizures represent an "acquired" or a "genetic" condition, there is now evidence that in many cases both factors may be responsible.

Depending on the particular patient population evaluated, there are varying frequencies of proven or suspected etiologies for absence seizures. Dalby (1969) determined an etiology in only 14% of the patients in a series of 346 patients with generalized spike-wave on the EEG. Patients with atypical absences have a much higher percentage of etiologic factors identified.

Genetics

Metrakos and Metrakos (1961) studied families of 211 probands with absence and/or GTC seizures and generalized spike-wave of their EEGs. In the probands, generalized spike-wave was seen in 37% of the siblings' EEGs, as opposed to 9% in the control group. The generalized spike-wave activity trait was age dependent. It was not present at birth but occurred in 45% of the siblings between the ages of $4\frac{1}{2}$ and $16\frac{1}{2}$ years. In older siblings the trait disappeared. It has been suggested that the EEG abnormality is the expression of an autosomal dominant gene with the unusual characteristic of a very low penetrance at birth, which increases rapidly to nearly complete penetrance during early childhood and the teenage years before decreasing rapidly. Other investigators have found a high rate of GTC seizures in other family members of children with absence seizures but argue that the mode of inheritance is not by an autosomal dominant pattern but rather is due to multiple genetic factors.

Evaluation

In patients who have typical absence seizures, an EEG with 3-Hz spike-wave activity, normal interictal EEGs, and normal neurologic examinations and intelligence, no further diagnostic studies are necessary. In patients with abnormal developmental histories, abnormal neurologic findings, or evidence on the EEG of a focal disease process, a CT scan is recommended. Although a treatable lesion is unlikely, the CT scan may give helpful information regarding etiology and prognosis.

Because absence seizures are brief and frequently subtle, their frequency can be grossly underestimated by parents. Each follow-up evaluation by the physician should include 3 to 5 minutes of hyperventilation. Ac-

---

Pearls and Perils: Absence Seizures

1. One of the best ways to determine if a child's absence seizures are controlled is to have the child hyperventilate for 3 to 5 minutes. Failure to induce an absence seizure indicates that the child's seizures are under satisfactory control.
2. Most patients that stare do not have seizures. Staring as the sole manifestation of absence seizures is unusual. Most children have other clinical changes during the seizure, such as eye blinking or clonic jerks of the arms.

---

tivation of a seizure by hyperventilation would indicate that the patient is probably continuing to have seizures, regardless of the history supplied by the patient and parents.

Treatment

The aim of AED therapy in typical absence seizures is to treat with a medication that reduces seizure frequency without producing drug toxicity. Care should be taken to avoid toxicity, which may make the treatment regimen worse than the seizures. The physician should aim for maximum seizure control with minimum toxicity.

Clonazepam, ethosuximide, and VPA are all useful in the treatment of absence seizures. An untreated child starting on any one of these three drugs will have greater than a 70% chance of having a significant reduction or total elimination of seizures. Ethosuximide is currently regarded by many neurologists as the drug of choice for the treatment of absence seizures. Comparison studies of ethosuximide and VPA demonstrated that both drugs are equally effective in controlling absence seizures. However, because of instances of severe and occasionally fatal hepatotoxicity and pancreatitis in patients taking VPA, this drug has been reserved for patients who do not respond to ethosuximide or who have side effects from it. VPA, however, should be considered the drug of choice in the patient who has both absence and GTC seizures. It appears to be as effective as phenytoin in the treatment of GTC seizures. Because of the relatively high incidence of adverse side effects, clonazepam is usually not used initially in absence seizures, although it is often used in refractory cases.

Patients who do not respond to either ethosuximide or VPA as a single agent may respond to the combination of the two drugs. This is one of the rare situations in the treatment of epilepsy in which two drugs may work better than one. As with other drug combinations, the patient should be watched closely for signs of toxicity.

There are no firm rules regarding when to withdraw medications. Although typical absence seizures have a favorable prognosis, the time when children go into remission is variable. Although it is often stated that children "outgrow" their seizures at puberty, this frequently is not true because some children do not go into remission until years after puberty. A general rule, therefore, is to withdraw AEDs slowly after the patient has been seizure free for 2 years and no longer has generalized spike-wave discharges on the EEG. Although the goal is to treat the patient rather than the EEG, spike-wave discharges on the routine EEG would be indicative of a high recurrence risk if medication were withdrawn.

ANNOTATED BIBLIOGRAPHY

Penry JK, Porter RJ, Dreifuss FE: Simultaneous recording of absence seizures with videotape and electroencephalography. A study of 374 seizures in 48 patients. *Brain* 98:427–440, 1975.

In this study the clinical features of absence seizures were studied using EEG and video monitoring.

Brown TR, Penry JK, Porter RJ, et al: Responsiveness before, during, and after spike-wave paroxysms. *Neurology* 24:659–665, 1974.

Porter RJ, Penry JK, Dreifuss FE: Responsiveness at the onset of spike-wave bursts. *Electroencephalogr Clin Neurophysiol* 34:239–245, 1973.

These two studies demonstrate that there may be impairment of function at the onset of spike-wave discharges. For practical purposes, absence seizures and spike-wave discharges on the EEG can be assumed to be overlapping phenomena.

Holmes GL, McKeever M, Adamson M: Absence seizures in children: Clinical and electroencephalographic features. *Ann Neurol* 21:268–273, 1987.

A review of typical and atypical absence seizures in children. The authors point out that the seizure types are not discrete entities but rather form a continuum.

LENNOX-GASTAUT SYNDROME

The Lennox-Gastaut syndrome presents one of the most difficult challenges to the physician dealing with children with seizures. The patients usually have very frequent, medically intractable seizures. In addition to the frequent seizures the children are usually, and often profoundly, retarded.

Classification

The Lennox-Gastaut syndrome can be operationally defined as having the following three characteristics: (1) a slow spike-wave EEG pattern during a portion of the awake EEG, (2) mental retardation, and (3) intractable seizures of various types. It should be noted that some authors do not require mental retardation to be a component of the syndrome.

Clinical Characteristics

The onset of seizures in the syndrome usually occurs between the ages of 1 and 6 years. Although a later age of

FEATURE TABLE 8-6. LENNOX-GASTAUT SYNDROME

Discriminating Feature	Consistent Features	Variable Features
1. Usually no difficulty in making diagnosis when the three consistent features are present.	1. Severe, mixed seizure disorder. 2. Mental retardation. 3. Slow spike-and-wave discharges on EEG.	1. Types of seizures (although usually consist of tonic, myoclonic, atypical absence, and generalized tonic-clonic). 2. Frequency of seizures. 3. Symptomatic or idiopathic etiology.

onset has been reported occasionally, it is unusual for seizures to begin after the age of 10 years. However, as the child matures the type of seizure may change in clinical characteristics.

The child with Lennox-Gastaut syndrome manifests a variety of seizure types. The most frequently occurring are tonic, atypical absences, tonic-clonic, and "head drops," which are either atonic, tonic, or myoclonic seizures.

Tonic seizures are very common in Lennox-Gastaut syndrome. These seizures consist of periods of tonic contraction of muscle groups and are accompanied by altered consciousness. Tonic seizures are especially common during sleep. The period of impaired consciousness during tonic seizures has an average duration of around 10 seconds and ranges from a few seconds to a minute. Postictal impairment, if present, is usually brief.

Atonic (astatic) seizures or drop attacks begin suddenly, without warning, and cause the patient, if standing, to fall quickly to the floor. Because there may be total loss of tone, the child has no means to protect himself or herself and head and facial injury often occur. In addition, a warning aura does not occur prior to the loss of tone. Although consciousness is momentarily impaired during the fall, the patient may regain alertness immediately on hitting the floor. If the patient is seated or standing, a fall forward can cause injury to the face. Children with uncontrolled atonic seizures often need to wear protective head and face gear. Atonic attacks are frequently associated with myoclonic jerks before the atonic seizure and are termed myoclonic-astatic seizures. Rather than always involving the entire body, the loss of tone may affect only the head. The resulting head drop can occur singly or in a series of head nods. Like body atonic seizures, the period of impaired consciousness is extremely brief and postictal impairment is rarely present.

Myoclonic jerks are sudden, extremely brief (under 1 second), shock-like contractions, which may be generalized or confined to the face and trunk or one or more extremities. When the entire body is involved, the sudden jerks may throw the patient to the floor and lead to significant injuries. When confined to the upper trunk, the movements are characterized by a head drop with associated arm extension. There is no postictal impairment. At times it may be difficult to differentiate myoclonic seizures from tonic and atonic seizures. In these cases, simultaneous EEG and electromyographic (EMG) monitoring is necessary. Decreased muscle activity occurs with atonic seizures, whereas increased EMG activity is seen with myoclonic seizures. Myoclonic seizures last less than 1 second; tonic seizures typically last at least 2 to 3 seconds. Myoclonic seizures may occur in isolation or as a component of an absence or atonic seizure.

Atypical absences occur in approximately half of the patients with the Lennox-Gastaut syndrome. As noted in the section on absence seizures, atypical absences are those seizures in which the onset or cessation is not as abrupt as in typical absences and in which changes in tone are more pronounced than in typical absences. Atypical absences, like typical absences, are frequently associated with clonic components, automatisms, and autonomic components as well as changes in tone. Prolonged absence seizures are characteristic of the Lennox-Gastaut syndrome. During these prolonged seizures, the child has a dull look on his or her face, drools, appears confused and disoriented, and is unable to perform skills of daily living. It is often difficult to tell when a given seizure actually begins and ends, because improvement in alertness and activity level may be minimal between the absences.

GTC seizures also occur frequently in the Lennox-Gastaut syndrome: 60% to 70% of the patients experience these seizures, which often occur at night, particularly around the time of going to sleep or awakening.

Patients with Lennox-Gastaut syndrome typically have very frequent seizures. Markand found that 60% of his patients had daily seizures while Papini and colleagues (1984), in a longitudinal study of 16 patients, found the mean daily frequency of seizures to range from 9 to 70. Some children with this syndrome have hundreds of seizures daily.

Seizure frequency may vary from day to day or even during the course of a day. Seizure frequency appears highest during drowsiness and inactivity. In addition, in many patients there is a weekly or monthly increase in seizure frequency unrelated to AED therapy. Periods of prolonged repetitive seizures of a mixed type are interspersed with periods of relative freedom from attacks. During the times when the child is seizure free, marked improvements in alertness, motivation, and academic progress can be seen. Unfortunately these periods are usually short, lasting only days to weeks. This feature of the syndrome leads to significant frustration for the child, parents, teachers, and medical professionals.

While some authors do not require mental retardation to be a component of the Lennox-Gastaut syndrome, all series report a very high incidence of mental retardation in this syndrome. Neurologic abnormalities have been reported in 40% to 88% of patients with the Lennox-Gastaut syndrome. In the series of patients reported by Markand, nearly 60% had definite motor signs, including quadriparesis, hemiparesis, paraparesis, monoparesis, or spasticity.

Electroencephalography

The characteristic EEG finding in the Lennox-Gastaut syndrome is the slow spike-wave discharge. The slow spike-wave or sharp and slow wave complexes consist of generalized discharges occurring at a frequency of 1.5 to 2.5 Hz. Typically, these discharges occur in long runs during the awake state. Although hyperventilation and photic stimulation do not activate these discharges, sleep increases their frequency.

The syndrome may arise in a previously well child or supervene in an already neurologically or mentally handicapped patient. The etiology of the Lennox-Gastaut syndrome has, therefore, been divided into primary and secondary cases. Primary refers to cases in which the etiology is idiopathic; secondary refers to cases where the syndrome is symptomatic of a definable etiology.

The majority of patients with Lennox-Gastaut syndrome with an established etiology have a static disorder. Rarely, degenerative disorders, such as ceroid lipofuscinosis, have presented as Lennox-Gastaut syndrome.

Evaluation

After making the diagnosis of Lennox-Gastaut syndrome, the physician should try to determine an etiology for the condition. In a number of children the etiology will be suggested from the medical history. In these cases no further workup is necessary. For example, the child with infantile spasms secondary to perinatal asphyxia who progresses into the Lennox-Gastaut syndrome does not need an extensive workup. However, the patient without a revealing medical history must be thoroughly evaluated.

Diagnostic studies ordered will be dependent on find-ings from the history and physical examination. In view of the devastating nature of the syndrome, every effort should be made to rule out any treatable disorders. Abnormalities on CT or MRI scans are common in Lennox-Gastaut syndrome. Of children with the syndrome, 80% were noted to have abnormal CT scans by Lagenstein and associates (1980). The most frequent abnormality associated with the syndrome is cortical or subcortical atrophy.

Treatment

Treatment of the child with Lennox-Gastaut syndrome is one of the more arduous tasks facing the physician. Because the syndrome is not heterogeneous, there is some variability in how children will respond to an antiepileptic regimen. Drug therapy should be individualized and standardized "cookbook" approaches to these children are not possible.

Because of the intractable nature of the seizures, there is a tendency to place the children on AED polytherapy. This approach usually results in children who are drug toxic and rarely in good seizure control. Combination drug therapy frequently results in additive effects of toxicity without any improvement in seizure control.

Prognosis

The poor prognosis in this syndrome has been reported by numerous authors. Although the natural course of the disorder is a decreasing frequency of atonic, myoclonic, and atypical absence seizures with increasing age, often there is an increase in GTC seizures and an emergence of partial seizures.

In addition, patients are often hindered in their attempt to lead independent lives because of intellectual impairment. Some patients have a progressive deterioration in mental function even though vigorous attempts have been made to control the seizures.

ANNOTATED BIBLIOGRAPHY

Blume WT, David RB, Gomez MR: Generalized sharp and slow wave complexes. Associated clinical features and long-term follow-up. *Brain* 96:289–306, 1973.

This is an excellent paper reviewing the clinical features of slow spike-wave discharges. The authors note the high incidence of mental retardation and the wide variety of seizures seen with this EEG pattern.

Markand ON: Slow spike-wave activity in EEG and associated clinical features: Often called "Lennox" or "Lennox-Gastaut" syndrome. *Neurology* 27:746–757, 1977.

Kurokara T, Goya N, Fukayama Y, et al: West syndrome and Lennox-Gastaut syndrome: A survey of natural history. *Pediatrics* 65:81–88, 1980.

These are two large series reviewing the clinical and EEG findings in Lennox-Gastaut syndrome.

Pearls and Perils:
Lennox-Gastaut Syndrome

1. Total seizure control in these patients is unlikely. Avoid the temptation to place the patient on multiple AEDs. Usually one or two drugs work better than three or four.

MYOCLONIC SEIZURES

Myoclonic jerks are sudden, brief, involuntary, lightning-like movements that are not associated with any obvious disturbance of consciousness. These brief involuntary contractions may affect one or several muscles. No common etiologic, anatomic, or physiologic features bind all types of myoclonus together. The condition has been reported in association with lesions of the cortex, cerebellum, brainstem, and spinal cord.

Multiple etiologic agents can lead to myoclonus. Myoclonic movements may be totally normal phenomena, such as hypnic jerks or sleep starts. Conversely, myoclonus may be associated with virtually any severe insult to the brain, whether toxic, metabolic, infectious, traumatic, or degenerative. Likewise, the pathophysiology of myoclonus varies. Some types of myoclonus are nonepileptic and are classified as movement disorders, similar to chorea, tics, athetosis, or tremors, whereas other types of myoclonus are epileptic phenomena.

Differential Diagnosis

Myoclonus may at times be difficult to differentiate from other movement disorders, including tics, chorea, and tremors. In children, tics consist of complex movements such as facial grimacing, eye blinking or rolling, head nodding or turning, and shrugging of the shoulders. Unlike myoclonus, tics can usually be suppressed, at least temporarily, by an effort of will. In chorea, movements are irregular and unpredictable and usually involve multiple muscle groups, whereas myoclonus is usually characterized by repetitive, stereotyped movements affecting the same muscle groups. Although at times the myoclonic jerks are irregular and less predictable, they do not have the characteristic continuous flow of movements that is so distinctive of chorea. When myoclonic jerks occur in a flurry, the movements may be confused with tremors. However, tremors can usually be differentiated from myoclonus by the smooth to-and-fro movements. Myoclonus is more abrupt and has a distinct interval between movements.

Classification

Table 8–9 is a classification of myoclonus that I have found helpful. The classification is based on both etiology and pathophysiology. Physiologically, myoclonus can be broadly divided into nonepileptic and epileptic types. The spectrum of nonepileptic myoclonus varies from normal physiologic events to severe disabling movements involving single or multiple muscle groups. Epileptic myoclonus may be either symptomatic or primary. In symptomatic cases, the myoclonus is secondary to a static insult or active disease process. In these cases, the myoclonus is usually only one of many neurologic symptoms. In

TABLE 8-9. CLASSIFICATION OF MYOCLONUS

I. **Nonepileptic myoclonus**
   A. Physiologic myoclonus
      1. Sleep starts
      2. Benign awake myoclonus
   B. Pathophysiologic myoclonus
      1. Hyperexplexia (startle disease)
      2. Shuddering attacks
      3. Periodic movements of sleep (sleep myoclonus)
      4. Restless leg syndrome
      5. Benign neonatal sleep myoclonus
      6. Benign myoclonus of early infancy
   C. Benign familial polymyoclonus
   D. Segmental myoclonus
      1. Brainstem
         a. Opsoclonus
         b. Palatal myoclonus
      2. Spinal cord

II. **Symptomatic epileptic myoclonus**
   A. Infections
      1. Subacute sclerosing panencephalitis
      2. Jakob-Creutzfeldt disease
      3. Encephalitis
   B. Congenital brain anomalies
   C. Toxins
   D. Systemic diseases
      1. Uremia
      2. Hepatic insufficiency
      3. Others
   E. Postanoxic
   F. Component of familial progressive neurologic disease
      1. Progressive myoclonic epilepsy with Lafora's bodies
      2. Progressive myoclonic epilepsy without Lafora's bodies
      3. Dyssnergia cerebellaris myoclonia (Ramsay-Hunt)
   G. Metabolic disorders
      1. Ceroid lipofuscinosis
      2. Juvenile form of Gaucher's disease
      3. Sialidosis (cherry-red spot–myoclonus syndrome)
      4. Gangliosidoses, including GM_2, GM_1
      5. Mitochondrial syndromes
         a. Myoclonus and ragged red fibers
         b. Mitochondrial myopathy, encephalopathy, lactic acidosis, and stroke-like episodes

III. **Primary epileptic myoclonus**
   A. Generalized epileptic myoclonus of early childhood
      1. Symptomatic myoclonic epilepsy
      2. Cryptogenic myoclonic epilepsy
   B. Juvenile myoclonic epilepsy of Janz
   C. Epilepsia partialis continua
   D. Focal cortical myoclonus
   E. As component of other seizure types
      1. Absence with myoclonic component
      2. Eyelid myoclonic seizures with absences
      3. Component of generalized tonic-clonic seizures
      4. Centrencephalic myoclonic-astatic absence
      5. Lennox-Gastaut syndrome

From Holmes (1987) with permission of the publisher.

primary epileptic myoclonus, the myoclonic seizures constitute the primary abnormality and the etiology is either familiar or idiopathic. Although this classification system is helpful in organizing myoclonus, some overlapping be-

FEATURE TABLE 8-7. MYOCLONIC SEIZURES

Discriminating Features	Consistent Features	Variable Features
1. May be confused with atonic seizures. EMG monitoring during seizure demonstrates increased EMG activity during myoclonic seizure and decreased EMG activity during atonic seizure. 2. May respond to VPA or clonazepam.	1. Very brief. 2. Sudden onset without aura or postictal impairment.	1. Distribution of muscle groups involved. 2. Frequency during day. 3. Severity varies greatly. Some myoclonic seizures are subtle and barely recognized by observer, while others may cause patient to fall to ground. 4. Association with structural brain lesions.

tween categories occurs. For example, although infantile spasms and Lennox-Gastaut syndrome are categorized under primary epileptic myoclonus, in some patients etiologic agents can be identified.

Etiology of Myoclonus

Nonepileptic Myoclonus

Physiologic myoclonus consists of phenomena that occur in normal children and adults. For example, "sleep starts" represent a form of physiologic myoclonus. These hypnic jerks are irregular movements, occur at sleep onset or awakening, and simultaneously involve the muscles of the trunk and extremities. This type of myoclonus is a normal physiologic response. In some infants and toddlers, however, the myoclonus can be quite striking. These movements are not associated with EEG abnormalities. In addition, many normal children will have an occasional, isolated, myoclonic jerk during the awake state.

Epileptic Myoclonus

Epileptic myoclonus may be secondary to a large number of entities. As a general rule, epileptic myoclonus is associated with severe central nervous system disorders. Epileptic myoclonus may occur in slow viral infections such as subacute sclerosing panencephalitis, following severe hypoxic-ischemic injuries, in severe metabolic abnormalities such as hepatic encephalopathy, as a component of a congenital brain anomaly such as porencephaly or hydranencephaly, as a feature of degenerative disorders such as ceroid lipofuscinosis, or as a familial disorder such as encephalitis with Lafora's bodies. Although space limitations prohibit a discussion of these disorders, one familial disorder, benign juvenile myoclonic epilepsy, occurs commonly in children and will be discussed separately. The interested reader should refer to the textbook by Holmes (1987) for a more detailed discussion of the etiologic factors associated with myoclonus.

Evaluation

Because of the diverse etiologies that can result in myoclonus, it is necessary to individualize the workup of each patient. The most important part of the initial evaluation of the patient with myoclonus is the history. In most patients the diagnosis can be surmised after a detailed history.

The history should include a detailed history of the pregnancy, labor and delivery, and perinatal periods; motor and mental development; and exposure to drugs, chemicals, and infectious diseases. A detailed family history is necessary because this may be a major clue to the diagnosis of the familial disorders.

Treatment

Myoclonic seizures are often difficult to treat. Although many AEDs have been used in the treatment of myoclonic seizures, only a few have been demonstrated to be effective. The current drugs of choice in the treatment of the myoclonic epilepsies are the benzodiazepines (clonazepam and Valium) and VPA. The ketogenic diet, adrenocorticotropic hormone (ACTH), and adrenal corticosteroids may also be effective in the treatment of these seizures, although they should be reserved for children with seizures refractory to the benzodiazepines and VPA. Myoclonic seizures are usually refractory to phenytoin, barbiturates, and carbamazepine.

Approximately 75% of patients with myoclonic seizures will improve on VPA, usually with no changes in alertness or behavior. The benzodiazepines, the ketogenic diet, and ACTH are sometimes effective in the treatment of myoclonic seizures.

Juvenile Myoclonic Epilepsy of Janz

Myoclonic seizures in children may occur as a component of juvenile myoclonic epilepsy of Janz (benign juvenile myoclonic epilepsy). The myoclonic seizures are usually mild to moderate in intensity and usually involve the neck and upper extremities. They may occur either singularly or in brief paroxysmal bursts and may cause the patient to drop or spill objects. Rarely are they severe enough to fling the patient to the ground. More commonly they are quite mild and the patient may pay little attention to them or attribute them to nervousness or clumsiness. Although the myoclonic seizures usually are most frequent after awakening from a night's sleep or nap, in some patients they may continue all day. The seizures are typically aggravated by sleep deprivation. Myoclonic status, a state in which the patient has myoclonic jerks every few seconds or in salvos of three to five jerks, may occur. Although consciousness is preserved, the patient is often incapacitated by the continuous myoclonic jerks.

In the vast majority of patients with this syndrome, tonic-clonic or clonic-tonic-clonic seizures occur. Like the myoclonic seizures, these seizures often occur shortly after awakening or during early-morning sleep. At times, patients have a series of myoclonic seizures, culminating in a GTC seizure. A significant number of patients will also have absence seizures. As with the myoclonic and tonic-clonic seizures, these usually occur on awakening.

Benign myoclonic epilepsy begins in the second decade in most patients. The average age of seizure onset was 13.6 years, with a range of 8 to 24 years, in a series of 43 patients studied by Delgado-Escueta and Enrile-Bascale (1984). The general physical and neurologic examinations and intelligence in these patients are usually normal. A positive family history of epilepsy is commonly obtained and the mode of inheritance appears to be polygenic, with females having a lower threshold than males.

The interictal EEG in this disorder is easily distinguished from that in other forms of generalized epilepsies. The characteristic features of the EEG are the fast (3.5- to 6-Hz) spike-wave or multiple spike-wave complexes, which contrast with the 3-Hz spike-wave complexes seen in classic absence seizures and the slow (1.5- to 2.5-Hz) spike-wave complexes of the Lennox-Gastaut syndrome. Photosensitivity may activate the epileptiform discharges. If the awake EEG is normal, a sleep-deprived EEG must be obtained because this may be the only time the abnormality is present.

VPA therapy is the treatment of choice in this disorder. In the series of 43 patients reported by Delgado-

Escueta and Enrile-Bascal, 86% were either seizure free or satisfactorily controlled either on VPA alone or on VPA with other AEDs. Asconape and Penry found that 73% of their patients had either complete control or a marked reduction in seizure frequency with VPA monotherapy.

Although seizures in patients with juvenile myoclonic epilepsy of Janz may be easily controlled with VPA, the treatment of the disorder is long-term. Attempts to withdraw the drug are usually not successful. Only rarely do the seizures remit spontaneously, and 90% of patients relapse after withdrawal of AEDs.

ANNOTATED BIBLIOGRAPHY

Asconape J, Penry JK: Some clinical and EEG aspects of benign juvenile myoclonic epilepsy. *Epilepsia* 25:108–114, 1984.
Delgado-Escueta AV, Enrile-Bascal FE: Juvenile myoclonic epilepsy of Janz. *Neurology* 34:285–294, 1984.

These are two articles that deal with juvenile myoclonic epilepsy of Janz. Clinical features, including associated seizure types, and EEG findings are reviewed.

INFANTILE SPASMS

Infantile spasms constitute an unusual seizure disorder that is confined to early childhood. Myoclonic seizures, hypsarrhythmic electroencephalograms, and mental retardation are characteristic features of the syndrome, and make up a triad sometimes referred to as West's syndrome. As will be seen, however, not all children with infantile spasms conform strictly to this definition. Other terms used for infantile spasms in the literature include massive spasms, salaam seizures, flexion spasms, jackknife seizures, massive myoclonic jerks, infantile myoclonic seizures, and, in the German literature, *Blitz-Nick-Salaam Krampfe*.

Infantile spasms are age specific with the disorder beginning during the first 2 years of life. The peak age of onset is between 4 and 6 months of age and approximately 90% of infantile spasms begin before 12 months of age. Infantile spasms rarely begin during the first 2 weeks of life or after 18 months.

Clinical Characteristics

Infantile spasms may vary considerably in their clinical manifestations. Some seizures are characterized by brief head nods whereas other seizures consist of violent flexion of the trunk, arms, and legs. The diagnosis may be delayed because the parents and even the family physician may not recognize spasms as seizures.

Infantile spasms may be classified into three major groups: flexor, extensor, and mixed flexor-extensor types. Flexor spasms consist of the neck, trunk, arms, and legs.

FEATURE TABLE 8-8. INFANTILE SPASMS

Discriminating Features	Consistent Features	Variable Feature
1. The clustering of spasms differentiates these from myoclonic or tonic spasms. 2. The EEG pattern usually demonstrates hypsarrhythmia or modified hypsarrhythmia. 3. Infantile spasms usually respond to treatment with ACTH.	1. Begin before the age of 2 years. 2. Seizures are brief, lasting less than 5 seconds.	1. Clinical spasms may be flex- or, extensor, or, most commonly, mixed.

Spasms of the muscles of the upper limbs result either in adduction of the arms in a self-hugging motion or in adduction of the arms to either side of the head with the arms flexed at the elbow. Extensor spasms consist of a predominance of extensor muscle contractions producing abrupt extension of the neck and trunk with extensor abduction or adduction of the arms, legs, or both. Mixed flexor-extensor spasms include flexion of the neck, trunk, and arms and extension of the legs or flexion of the legs and extension of the arms with varying degrees of flexion of the neck and trunk. Asymmetric spasms occasionally occur and consist of maintenance of a "fencing" posture. Infantile spasms are frequently associated with eye deviation or nystagmus.

Infantile spasms frequently occur in clusters. The intensity and frequency of the spasms in each cluster may increase to a peak before progressively decreasing. The seizures are very brief and are frequently overlooked. The number of clusters per day and seizures per cluster varies considerably. Some children have as many as 60 clusters per day. Clusters may occur during sleep or shortly after awakening.

Differential Diagnosis

The biggest error in the diagnosis of infantile spasms is not considering the possibility and diagnosing the spasms as bouts of colic or other nonepileptic phenomena. Occasionally, the clinical course will be atypical and the spasms will not occur in clusters or involve only slight movements or episodes of akinesia. In these patients the EEG will be useful, because in children with infantile spasms the EEG is invariably abnormal.

The one disorder that may be confused with infantile spasms is benign myoclonus of early infancy. In this disorder infants have clusters of tonic or myoclonic movements. The movements consist of rapid flexion and/or extension of either axial or limb musculature. Unlike those with infantile spasms, however, the infants are normal neurologically and developmentally and have normal EEGs. In all cases, the movements stop by age 18 months.

Electroencephalography

Infantile spasms are associated with markedly abnormal EEGs. The most commonly seen pattern is a hypsarrhythmic EEG one, consisting of very-high-voltage, random, slow waves and multifocal spikes in all cortical areas. The chaotic appearance of the EEG abnormality gives the impression of a nearly total disorganization of cortical voltage and regulation. Variations of this pattern have been described as modified hypsarrhythmia. Although a hypsarrhythmic or modified hypsarrhythmic EEG is the most common type of interictal abnormality seen in infantile spasm, these patterns may be absent in some children with infantile spasms. Some patients with infantile spasms do not have hypsarrhythmic EEGs early in the course but go on to develop this pattern. Although hypsarrhythmia is primarily associated with infantile spasms, it may occur in children with other disorders as well.

Etiology

Infantile spasms have been conventionally classified into those in which there is no apparent preceding neurologic disorder or identified etiologic factor (idiopathic) and those in which a preexisting presumptively responsible pathologic event or disorder is demonstrated (symptomatic cases).

Several disorders have been associated with infantile spasms. Common etiologic factors include hypoxic-ischemic encephalopathies, neonatal intracranial hemorrhages, congenital infections, encephalitis, meningitis, congenital abnormalities of the central nervous system, and metabolic diseases such as phenylketonuria.

Tuberous sclerosis is associated with a high incidence of infantile spasms. In three large series of cases of patients with tuberous sclerosis, 42% had a history of infantile spasms. Conversely, in reports of cases of infantile spasms, the frequency of patients with tuberous sclerosis has varied from 4% to 25%. Tuberous sclerosis may be overlooked during the first year of life because the characteristic skin lesion, adenoma sebaceum, is not present before the age of 3 years. However, infants may have hypopigmented areas on the skin, which can be seen well by using a Wood's lamp. Supporting evidence for the disorder may come from a CT scan, which may demonstrate intracranial calcifications; abdominal ultrasound, which may detect polycystic kidneys; or an echocardiogram, which may demonstrate cardiac tumors.

A controversy exists as to whether immunizations can cause infantile spasms. This argument has not only significant medical implications but also legal ones. Infantile spasms have been reported following immunization with several vaccines, including those for smallpox, influenza, Japanese encephalitis, and pertussis. However, most of the reports of the association of vaccines with infantile spasms have been based on anecdotal reports. The diphtheria-pertussis-tetanus vaccine has been the vaccine most frequently implicated. Of the three agents, pertussis has raised the most concern.

There are major problems in proving or disproving whether the pertussis vaccine results in infantile spasms. The time of peak incidence of infantile spasms corresponds to the time that the vaccine is given. A temporal coincidence would therefore be expected in a large number of cases. Yet because the onset of infantile spasms is often insidious it is difficult to determine the exact time of onset.

It remains possible that in a small number of patients, especially in cases in which a striking neurologic reaction occurs within 24 hours after the immunization, a causal relation exists. It may be possible that in some cases the vaccine acts in conjunction with other unidentified factors to precipitate infantile spasms in children already predisposed to the disease.

It is not known why some children develop infantile spasms. The fact that some infants have infantile spasms while other infants with similar brain disturbances do not develop then suggests that genetic factors may be important.

Evaluation

The infant who presents with infantile spasms requires a thorough evaluation, which includes a developmental assessment, neurologic examination, and laboratory studies to try to determine an etiology. In addition, the neurologic and developmental examinations at the time of diagnosis are important indicators of prognosis.

The skin should be closely inspected for hypopigmented lesions, which can occur in tuberous sclerosis. As noted previously, these lesions may be better seen using a Wood's lamp in a darkened room.

The laboratory studies to be ordered will be determined to a significant degree by the clinical history and physical examination Every child with a possible diagnosis of infantile spasms should have an EEG and a CT scan. A normal EEG would raise serious questions

about the diagnosis and suggest that the child instead has benign myoclonus of early infancy.

A CT or MRI scan is recommended because it may provide valuable information regarding the etiology. Abnormal CT scans occur in 70% to 80% of patients with infantile spasms. The most common abnormality on CT scan seen in large series has been diffuse cerebral atrophy. In addition, cranial calcifications may indicate tuberous sclerosis or a congenital infection. Brain anomalies such as agenesis of the corpus callosum, porencephaly, and hydranencephaly will also be apparent on the CT scan.

Prognosis for neurodevelopmental outcome and seizure control has also been related to CT scan results. Singer and associates (1982) reported that no children with infantile spasms with abnormal CT scans were normal in follow-up.

Because pyridoxine dependency has been associated with infantile spasms, in children in whom an etiology cannot be definitely established an infusion of 100 mg pyridoxine intravenously during EEG monitoring is indicated. Infants with pyridoxine dependency should have rapid improvement in their seizures and EEG. Infants with frequent vomiting, lethargy, failure to thrive, peculiar odors, and unexplained neurologic findings should have urine amino acid screening, serum ammonia measurements, and liver function tests. Because most children will be placed on ACTH, levels of electrolytes, calcium, phosphorus, and glucose should be obtained and a urine analysis performed. Examination of the cerebrospinal fluid is not usually necessary unless there is concern about an active infection.

Treatment

ACTH and corticosteroids are the effective drugs in the treatment of infantile spasms. No other drugs have been documented to be more effective, although a minority of infants respond to drugs such as clonazepam, nitrazepam, and sodium valproate. Although ACTH is currently the most frequently used drug in the treatment of infantile spasms, corticosteroids, such as hydrocortisone, prednisone/prednisolone, and dexamethasone, have been used.

Although ACTH and corticosteroids clearly decrease seizure frequency, their effect on long-term outcome re-

---

Pearls and Perils: Infantile Spasms

1. The majority of patients with infantile spasms who respond to ACTH will do so within several weeks.
2. Infantile spasms are often incorrectly diagnosed by primary care physicians as colic. A careful history should easily distinguish the two.

mains controversial. Several authors have found no developmental differences between patients who did or did not receive treatment. For the majority of infants who exhibit preexisting brain damage, it is unlikely that any form of therapy would greatly improve the long-range outcome in terms of mental and motor development. The important question is whether the type of treatment for infantile spasms can alter the outcome in children who were developmentally and intellectually normal before the onset of the spasms or in whom the cause of the spasms is cryptogenic. Lombroso did long-term assessments on infants with cryptogenic infantile spasms who received either ACTH, oral steroids, or other AEDs. He reported that the group that received ACTH had a lower incidence of seizures and better psychomotor development than infants treated with oral steroids or other agents.

There is some controversy in the literature as to whether the duration of the interval between the onset of infantile spasms and the initiation of ACTH or corticosteroids is a factor in determining outcome. Although no definite conclusions can be reached, it is recommended that ACTH or corticosteroids be started as soon as possible following the diagnosis.

The dosage and length of time for which a child should be treated with ACTH or corticosteroids has not been established. I recommend a starting dose of nonsynthetic ACTH of 60 IU per day given intramuscularly. The ACTH is given for a minimum of 1 month following the cessation of seizures. At that time it can begin to be tapered by 10 IU per week. If the seizures do not completely resolve after 2 weeks, the dose should be increased by 10 IU every week until the seizures cease or a maximum dose of 80 IU every day is reached. If at that point the seizures still persist, a trial of VPA or nitrazepam should be recommended. If patients relapse during tapering or after discontinuation of the ACTH, the ACTH should be restarted at the dose that originally stopped the spasms. Following control of the seizures, the ACTH should be continued for a minimum of 1 month before tapering is attempted again. The response to ACTH is sometimes very dramatic, with cessation of seizures and marked improvement of the EEG within a few days.

While ACTH and corticosteroids are effective in stopping spasms, there are many side effects, some of which are very serious. Steroid therapy is invariably associated with cushingoid obesity. In addition, growth retardation, development of acne, and irritability may ensue. These side effects are of no major concern with the short-term use of ACTH. However, more serious effects may include infection, arterial hypertension, intracerebral hemorrhages, osteoporosis, hypokalemic alkalosis, and other electrolyte disturbances.

Patients treated with ACTH or adrenal corticosteroids should be closely monitored, with twice-weekly blood pressure measurements and periodic checks of electrolyte levels. If the patient develops hypertension or hypokalemic alkalosis, a reduction in dosage is recommended. However, patients who have a relapse once the dosage is decreased may be restarted on the effective dose and managed with antihypertensives or salt restriction. If this strategy is not effective, it is better to change to synthetic glucocorticoids (e.g., methylprednisone), which have less of a sodium-retaining effect. Fever should be promptly investigated.

Clonzepam and VPA have also been used in the treatment of infantile spasms with moderate success. Because of the significant side effects of ACTH, some authors feel these drugs should be tried initially in children with significant neurologic or developmental abnormalities, in whom ACTH is unlikely to change the child's overall prognosis.

Some infantile spasms have a focal or partial onset and, if this focal onset can be consistently demonstrated, the infants may benefit from surgery. Often the children will have a structural lesion such as a hamartoma that coincides with the focal EEG and clinical features. However, Chugani and colleagues (1990) at UCLA have demonstrated that some infants with cryptogenic infantile spasms and normal MRI scans have deficits of cerebral metabolism (detected using positron emission tomographic scans). When this area of cortical hypometabolism is removed under the guidance of intraoperative corticography, the seizures are reduced or eliminated.

Prognosis

Infantile spasms are one of the most devastating seizure disorders to affect infants. The poor prognosis has been confirmed in virtually all follow-up studies. Fatalities occur in 6% to 22% of the cases and over two thirds of the patients are retarded. In addition, a significant number of patients have neurologic impairment in follow-up, with problems such as hemiplegia, diplegia, or quadriplegia. In a large number of cases myoclonic seizures, GTC seizures, or other seizure types are observed. Some patients develop the Lennox-Gastaut syndrome, already discussed. Because a large number of patients have neurologic impairment prior to the onset of the spasms, it is not surprising that the prognosis is so poor. In all likelihood these patients would have had similar neurologic outcomes regardless of the infantile spasms.

Prognosis is directly related to etiology. Authors who have coded their cases as symptomatic and cryptogenic have found that cryptogenic cases have a significantly better prognosis than symptomatic cases. Patients who are classified as doubtful usually have outcomes similar to those of the symptomatic cases. In view of the overwhelming evidence for the better outcome of cryptogenic cases, classification with respect to possible etiologic factors appears to be one of the most important prognostic indicators.

ANNOTATED BIBLIOGRAPHY

Bellman M: Infantile spasms, in Pedley TA, Meldrum BS (eds): *Recent Advances in Epileptology*, Vol 1. Edinburgh, Churchill Livingstone, 1983, p 113–138.

An excellent review of infantile spasms.

Kellaway P, Hrachovy RA, Frost JD, et al.: Precise characterization and quantification of infantile spasms. *Ann Neurol* 6:214–218, 1979.

This is a detailed study of the clinical manifestations of infantile spasms using long-term polygraphic and videotape monitoring.

Lombroso CT: A prospective study of infantile spasms: Clinical and therapeutic correlations. *Epilepsia* 24:135–158, 1983.

The author of this study reviews the clinical course of patients followed at Children's Hospital, Boston, Massachusetts.

Riikonen R, Donner M: ACTH therapy in infantile spasms: Side effects. *Arch Dis Child* 55:664–672, 1980.

The serious side effects of ACTH are reported in this study. Very high dosages were used in some patients.

Singer WD, Haller JS, Sullivan LR, et al: The value of neuroradiology in infantile spasms. *J Pediatr* 100:47–50, 1982.

The authors report that all infants who had abnormal neuroradiologic examinations prior to the onset of therapy showed mental retardation in follow-up.

Snead OC, Benton JW, Hosey LC, et al: Treatment of infantile spasms with high-dose ACTH: Efficacy and plasma levels of ACTH and cortisol. *Neurology* 39:1027–1031, 1989.

Of 15 infants with infantile spasms treated with high-dose ACTH (150 IU/m² per day), 14 (93.3%) were controlled and had normal EEGs. The authors speculate that sustained high levels of cortisol following high-dose ACTH were responsible for the improvement. Despite this paper, there is still controversy over whether high-dose ACTH offers advantages over prednisone or low-dose ACTH in the treatment of infantile spasms.

Chugani HT, Shields WD, Shewmon DA, Olsen DM, Phelps ME, Peacock WJ: Infantile spasm. I. PET identifies focal cortical dysgenesis in cryptogenic cases for surgical treatment. *Ann Neurol* 27:406–413, 1990.

The authors demonstrate that in some infants with cryptogenic infantile spasms focal lesions can be demonstrated using position emission tomography. Surgical ablations of areas of hypometabolism on PET resulted in elimination of the seizures. Although the MRI scans in these children were normal, EEGs and clinical seizures suggest focal pathology. In-

fants with medically intractable cryptogenic infantile spasms who have evidence of focality may benefit from surgery.

NEONATAL SEIZURES

Seizures in the newborn period usually indicate a significant insult to the immature nervous system. Because of the unique features of seizures in this age group, the physician caring for these children requires a thorough knowledge of neonatal physiology and medicine.

Clinical Characteristics

The International Classification of Epileptic Seizures is not applicable to newborns. Because of their lack of myelin and cortical organization, neonates are unable to sustain organized generalized discharges. GTC seizures are rarely if ever seen, and absence seizures never occur. The clinical characteristics of neonatal seizures are significantly different from manifestations in older children, making recognition of seizures in neonates difficult. Any type of unusual, repetitive, stereotyped behavior in a neonate may be a seizure. Until recently neonatal seizures were separated into five types based solely on clinical manifestations: subtle, tonic, clonic, and myoclonic. However, the use of simultaneous EEG and video monitoring of neonates has significantly changed our classification of seizures in this age group.

Mizrahi and Kellaway (1987), using simultaneous EEG and video monitoring, have developed the classification system in Table 8–10. These authors found that clonic seizures had the highest correlation with EEG ictal abnormalities. Focal clonic seizures consisted of rhythmic twitching of facial, limb, or axial muscles. Focal seizures were further subdivided into unifocal, multifocal, hemiconvulsive, and axial. Unifocal clonic seizures consisted of rhythmic jerking of one extremity or one side of the face, whereas in multifocal seizures the clonic movements shifted from limb to limb or from face to limb on the same or the opposite side in a random manner. In hemiconvulsive seizures one entire side of the body had rhythmic, clonic jerks. Axial seizures consisted of

FEATURE TABLE 8-9. NEONATAL SEIZURES

Discriminating Features	Consistent Feature	Variable Features
1. May be very difficult to differentiate from nonepileptic behavior without the aid of EEG monitoring. 2. Neonatal seizures usually respond to phenobarbital, phenytoin, or primidone.	1. Stereotyped activity with clear onset and cessation.	1. Clinical manifestations quite variable—may consist of focal clonic, multifocal clonic, tonic, or myoclonic seizures; subtle manifestations, or autonomic dysfunction. 2. Associated with virtually any insult to the neonatal brain.

TABLE 8–10. CLASSIFICATION OF NEONATAL SEIZURES

I. **Seizures with a close association to EEG seizure discharges**
- A. Focal clonic
    1. Unifocal
    2. Multifocal
        a. Alternating
        b. Migrating
    3. Hemiconvulsive
    4. Axial
- B. Myoclonic
    1. Generalized
    2. Focal
- C. Focal tonic
    1. Asymmetric truncal
    2. Eye deviation
- D. Apnea

II. **Seizures with an inconsistent or no relationship to EEG seizure discharges**
- A. Motor automatisms
    1. Oral-buccal-lingual movements
    2. Ocular signs
    3. Progression movements
        a. Pedaling
        b. Stepping
        c. Rotary arm movements
    4. Complex purposeless movements
- B. Generalized tonic
    1. Extensor
    2. Flexor
    3. Mixed extensor/flexor
- C. Myoclonic
    1. Generalized
    2. Focal
    3. Fragmentary

From Mizrahi and Kellaway (1987) with permission.

rhythmic jerking of the tongue, hips, or shoulders, or rapid, jerking respiratory movements. In focal clonic seizures there was usually a one-to-one relationship to EEG seizure discharges.

Many of the behaviors thought previously to be subtle seizures were not found by Mizrahi and Kellaway to be associated with EEG abnormalities. These activities include repetitive sucking and other oral-buccal-lingual movements; pedaling movements of the legs or paddling movements of the arms; blinking, momentary fixation of gaze with or without eye deviation; and nystagmus. Mizrahi and Kellaway have postulated that these behaviors are not epileptic in character.

Myoclonic and tonic events were variable in their relationship to EEG abnormalities. Focal tonic seizures consisting of sustained asymmetric posturing of the limbs or trunk, or sustained deviation of the eyes, were associated with EEG ictal abnormalities, whereas generalized tonic episodes did not have a consistent relationship to EEG ictal discharges. Myoclonic seizures, both focal and generalized, were sometimes associated with EEG ictal abnormalities.

Although apnea can occasionally occur as the sole manifestation of a neonatal seizure, it is usually associated with other seizure manifestations.

Differential Diagnosis

Jitteriness reflects central nervous system dysfunction and can be seen after hypoxic-ischemic insults and drug withdrawal, or with hypocalcemia and hypoglycemia. Jitteriness must be distinguished from seizures although at times this can be difficult. Helpful differentiating points are given in Table 8–11.

Coulter and Allen (1982) reported three infants with *benign sleep myoclonus* beginning in the first 2 weeks of life. There was bilateral, synchronous, repetitive jerking of the upper extremities, with two of the three infants also having lower extremity involvement. The myoclonus only occurred during sleep. EEGs and neurologic examinations were normal, and the babies had normal outcomes. As with benign familial neonatal seizures, this diagnosis is one of exclusion.

Electroencephalography

The EEG has now become accepted as a valuable, safe, and reliable test to assess cerebral function in newborns. Although the EEG is usually not specific for etiology, it may supply the physician with clues about the severity of central nervous system insults and indicate whether they are of a transient or permanent nature. In many instances, the EEG is superior to the clinical examination in determining neurologic prognosis. The EEG is valuable in supporting the clinical diagnosis of seizures in infants with atypical or minimal behavioral manifestations if the recording includes the episode in question. The EEG may also document seizure discharges that are not accompanied by overt clinical manifestations. In infants who are paralyzed and dependent on respiratory support, the EEG may be the only objective means of assessing

TABLE 8–11. CLINICAL COMPARISON OF JITTERINESS AND SEIZURES

Clinical Features	Jitteriness	Seizures
Stimulus sensitive	Usually	Rarely
Velocity of movements	Rapid	Slow
Four-extremity involvement	Frequently	Rarely
Duration of flexion-extension phase	Equal	Fast and slow component
Movements cease with passive flexion	Always	Rarely
Abnormality of gaze or eye movement	No	Often
Response to AEDs	Minimal to none	Frequent improvement

From Holmes (1987) with permission of the publisher.

cerebral function and monitoring the presence of seizure activity.

Etiology

Although an extensive array of neonatal disorders may be associated with seizures, only a few account for the majority. Because idiopathic seizures are rare in the first month of life, major efforts must be made to identify the cause of any seizures. Determining the etiology of the seizures is critical because this dictates therapy and is also highly correlated with outcome. Unfortunately, the ill neonate may present with a constellation of disturbances, each of which may contribute to the development of seizures. For example, asphyxia, hypoglycemia, hypocalcemia, and intraventricular hemorrhage, each sufficient alone to cause seizures, may all occur in the same infant.

Major causes of neonatal seizures include hypoxic-ischemic encephalopathy, hypocalcemia, hypoglycemia, hyponatremia and hypernatremia, intracranial hemorrhage, infection, congenital malformations, genetic factors, benign sleep myoclonus, inherited metabolic disorders, and drug withdrawal.

Hypoxic-Ischemic Encephalopathy

Hypoxic-ischemic encephalopathy is now the most common cause of neonatal seizures. Most asphyxia occurs before or during delivery, with only 10% of cases resulting from postnatal causes. Intrauterine factors causing asphyxia include both maternal considerations, such as hypotension, and placental disorders, such as infarcts, cord hematomas, placentae previae, or abruptio placentae. Events during delivery that may result in asphyxia include meconium aspiration and cord compression. Respiratory insufficiency, persistent fetal circulation, and severe right-to-left cardiac shunts are causes of asphyxia following birth.

In addition to being the major cause of seizures, hypoxia is a primary factor in periventricular-intraventricular and subarachnoid hemorrhages, both of which may also lead to seizures.

Hypocalcemia

Hypocalcemia (defined as calcium levels below 7.5 mg/dL in the preterm infant and 8 mg/dL in the term infant) was formerly among the most frequent causes of neonatal seizures. In more recent studies, however, hypocalcemia as a primary etiology is rare. Hypocalcemia has two major peaks of incidence in the newborn. The first occurs during the first 3 days of life and is associated with prenatal morbidity (small-for-date infants, maternal preeclampsia, diabetes, or polyhydramnios) or preinatal insults (asphyxia, intracranial hemorrhage, trauma). Late-onset hypocalcemia (5 to 14 days) occurs primarily in term infants consuming a nonhuman milk preparation with suboptimal ratios of phosphorus to calcium and phosphorus

to magnesium. In the United States, this type of hypocalcemia has become rare. Additionally, hypomagnesemia, defined as a level less than 1 mEq/L, may accompany or occur independently of hypocalcemia.

Hypoglycemia

Although there is no universal consensus regarding the definition of hypoglycemia, most authors cite levels under 20 mg/dL in preterm infants and under 30 mg/dL in term babies as indicating hypoglycemia. Like hypocalcemia, hypoglycemia is often associated with other neonatal disorders such as trauma, hemolytic disease, or asphyxia. Infants of diabetic and toxemic mothers, infants small for gestational age, and twins are particularly at risk. The duration of hypoglycemia is an important determinant in the development of neurologic signs, which typically include jitteriness, hypotonia, lethargy, and apnea in addition to seizures.

Hyponatremia and Hypernatremia

Both hyponatremia and hypernatremia are rare causes of neonatal seizures. Hyponatremia, like hypocalcemia, usually occurs in association with other disorders, such as intracranial hemorrhage or meningitis, and is secondary to inappropriate secretion of antidiuretic hormone. Hypernatremia is usually iatrogenic, most frequently secondary to improper mixing of formula.

Intracranial Hemorrhage

Primary subarachnoid hemorrhage (SAH) occurs in both term and preterm babies. Bleeding is from venous structures and is often associated with asphyxia or trauma. Although many SAHs are mild and inconsequential except for causing transient seizures, some result in a stormy course and result in hydrocephalus and parenchymal damage.

Intraventricular/periventricular hemorrhage is the most common type of intracranial hemorrhage and accounts for a large percentage of morbidity and mortality primarily, but not exclusively, in preterm infants. The hemorrhage usually occurs within 72 hours of birth, and the manifestations vary from no clinical signs to catastrophic deterioration with hypotonia, apnea, seizures, and a bulging fontanelle. The frequency with which seizures complicate this disorder is unclear, with estimates ranging from 15% to 50%.

Subdural hematomas are most common in term infants and usually follow traumatic deliveries. With improved obstetric techniques they have become rare. Seizures are usually associated with an underlying cerebral contusion.

Infection

Intrauterine or postnatal central nervous system infections may lead to seizures. Intrauterine transplacental causes include rubella, cytomegalovirus, herpes simplex, coxsackievirus B, and toxoplasmosis. Primary vaginal herpes simplex infection results in a devastating encephalitis with severe seizures and a characteristic EEG pattern. Intrauterine infections are usually associated with other systemic signs: microcephaly, jaundice, rash, hepatomegaly, and chorioretinitis. Common postnatal infections include those with *Escherichia coli* and group B beta-streptococcus. Meningitis must be suspected in any neonate with seizures, especially if there are additional risk factors such as prolonged rupture of the membranes. Any infant without a clear etiology of seizures requires prompt lumbar puncture. Sepsis without meningitis may also lead to seizures.

Congenital Malformations

Disorders of neuronal migration and organization may lead to severe neonatal seizures and offer great difficulties in diagnosis. Polymicrogyria, neuronal heterotopias, lissencephaly, holoprosencephaly, and hydranencephaly are all associated with seizures. Many of these dysgenetic central nervous system conditions occur in isolation with normal facies and without systemic abnormalities. Although CT scans and cranial ultrasound will detect the most severe abnormalities, microscopic brain anomalies usually go undetected.

Benign Autosomal Dominant Neonatal Seizures

Although rare, benign autosomal dominant neonatal seizures have been reported. The prognosis is usually excellent, although unexpected death can occur, and some patients develop seizures later in life. Regardless of the family history, this diagnosis should only be considered after other etiologies have been excluded.

Benign Neonatal Seizures

Benign neonatal seizures constitute a rare but increasingly recognized syndrome characterized by seizures in the neonatal or infantile period. Two forms are recognized: familial and nonfamilial. In both instances the seizures may be quite severe and status epilepticus is common. The nonfamilial form is characterized by idiopathic, self-limited seizures occurring in previously normal neonates. The seizures most commonly occur at day 5 and have been called "fifth-day fits" by some authors. Familial seizures most frequently have their onset during the first week of life but onset may occur as late as early infancy. These seizures may recur for several months before resolving. No cause is found for the seizures and during the interictal period the patient appears healthy. The family history reveals benign neonatal seizures in other family members. Although the prognosis is favorable in both syndromes, seizures may occasionally occur later in life in the familial form. The familial form of benign neonatal seizures is autosomal dominant and the gene has been localized to chromosome 20.

Inherited Metabolic Disorders

Although the differential diagnosis of neonatal seizures includes inherited metabolic disorders, these are fortunately rare and usually produce other significant symptoms, such as peculiar odors, protein intolerance, acidosis, alkalosis, lethargy, or stupor. In most cases of metabolic disease, pregnancy, labor, and delivery are normal. Whereas formula intolerance may be the earliest indication of a systemic abnormality, seizures are commonly the first specific clue to central nervous system involvement. If untreated, metabolic disorders commonly lead to lethargy, coma, and death. In surviving infants, weight loss, poor growth, and failure to thrive are common. Metabolic disorders that may lead to neonatal seizures include maple syrup urine disease, nonketotic hyperglycinemia, organic acidemias such as propionic acidemia and methylmalonic acidemia, and urea cycle defects such as carbamyl phosphate synthetase deficiency or ornithine transcarbamylase deficiency.

Vitamin B_6 or pyridoxine dependency is an extremely rare metabolic disturbance with variable clinical manifestations in which adequate quantities of ingested and circulatory B_6 fail to serve as a co-factor in metabolic pathways. Although pyridoxine dependency may be associated with intrauterine convulsions, this is not invariable. Because the clinical spectrum of abnormalities is quite broad, any child with unexplained seizures should receive an injection of 50 to 100 mg of pyridoxine intravenously during a seizure, preferably with EEG monitoring. Termination of the seizure would strongly suggest pyridoxine-dependent seizures.

Drug Withdrawal

A significant cause of neonatal seizures in urban hospitals is withdrawal from narcotic-analgesics, sedative-hypnotics, and alcohol. Infants born to heroin- or methadone-addicted mothers have an increased risk of seizures, although the most common neurologic findings are jitteriness and irritability. Infants of methadone-addicted mothers may have late withdrawal symptoms, with seizures occurring as long as 4 weeks after birth. Seizures may occur following administration of a short-acting barbiturate to the mother. These usually occur within the first 3 days of life in association with jitteriness and irritability. Longer-acting barbiturates such as phenobarbital are not associated with withdrawal seizures, although irritability, tremors, and hyperreflexia occur commonly. Seizures resulting from alcohol withdrawal are similar to those of short-acting barbiturates.

Although rare, seizures may be a prominent feature in infants poisoned with local anesthetics. Inadvertent fetal anesthetic injection usually occurs in deliveries at the time of local anesthesia administered for episiotomy. The infant presents at birth with bradycardia, apnea, and hypotonia. Seizures occur within the first 6 hours and are generally tonic in type. When anesthetic intoxication is suspected, the infant should be closely inspected for needle marks. The diagnosis can be confirmed by measuring serum levels of the offending drug. Treatment consists of maintaining adequate ventilation and facilitating elimination of the drug by inducing diuresis, acidifying the urine, or doing an exchange transfusion when renal impairment is present. AEDs are of questionable benefit, and seizures subside with clearance of the local anesthetic.

Treatment

Determining etiology is of upmost importance in the neonate with seizures. After ventilation and adequate glucose levels are assured, initial goals are to establish the underlying cause and institute appropriate therapy. The ready availability of accurate and timely chemistry screening panels has largely obviated the need for empirical infusions of glucose and calcium as the first steps in treatment. Chemical abnormalities should be corrected when documented and AEDs given to the infant with recurrent seizures.

Phenobarbital is the most widely used drug in the treatment of neonatal seizures. The half-life of phenobarbital varies widely, ranging from 45 to 173 hours in newborns. With maturation, the infant's ability to metabolize phenobarbital improves dramatically. The following dosage recommendations for phenobarbital have been formulated: the initial loading dose should be 15 to 20 mg/kg with a maintenance dose of 3 to 4 mg/kg daily. It is recommended that the loading dose be given intravenously. Neither the loading dose nor the maintenance dose of phenobarbital appears to be influenced by gestational age or birth weight. Because of its long half-life, phenobarbital can be given once or twice daily. Although therapeutic levels have not yet been established, most infants require serum levels between 10 and 40 μg/mL to suppress seizures. As with older children, levels above 40 μg/mL may result in lethargy.

Unfortunately, in a significant number of patients phenobarbital is ineffective in stopping seizures and a second drug must be added. The second drug of choice in neonatal seizures is phenytoin. As with phenobarbital, the range of half-lives for phenytoin is extremely large in newborns. The greatest variability and widest range of phenytoin half-life is encountered in the first week of life, varying in one study from 6 to 140 hours. The apparent half-life decreases with postnatal age from an average of 58 hours in the first week to 20 hours in the fourth week. As in older children phenytoin follows nonlinear kinetics in the newborn period. Loading doses of 15 to 20 mg/kg are required to achieve serum levels of 15 μg/mL. Unfortunately, phenytoin is not well absorbed in the gastrointestinal tract in newborns, and it is often difficult to obtain therapeutic levels using the oral route. Intramuscular administration of phenytoin is irritating and results in unpredictable plasma levels. Therefore, in the neonatal period the only reliable method of administering the drug is through the intravenous route. When phenytoin is administered intravenously, a recommended maintenance dose is 3 to 4 mg/kg per day, whereas, if oral treatment is attempted, 8 mg/kg per day is recommended. Data are not available concerning the clinical response with phenytoin alone in the treatment of neonatal seizures, although most neurologists and neonatologists agree that it is an effective medication in infants whose seizures are not controlled by phenobarbital.

Diazepam and lorazepam have been used in some centers to treat neonatal seizures. Like phenytoin and phenobarbital, diazepam has a wide range of half-lives in neonates. Although a dosage has not been established, Dodson (1984) recommends 0.5 mg/kg intravenously for the acute management of neonatal seizures. Owing to its short distribution phase diazepam has not been evaluated as a maintenance AED.

ANNOTATED BIBLIOGRAPHY

Brown JK, Minns RA: Epilepsy in neonates, in Tyrer JH (ed): *Current Status of Modern Therapy; Vol 5: The Treatment of Epilepsy.* Philadelphia, JB Lippincott, 1981, p 161–202.
Hill A, Volpe JJ: Seizures, hypoxic-ischemic brain injury and intraventricular hemorrhage in the newborn. *Ann Neurol* 10:109–121, 1981.
Holmes GL: Neonatal seizures, in Pedley TA, Meldrum, BS (eds): *Recent Advances in Epilepsy.* Vol. 2. New York, Churchill Livingstone, 1985, p 207–237.
    These three articles are all reviews dealing with neonatal seizures. With increasing use of simultaneous EEG and video monitoring of neonates it is very likely that our understanding or neonatal seizures will change in the future.

Pearls and Perils: Neonatal Seizures

1. All neonates with unexplained seizures must have a spinal tap to rule out the possibility of meningitis.
2. Pyridoxine should be given to every neonate with seizures when the etiologic agent has not been determined.
3. Although rare, apnea may be the sole manifestation of a seizure in a neonate.
4. Neonatal seizures may be as frequently overdiagnosed as underdiagnosed. When there is doubt it is better to withhold treatment with AEDs.
5. Worrying about the treatment of neonatal seizures instead of the etiology is a mistake. Determining the etiology of the seizures is much more important than trying to stop them with AEDs.

Dodson WE: Antiepileptic drug use in newborns and infants, in Pedley TW, Meldrum BS (eds): *Recent Advances in Epilepsy*, Vol 1. New York, Churchill Livingstone, 1983, p 231–248.

This is a review article describing the pharmacokinetics of AEDs in neonates. Metabolism of AEDs in neonates differs significantly from that in older children.

STATUS EPILEPTICUS

Status epilepticus is one of the most frequent and serious neurologic emergencies encountered by the physician working with children. There is unequivocal clinical and experimental evidence that status epilepticus can lead to brain damage and therefore must be stopped as quickly as possible. Fortunately, with prompt and appropriate treatment, most cases of status epilepticus can be quickly stopped.

In practical terms, status epilepticus is defined as continuous clinical or EEG seizures lasting at least 30 minutes. In addition, some authors extend the definition to include patients who have serial seizures in which consciousness is not regained between seizures and the series of seizures lasts 30 minutes or more.

The clinical manifestations of status epilepticus are as varied as the manifestations of seizures in general. The most dramatic and serious type of status epilepticus is the generalized convulsive form, and this chapter will deal with this type of status epilepticus.

Clinical Features

At the onset of the status, the seizure differs little from an isolated GTC seizure. Motor activity during the seizure usually involves both tonic and clonic phases. During generalized convulsive status, there are significant autonomic manifestations, including tachycardia, hyperpnea, mydriasis, and hypersecretion. If the seizure continues, the patient may develop fever, hypotension, acidosis, and respiratory depression.

Etiology

The etiologies of status epilepticus are as varied as the etiologies of epilepsy in general. Status epilepticus has generally been classified as either idiopathic or symptomatic, with symptomatic cases outnumbering idiopathic cases by a ratio of about 3:1. In series limited to children, nonspecific febrile illnesses, hypoxic-ischemic encephalopathies, and central nervous system infections account for the majority of cases of symptomatic status epilepticus, whereas in adults tumor- and trauma-related causes were most common.

In patients already being treated for epilepsy, status epilepticus can be precipitated by withdrawal of anticonvulsant medications, sleep deprivation, or intercurrent infection. Rapid discontinuation of AEDs, particularly the barbiturates and benzodiazepines, is likely to lead to status epilepticus. Sleep deprivation usually occurs in association with other precipitating factors and is unlikely to be the sole factor responsible for status epilepticus.

Prognosis

Although they have decreased significantly over the past 50 years, the mortality and morbidity from status epilepticus remain high. Death during status epilepticus may occur either as a result of the status epilepticus itself or because of the etiology of the status. Death is more likely to occur in symptomatic cases than idiopathic cases. In addition, the mortality rate is related to the duration of the convulsive status.

Treatment

While brain damage can occur in the absence of systemic abnormalities, it is clear that hyperpyrexia, hypoglycemia, hypotension, and hypoxia that may occur during status epilepticus can increase the cerebral damage. Although AEDs are essential for managing status epilepticus, systemic consequences of prolonged seizures must be recognized and treated. Failure to treat these systemic abnormalities quickly and successfully will likely result in neurologic sequelae or death. It is important, therefore, to achieve systemic metabolic stability as well as stop the seizures. As the status is being treated, it is also imperative for the physician to continue evaluating the patient for precipitating causes.

Initial treatment (Table 8–12) is aimed at providing

FEATURE TABLE 8-10. STATUS EPILEPTICUS

Discriminating Feature	Consistent Feature	Variable Features
1. Rarely is it difficult to diagnose convulsive status epilepticus. Nonconvulsive status epilepticus may be confused with drug intoxication, psychosis, or migraine and may require EEG monitoring for proper diagnosis.	1. Clinical and/or EEG seizure activity lasting 30 minutes or more.	1. Clinical seizures may be convulsive (i.e., tonic-clonic, clonic, or tonic) or nonconvulsive (i.e., absence or partial complex). 2. Etiologies for status epilepticus are as broad as those for epilepsy in general.

TABLE 8-12. SEQUENCE OF STEPS FOR EMERGENCY TREATMENT OF PATIENTS WITH STATUS EPILEPTICUS

1. Place patient in safe position.
2. Assess cardiorespiratory function.
3. Insert oral airway and administer oxygen. If there is any question of respiratory insufficiency, arrange for intubation.
4. Insert indwelling catheter.
5. Draw venous blood for measurement of AED levels; CBC; and determination of blood urea nitrogen, electrolytes, glucose, and ammonia.
6. Draw arterial blood gases.
7. Give 50% glucose solution (1–2 mL/kg).
8. Start maintenance fluids unless there is evidence of fluid overload, concern about increased intracranial pressure, or dehydration.
9. Give diazepam (0.2–0.4 mg/kg) at a rate of 1–2 mg/min. If seizures do not stop, repeat dose in 20 min.
10. If seizures stop, a longer-acting AED must be given to prevent a recurrence of seizures.
11. If status continues, give phenytoin (15–20 mg/kg) at a rate of 0.5–1.0 mg/kg per min. Blood pressure and electrocardiogram monitoring are mandatory during the infusion.
12. If status continues, give phenobarbital (15–20 mg/kg).
13. If status continues, give paraldehyde either intravenously or per rectum or start VPA per rectum.
14. If status continues, give general anesthesia.

satisfactory ventilation, maintaining adequate cardiac output and cerebral perfusion, and preventing injury as a result of the violent motor activity. Status epilepticus cannot be managed by one person, and a team approach in an emergency room or intensive care unit is imperative.

Immediate needs are to assess cardiorespiratory function and insert an oral airway. Oxygen should be administered by a nasal cannula or mask. Many patients in status epilepticus require intubation and the physician should not hesitate to do this any time respiratory compromise appears imminent. It is always better to intubate prior to respiratory compromise than after hypoxia and hypercapnia have occurred. While the patient is in status epilepticus arterial blood gas monitoring is essential.

A secure intravenous line, preferably a catheter, is essential for the treatment of status epilepticus. As soon as the line is established, blood should be obtained for chemical screening (electrolytes, blood urea nitrogen, glucose, ammonia), measurement of AED levels if the patient has a known seizure disorder, and toxic screening. After drawing the blood specimen, 25% or 50% glucose should be given by bolus injection to supply 0.5 to 1.0 g/kg (2 to 4 mL/kg of 25% or 1 to 2 mL/kg of 50%). This infusion may terminate the seizure if the status is due to hypoglycemia. Maintenance fluids should be started using 5% dextrose in half-normal or normal saline unless there is indication of fluid overload, increased intracranial pressure, or dehydration. Because prolonged seizures may result in hypoglycemia, it is important to

continue to monitor serum glucose. Rhabdomyolysis can result from excessive muscle activity and ischemia and the urine should be monitored for this complication.

Tissue hypoxia and excessive muscle contractions may lead to lactic acidosis and autonomic instability. Bicarbonate should be given intravenously to raise the pH if it is below 7.2. Temperature should be closely monitored, and if hyperthermia is present the patient should be rapidly cooled using a cooling blanket or ice packs. Hyperthermia may exacerbate electrolyte imbalance, hypertension, and cardiac arrhythmia.

No studies are available that adequately address the question of selection or order of administration of drugs for generalized tonic-clonic status epilepticus in children. Delgado-Escueta and Enrile-Bascal (1983) have proposed an empirical approach in adults that provides a rational guideline for therapy. The concurrent administration of diazepam and phenytoin at separate sites is recommended. The rationale for this treatment is that diazepam is quickly effective but has a short-lived effect while phenytoin is slower acting but has a longer-lasting effect. Although this combination would likely be effective in children, it is difficult to secure two intravenous lines in a young child in generalized convulsive status epilepticus. For that reason, most physicians have used single-drug infusions in children. Regardless of the drug used, it is critically important that the physician be aware of appropriate dosages and potential side effects.

Currently, four drugs are widely used initially in the treatment of status epilepticus in children: diazepam, lorazepam, phenytoin, and phenobarbital. All four drugs are highly efficacious.

Diazepam. Diazepam has gained wide acceptance as a first-line intravenous agent in the therapy of status epilepticus, with an efficacy of greater than 60%. However, the antiepileptic effect is often only temporary and administration of other longer-acting AEDs is required.

Peak brain concentrations following intravenous administration are reached within 12 minutes. Diazepam distributes quickly in lipoid tissues and rapidly crosses the blood-brain barrier, subsequently resulting in a rapid antiepileptic action. After the peak concentration has been reached, a biexponential decline of the plasma concentration is observed. A short distribution half-life of approximately 1 hour determines the rapid initial decline. Correspondingly, the plasma concentration may drop below therapeutic values within 15 to 20 minutes after intravenous injection, depending on the initial peak concentration. The subsequent slower decline results mainly from the elimination of the drug; its slope determines the elimination half-life.

The usual dosage is 0.2 to 0.4 mg/kg intravenously with a maximum dose of 10 mg. The drug should be administered at a rate of approximately 1 to 2 mg/min. When the initial administration produces no seizure control or the seizure only stops for a brief period, a second or third intravenous injection may be effective. An interval between injections of 10 to 20 minutes is recommended. As would be expected from the pharmacokinetics of the drug, diazepam is quick acting. Delgado-Escueta and Enrile-Bascal (1983) found that diazepam stops seizures within 3 minutes in 32%, within 5 minutes in 68%, and within 10 minutes in 80% of patients with status epilepticus. A longer-acting AED should be given if diazepam successfully stops the status.

Diazepam is widely known to lead to respiratory depression and hypotension. Many of the patients who developed these complications had received large doses of barbiturates prior to intravenous administration of diazepam or had evidence of severe acute brain lesions that could also lead to respiratory distress. Although it is likely that the dangers of using diazepam are over-emphasized, the physician must be aware that respiratory depression and hypotension may occur. These risks may be decreased by a slow infusion rate. Because of the possibility of respiratory depression, extreme care must be used in administering the drug to patients with pulmonary disease or those who have previously received sedative drugs such as phenobarbital. Because diazepam will depress consciousness, this drug should be avoided in situations in which neurologic signs must be followed closely, such as following head trauma. Diazepam is contraindicated in patients who are hypersensitive to the drug.

Lorazepam. Lorazepam is a relatively new benzodiazepine that is rapidly taking the place of diazepam in the treatment of status in both adults and children. The drug has a half-life of 13 to 15 hours, rapidly penetrates the central nervous system, and appears to produce minimal cardiovascular depression and less respiratory depression in patients than diazepam. Although the drug has a shorter half-life than diazepam, the longer distribution phase gives lorazepam a longer duration of action. The drug can also be used safely in patients on high doses of chronic barbiturates. The major side effect has been sedation. Although the optimal dosage has not yet been clearly established, Gilmore and colleagues (1984) used an initial dose of 0.05 mg/kg given at 1 mg/min with the dose repeated up to two times. The authors found that the mean time to seizure control was 10 minutes (range 6 to

15 minutes). Other clinicians have given higher dosages (0.1 mg/kg). Because of its prolonged antiepileptic effect and limited respiratory depression, the drug appears to be superior to diazepam.

Phenytoin. Phenytoin is an excellent first-line drug for the treatment of generalized status epilepticus. The drug reaches the brain rapidly, is effective in stopping GTC seizures in greater than 60% of patients, and can be safely given with minimal depression of consciousness or respirations.

Phenytoin loading for status epilepticus is achieved with a dose of 15 to 20 mg/kg administrated at a rate of 0.5 to 1.0 mg/kg per minute. Recent studies have indicated that phenytoin can be safely diluted in saline for infusion. Phenytoin enters the brain within minutes and reaches peak brain concentration in 15 to 30 minutes. Wilder and associates (1977), in a study of adult patients, found that the antiepileptic effect of phenytoin was evident as early as 10 minutes after the start of the infusion, with 30% of the patients having stopped at this time. Seizures were stopped within 20 minutes in more than 80% of the patients. This loading dose will result in a peak level greater than 10 μg/ml for over 24 hours in most patients. Therefore, if the seizures stop with this dose, maintenance AEDs may be started 12 hours after the loading dose. Intravenous phenytoin may also be used for status epilepticus even if the patient is on chronic phenytoin therapy.

With proper administration, side effects with phenytoin are unusual. Hypotension and cardiac arrhythmias have been reported, primarily in older patients. It is necessary to monitor both the electrocardiogram and blood pressure during the infusion of phenytoin. Contraindications to phenytoin include patients with a prior history of allergic response to phenytoin, porphyria, sinus bradycardia, sinoatrial block, second- and third-degree atrioventricular block, hypotension, and myocardial insufficiency.

Phenobarbital. Phenobarbital continues to be extensively used in some institutions for the treatment of childhood status epilepticus. The popularity of this drug is probably secondary to its efficacy, safety, and familiarity to pediatricians and family physicians. The drug should be given as an intravenous bolus in a dosage of 15 to 20 mg/kg at a rate no faster than 50 mg/min. Like phenytoin, phenobarbital enters the brain quickly but does not reach brain peak levels for approximately 30 to 60 minutes. Therapeutic responses, therefore, are usually slower than those observed with diazepam and the physician may have to wait 30 to 60 minutes to see the maximum effect of the drug. Major side effects include sedation, hypotension, and respiratory depression. The combination of diazepam and phenobarbital is particularly likely to lead to respiratory depression.

Like phenytoin, phenobarbital is long-lasting, and,

Pearls and Perils: Status Epilepticus

1. Phenytoin may be given to patients in status epilepticus even if they are on chronic phenytoin treatment.
2. Failure to give sufficient amounts of AEDs is one of the most common errors made in the treatment of status epilepticus.

if the seizures stop with the loading dose, maintenance drugs do not need to be started for 12 hours. Because phenobarbital may depress consciousness, the drug should be avoided when neurologic signs must be closely monitored.

In rare situations, general anesthesia may be necessary in patients refractory to all other AEDs. The use of general anesthesia serves to minimize the metabolic effects of prolonged seizure activity or suppress the process permanently. Unfortunately, few guidelines are available regarding the depth and duration of anesthesia. Some authors have recommended the use of halothane or enflurane, while others have recommended intravenous pentobarbital. There has not yet been a sufficient number of studies to enable one to make recommendations of one agent over the other. Unfortunately, some patients begin having seizures again following withdrawal of the anesthetic agent.

ANNOTATED BIBLIOGRAPHY

Aicardi J, Chevrie JJ: Convulsive status epilepticus in infants and children: A study of 239 cases. *Epilepsia* 11:187–197, 1970.
  This study of status epilepticus in children forms the basis of much of our knowledge about this disorder. The duration of status was longer (1 hour) than in many other studies, which might explain the high morbidity and mortality rate.
Bleck TP: Therapy for status epilepticus. *Clin Neuropharmacol* 6:255–259, 1983.
Camfield PR: Treatment of status epilepticus in children. *Can Med Assoc J* 128:671–672, 1983.
  Both of these articles are excellent, succinct reviews of the treatment of status epilepticus.
Delgado-Escueta AV, Wasterlain C, Treiman DM, et al: Management of status epilepticus. *N Engl J Med* 306:1137–1340, 1982.
  The simultaneous administration of diazepam and phenytoin is recommended in this article. No clinical trials using this method in children have been reported.

BIBLIOGRAPHY

Adams DJ, Lueders H: Hyperventilation and 6-hour EEG recording in evaluation of absence seizures. *Neurology* 31:1175–1177, 1981.
Adams RD, Lyon G: *Neurology of Hereditary Metabolic Diseases of Children.* New York, Hemisphere, 1982.
Aicardi J, Chevrie JJ: Myoclonic epilepsies of childhood. *Neuropaediatrie* 3:177–190, 1971.
Aicardi J, Chevrie JJ: Consequences of status epilepticus in infants and children, in Delgado-Escueta AV, Wasterlain CG, Treiman DM, et al (eds): *Advances in Neurology,* Vol 34: *Status Epilepticus.* New York, Raven Press, 1983, p 115–125.
Aicardi J, Amsili J, Chevrie JJ: Acute hemiplegia in infancy and childhood. *Dev Med Child Neurol* 11:162–173, 1969.

Aigner BR, Mulder DW: Myoclonus. *Arch Neurol* 2:600–615, 1960.
Ajmone-Marsan C, Lewis WR: Pathologic findings in patients with "centrencephalic" electroencephalographic patterns. *Neurology* 10:922–930, 1960.
Aminoff MJ, Simon RP, Wiedermann E: The hormonal response to generalized tonic-clonic seizures. *Brain* 107:569–578, 1984.
Andermann F, Robb JP: Absence status: A reappraisal following review of thirty-eight patients. *Epilepsia* 31:177–187, 1972.
Annegers JF, Hauser WA, Elveback LR: Remission of seizures and relapse in patients with epilepsy. *Epilepsia* 20:729–737, 1979.
Annegers JF, Grabow JD, Groover RV, et al: Seizures after head trauma: A population study. *Neurology* 30:683–689, 1980.
Bachman DS: Use of valproic acid in treatment of infantile spasms. *Arch Neurol* 39:49–52, 1982.
Bachman DS, Hodges FJ III, Freeman JM: Computerized axial tomography in chronic seizure disorders of childhood. *Pediatrics* 58:828–832, 1976.
Ballard RA, Vinocur B, Reynolds JW, et al: Transient hyperammonemia of the preterm infant. *N Engl J Med* 299:920–925, 1978.
Ballenger CE, King DW, Gallagher BB: Partial complex status epilepticus. *Neurology* 33:1545–1552, 1983.
Batshaw ML, Brusilow SW: Valproate-induced hyperammonemia. *Ann Neurol* 11:319–321, 1982.
Beaumanoir A, Ballis T, Varfis G, Ansari K: Benign epilepsy of childhood with Rolandic spikes. A clinical, electrophysiological and telencephalographic study. *Epilepsia* 15:301–315, 1974.
Beaussart M, Faou R: Evolution of epilepsy with Rolandic paroxysmal foci: A study of 324 cases. *Epilepsia* 19:337–342, 1978.
Belafsky MA, Carwille S, Miller P, et al: Prolonged epileptic twilight states: Continuous recordings with nasopharyngeal electrodes and videotape analysis. *Neurology* 28:239–245, 1978.
Bellman MH, Ross EM, Miller DL: Infantile spasms and pertussis immunization. *Lancet* 1:1031–1034, 1983.
Bergman I, Painter MJ, Hirsh RP, et al: Outcome in neonates with convulsions treated in an intensive care unit. *Ann Neurol* 14:642–647, 1983.
Bertoni JM, von Loh S, Allen RJ: The Aicardi syndrome: Report of 4 cases and review of the literature. *Ann Neurol* 5:475–482, 1979.
Bickford RG, Whelan JL, Klass DW, et al: Reading epilepsy: Clinical and electroencephalographic studies of a new syndrome. *Trans Am Neurol Assoc* 81:100–102, 1957.
Blom S, Heijbel J: Benign epilepsy of children with centrotemporal EEG foci: A follow-up study in adulthood of patients initially studied as children. *Epilepsia* 23:629–632, 1982.
Blom S, Heijbel J, Bergfors PG: Benign epilepsy of children with centro-temporal EEG foci. Prevalence and follow-up study of 40 patients. *Epilepsia* 13:609–619, 1972.
Blume WT, Girvin JP, Kaufman JCE: Childhood brain tumors presenting as chronic uncontrolled focal seizure disorders. *Ann Neurol* 12:538–541, 1982.
Booker HE: Phenobarbital: Relationship of plasma concentration to seizure control, in Woodbury DM, Penry JK, Pippenger CE (eds): *Antiepileptic Drugs.* New York, Raven Press, 1982, p 341–350.

Bray PF, Wiser WC: Evidence for a genetic etiology of temporal-central abnormalities in focal epilepsy. *N Engl J Med* 271:926–933, 1964.

Bray PF, Wiser WC: Hereditary characteristics of familial temporal-central focal epilepsy. *Pediatrics* 36:207–211, 1965.

Brown JK, Cockburn F, Forfar JO: Clinical and chemical correlates in convulsions of the newborn. *Lancet* 1:135–139, 1972.

Brown JK: Convulsions in the newborn period. *Dev Med Child Neurol* 15:823–846, 1973.

Browne TR: Clinical pharmacology of antiepileptic drugs. *Drug Ther Rev* 2:469–493, 1979.

Browne TR: Paraldehyde, chlormethiazole, and lidocaine for treatment of status epilepticus, in Delgado-Escueta AV, Wasterlain CG, Treiman DM, et al (eds): *Advances in Neurology*, Vol 34: *Status Epilepticus*. New York, Raven Press, 1983, p 509–517.

Browne TR, Pincus JH: Phenytoin (Dilantin) and other hydantoins, in Browne TR, Feldman RG (eds): *Epilepsy: Diagnosis and Management*. Boston, Little, Brown, 1983, p 175–189.

Browne TR, Dreifuss FE, Dyken PR, et al: Ethosuximide in the treatment of absence (petit mal) seizures. *Neurology* 25:515–524, 1975.

Bruni J, Albright P: Valproic acid therapy for complex partial seizures. Its efficacy and toxic effects. *Arch Neurol* 40:135–137, 1983.

Bruni J, Wilder BJ: Valproic acid: Review of a new antiepileptic drug. *Arch Neurol* 36:393–398, 1980.

Bruni J, Wilder BJ, Bauman AW, et al: Clinical efficacy and long-term effects of valproic acid therapy on spike-and-wave discharges. *Neurology* 30:42–46, 1980.

Callaghan N, O'Hare J, O'Driscoll D, et al: Comparative study of ethosuximide and sodium valproate in the treatment of typical absence seizures (petit mal). *Dev Med Child Neurol*, 24:830–836, 1982.

Camfield CS, Chaplin S, Doyle AB, et al: Side effects of phenobarbital in toddlers: Behavioral and cognitive aspects. *J Pediatr* 95:361–365, 1979.

Carter, CA, Helms RA, Boehm R: Ethotoin in seizures of childhood and adolescence. *Neurology* 34:791–795, 1984.

Chao, DHC, Plum RL: Diamox in epilepsy: A critical review of 178 cases. *J Pediatr* 58:211–218, 1961.

Charlton MH: *Myoclonic Seizures*. Princeton, Excerpta Medica, 1975.

Chevrie JJ, Aicardi J: Childhood epileptic encephalopathy with slow spike-wave. A statistical study of 80 cases. *Epilepsia* 13:259–272, 1972.

Chugani HT, Shields WD, Shewmon DA, Olsen DM, Phelps ME, Peacock WJ: Infantile spasms. I. PET identifies focal cortical dysgenesis in cryptogenic cases for surgical treatment. *Ann Neurol* 27:406–413, 1990.

Clarke TA, Saunders BS, Feldman B: Pyridoxine-dependent seizures requiring high doses of pyridoxine for control. *Am J Dis Child* 133:963–965, 1979.

Cloyd JC, Gummit RJ, McLain LW: Status epilepticus: The role of intravenous phenytoin. *JAMA* 244:1479–1481, 1980.

Cockburn F, Brown JK, Belton NR, et al: Neonatal convulsions associated with primary disturbance of calcium, phosphorus, and magnesium metabolism. *Arch Dis Child* 48:99–108, 1973.

Convers P, Bierme T, Ryvlin P, et al: Contribution of magnetic resonance imaging in 100 cases of refractory partial epilepsy with normal CT scans. *Rev Neurol* 146:330–337, 1990.

Coulter DL, Allen RJ: Hyperammonemia with valproic acid therapy. *J Pediatr* 99:317–319, 1981.

Coulter DL, Allen RJ: Benign neonatal sleep myoclonus. *Arch Neurol* 39:191–192, 1982.

Coulter DL, Wu H, Allen RJ: Valproic acid therapy in childhood epilepsy. *JAMA* 244:785–788, 1980.

Covanis A, Jeavons PM: Once-daily sodium valproate in the treatment of epilepsy. *Dev Med Child Neurol* 22:202–204, 1980.

Cranford RE, Leppik IE, Patrick B, et al: Intravenous phenytoin in acute treatment of seizures. *Neurology* 29:1474–1479, 1979.

Curless RG, Walson PD, Carter DE: Phenytoin kinetics in children. *Neurology* 26:715–720, 1976.

Dalby MA: Epilepsy and 3 per second spike and wave rhythms. A clinical electroencephalographic and prognostic analysis of 346 patients. *Acta Neurol Scand* 45(suppl 40):1–183, 1969.

Dam, M: Phenytoin: An update, in Pedley TA, Meldrum BS (eds): *Recent Advances in Epilepsy*, Vol 1. Edinburgh, Churchill Livingstone, 1983, p 25–33.

Davis AG, Mutchie KD, Thompson JA, et al: Once-daily dosing with phenobarbital in children with seizure disorders. *Pediatrics* 68:824–827, 1981.

de Jong JGY, Delleman JW, Houben M, et al: Agenesis of the corpus callosum, infantile spasms, ocular anomalies (Aicardi's syndrome). *Neurology* 26:1152–1158, 1976.

Delgado-Escueta AV, Bascal FE, Treiman DM: Complex partial seizures on closed-circuit television and EEG: A study of 691 attacks in 79 patients. *Ann Neurol* 11:292–300, 1982.

Delgado-Escueta AV, Enrile-Bascal F: Combination therapy for status epilepticus: Intravenous diazepam and phenytoin, in Delgado-Escueta AV, Wasterlain CG, Treiman DM, et al (eds): *Advances in Neurology*, Vol 34: *Status Epilepticus*. New York, Raven Press, 1983, p 537–541.

Dodrill CB: Diphenylhydantoin serum levels. Toxicity and neuropsychological performance in patients with epilepsy. *Epilepsia* 16:593–600, 1975.

Dodrill CB, Troupin AS: Psychotropic effects of carbamazepine in epilepsy: A double-blind comparison with phenytoin. *Neurology* 27:1023–1028, 1977.

Dodson, WE: Neonatal drug intoxication: Local anesthetics. *Pediatr Clin North Am* 23:399–411, 1976.

Dodson WE: Phenytoin elimination in childhood. Effect of concentration-dependent kinetics. *Neurology* 30:196–199, 1980.

Dodson WE: Antiepileptic drug use in newborns and infants, in Pedley TA, Meldrum BS (eds): *Recent Advances in Epilepsy*, Vol 1. Edinburgh, Churchill Livingstone, 1984, p 231–248.

Douglas FE, White PT: Abdominal epilepsy—A reappraisal *J Pediatr* 78:59–67, 1971.

Dreifuss FE: The differential diagnosis of partial seizures with complex symptomatology, in Penry JK, Dal DD (eds): *Advances in Neurology*, Vol 11: *Complex Partial Seizures and their Treatment*. New York, Raven Press, 1975, p 187–199.

Dreifuss FE: Proposal for revised clinical and electroencephalographic classification of epileptic seizures. *Epilepsia* 22:489–501, 1981.

Dreifuss FE: Sodium valproate: A reappraisal, in Pedley TA, Meldrum BS (eds): *Recent Advances in Epilepsy*, Vol 1, Edinburgh, Churchill Livingstone, 1983a, p 35–46.

Dreifuss FE: Treatment of the nonconvulsive epilepsies. *Epilepsia* 24(suppl 1):S45–S54, 1983b.

Dreifuss FE, Penry JK, Rose SW, et al: Serum clonazepam concentrations in children with absence seizures. *Neurology* 25:255–258, 1975.

Dreifuss FE, Langer DH, Moline KA, Maxwell BA: Valproate acid hepatic fatalities: II. US experience since 1984. *Neurology* 39:201–207, 1989.

Duncan R, Patterson J, Hadley DM, et al: CT, MR and SPECT imaging in temporal lobe epilepsy. *J Neurol Neurosurg Psychiatr* 53:11–15, 1990.

Dyken PR, DuRant RH, Minden DB, et al: Short term effects of valproate on infantile spasms. *Pediatr Neurol* 1:34–37, 1985.

Edwards R, Schmidley JW, Simon RP: How often does a CSF pleocytosis follow generalized convulsions? *Ann Neurol* 13:460–462, 1983.

Elliott FA: The episodic dyscontrol syndrome and aggression. *Neurol Clin* 2:113–125, 1984.

Fenichel GM, Greene HL: Valproate hepatotoxicity: Two new cases, a summary of others, and recommendations. *Pediatr Neurol* 1:109–113, 1985.

Fenichel GM, Olson BJ, Fitzpatrick JE: Heart rate changes in convulsive and nonconvulsive neonatal apnea. *Ann Neurol* 7:577–582, 1980.

Fincham RW, Schottelius DD: Primidone: Relation of plasma concentrations to seizure control, in Woodbury DM, Penry JK, Pippenger CE (eds): *Antiepileptic Drugs.* New York, Raven Press, 1982, p 429–440.

Fischer JH, Lockman LA, Zaske D, et al: Phenobarbital maintenance dose requirements in treating neonatal seizures. *Neurology* 31:1042–1044, 1981.

Flanigan H, King D, Gallagher B: Surgical treatment of epilepsy, in Pedley TA, Meldrum BS (eds): *Recent Advances in Epilepsy,* Vol 2. New York, Churchill Livingstone, 1985, 297–339.

Freeman JM: The clinical spectrum and early diagnosis of Dawson's encephalitis. With preliminary notes on treatment. *J Pediatr* 75:590–603, 1969.

Fukuyama Y, Tomori N, Sugitate M: Critical evaluation of the role of immunization as an etiological factor of infantile spasms. *Neuropaediatrie* 8:224–137, 1977.

Gal P, Toback J, Boer HR, et al: Efficacy of phenobarbital monotherapy in treatment of neonatal seizures—Relationship to blood levels. *Neurology* 32:1401–1404, 1982.

Gallagher BB, Baumel IP, Mattson RH, et al: Primidone, diphenylhydantoin and phenobarbital. Aspects of acute and chronic toxicity. *Neurology* 23:145–149, 1973.

Gastaut H: Clinical and electroencephalographic correlates of generalized spike and wave bursts occurring spontaneously in man. *Epilepsia* 9:179–184, 1968.

Gastaut H, Poirier F, Payan G, et al: H.H.E. syndrome: Hemiconvulsions, hemiplegia, epilepsy. *Epilepsia* 1:418–447, 1959/1960.

Gastaut H, Roger J, Ouahchi S, et al: An electro-clinical study of generalized epileptic seizures of tonic expression. *Epilepsia* 4:15–44, 1963.

Gastaut H, Roger J, Soulayrol R, et al: Childhood epileptic encephalopathy with diffuse slow spike-waves (otherwise known as "petit mal variant") or Lennox syndrome. *Epilepsia* 7:139–179, 1966.

Gastaut H, Gastaut JL, Regis H, et al: Computerized tomography in the study of West's syndrome. *Dev Med Child Neurol* 20:21–27, 1978.

Gates JR, Leppik IE, Yap J, et al: Corpus callosotomy: Clinical and electroencephalographic effects. *Epilepsia* 25:308–316, 1984.

Geoffroy G, Lassonde M, Delisle F, et al: Corpus callosotomy for control of intractable epilepsy in children. *Neurology* 33:891–897, 1983.

Gibbs EL, Fleming MM, Gibbs FA: Diagnosis and prognosis of hypsarrhythmia and infantile spasms. *Pediatrics* 13:66–73, 1954.

Gilmore HE, Veale LA, Darras BT, et al: Lorazepam treatment of childhood status epilepticus. *Ann Neurol* 16:376, 1984.

Gomez MR: Clinical experience at Mayo Clinic, in Gomez M (ed): *Tuberous Sclerosis.* New York, Raven Press, 1979, p 11–26.

Griffith PA, Karp HR: Lorazepam in therapy for status epilepticus. *Ann Neurol* 7:493, 1980.

Hallett M: Myoclonus: Relation to epilepsy. *Epilepsia* 26 (suppl 1):S67–S77, 1985.

Hauser WA, Kurland LT: The epidemiology of epilepsy in Rochester, Minnesota, 1935 through 1967. *Epilepsia* 16:1–66, 1975.

Hauser WA, Anderson VE, Lowenson RB, et al: Seizure recurrence after a first unprovoked seizure. *N Engl J Med* 307:522–528, 1982.

Hauser WA, Rich SS, Annegers JF, Anderson VE: Seizure recurrence after a first unprovoked seizure: An extended follow-up. *Neurology* 40:1163–1170, 1990.

Heijbel J, Blom S, Berfors PG: Benign epilepsy of children with centrotemporal EEG foci. A study of incidence rate in outpatient care. *Epilepsia* 16:657–664, 1975a.

Heijbel J, Blom S, Rasmuson M: Benign epilepsy of childhood with centrotemporal EEG foci: A genetic study. *Epilepsia* 16:285–293, 1975b.

Heinz ER, Heinz TR, Radtke R, et al: Efficacy of MR vs. CT in epilepsy. *AJR* 152:347–352, 1989.

Herzlinger RA, Kandall SR, Vaughan HG: Neonatal seizures associated with narcotic withdrawal. *J Pediatr* 91:638–641, 1977.

Hirtz DG, Ellenberg JH, Nelson KB: The risk of recurrence of nonfebrile seizures in children. *Neurology* 34:637–641, 1984.

Holden KR, Mellits ED, Freeman JM: Neonatal seizures. 1. Correlation of prenatal and perinatal events with outcomes. *Pediatrics* 70:165–176, 1982.

Holmes GL: *Diagnosis and Management of Seizures in Children.* Philadelphia, WB Saunders, 1987.

Holmes GL: Electroencephalographic and neuroradiologic evaluation of children with epilepsy. *Pediatr Clin* 36:395–420, 1989.

Holmes GL, Rowe J, Hafford J, et al: Prognostic value of the electroencephalogram in neonatal asphyxia. *Electroencephalogr Clin Neurophysiol* 53:60–72, 1982.

Hoppener RJ, Kuyer A, Meijer JWA, Hulsman J: Correlation between daily fluctuations of carbamazepine serum levels and intermittent side effects. *Epilepsia* 21:341–350, 1980.

Hrachovy RA, Frost JD Jr, Kellaway P, et al: A controlled study of prednisone therapy in infantile spasms. *Epilepsia* 20:403–407, 1979.

Hrachovy RA, Frost JD Jr, Kellaway P, et al: Double-blind study of ACTH vs. prednisone therapy in infantile spasms. *J Pediatr* 103:641–645, 1983.

Huf RL, Schain RJ: Liver functions in children receiving carbamazepine. *J Pediatr* 93:884, 1978.

Huf R, Schain RJ: Long-term experience with carbamazepine (Tegretol) in children with seizures. *J Pediatr* 97:310–312, 1980.

Huttenlocher PR, Wilbourn AJ, Signore JM: Medium chain triglyceride as a therapy for intractable childhood epilepsy. *Neurology* 21:1097–1103, 1971.

Iivanainen M, Himberg JJ: Valproate and clonazepam in the treatment of severe progressive myoclonus epilepsy. *Arch Neurol* 39:236–238, 1982.

Ito M, Takao T, Okuno T, et al: Sequential CT studies of 24 children with infantile spasms on ACTH therapy. *Dev Med Child Neurol* 25:475–480, 1983.

Jan JE, Riegl JA, Crichton JU, et al: Nitrazepam in the treatment of epilepsy in childhood. *Can Med Assoc J* 104:571–575, 1971.

Jeavons PM: Non-dose-related side effects of valproate. *Epilepsia* 25(suppl 1):850–855, 1984.

Jeavons PM, Bower BD: Infantile spasms: A review of the literature and a study of 112 cases. *Clin Dev Med* 15, 1964.

Jeavons PM, Bower BD, Dimitrakoudi M: Long-term prognosis of 150 cases of "West syndrome." *Epilepsia* 14:153–164, 1973.

Jeavons PM, Clark JE, Maheshwari MD: Treatment of generalized epilepsies of childhood and adolescence with sodium valproate (Epilim). *Dev Med Child Neurol* 19:9–25, 1977.

Kalff R, Houtkooper MA, Meyer JWA, et al: Carbamazepine and serum sodium levels. *Epilepsia* 25:390–397, 1984.

Kandall SR, Gartner LM: Late presentation of drug withdrawal symptoms in newborns. *Am J Dis Child* 127:58–61, 1974.

Kellaway P, Hrachovy RA: Status epilepticus in newborns: A perspective on neonatal seizures, in Delgado-Escueta AV, Wasterlain CG, Treiman DM, et al (eds): *Advances in Neurology*, Vol 34: *Status Epilepticus*. New York, Raven Press, 1983, p 93–99.

King DW, Ajmone-Marsan C: Clinical features and ictal patterns in epileptic patients with EEG temporal lobe foci. *Ann Neurol* 2:138–147, 1977.

Korberly BH, Mrazik TJ, Graziania LJ: Ethotoin use in pediatric seizure patients. *Am J Dis Child* 135:1139–1140, 1981.

Kurokawa T, Goya N, Fukuyama Y, et al: West syndrome and Lennox-Gastaut syndrome: A survey of natural history. *Pediatrics* 65:81–88, 1980.

Lacey DJ: Agenesis of the corpus callosum. Clinical features in 40 children. *Am J Dis Child* 139:953–955, 1985.

Lacey DJ, Singer WD, Horwitz SJ, et al: Lorazepam therapy of status epilepticus in children and adolescents. *J Pediatr* 108:771–774, 1986.

Lacy CR, Penry JK (eds): *Infantile Spasms*. New York, Raven Press, 1976.

Lagenstein I, Sternowsky HJ, Rothe M, et al: CCT in different epilepsies with grand mal and focal seizures in 309 children: Relation to clinical and electroencephalographic data. *Neuropediatrics* 11:323–328, 1980.

Lance JW, Adams RD: The syndrome of intention or action myoclonus as a sequel to hypoxic encephalopathy. *Brain* 86:111–136, 1983.

Lance JW, Anthony M: Sodium valproate and clonazepam in the treatment of intractable absence seizures in children. *Am J Dis Child* 136:526–629, 1982.

Landau WM, Kleffner FR: Syndrome of acquired aphasia with convulsive disorder in children. *Neurology* 7:523–530, 1957.

Laplante P, Saint-Hilare JM, Bouvier G: Headache as an epileptic manifestation. *Neurology* 33:1493–1495, 1983.

Levantine A, Almeyda J: Drug reactions XX—Cutaneous reactions to anticonvulsants. *Br J Dermatol* 87:646–649, 1972.

Levy RJ, Krall RL: Treatment of status epilepticus with lorazepam. *Arch Neurol* 41:605–611, 1984.

Lindsay J, Ounsted C, Richards P: Long-term outcome in children with temporal lobe seizures. I. Social outcome and childhood factors. *Dev Med Child Neurol* 21:285–298, 1979a.

Lindsay J, Ounsted C, Richards P: Long-term outcome in children with temporal lobe seizures. II. Marriage, parenthood, and sexual indifference. *Dev Med Child Neurol* 21:433–440, 1979b.

Lindsay J, Ounsted C, Richards P: Long-term outcome in children with temporal lobe seizures. III. Psychiatric aspects in childhood and adult life. *Dev Med Child Neurol* 21:630–636, 1979c.

Lindsay J, Ounsted C, Richards P: Long-term outcome in children with temporal lobe seizures. IV. Genetic factors, febrile convulsions, and the remission of seizures. *Dev Med Child Neurol* 21:429–439, 1980.

Lindsay J, Ounsted C, Richards P: Long-term outcome in children with temporal lobe seizures. V. Indications and contra-indications for neurosurgery. *Dev Med Child Neurol* 26:25–32, 1984.

Lockman LA, Kriel R, Zaske D, et al: Phenobarbital dosage for control of neonatal seizures. *Neurology* 29:1445–1449, 1979.

Loiseau P: Sodium valproate, platelet dysfunction, and bleeding. *Epilepsia* 22:141–146, 1981.

Loiseau P, Beaussart M: The seizures of benign childhood epilepsy with rolandic paroxysmal discharges. *Epilepsia* 14:381–389, 1973.

Loiseau P, Pestre M, Dartigues JF, Commenges D, Barberger-Gateau C, Cohadon S.: Long-term prognosis in two forms of childhood epilepsy: Typical absence seizures and epilepsy with rolandic (centrotemporal) EEG foci. *Ann Neurol* 13:642–648, 1983.

Lombroso CT: Prognosis in neonatal seizures, in Delgado-Escueta AV, Wasterlain CG, Treeman DM, et al (eds): *Advances in Neurology*, Vol 34: *Status Epilepticus*. New York, Raven Press, 1983, p 101–113.

Lombroso CT, Fejerman N: Benign myoclonus of early infancy. *Ann Neurol* 1:138–143, 1977.

Luders H, Lesser RP, Dinner DS, et al: Generalized epilepsies: A review. *Cleveland Clin Q* 51:205–226, 1984.

McAbee GN, Barasch ES, Kurfist LA: Results of computed tomography in "neurologically normal" children after initial onset of seizures. *Pediatr Neurol* 5:102–106, 1989.

McBride MC, Dooling EC, Oppenheimer EY: Complex partial status epilepticus in young children. *Ann Neurol* 9:526–530, 1981.

McKeever M, Holmes GL, Russman BS: Speech abnormalities in seizures: A comparison of absence and partial complex seizures. *Brain Lang* 19:25–32, 1983.

Markand ON, Wheeler GL, Pollack SL: Complex partial status epilepticus (psychomotor status). *Neurology* 28:189–196, 1978.

Matsumoto A, Watanabe K, Negoro T, et al: Long-term prognosis after infantile spasms: A statistical study of prognostic factors in 200 cases. *Dev Med Child Neurol* 23:51–65, 1981.

Matthews WB, Wright FK: Hereditary primary reading epilepsy. *Neurology* 17:919–921, 1967.

Mattson RH: Phenobarbital, primidone (Mysoline), and

mephobarbital (Mebaral), in Brown TR, Feldman RG (eds): *Epilepsy: Diagnosis and Management.* Boston, Little, Brown, 1983, 191-201.

Mattson RH, Cramer JA: Phenobarbital: Toxicity, in Levy R, Mattson R, Meldrum B, Penry JK, Dreifuss FE (eds): *Antiepileptic Drugs.* New York, Raven Press, 1989, p 341-355.

Mattson RH, Cramer JA, Williamson PD, et al: Valproic acid in epilepsy: Clinical and pharmacologic effects. *Ann Neurol* 3:20-25, 1978.

Mayeux R, Lueders H: Complex partial status epilepticus: Case report and proposal for diagnostic criteria. *Neurology* 28:957-961, 1978.

Melchior JC: Infantile spasms and early immunization against whooping cough. Danish survey from 1970 to 1975, *Arch Dis Child* 52:134-137, 1977.

Metrakos K, Metrakos JD: Genetics of convulsive disorders. II. Genetic and electroencephalographic studies in centrencephalic epilepsy. *Neurology* 11:474-483, 1961.

Mikati M: The newer antiepileptic drugs: Carbamazepine and valproic acid. *Pediatr Ann* 20:34-40, 1991.

Miles D, Holmes GL: Benign neonatal seizures. *J Clin Neurophysiol* 7:369-379, 1990.

Mitchell WG, Greenwood RS, Messenheimer JA: Abdominal epilepsy. Cyclic vomiting as the major symptom of simple partial seizures. *Arch Neurol* 40:251-252, 1983.

Mizrahi EM, Kellaway R: Characterization and classification of neonatal seizures. *Neurology* 37:1837-1844, 1987.

Morselli PL, Principi N, Tognoni G, et al: Diazepam elimination in premature and full term infants, and children. *J Perinat Med* 1:133-141, 1973.

Neophytides AN, Nutt JG, Lodish JR: Thrombocytopenia associated with sodium valproate treatment. *Ann Neurol* 5:389-390, 1979.

Opitz A, Marschall M, Degen R, et al: General anesthesia in patients with epilepsy and status epilepticus, in Delgado-Escueta AV, Wasterlain CG, Treiman DM, et al (eds): *Advances in Neurology,* Vol 34: *Status Epilepticus.* New York, Raven Press, 1983, p 531-535.

Painter MJ: How to use phenobarbital, in Morselli PL, Pippenger CE, Penry JK (eds): *Antiepileptic Drug Therapy in Pediatrics.* New York, Raven Press, 1983a, p 245-252.

Painter MJ: How to use primidone, in Morselli PL, Pippenger CE, Penry JK (eds): *Antiepileptic Drug Therapy in Pediatrics.* New York, Raven Press, 1983b, p 263-270.

Painter MJ, Pippenger C, MacDonald H, et al: Phenobarbital and diphenylhydantoin levels in neonates with seizures. *J Pediatr* 92:315-319, 1978.

Painter MJ, Pippenger C, Wasterlain C, et al: Phenobarbital and phenytoin in neonatal seizures: Metabolism and tissue distribution. *Neurology* 31:1107-1112, 1981.

Pampiglione G, Pugh E: Infantile spasms and subsequent appearance of tuberous sclerosis syndrome. *Lancet* 2:1046, 1975.

Papini M, Pasquinelli A, Armellini M, et al: Alertness and incidence of seizures in patients with Lennox-Gastaut syndrome. *Epilepsia* 25:161-167, 1984.

Parker WA, Shearer CA: Phenytoin hepatotoxicity: A case report and review. *Neurology* 29:175-178, 1979.

Pettit RE, Fenichel GM: Benign familial neonatal seizures. *Arch Neurol* 37:47-48, 1980.

Pinder RM, Brogden RN, Speight TM, et al: Sodium valproate: A review of its pharmacological properties and therapeutic efficacy in epilepsy. *Drugs* 13:81-123, 1977.

Porter RJ, Penry JK, Lacy JR: Diagnostic and therapeutic re-evaluation of patients with intractable epilepsy. *Neurology* 27:1006-1011, 1977.

Rasmussen T, Olszewski J, Lloyd-Smith D: Focal seizures due to chronic localized encephalitis. *Neurology* 8:435-445, 1958.

Redenbaugh JE, Sato S, Penry JK, et al: Sodium valproate: Pharmacokinetics and effectiveness in treating intractable seizures. *Neurology* 30:1-6, 1980.

Riikonen R: A long-term follow-up study of 214 children with the syndrome of infantile spasms. *Neuropediatrics* 13:14-23, 1982.

Rose AL, Lombroso CT: Neonatal seizure states. A study of clinical, pathological and electroencephalographic features in 137 full-term babies with a long-term followup. *Pediatrics* 45:404-425, 1970.

Rossi LN, Nino M, Principi N: Correlation between age and plasma level/dosage ratio for phenobarbital in infants and children. *Acta Paediatr Scand* 68:431-434, 1979.

Rowan AJ, Meijer JW, de Beer-Pawlikowski N, et al: Valproate-ethosuximide combination therapy for refractory absence seizures. *Arch Neurol* 40:797-802, 1983.

Rowe JC, Holmes GL, Hafford J, et al: Prognostic value of the electroencephalogram in term and preterm infants following neonatal seizures. *Electroencephalogr Clin Neurophysiol* 60:183-196, 1985.

Sarnat HB, Sarnat MS: Neonatal encephalopathy following fetal distress. A clinical and electroencephalographic study. *Arch Neurol* 33:696-705, 1976.

Sato S, Dreifuss FE, Penry JK: Prognostic factors in absence seizures. *Neurology* 26:788-796, 1976.

Sato S, Dreifuss FE, Penry JK, et al: Long-term follow-up of absence seizures. *Neurology* 33:1590-1595, 1983.

Schmidley KW, Simon RP: Postictal pleocytosis. *Ann Neurol* 9:81-84, 1981.

Schneider H, Vassella F, Karbowski K: The Lennox syndrome. A clinical study of 40 children. *Eur Neurol* 4:289-300, 1970.

Sherard ES, Steiman GS, Couri D: Treatment of childhood epilepsy with valproic acid: Results of the first 100 patients in a six-month trial. *Neurology* 30:31-35, 1980.

Shinnar S, Ballaban-Gil K: An approach to the child with a first unprovoked seizure. *Pediatr Ann* 20:29-33, 1991.

Shinnar S, Berg AT, Moshé SL, et al: Risk of seizure recurrence following a first unprovoked seizure in childhood: A prospective study. *Pediatrics* 85:1076-1085, 1990.

Simon D, Penry JK: Sodium di-n-propylacetae (DPA) in the treatment of epilepsy: A review. *Epilepsia* 16:549-573, 1975.

Singer WD, Rabe EF, Haller JS: The effect of ACTH therapy upon infantile spasms. *J Pediatr* 96:485-489, 1980.

Smith BT, Masotti E: Intravenous diazepam in the treatment of prolonged seizure activity in neonates and infants. *Dev Med Child Neurol* 13:630-634, 1971.

Smith DB, Mattson RH, Cramer JA, Collins JF, Novelly RA, Craft B: Results of a nationwide Veterans Administration Cooperative Study comparing the efficacy and toxicity of carbamazepine, phenobarbital, phenytoin, and primidone. *Epilepsia* 28:S50-S58, 1987.

Snead OC, Hosey LC: Exacerbation of seizures in children by carbamazepine. *N Engl J Med* 313:916-921, 1985.

Snodgrass GJAI, Stimmler L, Went J, et al: Interrelations of plasma calcium, inorganic phosphate, magnesium, and protein over the first week of life. *Arch Dis Child* 48:279-285, 1979.

Sofijanov NG: Clinical evolution and prognosis of childhood epilepsies. *Epilepsia* 23:61–69, 1982.

Spencer DD, Spencer SS, Mattson RH, et al: Intracerebral masses in patients with intractable partial epilepsy. *Neurology* 34:432–436, 1984.

Suchy FJ, Balistreri WF, Buchino JJ, et al: Acute hepatic failure associated with the use of sodium valproate. *N Engl J Med* 300:962–966, 1979.

Sussman NM, McLain LW: A direct hepatotoxic effect of valproic acid. *JAMA* 242:1173–1174, 1979.

Tassinari CA, Daniele O, Michelucci R, et al: Benzodiazepines: Efficacy in status epilepticus, in Delgado-Escueta AV, Wasterlain CB, Treiman DM, et al (eds): *Advances in Neurology*, Vol 34: *Status Epilepticus*. New York, Raven Press, 1983, p 465–475.

Thomas JE, Reagan TJ, Klass DW: Epilepsia partialis continua. *Arch Neurol* 34:266–275, 1977.

Thompson PJ, Trimble MR: Anticonvulsant drugs and cognitive functions. *Epilepsia* 23:531–544, 1982.

Thorpy MJ: Rectal valproate syrup and status epilepticus. *Neurology* 30:1113–1114, 1980.

Tibbles JAR: Dominant benign neonatal seizures. *Dev Med Child Neurol* 22:664–667, 1980.

Trimble MR: Anticonvulsant drugs and psychosocial development: Phenobarbitone, sodium valproate, and benzodiazepines, in Morselli PL, Pippenger CE, Penry JK (eds): *Antiepileptic Drug Therapy in Pediatrics*. New York, Raven Press, 1983, p 201–217.

Trimble MR, Thompson PJ: Sodium valproate and cognitive function. *Epilepsia* 25(suppl 1):S55–S63, 1985.

Troupin AS: Carbamazepine re-examined, in Pedley TA, and Meldrum BS (eds): *Recent Advances in Epilepsy*, Vol 1. Edinburgh, Churchill Livingstone, 1983, p 47–56.

Vajda FJE, Mihaly GW, Miles JL, et al: Rectal administration of sodium valproate in status epilepticus. *Neurology* 28:897–899, 1978.

Viani F, Jussi MI, Germano M: Rectal administration of sodium valproate for neonatal and infantile status epilepticus. *Dev Med Child Neurol* 26:677–680, 1984.

Villarreal HJ, Wilder BJ, Willmore LJ, et al: Effect of valproic acid on spike and wave discharges in patients with absence seizures. *Neurology* 28:886–891, 1978.

Volpe JJ: Neonatal seizures. *Clin Perinatol* 4:43–63, 1977.

Walker JE, Homan RW, Vasko MR, et al: Lorazepam in status epilepticus. *Ann Neurol* 6:207–213, 1979.

Walson PD, Mimaki T, Curless R, et al: Once daily doses of phenobarbital in children. *J Pediatr* 97:303–305, 1980.

Watanabe K, Harra K, Hakamada S: Seizures with apnea in children. *Pediatrics* 70:87–90, 1982.

Wilder BJ, Ramsey RE, Willmore LJ, et al: Efficacy of intravenous phenytoin in the treatment of status epilepticus. Kinetics of central nervous system penetration. *Ann Neurol* 1:511–518, 1977.

Wilder BJ, Karas BJ, Penry JK, et al: Gastrointestinal tolerance of divalproex sodium. *Neurology* 33:808–811, 1983a.

Wilder BJ, Ramsay RE, Murphy JV, et al: Comparison of valproic acid and phenytoin in newly diagnosed tonic-clonic seizures. *Neurology* 33:1474–1476, 1983b.

Williamson PD, Spencer DD, Spencer SS, et al: Complex partial seizures of frontal lobe origin. *Ann Neurol* 198:497–504, 1985.

Willmore LJ, Wilder BJ, Bruni J, et al: Effect of valproic acid on hepatic function. *Neurology* 28:961–964, 1978.

Wilson DH, Reeves AG, Gazzaniga MS: Division of the corpus callosum for uncontrollable epilepsy. *Neurology* 28:649–653, 1978.

Wilson DH, Reeves AG, Gazzaniga MS: "Central" commissurotomy for intractable generalized epilepsy: Series two. *Neurology* 32:687–697, 1982.

Wolf SM, Forsythe A, Stunden AA, et al: Long-term effect of phenobarbital on cognitive function in children with febrile convulsions. *Pediatrics* 68:820–823, 1981.

Yagi K, Mihara T, Tottori T, et al: Focal CT abnormality and epileptogenic focus. *Jpn J Psychiatr Neurol* 43:373–377, 1989.

Yang PJ, Berger PE, Cohen ME, et al: Computed tomography and childhood seizure disorders. *Neurology* 29:1084–1088, 1979.

Young AC, Costanzi JB, Mohr PD, et al: Is routine computerized axial tomography in epilepsy worthwhile? *Lancet* 2:1446–1447, 1982.

Zaret BS, Beckner RR, Marini AM, et al: Sodium valproate-induced hyperammonemia without clinical hepatic dysfunction. *Neurology* 32:206–208, 1982.

Movement Disorders

Raymond W.M. Chun
Steven M. Shapiro

Great strides have been made over the past three decades in elucidating the neurochemical and neurophysiologic mechanisms underlying several disorders of involuntary movement, most notably Parkinson's disease and Huntington's disease. The information acquired has significantly enhanced the understanding and management of cases of these disorders, most of which occur in adults. However, the basic pathophysiologic processes of movement disorders in children are not well characterized. Until data from research in this area become available, diagnostic and management decisions regarding children with movement disorders must be made on the basis of clinical information.

For the purpose of this discussion, movement disorders (dyskinesias) are defined as those characterized by involuntary movements, caused by extrapyramidal dysfunction, which interfere with normal motor function. Traditionally, diseases that affect only the cerebral cortex, pyramidal system, cerebellum, anterior horn cells, and neuromuscular systems are excluded from this group. However, it is difficult to provide a comprehensive classification of specific disorders and many diseases of the nervous system affect more than one system. Moreover, movement disorders caused by recognized biochemic or enzymatic defects are included in the classification of metabolic diseases. Others may present as pathology of an organ outside the nervous system and therefore may be classified with diseases specific to that organ. In this chapter, specific movement disorders are grouped with other conditions presenting with a particular dyskinesia. For diagnostic purposes, the dyskinesias are divided into five types: chorea or choreoathetosis, dystonia, tremor, tic, and myoclonus. Each has its own differential diagnosis.

ANATOMY AND FUNCTION

The extrapyramidal system plays an important role in the control and execution of motor movements. It consists of the basal ganglia, thalamus, subthalamic nuclei, substantia nigra, red nuclei, and brainstem reticular formation.

The basal ganglia are composed of the corpus striatum and the amygdaloid nuclear complex. The amygdala is not involved in movement and is not usually considered as part of the extrapyramidal system. The term *corpus striatum* refers to the caudate, putamen, and globus pallidus. *Neostriatum*, or just *striatum*, refers to the caudate and putamen; *pallidum* refers to the globus pallidus. The neostriatum and pallidum are phylogenetically, cytologically, and functionally distinct. *Lenticular nucleus*, a descriptive term, refers to the combination of the putamen and globus pallidus.

The extrapyramidal fiber pathways are complex and not completely understood. However, understanding the complexity of the extrapyramidal system is perhaps the key to understanding its function. A simplified discussion is presented here; for more detail the interested reader is referred to textbooks of neuroanatomy (Carpenter and Sutin, 1983; Gilman and Newman, 1987).

The neostriatum receives fibers from the cerebral cortex, the intralaminar nuclei of the thalamus nuclei, the substantia nigra, and the globus pallidus, and it sends fibers to the substantia nigra and globus pallidus (Figure 9-1).

Corticostriate fiber inputs from widespread areas of the cerebral cortex end on dendritic spines in the striatum. The anterior half of the hemisphere, including the sensorimotor cortex, is topographically related to a larger part of the striatum than is the posterior half of the hemisphere. The sensorimotor cortex projects ipsilaterally and contralaterally through the corpus callosum; the other cortical areas only project ipsilaterally.

The thalamostriate fibers from the intralaminar nuclei of the thalamus project profusely on the striatum with collaterals having diffuse cortical distribution. The centromedian-parafascicular nuclear complex projects to the putamen with precise topographic organization; smaller, more rostral intralaminar nuclei (medial central,

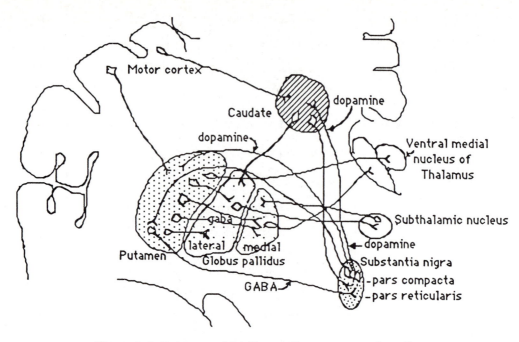

Figure 9-1. Extrapyramidal fiber pathways: coronal section.

paracentral, and lateral central) project to the caudate nucleus.

The pars compacta of the substantia nigra sends topographically arranged nigrostriatal fibers to the striatum. Nigrostriatal fibers traverse the inferior capsule and portions of the globus pallidus en route to dendritic spines in the putamen. With lesions in the substantia nigra or internal capsule, the dopamine content of striatum is markedly reduced.

Efferent pathways from the striatum include the striatonigral fibers to the substantia nigra and reciprocal and striatonigral fibers and striopallidal fibers to the

lateral and medial segments of the globus pallidus.

The major output from the basal ganglia is via pallidofugal pathways from the globus pallidus (Figure 9-2).

Fibers from the medial segment of the globus pallidus go to the ventrolateral, ventral anterior, and intralaminar nuclei of the thalamus through the ansa lenticularis and the lenticular fasciculus. Efferents from the lateral segment of the globus pallidus go to the subthalamic nucleus, which in turn sends fibers to the medial segment. Finally, the medial segment sends fibers to brainstem pontine nuclei (pedunculopontine tegmental nucleus). The

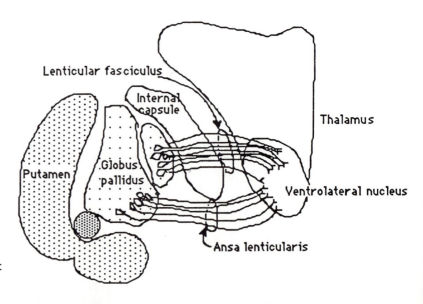

Figure 9-2. Extrapyramidal fiber pathways: horizontal section.

ventral nucleus of the thalamus also receives cerebellar input (dentatothalamic) and projects to the primary motor cortex. Fibers from the globus pallidus also project to the subthalamic nucleus and the brainstem tegmentum.

The extrapyramidal system can be thought of as a complex series of interconnected feedback loops that ultimately, through modulation of the direct corticospinal pyramidal pathways, influence movement. An example is a loop that connects cerebral cortex to striatum to globus pallidus to thalamus and back to cerebral cortex; another loops from striatum to substantia nigra and back again to striatum.

Striatal neurons fire prior to the onset of movement, suggesting that the basal ganglia participate in the initiation of movement. The extrapyramidal system also participates in control of ongoing movement, posture, and automatic and skilled volitional movement. Unilateral lesions in the subthalamic nuclei produce the wild flinging movements of hemiballismus; lesions elsewhere in the extrapyramidal system have generally not produced such clear effects.

Many extrapyramidal movement disorders are associated with disorders of neurotransmitter systems. Acetylcholine (ACh), glutamine, dopamine, and γ-aminobutyric acid (GABA) are important neurotransmitters in the extrapyramidal systems. Drug agonists and antagonists of these neurotransmitter systems may reproduce or ameliorate the symptoms of extrapyramidal movement disorders.

Cortical stimulation produces glutamate-mediated excitatory postsynaptic potentials in strial neurons, which are followed by inhibitory postsynaptic potentials owing to GABA-mediated striatal feedback inhibition. ACh is present in high concentration in the striatum, where it has an excitatory effect. Dopamine, an inhibitory neurotransmitter, is synthesized in the pars compacta of the substantia nigra and is present at the striatal endings of these fibers. GABA is present in the substantia nigra, striatum, and globus pallidus, where it probably has inhibitory functions.

A functional equilibrium exists between the excitatory ACh and the inhibitory dopamine systems. The reduction of dopamine in the striatum and substantia nigra in Parkinson's disease, and a relative increase in the cholinergic neurotransmitter system, are associated with akinesia or bradykinesia. The degeneration of GABA and cholinergic striatal neurons in Huntington's disease, with relatively preserved dopaminergic function, is associated with chorea.

The functional equilibrium between the ACh and dopaminergic systems is paralleled by symptomatology. Parkinsonian symptoms respond favorably to dopaminergic or anticholinergic drugs; an excess of these agents produces chorea and other hyperkinesias. The chorea of Huntington's disease is exacerbated by L-dopa, and treated with cholinergics or dopamine blockers.

DEFINITION AND DESCRIPTION OF MOVEMENTS

Because the precise pathologic, pharmacologic, and neurophysiologic mechanisms of movement disorders are not completely understood, clinical features provide the most reliable basis for their classification and differentiation. In childhood, the principal dyskinesias that occur as a dysfunction of the extrapyramidal system are athetosis, chorea, dystonia, tremors, and tics. Athetosis is characterized by slow, sinuous, writhing, and purposeless involuntary movements, which may flow into one another. The wrists are usually held in a flexed position, and the fingers, the shoulders, and much of the lower extremities are held in extension. Athetotic movements are exaggerated by voluntary activity and are not noted during sleep.

Choreic movements are single, quick, isolated muscle movements that result in uncoordinated jerks of the face, trunk, or extremities. Patients at times may attempt to conceal movements that occur distally by converting a sudden purposeless movement of the upper extremity into a purposeful act, such as pretending to straighten a tie. Often choreic movements occur in combination with athetosis, in which case the term *choreoathetosis* is used.

Dystonia refers to abnormal muscle tone in which there are slow, sustained contractions of the larger axial and some appendicular muscles, resulting in postural abnormalities. Patients with torsion dystonia (dystonia musculorum deformans) display contortions of the trunk and pelvic and shoulder girdles.

Tics are brief, sudden contractions of a muscle or muscle group. Children with Gilles de la Tourette syndrome have multiple tics, including vocal tics (throat clearing), shoulder shrugging, and grimacing. More often, however, tics are localized and affect only one muscle group, e.g., eye blinking.

The main abnormal movements that occur as a result of cerebellar dysfunction are tremor and ataxia. Tremors are involuntary, rhythmic, oscillatory movements caused by the alternate contractions of agonist and antagonist muscles. Intention tremor refers to the decomposition of movement that occurs during motion, such as on finger-to-nose testing.

Tremor may also result from an extrapyramidal disorder. The static tremor of adult Parkinson's disease occurs during rest. The cause of benign essential tremor is unknown.

Ataxia refers to uncoordination of motor function. When a child with cerebellar disease is asked to touch his or her nose with the tip of an index finger, the movement is performed in an unsteady, halting manner. Ataxic movements may occur in the extremities (appendicular) and/or in the axial musculature (truncal).

CLINICAL DESCRIPTIONS OF MOVEMENT DISORDERS

Disorders Presenting with Chorea, Athetosis, or Both

The differential diagnosis of disorders presenting with chorea or choreoathetosis primarily includes Sydenham's chorea, Huntington's disease, benign familial chorea, and the choreic conditions associated with static encephalopathy and systemic illnesses. While quick, uncoordinated, choreic jerks or choreoathetoid movements are seen during neurologic examination, this group of disorders is not similar in other aspects. The onset, duration, and progressive nature of the movement disorder provide important clues in the differential diagnosis. Each disorder must be recognized and treated individually.

Sydenham's Chorea

The child with Sydenham's chorea is punished three times before a diagnosis is made:

> Once for general fidgetiness, once for breaking crockery, and once for making faces at his grandmother.

> The unending profusion of quick purpose-like little movements, appearing at random mainly in distal segments and disfiguring the facies of childhood by a series of smirks or frowns, is pathognomonic. (Wilson and Bruce, 1955)

The choreic movements of Sydenham's chorea are quasipurposeful fragments of movements that occur in a disorderly fashion. Choreic movements are explosive and abrupt, increase with stress, and occasionally blend into athetosis. There is a disturbance of associated movements.

Rheumatic fever is a postinflammatory disease that may affect heart, joint, central nervous system, and subcutaneous tissue. It follows a group A β-hemolytic streptococcal pharyngitis. The incidence of Sydenham's chorea has gradually diminished over the years, in part owing to the introduction of antibiotics effective against this organism.

Pathology and Pathogenesis. Sydenham's chorea affects the caudate and subthalamic nuclei, cerebral cortex, trigeminal nerve, geniculate ganglion, and medullary hypoglossal nucleus. With neurologic symptoms there is arteritis of small meningeal and cortical vessels, embolism, and, rarely, meningoencephalitis with perivascular and diffuse round cell infiltration of gray and white matter.

There is experimental evidence that Sydenham's chorea is due to an autoimmune response. Serum γ-globulin from patients with Sydenham's chorea binds to caudate and subthalamus brain tissue in direct proportion to the clinical severity of the chorea (Husby et al., 1976). There is cross-reactivity between these central nervous system tissues and the bacteria, because binding activity can be abolished by preabsorption with group A streptococcal membranes.

Functional overactivity of the dopaminergic system in Sydenham's chorea is suggested by the finding of increased homovanillic acid (a dopamine metabolite) in cerebrospinal fluid (Naidu and Narasimhachari, 1980). Patients have an increased reaction to dopamine-active drugs (Nausieda et al., 1983). Drugs that release dopamine or sensitive postsynaptic dopamine receptors (e.g., amphetamines, L-dopa, decongestants, phenytoin, thyroid hormones) increase chorea; drugs that block dopamine receptors (e.g., haloperidol) decrease chorea.

Clinical Aspects. The onset of Sydenham's chorea is usually insidious, causing clumsiness, restlessness, fidgetiness, and fatigue. The abnormal movements begin in the face. Unlike Huntington's disease, Sydenham's chorea affects the upper extremities more than the lower extremities, and the distal muscles are more affected than the proximal. Speech is dysarthric and patients may even become mute. Onset occurs between 5 and 15 years of age and the sex ratio is about 50:50 until puberty, when females are affected twice as often as males. There may be a positive family history for rheumatic fever.

The physical signs associated with Sydenham's chorea are summarized in Table 9–1.

Chorea is most often generalized, but one out of five patients has hemichorea (Nausieda et al., 1980). Hemiparesis, seizures, or EEG abnormalities may occur rarely. Mental and emotional disturbances may occur before, during, or after the onset of the illness.

The natural history of the disorder is that one quarter to one third of patients with "pure" chorea who never have any other signs of rheumatic fever will eventually

FEATURE TABLE 9–1. SYDENHAM'S CHOREA

Discriminating Features	Consistent Features	Variable Features
1. Chorea 2. Chorea should be gone 2 years after onset	1. Generalized chorea 2. Subacute 3. Usually chorea disappears by 1 month	1. Insidious onset 2. Distal > proximal 3. Hemichorea 4. Mental and emotional disturbance 5. Recurrence within 2 years in 20% of cases

TABLE 9-1. PHYSICAL SIGNS ASSOCIATED WITH SYDENHAM'S CHOREA

Sign	Explanation
Milkmaid's grip	Inability to maintain a sustained handgrip contraction
Darting tongue	Inability to maintain tongue protrusion
Pronator sign	External rotation of the hands when arms are held over head
Choreic hand	"Dishing hand" or "spoon hand"
"Hung up" deep tendon reflexes	Evoked choreic movement when deep tendon reflex (e.g., knee jerk) is elicited, resulting in a slow return to original position
Pendular knee jerks	Antagonist hypotonia
Diffuse hypotonia	Floppy muscular tone
Abnormal speech	Indistinct, jerky, explosive, and irregular respiration

develop rheumatic heart disease. If other manifestations of rheumatic fever occur at any time, the risk of heart disease is greatly increased (Aron et al., 1965).

The course of the disease is *subacute*. Often chorea and associated findings disappear by 1 month, and invariably are gone by 2 years. About 20% of patients develop a second episode of chorea, usually within 2 years of the first attack (Nausieda et al., 1983).

Uncomplicated Sydenham's chorea is not necessarily a benign self-limited disorder of the central nervous system, though the neurologic sequelae are minimal. Mild motor abnormalities, such as choreiform movements, hypotonia, intention tremor, and impaired fine and gross motor abilities, have been found 20 years after the initial episode (M.T. Bird et al., 1976; Nausieda et al., 1983). Psychiatric symptoms are more frequent in patients evaluated two to three decades after the onset of Sydenham's chorea (Freeman et al., 1965).

Commonly prescribed drugs—such as phenytoin, female sex hormones and thyroid hormones (which sensitize postsynaptic striatal dopamine receptors), decongestants (sympathomimetic or anticholinergic), and *d*-amphetamine—may induce chorea at low doses in patients with a previous history of Sydenham's chorea. Nausieda et al. (1983) found dopaminergic hypersensitivity (adverse choreic reactions to these drugs) in about half of patients who had had Sydenham's chorea for an average of 22 years. These patients also had elevations in their Minnesota Multiphasic Personality Inventory scores, indicative of a potential for psychotic thought processes. These findings are consistent with the notion of chronic hypersensitivity of the dopaminergic system with effects on both motor and mental function in some patients following episodes of Sydenham's chorea.

Treatments for Sydenham's chorea have included bed rest, sedation, diazepam, haloperidol, chlorpromazine valproate, baclofen, and steroids, but their efficacy has not been well established. Neuroleptics such as chlor-

promazine decrease involuntary movements and are useful in other choreic disorders (Klawans and Weiner, 1976). Because of the high incidence of associated serious heart disease, penicillin or other antibiotic prophylaxis is indicated until adulthood.

Sydenham's chorea should be differentiated from other conditions in which chorea is a clinical manifestation, e.g., systemic lupus erythematosus, drug reactions, (phenothiazines, haloperidol, reserpine, isoniazid, L-dopa, phenytoin, oral contraceptives), Wilson's disease, Huntington's disease, paroxysmal choreoathetosis, familial benign choreoathetosis, static encephalopathy, attention deficit disorder and tic.

Huntington's Disease

In 1967, I sat reading in the National Airport in Washington, D.C., with tears streaming down my face. . . . My husband Woody lay dying in a mental hospital, his illness diagnosed as Huntington's chorea. My three little children were at home. I had no one to talk to, and when I finally boarded the plane to return to New York City I felt weak and the words "hopeless and helpless" were ringing in my ears. Reading the hereditary aspects troubled me the most. How could I live knowing that any or all of my children might inherit their father's disease? (Guthrie, 1982)

Huntington's disease is an autosomal, dominantly inherited, neurodegenerative disease. Juvenile-onset Huntington's disease, with onset at or before 10 years of age, occurs in about 5% of reported cases (Jervis, 1963; Osborne et al., 1982). The onset, presentation, and course of Huntington's disease differ in juveniles and adults.

Adult-onset Huntington's disease may present as (1) abnormal movements, especially chorea, (2) intellectual decline and dementia, (3) emotional instability, or (4) some combination of the foregoing. The course is slowly progressive, and unaffected by current treatment.

Juvenile-onset Huntington's disease most often presents with rigidity (the Westphal variant), speech defects, intellectual abnormalities, chorea or choreoathetosis, and tremor (Markham and Knox, 1965; Hansotia et al., 1968). Cerebellar signs and seizures are also frequent.

In contrast to patients with adult-onset Huntington's disease, seizures occur in up to 50% of children; the seizures are either grand mal or grand mal in combination with petit mal, myoclonic, astatic, or photosensitive seizures. The juvenile-onset disease progresses about twice as rapidly as the adult-onset version, with an average duration of 9.3 years (Osborne et al., 1982).

Table 9-2 presents a comparison of juvenile- and adult-onset Huntington's disease.

The pathologic findings include atrophy of the corpus striatum and, in contrast to adult-onset cases, severe gliosis of the globus pallidus and cerebellar atrophy. Involvement of the vestibular nuclei and the lateral corticospinal tracts has also been described. The damage to

TABLE 9-2. COMPARISON OF JUVENILE- AND ADULT-ONSET HUNTINGTON'S DISEASE

	Juvenile-Onset	Adult-Onset
Symptoms	Rigidity	Chorea
	Speech disorder	Dementia
	Behavioral abnormality	Emotional effects
	Seizures	Combinations
	Cerebellar signs	
Pathology	Striatum, globus pallidus, cerebellum	Striatum
Inheritance from:	Father in 80%–90% (Myers et al., 1983)	Mother in 55%–70% (Farrer and Connelly, 1985)

the globus pallidus has been proposed to be responsible for the prominence of rigidity in children (Byers and Dodge, 1967).

Diagnosis is difficult in the absence of a family history. Until recently, laboratory tests were not helpful. Computed tomograhic (CT) scans and magnetic resonance imaging (MRI) may show atrophy of the caudate nuclei, which often precedes clinical symptomatology (Terrence et al., 1977; Sax and Menzer, 1977). Additionally, cerebellar atrophy is seen in children. Positron emission tomographic scans show decreased glucose use in the caudate and putamen, which appears earlier than the tissue loss demonstrable by CT (Kuhl et al., 1982).

Recent studies have localized the defective genetic material in Huntington's disease to a single locus on the telomere of the short arm of chromosome 4. A genetic probe (G8) is now available, but its usefulness for presymptomatic testing is limited by its nonspecificity for the *HD* locus and the need for testing multiple family members. An overall 12% error rate for presymptomatic testing with this technique has been estimated (Folstein et al., 1985). Concern has been raised regarding the potentially damaging psychologic effects of presymptomatic testing for this devastating disease. However, studies show that 75% to 80% of people at risk for Huntington's disease wish to know this information in order to cope, plan, and prepare for the future (Koller and Davenport, 1984).

Management consists of symptomatic treatment and genetic counseling. The chorea may respond to such dopamine receptor blockers as haloperidol or dopamine depletors, e.g., reserpine. Supportive management by members of a multidisciplinary team is helpful.

Benign Familial Chorea

The condition of benign familial chorea was initially described in 1967 (Haerer et al., 1967). Several authors have stated that more cases of benign familial chorea exist than have been reported, so that it is difficult to estimate the prevalence of this syndrome (Chun et al., 1973; Sleigh and Lindenbaum, 1981). The syndrome is characterized by the early onset of nonprogressive chorea and is unassociated with intellectual deterioration. Lack of progressive dementia distinguishes it from Huntington's disease. The persistence of involuntary movements for many years distinguishes this condition from Sydenham's chorea. A history of familial occurrence makes the diagnosis of a choreic form of cerebral palsy unlikely.

The abnormal movements usually have their onset early, during infancy or childhood, and are often first noted when the child begins to walk. The gait of children with the syndrome is noticeably more lurching and halting than that of other children learning to walk. The abnormal movements persist throughout adulthood, and characteristically show little or no progression. On reaching middle age, some individuals use walking implements such as canes for greater gait stability. The severity of the choreic movements varies from mild jerking of the extremities to gross sudden jerks that interfere with ambulation and writing. Movements persist during the waking hours and invariably cease during sleep. As with other individuals with movement disorders, the chorea is aggravated by tension and anxiety. Some patients suffer varying degrees of dysarthria, the severity of which may be related to the extent of the chorea. The involuntary movements impair smooth air production during speech.

Progressive dementia is not a feature of this disorder. However, cognitive and academic skills may be impaired. One kindred was assessed for intellect malfunction; affected members were noted to have lower verbal intelligence and greater deficits in verbal abstract concept formation than unaffected family members (Leli et al., 1984). Some affected children have significant difficulty in learning to write legibly. This handicap may be due to the severity of the involuntary movements.

Virtually all of the reported pedigrees suggest autosomal dominant inheritance. It has been suggested

FEATURE TABLE 9-2. BENIGN FAMILIAL CHOREA

Discriminating Features	Consistent Features	Variable Features
1. Nonprogressive chorea 2. No intellectual deterioration or dementia 3. Persistence of involuntary movements for many years	1. Family history; autosomal dominant 2. Early onset 3. Lurching walk	1. Dysarthria 2. Mildly impaired cognitive skills

that penetrance of the gene is nearly 100% in males, but only 75% in females (Harper, 1978). Obligate but unaffected male and female carriers will transmit the syndrome. Examination of antecedents is important to assess accurately the inheritance pattern. There have been no complete neuropathologic studies reported.

No medication has been consistently effective in relieving the abnormal movements of these patients. It was discovered serendipitously that the movements were lessened by steroids in one instance (Robinson and Thornett, 1985). Some of our patients felt better while on short-term courses of haloperidol or other dopamine receptor blockers. Frequent hospitalizations for extended studies should be avoided. Genetic counseling, occupational and speech therapy, and educational guidance are important management measures.

Bilirubin Encephalopathy

Bilirubin encephalopathy in newborns is caused by a variety of conditions in which brain tissue is exposed to toxic levels of bilirubin. The clinical features of bilirubin encephalopathy range from severe athetoid cerebral palsy and deafness to mild mental retardation and subtle cognitive disturbances. The severity of bilirubin encephalopathy depends on the amount and duration of bilirubin exposure, as well as the maturational state of the exposed brain and factors that favor the net transfer of bilirubin into brain tissue (e.g., acidosis and hypoalbuminemia).

Autopsies of infants with severe bilirubin toxicity reveal the pathologic syndrome of kernicterus, consisting of bright yellow staining and neuronal necrosis of the basal ganglia, hippocampus, and brainstem nuclei, including oculomotor, cochlear, and inferior colliculi (Gerrard, 1952; Haymaker et al., 1961).

Kernicterus is mistakenly believed to be a disease of the past owing the decline of its best-known cause, Rh disease of the newborn. However, the prevalence of kernicterus in newborns with other conditions (e.g., prematurity, low birth weight, and associated conditions) is a continuing concern (Gartner et al., 1970).

The clinical symptoms of bilirubin toxicity can be classified into (1) acute bilirubin encephalopathy (2) chronic postkernicteric bilirubin encephalopathy and (3) chronic subtle bilirubin encephalopathy. Acute bilirubin encephalopathy in the neonate initially manifests with stupor, hypotonia, and poor suck, followed by hypertonia, retrocollis, opisthotonos, and, after the first week, diminishing tone.

After the first year of life, infants who survive significant bilirubin toxicity gradually develop the syndrome of chronic postkernicteric bilirubin encephalopathy. The clinical features of extrapyramidal abnormalities, gaze abnormalities, and auditory disturbances correlate with the pathologic findings of kernicterus (Byers et al., 1955; Perlstein, 1960). Dental enamel dysplasia is also commonly seen.

The extrapyramidal abnormalities are the most striking feature of this syndrome, occurring in over 90% of patients with severe neonatal jaundice (Perlstein, 1960). Athetosis is the principal manifestation, involving all limbs but usually with the upper limbs affected more than the lower. Abnormal swallowing, phonation, and facial movements are also present, and chorea, ballismus, dystonia, and, less often, tremor or rigidity may occur. In some cases the extrapyramidal abnormalities may be apparent only during attempted skilled movements. Gaze abnormalities occur because of oculomotor nuclear and supranuclear damage and primarily involve paresis of upgaze, though other directions may also be involved.

The auditory system is the neural system that is most sensitive to clinically overt bilirubin injury (Volpe, 1987); it can be assessed electrophysiologically with brainstem auditory evoked potentials in infants and children too young for reliable behavioral assessment. Auditory disturbances consist of bilateral high-frequency sensorineural loss with recruitment that is often severe, as well as central auditory disturbances, e.g., aphasia, auditory agnosia, and "deafness" to normal pure tone audiograms (Matkin and Carhart, 1966). The auditory disturbances correlate with lesions of the cochlear nuclei and inferior colliculi.

The less severe type of bilirubin encephalopathy may produce subtle cognitive disturbances, neurologic abnormalities, and hearing loss (Hyman et al., 1969; Odell et al., 1970; Johnson and Boggs, 1974; Naeye, 1978; Rubin et al., 1979), and may occur in premature infants without marked hyperbilirubinemia. Choreoathetosis and impaired upgaze are uncommon findings in this group of patients—about 60% having hearing loss as their only manifestation (Bergman et al., 1985). Thus, auditory dysfunction may be the principal manifestation of bilirubin neurotoxicity in the premature infant without marked hyperbilirubinemia (Volpe, 1987).

Chorea Associated with Static Encephalopathy

Extrapyramidal disorders are rarely observed before the end of the first year of life, possibly because the pyramidal tracts, which are necessary for the expression of movement disorders, have not yet fully myelinated. One fifth

FEATURE TABLE 9-3. BILIRUBIN ENCEPHALOPATHY

Discriminating Feature	Consistent Features	Variable Features
1. Unconjugated hyperbilirubinemia	1. Athetosis 2. Impairment of upgaze 3. Hearing loss	1. Dental enamel dysplasia 2. Impaired extraocular movements 3. Dysarthria

FEATURE TABLE 9–4. CHOREA ASSOCIATED WITH STATIC ENCEPHALOPATHY

Discriminating Features	Consistent Feature	Variable Feature
1. Choreoathetosis	1. Spasticity	1. Dysarthria
2. Dystonia		
3. Static encephalopathy caused by developmental defect brain injury		

of children with static encephalopathy caused by developmental defect or a brain injury acquired in the perinatal period develop movement disorders (Lagregran, 1983). Either athetosis or dystonia, or both, are most common, but chorea or choreoathetosis may also occur, usually in combination with pyramidal tract signs (spasticity, paresis).

Pure extrapyramidal syndromes (e.g., "athetotic cerebral palsy") are currently infrequent, probably owing to the rarity of pure bilirubin encephalopathy. The association of prematurity, hypoxia, ischemia, acidosis, and subependymal and intraventricular hemorrhage with increased susceptibility to bilirubin neurotoxicity may explain the frequent intermingling of pyramidal and extrapyramidal symptoms.

Chorea Associated with Systemic Illness

Chorea and other movement disorders, e.g., athetosis, myoclonus, tremor, and dystonia, may be associated with systemic illness. Chorea associated with systemic diseases such as systemic lupus erythematosus and anaphylactoid (Henoch-Schönlein) purpura may resemble Sydenham's chorea (Herd et al., 1978). Occasionally these diseases present with chorea. Chorea may be a manifestation of hyperthyroidism (or treatment of hypothyroidism), hypocalcemia or hypoparathyroidism (or treatment of

hypoparathyroidism), or hypocalcemia or hypoparathyroidism with cerebral calcification. Conditions that increase estrogen concentration, such as the taking of oral contraceptives, may be associated with chorea, presumably based on an estrogen-induced increase in dopamine receptor activity (Nausieda et al., 1979).

Chorea may also be a sequela of brain injury caused by head trauma or vascular disease. Various chronic, progressive metabolic and neurodegenerative disorders of childhood may be associated with chorea. These include infantile Leigh's syndrome, Pelizaeus-Merzbacher disease, Lesch-Nyhan disease, juvenile Niemann-Pick disease, ataxia-telangiectasia, and glutaric aciduria. Tumors of the basal ganglia are very rarely a cause of chorea, but should be considered in cases of unilateral chorea, even though other conditions are much more likely. Thus—in addition to the taking of clinical and family histories—a physical examination; tests such as blood and urine amino acid chromatograpy; measurements of lactate and pyruvate, uric acid and IgM, calcium, phosphorus, and thyroid and parathyroid hormones; lysosomal enzyme assays; and neuroradiologic imaging studies (CT and/or MRI) may be useful.

Disorders Presenting with Dystonia

The differential diagnosis of disorders that present with chronic and progressive dystonic movements include torsion dystonia and Hallervorden-Spatz syndrome. However, more than one type of abormal movement may regularly occur in specific disorders. Wilson's disease and hereditary progressive dystonia may manifest tremors as well as dystonic symptoms. The nature, course, and association of other types of movements, along with the presence or absence of significant dementia, provide significant differential diagnostic information. The diagnosis of a specific disorder is based on clinical and laboratory findings.

Torsion Dystonia

Dystonia, as a symptom, is characterized by slow sustained contortions of axial and appendicular muscles, and is found in a number of disorders. Dystonic syndromes may be classified into primary and secondary disorders. The primary dystonic states are familial and, in the past, have also been identified by such names as dystonia musculorum deformans, spasmodic torticollis, and progressive torsion spasm of childhood. The currently preferred term is torsion dystonia. Dystonia may be found in other familial or acquired disorders, including Wilson's disease and Hallervorden-Spatz syndrome, and as a

---

Pearls and Perils: Disorders Presenting with Chorea, Athetosis, or Both

1. Persistence of choreic movements over a 6-month period is uncommon in Sydenham's chorea.
2. In the assessment of the child who presents with chorea, a positive family history will distinguish Huntington's and benign familial chorea from Sydenham's chorea.
3. Metabolic studies and drug screening tests should be performed in all children with a new-onset movement disorder.
4. Children with progressive choreoathetosis and other neurologic manifestations should have a full diagnostic evaluation to rule out the possibility of a neurodegenerative disease. Young males with associated developmental delay should also have a uric acid determination and tests of renal function to rule out Lesch-Nyhan disease.

FEATURE TABLE 9-5. TORSION DYSTONIA

Discriminating Features	Consistent Features	Variable Features
1. Dystonic posturing	1. Autosomal dominant or recessive	1. X-linked recessive
2. Familial	2. Dystonic posturing of the neck and axial muscles	2. Dysphonia

sequela following perinatal brain injuries, encephalitis, and other conditions (Eldridge, 1970).

Torsion dystonia is a familial disorder most frequently transmitted as an autosomal dominant or as an autosomal recessive. A smaller number of cases may be X-linked recessive. While certain factors are more often noted in the recessive form (e.g., Jewish ancestry, consistent age of onset), and other factors are more frequently noted in the dominant form (e.g., non-Jewish ancestry), the differences are not sufficient to differentiate clinically between these forms in individual cases. There are no characteristic pathologic or biochemic abnormalities known (Zeman and Dyken, 1967; Zeman, 1970).

The age of onset in the recessive form is 10 years, while it varies in the dominant form from 1 to 40 years of age. The initial major symptom is dystonic posturing of the axial muscles, particularly the neck muscles. In some cases torticollis is the only manifestation of the disorder. Initial symptoms may be misdiagnosed as hysteria. Many other patients will have a variably progressive course in which dystonia affects other axial and limb muscles, resulting in segmental or generalized dystonia with contortions of the trunk, appendicular dystonia, and tortipelvis. Although dysphonia may develop in some cases, mental retardation is not a consistent associated finding. There is no convincing evidence of a decreased lifespan in individuals with torsion dystonia. The diagnosis is based on clinical findings. Laboratory studies delineate the secondary forms of dystonia.

Management of the patient with torsion dystonia requires attention to the physical and emotional aspects of the disorder. Severe emotional stress may impede the therapeutic progress in rehabilitation. The patient with generalized dystonia needs support from members of a multidisciplinary team, including physicians, counselors, physical and occupational therapists. No medications provide dramatic relief of the symptoms. L-Dopa has had limited success in controlling dystonia. Diazepam has been recommended but has not been universally beneficial. Neurosurgical procedures such as cryothalamectomy or chemothalamectomy have provided long-term improvement of some of the symptoms. Frequently, multiple procedures are necessary. Some patients who have undergone surgery have emerged in worse condition. There has been no uniformly accepted surgical procedure for the management of the child with torsion dystonia.

Hallervorden-Spatz Syndrome

The clinicopathologic findings of Hallervorden-Spatz syndrome (HSS) were initially described by Hallervorden and Spatz in 1922. They found pathologic amounts of iron stored in the globus pallidus and reticular zone of the substantia nigra of five siblings. After reviewing the literature of 64 pathologically verified cases, Dooling and co-workers reaffirmed that the condition had the following clinical and pathologic characteristics (Dooling et al., 1974). The clinical features include (1) occurrence at a young age, (2) motor disorder of the extrapyramidal type, (3) dementia, and (4) progressive course. The pathologic features are (1) symmetric lesions of the globus pallidus and pars reticulata of the substantia nigra with loss of myelinated fibers and neurons, (2) dissemination of round nonnucleated swollen axons (spheroids) in the central nervous system, and (3) accumulation of iron-containing pigments in the affected regions. HSS is an autosomal recessive condition.

The onset of the disease occurs during childhood and symptoms start by 10 years of age. A small number of cases may begin in adulthood. Posturing or movement abnormalities are the most frequent presenting symptoms. The changes lead to gait disorders. Motor symptoms include rigidity, dystonic posturing, choreoathetoid movements, and tremors. Dysarthria is present in most of the cases. The deep tendon reflexes tend to be hyperactive and the toe reflexes upgoing. Progressive intellectual

FEATURE TABLE 9-6. HALLERVORDEN-SPATZ DISEASE

Discriminating Features	Consistent Features	Variable Features
1. Symmetric pathologic lesions of globus pallidus and pars reticularis of the substantia nigra	1. Occurs at young age	1. Abnormal EEG, VEP
	2. Extrapyramidal motor disorder: rigidity, dystonia, choreoathetosis, and tremor	2. "Sea Blue" histiocytes and cytoplasmic inclusions in lymphocytes
2. Autosomal recessive	3. Dementia	3. Seizures
	4. Progressive course	4. Increased radioactive uptake of iron in the basal ganglia
	5. MRI findings of cortical atrophy, lesions of basal ganglia	

deterioration (dementia) is often present and the rate of its progression is variable. Seizures may occur. The mean duration of the illness is 11 years.

Because of the grave prognosis associated with the disease, the physician should make every effort to substantiate the diagnosis. Unfortunately, there are no pathognomonic laboratory findings. Electroencephalograms may be normal or show epileptic activity. Visual evoked potentials may be compatible with optic atrophy. CT has demonstrated cortical atrophy and ventricular enlargement of low-density lesions in the basal ganglia and MRI has demonstrated signal aberration in the lentiform nucleus—findings that are consistent with but not diagnostic of the disease (Littrup and Gebarski, 1985). Increased radioactive uptake of ^{59}Fe in the region of the basal ganglia has been reported (Vakili et al., 1977). Extraneural evidence of the disease was found when the presence of sea-blue histiocytes was demonstrated in the bone marrow cells and cytoplasmic inclusions of circulation lymphocytes (Swaiman et al., 1983) in two children with HSS. Further studies to substantiate these findings are needed.

Supportive and symptomatic therapy should be provided to children and their families. Emotional support and genetic counseling are important components of the management program. Anticonvulsants may be prescribed for children with seizures. Treatment with deferoxamine, an iron-chelating agent, has reduced the body stores of iron but not the deposits in the basal ganglia. Levodopa and anticholinesterase agents may help to relieve some of the clinical extrapyramidal symptomatology.

Childhood Tremor

The differential diagnoses of the group of disorders presenting with chronic tremors include familial tremor, juvenile parkinsonism, hereditary dystonia–parkinsonism syndrome of juvenile onset, and Wilson's disease. The presence or absence of other motor abnormalities, such as cogwheel rigidity or bradykinesia, along with tremor helps to differentiate the various conditions. Juvenile parkinsonism and hereditary progressive dystonia share many clinical and therapeutic characteristics. Children with Wilson's disease not only may have tremors but also may have dystonia and other features on neurologic examination.

Pearls and Perils: Disorders Presenting with Dystonia

1. Chronic progressive dystonia is a symptom complex that may be seen in children with a number of movement disorders. Treatable diseases such as hereditary progressive dystonia and Wilson's disease should be carefully ruled out.
2. As in other neurodegenerative diseases, extraneural tissue may provide supporting histologic evidence of Hallervorden-Spatz syndrome when the presence of sea-blue histiocytes and cytosomic inclusions can be demonstrated.
3. Early dystonia may be misinterpreted as a hysterical mannerism.

Juvenile Parkinsonism

Parkinson's disease (paralysis agitans) affecting individuals over 40 years old is a common disorder. However, parkinsonism in children is rare. In 1917, Hunt, and subsequently others (Martin et al., 1971), described a condition in which symptoms of parkinsonism appeared early in life. Juvenile parkinsonism shares some but not all of the clinical, pathologic, and pharmacologic properties of adult Parkinson's disease. Three pathologic studies of the childhood form of parkinsonism have been reported, with conflicting findings. Two studies reported a marked loss of neurons in the globus pallidus, caudate nucleus, and putamen, and no abnormalities in the substantia nigra (Hunt, 1917; VanBogaert, 1930). The other noted a loss of cells in the substantia nigra, similar to the major pathologic findings in Parkinson's disease (Davison, 1954). Nosologically, juvenile parkinsonism is an ill-defined disorder. Whereas it is clinically similar to the adult disorder, it also shares some characteristics with hereditary dystonia–parkinsonism syndrome of juvenile onset.

The most common form of Parkinson's disease is the idiopathic form. The clinical syndrome consists of tremor, rigidity, bradykinesias, and impaired postural stability. Other symptoms (e.g., oculogyric crisis, hyperhidrosis, and gait abnormalities) are often present. In children, the disorder is characterized by the early appearance of symptoms similar to those of the idiopathic form. Tremor, rigidity, and bradykinesia are also prominent in the

---

FEATURE TABLE 9–7. JUVENILE PARKINSONISM

Discriminating Features	Consistent Features	Variable Feature
1. Tremor, rigidity, bradykinesia, and impaired postural stability 2. Early onset	1. Gait abnormalities 2. Facial masking 3. Cogwheel rigidity 4. Autosomal dominant inheritance 5. Dramatic response to L-dopa, and other drug	1. Spasticity

juvenile form of the disorder. Facial masking, resting tremor, loss of associated movements, and cogwheel rigidity of the neck and limb muscles are prominent findings. The gait may be either dystonic or shuffling. Deep tendon reflexes are frequently brisk. The disorder in children and in some adults is familial. The mode of inheritance is autosomal dominant with incomplete penetrance, although sporadic cases have been reported. The diagnosis is made primarily by neurologic assessment.

Drug therapy in juvenile parkinsonism is similar to therapy for idiopathic parkinsonism. The cases reported in the literature have had dramatic response to relatively low doses of levodopa. Levodopa in combination with cabidopa may further reduce the total dose of L-dopa needed for control of symptoms (Naidu et al., 1978). Anticholinergic therapy has a beneficial effect in reducing the symptoms, but not to the extent of L-dopa.

Hereditary Dystonia–Parkinsonism Syndrome of Juvenile Onset

In children, this condition has also been called hereditary progressive dystonia with diurnal variation. The symptoms begin in childhood with dystonic manifestations and respond rapidly to L-dopa (Nygaard and Duvoisin, 1986). The syndrome is familial with an autosomal dominant mode of inheritance. There are reported sporadic cases.

Symptoms usually begin before the age of 10 years. Females are more frequently affected than males by a 2:1 ratio. A patient's presenting sign is often a gait disorder, with dystonia of the legs or with equinovarus posturing of a foot. As the disorder progresses, dystonia becomes more generalized and features of parkinsonism appear. There may be flexor and extensor posturing of the upper extremities and trunk musculature. Parkinsonian features include cogwheel rigidity, bradykinesia, and tremors. The deep tendon reflexes are often brisk with extensor toe responses. Diurnal variation, in which symptoms become more severe during the day and improve after sleeping, is a prominent feature especially noted in the cases reported from Japan (Segawa et al., 1976).

The diagnosis is based on clinical assessment. Routine laboratory studies are used to rule out such treatable disorders as Wilson's disease or to confirm the presence of dystonia or tremors. Cerebrospinal fluid homovanillic acid and 5-hydroxyindoleacetic acid levels have been reported as normal or low. One autopsy study revealed poorly pigmented cells in the substantia nigra (Yokochi et al., 1984).

The reduction of dystonic and parkinsonian features after the administration of L-dopa is rapid and marked. Function is often normalized within a day of initiation of medication. Small dosages of medication sometimes result in dramatic changes. Dosages should be individualized, but the daily dose seldom requires more than 3 g of L-dopa. Control with L-dopa is sustained, in some cases for more than 10 years. There has been no deterioration of the parkinsonian or dystonic symptoms while on medication. Anticholinergics (Allen and Knopp, 1976) are also beneficial in reducing the symptoms; however, the response is not as striking. Carbamazepine has also produced favorable therapeutic responses (Garg, 1982).

Wilson's Disease

Wilson's disease is a disorder of the copper-binding protein ceruloplasmin, resulting in the deposition of copper in the central nervous system and the liver. Early diagnosis and treatment of Wilson's diseases may prevent permanent neurologic damage.

Neurologic signs and symptoms may be the only early manifestations of the disease. Young children may present with dystonia followed by tremor and other findings. In such children, the onset of Wilson's disease is often rapid, presenting with tremor, coarse "flapping," or fine rhythmic tremor, whereas in adults the onset is usually insidious. Cerebellar and pseudobulbar signs, such as drooling, difficulty in swallowing, and dysarthria often occur. Rigidity develops later in the course of the disease. Dementia is not prominent in juvenile presentations. A Kayser-Fleischer ring (a brown to yellow to green discoloration in Descemet's membrane at the limbus of the iris) is pathognomonic of the disease.

Discussion of the diagnosis and a more detailed description of Wilson's disease may be found in Chapter 13. Because it is treatable, the diagnosis of Wilson's disease should be considered in all children with new onset of tremor or dystonia.

Benign Familial Tremor

Benign familial tremor is the most common persistent childhood tremor (Golden, 1984). It occurs at any age, generally after 8 years, without other evidence of neurologic disease. It involves the hands bilaterally, the head in 50% of cases (as titubation or fine head nodding), and the voice in about 35% of cases. Inheritance is autosomal dominant, with a positive family history in about 60% of cases.

The characteristic tremor is rapid (5 to 8 Hz) and

FEATURE TABLE 9–8. HEREDITARY DYSTONIA-PARKINSON SYNDROME OF JUVENILE ONSET

Discriminating Features	Consistent Features	Variable Features
1. Progressive dystonia 2. Diurnal variation	1. Gait disorder 2. Other parkinsonian symptoms 3. Marked and rapid response to L-dopa	1. Brisk deep tendon reflexes 2. Posturing

FEATURE TABLE 9–9. BENIGN FAMILIAL TREMOR

Discriminating Features	Consistent Features	Variable Feature
1. Intention tremor of the hands 2. Autosomal dominant	1. Positive family history 2. Dramatic response to alcohol	1. Shuddering

exacerbated by stress, anxiety, and antigravity posture. A component of intention tremor may be present. Tremor is absent at rest. Characteristically the tremor in adults responds dramatically to alcohol. The pathophysiology is unknown.

The condition is not usually debilitating, although slow progression with prolonged plateaus may occur. The judicious use of alcohol may control symptoms temporarily; however, patients should be cautioned about the increased risk of alcoholism in this group. Propranolol may be therapeutically useful in some cases.

Brief shuddering attacks of variable frequency, sometimes with posturing, may be seen in infancy or childhood in families with essential tremor (Vanasse et al., 1976). The shuddering attacks may be precipitated by emotional stimuli and disappear with time.

Hyperthyroidism

Hyperthyroidism is associated with tremor that is rapid, mainly involves the extremities, and is more prominent with the arms outstretched. Tremor secondary to hyperthyroidism can be ruled out by appropriate thyroid function tests.

Drug-Induced Tremor

Drugs—such as the β-adrenergic agnosists, valproic acid, lithium, heavy metals, alcohol, and "street drugs" can all produce tremor. The tremor stops when the drug is withdrawn.

**Pearls and Perils:
Childhood Tremor**

1. Benign essential tremor is the most common persistent tremor in childhood.
2. Alcohol dramatically decreases tremor in benign familial or essential tremor.
3. Shuddering attacks in infancy and childhood should prompt a careful history for the presence of familial tremor.
4. "Wing-beating tremor," which appears with the arms abducted and elbows flexed, suggests Wilson's disease.
5. A Kayser-Fleischer ring (a brown to yellow to green discoloration in Descemet's membrane at the limbus of the iris) is pathognomonic of Wilson's disease. This can be seen more readily in persons with blue eyes. It is definitively diagnosed by slit-lamp examination.

Tics

Tics are common in children. Often these involuntary movements are manifested in only one muscle group and occur transiently. The disorders described in this section represent a spectrum of movements occurring over a period of time.

Simple Tics

Tics are rapid involuntary rhythmic movements of individual muscle groups. Childhood tics are often simple, involving single muscle groups (e.g., eye blinking, facial grimacing) and are frequently transient. Transient tics may last for weeks or months and are not associated with other symptoms. Motor tics that persist over many years are defined as chronic tics. The muscle group affected may remain the same or other groups may be affected (chronic multiple tics).

Gilles de la Tourette Syndrome

Gilles de la Tourette syndrome (tic de Gilles de la Tourette, TS) is a disorder characterized by the early onset (2 to 15 years of age) of chronic motor and vocal tics. The tics involve multiple motor groups and vary in intensity, waxing and waning over a period of years. At times, remissions occur, usually during or after adolescence (Golden, 1986).

The motor tics may be simple or complex, with manifestations changing over time. Eye blinking and facial grimacing may occur in one period, writhing movements in the next. Vocal tics include simple sniffling sounds, barking, grunting, and throat-clearing sounds, and also more complex echolalia and coprolalia (Cohen et al., 1984), although coprolalia (the use of obscene language) is not often noted in children with TS.

Up to half of the children with this syndrome have behavioral disorders. Some manifest symptoms of attention deficit hyperactivity disorder (ADHD), with or without hyperactivity, and others display obsessive-compulsive or other behavioral disorders. Several recent reports correlate the use of stimulant medications (methylphenidate, dextroamphetamine, and pemoline) with the precipitation of TS or with increased incidence of tics. It has been recommended that children with ADHD should be monitored for the onset of tics while on stimulants, and that stimulant medication should be used cautiously in children with tics (Golden, 1985).

The etiology of this syndrome is incompletely understood. A number of neurotransmitter alterations have been implicated. The dramatic response of symptoms to dopamine-receptor-blocking agents like haloperidol and

FEATURE TABLE 9-10. GILLES DE LA TOURETTE SYNDROME

Discriminating Features	Consistent Features	Variable Features
1. Motor or vocal tics	1. Behavioral disorders	1. Coprolalia
2. Involves multiple motor groupings	2. ADHD	2. Remission in adolescense
3. Waxing and waning of symptoms	3. Response to dopamine receptor antagonists	
4. Early onset		

pimozide suggests a dopaminergic involvement. Baseline cerebrospinal fluid levels of homovanillic acid have been low, with levels increasing after the administration of haloperidol. Noradrenergic mechanisms have been implicated because symptoms of the syndrome are greatly reduced after the administration of clonidine, a drug that inhibits noradrenergic functioning. However, more information is needed to understand adequately these complex mechanisms.

Although the incidence of TS is unknown, it is no longer considered a rare disorder. Based on the genetic findings that chronic motor tics and TS occur in the same pedigree and that a patient may move from one condition to the other, it is estimated that the prevalence may be as common as 1 in 2000. With the currently available genetic information, no specific mode of transmission can be implicated. There are clear familial aggregations of TS and multiple tics. Males are more often affected. Twin studies show a lack of full concordance. Although there is evidence to suggest a strong genetic contribution, nongenetic factors, multifactorial gene effects, and multiple etiologies cannot be excluded.

Although there are drugs that can effectively reduce the symptoms of TS, the program of management of the children and their families is quite complex. The diagnosis should be based on firm data extending over a period of time. The severity of the symptoms and the extent to which these symptoms affect the development, self-image, and performance of the child in school and at home should be documented. Parents need to be educated about the disorder, counseled about its possible transmission, and reassured that the condition is not progressive.

Haloperidol has been prescribed for the treatment of TS symptoms for more than 20 years. In small doses, it is capable of eliminating the motor and vocal tics. In children, dosages start at 0.25 to 0.5 mg/day and are gradually increased to 4 or 5 mg/day as needed. On rare occasions, some children may require larger doses, and some may get by with smaller dosages. Of the patients with TS, 75% to 90% experience significant relief of their symptoms with this drug. Unfortunately, many patients experience side effects, including sleepiness, fatigue, weight gain, and other changes. There have been reports of tardive dyskinesias in some individuals following haloperidol therapy.

Pemozide, a potent dopamine-blocking agent, has been as effective as haloperidol in the treatment of TS. It is used in those patients who are unable to tolerate the side effects of haloperidol. It is started in 1-mg/day doses and gradually increased to 6 to 10 mg/day. It may cause electrocardiogram changes (primarily prolongation of the QT interval) and therefore periodic monitoring of the electrocardiogram has been recommended. Clonidine, an α-2-adrenergic agonist, is also effective in improving the motor and vocal tics, and has an effect on the associated behavioral problems. It is started at 0.05 mg/day and slowly increased to 0.125 to 0.3 mg/day. Improvement occurs at a slower rate than with haloperidol. Other agents, including phenothiazines and tetrabenazine, have been used less frequently to treat patients with TS.

Myoclonic Encephalopathy of Infancy

This rare syndrome has generated great interest because of its association with neuroblastoma. It consists of myoclonus and opsoclonus ("dancing eyes") in infants without other neurologic abnormalities, and appears in the literature with the names myoclonic encephalopathy of infancy, Kinsbourne's syndrome, infantile polymyoclonia, and "dancing eyes" syndrome. The syndrome may be idiopathic, viral, or neuroblastoma related. Idiopathic and neuroblastoma-related myoclonic encephalopathy of infancy may be distinct entities, or may represent immunologic reactions of varying effectiveness against neuroblastoma formation. The initial report of six cases (Kinsbourne, 1962) has been supplemented by over 100 additional case reports (Lott and Kinsbourne, 1986), some with long-term follow-up.

Onset usually occurs between the ages of 6 and 18 months but can occur at up to 36 months of age. The onset of myoclonus is acute, often occurring after a nonspecific respiratory or gastrointestinal illness, and reaches maximal intensity in 2 to 7 days. The myoclonic

Pearls and Perils: Tics

1. Children with ADHD on stimulant medication should be monitored for the onset of tics.
2. Because of the high incidence of behavior disorders in children with TS, psychologic or psychiatric consultation may be helpful.
3. TS and chronic multiple tics may be transmitted within the same family.

movements are intense, brief with continual shock-like muscular contractions, irregularly timed, and of variable amplitude. They are widely distributed across muscle groups, asymmetric, increased by startle, present at rest, and abolished only by deep sleep. Rarely, choreoathetosis may also be seen.

Abnormal eye movements (opsoclonus) temporally unrelated to the myoclonus consist of rapid (up to eight displacements or rotations per second), irregular, conjugate ocular movements, mainly horizontal but also vertical and diagonal. The eye movements are exacerbated by the same stimuli as the myoclonus, and some authors consider opsoclonus to be the ocular equivalent of myoclonus.

The diagnosis is clinical. Myoclonus should be distinguished from infantile spasms and myoclonic epilepsy (Table 9–3). Opsoclonus should be distinguished from nystagmus or the eye rotatory movements of Pelizaeus-Merzbacher disease.

In published literature the incidence of neuroblastoma associated with myoclonic encephalopathy of infancy is about 50%; however, because of a selection bias in favor of reporting cases associated with neuroblastoma, the true incidence of associated neuroblastoma is probably much lower (Lott and Kinsbourne, 1986). Neurologic symptoms may occur months before a tumor is found. Fifty percent of reported tumors are localized to the thorax. Plain chest x rays have the highest diagnostic yield, followed by abdominal films. Urinary catecholamines are rarely diagnostic. Electroencephalogram is normal. A virus (Coxsackie B3) has been cultured from cerebrospinal fluid and stool (Kuban et al., 1983).

Differential diagnoses include posterior fossa tumor, acute cerebellar ataxia, encephalitis, Pelizaeus-Merzbacher disease, and spasmus nutans.

Success of treatment ranges from complete recovery in 3 months to persistence over several years, and the latter course is more frequently noted. Incomplete recovery may be followed by relapse related to infection or discontinuation of effective therapy. Most cases show a remarkable response to adrenocorticotropic horomone (ACTH) or corticosteroid therapy, though it is not clear which treatment is more beneficial. Usually 20 to 40 units/day of ACTH, or 5 to 20 mg of prednisolone have been needed for therapeutic benefit, with the dose titrated downward to a level below which symptoms appear.

Pearls and Perils: Myoclonic Encephalopathy of Infancy

1. Myoclonic movements occur commonly in sleeping infants and are frequently misinterpreted as seizures.
2. Predominantly front-to-back head movements, the head appearing like a doll's head on a spring, occur in the "bobble head doll" syndrome, and should prompt a search for neuroblastoma, third ventricle cyst, dilatation, or tumor.

About half of patients are left with sequelae: mental retardation, dysarthria, learning disabilities, or ADHD. Patients with neuroblastoma have slightly less serious sequelae. Neuroblastoma associated with myoclonic encephalopathy has a more favorable prognosis than neuroblastoma without the neurologic syndrome (Altman and Bachner, 1976).

Myoclonic encephalopathy of infancy may be an important model of natural tumor regression. It has been postulated that neuroblastoma and cerebellum are joint targets of an immunologic attack. Leukocytes from children with neuroblastoma and children with myoclonic encephalopathy without neuroblastoma are inhibited by neuroblastoma in the capillary migration test (Stephenson et al., 1976). Because there is a high incidence of in situ neuroblastomas at autopsy, the "idiopathic" cases may actually have microscopic tumors.

Paroxysmal Movement Disorders

The movement disorders discussed thus far in this chapter have been persistent. The movements occur during the day and often disappear during sleep. However, some movement disorders only occur paroxysmally or intermittently. Paroxysmal movement disorders are characterized by sudden attacks of involuntary movements of the body without loss of consciousness. The movements may be choreic, athetotic, tonic, dystonic, or ataxic, or may occur in any combination. They may be unilateral or bilateral, or they may start in one extremity and then gradually spread to others. There is no loss of awareness during the episode; patients can hear and are conscious of pain and other sensations. However, many are unable

---

TABLE 9–3. MYOCLONIC ENCEPHALOPATHY OF INFANCY VERSUS MYOCLONIC EPILEPSY

Criterion	Myoclonic Epilepsy/Infantile Spasm	Myoclonic Encephalopathy of Infancy
Character of myoclonus	Bilateral, symmetric, synchronous, rhythmic	Asymmetric, arrhythmic, asynchronous
Dependence on stimuli	Not induced by movement	Induced by voluntary movement
State of consciousness	Loss of consciousness	No loss of consciousness
Electroencephalogram	Abnormal (hypsarrhythmia, atypical petit mal)	Normal

Modified from Adams and Lyon (1982).

to speak because of the severity of the movements. Paroxysmal movement disorders may be classified into (1) paroxysmal kinesigenic choreoathetosis, (2) paroxysmal dystonic choreoathetosis of Mount and Reback, (3) acquired forms of paroxysmal movement disorders, with neurologic disorders or metabolic disorders, and (4) familial periodic ataxia.

The differentiation of paroxysmal dyskinesia and tonic seizures induced by movements is not always readily discernible. Some cases of paroxysmal choreoathetosis are initially misdiagnosed as seizures. In reflex epilepsy, when the seizures are induced by movements, the differentiation may be particularly difficult. The state of consciousness is the most helpful distinguishing feature. When there is alteration or loss of consciousness the episode is more consistent with seizures. However, it may be necessary to obtain an electroencephalogram during the attack to confirm the diagnosis.

Paroxysmal Kinesigenic Choreoathetosis

Familial paroxysmal kinesigenic choreoathetosis has been called paroxysmal kinesigenic choreoathetosis, paroxysmal dystonic choreoathetosis, periodic dystonia, familial paroxysmal choreoathetosis, and periodic dystonia.

The most frequently reported familial paroxysmal choreoathetosis movement disorder is the kinesigenically induced one, in that the episodes are precipitated by movement. Characteristically, the precipitating movement is a brisk and sudden event such as a quick head turn, as might occur after a startle reaction. Attacks may be induced in the examination room by having the individual hop in place on one foot for a short period.

The episodes consist of choreoathetotic, dystonic, tonic, or mixed forms of movement occurring unilaterally or bilaterally (Goodenough et al., 1978). Characteristically, the movements are brief, with durations on the order of minutes, and may occur several times a day. Individuals with these episodes have noted the ability to abort some of the attacks by various maneuvers, such as grasping the involved extremity. Occasionally there is an aura of tightness or other vague sensation prior to the episode.

The attacks usually start in childhood and may increase in frequency during adolescence. The neurologic examination and history are otherwise normal. The electroencephalogram during the episodes is not different from that during an episode-free period. In most instances, electroencephalograms obtained during the episode are normal. There have been no consistent pathologic findings at autopsy. When the diagnosis is uncertain, videotaped recordings of the event may provide sufficient information to differentiate this condition from other types of paroxysmal movement disorders.

An autosomal dominant mode of inheritance with incomplete penetrance is described by a number of authors. Others have suggested an autosomal recessive inheritance pattern. Sporadic cases have been reported. However, a woman previously described as a sporadic case had a daughter 10 years later who not only inherited the disorder, but was more severely affected (T.D. Bird et al., 1978).

The response to anticonvulsant medication is dramatic in most instances. Phenytoin is the medication most commonly prescribed. The serum concentration necessary for control of the attacks is lower than that employed when phenytoin is prescribed for seizure control (Wang and Chang, 1985). Other anticonvulsants used include phenobarbital, carbamazepine, valproic acid, primidone, and clonazepam. Some cases have responded to medications not ordinarily used for seizure control (e.g., L-dopa).

Paroxysmal Dystonic Choreoathetosis of Mount and Reback

Paroxysmal dystonic choreoathetosis, initially described in 1940, occurs less frequently than the kinesigenic form (Mount and Reback, 1940). It has more recently been called familial paroxysmal dystonic choreoathetosis of Mount and Reback. Following the initial publication only a few case reports appeared until 1977, when Lance described four families (Lance, 1977). Since then a number of other families have been reported.

The attacks in many of the cases begin in infancy; a smaller number of patients do not exhibit attacks until adulthood. The paroxysmal attacks have been manifested as choreoathetotic or dystonic movements. Episodes invariably last longer than 5 minutes, and often last for more than an hour. They do not occur frequently and patients may go for months without one. The attacks are not precipitated by movements. More commonly, episodes are induced by excessive intake of alcohol, exhaustion, stress, or other factors. As in the kinesigenic form,

FEATURE TABLE 9-11. PAROXYSMAL KINESIGENIC CHOREOATHETOSIS

Discriminating Feature	Consistent Features	Variable Feature
1. Movement-induced paroxysmal episodes	1. Early onset 2. Brief duration of episodes 3. Choreoathetotic, dystonic, tonic, or mixed forms 4. Dramatic response to medication 5. No EEG changes during episode 6. Positive family history	1. None

FEATURE TABLE 9–12. PAROXYSMAL DYSTONIC CHOREOATHETOSIS OF MOUNT AND REBACK

Discriminating Features	Consistent Features	Variable Feature
1. Paroxysmal episodes of choreoathetosis or dystonia 2. Not induced by movement 3. Autosomal dominant	1. Early onset 2. Episodes of long duration 3. Inconsistent response to medication	1. Adult onset

there is no loss of consciousness during the attack.

Familial paroxysmal dystonic choreoathetosis is clearly transmitted through an autosomal dominant mode of inheritance. As in the kinesigenic form, more males are affected than females. Routine laboratory studies, including electroencephalograms during the attacks, have been normal. There have been no pathologic findings in the central nervous system. The pathophysiology of this disorder, like that of the kinesigenic form, is unknown. It has been suggested that a loss of cortical control of the neostriatum and thalamus owing to an unknown neurotransmitter defect may have a causative role.

Unlike results in the kinesigenic form, the frequency of the attacks has not been reduced by many different anticonvulsants. Clonazepam, however, has been an effective therapeutic agent in eliminating or significantly reducing the frequency of the episodes (Lance, 1977; Mayeux and Fahn, 1982). Alternate-day oxazepam therapy provided sustained relief of the attacks in another study (Kurlan and Shoulson, 1983), as did acetazolamide.

Acquired Forms of Paroxysmal Movement Disorders

Acquired forms of paroxysmal disorders occur in association with an underlying disease and are not the result of a genetic defect. The known underlying processes include neurologic and metabolic diseases. The nature of the involuntary movements during the attacks is similar to that in the kinesigenic forms of the disorder. The associated disease must be recognized and treated when possible.

The neurologic disorders most frequently associated with paroxysmal dyskinesia are static encephalopathy and multiple sclerosis. Paroxysmal movement disorders, particularly in children diagnosed as having had a static encephalopathy, are often misdiagnosed as seizures or hysteria. Because of their length, the episodes can be very painful and distressing to patients, families, and teachers. Correct diagnosis is important, because medication and treatment of the disease often reduce or eliminate the attacks.

The paroxysmal episodes that occur in individuals with a static encephalopathy syndrome often begin in childhood (Rosen, 1964). The attacks are usually brief, measured in minutes; however, in a number of cases the attacks have lasted for hours (Erickson and Chun, 1987). The movements can be dystonic, tonic, or choreoathetoid; occurrences range from several a day to once every several months.

Neurologic examination reflects the findings of the past encephalopathy. Some individuals have signs of spasticity or hemiparesis; others are severely hypotonic, or have persistent choreoathetosis. Electroencephalograms during the episode are no different than those recorded during the interictal period.

The response to anticonvulsants in the cases initially reported was variable. However, in our experience, the involuntary movements are eliminated or greatly reduced with phenytoin or clonazepam treatment.

The paroxysmal episodes of patients with multiple sclerosis are primarily flexor spasms (Miley and Forster, 1974). Because of the intensity, the attacks are often painful. They may be the initial symptoms of multiple sclerosis. The attacks are short, lasting minutes, and frequently stop after 1 or 2 months of symptoms. They respond to anticonvulsants.

Paroxysmal choreoathetotic episodes occur in individuals with endocrine diseases such as hyperparathyroidism (Arden, 1953), thyrotoxicosis (Fischbeck and Layzer, 1979), and diabetes during periods of hypoglycemia (Newman and Kinkel, 1984). The attacks consist of tonic or choreoathetoid movements, or both. Correction of the metabolic defect leads to cessation of the episodes. The etiology of the dyskinesia is unknown. It is postulated that striatal dysfunction may result from a neurotransmitter defect.

Pearls and Perils: Paroxysmal Movement Disorders

1. Neurologic examination of individuals with familial paroxysmal movement disorders is usually normal. Neurologic examination of individuals with acquired paroxysmal movement disorders is abnormal.
2. The kinesigenic form of paroxysmal choreoathetosis may also be manifested as bilateral or unilateral dystonic or tonic movements. Regardless of the type of abnormal movement, medication is uniformly effective.
3. Paroxysmal kinesigenic choreoathetosis attacks may be precipitated by sudden subtle movements. The precipitating event does not have to be a gross motor activity.
4. Attacks of familial periodic ataxia respond best to acetazolamide. Commonly used anticonvulsants have no effect on the frequency of these episodes.

Familial Periodic Ataxia

The syndrome of familial periodic ataxia has been called by a variety of other names, including familial periodic nystagmus and vertigo; familial intermittent ataxia; hereditary paroxysmal ataxia; dominant recurrent ataxia and vertigo of childhood; periodic ataxia; and vertibulocerebellar ataxia. It was initially described in 1946 (Parker, 1946). Since that time, 10 families with more than 100 affected individuals have been reported. It is an autosomal dominantly inherited disorder. The incidence of this disorder in the general population is unknown.

Familial periodic ataxia is distinguished by attacks of either cerebellar incoordination or vertigo without loss of consciousness. The episodes usually begin in infancy or childhood, but infrequently may start in adulthood (Tibbles et al., 1986).

The attacks of cerebellar incoordination are characterized by paroxysmal bouts of ataxia, dysarthria, and nystagmus. The frequency is variable; episodes may occur daily or may be separated by weeks or months. The duration of the episodes may be brief, but more often the episodes last for hours and sometimes days. Ataxia of the trunk and extremities is frequently so severe during the episodes that the patient cannot stand without assistance. Speech becomes dysarthric and difficult to understand, although receptive language function remains intact. Vertical or horizontal nystagmus may be present during the attack.

Vertiginous attacks are characterized by horizontal and vertical nystagmus, vertigo, and ataxia (White, 1969). When vertigo is severe, walking is impossible, and vomiting is frequent. As in the cerebellar incoordination form, there is no loss of consciousness and attacks may be precipitated by physical or emotional stress. Manifestations of the incoordination and vertiginous forms may occur during different attacks in some individuals. Mild episodes may occur in either form with brief attacks of dizziness or ataxia.

Slight cerebellar signs are often noted during interim neurologic examination. Horizontal and sometimes vertical nystagmus and mild ataxia on finger-to-nose and heel-to-shin testing are typical findings. Although some authors found no progressive neurologic involvement, others reported a slow progression of ataxia.

Routine laboratory studies have not revealed any consistent abnormalities. In one report, a defect in pyruvate metabolism was noted (Livingstone et al., 1984). Between episodes, electroencephalograms, caloric testing of vestibular function, and routine serum chemistries have been normal (Donat and Auger, 1979).

Cerebellar degeneration of the olivo-ponto-cerebellar system and histologic findings similar to those of Leigh's disease were noted on postmortem examination of one patient (Livingstone et al., 1984). In our experience, CT and MRI studies are usually unremarkable; however, in individuals whose symptoms persist over a prolonged period, neuroimaging will frequently reveal cerebellar atrophy, especially of the vermis.

Acetazolamide in many cases completely eliminates or greatly reduces the number of episodes within 24 hours of its administration (Griggs et al., 1978). Some patients on medication have remained attack free for many years. Other authors report a less complete response to this drug. Renal stones may occur in individuals on continuous acetazolamide therapy. Contrary to results observed in therapy of individuals with familial kinesigenic choreoathetosis, commonly used anticonvulsants such as phenytoin and phenobarbital have no effect on these paroxysmal attacks.

As in paroxysmal dyskinesia, episodic or intermittent ataxia may be caused by a heterogenous group of diseases. Patients with recessively inherited errors of metabolism such as Hartnup's disease, Leigh's disease, and maple syrup urine disease may intermittently be ataxic. Individuals with acquired diseases could possibly manifest periodic ataxia as part of the clinical spectrum.

ANNOTATED BIBLIOGRAPHY

Dooling E, Schoene WC, Richardson EP: Hallervorden-Spatz syndrome. *Arch Neurol* 30:70–83, 1974.
   An extensive review of the literature, including suggested clinical and pathologic criteria for diagnosis.
Eldridge R: The torsion dystonias: Literature review and genetic and clinical studies. *Neurology* 20(no 11, pt 2):1–78, 1970.
   An extensive discussion of the history and genetic and clinical manifestations of the inherited torsion dystonias.
Swaiman KF, Smith SA, Trock GL, Siddiqui AR: Sea-blue histiocytes, lymphocytic cytosomes, movement disorder and ^{59}Fe uptake in basal ganglia: Hallervorden-Spatz disease or ceroid storage disease with abnormal isotope scan? *Neurology* 33:301–305, 1983.
   The initial demonstration of sea-blue histiocytes and electron microscopic findings of lymphocytic cytosomes as extraneural evidence of HSS.
Vakili S, Drew AL, Von Schuching S, Becker D, Zeman W:

FEATURE TABLE 9–13. FAMILIAL PERIODIC ATAXIA

Discriminating Features	Consistent Features	Variable Feature
1. Periodic episodes of ataxia or vertigo	1. Difficulty walking during ataxia or vertiginous attacks	1. Cerebellar degeneration
2. Autosomal dominant	2. Precipitated by physical or emotional stress	
3. No loss of consciousness	3. Cerebellar signs on neurologic examination	
	4. Responds to acetazolamide	

Hallervorden-Spatz syndrome. *Arch Neurol* 34:729–738, 1977.

Summarizes radioactive studies demonstrating high uptake of iron in the basal ganglia region in a patient with HSS.

REFERENCES

Adams RD, Lyon G: *Neurology of Hereditary Metabolic Diseases of Children.* Washington/New York, Hemisphere/McGraw-Hill, 1982.

Allen N, Knopp W: Hereditary parkinsonism–dystonia with sustained control by L-dopa and anticholinergic medication. *Adv Neurol* 14:201–213, 1976.

Altman AJ, Bachner RL: Favorable prognosis for survival in children with coincident opsomyoclonus and neuroblastoma. *Cancer* 37:846–852, 1976.

Arden F: Idiopathic hypoparathyroidism. *Med J Aust* 2:217–219, 1953.

Aron AM, Freeman JM, Carter S: The natural history of Sydenham's chorea. *Am J Med* 38:83–95, 1965.

Bergman I, Hirsch RP, Fria TJ, Shapiro SM, Holzman I, Painter MJ: Cause of hearing loss in the high-risk premature infant. *J Pediatr* 106:95–101, 1985.

Bird MT, Palkes HP, Prensky AL: A follow-up study of Sydenham's chorea. *Neurology* 26:601–606, 1976.

Bird TD, Carlson CB, Horning M: Ten year follow-up of choreoathetosis: A sporadic case becomes familial. *Epilepsia* 19:129–132, 1978.

Byers RK, Dodge PA: Huntington's chorea in children. *Neurology* 17:587–596, 1967.

Byers RK, Paine PS, Crothers B: Extrapyramidal cerebral palsy with hearing loss following erythroblastosis. *Pediatrics* 15:248–254, 1955.

Carpenter MB, Sutin J: *Human Neuroanatomy,* 8th ed. Baltimore, Md, Williams & Wilkins, 1983, p 579–611.

Chun RWM, Daly RF, Mansheim BJ Jr, Wolcott GJ: Benign familial chorea with onset in childhood. *JAMA* 225:1603–1607, 1973.

Cohen DJ, Leckman JF, Shaywitz B: A physician's guide to diagnosis and treatment of Tourette syndrome. A neurological multiple tic disorder. Bayside, NY, Tourette Syndrome Association, 1984.

Davison C: Pallido-pyramidal disease. *J Neurol* 13:50–59, 1954.

Donat JR, Auger R: Familial periodic ataxia. *Arch Neurol* 36:568–569, 1979.

Dooling E, Schoene WC, Richardson EP: Hallervorden-Spatz syndrome. *Arch Neurol* 30:70–83, 1974.

Eldridge R: The torsion dystonias: Literature review and genetic and clinical studies. *Neurology* 20(no 11, pt 2):1–78, 1970.

Erickson GR, Chun RWM: Acquired paroxysmal movement disorders. *Pediatr Neurol* 3:226–229, 1987.

Farrer LA, Conneally PM: A genetic model for age of onset in Huntington's disease. *Am J Hum Genet* 37:350–357, 1985.

Fischbeck KH, Layzer RB: Paroxysmal choreoathetosis due to hypoglycemia. *Arch Neurol* 6:453–454, 1979.

Folstein SE, Phillips JA, Meyers DA, et al: HD: Two families with differing clinical features show linkage to the G8 probe. *Science* 229:776–779, 1985.

Freeman JM, Aron AM, Collard JE, MacKay MC: The emotional correlates of Sydenham's chorea. *Pediatrics* 35:42–48, 1965.

Garg BP: Dystonia musculorum deformans. Implications of therapeutic response to levodopa and carbamazepine. *Arch Neurol* 39:376–377, 1982.

Gartner LM, Snyder RN, Chabon RS, Bernstein J: Kernicterus: High incidence in premature infants with low serum bilirubin concentrations. *Pediatrics* 45:906–917, 1970.

Gerrard J: Nuclear jaundice and deafness. *J Laryngol Otol* 66:39–46, 1952.

Gilman S, Newman SW: *Manter and Gatz's Essentials of Clinical Neuroanatomy and Neurophysiology,* 7th ed. Philadelphia, FA Davis, 1987.

Golden GS: Movement disorders in children, in Kelley VC (ed): *Practice of Pediatrics,* Vol 9, Philadelphia, Harper & Row, 1984, p 1–24.

Golden GS: Tardive dyskinesia in Tourette syndrome. *Pediatr Neurol* 1:192–194, 1985.

Golden GS: Tourette syndrome: Recent advances. *Pediatr Neurol* 2:189–192, 1986.

Goodenough DJ, Fariello RG, Annis BJ, Chun RWM: Familial and acquired paroxysmal dyskinesias. A proposed classification with delineation of clinical features. *Arch Neurol* 35:827–831, 1978.

Griggs RC, Moxley RT III, Lafrance RA, McQuillen J: Hereditary paroxysmal ataxia: Response to acetazolamide. *Neurology* 28:1259–1264, 1978.

Guthrie M: Foreword, in Phillips DH (ed): *Living with Huntington's Disease.* Madison, University of Wisconsin Press, 1982, p xi.

Haerer AF, Currier RC, Jackson JF: Hereditary unprogressive chorea of early onset. *N Engl J Med* 276:1220–1224, 1967.

Hallervorden J, Spatz H: Eigenartige Erkrankung in extrapyramidalen System mit besonderer Beteiligung des Globus pallidus und der Substantia nigra. *Z Neurol Psychiatr* 79:254–302, 1922.

Hansotia P, Cleeland CS, Chun RWM: Juvenile Huntington's chorea. *Neurology* 18:217–224, 1968.

Harper PS: Benign hereditary chorea: Clinical and genetic aspects. *Clin Genet* 13:85–95, 1978.

Haymaker W, Margles C, Pentshew A, et al: Pathology of kernicterus and posticteric encephalopathy, in Swinyeard CA (ed): *Kernicterus and Its Importance in Cerebral Palsy.* Springfield, Ill, Charles C Thomas, 1961, p 21–228.

Herd JK, Medhi M, Uzendoski DM, Sadivar VA: Chorea associated with systemic lupus erythematosus: Report of two cases and review of the literature. *Pediatrics* 61:308–315, 1978.

Hunt JR: Progressive atrophy of the globus pallidus. (Primary atrophy of the pallidal system). A system disease of the paralysis agitans type, characterized by atrophy of the motor cells of the corpus striatum. *Brain* 40:58–148, 1917.

Husby G, Rijn IVD, Zabriskie JB, Abdin ZH, Williams RC: Antibodies reacting with cytoplasm of subthalamic and caudate nuclei neurons in chorea and acute rheumatic fever. *J Exp Med* 144:1094–1110, 1976.

Hyman CB, Keaster J, Hanson V, et al: CNS abnormalities after neonatal hemolytic disease or hyperbilirubinemia. A prospective study of 405 patients. *Am J Dis Child* 117:395–405, 1969.

Jervis JA: Huntington's chorea in childhood. *Arch Neurol* 9:244–256, 1963.

Johnson L, Boggs TR: Bilirubin-dependent brain damage: Incidence and indications for treatment, in Odell GB, Schalffer R, Sionpoulous AP (eds): *Phototherapy in the Newborn: An Overview.* Washington, DC, National Academy of Sciences, 1974, p 122–149.

Kinsbourne M: Myoclonic encephalopathy of infants. *J Neurol Neurosurg Psychiatr* 25:271–276, 1962.

Klawans HL, Weiner WJ: The pharmacology of choreatic movement disorders. *Prog Neurobiol* 6:49–80, 1976.

Koller WC, Davenport J: Genetic testing in HD. *Ann Neurol* 16:511–513, 1984.

Kuban KC, Moshe AE, Freeman RL, Laffell LB, Bresnan MJ: Syndrome of opsoclonus-myoclonus caused by Coxsackie B3 infection. *Ann Neurol* 13:69–71, 1983.

Kuhl DE, Phelps ME, Markham CH, et al: Cerebral metabolism and atrophy in Huntington's Disease determined by ^{18}FDG and computed tomographic scan. *Ann Neurol* 12:425–434, 1982.

Kurlan R and Shoulson I: Familial dystonic choreoathetosis and response to alternate day oxazepam therapy. *Ann Neurol* 13:456–457, 1983.

Lagregran J: Children with motor handicaps. *Acta Pediatr Scand (Suppl)* 289:1–71, 1981.

Lance JW: Familial dystonic choreoathetosis and its differentiation from related syndromes. *Ann Neurol* 2:285–293, 1977.

Leli DA, Furlow TW Jr, Falgout JC: Benign familial chorea: An association with intellectual impairment. *J Neurol Neurosurg Psychiatr* 47:471–474, 1984.

Littrup PL, Gebarski SS: MR imaging of Hallervorden-Spatz disease. *J Comput Assist Tomogr* 9:491–493, 1985.

Livingstone JR, Gardner-Medwin D, and Pennington RJT: Familial intermittent ataxia with possible X-linked recessive inheritance. Two patients with abnormal pyruvate metabolism and a response to acetazolamide. *J Neurol Sci* 64:89–97, 1984.

Lott I, Kinsbourne M: Myoclonic encephalopathy of infants. *Adv Neurol* 43:127–136, 1986.

Markham CH, Knox JW: Observations on Huntington's chorea in childhood. *J Pediatr* 67:46–56, 1965.

Martin WE, Resch JA, Baker AB: Juvenile parkinsonism. *Arch Neurol* 25:494–500, 1971.

Matkin ND, Carhart R: Auditory profiles associated with Rh incompatibility. *Arch Otolaryngol* 84:502–513, 1966.

Mayeux R, Fahn S: Paroxysmal dystonic choreoathetosis in a patient with familial ataxia. *Neurology* 32:1184–1186, 1982.

Miley CE, Forster FM: Paroxysmal signs and symptoms in multiple sclerosis. *Neurology* 24:458–461, 1974.

Mount LA, Reback S: Familial paroxysmal choreoathetosis; preliminary report on a hitherto undescribed clinical syndrome. *Arch Neurol Psychiatr* 44:841–847, 1940.

Myers RH, Goldman D, Bird ED, et al: Maternal transmission in Huntington's disease. *Lancet* 1:208–210, 1983.

Naeye RL: Amniotic fluid infections, neonatal hyperbilirubinemia and psychomotor impairment. *Pediatrics* 62:497–503, 1978.

Naidu S, Narasimhachari N: Sydenham's chorea: A possible presynaptic dopaminergic dysfunction initially. *Ann Neurol* 8:445–447, 1980.

Naidu S, Wolfson LI, Sharpless NS: Juvenile parkinsonism: A patient with possible primary striatal dysfunction. *Ann Neurol* 3:453–455, 1978.

Nausieda PA, Koller WC, Weiner WJ, Klawans HL: Chorea induced by oral contraceptives. *Neurology* 29:1605–1609, 1979.

Nausieda PA, Grossman BJ, Koller WC, Weiner WJ, Klawans HL: Sydenham chorea: An update. *Neurology* 30:331–334, 1980.

Nausieda PA, Bieliauskas LA, Bacon LD, Magerty M, Koller WC, Glantz RN: Chronic dopaminergic sensitivity after Sydenham's chorea. *Neurology* 33:750–754, 1983.

Newman RP, Kinkel WR: Paroxysmal choreoathetosis due to hypoglycemia. *Arch Neurol* 41:341–342, 1984.

Nygaard TG, Duvoisin RC: Hereditary dystonia–parkinsonism syndrome of juvenile onset. *Neurology* 36:1424–1428, 1986.

Odell GB, Storey GN, Rosenberg LA: Studies in kernicterus. III. The saturation of serum proteins with bilirubin during neonatal life and its relationship to brain damage at five years. *J Pediatr* 76:12–21, 1970.

Osborne JP, Munson P, Burman D: Huntington's chorea: Report of 3 cases and review of literature. *Arch Dis Child* 57:99–103, 1982.

Parker HL: Periodic ataxia. *Mayo Clin Proc* 38:642–645, 1946.

Perlstein MA: The late clinical syndrome of posticteric encephalopathy. *Pediatr Clin North Am* 7:665–687, 1960.

Robinson RO, Thornett CEE: Benign hereditary chorea—Response to steroids. *Dev Med Child Neurol* 27:814–821, 1985.

Rosen JA: Paroxysmal choreoathetosis associated with perinatal hypoxic encephalopathy. *Arch Neurol* 11:385–387, 1964.

Rubin RA, et al: Neonatal serum bilirubin levels related to cognitive development at ages 4–7 years. *J Pediatr* 94:601–604, 1979.

Sax DS, Menzer L: Computerized tomography in Huntington's disease. *Neurology* 27:388, 1977.

Segawa M, Hosaka A, Miyagawa F, et al: Hereditary progressive dystonia with marked diurnal fluctuation. *Adv Neurol* 14:215–233, 1976.

Sleigh G, Lindenbaum R: Benign (nonparoxysmal) familial chorea. Paediatric perspectives. *Arch Dis Child* 56:616–621, 1981.

Stephenson JBP, Graham-Pole J, Ogg L, Cochran AJ: Reactivity to neuroblastoma extracts in childhood cerebellar encephalopathy ("dancing eyes" syndrome). *Lancet* 2:976–976, 1976.

Swaiman KF, Smith SA, Trock GL, Siddiqui AR: Sea-blue histiocytes, lymphocytic cytosomes, movement disorder and ^{59}Fe uptake in basal ganglia: Hallervorden-Spatz disease or ceroid storage disease with abnormal isotope scan? *Neurology* 33:301–305, 1983.

Terrence CF, Delaney JF, Alberts MC: Computed tomography for Huntington's disease. *Neuroradiology* 13:173–175, 1977.

Tibbles JAR, Camfield PR, Cron CC, and Farrell K: Dominant recurrent ataxia and vertigo of childhood. *Pediatr Neurol* 2:35–38, 1986.

Vakili S, Drew AL, Von Schuching S, Becker D, Zeman W: Hallervorden-Spatz syndrome. *Arch Neurol* 34:729–738, 1977.

Vanasse M, Bedard P, Andemann F: Shuddering attacks in children: An early clinical manifestation of essential tremor. *Neurology* 26:1027–1030, 1976.

VanBogaert L: Contribution clinique et anatomique à l'étude de la paralysie agitante juvenile primitive. *Rev Neurol (Paris)* 37:315–326, 1930.

Volpe JJ: Bilirubin and brain injury, in Volpe JJ (ed): *Neurology of the Newborn*, 2nd ed. Major Problems in Clinical Pediatrics, Vol 22. Philadelphia, WB Saunders, 1987, p 386–408.

Wang BJ, Chang YC: Therapeutic blood levels of phenytoin in treatment of paroxysmal choreoathetosis. *Ther Drug Monitor* 7:81–82, 1985.

White JC: Familial periodic nystagmus, vertigo, and ataxia.

Arch Neurol 20:276–280, 1969.

Wilson SAK, Bruce BA: *Neurology*, 2nd ed, Vol 2, Baltimore, Md, Williams & Wilkins, 1955, p 709, 719.

Yokochi M, Narabayashi H, Lizuka R, Nagatsu T: Juvenile parkinsonism: Some clinical, pharmacological, and neuropathological aspects. *Adv Neurol* 40:407–413, 1984.

Zeman W: Pathology of the torsion dystonias (dystonia musculorum deformans) *Neurology* 20(no 11, pt 2):79–88, 1970.

Zeman W, Dyken P: Dystonia musculorum deformans. Clinical, genetic and pathoanatomic studies. *Psychiatr Neurol Neurochir (Amsterdam)* 70:77–121, 1967.

Chapter Ten

Infectious Diseases

Marvin A. Fishman

This chapter is organized according to the location of the infection within the nervous system or surrounding tissues. Descriptions of clinical syndromes are reviewed in the manner in which patients present to physicians. Detailed discussions of all etiologic agents that may cause a particular syndrome are not included but references are supplied for the interested reader.

Discriminating features point to specific location of infection along with the exclusion of other encephalopathic causes of the same entity.

SUBDURAL EMPYEMA

A subdural empyema is a collection of pus located between the dura and the arachnoid. It is usually located over the convexity of one or both cerebal hemispheres or in the parafalcine region between the two hemispheres, rarely beneath the tentorium. Predisposing conditions include infections of the middle ear and paranasal sinuses or a contiguous site of osteomyelitis. Occasionally empyemas may be complications of trauma or neurosurgical procedures. In infants and young children, the empyema can accompany meningitis.

Symptoms and Signs

The symptoms and signs are produced either by the underlying infection (i.e., sinusitis or otitis, previous surgery, or trauma) or intracranial complications. The latter may be produced by focal cortical inflammation corresponding to the location of the empyema or meningeal irritation and increased intracranial pressure. The disease is usually severe and rapidly progressive, but cases have been noted in which the symptoms have been present for several weeks before the diagnosis has been made. Fever is present in the majority of cases. In infants, findings often may be those related to meningitis or otitis and will include a bulging fontanelle, vomiting, lethargy, stiff neck, and seizures, which may be focal or generalized. Focal neurologic deficits are less common than in older children and adults. Headache is a prominent and frequent complaint in older children and adults. Lethargy is often present and hemiparesis or focal neurologic deficits are common. Seizures occur frequently and, when the empyema is parafalcine in location, focal seizures involving the leg are often present. Other findings include ocular palsies, dysphasia, homonymous hemianopia, dilated pupils, and cerebellar signs. Some of these are obviously related to increased intracranial pressure. The meningeal irritation may produce a stiff neck in the absence of meningitis.

Laboratory Findings

A peripheral leukocytosis may be present. The cerebrospinal fluid (CSF) shows nonspecific abnormalities unless meningitis is present. Because of the risk of cerebral herniation, lumbar puncture may be contraindicated. When the fluid is examined it is often under increased pressure and has an increased protein content and a moderate pleocytosis, which may have a polymorphonuclear predominance. The glucose is normal and the cultures are negative unless there is meninigitis.

Computed tomographic (CT) scanning or magnetic resonance imaging (MRI) are the methods of choice for making the diagnosis. These procedures will often define the location and extent of the subdural empyema. The findings include extra-axial crescentic or lentiform collections. There is usually a prominent, sharp medial rim of enhancement (Figure 10–1). Enhancement of the adjacent cerebral cortex is often present. Mass effect may be predominant. If the study is positive, no further imaging procedures are usually necessary. In rare instances, particularly early in the course of the illness, the CT scan may be nonspecific and only demonstrate findings consistent with a cerebritis. Rarely no abnormal findings will be found. In these cases repeat imaging procedures may be necessary. In infants, subdural paracentesis may be performed; the fluid will have a high protein content, a polymorphonuclear pleocytosis, low sugar, and positive bacterial culture.

FEATURE TABLE 10-1. SUBDURAL EMPYEMA

Discriminating Feature	Consistent Features	Variable Features
1. MRI/CT scan appearance and laboratory examination of fluid aspirated from subdural space	1. Fever 2. Headache (older children)	1. Focal neurologic deficits 2. Seizures

Etiology

The predisposing causes have been previously mentioned. These include sinusitis, otitis, trauma, neurosurgical procedures, osteomyelitis, and, in infants, meningitis. Occasionally, there may be a hematogenous spread of organisms from distant sites of infection.

The organisms isolated from subdural empyemas are similar to those associated with chronic sinusitis and cerebral abscesses. Aerobic streptococci are the most commonly isolated organisms. Staphylococci and microaerophilic and anaerobic streptococci are also frequently found. Aerobic Gram-negative rods and other anaerobes are found less frequently. A variety of other organisms have been isolated. In infants, the pathogens are those often found with meningitis and include *Hemophilus influenzae*, *Streptococcus pneumoniae*, Enterobacteriaceae, *Neisseria meningitidis*, and Group B Streptococci.

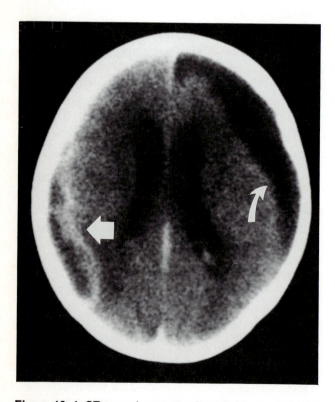

Figure 10-1. CT scan demonstrating bilateral extra-axial fluid collections. The straight arrow indicates an enhancing lesion, a subdural empyema, and the curved arrow points to a subdural effusion.

Pathology

The pathology is that which would be expected to be found with a localized empyema. There is often neovascularization and capsule formation. The adjacent normal brain is hyperemic. Other changes may include cortical vein thrombosis, cerebral arteritis, cerebritis with brain softening and necrosis, and abscess formation.

Course

Mortality and morbidity have been significantly reduced since the advent of CT and MRI, which have provided means for early diagnosis and noninvasive methods for following the course of the illness. Mortality is now under 10%. Early intervention with antibiotics, antiedema therapy, and surgical intervention have reduced the morbidity. Many of the deficits existing early in the course of the illness will show remarkable recovery. The late sequelae include epilepsy and persistent focal neurologic deficits, such as hemiparesis and dysphasia.

Treatment

Specific treatment of the bacterial infection is important. Until an etiologic diagnosis can be made, broad coverage with antibiotics that penetrate the blood-brain barrier well should be undertaken. This strategy might include the use of third-generation cephalosporins administered intravenously in doses appropriate to treat meningitis. Whenever possible, material for direct culture should be obtained and handled according to procedures similar to those used to isolate organisms from brain abscesses. Treatment of seizures with antiepileptic drugs and of cerebral edema with corticosteroids is appropriate. The

---

Pearls and Perils: Subdural Empyema

1. The clinical presentation of some patients with subdural empyemas, fever and focal seizures, may be similar to those caused by an encephalitis. Patients with meningismus who do not have meningitis may have a subdural empyema.
2. The CT scan may be negative early in the course of the illness. Therefore a normal scan at that time does not exclude the diagnosis.

majority of patients are also treated with surgical procedures, either multiple burr holes to access the subdural space or a large craniotomy for irrigation and removal of pus. There have been case reports of successful medical management. This may be considered in patients with small collections of fluid and with minimal symptomatology and signs who improve and stabilize with antibiotic therapy and in whom serial imaging shows resolution of the inflammatory process.

ENCEPHALITIS

Encephalitis will be defined in this chapter as an infection of brain parenchyma usually manifested by an altered state of consciousness, headache, neurologic signs, and fever. The diagnosis can often be confirmed by laboratory and neuroradiologic procedures. A variety of infectious agents can cause encephalitis, but this chapter will primarily focus on viral causes. Clinical syndromes resulting from acute, persistent, latent, chronic, and slow viral infections have been defined. The main focus of this discussion will be on acute syndromes.

The involvement of the nervous system may be confined primarily to the cerebrum, but predominant involvement of other areas of the central nervous system (CNS), such as the cerebellum, brainstem, and spinal cord has been noted. The clinical manifestations of the illness will depend on which part(s) of the CNS are affected. In addition, the viral infection may involve other organs of the body, such as the lungs, liver, heart, or skin, and this will also influence the clinical manifestations of the disease. The spectrum of illness may extend from short, relatively benign illness to a devastating one in which there are permanent neurologic sequelae or death.

Symptoms and Signs

The encephalitis may be part of a systemic illness such as measles or varicella, and thus the initial manifestations will be those of the initial illness. When the encephalitis is not part of a generalized viral infection there may be symptoms preceding the neurologic syndrome. These often include headache, malaise, myalgia, upper respiratory symptoms, and fever. Nausea, vomiting, and a stiff neck may be present. Direct involvement of the brain is heralded by lethargy, drowsiness, or stupor, which may progress to coma. Confusion, hallucinations and disorientation may be detected if consciousness is not too depressed. Seizures, either generalized or focal, may occur. Other neurologic findings include hemiplegia, papilledema, nystagmus, ataxia, anisocoria, dysphasia, diplopia, dysarthria, and hemianopia. Some of these findings may be produced by increased intracranial pressure and herniation syndromes rather than direct involvement of specific parts of the brain by the virus.

With predominant involvement of the brainstem, pupillary and oculovestibular reflexes may be altered. Cranial nerve deficits and changes in respiratory pattern occur. There may also be signs of ataxia, tremor, and coordinaton deficits related to dysfunction of cerebellar connections. Paraplegia, sensory levels, and involvement of bowel and bladder sphincters may be present with predominant involvement of the spinal cord. Involvement of the anterior horn cell is manifested by flaccid paralysis, hypotonia, and a loss of deep tendon reflexes without significant sensory signs. Predominant cerebellar involvement may be manifested by ataxia, nystagmus, dysarthria, and tremors.

Specific Syndromes

A complete review of the various viral agents that affect the nervous system is beyond the scope of this chapter; however, a few will be discussed. The most common cause of nonepidemic acute viral encephalitis is herpes simplex virus (HSV) type I. Illness in the neonate, including disseminated herpes infection, is often caused by HSV type II. In children, the encephalitis may be preceded by a vague prodrome of fever, headache, and malaise. There is usually a rapid progression of the illness with development of prominant neurologic signs, such as behavioral abnormalities, clouding and diminished levels of consciousness, seizures, and focal neurologic deficits. The HSV shows a propensity for affecting the temporal lobes and thus many of the neurologic signs may be associated with dysfunction of these areas of the brain. The involvement is often asymmetric and the neurologic dysfunction may be related to one hemisphere. Fever occurs in almost all cases and may be marked. The clinical signs are not specific for herpes simplex encephalitis but a focal encephalitis with involvement of temporal lobes strongly suggests that the illness is due to HSV. The ex-

FEATURE TABLE 10-2. ENCEPHALITIS

Discriminating Feature	Consistent Features	Variable Features
1. Evidence of diffuse cerebral dysfunction in absence of infection localized to other CNS location(s) and/or toxic metabolic encephalopathies	1. Characteristic CSF findings 2. Abnormal EEG 3. Fever	1. Change in sensorium 2. Focal neurologic signs 3. Seizures

act pathogenesis of the infection is not totally understood but the majority of the cases do not appear to be related to primary infection with the virus. The illness is thought to be due to activation of a latent infection during which the viral genome is sequestered in neurons of various portions of the nervous system, including the trigeminal ganglia. Early diagnosis and institution of therapy are important because the prognosis is best in younger patients who have the least depression of level of consciousness.

Subacute sclerosing panencephalitis (SSPE) is caused by a chronic infection of the brain with a measles virus that is defective in relation to the matrix protein. The disease usually occurs in children between 5 and 17 years of age, and most of the patients have had exposure to natural measles infection early in life. The incidence of this disease has been drastically reduced following the institution of measles immunizations. The symptoms usually begin with a decline in intellectual function and a decrease in school performance. There may be forgetfulness, irritability, lethargy, and slurred speech. The second phase of the illness is characterized by convulsions and motor signs, including dyskinesias, choreoathetoid movements, incoordination, and myoclonus of the head, limbs, or trunk. Progression of the disease leads to coma, and opisthotonus with decerebrate rigidity, extensor hypertonus, and lack of responsiveness to stimuli. The final stage of the disease is that of vegetative mutism, with quadriparesis, myoclonus, and startle responses. Ophthalmologic abnormalities found during the course of the disease include optic atrophy or pallor, occasionally papilledema, and macular pigmentary abnormalities.

Progressive rubella panencephalitis is a slowly progressive illness caused by the rubella virus. It occurs in patients who have had congenital as well as postnatally acquired rubella. The disease has its onset in childhood in patients who have static neurologic deficits related to congenital rubella or who are free of symptoms. The manifestations include the insidious onset of intellectual deterioration, ataxia, and seizures. The findings on examination include dementia, spasticity, deficits in coordination, and abnormal ophthalmologic findings, including optic atrophy and retinitis.

Infection of brain with the human immunodeficiency virus (HIV) is becoming one of the most common causes of progressive neurologic syndromes in children. The majority of children are infected during the prenatal or perinatal period. After a latency, which is most often several years and may be as long as 10 years, neurologic signs and symptoms develop. Neurologic involvement tends to parallel the immune system dysfunction but on occasion may be the first manifestation of HIV infection.

Involvement by the nervous system is manifest by a variety of neurologic syndromes, developmental disturbances, and behavioral abnormalities. The neurologic manifestations include loss of intellectual abilities or motor milestones, accompanied by weakness, pyramidal signs, pseudobulbar palsy, ataxia, seizures, myoclonus, and extrapyramidal rigidity. There is often secondary microcephaly. Several clinical courses have been noted. The most severe is subacute and relentlessly progressive, resulting in death within several months. A more indolent course with an insidious onset has also been described. Developmental progress plateaus but, after a period of quiescence, neurologic deterioration results and death usually occurs within a year. In some children the course may appear to plateau and a static phase may persist for several years. Unusually, a progressive neurologic syndrome, subacute in nature, may be the first manifestation of HIV infection. This may be manifest by personality changes, lethargy, loss of previously acquired cognitive and motor skills, and seizures.

The developmental manifestations may be characterized by normal acquisition of early developmental milestones followed by mild or moderate delays. The symptoms usually appear between 2 months and 5 years of age. The course may be static, slowly progressive, or in the form of a rapid dementia. In infancy, the most profound delays tend to occur in the acquisiton of motor skills. In older children, perceptual motor deficits, impairment of gross and fine motor skills, and expressive language delay are prominent.

Behavioral changes may be the first symptoms. Syndromes of aggressiveness and hyperactivity have been noted. Cognitive and motor deficits may follow the initial manifestations of the behavioral disorder.

The encephalopathy is thought to be due to direct involvement of the brain by the HIV. Opportunistic infections of the CNS are much less common in children compared to adults.

Routine analysis of the CSF is usually normal. Occasionally, increased protein content and modest pleocytosis may be present. Intrathecal antibody synthesis against HIV or the presence of HIV antigens may be demonstrated. Neuroimaging of the brain may reveal progressive atrophy and abnormalities of the white matter. Bilateral symmetric calcifications have been noted in the basal ganglia and frontal lobe white matter.

Patients with acquired immunodeficiency syndrome are susceptible to multiple opportunistic infections. Many of these can affect the nervous system, and involvement with cytomegalovirus, echovirus, *Mycobacterium, Pneumocystis, Toxoplasma, Cryptococcus, Candida,* papovavirus, and HSV, among others, has been documented.

Many agents can affect the developing nervous system in utero and have devastating effects. Depending on the gestational age at the time of infection, multiple organ systems may be involved. Infection with rubella virus often results in cataracts, congenital heart disease, and deafness. Microcephaly, mental retardation, and seizures may result from intrauterine infection. Other manifestations include microphthalmia, glaucoma, and chorioretinitis. Congenital herpes simplex encephalitis

(HSE) produces a severe encephaloclastic process resulting in microcephaly and marked motor and developmental impairment. Congenital cytomegalovirus infection may affect the developing nervous system and produce a severe picture of meningoencephalitis, either hydrocephalus or microcephaly, seizures, mental retardation, and deafness. In the fulminant form of the disease other organ systems may be involved and hepatosplenomegaly, thrombocytopenia, and jaundice are often present. The manifestations may be much less severe without overt signs of generalized infection and children may present later in infancy or childhood with seizures or hearing loss.

Congenital toxoplasmosis, a parasitic infection, may also produce disseminated disease in the fetus. The clinical picture may be similar to that of congenital cytomegalovirus disease. Hydrocephalus, increased intracranial pressure, and opisthotonic posturing may be present. Chorioretinitis, seizures, and microcephaly are noted sequelae. The clinical manifestations may be less severe and manifest as only mild intellectual impairment.

Laboratory Findings

Examination of the CSF may show variable results. The pressure may be elevated. If signs of increased intracranial pressure are present, the etiology of the symptoms may be due to a space-occupying lesion. The performance of emergency imaging procedures such as CT scans should be considered before doing a lumbar puncture. The usual findings in the CSF with viral infections of the nervous system include increased protein content, normal glucose content, and a pleocytosis with predominantly mononuclear cells. However, early in the course of the illness there may be a predominance of polymorphonuclear cells and a low glucose concentration. Rarely the CSF may be normal. Antibodies to viruses may be found in the CSF and the titers may increase during the course of the illness or during the recovery phase. The ratio of serum to CSF antibodies may be helpful in demonstrating intrathecal synthesis of immune globulins, as opposed to the nonspecific passive transfer of antibodies from serum to CSF through a damaged blood-brain barrier. In chronic infections such as SSPE and progressive rubella panencephalitis, the titer may be abnormally high and diagnostic at the time of the initial CSF evaluation. Nonspecific elevations of CSF IgG are also found in these latter conditions. Attempts to isolate virus from the CSF may be undertaken. However, even with proven viral infections of the brain, the agent may not be recovered. This is particularly true for HSE, in which the virus can be isolated from the brain but not from the CSF.

The electroencephalogram may show nonspecific abnormalities. Focal abnormalities may be helpful in selecting an appropriate site for brain biopsy if this is being considered. The electroencephalogram may reveal patterns that are characteristic but not necesssarily diagnostic of certain types of encephalitides. In HSE there may be periodic lateralized discharges or slowing over temporal lobe regions. In SSPE the electroencephalogram may reveal periodic bursts followed by periods of electrical inactivity. These may correlate with myoclonic jerks.

Imaging of the brain should be performed in all children with a clinical diagnosis of encephalitis. Other diagnoses that may produce similar clinical findings include abscesses, tumors, strokes, and subarachnoid hemorrhage. Focal temporal lobe abnormalities when present suggest HSE, but these changes may not be present early in the course of the disease. The finding of intracranial calcifications may suggest infection with cytomegalovirus or toxoplasmosis. The imaging may also suggest other diagnoses such as tuberculosis or cysticercosis.

Brain biopsy may rarely need to be considered to establish a definitive diagnosis, particularly in HSE, or to help establish an alternate diagnosis. In addition to routine histochemical studies, electron microscopy, immunofluorescent studies, and culture should be performed.

Demonstration of rises in serum antibody titers to specific viral agents may be suggestive of an etiologic agent for the encephalitic illness. This may be very helpful in illnesses associated with Epstein-Barr virus infection or *Mycoplasma pneumoniae* infection.

Other laboratory tests can be helpful in excluding other conditions or documenting involvement of other organ systems. In addition to routine serum chemistries, tests of liver function and serum ammonia should be obtained. Toxicologic screens of urine and serum should be considered. Chest x rays and electrocardiograms may be appropriate when pulmonary or myocardial involvement is suspected. Determination of cold agglutinin and heterophil antibody titers, in addition to specific serologies, may be helpful.

Etiology

Table 10-1 lists viruses responsible for acute encephalitis in children. In addition to viral infections of the brain, a number of nonviral agents can involve the

TABLE 10-1. VIRUSES PRODUCING ACUTE ENCEPHALITIS IN CHILDREN

Adenovirus	Influenza
California group	Lymphocytic choreomeningitis
Coxsackie virus	Measles
Cytomegalovirus	Mumps
Eastern equine	Poliovirus
Echo virus	Rubella
Epstein-Barr	St. Louis
Herpes simplex	Varicella-Zoster
HIV	Western equine

TABLE 10-2. INFECTIONS THAT MAY MIMIC VIRAL ENCEPHALITIS

Bacterial infections	Parasitic infections
Brain abscess	Cysticercosis
Meningitis	Naegleria
Mycoplasma pneumoniae	Toxoplasmosis
infection	Rickettsial infections
Shigellosis	Rocky Mountain spotted
Subacute bacterial	fever
endocarditis	Spirochaetal infections
Tuberculosis	Leptospirosis
Fungal infections	Syphilis
Candida infection	
Coccidioidomyosis	
Cryptococcosis	
Histoplasmosis	

nervous system and produce clinical illnesses that mimic the symptomatolgy and signs of viral encephalitis. The more common infections are listed in Table 10-2. In addition to infectious agents involving the nervous system, the clinical symptomatology of a number of other noninfectious illnesses may also mimic that of an acute encephalitis. The more common conditions are listed in Table 10-3.

Pathology

The changes found in the brains of patients with encephalitis will vary depending on the causative agent. The basic pathology in acute viral encephalitides consists of a predominantly mononuclear perivascular inflammatory response, which may be associated with inflammation of the meninges. The neurons may show degenerative changes with neuronophagia. Gross areas of hemorrhage and necrosis may occur and are particularly common with infection by HSV. Inclusion bodies may be found in infections caused by HSV and cytomegalovirus, measles, SSPE, polio, and rabies.

Course

The course of the illness is quite variable and depends in part on the infectious agent, the age of the patient, and any underlying medical conditions. Severe involvement

TABLE 10-3. NONINFECTIOUS DISORDERS THAT MAY MIMIC VIRAL ENCEPHALITIS

Intoxications	Neoplastic disorders
Drug	Brain tumor
Lead	CNS leukemia, lymphoma
Endocrine-metabolic	Psychoses
disorders	Acute psychosis
Electrolytes, glucose,	Vascular disorders
organic acids	Hypertensive
Hepatic encephalopathies	encephalopathy
Pulmonary (hypoxic)	Stroke (thrombotic or
encephalopathies	hemorrhagic)
Renal encephalopathies	Vasculitis, including lupus
Reye's syndrome	erythematosus

of the developing brain in utero will obviously cause permanent sequelae, including motor and mental deficits, blindness, deafness, and epilepsy. Some illnesses, such as SSPE, are universally fatal but their course may extend from months to years. Occasionally there may be a smoldering course over a prolonged period of time, such as with progressive rubella encephalitis. Remitting and relapsing courses have been noted in patients infected with HSV. Early treatment of patients who have HSV with appropriate antiviral chemotherapeutic agents, such as acyclovir, reduces the morbidity and mortality.

Treatment

Infections such as those listed in Table 10-2 may respond to specific therapy. Acyclovir has been demonstrated to be effective in the treatment of patients with HSE. At the present time this is the only viral encephalitis that definitely responds to treatment. Therefore, diagnosis and early initiation of therapy are of paramount importance. Studies using other agents to treat various encephalitides are underway but definitive results are not yet available. Recently, zidovudine has been shown to increase brain growth and cognitive function of children with HIV.

Increased intracranial pressure is often a problem. Treatment would include elevation of the head of the patient to approximately 30°, fluid restriction when appropriate, and hyperventilation with maintaining the PCO_2 at approximately 25 mm Hg. The use of mannitol and other hyperosmotic agents as well as diuretics should be considered. The use of corticosteroids in the treatment of viral encephalitis appears to be of no value.

Seizures are often a problem and one should be prepared to treat patients with serial seizures or status epilepticus. The intravenous use of antiepileptic agents, such as diazepam, phenytoin, and phenobarbital may be necessary.

Good supportive care is essential for improving the survival and decreasing the morbidity of patients with acute encephalopathies.

Pearls and Perils: Encephalitis

1. The symptoms and signs produced by viral encephalitides may be similar to those produced by other processes affecting the CNS. These include infections, such as subdural empyema and brain abscess, and noninfectious causes, such as strokes and intoxications.
2. The CT scan is often normal during the early stages of HSE.
3. A lumbar puncture may promote the development of a herniation syndrome in patients with symptoms or signs of acute increased intracranial pressure. There should be sound clinical or imaging evidence excluding intracranial masses before a lumbar puncture is undertaken.

BRAIN ABSCESS

Local suppurative infection within the brain parenchyma results in abscess formation. Most often there is a single abscess but multiple foci do occur. Brain abscesses are unusual in children under 2 years of age. Males are affected more frequently than females. In the majority of instances an underlying predisposing cause is present. Possible causes include chronic otitis media, sinusitis, and facial cellulitis. Often direct extension from these areas or extension along the vascular channels is responsible for the spread of the infection into the brain. Hematogenous spread occurs after dental work, in the presence of congenital heart disease (especially cyanotic heart disease), and in the presence of pulmonary infection, including cystic fibrosis. Direct infection of the brain can occur after neurosurgical procedures or head trauma, including such relatively minor clinical events as penetration of the skull by a pencil tip or a rose thorn. In approximately 25% of the cases, no predisposing factor can be identified.

Symptoms and Signs

Symptoms and signs are produced by a number of mechanisms. These would include those attributable to the predisposing condition, that is, sinusitis, chronic otitis, heart disease, and pulmonary disease; those attributed to an intracranial mass and thus dependent on the location of the abscess; and those that are due to brain edema and increased intracranial pressure. Symptoms and signs related to the predisposing condition will not be discussed. Fever is not present in the majority of the patients. During the early stages the symptoms are often nonspecific and include headache, lethargy, changes in sensorium, or seizures. In early infancy, vomiting and seizures may be the initial manifestations and the symptoms are often related to increased intracranial pressure rather than focal neurologic deficits. As the disease progresses, headache and lethargy become more prominent and focal neurologic dysfunction becomes apparent. Signs may include hemipareses, focal seizures, and coordination and balance difficulties related to cerebellar dysfunction when the abscess is in the posterior fossa. Most unusually cranial nerve deficits, nystagmus, ataxia, and long tract signs may be present when the abscess is located in the brainstem. If the disease continues to progress increased intracranial pressure and herniation syndromes develop. Deficits include papilledema; diplopia owing to paresis of the third or sixth cranial nerve; abnormal pupillary findings; ptosis; hemiparesis; posturing; changes in respiration, blood pressure, and heart rate; and coma caused by herniation syndromes. Sudden deterioration can also occur owing to rupture of an abscess into the ventricular system.

Laboratory Findings

There may be nonspecific findings such as a leukocytosis and elevated sedimentation rate. Examination of the CSF may reveal abnormalities. The pressure is almost always elevated and the majority of specimens will have an elevated protein content or an increased number of white cells, which may be lymphocytic or polymorphonuclear leukocytes. Markedly elevated white blood cell counts with a predominance of polymorphonuclear leukocytes may indicate an associated meningitis or rupture of the abscess into the ventricular system. In the absence of the latter events, cultures are rarely positive. Performance of a lumbar puncture in a patient who has a brain abscess may not be safe. The presence of a localized mass lesion and increased intracranial pressure may predispose to herniation syndromes, which can be precipitated by removal of CSF at the time of the lumbar puncture or by continued leakage of CSF through the dura after the tap. Therefore, whenever the possibility of a brain abscess exists, an imaging procedure, such as CT or MRI of the brain, should be performed and, if an abscess is found, examination of the CSF should not be undertaken.

Radiographs of the skull in most instances are not helpful. They may show nonspecific signs of increased intracranial pressure. Evidence of chronic otitis media, mastoiditis, or sinusitis may be present. However, the same information can often be obtained by CT or MRI examination. The skull radiographs may be more useful after significant head trauma. Radiographs of the chest may reveal the presence of cardiac or pulmonary disease.

CT and MRI scanning have significantly increased the ability to diagnose and manage patients with brain abscesses. They have a high degree of sensitivity and when used in conjunction with contrast enhancement will provide information regarding localization, presence of multiple lesions, and stage of the infection, and be useful in following the effectiveness of therapeutic interventions. Early in the course of the disease only a pattern of cerebritis may be present. This includes the finding of a patchy, nonuniform enhancement pattern in which there is not definite encapsulation. The abscess may appear as

FEATURE TABLE 10-3. BRAIN ABSCESS

Discriminating Feature	Consistent Feature	Variable Features
1. CT scan appearance with laboratory or pathologic confirmation of infection	1. Headache	1. Focal neurologic deficits 2. Increased intracranial pressure

a dense nodule with a surrounding lucent zone, a faint dense ring with surrounding lucent zone, or a purely radiolucent lesion. After administration of contrast material, there may be enhancement of the nodule or the ring around the lucent lesion and the edema surrounding the site of infection may be more apparent (Figure 10–2). Enhancement of the ependyma indicates the presence of an associated ventriculitis. Use of CT has led to a significant decrease in the mortality associated with brain abscesses. The CT findings with an abscess may be similar to those with gliomas, infarcts, or metastatic tumors.

Etiology

The bacterial organism(s) in and location of abscesses are influenced by the presence of predisposing diseases. Abscesses associated with chronic otitis or mastoiditis are often located in the temporal lobe or cerebellar hemisphere. Those associated with sinusitis are commonly found in the frontal areas. Tetralogy of Fallot is the most common cyanotic heart lesion predisposing to abscess formation. Right-to-left shunts allow venous blood to circulate directly to the brain and thus bypass the filtering effect of the lungs. Abscesses associated with hematogenous spread are distributed among the frontal, temporal, and parietal lobes. The organisms most commonly found include various species of streptococci, a staphylococci, and *Hemophilus*. A variety of other organisms, including Gram-negative bacteria, may be present. Often more than one organism may be found in a culture. The organisms include both aerobic and anaerobic bacteria and particular care must be taken by the bacteriology laboratory to culture for all possible types of species. Less commonly found organisms include species of *Candida*, *Nocardia*, and *Amoeba.* Localized parenchymal infections can also be caused by the tubercle bacillus and various parasitic organisms.

Pathology

The earliest stage in abscess formation is cerebritis. There is softening and hyperemia of the brain parenchyma accompanied by an infiltration of inflammatory cells. Necrosis occurs in the center of the lesion, which undergoes liquefaction during pus formation. Fibroblastic activity occurs around the circumference of the abscess and gliosis develops in the surrounding brain tissue. The lesion thus becomes encapsulated. There is considerable reaction in the brain tissue surrounding the abscess; often marked edema of the white matter is present and may extend some distance from the center of the abscess (Figure 10–3). This adds to the mass effect. The capsule is often thicker on the lateral side of the lesion compared to the medial side. Thus when the abscess is near the ventricular system rupture results in the spillage of pus into the CSF.

Course

The progression of the clinical symptomatology has already been outlined. In children, nonspecific signs and symptoms, such as headache and lethargy, may progress to localizing signs, such as hemiparesis, hemianopia, focal seizures, or cerebellar deficits. Eventually signs of increased intracranial pressure and herniation develop.

The findings on CT reflect the stages of development of the abscess, which can be divided into cerebritis and capsule phases. In the cerebritis phase, the nonenhanced scan shows areas of low density that initially show nodular patchy or ring-like enhancement. As the cerebritis progresses, typical ring enhancement is present, which is often diffuse and thick. A delayed scan may demonstrate diffusion of the contrast material into the center of the lesion with persistent ring-like enhancement. In the capsular stage, the nonenhanced scan will reveal the presence of the capsule, which is visualized as a faint ring surrounding the necrotic center. Edema is present outside the capsule. The enhancement forms a definite ring, which may be thin to thick, depending on the degree of encapsulation. On delayed scans there is decay in the contrast enhancement and no diffusion into the center of the abscess. The ability to image the brain in a noninvasive

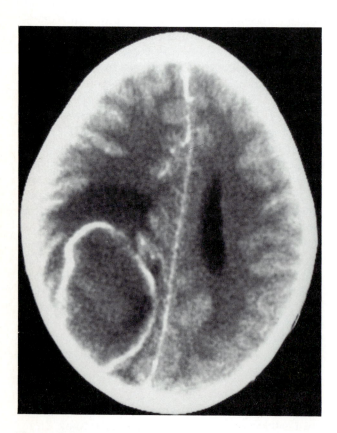

Figure 10–2. CT scan demonstrating an enhancing brain abscess. There is associated edema and mass effect with compression of the ventricle and shift of the midline.

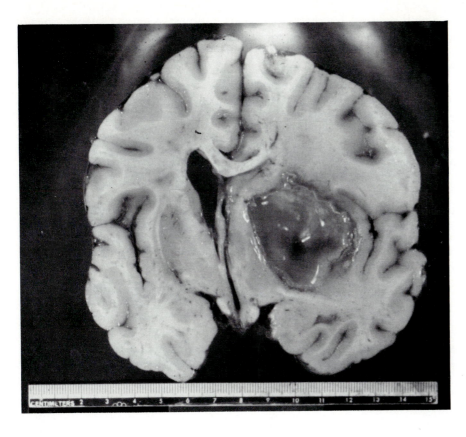

Figure 10-3. Coronal section of a brain demonstrating an abscess with a necrotic center and surrounding gliosis. There is edema of the white matter, compression of the adjacent ventricle, and shift of the midline.

fashion and the sensitivity of the CT scan for brain abscesses have resulted in significant improvement in the management of this problem. Earlier diagnosis in the cerebritis stage and the earlier institution of appropriate therapy are now possible, and this has resulted in a decrease in morbidity and mortality. Use of serial CT scans has allowed monitoring of the size of the abscess during treatment and has resulted in a decreased need for attempts at early surgical excision or repeated aspirations.

The long-term sequelae of brain abscess are variable. Difficulty with academic achievement has been noted as well as residual emotional problems. There may be deficits related to motor functions, such as hemiparesis and coordination difficulties, as well as visual field defects. Epilepsy is often a late sequela.

Treatment

The treatment can be divided into various aspects. Once the diagnosis of brain abscess has been made, treatment with antibiotics should be initiated. Broad-spectrum coverage may be initiated in doses similar to those used to treat meningitis. If one suspects a fungal etiology, then additional therapeutic agents may be required. Whenever possible the abscess should be aspirated and appropriate cultures obtained for a variety of organisms, as discussed under Etiology. When results become available, specific antibiotic therapy can be continued or initiated. If the neurologic condition of the patient is stable, conservative management with intravenous antibiotics is preferred. Repeated aspiration may be necessary to reduce the size of the abscess if the lesion does not spontaneously stabilize or become smaller with medical therapy. This strategy allows the pus to be recultured, so that the effectiveness of antibiotic therapies can be monitored. Attempts to ex-

---

Pearls and Perils: Brain Abscess

1. Findings related to infection, that is, fever and leukocytosis, are often absent in patients with brain abscesses, and their absence should not dissuade one from the possibility of a brain abscess being present.
2. In children with congenital heart disease under 2 years of age who develop focal neurologic deficits, the etiology is more likely to be vascular events than brain abscesses.
3. The onset of focal neurologic symptoms or signs in a patient with cystic fibrosis should suggest the possibility of a brain abscess.
4. Lumbar punctures are not helpful in establishing the bacterial etiology of a brain abscess unless there is an associated meningitis. The performance of a lumbar puncture may cause neurologic deterioration and thus should be avoided.

cise the abscess totally are rarely required with current management strategies. Antibiotic therapy may be required for many weeks.

Cerebral edema associated with brain abscess responds readily to steroid administration. If significant edema and mass effect are found on CT examination intravenous steroids should be employed. Their use will decrease the degree of contrast enhancement seen on CT scans. This is more obvious in the cerebritis and early capsule stages but is less apparent with well-encapsulated lesions.

Many neurologists would routinely institute antiepileptic drug therapy because of the high epileptogenicity of brain abscesses. Therapy with appropriate doses of phenytoin can be initiated intravenously and later continued orally, or other anticonvulsants may be used.

ACUTE CEREBELLAR ATAXIA

Acute cerebellar ataxia usually occurs in pre-school-age children following a variety of acute infectious diseases. In some instances, no history of preceding illness exists and the syndrome occurs in otherwise previously well children. Most of the signs and symptoms are related to cerebellar dysfunction; however, there may be more diffuse involvement of the nervous system and the clinical picture may not be one of ataxia alone.

Symptoms and Signs

The prodrome may be a nonspecific illness occurring anywhere from 1 day to 3 weeks prior to the onset of neurologic symptoms. The preceding infection may be respiratory or gastrointestinal, or one of the childhood exanthems (especially varicella). The most common neurologic symptom is rapid deterioration of gait. The child may stagger or fall. Truncal ataxia may be present and interfere with standing or sitting. In severe cases he or she may be confined to bed. Ataxia of the upper extremities may occur. Tremors of the head, trunk, and axial musculature may be present, which may be apparent at rest or during volitional movement. Abnormal eye movements are often present, and these may consist of nystagmus or abnormalities of gaze. Ocular dysmetria or flutter and opsoclonus have been noted. Other symptoms include vomiting, headache, photophobia, and ir-

ritability. Rarely do seizures occur. This latter group of symptoms may not be explained only on the basis of cerebellar dysfunction. The disability usually reaches its maximum within 1 to 2 days from onset but may progress more slowly.

The most significant findings on examination are related to the neurologic dysfunction. However, there may be findings related to the prodromal illness. The majority of children are afebrile. Residue of the previous exanthems may be noted. The findings on neurologic examination include truncal and limb ataxia, abnormal eye movements, tremors, and hypotonia. The deep tendon reflexes are variable and may be either increased or decreased. The fundi are normal. Rarely hemipareses have been noted.

Laboratory Findings

No characteristic abnormalities are present. Evidence of preceding infection may be present. The CSF in most instances is normal. Occasionally there may be slight CSF pleocytosis or an occasional mild elevation of the protein content. Magnetic resonance imaging of the brain will exclude the presence of a posterior fossa mass lesion or hydrocephalus, which could cause similar symptoms.

Etiology

A variety of preceding infections have been associated with the development of acute cerebellar ataxia. These have included varicella, measles, scarlet fever, influenza, polio, rubeola, rubella, mumps, *Mycoplasma pneumoniae infection*, Epstein-Barr virus infection, and possibly legionellosis and enterovirus infection.

Pathology

The disease is not fatal unless death occurs because of an underlying preceding infection. Therefore, there are no specific studies of the neuropathology of this syndrome.

Course

The majority of the patients will show spontaneous improvement and resolution of symptoms within a week to months after the onset. However, those patients who are most severely affected initially may show persistent deficits, including unsteadiness of gait, extremity ataxia, and tremor. Occasionally speech problems may persist.

FEATURE TABLE 10–4. ACUTE CEREBELLAR ATAXIA

Discriminating Feature	Consistent Feature	Variable Features
1. Ataxia in association with acute preceding infection in the absence of symptoms of elevated intracranial pressure or toxic or metabolic disorders	1. Tremor	1. Abnormal eye movements 2. "Noncerebellar" deficits 3. Seizures

Pearls and Perils: Acute Cerebellar Ataxia

1. Varicella is the most common exanthem preceding acute cerebellar ataxia. Occasionally the ataxia may precede the appearance of a rash.
2. Children with the Guillain-Barré syndrome may present with gait difficulty that at times can be confused with ataxia. The findings of distinct muscle weakness and areflexia, which occur in the Guillain-Barré syndrome, should distinguish that disorder from acute cerebellar ataxia.
3. Acute ataxia may be a manifestation of an intoxication. Appropriate laboratory tests should be considered to exclude the possibility of toxin or drug ingestion.
4. Acute illness often results in closer observation of children by their parents. A preexisting deficit may first be noted or the intercurrent illness may exacerbate preexisting symptoms. Therefore, one should always consider the possibility of structural lesions such as tumors or hydrocephalus being present. Posterior fossa mass lesions such as hematomas may also present with ataxia.
5. Other conditions, such as bacterial meningitis, underlying metabolic disorders, and infantile polymyoclonia associated with neuroblastoma, must be considered.

Treatment

Supportive treatment is appropriate. There is no specific therapy.

ACUTE TRANSVERSE MYELITIS

Acute transverse myelitis is characterized by intramedullary bilateral dysfunction of the spinal cord occurring in patients who have not had any previous history of similar neurologic diseases. Motor, sensory, and sphincter disturbances are present. In children, there is often a history of a preceding infectious disease. The syndrome occurs in children of all ages, including infancy.

Symptoms and Signs

The symptoms usually develop rapidly and reach their maximum extent within 3 to 4 days. Occasionally the course is subacute with progression over days to weeks. The initial symptom usually consists of pain or paresthesia involving the legs and trunk. Weakness begins in the legs and may ascend up the trunk. Occasionally the arms are involved as well. Rarely urinary retention may be the presenting symptom.

Examination reveals a flaccid weakness of the lower extremities with loss of reflexes. In patients with an ascending pattern the upper extremities may be involved. A sensory level occurs over the trunk, usually in the lower thoracic region. Occasionally, the sensory findings are dissociated, but loss of pinprick sensation is the most consistent finding. The levels of vibratory and proprioception losses are often below that of the analgesia. Occasionally posterior column function is spared. Neck stiffness or pain on straight leg raising may be present. Tenderness over the spine is occasionally noted. The flaccid weakness may become spastic over a period of weeks to months.

Laboratory Findings

There are no characteristic laboratory tests. The CSF may show a pleocytosis with a variable portion of polymorphonuclear cells. Elevated protein content may be present and the γ-globulin fraction may be increased. MRI is now the procedure of choice to exclude such conditions as an acute spinal epidural abscess, spinal cord tumor, or vascular malformation. If MRI is unavailable or inconclusive, myelography may be necessary. Typical MRI findings include edema and increased signal intensity at the levels of the lesion on T_2-weighted images.

Etiology

A variety of preceding illnesses have been associated with acute transverse myelitis. These include measles, mumps, rubella, herpes zoster, varicella, infectious mononucleosis, and other nonspecific viral illnesses involving the respiratory and gastrointestinal systems. Picornaviruses and retroviruses, including HIV, have been associated with the development of myelitis.

Pathology

There is nonspecific necrosis affecting the gray and white matter of the spinal cord and the distribution is not confined to the area of blood supply of a single artery. Axons, cell bodies, and myelin sheaths are destroyed. The area of involvement may be focal and transverse or extend over a more longitudinal section of the spinal cord.

FEATURE TABLE 10-5. ACUTE TRANSVERSE MYELITIS

Discriminating Feature	Consistent Feature	Variable Features
1. Imaging and laboratory procedures excluding other pathology	1. Motor and sensory deficits owing to spinal cord dysfunction	1. Neck stiffness 2. Spine tenderness

Pearls and Perils: Acute Transverse Myelitis

1. Acute transverse myelitis may be the first sign of multiple sclerosis. Patients who later develop acute optic or retrobulbar neuritis after the presence of a transverse myelitis have an illness known as Devic's syndrome, which is a demyelinating disease and probably a variant of multiple sclerosis.
2. A surgically treatable lesion such as an epidural abscess must be excluded.
3. Occasionally acute transverse myelitis may be a manifestation of other conditions, including syphilis and systemic lupus erythematosus; these must be remembered because of additional therapeutic considerations.

Course

The outcome is variable and ranges from almost total recovery to severe permanent paralysis and disability. Approximately one third of the patients will have a good recovery, one third have a fair recovery, and one third will show no significant improvement. Those patients who have a more catastrophic onset tend to have worse prognoses. There is no correlation between the abnormalities found in the CSF and the eventual outcome.

Treatment

Good supportive care is extremely important. The rapid detection and treatment of urinary tract infections and the prevention of decubiti will reduce the morbidity. Corticosteroids have been used but it is unclear whether this strategy has modified the natural history of the disorder. Rehabilitation will help improve the functional recovery.

MENINGITIS

Bacterial meningitis is a life-threatening infection that occurs more often in the pediatric age group than in any other population. Children under 1 year of age have the highest age-specific attack rate. More than 20,000 cases of bacterial meningitis occur per year in the United States and the most common etiologic agent is *Hemophilus influenzae* type B. Different organisms are more likely to cause disease at various ages; this pattern will be further discussed under Etiology. Many bacteria are thought to affect the epithelial cells of mucosal surfaces and colonize in the nasopharynx. Thus there is often a history of preceding upper respiratory viral infection. Bacteremia is thought to be the next step. A concomitant viral infection may contribute to the disruption of local barriers and promote the occurrence of bacteremia. The bacteria may enter the CSF from the blood via the choroid plexus. They are then not cleared from the CSF and invade the meninges over the cerebral cortex, resulting in a leptomeningitis. The bacteria may follow the course of vessels connecting the meninges and superfical surfaces of the brain, producing a penetrating thrombophlebitis and cerebritis.

Symptoms and Signs

The clinical picture of bacterial meningitis in children is quite variable and depends on the age of the child and the duration of the illness prior to diagnosis. In older children, specific symptoms include fever, nausea, vomiting, anorexia, listlessness, and lethargy. Headache, myalgia, neck stiffness, and sensitivity to light may be present. In young infants the symptoms may be nonspecific and the diagnosis of meningitis requires a high index of suspicion by the physician. Lethargy, irritability, vomiting, and poor feeding may be the only symptoms. Fever may not be present. Seizures tend to be more common in this age group. Physical examination in older children may reveal neck stiffness and positive Brudzinski's and Kernig's signs. Signs of increased intracranial pressure may be present and be manifest as sixth-nerve palsies. Other cranial nerves may be involved, including the third and the seventh. Hearing may be affected and may be absent when the child is first examined. Papilledema is unusual and often suggests a complication of meningitis, such as cortical thrombophlebitis, venous thrombosis, subdural empyema, or brain abscess. In young infants, papilledema may be less common but bulging of the anterior fontanelle is often present. Occasionally, focal cerebral deficits, including hemiparesis or ataxia, may be present.

The general physical examination may reveal cutaneous lesions, which may be a sign of sepsis. These would include petechiae and hemorrhagic rashes; less

FEATURE TABLE 10-6. MENINGITIS

Discriminating Feature	Consistent Features	Variable Features
1. Characteristically abnormal CSF	1. Drowsiness 2. Headache 3. Increased intracranial pressure	1. Focal neurologic deficits 2. Ataxia 3. Deafness 4. Seizures 5. Hyponatremia

commonly hemorrhagic bullous lesions may be present. Rarely necrosis or gangrene of extremities occurs. Other manifestations of the bacterial illness may include otitis media, cellulitis, septic arthritis, pneumonia, and pericarditis.

Laboratory Findings

The hallmark of bacterial meningitis in the CSF includes a pleocytosis with predominantly polymorphonuclear cells, an elevated protein content, and a decreased glucose content. However, these findings may not be present early in the course of the illness, at which time the pleocytosis may have a predominance of mononuclear cells and a normal glucose content. Therefore, bacterial meningitis cannot be excluded solely on the basis of the CSF findings. A Gram stain may be helpful in identifying the etiologic agent. The majority of children with bacterial meningitis will have positive Gram stains of their CSF. However, cultures of the CSF remain the key to diagnosis and also help establish the bacterial sensitivity of the causative organism. Rapid diagnostic tests may be helpful in identifying bacterial antigen in the CSF prior to the availability of culture results. Various techniques have been used, including countercurrent immunoelectrophoresis, latex particle agglutination, enzyme-linked immunosorbent assay, and enzyme-multiplied immunoassay.

Blood cultures are often positive in children with meningitis. Other foci of infection, such as joints, skin, and pericardium, should be cultured when possible.

Appropriate radiographic and imaging procedures should be used when sources of infection outside the nervous system are suspected. Routine laboratory tests, such as a complete blood count and urinalysis and the measurement of serum glucose and electrolytes, are helpful in managing fluid therapy as well as detecting hyponatremia (which may indicate inappropriate antidiuretic hormone secretion). Tests of liver and kidney function should also be performed. Other studies—such as coagulation function measures, blood and urine osmolalities, electrocardiograms, electroencephalograms, and CT or MRI of the brain—should be obtained when indicated (Figure 10–4).

Etiology

The organism most likely to cause meningitis varies with the age of the patient. In the newborn, *Streptococcus* group B, *Staphylococcus*, and Gram-negative bacteria including *E. coli* are the most common agents. In infants, *Hemophilus influenzae*, *Neisseria meningitides*, and *Streptococcus pneumoniae* are the most common agents. In older children *Neisseria meningitides* and *Streptococcus pneumoniae* are the most common organisms. Almost all bacteria can cause meningitis, and these would include *Staphylococcus aureus*, *Staphylococcus epidermidis*, and Gram-negative enteric and aerobic organisms. Predispos-

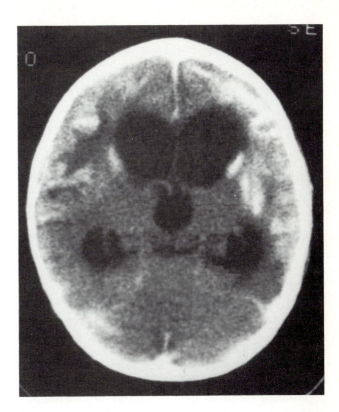

Figure 10–4. CT scan demonstrating acute hydrocephalus, contrast enhancement of areas of the cortex indicating a cerebritis, and small areas of lucency indicating infarctions.

ing conditions to meningitis might include basilar skull fractures, ventricular shunt systems, congenital dermoid sinuses, and immunodeficiency syndromes. Other infectious agents that may simulate the clinical features and laboratory findings include infections with viruses, fungi, and parasites. Tuberculous meningitis should also be considered and skin tests applied. Parameningeal infections in the brain and the subdural, epidural, and paraspinal spaces should also be considered. Noninfectious illnesses such as lead intoxication, chemical meningitis, and vasculitis, must not be overlooked.

Pathology

Examination of the brain reveals the meninges to be thickened, and the surface and base of the brain may be covered with a purulent exudate. The cortex may appear congested. Pus may also be found in the ventricles or on the ventricular walls. The exudate is also found in the spinal subarachnoid space. The brain is often edematous, predominantly affecting the white matter. Small cortical infarcts may be seen. Inflammatory cells may infiltrate along the Virchow-Robin spaces of the cortical veins. Microglial reaction may be present in the outer cortical layers. Involvement of blood vessels may occur, causing a vasculitis involving the small arteries and arterioles as well as cortical vein thromboses. When obstruction to CSF flow exists, ventricular dilatation resulting in hydrocephalus occurs. The obstruction to CSF flow is often related to adhesions and meningeal thickening at the base of the brain.

Course

Seizures occur in approximately one third of the children with meningitis and are more prevalent in infants than older children. Generalized or brief multifocal seizures occurring early in the course of the illness usually do not signify significant complications and often do not lead to epilepsy. Focal seizures occurring after 48 to 72 hours may indicate an underlying complication, such as cortical thrombophlebitis, arterial occlusion, focal cerebritis, or empyema. Focal findings on neurologic examination or a focal seizure during the course of treatment are indications for performing CT or MRI of the brain. Subdural effusions occur in up to 30% of children with bacterial meningitis. They may be detected by CT scan in older children or by transillumination in children under 1 year of age. They often resolve spontaneously and do not require intervention. A subdural tap is indicated in the face of persistent fever or relapsing of meningitis, symptomatic increased intracranial pressure, or abnormal increases in head size, or if the effusion produces focal neurologic signs. Hearing loss owing to infection of the cochlea may occur, more often in children with pneumococcal meningitis but also with *Hemophilus influenza* type B infections. Ataxia may be an associated finding. Other neurologic complications include strokes, hydrocephalus, and cortical blindness. Long-term follow-up may reveal the presence of language delays, mental retardation, or learning disabilities. Behavioral problems also have been noted.

The mortality varies with the organism and the age of the patient. The mortality rate is higher in neonatal meningitis compared to that in older children, in which it is in the 5% to 10% range. Tuberculous meningitis has a higher morbidity and mortality compared to other bacterial infections.

Treatment

Effective treatment of bacterial meningitis includes the use of appropriate antibiotics. These should be administered intravenously and in doses appropriate for the patient's weight. In children older than 6 weeks of age, therapy may be initiated with third-generation cephalosporins. Therapy may be changed when the results of cultures, including antibiotic sensitivities, become available. Table 10-4 lists the more common antibiotics used and their average daily dose in infants and older children. Meningitis in the neonate requires special consideration because of the different organisms commonly found in that age group. Antibiotic coverage to include Gram-negative bacteria is essential and one also has to consider the toxicity of certain antibiotics such as chlor-

TABLE 10-4. ANTIBIOTICS USED IN THE TREATMENT OF BACTERIAL MENINGITIS

Antibiotic	Average dose per day
Ampicillin	300 mg/kg
Cefotaxime	25–50 mg/kg
Chloramphenicol	100 mg/kg
Moxalactum	50 mg/kg
Nafcillin	200 mg/kg
Penicillin	250,000 U/kg
Sulfamethoxazole	50 mg/kg
Trimethoprim	10 mg/kg
Vancomycin	10–15 mg/kg

amphenicol as well as the ability of various antibiotics to penetrate into the CSF.

Seizures should be treated with antiepileptic medications such as diazepam (0.25 mg/kg intravenously) as well as phenytoin (10 to 15 mg/kg intravenously). Therapy during the course of the hospitalization can be maintained with phenytoin and the need for long-term treatment can be assessed based on the duration and type of seizures, the time of onset in relation to the course of the disease, and the persistence of neurologic sequelae. Fluid restriction may be necessary initially. In the absence of poor perfusion or dehydration 800 to 1000 mL/m² per

---

Pearls and Perils: Meningitis

1. Hearing loss may be present when the meningitis is first diagnosed and is not necessarily related to delayed diagnosis or therapy.
2. Otitis media associated with meningitis may be caused by retrograde infection from the meninges to the ear.
3. Inappropriate secretion of antidiuretic hormone often occurs in meningitis and can result in hyponatremia.
4. The administration of excessive amounts of fluid to children with meningitis, particularly in the presence of inappropriate antidiuretic hormone secretion, may contribute to the production of increased intracranial pressure.
5. Lumbar punctures should not be carried out prior to performing a brain imaging procedure in older patients with suspected meningitis who have increased intracranial pressure or focal signs, for herniation syndromes can be precipitated. Antimicrobial therapy may be instituted and the lumbar puncture performed several hours later, after the radiologic study. Culture results will not be affected by this delay and other tests for the detection of the etiologic agents can be performed.

day may be administered. Hyponatremia secondary to inappropriate antidiuretic hormone secretion is common and may influence the volume and electrolyte content of the intravenous fluids. Within a short period of time (36 to 48 hours), most children can have their fluids increased to 1500 to 1700 mL/m² per day. Hypoxemia and hypoglycemia should be avoided. Cerbral edema can be treated by fluid restriction (if peripheral perfusion is adequate), hyperventilation, and osmotic agents. Temperature control with antipyretics and sponging may be necessary. In patients who are lethargic or comatose and are unable to swallow, nutrition should be maintained and nasogastric feedings may be necessary once the danger of vomiting and aspiration is not great.

Close contacts of patients with meningitis caused by *Neisseria meningitides* or *Hemophilus influenzae* type B should be considered for prophylactic therapy with rifampin. Current guidelines of the Committee on Infectious Diseases of the American Academy of Pediatrics should be consulted. In addition, vaccines against common bacterial infections such as *Hemophilus influenzae* type B are being developed. Certain high-risk populations may benefit from this immunization.

PARASPINOUS INFECTIONS

Spinal epidural abscesses and spinal subdural empyemas are unusual infections in children. Of the two, the epidural abscess is the more common. The epidural infection is usually hematogenous in origin and there may be a history of a preceeding infection elsewhere in the body. A history of mild preceding trauma to the spine, which is thought to create a nidus for hematogenously born infection, may be present. Spinal osteomyelitis by continuous spread may result in an epidural abscess. The subdural emypema is usually of hematogenous origin. Both may lead to spinal cord compression and severe neurologic disability if unrecognized and untreated.

Symptoms and Signs

The initial symptoms in infants may be nonspecific and include fever, irritability, and excessive crying. In older children back pain is a common complaint. Because of the severe pain, the child may refuse to walk. If the infection continues, the nonspecific back pain may be replaced by radicular pain and eventual weakness of the legs. Sensory deficits or hyperesthesia in the lower extremities may be present and eventually bladder function becomes impaired. The findings on examination are variable. Tenderness to percussion over the spine occurs more frequently with an epidural abscess than with a subdural empyema. Spinal rigidity results from spasm of the paraspinal muscles. The child may be reluctant to lie prone or stand. The findings on neurologic examination are variable. Most abscesses are located in the thoracic and lower lumbar regions. The thoracic abscesses may be associated with a loss of reflexes and flaccidity of the lower extremities but also may cause hyperreflexia with Babinski signs in some patients. Abscesses in the lumbar region result in diminished deep tendon reflexes and sensory deficits following root distributions.

Laboratory Findings

A complete blood count may demonstrate a leukocytosis. Radiographs of the spine are most often normal and are only helpful if they demonstrate an osteomyelitis. Cultures of the blood may reveal the etiologic organism but the incidence of septicemia is low. Examination of the CSF is helpful. This should be done cautiously so as not to introduce infection into the subarachnoid space from the lumbar epidural space. If the site of infection is above the level of the lumbar puncture, the CSF may have an elevated protein content, which, if marked, will cause the fluid to appear xanthochromic. Pleocytosis, with lymphocytes and polymorphonuclear leukocytes, is often present. Before performing the lumbar puncture, one should consider the need to perform MRI of the spine. If there is a high index of suspicion that the infection is under the preferred site of the lumbar puncture, then the performance of a cervical or cisternal tap to obtain CSF and perform a myelogram is necessary after a MRI examination.

Etiology

There is often a history of a preceding bacterial infection or an injury with blunt trauma to the back. Antecedent infections have included upper respiratory tract infections, otitis media, tonsillitis, secondarily infected varicella lesions, pyelitis, sinusitis, skin infections, and osteomyelitis of bones other than the spine. The most common bacteria is *Staphylococcus aureus*. However, many other organisms have been responsible and these include *Pseudomonas, Pneumococcus, Streptococcus,*

FEATURE TABLE 10-7. PARASPINOUS INFECTIONS

Discriminating Feature	Consistent Feature	Variable Features
1. Abnormal MRI, myelogram, or CT exam	1. Back pain	1. Weakness of legs 2. Sensory deficits 3. Impaired bladder function

---

Pearls and Perils:
Paraspinous Infections

1. The diagnosis should be considered in children who develop symptoms and signs out of proportion to a preceding mild trauma to the spine.
2. There may not be signs of systemic infection, fever, or leukocytosis, but this absence of symptoms should not mitigate against considering an epidural abscess as a cause.
3. Epidural abscess has been noted following repeated lumbar punctures in infants.

Proteus, Enterobacter, Salmonella, Nocardia, Coccidioides, Actinomyces, Aspergillus, and *Mycobacterium tuberculosis.*

Pathology

At the time of surgery the findings are typical of those with an abscess composed of purulent material and thick granulation tissue. In fatal cases, the spinal cord has shown areas of softening and hemorrhagic necrosis.

Course

In those patients diagnosed early and treated appropriately, complete recovery can occur. If there has been significant progression of the neurologic syndrome before the institution of therapy, residual paraparesis will occur.

Treatment

An acute spinal epidural abscess with progressive neurologic findings is an emergency. Laminectomy and drainage should be promptly performed. At that time appropriate culture material may be obtained and specific antibiotic therapy instituted. If paralysis has been present for more than 48 hours, recovery becomes less likely. In those patients in whom there is osteomyelitis, a long course of antibiotic therapy is indicated. Recently, success has been reported with conservative medical management, that is, no laminectomy. Management has been aided by the use of repeated CT examinations. This approach may be considered if the diagnosis is made very early, before any neurologic signs are present, and if no evidence of root or cord compression develops during the course of therapy.

INTERVERTEBRAL DISK INFECTION (DISKITIS)

Diskitis is an inflammatory process of the intervertebral disk space. It is generally considered to be due to a low-grade viral or bacterial infection, the pathogenesis of which remains uncertain. A striking and often distinctive clinical syndrome is present and familiarity with the problem enables the diagnosis to be established.

Symptoms and Signs

There may be a history of a preceding mild, systemic febrile illness or of blunt trauma to the back. However, in many children the onset of the illness is related to the symptoms of diskitis itself. Major complaints can be divided into various categories: (1) back, hip, and leg pain; (2) irritability; (3) meningeal irritation; and (4) abdominal discomfort. Symptoms referable to the back often begin with complaints of vague pain, which may be accompanied by a limp. As the disease progresses there may be refusal to walk, stand, or even sit. The child is relatively comfortable when lying in bed. There may be splinting of paraspinus muscles and tenderness to spine percussion or compression. There may be pain in the hip or leg that appears to be nonspecific. However, the pain may have a radicular quality and be referred to the thigh or lower leg. It is usually not well localized. Back pain and muscle splinting are present when specifically looked for. There may be loss of normal lumbar lordosis. In young infants irritability may be the only symptom and may be accompanied by excessive crying and low-grade fever. When meningeal irritation is present, Kernig's and Brudzinski's signs may be present. Hyperreflexia and even clonus may occur. The symptoms often suggest an intradural tumor. In some children the syndrome is characterized by abdominal pain, anorexia, and vomiting. This symptom complex occurs when the lower thoracic or upper lumbar spine is involved. Local findings may be elicited. The character of the complaints often suggests an acute abdominal process.

Laboratory Findings

Mild pleocytosis and elevated sedimentation rate often occur. The CSF examination is normal. Plain radiographs of the spine reveal narrowing of the disk space; however, these findings may not occur until weeks after the onset of the illness. Thus plain x-ray studies may not be helpful early in the course of the illness. As the disease progresses

---

FEATURE TABLE 10-8. INTERVERTEBRAL DISK INFECTION (DISKITIS)

Discriminating Feature	Consistent Feature	Variable Features
1. Abnormal appearance of disk space on CT or MRI scan	1. Abnormal bone scans	1. Back pain 2. Abdominal pain 3. Refusal to walk 4. Radicular pain

there may be involvement of the adjacent vertebral bodies and the vertebral endplates may show erosion, producing a saw tooth appearance. Vertebral body wedging and compression are not common. Follow-up studies may reveal permanent collapse of the disk space; however, on occasion the findings may revert to normal. Myelography often yields a normal examination unless there is extrusion of the disk space material. MRI may demonstrate abnormal signals in the disk. Involvement is most common in the lower thoracic and lumbar areas but involvement of the cervical spine has been reported.

Radionuclide scanning with either technetium or gallium may reveal abnormalities long before there are changes in the plain radiographs. These scans often become positive within 1 to 2 weeks of the onset of the illness and help establish the diagnosis.

Direct aspiration of the disk may occasionally reveal positive cultures for *Staphylococcus aureus*. Occasionally the staphylococci have been isolated from blood. Other bacteria found have included *Diplococcus pneumoniae* and diphtheroids. In the majority of cases, no bacterial etiology is determined.

Etiology

The exact pathogenesis of the syndrome is unclear. A hematogenous route of infection is the most likely cause. In young children, in whom this syndrome is most prevalent, the disk has an intact direct blood supply. In older children and adults, the blood vessels to the disk gradually involute and the disk becomes avascular. This may explain why the majority of the children affected are under 2 years of age.

Pathology

The condition is relatively benign with a good outlook, and surgical intervention is not warranted. Therefore, there have not been any reports of pathologic examination of tissue.

Course

The majority of children will respond to bed rest. Splinting or bracing may also be helpful. Recovery has occurred both with and without antibiotic therapy. The illness may run its course over several weeks or longer. Even in those children in whom there is permanent narrowing of the disk space or involvement in the adjacent vertebral bodies, symptoms abate and a return to full activity is the usual course.

Treatment

As indicated previously, bed rest with or without immobilization is often employed. It is unclear whether this treatment affects the eventual outcome of the disease and most children will regulate their own activity. Because of occasional positive cultures from either blood or disk

---

Pearls and Perils: Intervertebral Disk Infection (Diskitis)

1. The symptoms and signs of diskitis may mimic an intradural tumor or an acute abdomen. Isotope scans are more sensitive than plain x-ray studies in establishing the diagnosis.
2. Plain radiograph studies of the spine are often normal early in the course of the illness.

---

material, antibiotic therapy seems indicated. If the treatment is empirical, drugs that provide coverage for coagulase-positive *Staphylococcus aureus* would seem to be indicated. if there is progression of the disease one would have to consider obtaining material for culture and possibly introducing therapy to cover Gram-negative bacteria.

ANNOTATED BIBLIOGRAPHY

Baker AS, Ojemann RG, Swartz MN, et al: Spinal epidural abscess. *N Eng J Med* 293:463–468, 1975.

The authors report 39 cases and describe the clinical progression of the symptoms and signs. The most common sources of infection were osteomyelitis, bacteremia, and postoperative infections.

Baker CJ: Primary spinal epidural abscess. *Am J Dis Child* 121:337–339, 1971.

The author reviews the literature and reports that the most frequent cause of infection was *Staphylococcus aureus* spread via the hematogenous route from infections of skin, respiratory tract, or urinary tract.

Viral infections of the nervous system, in Bell WE, McCormick WF (eds): *Neurologic Infections in Children.* Major Problems in Clinical Pediatrics, Vol XII. Philadelphia, WB Saunders, 1975, p 143–301.

This chapter offers comprehensive, well-illustrated discussions of viral infections of the CNS organized by etiologic agent. The nonneurologic aspects of infections are included in the text.

Bell WE, Chun RWM, Jabbour JT, et al: Infections of the brain and spinal cord, in Swaiman KF, Wright FS (eds): *The Practice of Pediatric Neurology,* 2nd ed. St. Louis, CV Mosby, 1982, p 659–765.

This is a comprehensive discussion of infections of the nervous system caused by bacteria, viruses, rickettsiae, fungi, and parasites. An extensive bibliography is included.

Britt RH, Enzmann DR: Clinical stages of human brain abscesses on serial CT scans after contrast infusion. *J Neurosurg* 59:972–989, 1983.

The CT criteria for categorizing brain abscesses into cerebritis and capsule stages are discussed. Corticosteroid administration reduced contrast enhancement in the cerebritis stage.

Cottom DG: Acute cerebellar ataxia. *Arch Dis Child* 32:181–188, 1957.

This study provides a good description of the spectrum of the clinical picture and CSF findings.

Fischer EG, McLennon JE, Suzuki Y: Cerebral abscess in children. *Am J Dis Child* 135:746–749, 1981.

The authors review 94 episodes of pyogenic brain abscesses. Predisposing factors included congenital heart disease, otitic and sinus infections, closed-head injury, and cystic fibrosis. Mortality correlated with presence of coma on admission.

Fraser RAR, Ratzan K, Wolpert S, et al: Spinal subdural empyema. *Arch Neurol* 28:235–238, 1973.

The majority of patients had a history of preceding or concurrent bacterial infection, absence of vertebral percussion tenderness, slowly evolving neurologic deficits, and CSF and myelographic abnormalities compatible with parameningeal inflammation.

Jacobson PL, Farmer TW: Subdural empyema complicating meningitis in infants: Improved prognosis. *Neurology* 31: 190–193,1981.

There has been a recent significant decrease in the mortality rate in treating infants with subdural empyemas compared to past experiences. The improved outcome is related to early diagnoses provided by the use of CT scanning and subdural punctures.

Kaplan SL: Meningitis, in Fishman MA (ed): *Pediatric Neurology*. Orlando, Fla, Grune & Stratton, 1986, p 153–171.

A comprehensive review of bacterial meningitis in children. Included are dicussions regarding pathogenesis, diagnosis, therapy, complications, and prognosis.

Rocco HD, Eyring EJ: Intervertebral disk infections in children. *Am J Dis Child* 123:448–451, 1972.

The authors review 155 cases from the literature and their own experience. Clinical symptom complexes are defined: back, hip, leg, meninges, abdomen, and irritable child.

Smith HP, Hendrick EB: Subdural empyema and epidural abscess in children. *J Neurosurg* 58:392–397, 1983.

The authors report their experiences with 31 children. Older children tended to be sicker and more likely to present with focal seizures compared to infants. Streptococci and staphylococci were the organisms most frequently responsible for the infections.

Taber LH: Encephalitis, in Fishman MA (ed): *Pediatric Neurology*. Orlando, Fla, Grune & Stratton, 1986, p 173–202.

A general review of the more common viral agents causing encephalitis in children. Helpful tables regarding nonviral infections with CNS involvement, noninfectious diseases with CNS involvement, and diagnostic studies indicated in children with acute viral encephalitis are included.

Weiss S, Carter S: Course and prognosis of acute cerebellar ataxia in children. *Neurology* 9:711–721, 1959.

This study reports the long-term follow-up of patients hospitalized for acute ataxia and documents persistent disabilities in some patients, especially those with severe deficits at the onset of the illness.

BIBLIOGRAPHY

Altrocchi PH: Acute transverse myelopathy. *Arch Neurol* 9:111–119, 1963.

Awerbuch G, Feinberg W, Ferry P, et al: Demonstration of acute postviral myelitis with magnetic resonance imaging. *Pediatr Neurol* 3:367–369, 1987.

Bannister GB, Williams B, Smith S: Treatment of subdural empyema. *J Neurosurg* 55:82–88, 1981.

Bell WE: Treatment of bacterial infections of the central nervous system. *Ann Neurol* 9:313–327, 1981.

Belman AL, Ultmann MH, Horoupian D, et al: Neurological complications in infants and children with acquired immune deficiency syndrome. *Ann Neurol* 18:560–566, 1985.

Bergman I, Wald ER, Meyer JD, et al: Epidural abscess and vertebral osteomyelitis following serial lumbar punctures. *Pediatrics* 72:476–480, 1983.

Brown P: Viral encephalitis and encephalopathy, in Conn HF, Conn RB (eds): *Current Diagnosis*, 6th ed. Philadelphia, WB Saunders, 1980, p 884–894.

Carey ME, Chou SN, French LA: Long-term neurological residua in patients surviving brain abscess with surgery. *J Neurosurg* 34:652–656, 1971.

Curless RG: Subdural empyema in infant meningitis: Diagnosis, therapy and prognosis. *Child's Nerv Syst* 1:211–214, 1985.

Dodge PR, Davis H, Feigin RD et al: Prospective evaluation of hearing impairment as a sequela of acute bacterial meningitis. *N Engl J Med* 311:869–874, 1984.

Eavey RD, Gao Y-Z, Schuknecht HF, et al: Otologic features of bacterial meningitis of childhood. *J Pediatr* 106:402–407, 1985.

Enberg RN, Kaplan RJ: Spinal epidural abscess in children. *Clin Pediatr* 13:247–253, 1974.

Epstein LG, Sharer LR, Joshi VV, et al: Progressive encephalopathy in children with acquired immune deficiency syndrome. *Ann Neurol* 17:488–496, 1985.

Farmer TW, Wise GR: Subdural empyema in infants, children and adults. *Neurology* 23:254–261, 1973.

Fischer GW, Papich GA, Sullivan DE, et al: Diskitis: A prospective diagnostic analysis. *Pediatrics* 62:543–547, 1978.

Fishman MA, Lifschitz MH, Wilson GS: Pediatric acquired immunodeficiency syndrome. *Neurodev Abnormal* 1:107–111, 1990.

Galil A, Gorodischer R, Bar-Ziv J, et al: Intervertebral disc infection (discitis) in childhood. *Eur J Pediatr* 139:66–70, 1982.

Goitein KJ, Amit Y, Mussaffi H: Intracranial pressure in central nervous system infection and cerebral ischaemia of infancy. *Arch Dis Child* 58:184–186, 1983.

Horowitz SJ, Boxerbaum B, O'Bell J: Cerebral herniation in bacterial meningitis in childhood. *Ann Neurol* 7:524–528, 1980.

Kagawa M, Tukeshita M, Yato S, et al: Brain abscess in congenital heart disease. *J Neurosurg* 58:913–917, 1983.

Kaplan SL, Feigin RD: The syndrome of inappropriate secretion of antidiuretic hormone in children with bacterial meningitis. *J Pediatr* 92:758–761, 1978.

Kaplan SL, Goddard J, VanKleeck M, et al: Ataxia and deafness in children due to bacterial meningitis. *Pediatrics* 68:8–13, 1981.

Kaplan SL, Catlin FI, Weaver T, et al: Onset of hearing loss in children with bacterial meningitis. *Pediatrics* 73:575–578, 1984.

Kaufman DM, Kaplan JG, Litman N: Infectious agents in spinal epidural abscesses. *Neurology* 30:844–850, 1980.

Kaufman DM, Litman N, Miller MH: Sinusitis induced subdural empyema. *Neurology* 33:123–132, 1983.

Kennard C, Swash M: Acute viral encephalitis—Its diagnosis and outcome. *Brain* 104:129–148, 1981.

Lascari AD, Graham MH, MacQueen JC: Intervertebral disk infection in children. *J Pediatr* 70:751–757, 1967.

Legg NJ, Gupta PC, Scott DF: Epilepsy following cerebral abscess—A clinical and EEG study of 70 patients. *Brain* 96:259–268, 1973.

Leys D, Lesoin F, Viaud C, et al: Decreased morbidity from acute bacterial spinal epidural abscesses using computed tomography and non-surgical treatment in selected patients. *Ann Neurol* 17:350–355, 1985.

Leys D, Destee A, Petit H, et al: Management of subdural intracranial empyemas should not always require surgery. *J Neurol Neurosurg Psychiatr* 49:635–639, 1986.

Luken MG, Whelan MA: Recent diagnostic experience with subdural empyema. *J Neurosurg* 52:764–771, 1980.

McMenamin JB, Volpe JJ: Bacterial meningitis in infancy: Effects on intracranial pressure and cerebral blood flow velocity. *Neurology* 34:500–504, 1984.

Mathisen GE, Meyer RD, George WL, et al: Brain abscess and cerebritis. *Rev Infect Dis* 6:5101–5106, 1984.

Mauser HW, Ravijst RA, Elderson A, et al: Nonsurgical treatment of subdural empyema. *J Neurosurg* 63:128–130, 1985.

Nelson JD: Emerging role of cephalosporins in bacterial meningitis. *Am J Med* 79(S2A):47–51, 1985.

Nigro G, Pastoris MC, Fantasia MM, et al: Acute cerebellar ataxia in pediatric legionellosis. *Pediatrics* 72:847–849, 1983.

Paine RS, Byers RK: Transverse myelopathy in childhood. *Arch Dis Child* 85:151–163, 1953.

Rosenblum ML, Hoff JT, Norman D, et al: Nonoperative treatment of brain abscesses in selected high risk patients. *J Neurosurg* 52:217–225, 1980.

Rubia RC, Jacobs GB, Cooper PR, et al: Disc space infections in children. *Child's Brain* 3:180–190, 1977.

Silverberg AL, DiNubile MJ: Subdural empyema and cranial epidural abscess. *Med Clin North Am* 69:361–374, 1985.

Snyder RD, Stovring J, Cushing AH, et al: Cerebral infarction in childhood bacterial meningitis. *J Neurol Neurosurg Psychiatr* 44:581–585, 1981.

Steele JC, Gladstone RM, Thanasophon S, et al: Acute cerebellar ataxia and concomitant infection with *Mycoplasma pneumoniae*. *J Pediatr* 80:467–469, 1972.

Swartz MN, Dodge PR: Bacterial meningitis—A review of selected aspects. I, II. *N Engl J Med* 272:725–731, 779–787, 842–848, 898–902, 954–960, 1003–1010, 1965.

Ultmann MH, Belman AL, Ruff HA, et al: Developmental abnormalities in infants and children with acquired immune deficiency syndrome (AIDS) and AIDS related complex. *Dev Med Child Neurol* 27:563–571, 1985.

Vienny H, Desplond PA, Lutschg J, et al: Early diagnosis and evaluation of deafness in childhood bacterial meningitis: A study using brainstem auditory evoked potentials. *Pediatrics* 73:579–586, 1984.

Wang D, Bortolussi R: Acute viral infection of the central nervous system in children: An 8 year review. *Can Med Assoc J* 125:585–589, 1981.

Weiner LP, Fleming JO: Viral infections of the nervous system. *J Neurosurg* 61:207–224, 1984.

Whelan MA, Hilal SK: Computed tomography as a guide in the diagnosis and follow-up of brain abscesses. *Radiology* 135:663–671, 1980.

Whitby M, Finch R: Bacterial meningitis—Rational selection and use of antibacterial drugs. *Drugs* 31:266–278, 1986.

Wise GR, Farmer TW: Bacterial cerebral vasculitis. *Neurology* 21:195–200, 1971.

Yamashima T, Kashihara K, Ikeda K, et al: Three phases of cerebral arteriopathy in meningitis: Vasospasm and vasodilatation followed by organic stenosis. *Neurosurgery* 16:546–553, 1985.

Yang S-Y: Brain abscess: A review of 400 cases. *J Neurosurg* 55:794–799, 1981.

Zimmerman RD, Leeds NE, Danziger A: Subdural empyema: CT findings. *Radiology* 150:417–422, 1984.

Neuroimmunologic Disorders

Richard J. Allen

Pediatric neuroimmunologic disorders have unique clinical presentations. The phenotypes and etiologies also vary significantly from the newborn to the adult. Neurologic signs may indicate an underlying immunologic defect or immunologic laboratory data may define the disorder. Both chronic and acute neurologic events occur; some are catastrophic in presentation whereas others evolve slowly over months or years. In recent years therapeutic approaches to immunologic disorders have often changed following advances in the molecular sciences.

At any age, seizure disorders, disabilities in motor function of either the central (CNS) or peripheral nervous system (PNS), altered states of consciousness, and movement disorders such as Sydenham's chorea are common presentations. Especially in children serious syndromes appear after bacterial or viral infections or after common exanthematous diseases and immunizations. Bacterial infections such as *Hemophilus influenzae* meningitis in young children involve bacterial polysaccharide antigens capable of inducing pathophysiologic neurocellular effects associated with serious brain damage. In this group of disorders, neurologic localization should be supplemented with selected immunologic studies aimed at sorting out etiologies and disease mechanisms, even though primary and secondary roles are difficult to define in many immunoregulatory disorders.

Children have special mechanisms for self-protection. The placenta protects the fetus from antigenic stimulation and the neurologic consequences of infection; it also limits the transport of immunoglobulins to IgG, providing neonatal immunoprotection. Fetal immune responses are different from those in the mature adult and follow adaptive developmental ontogenic stages, however, without a precise relationship to the development of most neurologic disorders. Young children are resistant to certain immunoregulatory disorders, such as adult demyelinating diseases. Multiple sclerosis is uncommon in childhood.

Even in their fully developed clinical form, recognized immunoregulatory disturbances are diagnostically and therapeutically complex. Clinical or therapeutic studies employing randomized controlled trials constitute an application problem for pediatric cohorts even when large patient groups participate. Neuroimmunologic evidence provides the opportunity to identify disorders through laboratory studies, and treatment often provides symptomatic relief or occasionally complete clinical reversal of neurologic findings. Intravenous immunoglobulin (IVIG), for example, may modify autoimmune hematologic and systemic diseases. In several neurologic autoimmune disorders there are reports of the effectiveness of IVIG, including myasthenia gravis, multiple sclerosis, and inflammatory polyneuropathy. In seizure disorders the beneficial effect of IVIG is less clearly established, although some types of seizures respond to immunosuppressive drugs, such as adrenocorticotropic hormone and corticosteroids. Recent consensus conference reports summarize the recommended usage of IVIG for all ages. In pediatrics the prevention of systemic infections and the subsequent neurologic disability by immunization is well established. Experimentally T-cell reactivity, the basis of autoimmune disorders, can be suppressed by vaccination, and this strategy could prove to have a similar benefit in clinical situations.

Epidemiologically the treatment of neuroimmunologic disorders related to viral infections is especially important during childhood. Acquired immunodeficiency syndrome has demonstrated an enormous growth in the last decade. This group of diseases, growing rapidly in younger age groups, now constitutes a major socioeconomic and scientific challenge.

ANNOTATED BIBLIOGRAPHY

Ellison GW, Mickey MR, Myers LW: Alternatives to randomized clinical trials. *Neurology* 38:73–75, 1988.

Intravenous immunoglobulin: Prevention and treatment of disease. NIH Consensus Conference. *JAMA* 264:3189–3193, 1990.

Lawton AR, Cooper MD: *Ontogeny of Immunity*. Gainesville: University of Florida Press, 1967, pp 39–51.

Noseworthy JH: There are no alternatives to double-blind, controlled trials. *Neurology* 38:76–79, 1988.

Schiffer MS, Oliviera E, Glode MP, et al: Relation between invasiveness and the K-1 capsular polysaccharide of *Escherichia coli. Pediatr Res* 10:82–87, 1976.

Schwartz SA: Intravenous immunoglobulin (IVIG) for the therapy of autoimmune disorders. *J Clin Immunol* 10:81–89, 1990.

Schwartz SA, Gordon KE, Johnson MN, Goldstein GW: Use of intravenous immune globulin in the treatment of seizure disorders. *J Allergy Clin Immunol* 84:603–607, 1989.

A recent review by Schwartz provides a brief but substantial overview of immunoregulatory disorders of special interest in childhood neurologic disease. Other topics of recent scientific interest are represented in several additional papers, such as the reports on IVIG.

There are several categories of immunologic disorders to consider in establishing clinical neurologic diagnoses. One group, the *primary immunodeficiency syndromes*, present as generalized infections involving lymphoid, phagocytic cells and complement. Ataxia-telangiectasia, as an example, presents with severe progressive motor neurologic disability in the first years of life, with a poorly understood relationship to immunologic deficiencies and with prominent systemic symptoms owing to infections. This genetic disease is characterized by combined nervous system, vascular, and immunologic effects. Immunodeficiency may also appear secondarily to viral infections, as in acquired immunodeficiency syndrome (AIDS). Most primary immunodeficiency diseases appear as systemic disorders with generalized infections. The *autoimmune diseases* present as collagen-vascular disorders or vasculitides with inflammatory reactions, with antibody-mediated reactions in the CNS and PNS possibly causing the symptom complex. One special group with neoplastic proliferation of plasma cells, the end stage of mature activated B cells, synthesizes classes of immunoglobulins; these plasma cell dyscrasias occur predominantly in adults.

Autoimmune diseases are caused by "self-reactivity" or autoreactivity in T- and B-cell functions. Immunoregulatory mechanisms overlap, so precise classification related to molecular mechanisms is only possible in a select group. Fundamental biologic errors are unknown, although some appear to be genetic in origin, with defects located on the X chromosome. The CNS effects—in childhood neuroblastoma and adult cancer with ataxia, opsoclonus-myoclonus, or muscle weakness as in "paraneoplastic syndromes"—are manifested at sites distant from the neoplasia. Recent evidence suggests circulating antibodies leading to an autoimmune pathogenesis for these "remote" effects.

A subgroup of primarily systemic autoimmune diseases is represented by collagen vascular disease with characteristic immunologic abnormalities, and neurologic symptoms. Another group has relatively specific effects on the CNS, with acute or chronic presentation at any age. "Central" CNS localization affecting neurologic structures and functions, alters consciousness with coma, and produces seizures, and opisthotonus as initial signs. After recovery, disorders involving dementia, mental impairment, spasticity, ataxia, or movement deficits may persist. "Peripheral" CNS localization is associated with generalized or localized muscle or nerve weakness. Multiple sclerosis and myasthenia gravis reflect such neurologic-autoimmune localizations in children as well as adults.

The major features of cell-mediated immunity involve the complex cell activities of specific T lymphocytes (the cellular immune system) and B lymphocytes (the humoral immune system). A virus, for example, may initially activate myelin-reactive T cells that then gain entry to brain parenchyma through the blood-brain barrier (BBB) and induce demyelination, a characteristic pathologic myelin breakdown with preservation of axons. This occurs in multiple sclerosis as well as a similar autoimmune disorder, experimental allergic encephalomyelitis, found in animals. In order for myelin basic protein (MBP), a normal constituent of myelin, to be recognized by T cells, the antigenic peptide must be associated with mouse histocompatibility complex (MHC) class II antigens (DR and DQ phenotypes), located in a molecular complex including the T-cell receptor. Regulation of these immune system activities is in part genetic when linked to MHC proteins. Clinical therapies attempt to alter T-cell functions at different sites in the complex. In humoral B-cell immunodeficiencies, clinical improvement may follow the therapeutic use of γ-globulin. Nonspecific cell functions also amplify and modify tissue responses to humoral factors. Systemic immunoregulatory diseases affect the CNS centrally or peripherally (or both) through these components of the immune system.

This chapter focuses on the CNS as the major organ system in disordered immunoregulation in children. Although basic knowledge in immunoregulatory mechanisms has expanded in recent years, only in a few of the associated pediatric neurologic disorders has a relationship between specific cellular and humoral mechanisms and clinical symptomatology been clearly established. Reference to basic molecular mechanisms is necessary in separating disorders with overlapping clinical symptoms. Many neurologic effects in children are simply secondary to a basic illness in which systemic effects of malnutrition and dehydration accompany infection. In many, however, CNS or PNS localization is important in defining an accurate clinical diagnosis.

ANNOTATED BIBLIOGRAPHY

Buckley RH: Humoral immunodeficiency. *Clin Immunol Immunopathol* 40:13–24, 1986.

De Shazo RD, Lopez M, Salvaggio JE: Use and interpretation

of diagnostic immunologic laboratory tests. *JAMA* 258:3011–3031, 1987.

Haynes BF, Warren RW, Buckley RH, et al: Demonstration of abnormalities in expression of thymic epithelial surface antigens in severe cellular immunodeficiency diseases. *J Immunol* 130:1182–1188, 1983.

Nihei K, Naitoh H, Ikeda K: Poliomyelitis-like syndrome following asthma attack (Hopkins syndrome). *Pediatr Neurol* 3:166–170, 1987.

White CJ, Gallin JI: Phagocyte defects. *Clin Immunol Immunopathol* 40:50–61, 1986.

The review by Buckley is a useful overview of immunoregulatory disorders, with particular attention to neurologic effects. The other reports address important special aspects of pediatric immunoregulation and clinical disease.

PRIMARY IMMUNODEFICIENCY SYNDROMES

Disorders with Limited CNS Involvement

In some immunodeficiency syndromes there is relatively little CNS involvement and the neurobiology is not well understood. Agammaglobulinemia (X-linked or Bruton's), thymic hypoplasia (DiGeorge's syndrome), severe combined immunodeficiency disorders (SCID), and Chediak-Higashi-Steinbrink syndrome deserve brief comment. These primary defects are not linked to specific genes on chromosome 6 (HLA sites) because none are related to deficiencies of particular HLA antigens. X-linked or Bruton's agammaglobulinemia as well as acquired forms is related to B-cell maturational arrests. The arrests are often associated with CNS infections, and enterovirus invasion with echovirus meningoencephalitis is especially common in the X-linked type. Anterior horn cell destruction causing typical muscle paralysis occurs in some patients after receipt of a polio vaccine, possibly because of neurotropic activation of the virus. An apparently unrelated poliomyelitis-like syndrome (Hopkins's syndrome), following allergic asthma attacks in children, occurs without known etiology. Combined forms affect other elements, such as T cells. In thymic hypoplasia a characteristic dysmorphogenesis is associated with neonatal hypocalcemic seizures. As in any immunologically compromised state, the CNS may be af-

fected in congenital-genetic forms of SCID. Although different humoral and cellular elements are altered in the Cediak-Higashi-Steinbrink syndrome, neurologic symptoms are due to cerebral atrophy and abnormal Schwann cells. Major immunodeficiency syndromes include neurologic symptoms related to single or combined antibody and immune cell deficiencies.

Acquired Immunodeficiency Syndrome

Viral induction of neurologic dysfunction is currently a major clinical pediatric concern, especially that resulting from AIDS, a disease caused by the human immunodeficiency virus (HIV) and recognized first in adults in 1978. This is a lethal epidemic disorder that causes severe cellular immune deficiency. An increasing number of children born to affected women have been observed in recent years to have neurologic abnormalities. The CNS effects, different in children than in adults, are due either to primary HIV infection or to secondary immunodeficiency. Seropositivity prevalence rates among newborn infants in one cohort analysis suggested that 1 in 200 infants is born to an HIV-infected mother; one-third of seropositive infants develop active HIV infection.

Signs and Symptoms

Primary CNS HIV infection, meeting Centers for Disease Control criteria for AIDS in children, is the cause of an HIV-related progressive encephalopathy with dementia or myelopathy. In HIV-seropositive infants the progressive encephalopathy generally develops in the first 2 years, but the age of onset may vary from 2 months to 5 years. Secondary CNS complications of immunodeficiency consist of neoplasms or opportunistic infections. *Pneumocystis carinii* infection is a leading cause of serious morbidity and mortality. Hemorrhagic or nonhemorrhagic stroke occurs in nearly one-quarter of this age group. In adults the incidence of vascular complications in AIDS is lower.

Neurologic symptoms include generalized tonic-clonic seizures, aphasia, and focal motor paresis with hypotonia, weakness, and dystonia from vascular localization. A subacute necrotizing encephalomyelopathy, resembling the mitochrondrial cytopathy of Leigh's syndrome, has been observed in children. In some groups

FEATURE TABLE 11-1. ACQUIRED IMMUNODEFICIENCY SYNDROME

Discriminating Feature	Consistent Features	Variable Features
1. HIV virus in brain or CSF	1. Progressive neurologic deterioration 2. Strokes in HIV-seropositive infants 3. HIV monoclonal antibodies 4. CSF neopterin/biopterin ratio	1. Progressive cardiomyopathy with neurologic signs 2. Infective dermatitis

of children infected with HLV-1, an infective dermatitis is a clinical marker.

Diagnostic Evaluation

Many laboratory tests are available for antibodies to viral antigens, for the detection of the HIV virus in specific tissues, or for the culture of the virus. Evidence of HIV infection of the brain in children includes brain tissue transmission of infection to chimpanzees, identification of an HIV genome in brain, isolation of HIV from brain or cerebrospinal fluid (CSF), or detection of specific HIV antibody and antigen in CSF, as well as the neuropathologic features. Immunologic laboratory studies offer a wide variety of diagnostic tests to detect cellular and humoral abnormalities associated with this group of diseases. None are specific for the associated neurologic disorders except in those cases in which a particular organism or virus (i.e., HIV) can be detected. Recent evidence suggests that the CSF neopterin/bioipterin ratio may be an indicator of brain macrophage invasion and thus may serve as a useful diagnostic test as well as a means of evaluating therapeutic interventions. An absolute lymphopenia owing to T- and B-cell defects is associated with humoral abnormalities in immunoglobulins and elevated antibodies to many antigens. B-cell dysfunction may precede T-cell defects in pediatric patients with elevated circulating immune complexes present. A reversal in the T-helper (CD 4) to T-suppressor (CD8) cell ratio differs from findings in SCID patients, who have histologically normal thymic epithelium compared with that in patients with AIDS. Pro-inflammatory CD4 cells react with specific monoclonal antibodies and recognized antigen in the context of class II components of the MHC (HLA-DR).

Treatment

Zidovudine (AZT) decreases morbidity in adults and children but intolerance, toxicity, and refractory disease occur. Dideoxyinosine in symptomatic HIV infection in children may also be beneficial. Supportive care predominates for the long term. Guidelines for children have recently been published.

ANNOTATED BIBLIOGRAPHY

Belman AL, Ultmann MH, Horoupian D, et al: Neurological complications in infants and children with acquired immune deficiency syndrome. *Ann Neurol* 18:560–566, 1985.

Blanche S, Rouzioux C, Moscato ML, et al: A prospective study of infants born to women seropositive for human immunodeficiency virus type 1. *N Engl J Med* 320:1643–1648, 1989.

Bowen DL, Lane HC, Fauci AS: Immunologic abnormalities in the acquired immunodeficiency syndrome. *Prog Allergy* 37:207–223, 1986.

Brew BJ, Bhalla RB, Paul M, et al: CSF neopterin in human immunodeficiency virus type 1 infection. *Ann Neurol* 28:556–560, 1990.

Butler KM, Husson RN, Balis FM, et al: Dideoxyinosine in children with symptomatic human immunodeficiency virus infection. *N Engl J Med* 324:137–144, 1991.

Centers for Disease Control: Classification system for human immunodeficiency virus (HIV) infection in children under 13 years of age. *MMWR* 36:225–230, 1987.

Cooper ER: AIDS in children: An overview of the medical, epidemiological, and public health problems, in O'Malley P (ed): *The Aids Epidemic: Private Rights and the Public Interest.* Boston: Beacon Press, 1989, pp. 121–133.

Edelson PJ (ed): *The Pediatric Clinics of North America, Childhood AIDS.* Philadelphia: WB Saunders, 1991.

Ellaurie M, Cavelli T, Rubinstein A: Immune complexes in pediatric human immunodeficiency virus infections. *Am J Dis Child* 144: 1207–1209, 1990.

Epstein LG, Sharer LR, Goudsmit J: Neurological and neuropathological features of human immunodeficiency virus infection in children. *Ann Neurol* 23(suppl):S19–S23, 1988.

Fischl MA, Richman DD, Causey DM, et al: Prolonged zidovudine therapy in patients with AIDS and advanced AIDS-related complex. *JAMA* 262:2405–2410, 1989.

Griffin DE, McArthur JC, Cornblath DR: Neopterin and interferon-gamma in serum and CSF of patients with HIV-associated neurologic disease. *Neurology* 41:69–744, 1991.

Grimaldi LME, Martino GV, Franciotta DM, et al: Elevated alpha-tumor necrosis factor levels in spinal fluid from HIV-1-infected patients with CNS involvement. *Ann Neurol* 29:21–25, 1991.

Hauger SB, Nicholas SW, Caspe WB: Guidelines for the care of children and adolescents with HIV infection. *Lancet* 336:1345–1347, 1990.

LaGrenade L, et al: Infective dermatitis of Jamaican children: A marker for HTLV-1 infection. *Lancet* 1:1345–1347, 1990.

Laverda AM, Cogo P, Condini A, et al: How frequent and how early does the neurological involvement in HIV-positive children occur? *Child Nerv Syst* 6:406–408, 1990.

Levy RM, et al: Central nervous system dysfunction in acquired immunodeficiency syndrome, in: Rosenblum ML, Levy RM, Bredesen DE, et al (eds): *AIDS and the Nervous System.* New York, Raven Press, 1988, pp. 29–63.

Pizzo PA, Eddy J, Falloon J, et al: Effect of continuous IV infu-

---

Pearls and Perils: Acquired Immunodeficiency Syndrome

1. Maternal antibodies persisting in the neonate for up to 15 months after birth delay the detection of neonatal AIDS.
2. Cerebral vascular strokes with progressive dementing neurologic deterioration are major clinical findings.
3. Unusual neurologic manifestations—as observed in subacute necrotizing encephalomyelitis, similar to Leigh's disease, a mitochondrial cytopathy—may be diagnostically misleading.
4. CSF analysis of pterins for the neopterin/biopterin ratio may be useful as early evidence of CNS infection.

sion of AZT in children with symptomatic HIV infection. *N Engl J Med* 319:889–896, 1988.

Pizzo PA: Emerging concepts in the treatment of HIV infection in children. *JAMA* 262:1989–1992, 1989.

Primary immunodeficiency diseases: Report of a World Health Organization scientific group. *Clin Immunol Immunopathol* 40:166–196, 1986.

Sever JL, Madden DL: Serologic tests for AIDS. *Clin Immunol Newsl* 7:137–140, 1986.

Shahar EM, Hwang PA, Niesen CE, Murphy EG: Poliomyelitis-like paralysis during recovery from acute bronchial asthma: Possible etiology and risk factors. *Pediatrics* 88:276–279, 1991.

Yong D, et al: Stroke in pediatric acquired immunodeficiency syndrome. *Ann Neurol* 28:303–311, 1990.

New sources of information appear frequently, requiring continuous updating of our knowledge of the epidemiology of, clinical characteristics of, and especially available drug treatments for immunodeficiency syndromes. The report by Cooper provides an excellent overview before researching individual aspects of this increasingly important disorder in infants and children. The paper by Yong and associates is an important update on neurologic localization of HIV infections in children. The volume edited by Edelson provides a general review of childhood AIDS.

Ataxia-Telangiectasia

Ataxia-telangiectasia (AT) or Louis-Bar Syndrome should be an initial consideration in young children with the onset of ataxia and choreoathetosis in the first 2 to 3 years of life. The disorder was first reported by Syllaba and Henner in 1926 and established as a clinical entity by Boder and Sedgwick in 1957. Early neurologic diagnosis may be obscured by a toddler's uncertain gait, but all motor milestones are delayed in appearance. Very frequent upper respiratory tract infections should suggest the diagnosis, especially if bulbar conjunctivae appear unusually vascular. In girls, delayed motor skills and a movement disorder may suggest Rett's syndrome. The important immunologic abnormalities in AT may remain undetected owing to initial concern for the many causes of ataxia in children (such as Friedreich's ataxia, a combined immunodeficiency with reduced circulating immunoglobulins as well as autoimmune phenomena); the presence of neurologic involvement is determined by specific immunologic testing. The molecular mechanisms underlying the ataxia are unknown, but the neuropathologic findings differ from those in Freidreich's ataxia, which, although common in children, is usually of later onset. There is no direct treatment.

Signs and Symptoms

In this autosomal recessive disorder, the child generally develops ocular bulbar conjunctival telangiectasia after the recognition of the cerebellar gait ataxia; however, frequent sino-pulmonary infections predominate in the first few years. The extrapyramidal postures, upper extremity intention dysmetria, dysarthria, and abnormal ocular following and volitional saccades develop in a progressive course of deterioration. At birth the infant is normal. Careful neurologic examination eventually reveals the extrapyramidal signs of a subtle choreoathetosis if the child is observed over time. The early delay in development could suggest a diagnosis of cerebral palsy. These children are generally mentally normal early in life, without the signs of brain damage present in perinatal static encephalopathies. A cluster of large blood vessels between the lateral or medial limbus and the canthal angle is distinctive in the fully developed form. Areas of cutaneous telangiectasis about the face and trunk and a variety of less diagnostic skin lesions, including scleroderma, have been observed to develop later. These findings are frequently preceded by a history of repeated sinopulmonary disease, which may have an onset in early infancy as respiratory infections, eventually leading to bronchiectasis. Muscle weakness and atrophy, possibly caused by disuse, occur in some patients.

In about 70% of the patients there is defective cell-mediated immunity (described in 1961 by the absence of serum IgA and in 1969 by a deficiency of IgE) and more recently associated with an increased level of plasma α-fetoprotein. Failure to develop secondary sex characteristics, irregular menses, testicular atrophy, and growth failure are common in the long term. A propensity for various malignancies has been described, including leukemia, adenocarcinoma, and medulloblastoma. Family members also appear to be at increased risk for the development of malignancy.

FEATURE TABLE 11-2. ATAXIA-TELANGIECTASIA

Discriminating Features	Consistent Features	Variable Features
1. Conjunctival and cutaneous telangiectasia	1. Thymic hypoplasia	1. Leukemia, lymphoma
2. Progressive cerebellar ataxia	2. CD3$^+$/CD4$^+$ lymphocyte deficiency	2. Solid tumors of breast, pancreas, stomach, bladder, and ovary
3. Increased chromosomal sensitivity to radiation-induced breakage	3. Sinopulmonary infections	3. High α-fetoprotein levels
4. Low serum IgA levels		4. Ovarian dysgenesis
		5. Endocrine disorders

This Feature Table courtesy of Daniel W. Stowens, MD.

Diagnostic Evaluation

The neurologic symptoms of AT are to be differentiated from those of other disorders leading to childhood ataxia, such as early-onset Friedreich's ataxia, which also progresses to nonambulatory disability by the second decade. Clinical neurologic examination may determine normal posterior column sensory findings with the appropriate immunologic laboratory studies if the older child is able to cooperate. The elevation of serum α-fetoprotein is a useful indicator, but it must be differentiated from the physiologic elevation normally present in the first months of life, and at times the α-fetoprotein level is normal. Levels of other immunoglobulins, such as IgE, have variably been reported to be increased or decreased. Monoclonal antibody studies of T cells show altered numbers of CD3/CD4 phenotypes. Studies of immunoglobulin synthesis suggest defects in both helper T and intrinsic B cells. Antibody responses to viral and bacterial antigens may be deficient. Excessive chromosomal breakage and structural abnormalities of chromosomes 14 and 7 have been reported. Radioresistant DNA synthesis in fibroblast cell strains is a consistent finding. Nonspecific widespread changes in endocrine function include urinary steroid excretion, abnormal insulin responses, hyperglycemia, and abnormal liver function. Computed tomographic scanning (CT) or magnetic resonance imaging (MRI) is useful to exclude intracranial neoplasms, especially posterior fossa mass lesions, of which ataxia is also an early neurologic symptom.

In cases in which they are sought, systemic histopathologic changes are widespread in the endocrine organs, including the anterior pituitary. In the CNS, there is significant loss of Purkinje and granular cells in the cerebellum and in the spinal cord, and anterior horn cell degeneration. Posterior column regions of demyelination have been observed.

Treatment

An awareness of a variable prognosis may be helpful, since the longest reported survival was to the age of 41 years. Supportive measures to manage and avoid infections as well as physical rehabilitative interventions for ataxia are useful. Treatment is largely supportive. Early diagnostic confirmation should be followed by genetic and family counseling for family planning purposes, and to advise regarding the risk of neoplasia and a sensitivity to radiation exposure.

(*Ataxia-telangiectasia is further discussed on pages 454 and 455.*)

ANNOTATED BIBLIOGRAPHY

Ammann AJ, Hong R: Disorders of the T-cell system, in Stiehm ER, Fulginiti VA (eds): *Immunologic Disorders in Infants and Children*, 2nd ed. Philadelphia, WB Saunders 1980a, p 286.

Ammann AJ, Hong R: Immunodeficiency with ataxia-telangiectasia, in Stiehm ER, Fulginiti VA (eds): *Immunologic Disorders in Infants and Children*, 2nd ed. Philadelphia, WB Saunders, 1980b, pp 310–315.

Boder E, Sedgwick RP: Ataxia-telangiectasia: A familial disorder of progressive cerebellar ataxia, oculo-cutaneous telangiectasia and frequent pulmonary infection. *Pediatrics* 21:526, 1958.

Gatti RA, Boder E, Vinters HV, Sparkes RS, Norman A, Lange K: Ataxia-telangiectasia: An interdisciplinary approach to pathogenesis. *Medicine* 70(2):99–117, 1991.

Painter RB: Radioresistant DNA synthesis: An intrinsic feature of ataxia-telangiectasia. *Mutat Res* 84:183–190, 1981.

Swift M, Reitnauer PJ, Morrell D, Chase CL: Breast and other cancers in families with ataxia-telangiectasia. *N Engl J Med* 316:1289–1294, 1987.

The chapter by Ammann and Hong (1980a) is an excellent and comprehensive review of all aspects of immunoregulatory abnormalities in AT, but unfortunately it has not been recently updated.

AUTOIMMUNE DISEASES

Acute Rheumatic Fever

Acute rheumatic fever (ARF) is one of several general systemic disorders with neurologically important symptoms, which include the collagen-vascular (rheumatic) diseases, systemic lupus erythematosus, juvenile rheumatoid arthritis (JRA), childhood dermatomyositis and polymyositis, and the vasculitides. Rheumatic fever is caused by immunologic defects in the basal ganglia. The Jones diagnostic criteria include chorea (often a subtle movement disorder in children) as one of five major manifestations. This multisystem, primarily cardiovascular, inflammatory disorder is related to group A streptococcal infection, without a known neurologic immunopathophysiology. The cardiac injury may be permanent. The choreic movement disorder causes weakness and muscular hypotonia but is self-limiting and may be controlled with specific medications. The loss of motor skills and emotional lability often initially disguise the acute-onset movement disorder in young children (most often between the ages of 3 and 10 years). An antibody mechanism for this combined involvement of the vasculature and striatum is supported by experimental

---

Pearls and Perils:
Ataxia-Telangiectasia

1. AT is the earliest-onset childhood ataxia syndrome and may be confused with many nongenetic causes of motor system disability.

2. Because brain tumors in children cause gait and head posture abnormalities, mass lesions are to be excluded by head neuroimaging as immunologic studies proceed.

3. The clinical diagnosis may be supported in the early stages by a low plasma IgA level and increased α-fetoprotein levels.

evidence. High-signal striatal lesions have been detected by MRI in JRA and ARF that suggest mass lesions but that disappear in time, similar to those observed in post-infectious encephalomyelitis.

Systemic Lupus Erythematosus

Several predominantly adult autoimmune diseases occasionally present as pediatric neurologic disorders. The eleven 1982 criteria for the classification of systemic lupus erythematosus (SLE) include the neurologic symptoms, seizures, and psychosis, especially in women over the age of 20 years. When peripheral neuropathies, Raynaud's phenomenon, and myalgia are included, over 50% of patients show neurologic effects. SLE is a particularly important consideration at younger ages, when medications—especially anticonvulsants used in treatment of the epilepsies and systemic disorders—may cause drug-induced forms of SLE. There are also immunologic differences in levels of detectable antinuclear antibodies (ANA). Histone-dependent ANA reactions occur frequently in drug-induced SLE compared to idiopathic SLE. Neonatal SLE may be especially difficult to recognize with a presentation of seizures and hypotonia.

Juvenile Rheumatoid Arthritis

In children and adolescents below the age of 16 years, most of the members of this group of autoimmune disorders are clinically classified by mode of onset. Immunologic findings may assist the diagnosis in some patients, but positive rheumatoid factors generally are more suggestive of adult disease. Cellular immunity plays a role in dermatomyositis and polymyositis, causing proximal muscle weakness syndromes in childhood. Males are more commonly affected than females, creating difficulty in the differential diagnosis from other types of childhood myopathies and dystrophies. Immunologic features are not specific and many are associated with elevations of creatinine phosphokinase (CK). Muscle biopsies may not be entirely distinctive because cellular infiltrations, muscle degeneration, and phagocytosis may be observed at different times and in different sites in the course of other diseases. Many forms of vascular disease may be grouped with these disorders, related to immune complex depositions, as in polyarteritis nodosa. Hypersensitivity vasculitis (related to cell-mediated mechanisms with round cell granuloma formation, as seen in giant cell arteritis) and a diverse, less specific group of disorders, such as Kawasaki's disease (a mucocutaneous lymph node syndrome seen in children) only occasionally affect the nervous system, usually as a meningoencephalitis.

The neurologic manifestations of vasculitis may be associated with cerebrovascular accidents, seizures, altered mental status, and cranial and peripheral neuropathies. Arteritis may be entirely limited to the nervous system. Hypersensitivity vasculitis, as in Henoch-Schönlein purpura, is commonly observed in children

with infections, although the CNS is rarely involved. The mechanism of CNS involvement in this group of diseases is unknown. Treatment includes steroids and cytotoxic drugs and supportive measures.

ANNOTATED BIBLIOGRAPHY

Blomgren SF, Condemi JJ, Vaughan JH: Procainamide induced lupus erythematosus: Clinical and laboratory observations. *Am J Med* 52:338–348, 1972.

Bohan A, Peter JB: Polymyositis and dermatomyositis. *N Engl J Med* 292:344–348, 403–408, 1975.

Cassidy TJ: Juvenile rheumatoid arthritis, in Kelley WN, Harris ED, Ruddy S, et al (eds): *Textbook of Rheumatology*, 2nd ed. Philadelphia, WB Saunders, 1985, pp 1247–1277.

Cupps TR, Fauci AS: The vasculitides, in Smith LH (ed): *Major Problems in Internal Medicine*, Vol 21. Philadelphia, WB Saunders, 1981, pp 1–211.

Cupps TR, Moore PM, Fauci AS: Isolated angiitis of the central nervous system: Prospective diagnostic and therapeutic experience. *Am J Med* 74:97–105, 1983.

Donovan MK, Lenn NJ: Postinfectious encephalomyelitis with localized basal ganglia involvement. *Pediatr Neurol* 5:311–313, 1989.

Fauci AS, Katz P, Haynes BF, et al: Cyclophosphamide therapy of severe systemic necrotiziung vasculitis. *N Engl J Med* 301:235–238, 1979.

Hirabayashi S, Kasai S, Tsukahara T, Fujisawa N, Watanabe T: Basal ganglia mass lesions in juvenile rheumatoid arthritis. *Pediatr Neurol* 7:141–143, 1991.

Husby G, Vande Rijn I, Zabriskie JB, et al: Antibodies reacting with cytoplasm of subthalamic and caudate nuclei neurons in chorea and acute rheumatic fever. *J Exp Med* 144:1094–1110, 1976.

Jones criteria (revised) for guidance in the diagnosis of rheumatic fever. *Circulation* 32:664–668, 1965.

Tan EM, Cohen AS, Fries JF, et al: The 1982 revised criteria for the classification of systemic lupus erythematosus. *Arthritis Rheum* 25:1271–1277, 1982.

Zabriskie JB, Friedman JE: The role of heart binding antibodies in rheumatic fever, in Spitzer JJ (ed): *Myocardial Injury*. Advances in Experimental Medicine and Biology, Vol 161. New York, Plenum Press, 1983, pp 457–470.

Multiple Sclerosis

In contrast to the primarily systemic immunoregulatory defects of the diseases discussed thus far, other disorders of both children and adults predominantly affect the CNS, with few systemic effects. The neuromuscular disease myasthenia gravis (MG) causes muscle weakness at any time from the neonatal period through adult life. One form of adult MG, seen during pregnancy, represents a prototypic autoimmune disorder and is caused by the pathogenic effect of anti-acetylcholine receptor antibodies transported to the fetus, causing temporary neonatal muscle weakness. MG will be discussed in detail in Chapter 16.

Other common nervous system disorders are related to immunoregulatory effects on central CNS and peripheral CNS myelin, causing encephalomyelitides, neuropathies, and multiple sclerosis (MS). Although MS is predominantly an adult disorder, the very young are not completely unaffected. An autopsy-proven infant developed symptoms at 10 months of age. MS is more benign in children, with 60% showing no deficits after 10 years. Demyelination and dysmyelination in children also occur in the lysosomal diseases and may suggest a clinical diagnosis of MS before definitive laboratory diagnostic studies have been undertaken. For example, metachromatic leukodystrophy, a disorder of myelin dysmetabolism (rather than demyelination of formed normal myelin) that is due to a specific lysosomal enzyme deficiency, may have clinical similarities to adolescent MS.

Common exanthematous and viral infections in children involve immunoregulatory mechanisms causing both central and peripheral nerve demyelination. In 1933 Rivers, after repeated injections of spinal cord material into animals, demonstrated a prototypic postimmunization demyelinating encephalomyelitis known as experimental allergic encephalomyelitis (EAE). This disorder forms the basis for modern-day comparisons to human demyelinating diseases, in particular MS. The antigen may be MBP, found normally in central brain myelin and in smaller amounts in peripheral myelin. The disorder may be mediated by MBP-reactive T cells because the antibody to MBP will not transfer the disease. Some proposed experimental therapies affect T-cell function or receptors. Other forms of demyelination occur in acute disseminated encephalomyelitis (ADEM) as parainfectious or postinfectious or postvaccinal encephalomyelitis. Upper and lower motor neuron paralytic effects following vaccination or infection are typical human models indistinguishable from the monophasic animal EAE mode.

MS is multiphasic, with scattered lesions occurring irregularly throughout the nervous system in time and location. Some monophasic demyelinating disorders in children, such as optic neuritis, are considered to be an early stage of MS. When optic neuritis is combined with a transverse myelitis, as in neuromyelitis optica or Devic's disease, the condition may be considered childhood-onset MS and may respond to steroid treatment. Some forms

of subacute myelo-optic neuropathy have a similar course but are related to toxic compounds.

Immunoregulatory etiologies have also been suggested for experimental allergic neuritis, Guillain-Barré syndrome, Lambert-Eaton syndrome in adults, and certain paraneoplastic syndromes affecting cerebral or cerebellar neurons. The response of some of these disorders to plasmapheresis suggests that a humoral factor is involved. Postinfectious encephalomyelitis or acute disseminated encephalomyelitis, an important disorder in children, is frequently associated with contagious exanthematous diseases, such as measles, chickenpox, and rubella. Mumps causes a viral parainfectious meningoencephalitis. Postimmunization disorders occur following routine vaccination for vaccinia, rabies, influenza, and pertussis and are similar to other immunoregulatory encephalomyelitic syndromes.

Myelin injury in immunoregulatory diseases may be reversible or may improve spontaneously with or without certain treatments. However, central myelin formed by oligodendrocytes is unable to regenerate after damage, whereas Schwann cells in the PNS retain a greater capacity for repair. Remyelination may be inducible but axonal regeneration is anatomically much more complex. Astrocytes also play a role in the central remyelination process. Experimentally glial cell grafts induce remyelination. At remyelination sites, myelin is thin with a reduced distance between neighboring nodes of Ranvier.

MS and ADEM patients show experimental similarities in CSF lymphocyte activity. Autoantibodies, humoral factors, and B and T lymphocytes all play an uncertain role in the pathogenesis of demyelination. Treatment trials support a role for an immune pathogenesis of MS because improvement occurs with lymphoid irradiation, causing global immunosuppression and worsening with γ-interferon, which augments immune function. There is no direct evidence for an effective specific therapy. The different stages of MS, with acute remitting disease in some and a chronic progressive form in others, may relate to different immune mechanisms. Different immunopharmacologic responses to cyclophosphamide in chronic progressive MS, and corticosteroids, azathioprine, and cyclosporine in the active disease, are supported by these reports of immunoregulatory mechanisms. Cyclophospha-

FEATURE TABLE 11-3. MULTIPLE SCLEROSIS

Discriminating Features	Consistent Features	Variable Features
1. Remitting and exacerbating clinical symptomatic course over time, affecting different CNS topographic regions 2. MRI (Gd-enhanced) of CNS demyelination, changing over time	1. Sudden visual loss, ataxia, vertigo, sensory symptoms 2. No apparent etiology for the sudden onset	1. Headache and emesis, suggesting an intracranial mass lesion 2. Sudden transverse myelitis with delayed-onset optic neuritis

mide is an agent capable of preventing EAE in animals, although exacerbations occur when the drug is stopped. Experimental evidence implies a T-cell–mediated disease since monoclonal antibodies bind to lymphocytes and act as immunosuppressive agents, with uncertain BBB transport. Intra-BBB IgG synthesis suggests an autoantibody mechanism. Employing these immunopharmacologic therapies, a beneficial response has been reported in chronic progressive MS. Preliminary reports are inconsistent but systemic interferon and copolymer 1 therapy, stimulating elements of the immune system, may also be ineffective.

Treatment in most demyelinating diseases is nonspecific, although recurrent claims of success mark the history of many of these disabling conditions.

Signs and Symptoms

MS affects cerebral, cerebellar, brainstem, spinal cord, and peripheral myelin, and pathologically characteristic plaques of demyelination appear in the brain. The clinical course is characterized by exacerbations and remissions but a chronic progressive course is not unusual. Genetic factors also play a role in MS because there is an increased incidence in families and an association with certain histocompatibility haplotypes. There is also an increased incidence of MS in colder climates, suggesting a role for viral infection.

Ataxia, visual disturbances, cranial nerve palsies, myelopathies, peripheral sensory symptoms, dizziness, vertigo, headache, and vomiting are major symptoms. The onset in children may appear monophasic because recurrences may be delayed for years. However, before the diagnosis of a monophasic disorder suggests MS, common neoplasms of childhood must be excluded by CT or MRI. MRI with gadolinium diethylenetriamine acetic acid enhancement of BBB permeability may be useful in evaluating therapeutic interventions. Because children do not readily admit visual loss or visual field defects, MRI enables the detection of MS lesions in the absence of reported symptoms. A careful neurologic examination establishing subtle bilateral upper motor neuron signs, dystaxia, and sensory changes favors the diagnosis of a demyelinating process. Transitional severe forms of MS have been described in adolescents.

Diagnostic Evaluation

CT and MRI studies to exclude mass lesions may suggest a demyelinating disorder after clinical neurologic examination. Special studies of blood and CSF cells may identify T-lymphocyte subpopulations and other humoral relations. In a clinical setting CSF examination in nearly all patients will eventually show a modest pleocytosis, elevated total protein, an abnormal colloidal gold curve if results are available, an increase in γ-globulin levels, increased IgG and oligoclonal bands, and increased levels of MBP. Visual evoked responses and brainstem auditory responses are helpful diagnostically but are not specific.

Pearls and Perils: Multiple Sclerosis

1. Multiple sclerosis occurs uncommonly below the age of 10 years and can simulate many neurologic disorders.
2. Brain tumors in children affect the optic nerves, with resultant visual deficits, and, if located in the posterior fossa, cause ataxia and cranial nerve dysfunction, simulating MS.
3. MRI with Gd is useful in identifying demyelination within brain and spinal cord.
4. There are few specific discriminating features in childhood MS, so alternative diagnoses should be considered after careful neurologic examination and laboratory studies.

Treatment

Conservative supportive treatment programs are encouraged, especially in children, in whom the course is often benign and the disease may remit spontaneously. Many treatment plans claim success only to cause disappointment as the disease follows a progressive course.

ANNOTATED BIBLIOGRAPHY

Duquette P, Muray TJ, Pleines J, et al: Multiple sclerosis in childhood: Clinical profile in 125 patients. *J Pediatr* 111:359–363, 1987.

Lisak RP: Immunopathogenic mechanisms, abnormal immunoregulation, and immunomodulating therapy in multiple sclerosis. *Clin Aspects Autoimmun* 1:14–21, 1987.

Lisak RP: Overview of the rationale for immunomodulating therapies in multiple sclerosis. *Neurology* 38(suppl 2):5–8, 1988.

Low NL, Carter S: Multiple sclerosis in children. *Pediatrics* 18:24–30, 1956.

Mechanisms of demyelination (editorial review). *Lancet* 1:495–496, 1985.

Riikonen R, Donner M, Erkkila H: Optic neuritis in children and its relationship to multiple sclerosis: A clinical study of 21 children. *Dev Med Child Neurol* 30:349–359, 1988.

The utility of therapeutic plasmapheresis for neurological disorders: Consensus Development Conference, NINCDS. *JAMA* 256:1333–1337, 1986.

Shaw CM, Alvord EC Jr: Multiple sclerosis beginning in infancy. *J Child Neurol* 2:252–256, 1987.

Willoughby EW, Grochowski E, Li D, et al: Serial magnetic resonance scanning in multiple sclerosis: A second prospective study in relapsing patients. *Ann Neurol* 25:43–49, 1989.

Zweiman B, Arnason BGW: Immunologic aspects of neurological and neuromuscular diseases. *JAMA* 258:2970–2973, 1987.

The paper by Zweiman and Arnason is an excellent brief review of neuroimmunologic disorders but is not confined to children.

FEATURE TABLE 11-4. GUILLAIN-BARRÉ SYNDROME

Discriminating Features	Consistent Features	Variable Features
1. Symmetric, bilateral, subacute, distal onset of weakness with loss of tendon reflexes 2. Minimal sensory loss 3. Cranial nerve pareses of facial and pharyngeal muscles	1. Normal CSF cell count 2. Elevated CSF protein level after the acute phase	1. Dysphagia 2. Respiratory arrest 3. Autonomic dysfunction 4. Antecedent infection

Guillain-Barré Syndrome

Signs and Symptoms

Idiopathic polyneuritis or Guillain-Barré syndrome (GBS), an acute polyneuropathy causing subacute progressive lower motor neuron muscle paralysis of varying degrees, is characterized by the destruction of peripheral myelin and Schwann cells by a cellular inflammatory infiltration. Although the triggering mechanisms are uncertain, the onset may be preceded by respiratory viral infection. The fact that plasmapheresis is therapeutically effective in certain stages of this disorder suggests a humoral immunodeficiency. GBS may lead to symmetric quadriparesis with ventilatory and autonomic nervous system failure. All ages are affected but in childhood the disorder peaks at between 4 and 9 years. Paralysis often begins in the lower extremities with variable sensory symptoms; eventually the loss of cranial nerve function causes dysphagia, which is followed by respiratory difficulty and autonomic dysfunction in the severe form of the disorder encountered in 3% to 14% of patients. The overall mortality is 5% to 20%, while autonomic, sympathetic, and parasympathetic dysfunction is evident in 65% of clinical reports. The disorder is generally self-limited, with most children making a complete recovery, although relapses with residual paresis may occur. Increased levels of circulating catecholamines and renin, with exaggerated responses reported to drugs causing hypotensive or hypertensive effects, arrhythmias, and cardiac arrest may account for sudden death in certain cases.

Pathologically a cellular infiltration of the PNS, including the sympathetic nerves and ganglia, takes place along with destruction of myelin. Central brainstem and medullary lesions have also been suggested from clinical signs. Although the pathogenesis is unknown, an immunoregulatory disorder is suggested by the antecedent viral infections or preceding immunizations, especially in children. There are similarities to experimental allergic neuritis produced by peripheral nerve myelin. Both cellular and humoral immune responses are affected. There is a marked increase in CSF immunoglobulin levels and some changes in T-lymphocyte subsets. A therapeutic response to corticosteroid therapy and plasmapheresis in chronic forms or those patients with ventilatory difficulties is also suggestive of an immune mechanism.

Diagnosis

Neurologic examination initially establishes the symmetric involvement of peripheral nerves with distal, occasionally ascending, weakness, peripheral sensory deficits, reduced to absent tendon reflexes, and flexor toe signs. The onset may be rapid, with quadriparesis appearing within several hours, or prolonged over several days. Subtle blunting of superficial modalities may occur, but vibration and joint position is reduced. Cranial nerve (especially facial) weakness and pharyngeal paresis affect respiration, speech, and swallowing. The mental status remains intact until severe autonomic dysfunction intervenes with ileus and urinary retention. Meningeal irritation with nuchal rigidity in young children is not uncommon. Occasionally papilledema is acutely evident, suggesting increased intracranial pressure. CSF examinations rule out other CNS infections while increased CSF

Pearls and Perils: Guillain-Barré Syndrome

1. There is symmetric peripheral, slowly or rapidly ascending lower motor neuron paresis, especially with cranial nerve paralysis, causing swallowing and respiratory compromise. Some clinical features are similar in onset to those of MG.
2. Facial weakness is reported in about one-half of affected children. This requires careful examination, because bilateral facial nerve involvement is difficult to recognize compared to a unilateral palsy. In the absence of cranial nerve dysfunction, neurologic localization could suggest a cord level syndrome, especially in a young child in whom the examination is limited. Myelopathies may present lower motor neuron findings, especially at the level of the lesion, so sensory testing is important in neurologic localization.
3. Papilledema occasionally occurs suggesting an intracranial mass lesion.
4. The acute-onset lower extremity weakness may also have the appearance of astasia abasia with inconsistent neurologic findings in early stages.

protein and immunoglobulin levels measured after the acute phase of the disorder are helpful in making the diagnosis. Nerve conduction studies and distal latencies suggest demyelination in later stages and are seldom useful in the acute phase.

Treatment

Primarily supportive measures are indicated because there is no specific therapy. Steroids and plasmapheresis should be reserved for special stages and courses of the disorder. Swan-Ganz monitoring appears to be especially helpful in those with autonomic dysfunction. Intravenous γ-globulin may be useful.

ANNOTATED BIBLIOGRAPHY

Arnason BG: Acute inflammatory demyelinating polyradiculo-neuropathies, in Dyck PJ, Thomas PK, Lambert EH, et al (eds): *Peripheral Neuropathy.* Philadelphia, WB Saunders, 1984, pp 2050–2100.

Asbury AK, Gibbs CJ (eds): Autoimmune Neuropathies: Guillain-Barré Syndrome. *Ann Neurol (Suppl.)* 2:1990.

Dalos NP, Borel C, Hanley DF: Cardiovascular autonomic dysfunction in Guillain-Barré syndrome. *Arch Neurol* 45:115, 1988.

Levinson AI, Zweiman B, Lisak RP: Immunopathogenesis and treatment of myasthenia gravis. *J Clin Immunol* 7:187–195, 1987.

The utility of therapeutic plasmapheresis for neurological disorders. Consensus conference. *JAMA* 256:1333–1337, 1986.

The special issue edited by Asbury and Gibbs is an excellent review of all aspects of this syndrome, including pediatric aspects.

Acute Disseminated Encephalomyelitis

Postinfectious or postvaccinal encephalomyelitis is the name given to immunoregulatory neurologic disorders related to somewhat more specific etiologies than those conditions discussed earlier, but with clinical and pathologic similarities. Postinfectious encephalomyelitis may follow viral or bacterial infections, immunizations, or drug and serum administrations. An acute hemorrhagic necrotizing leukoencephalitis is a severe form of postinfectious encephalomyelitis. There is great variation in the incidence of postinfectious encephalomyelitis after natural infection such as measles (virtually unknown below 1 year of age) or after immunizations for common pediatric infectious diseases since in the last decade vaccination for mumps, measles, and rubella has essentially eradicated the associated encephalitides. MRI of the brain may be helpful in identifying leukodystrophic changes owing to these various causes. Recent MRI studies suggest that there are brain changes in children, representing the earliest stages of demyelination, not recognizable by clinical examination.

Natural measles postinfectious encephalomyelitis is similar to EAE. There are, however, several CNS syndromes that follow measles infection and immunization, such as "allergic" postinfectious encephalomyelitis resulting from natural infection or "acute measles encephalitis" owing to direct viral invasion of the brain. Subacute sclerosing panencephalitis (SSPE) represents a late onset of brain invasion by the virus, in contrast to the acute postinfectious variety. Postinfectious encephalomyelitis may be associated with the exanthematous viral infections varicella, vaccinia, and rubella. An encephalopathy or neuropathy also may occur after rabies, influenza, and pertussis vaccination. This group of inflammatory demyelinating diseases are primarily immunoregulatory responses to infections and vaccines.

The recognized causes of the encephalitides in children have changed in recent years. Below 1 year of age, enteroviruses and HSV are especially prominent. Respiratory viruses predominate in very young children and varicella-zoster virus (VZV) in older children (5–9 years). There are important seasonal- and age-related frequencies for pediatric encephalitides and acute disseminated encephalomyelitis that may assist early diagnostic considerations. In addition to VZV, HVS, influenza A and B, parainfluenza 1 and 3, respiratory syncytial (RSV), and adenoviruses must be considered. Unfortunately, an unknown etiology is much more common at the youngest ages where the damage is the greatest.

Signs and Symptoms

An abrupt onset of fever, seizures with obtundation, and multifocal neurologic signs after an exanthem or an identifiable "viral" exposure are commonly observed. Headaches and cervical neck pain may simulate a posterior fossa tumor but may also be observed in these acute immunologic disorders. Prior nonspecific respiratory infections are too common to be diagnostically helpful. The effects of vaccinia and smallpox vaccination are now only of historic interest.

Acute measles encephalitis may be either immunologic in origin or related to viral CNS invasion. In either case an acute encephalopathy, transverse myelitis, generalized ataxia, or stroke-like picture with hemiparesis may evolve. The symptoms appear several days after the rash but may occur before or during eruption. A variable alteration in mentation occurs, ranging from delirium to coma with or without frequent generalized and multifocal seizures. Of the children with severe encephalopathies, 20% do not survive. Many studies have suggested long-term neuropsychiatric effects from subtle CNS involvement in measles. SSPE is a delayed-onset progressive CNS invasion, with immunoregulatory effects manifesting themselves in children often years after natural measles infection. Varicella encephalopathy is similar to that associated with measles but ataxia is more common. The acute toxic encephalopathy, Reye's syndrome, follows infection but is now seen very infrequently since the limitation of aspirin use in children with acute illnesses. Except for Reye's syndrome, the prognosis is generally better in varicella than in measles postinfectious syndromes. Rubella may present with a similar, often more benign, nonspecific neurologic syndrome, although a progressive SSPE course also occurs.

Diagnostic Evaluation

The age of the affected infant or child and the time of year are initially important because of known seasonal and age frequencies. In clinical diagnosis a focal onset (ie., partial seizures) may be helpful in differentiation from a more generalized disseminated process. However, HVS encephalitis mimics many disorders so that a more specific diagnosis must be sought through laboratory testing. A gadolinium-enhanced MRI and an EEG or other electrophysiologic-evoked potential studies may assist localization. The microbiologic diagnosis requires recognition of virus or antigen in CNS tissue or CSF or an increased serum/CSF antibody ratio (detected in 2% in the Koskiniemi and associates report); in children with "clinical encephalitis" a significant rise of antibody titer in paired specimens occurs in 40%; very high titers, positive virus cultures, or specific antigen detection is observed in another 35%. Antigen detection of specific viruses (ie., HSV, VZV) by immunofluorescence (IF) is necessary. CSF pleocytosis, increased IgG or oligoclonal bands, and MBP levels are nonspecific but may be helpful with associated presence of immunoregulatory disturbances.

Treatment

The use of antiviral compounds may be considered when the diagnosis is uncertain. However, there are many disorders that mimic HSV encephalitis. In the long term, prevention is the best treatment. Vaccines have proven effective in avoiding the serious CNS involvement of exanthematous childhood disorders. The delayed onset of SSPE is a serious untreatable terminal complication. Routine immunizations avoid the deafness and mental impairment associated with these infections. General supportive treatment is the standard of care. There is no substantive evidence that steroid treatment or immunosuppressive drugs alter the outcome.

ANNOTATED BIBLIOGRAPHY

Johnson RT, Griffin DE, Hirsch RL, et al: Measles encephalomyelitis—Clinical and immunologic studies. N Engl J Med 310:137–141, 1984.

Johnson RT, Griffin DE, Gendelman HE: Postinfectious encephalomyelitis. Semin Neurol 5:180–190, 1985.

Kipps A, Dick G, Moodie JW: Measles and the central nervous system. Lancet 2:1406–1410, 1983.

Koskiniemi M, Raautonen J, Lehtokoski-Lehtiniemi E, Vaheri A: Epidemiology of encephalitis in children: A 20-year survey. Ann Neurol 29:492–497, 1991.

Whitley RJ, Cobbs CB, Alford CA, et al: Diseases that mimic herpes simplex encephalitis: Diagnosis, presentation and outcome. JAMA 262:234–239, 1989.

The 1985 paper by Johnson and associates is a review of disorders included in this group, including immunoregulatory, histopathologic, and clinical symptoms.

Lyme Disease

Autoimmune neurologic disorders may involve viral CNS invasion with immunoregulatory humoral and monocytic cell effects. SSPE is the delayed onset after natural measles of a progressively fatal encephalitis. Progressive multifocal leukoencephalopathy usually affects oligodendrocytes in immunosuppressed individuals infected with the papovaviruses SV40 or JC. Lyme disease is a recently recognized multisystem disease resulting from spirochetal infection with a delayed-onset neurologic syndrome involving immunoregulatory mechanisms.

This disorder was first reported in 1970 but first came to widespread attention in 1975 as Lyme disease (named after a community in Connecticut) because of an unusual number of affected children. Several endemic areas are recognized in the United States, predominantly along the east and west coasts and the northern Great Lakes. Lyme disease requires a vector life cycle through mammalian and avian hosts, and children are infected after the bite of one of several species of deer or bear ticks. The disease is now known to be caused by the spirochete *Borrelia burgdorferi*.

Signs and Symptoms

Lyme disease may be specific, subtle, elusive, and simulate other disorders. A dermatologic first stage (erythema chronicum migrans) in about 50% of the cases is followed by two later stages affecting other organ systems. The earliest stage passes into a middle stage involving variable neurologic symptoms and findings, some suggesting MS and appearing weeks or months after the first stage. The third stage consists of rheumatologic symptoms and must be differentiated from JRA.

Pearls and Perils: Acute Disseminated Encephalomyelitis

1. The diagnosis of postinfectious encephalomyelitis depends on identifying the exanthem or a history of a definite exposure. Differential diagnosis is difficult because many agents or exposures to infective agents cause a similar clinical picture.

2. The similar clinical presentation of a treatment-responsive disorder, such as herpes encephalitis, may be difficult to differentiate initially from acute disseminated encephalomyelitis.

Specific neurologic symptoms include neuropathies affecting cranial nerves III through IV and not uncommonly unilateral or bilateral Bell's palsy (cranial nerve VII). Radiculopathies, unilateral or bilateral, affecting predominantly the cervical dorsal junctional plexus, as in other forms of brachial neuritis, are observed. Aseptic meningitis, encephalitis with seizures and/or psychosis, and encephalomyelitis with a transverse myelitis have been reported. Demyelinating lesions may be observed by CT and MRI. Much less commonly, manifestations of a demyelinating polyneuropathy (Guillain-Barré syndrome), pseudotumor cerebri, chorea, or an axonal neuropathy in mononeuritis multiplex are observed. While in utero, placental transmission of the spirochete is known; fetal effects during pregnancy are uncertain.

Spirochetal invasion of the CNS occurs in an "aseptic" meningitis with a lymphocytic and plasma cell pleocytosis. The organism has been demonstrated in several tissues. Immunoregulatory mechanisms probably account for the demyelinating features. Intra-BBB IgM and IgG have been demonstrated. CSF IgM levels are elevated, altering the IgM and IgG indexes. There is an increase in IgG synthesis, CSF protein is increased, and oligoclonal immunoglobulins may be present.

Diagnostic Evaluation

A history relating the child to locations where tick bites might occur is important. The neurologic symptoms follow the characteristic skin lesions by several weeks. These symptoms and findings are nonspecific because most can be related to other etiologies. Considerable reliance on a variety of special laboratory tests will be important to allow the initiation of early antibiotic treatment.

Detection of spirochete-specific IgM antibodies may occur a few weeks after the first symptoms, with additional time necessary for IgG antibodies. Early in the disease the antibody responses are more specific since IgG antibodies to many spirochetal antigens appear in the chronic stages. An immunofluorescence assay (IFA) and an immunosorbent enzyme-linked assay (ELISA) are available, but both false-negative and false-positive responses have been reported. ELISA is generally more reliable than the IFA, but there is interlaboratory variability. A PCR test has also been developed.

Treatment

The selection of an antibiotic depends on the age of the patient and the stage of the disease. Perhaps 95% of patients achieve full recovery if properly treated. As experience is gained, the selection of antibiotic and route

---

Pearls and Perils: Lyme Disease

1. Lyme disease may be considered when a number of children develop a similar variety of neurologic symptoms in a region with the necessary vector ticks present.
2. The delay in appearance of neurologic symptoms may be too long to permit recall of the characteristic skin lesion.
3. Diagnosis of early stages is important for commencement of necessary antibiotic treatment to avoid late neurologic manifestations.

---

of administration change. Oral doxycycline hyclate (100 mg 2 times a day) for 2 to 3 weeks in older children and adults in early stages of Lyme disease is effective. Amoxicillin orally for 2 to 3 weeks in early stages and especially in young children (20–40 mg/kg/day) may also be employed. Alternatives include erythromycin, tetracycline, or penicillin. IV administration of ceftriaxone sodium (2 gm/day) is recommended for neurologic manifestations, also for 2 to 3 weeks; this route should be considered if CSF abnormalities are detected. With either oral or IV therapy, intensified symptoms in the Jarisch–Herxheimer reaction may occur in the first day or two of treatment. The use of corticosteriods is uncertain even for the arthritis of advanced disease.

ANNOTATED BIBLIOGRAPHY

Committee on Infectious Diseases of the American Academy of Pediatrics: Treatment of Lyme borreliosis. *Pediatrics* 88:176–179, 1991.

Duffy J, Schoen RT, Sigal LH: 1991 update on Lyme disease. *Patient Care* 25:24–51, 1991.

Finkel MF: Lyme disease and its neurologic complications. *Arch Neurol* 45:99–104, 1988.

Luger SW, Krausse: Serologic tests for Lyme disease: Interlaboratory variability. *Arch Intern Med* 150:761–763, 1990.

Rosa PA, Schwan TG: A specific and sensitive assay for the Lyme disease spirochete *Borrelia burgdorferi* using the polymerase chain reaction. *J Infect Dis* 160:1018–1029, 1989.

Szer IS, Taylor E, Steere AC: The long-term course of Lyme arthritis in children. *N Eng J Med* 325:159–163, 1991.

The Finkel article presents a brief, comprehensive review of Lyme disease focusing on the neurologic manifestations. Duffy and colleagues give a very recent summary, particularly of antibiotic therapy, of the ever changing recommendations for inpatient or outpatient therapy. The Szer study also mentions the long-term appearance of keratitis and the chronic encephalopathy.

Chapter Twelve

Vascular Disease

Nicholas J. Lenn
Richard H. Haas

Cerebrovascular disease in children is important and deserves greater clinical and investigative attention than it has thus far received. Every year in the United States an estimated 2000 children suffer from a major cerebrovascular event. This figure is surely an underestimate. Although perhaps 90% of these children survive the acute insult, most have residual disability. Thus, the importance of this condition is related more to its high prevalence than to its relatively low incidence. The fact that there is a wide range of etiologic and pathologic factors has also contributed to the perception that childhood vascular disease is rare. By contrast, cerebrovascular disease in adult life has a high incidence, but a generally shorter survival time and a small number of causes.

In this chapter, the prenatal and perinatal periods are grouped together and considered separately from the remainder of childhood. For each age group, ischemic and hemorrhagic lesions are discussed separately, in a clinico-anatomic framework.

PRENATAL AND PERINATAL ISCHEMIC DISEASE

It has long been recognized by pathologists that some congenital brain injuries are the result of cerebrovascular events that occur during gestation (Vogel, 1961; Larroche and Amiel, 1966; Lyon and Robain, 1967; Friede, 1973). Anencephaly (owing to lesions at 6 to 7 weeks gestation), hydranencephaly and some porencephalic cysts (3 to 6 months), and some focal lesions had either a distribution or pathologic feature(s) suggestive of a vascular pathogenesis. The "watershed" appearance of this last group suggested that infarcts were related to circulatory failure. All of these cases are recognized as prenatal in origin (Goutieres et al., 1972). The clinical importance of focal and multifocal ischemic infarcts has acquired new emphasis in recent years as a result of intensive care of neonates and the availability of newer imaging methods.

Pathophysiology

Although there is a similarity of histopathology between cerebral infarcts in the immature brain and later in life, there are a number of differences. Both groups show ischemic and hemorrhagic infarcts of venous and arterial origin. Criteria for dating lesions are tenuous; however, acute clinical presentation occurring postnatally, enhancement of the infarct on the computed tomographic (CT) scan, and the temporal relationship of these findings to the histopathology suggest that the dating of such events is similar to that for older individuals (Larroche, 1977, pp. 421–430; Lenn, 1987). Infarcts in neonates have greatly accelerated clearing of debris, early calcification, and differences in distribution related to immature features of vascular anatomy.

Pathologic studies have provided some of the most reliable data, but are biased for acutely ill babies (Banker, 1961; Ahdab-Barmada et al., 1981). Cerebral infarcts, excluding venous infarcts and periventricular leukomalacia (PVL) secondary to vascular disease, occur in at least 5.4% of autopsied neonates. Both clinical and pathologic series usually show more left than right cerebral infarcts and a high incidence of multiple infarcts. Arterial occlusions are more common than venous in neonates. The reverse is true in infants and children. Arterial occlusions are more often embolic and occur in the presence of sepsis and disseminated intravascular coagulopathy (DIC). Focal infarcts can be seen in a variety of systemic disturbances, including apnea, bradycardia, hypotension, acidosis, hypoglycemia, DIC, respiratory distress syndrome, sepsis, surgery, congenital heart disease, germinal matrix hemorrhage, PVL, and autonomic instability. A specific etiology will not be demonstrable in most prenatal and in many perinatal cases of vascular occlusion. Maternal trauma must be massive, as in motor vehicle accidents with pelvic fracture and visceral damage, to affect the fetus. Maternal infection or chemical exposure is a doubtful cause, although indirect effects remain a possibility. Perinatal infarcts occasionally are due to amniotic fluid

283

embolization. Acute massive maternal exposure to cocaine has been incriminated as an etiology of infarction (Chasnoff et al., 1986), raising questions about smaller amounts of cocaine and other maternal drug exposures in the etiology of neonatal infarction.

A number of factors may contribute pathogenetically to prenatal and perinatal infarction. DIC and intracardiac thrombosis may produce increased factor VIII and free fatty acids, which increase platelet aggregation (Favara et al., 1974; McDonald et al., 1984). DIC or meningitis with arteritis has been observed when sepsis is associated with cerebral infarction. Up to 30% of autopsies in neonates with meningitis show infarcts, many hemorrhagic (Friede, 1973). Phlebothrombosis and thrombophlebitis occur more often than endarteritis in meningitis and congenital heart disease.

PVL presents a somewhat different picture. These ischemic lesions are usually symmetric and are located in the white matter adjacent to the lateral ventricles. The lesions vary in degree and size. They occur predominantly in premature infants who have survived several days or more and have had severe systemic illness, such as cardiorespiratory dysfunction and bacteremia (Leviton and Gilles, 1984). PVL is often associated with intraventricular hemorrhage (Volpe, 1987). The location of the lesions is related to the extensive periventricular vascular (mainly venous) plexus that is prominent at 28 to 32 weeks, which arises from penetrating cortical arteries (Ahdab-Barmada and Moossy, 1985).

Signs and Symptoms

The baby with a prenatal lesion will most often present with developmental abnormalities at 6 to 12 months of age (Byers, 1941). The mother or physician will note either asymmetry of motor function or developmental delay. Even when an infant has a known cerebral infarct, his or her development and examination may be normal for several weeks. The reasons for such delay of symptoms and signs, and for their failure to occur in some cases, are not well understood. With prenatal vascular lesions, hemiparesis almost always spares the face, and facial involvement is often mild with early postnatal lesions (Lenn and Thurston, 1983). Obviously, cognitive function may suffer, but this may not be noted until language development or school performance is affected. This is especially true with left hemisphere lesions. It is also important to realize that 50% of children showing

motor dysfunction at 1 year of age may be *normal* by 7 years, especially if the earlier involvement was not severe (Nelson and Ellenberg, 1982).

Seizures are the other major symptom of prenatal and perinatal cerebral infarcts (Ment et al., 1984; Clancy et al., 1985). A large proportion of cases diagnosed in the perinatal period come to attention because of focal seizures. Such cases are not particularly associated with marked prematurity, so that the apparent increase in incidence since 1980 is probably due to increased diagnosis, related to more frequent neuroimaging. The cocaine "epidemic" may be another factor. The seizures may be focal, focal plus secondarily generalized, or generalized. Persistent focal seizures in the newborn, or persistent generalized seizures in the absence of infectious or metabolic etiologies, suggest a stroke.

Diagnostic Studies

Diagnostic studies can be considered by time of diagnosis relative to the infarct. A specific diagnosis, which may be specifically treatable, is found by thorough evaluation in 80% of newborns with seizures. The yield is also high when examination or electroencephalography (EEG) demonstrate focality. Head ultrasound and often contrast-enhanced head CT or magnetic resonance imaging (MRI) scan are needed to recognize a recent infarct or other focal lesion. If a cerebral lesion is demonstrated, etiology may be pursued with lumbar puncture and antibody titers if possibly infectious, or with biopsy if it is neoplastic.

There is limited information about the safety or the yield of information from angiographic studies; they are rarely done and should be limited to specific indications. Although safe, the clinical value of noninvasive vascular studies such as directional doppler through the anterior fontanelle and carotid studies are not yet known. Positron emission tomography remains an experimental rather than a clinical tool.

In both groups, those with focal seizures and those with focal neurologic dysfunction, one should seek the etiologic factors described under Pathophysiology. These include sepsis, DIC, apnea, bradycardia, hypotension, acidosis, hypoglycemia, congenital heart disease, germinal matrix hemorrhage, periventricular leukomalacia, and autonomic instability. In many cases the cause will not be identified; in many others, more than one etiologic factor will be present, producing a combination of

FEATURE TABLE 12-1. PRENATAL AND PERINATAL ISCHEMIC DISEASE

Discriminating Feature	Consistent Feature	Variable Features
1. Focal infarction on CT or MRI	1. Hemiparesis or other focal dysfunction by 1 year of age	1. Focal seizures in the neonatal period 2. Focal EEG abnormalities

Pearls and Perils: Prenatal and Perinatal Ischemic Disease

1. Focal seizures in the neonate suggest infarction, even more so if such seizures persist.
2. Facial sparing in an infant with hemiparesis suggests a prenatal onset.
3. Strabismus in an infant raises the question of other cerebral lesions.
4. The development of hand preference under 1 year of age suggests dysfunction of the opposite upper extremity.
5. Persistent electrographic status epilepticus may be due to perinatal infarction, but may not be evident clinically in a generally ill neonate.

interacting causes. If no cerebral lesion is found on CT or MRI, consideration of spinal cord disease may require spine x rays or a myelogram. Peripheral nerve injury should be considered, but will usually be readily differentiated from central lesions.

If motor deficit of definite cerebral origin or seizures are first recognized later in the first year or two of life, and there is no indication of acute onset or acquired etiology, and especially if there are other indicators of early occurrence, the workup may be limited or omitted. Careful clinical followup to avoid failure to detect progressive diseases is essential. If there is doubt, workup for structural lesions with CT or MRI scans or for functional lesions with EEG and etiologic tests such as metabolic studies are warranted.

Healed PVL has a characteristic CT appearance (Hill et al., 1986). Because the white matter is deficient, the lateral wall of the lateral ventricle has a scalloped contour, and the gray matter at the depth of the Sylvian fissure nearly touches the ventricular wall.

Treatment

There is no specific treatment for cerebral infarcts. Recurrent infarcts are not expected in neonates. Seizures should be treated vigorously with the usual drugs. The child should have close follow-up and early physical, occupational, and language therapy.

ANNOTATED BIBLIOGRAPHY

Ahdab-Barmada MA, Moossy J, Shuman RM: Cerebral infarcts with arterial occlusion in neonates. *Ann Neurol* 6:495–502, 1981.
 This is a large and focused review. Although most of the case reports have appeared since this article was published, most issues in this so far poorly understood area are presented well, along with a good review of the preceding literature.

REFERENCES

Ahdab-Barmada M, Moossy J: Cerebrovascular lesions in the neonate: Clinical, anatomical, and developmental correlates, in Plum F, Pulsinelli W (eds): *Cerebrovascular Diseases.* New York, Raven Press, 1985, p 133–142.
Banker BQ: Cerebral vascular disease in infancy and childhood. I. Occlusive vascular diseases. *J Neuropathol Exp Neurol* 20:127–140, 1961.
Byers RK: Evolution of hemiplegias in infancy. *Am J Dis Child* 61:915–927, 1941.
Chasnoff IJ, Bussey ME, Savich R, Stack CM: Perinatal cerebral infarction and maternal cocaine use. *J Pediatr* 108:456–459, 1986.
Clancy R, Malin S, Laraque D, Baumgart S, Younkin D: Focal motor seizures heralding stroke in full-term neonates. *Am J Dis Child* 139:601–606, 1985.
Favara BE, Franciosi RA, Butterfield LJ: Disseminated intravascular and cardiac thrombosis of the neonate. *Am J Dis Child* 127:197–204, 1974.
Friede RL: Cerebral infarcts complicating neonatal leptomeningitis. *Acta Neuropathol* 23:245–253, 1973.
Goutieres F, Challamel MJ, Aicardi J, Gilly R: Les hemiplegies congenitales. *Arch Fr Pediatr* 29:839–851, 1972.
Hill A, Flodmark O, Roland EH, Whitfield MF: New and characteristic diagnostic features of periventricular leukomalacia on CT scan. *Ann Neurol* 20:394, 1986.
Larroche JC: *Developmental Pathology of the Neonate.* Amsterdam, Excerpta Medica, 1977.
Larroche JC, Amiel C: Thrombose de l'artère Sylvienne à la période néonatale. *Arch Fr Pediatr* 23:257–274, 1966.
Lenn NJ: Plasticity and responses of the immature nervous system to injury. *Semin Perinatol* 11:117–131, 1987.
Lenn NJ, Thurston S: Is facial sparing in children with prenatal hemiparesis evidence for neuronal plasticity? *Ann Neurol* 14:371, 1983.
Leviton A, Gilles FH: Acquired perinatal leukencephalopathy. *Ann Neurol* 16:1–8, 1984.
Lyon G, Robain O: Etude comparative des encephalopathies circulatoires prénatales et para-natales (hydrancephalies, porencephalies et encephalomalacies kystiques de la substance blance). *Acta Neuropathol* 9:79–98, 1967.
McDonald MM, Johnson ML, Rumack CM, et al: Role of coagulopathy in newborn intracranial hemorrhage. *Pediatrics* 74:26–31, 1984.
Ment LR, Duncan CC, Ehrenkranz RA: Perinatal cerebral infarction. *Ann Neurol* 16:559–568, 1984.
Nelson KB, Ellenberg JH: Children who "outgrew" cerebral palsy. *Pediatrics* 69:529–536, 1982.
Vogel FS: The anatomic character of the vascular anomalies associated with anencephaly. *Am J Pathol* 39:163–174, 1961.
Volpe JJ: *Neurology of the Newborn,* 2nd ed. Major Problems in Clinical Pediatrics, Vol 22. Philadelphia, WB Saunders, 1987.

INTRAVENTRICULAR HEMORRHAGE

Intraventricular hemorrhage (IVH) is the major type of intracranial hemorrhage in the newborn. Probably no subject has produced more intense effort and study in modern child neurology than this frequent and devastating group of conditions, which includes germinal matrix hemorrhage, subependymal hemorrhage, and choroid plexus hemorrhage (Volpe, 1987).

Clarification of the pathogenesis of IVH is in progress, and new approaches to reducing occurrence and improving outcome have resulted (Goddard-Finegold and Mizrahi, 1987). Birth-related hypoxic-ischemic insult, fluctuations in cerebral blood flow, and many secondarily correlated effects of these parameters are the major focus of these efforts.

Pathophysiology

The weight-specific rates of IVH, like other neonatal morbidity rates, are probably still changing. Through the 1980s, IVH occurred in 40% of infants below 35 weeks gestation and in 13% of those weighing between 1501 and 2000 grams at birth (Ahmann et al., 1980; McGuinness and Smith, 1984). IVH lesions are usually graded on sonographic or radiologic criteria as (Papile et al., 1978a):

Grade I	Subependymal only
Grade II	Intraventricular blood
Grade III	Intraventricular blood and ventricular dilatation
Grade IV	Intraventricular blood with parenchymal hemorrhage

The normal germinal matrix vasculature undergoes major changes late in gestation. In nonhuman primates these changes include enlargement of veins during the period corresponding to susceptibility to IVH, followed by thickening and strengthening of their walls near term (Lenn and Whitmore, 1985). In spite of this lack of morphologic change in capillaries from midgestation, pathologic examination of human IVH suggests that hemorrhage may begin at capillary-venous junctions (Pape and Wigglesworth, 1979). In any case, a prominent role of physiologic parameters in the pathogenesis of IVH is universally acknowledged, and is the principal target of preventive efforts. These include taking the utmost care not only to normalize but also to avoid extremes in cardiovascular, respiratory, and fluid/electrolyte status. Stimulation is also to be avoided. Labor,

whether completed or not, is a risk factor for IVH in babies under 2000 g (Tejani et al., 1984). Defective or pressure-passive regulation of cerebral blood flow is a major risk factor (Lou et al., 1979). Prevention of fluctuations in cerebral blood flow velocity is important (Perlman et al., 1983, 1985).

Histopathologically, germinal matrix hemorrhage is associated with primary or secondary infarcts, edema, parenchymal extension beyond the germinal matrix, rupture of overlying ependyma, and intraventricular blood clots. Blood in the subarachnoid space may contribute to the occurrence of hydrocephalus by interfering with cerebrospinal fluid (CSF) absorption through the arachnoid granulations. Later evolution of the lesions produces porencephaly in up to two thirds of long-term survivors of grade III and IV hemorrhages. These multicystic or confluent areas result from associated leukomalacia and infarction. Volpe (1987) has presented the concept that asymmetric hemorrhagic lesions are infarcts rather than extensions of the germinal matrix hematoma.

Short-term mortality from all causes varies with grade of IVH, birth weight, Apgar score, and many other factors. It is about 20%, and occurs largely with grade III and IV lesions (McGuinness and Smith, 1984). Progressive ventricular dilatation occurs in approximately half of the babies with IVH (usually 1 to 3 weeks following the hemorrhage), more often with higher grade, and in only 10% of grade I cases (Allan et al., 1982). Up to half of the patients will have spontaneous resolution of this problem and not require shunting.

The later clinical picture or long-term outcome for infants with IVH is one of markedly increased incidence of all major neurologic handicaps. With grade III and IV hemorrhages, this increase is three- to sevenfold (Papile et al., 1983; Catto-Smith et al., 1985). Survivors of grade I and II IVH do not clearly have a worse outcome than similar-weight babies without IVH (Ment et al., 1985).

Signs and Symptoms

IVH occurs in the first 2 days of life in 70% of cases. It may occur by 12 hours of age, and 35% to 50% of cases occur by 24 hours (Rumack et al., 1985). There are several clinical profiles, dependent in part on the gestational age and on the general condition of the infant. In severely

FEATURE TABLE 12-2. INTRAVENTRICULAR HEMORRHAGE

Discriminating Feature	Consistent Features	Variable Feature
1. Demonstration of the hemorrhage with head ultrasound and/or CT scan	1. Prematurity (in germinal matrix hemorrhage) 2. Associated with hypoxia-ischemia or major cerebrovascular disturbance 3. Blood in brain parenchyma and/or ventricles on CT scan	1. Associated parenchymal damage from periventricular leukomalacia, hemorrhagic infarction, or hematoma

Pearls and Perils:
Intraventricular Hemorrhage

1. IVH may occur in the absence of signs or symptoms, justifying the use of routine head ultrasound for detection of IVH in sick prematures.
2. Serial ultrasound and head measurements should be made in all cases of IVH to follow ventricular size and hydrocephalus.
3. Subtle seizures may occur and require EEG confirmation.
4. Serial ultrasounds and head measurements are useful in following ventricular size and helping to distinguish between cerebral atrophy secondary to encephalomalacia and hydrocephalus.

ill neonates, no specific clinical change may be noted. The IVH is discovered on sonography or CT, or at autopsy. In initially stable babies an abrupt, often marked deterioration in activity, feeding, temperature control, hematocrit, brainstem reflexes, or respiratory function, or the onset of seizures, may occur at the time of acute hemorrhage. Most often the situation lies between the subtle and the more abrupt modes of onset. There can also be considerable overlap between the profiles of premature infants with and without IVH (Papile et al., 1978a). Although clinical signs, such as decreased tracking, abnormal popliteal angle, and decreases in tone or motility, are correlated with IVH in infants under 36 weeks gestation (Dubowitz et al., 1981), the problem of overlap obscures diagnosis of the individual baby.

Diagnostic Studies

Current technology has made ultrasound scanning the mainstay of diagnosis and follow-up for both IVH and its consequences. In some units, high-risk babies are scanned routinely at 2 to 3 days of age, and surely at any time suggestive symptoms occur. Once IVH has been diagnosed, subsequent scans provide information on the resolution of the hemorrhage, the development of hydrocephalus, the effect of treatment, if any, and the development of encephalomalacia or porencephaly.

CT may be preferred if subdural hematoma or infarction is suspected, and is equally good for detecting IVH. MRI is indicated if a major malformation is suspected, or if other concerns remain. CT is also helpful to assess hypoxic-ischemic injury to subcortical white matter and other lesions, but is clearly inferior to MRI for detecting malformations. EEG is helpful in detecting unrecognized seizures and in providing electrographic confirmation of questionable spells. It also has some prognostic importance. Spinal fluid examination is poorly discriminating for IVH, but often important to evaluate the possibility of bacterial meningitis.

Active areas of investigation include the role of cerebral blood flow velocity measurements, evoked potentials, and cerebral metabolism, as measured by magnetic resonance spectroscopy and positron emission tomography.

Treatment

A reduction in both premature births and IVH is a major goal. Means of achieving a reduction in IVH include prenatal and postnatal measures. When premature birth is imminent, tocolytic agents, steroids, and phenobarbital may be helpful, although investigations continue. Details of postnatal care are of great importance. The goals of avoiding hypoxia, hypertension, volume expansion, and seizures (Papile et al., 1978b) are now more obtainable, and remain important even after IVH has occurred.

The treatment of hydrocephalus after IVH is complex because of clinical variables, limitations of the data available for individual patients, and limited knowledge of the risks and benefits of various approaches. There are two main groups of patients: those with rapidly progressive ventriculomegaly with increased pressure, and those without one or both of these features. Repeated lumbar puncture is a temporizing measure in both groups (Kreusser et al., 1985). This strategy is particularly indicated when systemic blood pressure is low at the same time. In the former group, if CSF protein content is greater than 200 mg/dL, serial lumbar punctures are often sufficient to avoid external ventricular drainage, with its higher risk of infection (Mayhall et al., 1984). When the CSF protein level falls, a ventriculoperitoneal shunt may be placed if hydrocephalus is still present, as it usually is. Many of the remaining infants with less severe hydrocephalus, if managed with serial lumbar punctures and monitored with ultrasound examinations, will have resolution of the problem with no need for a CSF shunt. Similar efficacy has been reported in a limited number of patients treated with acetazolamide (100 mg/kg per day) and furosemide (1 mg/kg per day) (Shinnar et al., 1985). However, unless this finding is confirmed in larger series, this drug regimen should probably be reserved for special cases. With either regimen, close surveillance for the development of progressive hydrocephalus is essential.

ANNOTATED BIBLIOGRAPHY

Volpe JJ: *Neurology of the Newborn,* 2nd ed. Philadelphia, WB Saunders, 1987, p 311–361.
    A detailed review of this subject with a balanced presentation of the many controversies.
Goddard-Finegold J, Mizrahi EM: Understanding and preventing perinatal, intracerebral, and intraventricular hemorrhages. *J Child Neurol* 2:170–185, 1987.
    This review emphasizes the application of current concepts of pathogenesis in seeking approaches to the prevention of IVH.

REFERENCES

Ahmann PA, Lazzara A, Dykes FD, et al: Intraventricular hemorrhage in the high-risk preterm infant: Incidence and outcome. *Ann Neurol* 7:118–124, 1980.

Allan WC, Holt PJ, Savage LP, Tito AM, Meade SK: Ventricular dilatation after neonatal periventricular-intraventricular hemorrhage. *Am J Dis Child* 136:589–593, 1982.

Catto-Smith AG, Yu VYG, Bajuk B, Orgill AA, Astbury J: Effect of neonatal periventricular hemorrhage on neurodevelopmental outcome. *Arch Dis Child* 60:8–11, 1985.

Dubowitz LMS, Levene MI, Morante A, et al: Neurologic signs of neonatal intraventricular hemorrhage: A correlation with real-time ultrasound. *J Pediatr* 99:127–133, 1981.

Kreusser KL, Tarby TJ, Kovnar E, Taylor DA, Hill A, Volpe JJ: Serial lumbar punctures for at least temporary amelioration of neonatal posthemorrhagic hydrocephalus. *Pediatrics* 75:719–724, 1985.

Lenn NJ, Whitmore L: Gestational changes in the germinal matrix of the normal rhesus monkey fetus. *Pediatr Res* 19:130–135, 1985.

Lou HC, Lassen NA, Friis-Hansen B: Impaired autoregulation of cerebral blood flow in the distressed newborn infant. *J Pediatr* 94:118–121, 1979.

McGuinness GA, Smith WL: Head ultrasound screening in premature neonates weighing more than 1500 grams at birth. *Am J Dis Child* 138:817–820, 1984.

Mayhall CG, Archer NH, Lamb VA, et al: Ventriculostomy-related infections. A prospective epidemiologic study. *N Engl J Med* 310:553–559, 1984.

Ment LR, Scott DT, Ehrenkranz RA, Duncan CC: Neurodevelopmental assessment of very low birth weight neonates: Effect of germinal matrix and intraventricular hemorrhage. *Pediatr Neurol* 1:164–168, 1985.

Pape KE, Wigglesworth JS: *Hemorrhage, Ischaemia, and the Perinatal Brain.* Philadelphia, JB Lippincott, 1979.

Papile L, Burstein J, Burstein R, Koffler H: Incidence and evolution of subependymal and intraventricular hemorrhage: A study of infants with birth weight less than 1500 grams. *J Pediatr* 92:529–534, 1978a.

Papile L, Burstein J, Burstein R, Koffler H, Koops B: Relationship of intravenous sodium bicarbonate infusions and cerebral intraventricular hemorrhage. *J Pediatr* 93:834–836, 1978b.

Papile L, Munsick-Bruno G, Shaefer A: Relationship of cerebral intraventricular hemorrhage and early childhood neurologic handicaps. *J Pediatr* 103:273–277, 1983.

Perlman JM, McMenamin JB, Volpe JJ: Fluctuating cerebral blood-flow velocity in respiratory-distress syndrome. *N Engl J Med* 309:204–209, 1983.

Perlman JM, Goodman S, Kreusser KL, Volpe JJ: Reduction in intraventricular hemorrhage by elimination of fluctuating cerebral blood-flow velocity in preterm infants with respiratory distress syndrome. *N Engl J Med* 312:1353–1357, 1985.

Rumack CM, Manco-Johnson MD, Manco-Johnson MJ, Koops BL, Hathaway WE, Appareti K: Timing and course of neonatal intracranial hemorrhage using real-time ultrasound. *Radiology* 154:101–105, 1985.

Shinnar S, Gammon K, Bergman EW Jr, Epstein M, Freeman JM: Use of acetazolamide and furosemide to avoid cerebrospinal fluid shunts. *J Pediatr* 107:31–37, 1985.

Tejani N, Rebold B, Tuck S, Ditroia D, Sutro W, Verma U: Obstetric factors in the causation of early periventricular-intraventricular hemorrhage. *Obstet Gynecol* 64:510–515, 1984.

INFANT, CHILD, AND ADOLESCENT ISCHEMIC DISEASE

Our approach to arterial or venous ischemic disease in this section will be anatomic, because localizing information can often be obtained from the history and examination as well as from the sophisticated neuroimaging procedures available today. The ready availability of CT and increasingly of MRI technologies allows a diagnosis of even small ischemic and hemorrhagic strokes in adults and children. Many of these would have remained unsuspected clinically. Incidence and prevalence figures produced in the past largely from clinical data underestimate the true incidence of childhood stroke.

Arterial Disease

Pathophysiology

The pathophysiologic mechanisms involving the major cerebral arteries include thrombosis, embolism, and vasculitis. Thrombotic events are the most common. Accurate epidemiologic data are not available, but based on autopsy data from Japan (Kurtze, 1969) the death rate from thrombotic and embolic events combined is 3 per 1 million children under age 14 years per year. Fortunately, the mortality from childhood stroke is low, so that the prevalence of this condition is far higher than the mortality figures would suggest. In one community study (Health Statistics from the U.S. National Health Survey) the prevalence of "hemiplegia due to stroke" was 24.8 per 100,000 children under the age of 15.

The incidence of childhood stroke has dramatically fallen since the early part of the century (Kurtzke, 1969). Much of this decline is thought to be due to a decrease in serious infections in the pediatric population. Meningitis in particular can produce intense basilar inflammation, locally damaging vessels in the circle of Willis and the anterior and posterior circulations. Tuberculous meningitis, which often produces this complication, has dramatically decreased in incidence (although in recent years tuberculosis is again on the increase).

Thrombotic carotid artery or carotid branch occlusion is responsible for most cases of acute childhood hemiplegia. In one third of cases a preceding infection is noted, often in the pharynx or cervical area. Pharyngitis, cervical adenitis, tonsillitis, sinusitis, and retropharyngeal abscess are all reported precursors of internal carotid artery thrombosis. The mechanism is thought to be local inflammation of the wall of the artery. Trauma to the neck may result in carotid thrombosis. Falling with a pencil in the mouth can produce local carotid trauma and a subsequent thrombus.

Vertebrobasilar thrombotic occlusion is less common

than thrombosis affecting the anterior distribution (McRae, 1953; DeVivo and Farrell, 1972). Cervical spine anomalies (Singer et al., 1975) and systemic diseases with trauma to the vertebral arteries are an uncommon cause. When they occur they are usually at the C_2 level (Fraser and Zimbler, 1975).

The causes of thrombosis involving smaller arteries and arterioles in both carotid and vertebrobasilar areas are somewhat different. These can include mucocutaneous lymph node syndrome (Kawasaki's syndrome), general coagulopathies, and disseminated intravascular coagulation. Polycythemia associated with cyanotic congenital heart disease, sickle cell disease, other hemoglobinopathies, leukemia, and the hemolytic-uremic syndrome may all produce cerebral thrombosis, usually affecting smaller vessels. Many serious metabolic disorders produce cortical infarction, which is often multifocal. In lactic acidemia, the organic acidemias, and hyperammonemic states, cerebral ischemia and infarction may occur particularly during episodes of severe metabolic decompensation. Homocystinuria may present as a thrombotic syndrome that may involve cerebral vasculature. Basal ganglion infarction is often seen in disorders of oxidative metabolism such as Leigh's syndrome, methylmalonic acidemia, and glutaric aciduria type II (Bousounis, 1988; Rutledge et al., 1988). Stroke-like episodes in a nonvascular distribution are seen in mitochondrial encephalomyopathy with lactic acidemia and stroke-like episodes (MELAS) (Allard et al, 1988).

Hypoxic-ischemic injury is the commonest cause of more widespread ischemic brain injury in childhood. Causal events include cardiorespiratory arrest, asphyxia, near-drowning, and hypotension. Damage tends to be widespread and bilateral, although preexisting variants in collateral blood supply may result in asymmetric lesions. Areas of the brain particularly susceptible to damage are those with a "watershed" or terminal arterial supply. Medial hemisphere infarctions occur in the border zone between the anterior and middle cerebral artery distributions. Occipital infarcts producing cortical blindness are a common result of ischemia in the watershed at the boundary of the middle and posterior cerebral artery distributions. Multiple rounded infarcts, which tend to be symmetric, are often found scattered throughout gray and white matter in these circumstances. The basal ganglia are largely supplied by the distal portions of small perforating arteries originating at the anterior portion of the circle of Willis, producing additional sites of enhanced susceptibility to hypoxic-ischemic change. The spinal cord may be damaged by generalized or focal hypoxic-ischemic injury, leading to paraplegia or quadriplegia.

Embolic events are apparently uncommon causes of cerebral arterial occlusion in childhood. Fungal (mycotic) or tumor-associated emboli are occasional causes. Acquired immunodeficiency syndrome is now responsible for an increasing number of exotic systemic and central nervous system infections, which may produce embolic occlusion. Subacute bacterial endocarditis is an occasional cause, as are mural and atrial cardiac thrombi in patients with cardiomyopathies. Atrial fibrillation is an uncommon cause of stroke in childhood. Intravenous drug use is now a common cause of infective embolic stroke in adolescents. Iatrogenic causes include emboli from indwelling long venous catheters, fat emboli from parenteral nutrition, and accidental air emboli. In these cases, a cardiac right-to-left shunt must be present for emboli to find their way to the cerebral circulation. MRI and CT scanning confirm that small emboli occur after cardiac catheterization and cardiac surgical procedures more frequently than was previously thought. These embolic events may involve carotid or vertebrobasilar distributions.

Systemic vasculitic diseases may involve the central nervous system. Vasculitic damage to the arterial wall results in the development of local thrombi and the potential for occlusion and embolization. Small arterioles are generally involved in this process but larger vessels may also be damaged. Both carotid and vertebrobasilar arterial distributions may be affected. In the case of systemic lupus erythematosus, neurologic involvement is seen in over 50% of patients. Arterioles are predominantly involved in this disease, with the production of microinfarcts leading to cortical atrophy. Polyarteritis nodosa, Wegener's granulomatosis, and the determatomyositis/ polymyositis complex are rare causes of childhood ischemic stroke. Fibromuscular dysplasia is a systemic arterial disease that commonly affects the renal arteries. When the internal carotid arteries are involved, aneurysms, thrombosis, and embolism may occur. Pathologically, there is fibrosis in the media with associated hyperplasia of intima or adventitia. Moyamoya disease (a rare condition of unknown etiology; Suzuki and Takaku, 1969) and the similar syndrome associated with a number of other diseases (Pearson et al., 1985) are characterized by progressive unilateral or bilateral carotid arterial occlusion and the development of a fine web-like collection of abnormal anastomotic vessels at the base of the brain (Figure 12-1). The large vessel vasculitis of Takayasu's disease or "pulseless" disease has been reported in Japanese teenage women, but is rarely seen in younger children.

Signs and Symptoms

Occlusion of the internal carotid artery results in most cases in the sudden onset of hemiplegia. In the acute phase there may be seizures, lethargy, or coma. Occasionally, a more gradual occlusive process will produce the syndrome of "stroke in evolution." Recurrent transient ischemic attacks will rarely precede a completed stroke in childhood. Although a profound motor weakness (initially flaccid and later becoming spastic) is the most striking presentation, some children have no clinical manifestations of major arterial occlusive disease (Prensky and

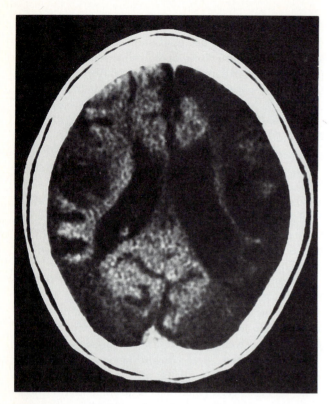

Figure 12-1. Brain CT scan from a 10-year-old girl with moyamoya disease. There is bilateral extensive loss of brain tissue as a result of ischemic stroke following occlusion of both middle cerebral arteries.

David, 1970). In these cases, it may be that the occlusion is gradual, allowing adequate arterial anastomotic channels to open so that infarction does not occur. Second, the potential for recovery is so great that children may be seen without major deficit months or years after an ischemic event, despite large areas of brain infarction. A third factor is the delay in the identification of clinical signs, which may occur until brain maturation reaches a stage allowing expression of the clinical deficit.

Sensory symptoms and signs often accompany hemiplegia, and may include loss of half of the visual field and loss of all modalities of sensation in affected limbs. These signs will usually be unilateral. Speech will often become slurred (dysarthria) and language involvement is often seen when the language-dominant hemisphere is involved. Receptive and expressive dysphasias as well as difficulty with reading, writing, and naming objects may be demonstrated in older children. When arterioles or small arteries are involved in a thrombotic or embolic process, symptoms and signs are often quite subtle. This is particularly the case if the "silent" areas of the brain, such as the posterior parietal lobes and the frontal lobes, are involved. Transient headache often accompanies ischemic cortical infarction. If only the vertebrobasilar system is involved the child will present any combination of brainstem, cerebellar, and occipital lobe dysfunction. Symptoms may include drowsiness, ataxia, vertigo, and visual loss. Signs may include eye movement disorders including internuclear ophthalmoplegia and are referable to cranial nerves III, IV, and VI or their central connections. Ataxia and dysarthria are common in brainstem ischemia. Long tract motor signs and sensory loss may occur. Respiratory abnormalities, including apnea, apneustic breathing, hyperventilation, and gasping or ataxic breathing patterns, may be seen. Children with large brainstem infarcts will usually be comatose.

Alternating hemiplegia suggests a more widespread vascular process, such as moyamoya disease or a vasculitis; however, idiopathic alternating hemiplegia of infancy also occurs (Aicardi, 1987). It is not surprising that migraine attacks are seen coincidentally in patients who later develop stroke syndromes. Complicated migraine, however, may be associated with a very small increase in the incidence of ischemic stroke.

Diagnostic Studies
Diagnosis of cerebral arterial ischemia is easier when the sudden onset of persistent neurologic signs develops in

FEATURE TABLE 12-3. INFANT, CHILD, AND ADOLESCENT ISCHEMIC DISEASE

Discriminating Feature	Consistent Features	Variable Features
1. The discriminating features of cerebral ischemia are included in Table 12-1.	1. Children with cerebral ischemia lose neurologic function in ischemic areas of brain. This loss may be temporary or permanent. It may not be detectable clinically or by neuroimaging. Thus there are no consistent features of cerebral ischemia. 2. Spinal cord ischemia produces dramatic signs as there is little redundancy in the spinal cord.	1. Headache in cerebral ischemia. 2. Predisposing disease. 3. The clinical presentation of brain ischemia ranges from very subtle changes in mentation to gross motor deficit with or without coma. 4. Small lesions may not be seen on neuroimaging studies.

a child with a predisposing systemic disease or precipitating cause. Often, however, these events occur in previously normal children and in as many as 50% of children the cause will remain unknown in spite of extensive investigation. The physical signs may be subtle with small lesions, and a high index of suspicion is needed in high-risk situations, such as sickle cell disease and after cardiac procedures. Subtle changes on the examination or a history of transient loss of function should be evaluated by a neuroimaging study in these situations. The MRI scan is the most sensitive method for detection of small or early ischemic lesions. Brainstem lesions are much more reliably seen on MRI than on CT. CT scanning, however, is more readily available and more suitable for seriously ill patients. It will detect most hemorrhagic and many ischemic lesions. In Figure 12–2, an MRI scan from a 9-month-old infant shows an idiopathic extensive infarction in the right hemisphere in the middle cerebral artery territory, and illustrates the anatomic information available with this technology. This infant had a moderately severe left hemiparesis predominantly affecting the left arm and hand. A rapid improvement in the function of this limb has occurred over a 6-month-period and ultimately full recovery of function may occur. The differential diagnosis of an acute focal loss of neurologic function in a child is listed in Table 12–1.

In infancy signs of even a major cerebral ischemic event may be subtle. Parents may report the early development of handedness, motor or intellectual delay, or actual focal loss of function. A higher index of suspicion is necessary in this age group to identify vascular accidents.

Migraine in the child is often atypical and can be temporarily confused with stroke, particularly when the basilar artery is involved. In a review of eight such cases symptoms varied from ataxia to alternating hemipareses and vertigo. None of these children had progressive neurologic disease or persistent signs. Most of the patients were girls with onset before age 4 years (Golden and French, 1975).

Diagnosis of a cerebral ischemic event in the carotid or vertebrobasilar territory requires a detailed history and family history, and a careful general examination, including the skin and particularly the cardiovascular system. Coarctation, hypertension, and cardiomyopathy are all predisposing causes. Extensive neurologic examination is essential. Usually an EEG and a neuroimaging study (preferably MRI) as well as extensive laboratory testing will be needed.

Identification of the etiology requires a search for systemic disease, including tumor, leukemia, lymphoma, infection, vasculitis, and metabolic disease (Table 12–2). The EEG may help identify focal, multifocal, ischemic, and irritative lesions. A skull x ray may reveal abnor-

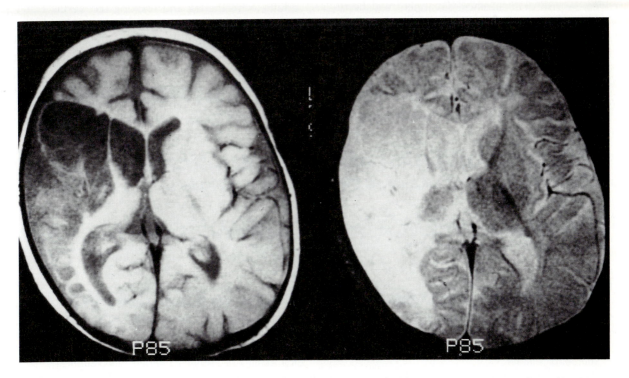

Figure 12–2. MRI scan from a 9-month-old infant with a moderately severe left hemiparesis owing to an idiopathic extensive infarction of the right cerebral hemisphere in the middle cerebral artery territory. The image on the left is T_1 weighted and shows the large porencephalic area as low signal intensity (*dark*). The image on the right is T_2 weighted and shows the abnormal area with a high water content as high signal intensity (*white*).

TABLE 12–1. DIFFERENTIAL DIAGNOSIS AND DISCRIMINATING FEATURES OF ACUTE FOCAL LOSS OF NEUROLOGIC FUNCTION IN CHILDHOOD

Condition	Discriminating Features
Focal cerebral ischemia	History, neurologic exam, neuroimaging features
Primary intracerebral hemorrhage	Neuroimaging features
Traumatic epidural or subdural hematoma	Neuroimaging features, neurologic exam, history
Traumatic contusion	Neuroimaging features, neurologic exam, history
Subarachnoid hemorrhage	History, blood in cerebrospinal fluid, neuroimaging procedures
Cerebral abscess	History, fever, neuroimaging features
Focal seizure with a postictal Todd's paresis	History, recovery, EEG
Cerebral tumor	History, neuroimaging features
Focal encephalitis	History, EEG, neuroimaging features, CSF
Metabolic disease	Blood or urine abnormalities, neuroimaging features
Complicated migraine	History, transient signs, negative imaging studies
Malingering/hysteria (very rare)	History, examination, exclusion of organic disease

mal calcification in intracranial infection and arteriovenous malformation, but CT is more sensitive. A cerebral angiogram may be needed to define local lesions in the intracranial vessels and exclude arteriovenous malformations, but this most often is now satisfactorily evaluated by MRI.

Treatment

The acute treatment of cerebral ischemia is largely supportive. If an underlying disease is identified, it is treated to reduce the risk of recurrence. Treatment will be required for each of the specific disorders listed in Table 12–2. Thus, an aggressive approach to investigation is based on prevention of future episodes, not on the present event. The use of anticoagulation in ischemic stroke is controversial and risky, although it may be indicated in the presence of a continuing source of emboli. Rehabilitation through aggressive physical, occupational, and speech therapy is essential.

The prognosis for cerebral ischemia caused by arterial thrombosis is surprisingly good in infants and young children. Virtually complete recovery can occur from even extensive infarctions, especially for language function. However, most often functional recovery is partial. The experience from the Mayo Clinic from 1965 to 1974 (Schoenberg et al., 1978) indicates that 80% of children are surviving 10 years after an ischemic stroke, although most have residual hemiparesis. Recovery from hemiparesis follows the same pattern in children and adults, with the leg and walking recovering faster and more completely, and the fine movements of the hand least. The earlier studies of Solomon and colleagues (1970) highlighted the prognostic importance of seizures occurring with the onset of acute hemiplegia. Children without seizures early on were more likely to have a good motor and intellectual outcome. Dusser and associates (1986) reported a better overall outcome in idiopathic ischemic strokes but a high incidence of residual dystonia and

TABLE 12–2. INVESTIGATIVE STUDIES FOR SYSTEMIC DISEASE IN CEREBRAL ISCHEMIA

Disorder	Test
Infection; leukemia; polycythemia, thrombocytosis, and thrombocytopenia; hemoglobinopathies	CBC, differential, platelet count
Hemoglobinopathies	Sickle test, hemoglobin electrophoresis
Vasculitis and autoimmune diseases	Sedimentation rate, antinuclear antibody
Syphilis	Venereal disease reaction level (VDRL)
Renal disease (hemolytic uremic syndrome; renal causes of hypertension) systemic vasculitis, diabetes mellitus	Blood urea, creatinine, electrolytes, calcium, phosphorus, glucose, urine microscopy, urinalysis
Coagulopathies; DIC	Blood platelets, prothrombin, partial thromboplastin time, fibrin split products
Cardiac source for emboli	EKG, chest x ray, echocardiogram, blood cultures
Lactic acidemia, homocystinuria, organic acidemias	Blood and CSF lactic acid, pyruvic acid and amino acids, quantitative urine amino and organic acids
Chromosomal syndromes	Karyotype
Hyperlipidemia	Blood triglycerides and cholesterol

Pearls and Perils: Infant, Child, and Adolescent Ischemic Disease

1. In younger children the symptoms and signs of cerebral ischemia may be subtle. A high index of suspicion is needed.
2. Neuroimaging studies may be needed to diagnose small ischemic lesions and define the extent of larger lesions. Exclusion of many other serious cerebral disorders requires neuroimaging. MRI is the single best test. MRI or CT should be obtained in virtually all cases.
3. A history of previous transient neurologic loss suggests the possibility of complicated migraine, seizures, hysteria, or rarely demyelinating disease.
4. Learning disability may be the only residual manifestation of childhood stroke.
5. Delay in identification of underlying disease may allow further ischemic episodes.
6. Without neuroimaging small ischemic infarcts may be missed.
7. Anticoagulation treatment should only be used after very careful consideration and generally only in cases with clear evidence for continuing thrombosis or embolization.
8. Lumbar puncture should only be performed after neuroimaging studies unless meningitis is seriously suspected.
9. In any acute spinal cord syndrome treatable causes of cord compression must be urgently excluded.

dyskinesia in this group. However, to date there have been no large studies in which the natural history and prognosis of childhood stroke have been adequately studied.

Atherosclerosis begins in infancy and so the most effective approach to the prevention of stroke in adulthood may lie in the early institution of healthy dietary practices, the encouragement of regular exercise, and the abolition of smoking. These life-styles can be encouraged in the early school years (Cresanta et al., 1986).

Spinal Cord Ischemia

Pathophysiology

In theory the spinal cord is susceptible to the same systemic disorders that produce vasculitis and thrombosis in cerebral arteries (Table 12–2). In practice, however, spinal cord ischemia is rare in childhood. This may in part be due to the extensive blood supply of the spinal cord. The anterior and posterior spinal arteries enjoy a limited anastomosis and are supplied by several arterial branches at various levels of the cord. The anterior two thirds of the spinal cord is supplied largely from branches of the anterior spinal artery. The levels of maximal susceptibility to generalized ischemia lie at arterial watersheds usually located at the lower cervical and lower thoracic levels of the spinal cord. Tumor and arteriovenous malformation are the commonest lesions causing cord ischemia. Cord compression and/or vascular steal reduces blood supply, resulting in ischemia. Scoliosis can compromise flow in the anterior spinal artery but actual cord ischemia is rare in scoliotic patients. Traumatic lesions to the spinal cord generally produce contusion without arterial or venous thrombosis, although epidural and subdural hematomas can produce cord ischemia by vascular compromise. Iatrogenic causes of spinal cord ischemia are important but fortunately rare. Umbilical artery catheterization in the newborn is associated with a significant risk of aortic, iliac, and femoral artery thrombosis. In some of these infants the arterial supply to the spinal cord is in jeopardy. Surgery for aortic coarctation is associated with symptoms of cord ischemia in some patients. Usually this is reversible but some patients are left with irreversible cord infarction.

Signs and Symptoms

The clinical signs of spinal cord ischemia depend on the level of the lesion. Initially a cord "shock" syndrome will be seen at and below the level of the lesion. Later this evolves into upper motor neuron signs of spasticity below the level of the lesion, with flaccidity and areflexia confined to the level of the cord infarction itself. Bladder and bowel function will often be affected, with urinary retention most common. An anterior spinal artery syndrome is quite characteristic with loss of anterior cord function and preservation of the dorsal column functions of light touch, vibration, and joint position sense.

Diagnosis and Treatment

Diagnosis of spinal cord ischemia in childhood is made when signs of partial or complete ischemic damage to the cord appear and a predisposing cause is apparent. Cord ischemia is usually a sudden event, although a more stuttering progression of symptoms and signs may be seen and clinical presentation may be delayed for some hours (Lenn, 1977). Causes of spinal cord compression and ischemia—including arteriovenous malformation, tumor, abscess, or myelitis—must be identified. MRI imaging provides an excellent view of the spinal cord without bony artifact but myelography is still necessary in selected cases.

Treatment is supportive. Hypotension, which may further damage the ischemic cord, must be avoided. A full, organized spinal cord injury protocol should be instituted at once. Urinary retention requires catheterization. Early passive and later active physical therapy is important to prevent joint contractures and improve residual function. The prognosis depends on the extent and duration of the ischemic insult.

ANNOTATED BIBLIOGRAPHY

Mueller SM, Golden GS, Swaiman KF, Aswal S, Schneide S, Fenichel GM: Vascular diseases of the brain and spinal cord, in Swaiman KF, Wright, FS (eds): *The Practice of Pediatric Neurology*, 2nd ed. St. Louis, CV Mosby, 1982, p 765–822.

 A good review covering most types of vascular disease in infancy and childhood.

Sahs AL, Hartman EC (eds): Fundamentals of Stroke Care. DHEW Publ No (HRA) 76-14016, 1976.

 Chapter IX collates most aspects of the epidemiologic data available in 1976 and also summarizes diagnosis and treatment possibilities.

REFERENCES

Aicardi J: Alternating hemiplegia of childhood. *Int Pediatr* 2:115–119, 1987.

Allard JC, Tilak S, Carter AP: CT and MR of MELAS syndrome. *AJNR* 9:1234–1238, 1988.

Bousounis DP: Methylmalonic aciduria resulting in globus pallidus necrosis. *Ann Neurol* 24(2):302–303, 1988.

Cresanta JL, Hyg MS, Burke GL: Prevention of atherosclerosis in childhood. *Pediatr Clin North Am* 33(4):835–858, 1986.

DeVivo DC, Farrell FW Jr: Vertebrobasilar occlusive disease in children: A recognizable clinical entity. *Arch Neurol* 26:278–281, 1972.

Dusser A, Goutieres F, Aicardi J: Ischemic strokes in children. *J Child Neurol* 1:131–136, 1986.

Fraser RAR, Zimbler SM: Hindbrain stroke in children caused by extracranial vertebral artery trauma. *Stroke* 6:153–159, 1975.

Golden GS, French JH: Basilar artery migraine in young children. *Pediatrics* 56(5):722–726, 1975.

Health Statistics from the US National Health Survey. Origin and program of the US National Health Survey. PHS Publ No 584, Series A1.

Kurtzke JF: *Epidemiology of Cerebrovascular Disease*. Berlin, Springer-Verlag, 1969.

Lenn NJ: Spinal cord infarction due to minor trauma. *Neurology* 27:999, 1977.

McRae DL: Bony abnormalities in the region of the foramen magnum: Correlations of the anatomic and neurological findings. *Acta Radiol* 40:335–354, 1953.

Pearson E, Lenn NJ, Cail WS: Moyamoya and other causes of stroke in Down syndrome. *Pediatr Neurol* 1:174–179, 1985.

Prensky AL, David DO: Obstruction of major cerebral vessels in early childhood without neurological signs. *Neurology* 20:945–953, 1970.

Rutledge JN, Hilal SK, Silver AJ, Defendini R, Fahn S: Magnetic resonance imaging of dystonic states. *Adv Neurol* 50:265–275, 1988.

Schoenberg BS, Mellinger JF, Schoenberg DG: Cerebrovascular disease in infants and children: A study of incidence, clinical features, and survival. *Neurology* 28:763–768, 1978.

Singer WD, Haller JS, Wolpert SM: Occlusive vertebrobasilar artery disease associated with cervical spine anomaly. *Am J Dis Child* 129:492–495, 1975.

Solomon GE, Hilal SK, Gold AP, Carter S: Natural history of acute hemiplegia of childhood. *Brain* 93:107–120, 1970.

Suzuki J, Takaku A: Cerebrovascular "Moyamoya" disease. Disease showing abnormal net-like vessels in base of brain. *Arch Neurol* 20:288–299, 1969.

Cerebral Veins and Sinuses

Pathophysiology

The pathophysiologic mechanisms affecting the cerebral venous system can be divided into those related to local infection of the head or neck and "primary" cerebral venous or dural sinus occlusions, which usually occur in a child with a systemic illness (Bailey and Hass, 1937; Yang et al., 1969; Scotti et al., 1974). Many of the systemic diseases that cause arterial occlusion also affect the venous system. Coagulopathies, blood dyscrasias, and hemoglobinopathies (particularly sickle cell disease) may produce venous occlusion. Infection or tumor in areas adjacent to veins or dural sinuses may involve the wall of the vessel and produce local inflammation and thrombosis. The most common cause of cerebral vein thrombosis is purulent meningitis. Cortical vessels running through the subarachnoid space are particularly susceptible to injury in meningitis. Trauma may produce local venous or dural sinus damage, leading to thrombosis. Infection secondary to trauma produces an additional risk of thrombosis. Children with cyanotic congenital heart disease are at increased risk for cerebral venous thrombosis. Often these children will have polycythemia with a high hematocrit and a low hemoglobin owing to iron deficiency. The most common cause of dural sinus thrombosis is dehydration. This is a problem generally occurring in infants and young children with gastroenteritis. The thrombosis results from a hypercoagulable state. Such children are often hypotensive and acidotic, compounding the ischemic insult. Infective causes of dural sinus thrombosis tend to produce local effects. Otitis media and mastoiditis may cause lateral sinus thrombosis. Facial soft tissue, paranasal, or frontal sinus infections may produce cavernous sinus thrombosis. This rare complication occurs more commonly in older children. Sagittal sinus thrombosis usually arises from retrograde infection spread from adjacent dural sinuses involved in a head or neck infection. Tumor may cause local cerebral venous or dural sinus occlusion. Both primary central nervous system tumors and secondary tumors, particularly neuroblastoma, can cause thrombotic complications. Radiotherapy can cause venous thrombosis.

 Venous occlusion produces ischemia in the area of the brain drained by the affected vein or sinus, with accompanying microscopic and larger areas of hemorrhage. In these hemorrhagic infarctions edema is often more marked than with arterial occlusive disease, and thus raised intracranial pressure is a common problem. The edematous phase can last for several days and presents a major management challenge. Neuronal and glial necrosis occurs in the infarcted area and ultimately macrophages remove necrotic material, leaving a cystic cavity. Cerebral veins and dural sinuses tend to recanalize rapidly after thrombotic occlusion, making early radiologic study important if the diagnosis is to be confirmed.

Signs and Symptoms

Generalized or extensive cerebral vein or dural sinus thrombosis is usually rapidly fatal. The child presents with a rapidly evolving encephalitic picture consisting of confusion, headache, irritability, seizures, and increasing lethargy as the intracranial pressure rises secondary to brain edema. Less extensive thrombosis of cerebral veins or dural sinuses can produce more focal central nervous system signs resulting from hemorrhagic infarction and edema of the affected area of the brain. The most dramatic constellation of signs arises from cavernous sinus thrombosis, which is fortunately rare. Impaired drainage of the ophthalmic veins and direct involvement of cranial nerves III, IV, and VI lead to an initially unilateral eye edema, chemosis, exophthalmos, ptosis, and strabismus with a severe headache and eye pain. Sagittal sinus thrombosis and the resultant impairment of parasagittal cortical vein drainage tend to produce bilateral cortical signs with alternating hemiplegia, seizures, and deepening coma. Lateral sinus thrombosis impairs venous drainage from the ipsilateral cerebellum and occipital lobe, producing visual field loss and ataxia along with headache. A more generalized increase in intracranial pressure may be seen with lateral sinus occlusion and is one cause of the syndrome of pseudotumor cerebri.

Diagnosis and Treatment

Diagnosis of cerebral vein or dural sinus thrombosis is usually difficult. Only in the case of cavernous sinus thrombosis are there characteristic symptoms and signs, proptosis and chemosis. The clinical features of cerebral venous and dural sinus thrombosis depend on the location and extent of the thrombotic event. Widespread or extensive thromboses often present with a history of headache, confusion, and seizures rapidly followed by

---

Pearls and Perils: Cerebral Veins and Sinuses

1. Severe headache with a rapid deterioration in consciousness is a common presentation of extensive cerebral venous or dural sinus thrombosis.
2. An urgent CT scan will help exclude other causes and may confirm the diagnosis.
3. An urgent MRI scan provides the best non-invasive test for cerebral venous or dural sinus thrombosis, but risks of transport and difficulties with patient monitoring in the scanner may be contraindications for MRI in sick and unstable patients.
4. Urgent treatment of the precipitating cause and of raised intracranial pressure is essential.
5. Anticoagulation therapy is risky and contraindicated in patients with hemorrhage.
6. Untreated seizures, hypoxia, or hypotension will increase the cerebral insult.

---

coma. Differential diagnosis includes toxic and metabolic causes of coma, viral encephalitis, bacterial meningitis, and cerebral abscess, as well as the various causes of intracranial hemorrhage. Lumbar puncture will reveal raised pressure and CSF will often be xanthochromic or blood tinged.

Neuroimaging studies are generally warranted. Because of the tendency for occluded veins and sinuses to recanalize, studies must be carried out early—preferably within 48 hours for maximal information. Dural sinus thrombosis is usually well visualized on MRI scan, where an area of high signal intensity on the T_2-weighted image replaces the normally low-signal sinus. Edema and hemorrhage are also well visualized on MRI. With CT scanning hemorrhagic infarctions are well seen and edema is usually obvious. A ring sign on contrast-enhanced CT scanning may identify a dural sinus or large venous occlusion. Angiography, if warranted, may confirm cere-

---

FEATURE TABLE 12–4. CEREBRAL VEINS AND SINUSES

Discriminating Features	Consistent Features	Variable Features
1. History of gradual deterioration helps discriminate between arterial ischemia and cerebral venous or dural sinus thrombosis.	1. The location and extent of both cerebral venous thrombosis and dural sinus thrombosis determine the physical findings.	1. Focal findings may be seen in localized cerebral vein or dural sinus thrombosis.
2. Cerebral edema is often severe in venous infarction.	2. Headache is generally present.	2. Usually irritability, lethargy, and generalized symptoms of increasing intracranial pressure are seen.
3. Neuroimaging studies provide the best differential diagnostic test.	3. Raised intracranial pressure is usual.	3. In some patients fluctuating neurologic signs are found.

bral vein occlusion or identify localized dural sinus occlusion.

Treatment of both cerebral vein occlusion and dural sinus thrombosis is directed at control of intracranial pressure, cerebral edema, and the predisposing cause of the thrombosis, whether local infection or a systemic disorder such as dehydration. Corticosteroids, such as dexamethasone (0.25 to 0.5 mg/kg per day, up to 40 kg weight) given every 6 hours may be helpful in controlling edema. A pressure bolt or ventricular catheter allows accurate intracranial pressure monitoring and may be useful. Mannitol is generally to be avoided—particularly in patients who are dehydrated. Intubation and hyperventilation will often be needed. Antibiotics are usually necessary, definitely if infection is the probable cause of the occlusion. The infarction is generally hemorrhagic and thus anticoagulants are usually contraindicated. Their use has not been established to benefit any of the childhood patients. In patients with the syndrome of pseudotumor cerebri, repeated lumbar puncture may save vision and should not be delayed if visual impairment is present or if there is any concern that medical therapy is not working.

ANNOTATED BIBLIOGRAPHY

Mueller SM, Golden GS, Swaiman KF, et al: Vascular diseases of the brain and spinal cord, in Swaiman KF, Wright FS, (eds): *The Practice of Pediatric Neurology,* 2nd ed. St. Louis, CV Mosby, 1982, p 765–822.
    A good review covering most types of vascular disease in infancy and childhood.

REFERENCES

Bailey OT, Hass GM: Dural sinus thrombosis in early life. I. The clinical manifestations and extent of brain injury in acute sinus thrombosis. *J Pediatr* 11:755–771, 1937.
Scotti LN, Goldman RL, Hardman DR, Heinz ER: Venous thrombosis in infants and children. *Radiology* 112:393–399, 1974.
Yang DC, Sohn D, Anand MK: Thrombosis of the superior longitudinal sinus during infancy. *J Pediatr* 74:570–575, 1969.

INTRACRANIAL HEMORRHAGE IN INFANCY AND CHILDHOOD

Aneurysms

In this and the following sections, which consider additional conditions predominantly associated with intracranial hemorrhage, infants and children are considered together. Unlike the situation for ischemic disease and IVH of prematurity, these causes of intracranial hemorrhages are for the most part similar across this age spec-

trum, and most of these events are rare in neonates, precluding detailed presentation. Certain controversial issues in the classification of aneurysms and vascular malformations do not have clinical application at this time, and are not discussed. For example, vein of Galen "aneurysms" are complex vascular malformations with considerable variation from case to case.

Most aneurysms and vascular malformations in adults—in whom clinical presentation of these lesions is far more common—no doubt have antecedents earlier in life. However, there is no clinical expression of these lesions during childhood and no current approach to preventing or delaying the future manifestations.

The incidence of intracranial hemorrhage is approximately three times the incidence of ischemic infarction. Extensive data are available concerning primary subarachnoid hemorrhage (SAH). Considering all ages and almost 11,000 patients, 60% of such hemorrhages were due to aneurysms and 7% to vascular malformation, with the causes of the rest undetermined. However, only 4% of these cases presented at between 0 and 19 years of age; of those, 90% occurred in the second decade, and 10% in the first decade. The incidence is higher and similar in the first year of life and from 8 to 15 years of age, with the lowest incidence from ages 1 to 8 years. Of children with primary SAH, 40% are due to aneurysm, 30% to arteriovenous malformations, and 30% to unknown causes (Sedzimir and Robinson, 1973).

Pathophysiology

Intracranial aneurysms in all age groups can be divided into three types: congenital, traumatic, and mycotic (resulting from infection, especially in congenital heart disease in children). These types occur in the proportions of 75%, 15%, and 10%, respectively, during childhood. Childhood aneurysms are more variable and more peripheral in location when compared to those in adults (Amacher and Drake, 1975). Giant aneurysms represent one third or more of diagnosed lesions in childhood, mostly occurring in the first year of life and presenting as mass lesions, with seizures in half the cases. Similar aneurysms have presented in only a few neonates (Lee et al., 1978). Another one third of aneurysms present clinically between 1 and 12 years of age. They are often located on the terminal portion of the carotid artery or anterior cerebral complex, and therefore are usually surgically accessible. The remaining one third present in adolescence, generally with acute hemorrhage.

The main histopathologic features are abnormalities of the arterial wall, especially of the elastica and media, with inflammatory changes in mycotic cases. The aneurysmal region may be saccular, fusiform, or irregular. Clotting is usually present in some portion of the lumen. A defect responsible for hemorrhage can often be found. Perivascular and extensive subarachnoid blood is the rule.

Traumatic aneurysms are relatively less common in

children, occurring mainly in adolescence, and then more often in boys (Epstein, 1982). In infants, an aneurysm may be induced by a subdural tap.

Mycotic aneurysms have a far higher relative incidence in children than in adults (Shapiro, 1985). They occur in bacterial endocarditis and thrombophlebitis, and 60% present hemorrhagically. Mortality is 18%, but morbidity in the remainder is said to be low, probably on the basis of informal observations of short duration.

Intracerebral hemorrhage complicates aneurysmal SAH in 25% to 50% of cases, and the proportion in children is probably similar. Although vasospasm complicates SAH in 30% or more of children, it does not seem to affect outcome as it does in adults.

Signs and Symptoms

In the majority of cases of aneurysms that present with hemorrhage, onset is apoplectic. There is a retrospective history of headache in 20%. The sudden onset of severe, sometimes localized headache—at times associated with focal neurologic deficits and frequently followed by diffuse cerebral dysfunction of mild to profound extent—represents a clinical picture as characteristic in children as in adults. Because some children will bleed at the time of or soon after head trauma of variable severity, aneurysm may not be considered, and may be missed on angiogram as a result of an incomplete study, vasospasm, or obliteration of the aneurysm. Mass effect from enlarging giant aneurysms has been described as producing progressive lower cranial nerve, brainstem, and oculomotor nerve dysfunction; trigeminal distribution pain and sensory loss; and hydrocephalus owing to aqueductal stenosis. Seizures may occur at the onset or during the first days, but are uncommon except in infancy. Meningismus, fever, leukocytosis, nausea, and vomiting are the principal systemic symptoms. Examination may show nuchal rigidity, alteration of consciousness, and focal deficits referable to cranial nerves or any portion of the cerebrum or brainstem. Although intracranial pressure is generally elevated, and the fontanelle will reflect this in infants, papilledema is uncommon. If the patient is seen early, progression of these findings is frequent, may be very rapid, and is of ominous significance.

Diagnostic Studies

Two problems must be considered. In the case of symptomatic patients, establishment of the diagnosis will be by MRI or cerebral angiography in virtually all cases. The

hemorrhage will be demonstrable in some infants by sonography, and in many children by CT; however, the angiogram is the confirmatory test, which is the firm basis for diagnosis and planning surgery. As mentioned previously, the study should be complete, especially if negative. The timing of the initial studies is based first on the need to establish a diagnosis in an acutely ill child in whom the differential diagnosis includes not only aneurysm and arteriovenous malformation, but also neoplasm, hemorrhagic encephalitis, hemorrhagic infarction, and trauma. Additionally, the timing, especially of angiography, should be related to the total management approach to the lesion, in coordination with the neurosurgical consultant. Factors to be considered are time since bleeding, condition of the patient, medical therapy modalities, and preferred time of surgery. Probably the most common current approach in cases arriving within 24 hours of the event is early angiography, with subsequent management planned thereafter. In the case of unruptured aneurysms, this study helps define prognosis, because the probability of rupture is proportional to size, if the diameter is greater than 5 mm.

There are several situations in which cerebral aneurysms are sufficiently increased in frequency to suggest a causal association (Epstein, 1982). The coexistence with an underlying condition is much more common in children than in adults. These include polycystic kidney disease (which is associated with 5% of intracranial aneurysms); fibromuscular dysplasia; and possibly coarctation of the aorta (12% of cases in Patel and Richardson [1971]), Ehlers-Danlos syndrome, Marfan's syndrome, pseudoxanthoma elasticum, tuberous sclerosis, and Klinefelter's syndrome. These latter disorders require better data to support the suggested association (Torner, 1984). The association of aneurysms with developmental cysts and malformations, such as agenesis of the corpus callosum, suggests a basis for some aneurysms (Shuangshoti et al., 1978).

In many ways more difficult for the physician is the approach to the unfounded anxiety that parents sometimes have about the possibility of an unruptured aneurysm. This fear is often based on the occurrence of rupture in an acquaintance or a relative, and is precipitated by headache in the child. The associated conditions listed earlier should be considered. Barring evidence for these, clearly reassurance rather than MRI or angiography is appropriate. Reports of familial occurrence of aneurysms are rare, with as few as six cases reported. The

FEATURE TABLE 12–5. ANEURYSMS

Discriminating Feature	Consistent Feature	Variable Features
1. Angiographic demonstration of the aneurysm	1. Symptoms or signs of acute SAH in most cases	1. Antecedent headache (20% of patients) 2. Focal cerebral ischemia secondary to vasospasm

familial cases seem to present earlier, and have more variable location. These facts may help with reassurance. CT scan with contrast may offer reassurance beyond its true value, but ordering it may reinforce the fears of an anxious parent. The true sensitivity of MRI is uncertain, but it is increasing with the use of advanced software. Clearly, clinicians sometimes decide that the low risk of MRI or an angiogram in a healthy young person is better than continued anxiety, but one hopes that this impasse is rarely reached.

Treatment

The improved treatment of ruptured aneurysms appears to have lowered mortality. For instance, mortality in the first 24 hours has been reduced considerably. However, nearly 60% of adult patients still die or survive disabled (Torner, 1984). An estimated 11% die suddenly, and 25% die or are disabled in association with delayed rebleeding, 11% with vasospasm, 3% with medical complications, and 3% with surgical complications. The 40% of functional survivors are predominantly from the early-diagnosis group hospitalized in a neurologic center. Children apparently do better than these averages. Surgical mortality for clipping is much less than 10%. In one series of 33 children, surgical mortality was 3%, and 80% of patients had no deficit except on psychometric testing (Heiskanen and Vilkki, 1981). Given this and the high mortality from rebleeding, surgery is surely indicated for alert patients (Patel and Richardson, 1971; Storrs et al., 1982). Authors disagree about the benefit of surgery for the moribund child. Treatment advances have largely been in the care of intracranial hypertension, supportive intensive care, and prevention of rebleeding by surgical means. The treatment of vasospasm continues to be an active area for research. The significant and lifelong risk of rebleeding, which is 1% to 2% per year beginning 6 months after the first bleed, is also reduced by surgery (Jane et al., 1985).

Pearls and Perils: Aneurysms

1. There is a high incidence of associated medical conditions in children with aneurysms.
2. Unusual sudden-onset headache in children deserves attention, especially if persistent for hours.
3. Prognosis for a child with an aneurysm is better than that for an adult with similar involvement.
4. Consider mycotic aneurysm if bacterial infection or congenital heart disease is present.
5. Ruptured aneurysm should be considered in closed-head injury.
6. An unruptured aneurysm may produce a mass effect.

Mycotic aneurysms are treated with antibiotics. Half will resolve and one third will decrease in size with this approach (Epstein, 1982). Surgery is indicated if the aneurysm is unchanged or larger on repeat angiogram 2 weeks after diagnosis.

ANNOTATED BIBLIOGRAPHY

Shapiro K: Subarachnoid hemorrhage in children, in Fein JM, Flamm, ES (eds): *Cerebrovascular Surgery*, Vol III. New York, Springer-Verlag, 1985, p 941–965.
A balanced review that tempers the literature with reason and experience to derive practical conclusions.

REFERENCES

Amacher AL, Drake CG: Cerebral artery aneurysms in infancy, childhood and adolescence. *Child's Brain* 1:72–80, 1975.
Epstein MH: Subarachnoid hemorrhage in children, in Hopkins LN, Long DM (eds): *Clinical Management of Intracranial Aneurysms*. New York, Raven Press, 1982, p 177–181.
Heiskanen O, Vilkki J: Intracranial arterial aneurysms in children and adolescents. *Acta Neurochir* 59:55–63, 1981.
Jane JA, Kassell NF, Torner JC, Winn HR: The natural history of aneurysms and arteriovenous malformations. *J Neurosurg* 62:321–323, 1985.
Lee YJ, Kandall SR, Ghali VS: Intracerebral arterial aneurysm in a newborn. *Arch Neurol* 35:171–172, 1978.
Patel AN, Richardson AE: Ruptured intracranial aneurysm in the first two decades of life. *J Neurosurg* 35:571–576, 1971.
Sedzimir CB, Robinson J: Intracranial hemorrhage in children and adolescents. *J Neurosurg* 38:269–281, 1973.
Shuangshoti S, Netsky MG, Switter DJ: Combined congenital vascular anomalies and neuroepithelial (colloid) cysts. *Neurology* 28:552–555, 1978.
Storrs BB, Humphreys CP, Hendrick EB, Hoffman HJ: Intracranial aneurysms in the pediatric age-group. *Child's Brain* 9:358–361, 1982.
Torner JC: Epidemiology of subarachnoid hemorrhage. *Semin Neurol* 4:354–369, 1984.

Arteriovenous Malformations

The prevalence of arteriovenous malformations (AVMs) based on cases with hemorrhage is estimated at one tenth that of aneurysms. There is a suggestion that a higher proportion of AVMs compared to aneurysms bleed, and at earlier ages (Torner, 1984). They are rarely familial. In a large series of first bleeds from AVMs, the peak age was in the second decade; 7% bled in the first decade and 25% in the second. Mortality of the first bleed is 5% to 25%, morbidity 50%. Rebleeding occurs in 25% to 50% of cases, with a higher mortality of 28% to 41%. Thus, this is a very serious lesion, although the more favorable figures suggest that both mortality from hemorrhage and risk of rebleeding are less than with aneurysms.

Pathophysiology

The lesions vary greatly in location, size, number of arteries, character of the abnormal vessels, and changes over time. A great deal of interest has centered on these issues, but their clinical application is limited to broad groupings. The most common lesion is the AVM "proper" (Stein and Wolpert, 1980a). In this lesion one (60%) or several (average of two) arteries drain directly into venous channels. Both the arteries and the veins may be either enlarged normal or anomalous vessels. The presence of a limited capillary bed does not seem to be clinically important. Locations are parietal in 30% of cases, frontal in 17%, occipital in 10%, temporal in 10%, and in the basal ganglia in 16%. Specimens show unsuspected old hemorrhage in 10% of cases. Venous angiomas are pathologically distinct, but clinically similar to AVMs. Vein of Galen malformations differ in that the venous side of the AVM is the vein of Galen enlarged and in some cases itself malformed.

Cavernous hemangiomas are nonneoplastic malformations in which large, venous channels form a complex meshwork. They occur predominantly in frontal and parietal regions, and are much less frequent than AVMs. Capillary angiomas occur in the posterior fossa and in the subependymal region in the cerebral hemispheres.

Spinal vascular malformations present with sudden motor impairment and/or SAH in most cases, often with premonitory attacks, which include severe pain (Buchanan and Walker, 1941; Riche et al., 1982). CSF is abnormal in over 80% of cases. MRI is often diagnostic. Myelogram is abnormal in 95%, but diagnostic in fewer. In addition to establishing the diagnosis, a preoperative angiogram improves the surgical attack. An alternative to direct angiography is digital subtraction, if available. The location of these lesions is cervical in 30% of cases, and these have the slowest clinical evolution. Thoracic AVMs (20% of cases) have the worst prognosis, frequently being associated with early necrosis of the cord. The 50% of cases with thoracolumbar lesions have a variable clinical course. Half of the lesions are intramedullary, 20% are extramedullary, and 30% are mixed. Associated skin lesions have been described in 20% to 35% of cases, consisting of port wine stain or the cutaneous manifestations of Osler-Weber-Rendu disease, Klippel-Trénaunay syndrome, familial hereditary cutaneous hemangioma, or Cobb's syndrome (Barek et al., 1982). When a spinal AVM and cutaneous hemangioma are both present (20% to 30% of cases), they are in the same dermatome in almost half the cases.

"Cryptic" vascular malformations are sometimes found on pathologic examination. They are hypothesized when a patient presents with intracerebral and/or SAH, but angiogram, surgical specimen, or autopsy fail to demonstrate a source. The same may be said of apparently spontaneous spinal epidural hematoma (Posnikoff, 1968).

AVMs may present with acute intracranial hemorrhage, ischemia, or a bruit. Peak age is 8 to 12 years (58%); 20% of cases each present at 1 to 7 and 14 to 17 years of age. The rare case diagnosed in infancy has usually presented with heart failure (Holden et al., 1972). AVMs are occasionally discovered incidentally or during evaluation of massive cutaneous hemangiomas. If a primary SAH occurs, the signs and symptoms will be the same as for aneurysms. If it is intracerebral, the picture will be that of any intracerebral bleed. The role of AVMs in producing the headaches that sometimes lead to diagnosis is moot. SAH, the presenting symptom in 60% of AVMs, is due to AVM in 30% to 60% of cases in children. Seizure is the first symptom in one third of AVMs, and occurs at some point in 60% of cases (Shapiro, 1985). Of patients presenting with seizure, 20% to 70% will hemorrhage before diagnosis of their AVM. Focal and secondarily generalized seizures are approximately equally common. They are probably successfully treated with anticonvulsants as often as seizures with other etiologies. EEG is not discriminating. Headache is an initial symptom in 70% of cases, altered state of consciousness in 35%. Ischemia may result from a distal thrombotic infarction, in which case it may produce focal signs related to the location involved. A "steal" syndrome can produce ischemia of variable degree, with reversible dysfunction, but at times resulting in hypoplasia or infarction of deprived areas. After bleeding, vasospasm may of course produce ischemia as well.

Cranial bruits are common in childhood. Authors

FEATURE TABLE 12-6. ARTERIOVENOUS MALFORMATIONS

Discriminating Feature	Consistent Feature	Variable Features
1. Radiologic demonstration, angiography	1. None	1. Occurrence of headache, seizure, bruit, signs and symptoms of hemorrhage 2. Neurologic symptoms and signs and depending on size and location of lesions 3. Natural history and surgical risks

who have systematically sought them report figures that are much higher than most physicians find in general or neurologic practice: 60% in 4- to 5-year-olds and 10% in 10- to 15-year-olds, versus 1% in adults. All of these incidence figures double during contralateral carotid compression (Wadia and Monckton, 1957). Occasionally they are reported by the child. The vast majority are not due to AVMs. Bruits over the great vessels of the neck, which are particularly common, are usually markedly modified by turning the head in various directions, and rarely indicate pathology. Conversely, however, large AVMs may produce bruits that may be heard widely or only over a tiny area of the head. Bruit over a spinal AVM is rare (Ommaya, 1985).

Vein of Galen malformations are AVMs with markedly variable size and blood flow, features which correlate with both age and mode of onset (Gold et al., 1964; Massey et al., 1982). They comprise 63% of AVMs presenting before 6 months of age. The largest lesions cause massive shunting of blood flow. This is responsible for high-output cardiac failure, which presents as early as the day of birth. The shunt also produces a cerebral "steal" syndrome sufficient to produce cerebral ischemia, and we have observed marked cerebral atrophy on neonatal CT scan, sufficient to predict a poor neurologic outcome in some if not all such cases by the time of birth. However, since survival to more than a few weeks as a result of interventional neuroradiology is such a recent phenomenon, the reversibility of the cerebral deficit is an unanswered question. Diagnosis depends on hearing the cranial bruit, usually near the inion, the absence of cardiac malformation, rhabdomyoma of the heart, and Pompe's disease. Cardiac catheterization is appropriate, but should be avoidable with typical findings and MRI or CT. Smaller lesions produce proportionately less shunting and milder, later presentation. Presentation in infancy is usually due to some combination of hydrocephalus, seizures, dilated scalp veins with bruit, and SAH. Mortality is extremely high. Presentation and prognosis in the rest of childhood and into adulthood is like that of other AVMs.

Diagnostic Studies

Angiography not only makes the diagnosis of AVM certain, but also defines the vascular anatomy. This is essential for determining if the lesion is surgically approachable. CT will show many, especially if they have bled or with contrast enhancement, as will MRI. Sonography will detect very large lesions. Myelography will demonstrate some abnormality in almost all spinal AVMs, but often will not discriminate the nature of the lesion; CT metrisemide myelography and MRI afford superior results. Digital subtraction angiography is not optimal for intracranial lesions, but spinal AVMs have been demonstrated by this technique, and it is an attractive alternative to spinal angiography in centers with less experience, especially in infants (Smith et al., 1982).

Pearls and Perils: Arteriovenous Malformations

1. Bruits over AVMs may be limited to a 1-cm-diameter spot on the skull; one may have to search to find the spot.
2. Most neck and cranial bruits in children are of no significance.
3. It is easy to confuse the clinical manifestations and CSF findings of aseptic meningoencephalitis with traumatic tap on the one hand, and SAH, especially from AVM, on the other. Care to observe the color of spun CSF for the presence or absence of xanthochromia and to compare red and white blood cell counts in two tubes will usually prevent this error.
4. It is easy to confuse the presentation of AVM with epilepsy or with stroke of other etiology. This again emphasizes the need for thorough work-up in cerebrovascular disease of childhood.

Treatment

Even though the natural history is unfavorable and morbidity is high, the decision to treat must be based on the size and location of the lesion. Surgery gives excellent results in selected cases with little morbidity or mortality. Conservative treatment has a high long-term risk: roughly 20% mortality, 30% of patients disabled, and 11% of patients with moderate dysfunction in variable follow-up periods in reported series. Rebleeding occurs in 6% of patients in the first year, and in 2% per year thereafter. Results are better if there are fewer arterial feeders. Surgical approaches vary from occlusion of feeding arteries to total excision, and both strategies may be implemented in stages. Interventional neuroradiology is currently in development, with embolization aiming to occlude feeders. A flexible approach that includes combinations of methods has been advocated (Stein and Wolpert, 1980b). Highly focused gamma radiation has been reported to be relatively safe and effective by its developers.

Treatment of seizures, rehabilitation of deficits, and control of systemic problems such as hypertension are of course necessary.

ANNOTATED BIBLIOGRAPHY

Smith RR, Haerer AF, Russell WF (eds): *Vascular Malformations and Fistulas of the Brain.* Seminars in Neurological Surgery. New York, Raven Press, 1982.
  Although largely concerned with the more frequent cases in adulthood, this is a general review including children.

REFERENCES

Barek L, Ledor S, Ledor K: The Klippel-Trénaunay syndrome: A case report and review of the literature. *Mt Sinai J Med, NY* 49:66–70, 1982.

Buchanan DN, Walker AE: Vascular anomalies of the spinal cord in children. *Am J Dis Child* 61:928–932, 1941.

Gold AP, Ransohoff J, Carter S: Vein of Galen malformation. *Acta Neurol Scand* 40(suppl 11):1–32, 1984.

Holden AM, Fyler DC, Shillito J Jr, Nadas AS: Congenital heart failure from intracranial arteriovenous fistula in infancy. *Pediatrics* 49:30–39, 1972.

Massey CE, Carson LV, Beveridge WD, Allen MB Jr, Brooks B, Yaghmai F: Aneurysms of the great vein of Galen: report of two cases and review of the literature, in Smith RR, Haerer AR, Russell WF (eds): *Vascular Malformations and Fistulas of the Brain.* New York, Raven Press, 1982, p 163–179.

Ommaya AK: Spinal cord arteriovenous malformations, in Fein JM, Flamm ES (eds): *Cerebrovascular Surgery,* Vol IV. New York, Springer-Verlag, 1985, p 217–228.

Posnikoff J: Spontaneous spinal epidural hematoma of childhood. *J Pediatr* 73:178–183, 1968.

Riche MC, Modenesi J, Djindjian M, Merland JJ: Arteriovenous malformations (AVM) of the spinal cord in children. A review of 38 cases. *Neuroradiology* 22:171–180, 1982.

Shapiro K: Subarachnoid hemorrhage in children, in Fein JM, Flamm, ES (eds): *Cerebrovascular Surgery,* Vol III. New York, Springer-Verlag, 1985, p 941–965.

Stein BM, Wolpert SM: Arteriovenous malformations of the brain. II. Current concepts and treatment. *Arch Neurol* 37:1–5, 1980a.

Stein BM, Wolpert SM: Arteriovenous malformations of the brain. II. Current concepts and treatment. *Arch Neurol* 37:69–75, 1980b.

Torner JC: Epidemiology of subarachnoid hemorrhage. *Semin Neurol* 4:354–369, 1984.

Wadia NH, Monckton G: Intracranial bruits in health and disease. *Brain* 80:492–509, 1957.

Other Intracranial Hemorrhages in Childhood

The previous sections have presented intracranial hemorrhages that occur in the settings of IVH or asphyxia, as hemorrhagic infarcts, with aneurysms, and with vascular malformations. The remaining causes of intracranial hemorrhage in childhood are discussed here (Shapiro, 1985).

Intracerebellar hemorrhage is similar to posterior fossa subdural hematoma in newborns as regards pre-

---

Pearls and Perils: Other Intracranial Hemorrhages in Childhood

1. It is essential in the early hours after onset to distinguish between concussion (general cerebral symptoms without parenchymal injury) and more serious injury.
2. In cases of child abuse, the history is usually factitious, and there may be no external sign of trauma because of lack of impact. Retinal hemorrhages, if present, are a suggestive sign.
3. Consider both encephalitis and various causes of intracerebral hemorrhage when multifocal dysfunction and multiple lesions on imaging are present.
4. Do not fail to diagnose the underlying cause of the hemorrhage.
5. Transfer the patient with serious injury to a neurosurgical center.

---

disposing factors and the clinical picture. However, neurologic outcome is much poorer. Clinical features indicative of the coexistence of significant cerebral insult may be present, and they may lead to incidental discovery of this lesion (Williamson et al., 1985). Recent reports and personal experience indicate that, even with no specific therapy, the outcome can be good (Koch et al., 1985).

The hematologic causes of intracranial hemorrhage are sickle cell disease (Hoff et al., 1985) and those conditions that are associated with coagulopathy, primarily the hemophilias and idiopathic thrombocytopenic purpura (Woerner et al., 1981). In hemophilia, 40% of deaths and 10% of all bleeding episodes involve intracranial bleeds, especially subdural and intracerebral. The secondary causes are hepatic dysfunction, DIC, bone marrow depression, and various hypercoagulation states, including those in dehydration of infancy, diabetic ketoacidosis (Atluru, 1986), collagen vascular diseases, dysproteinemias, parasitic infections, poststreptococcal glomerulonephritis, and moyamoya disease. The bleeding sites are apparently random, reflecting only the relative mass of the various parts of the brain.

FEATURE TABLE 12-7. OTHER INTRACRANIAL HEMORRHAGES IN CHILDHOOD

Discriminating Features	Consistent Feature	Variable Features
1. Results of neuroimaging studies 2. Laboratory tests for the various underlying medical conditions	1. These conditions will have a predisposing traumatic or medical basis	1. Size of hematoma or amount of cerebral damage, even in apparently similar circumstances 2. Early clinical course in cases with life-threatening lesions

Bleeding into neoplasms occurs at all ages, its low frequency representing a fraction of the low prevalence of cerebral neoplasms in childhood. Leukemic masses in brain are one such instance, but reports of these have declined markedly in recent years.

Separate mention should be made of the potential confusion clinically and on imaging studies of hemorrhage in necrotizing encephalitis as opposed to bleeding from the vascular lesions or the other causes listed. Careful examination of the CT scan, with appropriate window selection, may show multiple lesions in cases of encephalitis. MRI is the most useful early test for encephalitis.

ANNOTATED BIBLIOGRAPHY

Shapiro K: Subarachnoid hemorrhage in children, in Fein JM, Flamm ES (eds): *Cerebrovascular Surgery*, Vol III. New York, Springer-Verlag, 1985, p 941–965.

The portion of this chapter dealing with hemorrhages, like all of the chapter, gives a balanced review that tempers the literature with reason and experience to derive useful generalizations.

REFERENCES

Atluru VL: Spontaneous intracerebral hematomas in juvenile diabetic ketoacidosis. *Pediatr Neurol* 2:167–169, 1986.

Hoff JV, Ritchey AK, Shaywitz BA: Intracranial hemorrhage in children with sickle cell disease. *Am J Dis Child* 139:1120–1123, 1985.

Koch TK, Jahnke SE, Edwards MSB, Davis SL: Posterior fossa hemorrhage in term newborns. *Pediatr Neurol* 1:96–99, 1985.

Williamson WD, Percy AK, Fishman MA, et al: Cerebellar hemorrhage in the term neonate: Developmental and neurologic outcome. *Pediatr Neurol* 1:356–360, 1985.

Woener SJ, Abildgaard CF, French BN: Intracranial hemorrhage in children with idiopathic thrombocytopenic purpura. *Pediatrics* 67:453–460, 1981.

Inborn Errors of Metabolism I Neurologic Degenerative Diseases

Paul Maertens
Paul R. Dyken

Neurodegenerative diseases with onset in infancy, childhood, or adolescence make up a sizeable portion of the practice of pediatric neurology. The extent or incidence of such disorders is inexact and varies from one reporter to the next. This variation is explained, perhaps, by inexact definitions as to what is progression, and by the semantics of traditional classification. The majority of the diseases discussed in this book are progressive. Yet because of the acceptance of another system of classification many of these diseases are included within other chapters. What is more typically progressive than subacute sclerosing panencephalitis? This disorder is not discussed in this chapter but rather in Chapter 10, on infectious disease. Many other diseases of typical degenerative nature are discussed in other chapters.

We have organized this chapter into an overview of some of the more characteristic neurologic degenerative diseases encountered in pediatric neurology that are not included in other chapters. We will attempt to present them in the manner suggested by Dyken and Krawiecki in 1983. These authors used a pathoanatomic classification of the neurodegenerative diseases of infancy, childhood, and adolescence based on clinical phenomena and on pathologic findings that suggested the maximum or most obvious site of anatomic involvement. Roughly speaking, all neurodegenerative diseases were classified into one of the following subtypes, regardless of whether a genetic mechanism or a metabolic basis was suspected: (1) polioencephalopathy, (2) leukoencephalopathy, (3) corencephalopathy, (4) spinocerebellopathy, and (5) diffuse encephalopathy or miscellaneous. In polioencephalopathies the maximum clinical and pathologic features included involvement of the cerebral cortex. In the leukoencephalopathies clinical and pathologic features were maximum in the subcortical white matter. In the corencephalopathies involvement of the subcortical gray matter, including structures of the basal ganglion, thalamus, and midbrain, was maximum. In the spinocerebellopathies the maximum clinical and pathologic features included involvement of the cerebellum, spinal cord, and sometimes medulla and pons regardless of whether gray or white matter was affected. In many of the neurodegenerative diseases both clinical and pathologic studies failed to characterize a maximal central nervous system (CNS) involvement; or studies were such that diffuse, nonlocalized symptoms or pathologic findings were present; or (fortunately only rarely) the disease investigation was incomplete so that no characterization could be made. These disorders were classified as diffuse encephalopathies. We eliminate here discussion of many of the rarer disorders listed in the Dyken and Krawiecki study and some of those discussed in more detail in other portions of this volume.

REFERENCE

Dyken P, Krawiecki N: Neurodegenerative diseases of infancy and childhood. *Ann Neurol* 13(4):351–364, 1983.

Polioencephalopathies

NEURONAL CEROID LIPOFUSCINOSES

The neuronal ceroid lipofuscinoses (NCLs) are a group of diseases characterized by neurologic symptomatology and the accumulation of the autofluorescent lipopigments, ceroid and lipofuscin, within lysosomes of the cells of the nervous system and other tissues.

The clinical presentation of NCL is dependent on the specific syndrome represented. The most commonly encountered form of NCL has been described as chronic juvenile NCL or Batten disease. As the descriptive name implies, onset is usually during a period between 4 and 12 years of life and takes on a chronic course. Initial symptoms are usually either visual failure, behavioral reaction, or intellectual failure. These symptoms are slowly progressive, usually over a period of years. Within this framework neurologic symptoms owing to slowly progressive pyramidal and extrapyramidal dysfunction are seen. Seizures are at first uncommon but then later become much more frequent. Early clinical diagnosis can often be made by the typical retinal picture, which shows attenuation of retinal vessels, macular degenerative changes, patches of retinal atrophy, and a so-called waxy, yellow type of optic atrophy. Later, minimal peripheral retinitis pigmentosa may be seen. Because the disease is slowly progressive, a monophasic staging process can be identified over years of follow-up. The results of laboratory investigations—including electroencephalogram (EEG), computed tomographic (CT) scan, magnetic resonance imaging (MRI), measurement of evoked potentials, and cerebrospinal fluid (CSF) analysis—are greatly dependent on the stage of the disease. The electroretinogram (ERG) is consistently abnormal once retinopathy and visual failure have begun clinically. Even early in the development of the disease, the ERG is often absent if not attenuated. Pathohistologic confirmation of the disease is by electron microscopic examination of lymphocytes, which are excessively vacuolated even on light microscopy. Within the vacuoles highly characteristic osmophilic cytosomes are identified, with the so-called fingerprint profile predominating. Other tissues also show these cytosomes, including many cells of the brain, muscle, skin, conjunctiva, and rectum. The pathologic reaction is of accumulation of autofluorescent lipopigments within cells, particularly neurons. This reaction is not as obvious within the retina, where the major brunt of the disease appears to be a primary loss of cells in the rod and cone layer. Retinal ganglion cells do show less dramatic accumulation of intracellular lipopigments. Some patients have excessive excretion of dolichols in the urine. Batten disease is inherited as an autosomal recessive trait. The causes of the disorder are still speculative.

The next most common type of NCL has been called the acute late infantile type or Bielschowsky disease. In this variety, the onset of the disease occurs between 2 and 4 years of age. Initial symptoms are overwhelmingly of seizures, of a wide variety. If a seizure is not the first complaint, progressive psychomotor regression is encountered. In yet a smaller number of cases, sudden onset of incoordination as frank ataxia is seen. These early symptoms often occur together. The course is dramatically downhill so that within months the patient is often nonambulatory if not bedridden. In this condition, mental and motor regression has been so severe that visual failure is often unnoticed. The retinal picture is similar to the findings in Batten disease if the disease has become well developed. In the early stages, however, the retina may be normal, only to be characterized within weeks by severe pigmentary disturbances. Laboratory findings are also variable depending on the stage of the disease. The EEG is almost always severely abnormal and of an epileptogenic type, especially early in the course or at the onset of the disease. Evoked potential studies may show an early exaggerated response, which is replaced by poor or absent responses later. The ERG may also be absent. CT scans and MRI may show atrophic changes more readily than in Batten disease even early in the course. These changes are especially located in the cerebellum and brain-

FEATURE TABLE 13-1. NEURONAL CEROID LIPOFUSCINOSES

Discriminating Feature	Consistent Features	Variable Features
1. Vacuolar or avacuolar osmophilic cytosomes in lymphocytes, conjunctiva, skin, rectum, muscle, and brain	1. Waxy, yellow type of optic atrophy 2. Peripheral retinitis pigmentosa 3. Abnormal ERG	1. Progressive dementia 2. Seizures, myoclonia 3. Ataxia 4. Early blindness 5. Mental changes (disruptive behavior, psychosis, neurosis) 6. Basal ganglia symptoms 7. Rett-like symptoms

stem. CSF analysis may be normal. Pathohistologic study of lymphocytes is often abnormal, showing excessive vacuolation with electron microscopic cytosomal osmophilic profiles within the vacuoles. These show more curvilinear bodies than in Batten disease, even though fingerprint and other types of cytosomes are also seen. Other tissues also show the ultrastructural diagnostic bodies, including a variety of cells in brain, skin, muscle, conjunctiva, and rectum. Pathologic study of the nervous system and other tissues shows changes very similar to those encountered in the chronic juvenile variant of NCL, although in the acute late infantile form, there are usually more atrophic changes and less dominant storage. Some patients with Bielschowsky disease show excessive dolicholuria. Acute late infantile NCL is inherited as an autosomal recessive trait. The cause is unknown. Variants of the acute form of NCL include adult-onset and childhood-onset variations. These have similar features to the acute late infantile form clinically, dynamically, and pathologically.

All other types of NCL are less common and can be summarized by differences in their clinical course, age of onset, morphologic picture, and genetics. An acute infantile form of the disease was stressed by Finnish workers in 1975. This syndrome deviates from the other acute NCL disorders by occurring within the first 2 years of life, and by a rapidly downhill course characterized by severe seizures or myoclonia, severe mental-motor regression, and blindness. The laboratory picture is much more variable than in the other forms of NCL. Distinct differences in such studies as EEG and evoked potential measurements may represent developmental changes, as might be expected in a more devastating disease with an earlier onset. The ultramorphologic picture is quite different in the Santouroni-Haltia syndrome. Granular electron microscopic cytosomes are characteristic and rarely are the other electron microscopic cytosomes encountered. Pathologic reaction is characterized by a more severe atrophic picture, more signs of acute cellular destruction, and a severe, almost diagnostic, macrophagocytosis.

Another rare variety of NCL is represented by an adult onset and chronic course. There are probably at least two varieties of what has been called the chronic adult-onset type of NCL. One of the subtypes is an autosomal-dominant-inherited disease characterized by seizures and myoclonia as early features, which are followed even years later by dementia. The other chronic adult subtype is an autosomal recessive disease with early dementia with or closely followed by prominent motor symptoms. The motor features are usually either a pure cerebellar syndrome or a pure basal ganglion deterioration. In families, the subtypes show homotypism (some characteristics) and homochronism (same onset and course). In the uncommon instances when this disorder has been studied, granular cytosomes have been identified ultrastructurally in the lymphocytes. Pathologic study of the CNS shows less striking storage. The classic type of lipofuscin, which is seen in the aging process, is encountered, as well as membrane-bound granular osmophilic profiles.

A congenital type of NCL is now postulated, as examples of NCL are clearly delineated in the light of modern investigations. Many of the original NCL reports have now been shown to be examples of gangliosidoses. The congenital form of NCL is a fulminating disease of the newborn period, associated with refractive seizures and often early death. Three of four well-documented patients with this disease died in the first few months of life. Yet one survived to 4½ years of age. This protracted course, brought about by vigorous supportive care, allows one to document the true chronic nature of the disease. It has been proposed to identify the congenital form as a chronic type. In the uncommon examples studied, continued myoclonic, tonic, clonic, atonic, and astatic seizures occur with severe incapacitation to the level of vegetation. Blindness and deafness are common and total care is necessary.

Recently isolated case reports of even more atypical forms of NCL have certain common characteristics but can be differentiated from each other. One type of particular interest is a chronic infantile-onset disorder resembling Rett disease with features of infantile autism. Another rare atypical form of NCL is a chronic childhood-onset disorder appearing as a pervasive psychotic reaction. A third atypical type of NCL is a chronic juvenile-onset disorder presenting as a fairly pure cerebellar ataxia with hyperreflexia and psychoneurotic symptoms.

In the chronic infantile syndrome a relatively normal period between birth and the later part of the first year of life is typical. Thereafter retardation in developmental milestones occurs, especially concerning language development. Behavior slowly becomes bizarre and is characterized by irritability, withdrawal, and progressively repetitive, sometimes destructively oriented, behavior. Coexistent with this abnormal behavior are progressively worsening peculiar hand and arm movements and posture. All of these features are extremely variable but over the years a homogeneous worsening is obvious. Regression in previously acquired milestones occurs in the early stages. Other neurologic deficits develop slowly, including frank pyramidal, extrapyramidal, and cerebellar symptoms. Seizures may occur but these are less of a problem than in other forms of NCL, such as the Bielschowsky variant. Retinal lesions are not typical in this atypical Rett-like syndrome. Yet careful study of lymphocytes and other tissues reveals the characteristic ultrastructural cytosomes, with fingerprint and lamellar patterns predominating. No autopsy material has been studied.

In the chronic childhood syndrome, a normal period of early psychomotor development occurs, although this period may be associated with what has been interpreted as benign single seizures. In late infancy or early childhood, a prominent psychiatric presentation develops that is characterized by frank psychotic behavior. One sees severe withdrawal, autistic behavior, alternating violent and lethargic behavior, overactivity alternating with underactivity, hallucinations, and delirium. Neurologic symptomatology in these early stages is not severe. Later children show mild pyramidal, then extrapyramidal, and then cerebellar symptoms. These symptoms and signs are never as severe as the more obvious behavioral features and never follow the usual time frame seen in the classic types of the disease. Even years after onset, the retinal picture remains normal. Yet ultrastructural study of lymphocytes shows consistently abnormal diagnostic cytosomes, with fingerprint profiles being the most prominent. Autopsy material has not been available for study.

In the chronic juvenile atypical syndrome of NCL, the infantile and early childhood periods are normal. In one such case mild behavioral symptoms have been identified in childhood. The youngsters are usually described as awkward. It is not until the teenage years, however, that gait and station disturbances become so obvious that a neurologic disease is first considered in the differential diagnosis. Then patients develop definite cerebellar symptoms and signs, consisting of both trunkal and appendicular involvement. Ataxia, dyssynergia, dysmetria, dysdiadochokinesis, scanning speech, and nystagmus may develop. Although the mental symptomatology is less obvious than the neurologic, psychoneurotic features of illness are also observed, usually in coexistence with the neurologic ones. Never have the psychiatric symptoms been of the severity or nature of those in the previously described atypical NCL syndromes. Hyperreflexia is common throughout the course of the disease, even early in the course. The retina does not show the typical picture believed to be diagnostic of NCL, although vague ocular abnormalities have been

---

Pearls and Perils:
Neuronal Ceroid Lipofuscinoses

1. If the presentation and course are chronic and if behavioral and visual symptoms are present, it is probably Batten disease (chronic juvenile NCL).
2. Look at the retina for the most important diagnostic feature in Batten disease.
3. If the disease is acute with seizures, it is probably Bielschowsky disease (acute late infantile NCL).
4. The presence of early incoordination and abnormal EEG are the most important clinical features of Bielschowsky disease.
5. Pathologic reports on tissues studied by electron microscopic methods may be misleading owing to lack of experience in searching for the bodies and naivite in recognizing them.
6. In some of the less common forms of NCL, pure autism, pure pervasive psychosis, and pure cerebellar ataxia are prominent atypical findings.

---

seen. These usually represent the retinal picture that can be seen in severe refractive errors and are not diagnostic of retinal NCL. Progression of neurologic symptoms is slow, covering a period of many years. The slow progression is out of proportion to the course in all the other syndromes of NCL. Ultrastructural study of lymphocytes and skin shows accumulation of a wide variety of osmophilic cytosomal profiles with fingerprint lamellar patterns predominating.

In none of the NCLs has there been a consistent beneficial therapy. Antioxidant treatment programs using vitamin E, vitamin C, D,L-methionine and butylated

---

TABLE 13–1. THE NEURONAL-CEROID LIPOFUSCINOSES

	Major Clinical Features	Prominent Morphologic Features
Acute forms		
Infantile	Seizures	Granular
Late infantile	Seizures	Curvilinear
Childhood	Seizures	Mixed
Adult	Seizures	Mixed
Chronic forms		
Congenital	Seizures, amentia	Curvilinear
Infantile (atypical with autism)	Autism, no visual loss	Mixed
Childhood (atypical with pervasiveness)	Pervasiveness, no visual loss	Mixed
Juvenile (classic)	Visual loss, dementia	Fingerprint
Juvenile (atypical with ataxia)	Ataxia, no visual loss	Mixed
Adult (dominant with seizures)	Seizures, myoclonia	Granular
Adult (recessive with dementia)	Dementia, motor loss	Granular

hydroxytoluene, or vitamin E and selenium in large dosages have shown some promise in arresting progression, especially in the chronic forms of the disease, but have been ineffective in the acute forms. Key features of the NCLs are summarized in Table 13–1.

ANNOTATED BIBLIOGRAPHY

Zeman W, Dyken P: Neuronal ceroid-lipofuscinosis (Batten's disease): Relationship to amaurotic family idiocy? *Pediatrics* 44:570–583, 1969.

 This paper contained the original use of the term *neuronal ceroid lipofuscinosis*. The differentiation between these diseases and amaurotic familial idiocies was established.

Dyken P: Neuronal ceroid-lipofuscinosis, in Swaiman K, Wright F (eds): *The Practice of Pediatric Neurology*. St Louis, CV Mosby, 1982, p 902–914.

 An updated description and current classification of the neuronal ceroid lipofuscinoses.

Dyken P: Reconsideration of the classification of the neuronal ceroid-lipofuscinoses (NCL). *Am J Med Genet* 5(suppl): 69–84, 1988.

 A description of newer forms of the disorders and a revised classification.

GM₂ GANGLIOSIDOSES

The GM_2 gangliosidoses are neuronal lipidoses in which lysosomal catabolism of a sialic-acid-containing lipid, ganglioside GM_2, is deficient, leading to progressive mental and motor deterioration. Two proteins are involved in the degradation of ganglioside GM_2: The GM_2 activator protein and hexosaminidase A (hex A). GM_2 activator (encoded on chromosome 5) is a specific, nonenzymatic protein that binds to ganglioside GM_2 with the motor stoichiometry of 1:1, and extracts GM_2 ganglioside from the membranes and solubilizes it. The resultant complex is then recognized by lysosomal hex A, which hydrolyzes the ganglioside GM_2. Hex A consists of two different polypeptide chains, α and β, in the combination α_1 and β_2. The α chain, encoded on chromsome 15, is only found in hex A. The β chain, encoded on chromsome 5, is found in hex A and hexosaminidase B (hex B), a homopolymer of β subunits with the structure $\beta_2\beta_2$. Hex A is acid and heat labile, whereas $\alpha_1\beta_2$ is stable under the same conditions. Hex B but not hex A is active on dermatan sulfate. Three types of GM_2 gangliosidoses are distinguished biochemically. Mutations in the α subunit lead to various forms of type I GM_2 gangliosidosis (hex A deficiency). Mutations in the β subunit lead to various forms of type II GM_2 gangliosidosis (hex A and B deficiency). Type III GM_2 gangliosidosis is a rare variant characterized by a GM_2 activator deficiency.

 The clinical features of the three types of GM_2 gangliosidoses are essentially identical. Infantile, juvenile, and adult forms of GM_2 gangliosidosis can be distinguished according to age of onset. The infantile form (Tay-Sachs and Sandhoff's diseases) is characterized by an early onset of symptoms. Infants appear normal at birth and develop normally, but by 6 months of age psychomotor retardation becomes apparent. During the first few months of life, irritability and hyperacusia (i.e., an exaggerated startle response to a relatively modest sound) dominate the clinical picture. The onset of motor weakness usually begins between 3 and 6 months. After 6 months of age, motor weakness becomes obvious, with a flaccid paralysis, hyporeflexia, and hypotonia. Visual acuity deteriorates. The patient lacks the ability to fixate and frequently presents with searching eye movements. The characteristic cherry-red spot is present in the macula. Blindness usually occurs before 1 year of age. Sometimes, the cherry-red spot disappears, leaving optic and retinal atrophy as the only visible funduscopic defect. The visual loss may be due to cortical abnormalities in some patients who present brisk pupillary responses despite the blindness. After 1 year of age, the symptoms continue to progress and the hyporeflexia and hypotonia give way to generalized spastic paralysis with hyperreflexia and opisthotonos. The child becomes pro-

FEATURE TABLE 13–2. TAY-SACHS DISEASE

Discriminating Feature	Consistent Features	Variable Features
1. Hexosaminidase A deficiency in serum and fibroblasts	1. Startle response to noise 2. Cherry-red spot	1. Nystagmus 2. Blindness 3. Megalencephaly 4. Hypotonia (early) and opisthotonos (late) 5. Hyporeflexia (early) and hyperreflexia (late) 6. Difficulty swallowing 7. Seizures 8. Deafness 9. Blindness

FEATURE TABLE 13–3. SANDHOFF'S DISEASE

Discriminating Feature	Consistent Features	Variable Features
1. Hexosaminidase A and B deficiency in serum and fibroblasts	1. Startle response to noise 2. Cherry-red spot 3. Oligosaccharides in urine	1. Nystagmus 2. Blindness 3. Megalencephaly 4. Hypotonia (early) and opisthotonos (late) 5. Hyporeflexia (early) and hyperreflexia (late) 6. Difficulty swallowing 7. Seizures 8. Deafness 9. Blindness 10. Splenomegaly 11. Bony deformities

gressively deaf. The occipitofrontal circumference increases at an abnormal rate, but because of hydrocephalus but chiefly because of megalencephaly. Various major and minor seizures occur; some seizures may begin with an inappropriate laughter (gelastic seizures). Feeding difficulties, owing to ineffective swallowing, lead to a progressive weight loss and cachexia. Late in the disease, a state of decerebrate rigidity is reached. The patient usually expires from a respiratory infection before the age of 5 years. Tay-Sachs disease (infantile type I GM_2 gangliosidosis), Sandhoff's disease (infantile type II GM_2 gangliosidosis), and GM_2 activator protein deficiency (infantile type III GM_2 gangliosidosis) are clinically similar. A mild splenomegaly, when present, is characteristic of Sandhoff's disease. Occasional infants with Sandhoff's disease have bony deformities similar to those in type I GM_1 gangliosidosis.

Juvenile GM_2 gangliosidosis has an onset between 2 and 6 years of age and progresses more slowly than the infantile GM_2 gangliosidosis. Ataxia, dysarthria, and loss of speech are frequently the initial symptoms. Dysphagia tends to appear later in the illness. Dementia is a universal feature but frequently is not apparent during the first year or two of the illness. Movement disorders, such as choreoathetosis, dystonia, and oculogyric crisis, may occur early or late in the course of the disease. Often, a progressive spasticity, leading to a decerebrate rigidity, is reported. Seizures are not always present. Cherry-red spots are uncommon and not well defined when they are present. Blindness occurs late in the disease. Megalencephaly does not develop. Death occurs up to 10 years from the onset of clinical symptoms.

The onset of adult GM_2 gangliosidosis is variable. Those with onset in childhood have a protracted juvenile form with long survival. They present with a spinocerebellar disorder masquerading as a spinocerebellar ataxia. Dystonia and spasticity are frequent findings. Seizures and ocular abnormalities do not occur. Mental retardation may only be slight. Those with onset in the second to fourth decade have a more variable clinical picture. Presenting symptoms include dementia, psychosis, progressive muscle weakness with atrophy (with clinical course similar to that of Kugelberg-Welander disease), seizures, ataxia, dystonia, rubral tremor, and supranuclear ophthalmoplegia, either alone or in various combinations. A slow, progressive ataxia with dysarthria is not always present. Intellectual function is normal or mildly impaired. Seizures rarely occur. Funduscopic exam is frequently normal.

In the various forms of GM_2 gangliosidoses, the ERG is normal. The amplitude, latency, and waveform remain normal throughout the course of the disease. GM_2 gangliosidoses involve only the ganglion cell layer and the electrical activity generated by the outer nuclear layer is not affected. In the infantile form of GM_2 gangliosidosis, the visual evoked potential is preserved in the early stages of the disease, but after 3 to 12 months the various components become increasingly poorly defined. Visual evoked responses may become abnormal late in the course of juvenile GM_2 gangliosidosis. In the various forms of GM_2 gangliosidoses, auditory evoked potentials may be abnormal in morphology and latency. EEG becomes abnormal early after birth in infantile GM_2 gangliosidosis. Hypsarrhythmia and multifocal cortical spikes are frequently recorded. In the juvenile form, the EEG is usually diffusely abnormal with occasional epileptiform activity. In the adult form, EEG may be normal or show nonspecific diffuse electric abnormalities. EMG in the protracted juvenile form and in adult-onset GM_2 gangliosidosis frequently shows evidence of denervation. Sensory nerve conduction is rarely decreased. CT scan of the head may show a diffuse atrophy or a gross cerebellar and brainstem atrophy in some patients with juvenile or adult forms of GM_2 gangliosidosis.

CSF is usually unremarkable. An important urinary excretion of oligosaccharides containing N-acetylglucosamine and mannose has been observed in Sandhoff's disease. The diagnosis of GM_2 gangliosidoses is confirmed by enzyme assay of hex A and B in serum, separated white blood cells, fibroblasts, or amniotic cells. Assays for hex A and B employing synthetic substrates (sulfated or nonsulfated) are generally sufficient to diagnose defects in the α or β chains. Hex A activity is usually calculated from the difference between total hexosaminidase activity and activity left after heat inactivation of hex A. Hex A and B deficiency in Sandhoff's disease and hex A deficiency in Tay-Sachs disease are demonstrated. However, mutations in the β subunit leading to heat-labile hex B may be misdiagnosed. Furthermore, this assay procedure cannot diagnose the GM_2 activator deficiency or hex A mutations resulting in a decreased responsiveness to activator protein. In those cases, activity toward artificial substrates, which do not need activator protein, may be normal. Feeding experiments with radiolabeled GM_2 ganglioside to mutant cells clearly identify the presence of a block in the metabolism of GM_2 and should be the preferred screening procedure whenever an atypical case of hexosaminidase deficiency is suspected.

There is no vacuolation in lymphocytes and in these cells no storage can be reliably detected by electron microscopy. The bone marrow contains no storage cells, although occasional foamy cells may be found in the Sandhoff variant. Neuropathologic examination reveals histologic evidence of ganglioside storage in neurons and glial cells. In paraffin sections, the stored ganglioside is extracted from the neurons during processing and periodic acid–Schiff (PAS) reaction is negative while the glial cells remain strongly positive. In cryostat sections, neurons are strongly PAS positive. Electron microscopy of the stored material demonstrates a great number of round or oval laminated membrane-bound structures, referred to as membranous cytoplasmic bodies (MCBs). MCBs measure 0.5 to $2\mu m$ in diameter. The limiting membrane of the MCB does not differ from the layers making up the interior. Characteristically, lamellae of 5-nm thickness are arranged in a regular fashion. Three forms of MCB are described: concentric, compound, and zebra bodies. In concentric bodies, the lamellae are arranged concentrically with a homogeneous or firmly granular zone in the center. In compound bodies, several outer concentric layers surround an inner zone filled with straight elements. In zebra bodies, a dense, double-layer, oval shell is filled with flat layers. The MCBs have been isolated by differential gradient centrifugation and shown to contain GM_2 ganglioside, cholesterol, and phospholipid. These bodies are found not only in the cerebrum, cerebellum, and spinal cord, but also wherever the neurons are distended, i.e., the ganglion cells of the retina, the spiral ganglia of the inner ear, the myenteric plexuses, and the autonomic nerve ganglia. Axonal terminals may accumulate disease-specific MCBs (in Schwann cells MCBs are nonspecific). Therefore, skin and rectal biopsy may provide diagnostic clues. Intralysosomal

storage progressively results in death of nerve cells with subsequent Wallerian degeneration of myelin.

Specific neuropathologic findings allow distinction of various forms of GM_2 gangliosidoses. In infantile GM_2 gangliosidosis, extensive gliosis and edema contribute to the megalencephaly. The cerebellum is atrophic with depletion of Purkinje cells and granules. In juvenile and adult GM_2 gangliosidoses, involvement of certain nerve cell groups is not unusual, i.e., basal ganglia with sparing of the cerebral cortex, and granular layer with sparing of Purkinje cells in the cerebellum (centripetal atrophy). The electron microscopic examination of the neurons in juvenile and adult GM_2 gangliosidoses show many kinds of abnormal inclusions. In addition to the disease-specific MCBs, poorly defined lamellar structures, lipofuscin bodies (fingerprint-like structures or granular material), and large conglomerates formed by all of these inclusions are found. Whether these lipopigments are identical in their composition to those formed in primary neuronal ceroid lipofuscinosis has not yet been elucidated. GM_2 ganglioside is already increased in the fetal brain. Before 12 weeks gestation, the immature subcortical neurons contain inclusion bodies that are not membrane bound and have a negative acid phosphatase reaction. This finding suggests that biochemical changes in Tay-Sachs disease precede lysosomal formation.

GM_2 gangliosidoses are autosomal recessive inherited disorders. The infantile Tay-Sachs disease is much more

---

Pearls and Perils:
GM_2 Gangliosidoses

1. Patients with GM_2 gangliosidosis do not develop bony changes, macroglossia, cataracts, or retinitis pigmentosa. Hepatosplenomegaly is only found in the infantile form or Sandhoff's disease.
2. Juvenile and adult hex A deficiency may present as an atypical spinocerebellar degeneration.
3. Adult hex A deficiency may present as juvenile cerebellar ataxia (Ramsey-Hunt), Kugelberg-Welander disease, or dystonia musculorum deformans.
4. Cherry-red spots may disappear with age.
5. If assay for hex A and B is performed with artificial substrates, false negative results may be obtained.
6. Juvenile GM_2 gangliosidosis is clinically similar to chronic juvenile NCL. Important differentiating features include prominent visual disturbances and pigmentary retinal degeneration early in the course of chronic juvenile NCL, and absent or late retinal involvement in juvenile GM_2 gangliosidosis.
7. In Tay-Sachs disease, cytoplasmic lamellar inclusions are only found in the brain.

frequent among Ashkenazi Jews than in other ethnic groups. It has been suggested that approximately 80% of all infantile Tay-Sachs patients are of Jewish ancestry. The incidence of infantile Tay-Sachs disease is about 1 in 3600 among Ashkenazi Jews. Gene frequency in Jews is approximately tenfold higher than in the general population. Non-Jewish French Canadians also have a high incidence of infantile Tay-Sachs disease. The juvenile and adult forms of GM_2 gangliosidoses have no ethnic predilection. Heterozygotes for GM_2 gangliosidoses can be detected through analysis of serum, leukocytes, and tears. Prenatal diagnosis of Tay-Sachs disease can be established by lack of hex A and increase of GM_2 in cultured amniotic cells or fresh chorionic villi. Management is entirely supportive. There are no well-documented studies to indicate that the pathology can be reversed by enzyme replacement. If such a therapy is to be considered it should be started in utero.

ANNOTATED BIBLIOGRAPHY

Sandhoff K, Conzelmann E: The biochemical basis of gangliosidoses. *Neuropediatrics* 15(suppl):85–92, 1984.

The protein defects underlying GM_2 gangliosidosis are reviewed. The processing of lysosomal enzymes may sometimes be deficient. In general, it seems to be impossible to design a synthetic substrate for the diagnosis of all variants of GM_2 gangliosidosis.

Okada S, McCrea M, O'Brien JS: Sandhoff's disease (GM_2 gangliosidosis type II): Clinical, chemical, and enzyme studies in five patients. *Pediatr Res* 6:606–615, 1972.

The phenotypic similarities between Sandhoff's disease and Tay-Sachs disease are so great that clinical or pathologic differentiation between the two is not reliable. Some patients with either disease have doll-like facial appearances, with pale, translucent skin, long eyelashes, and fine hair. Rectal biopsy demonstrates in both phenotypes conspicuous neuronal lipidosis.

Conzelmann E, Sandhoff K: AB variant of infantile GM_2-gangliosidosis: Deficiency of a factor necessary for stimulation of hexosaminidase A-catalyzed degradation of ganglioside GM_2 and glycolipid GA_2. *Proc Natl Acad Sci* 75:3979–3983, 1978.

An activating factor is necessary for the interaction of lipid substrates and the water-soluble hydrolase hex A. This activating factor is defective in the AB variant.

Meek D, Wolfe L, Andermann E, Andermann F: Juvenile progressive dystonia: A new phenotype of GM_2 gangliosidosis. *Ann Neuron* 15:348–352, 1984.

The clinical features in patients with late infantile and juvenile GM_2 gangliosidosis are reviewed. GM_2 gangliosidosis is added to the list of causes of progressive juvenile dystonia.

Wood S: Juvenile Sandhoff disease: Complementation tests with Sandhoff and Tay-Sachs disease using polyethylene glycol-induced cell fusion. *Hum Genet* 41:325–329, 1978.

In a 10-year-old male with progressive cerebellar ataxia and psychomotor retardation and almost complete deficiency of hex A and B, no complementation of Sandhoff and juvenile Sandhoff cells is found, suggesting allelism.

Johnson WG: The clinical spectrum of hexosaminidase deficiency diseases. *Neurology* 31:1453–1456, 1981.

Hexosaminidase deficiencies may masquerade under various phenotypes, such as dystonia or motor neuron disease or as spinocerebellar degenerations, including the various forms of ataxia.

Barbeau A, Plasse L, Cloutier T, Paris S, Roy M: Lysosomal enzymes in ataxia: Discovery of two new cases of late onset hexosaminidase A and B deficiency (adult Sandhoff disease) in French-Canadians. *Can J Neurol Sci* 11:601–606, 1984.

Two brothers presenting with progressive ataxia since childhood developed dystonic postures and the clinical phenotype of Kugelberg-Welander disease during adulthood. Funduscopic exam and intelligence were normal. Both showed a low activity of hex A and B in leukocytes.

Johnson WG, Wigger HJ, Karp HR, Glaubiger LM, Rowland LP: Juvenile spinal muscular atrophy: A new hexosaminidase deficiency phenotype. *Ann Neurol* 11:11–16, 1982.

A 24-year-old Ashkenazi man with a 9-year history of progressive leg weakness and fasciculations had marked hex A deficiency.

Rapin I, Suzuki K, Suzuki K, Valsamis MP: Adult (chronic) GM_2 gangliosidosis. *Arch Neurol* 33:120–130, 1976.

A brother and two sisters of Ashkenazic extraction showed progressive deterioration of gait and posture beginning in childhood, muscle atrophy beginning distally, pes cavus, foot drop, spasticity, mild ataxia of limbs and trunk, dystonia, and dysarthria. Intelligence was little affected. No seizures occurred. Vision and optic fundi were normal. Hex A was decreased in the serum and leukocytes.

Mitsumoto H, Sliman RJ, Schafer IA et al: Motor neuron disease and adult hexosaminidase A deficiency in two families. *Ann Neurol* 17:378–385, 1985.

Three patients from two unrelated families presented with marked cerebellar atrophy. Dementia was found in two brothers. Juvenile spinal muscular atrophy was absent in the older brother. Hex A deficiency was in the range of that in Tay-Sachs disease homozygotes, but was higher when the natural substrate was used.

Harding AE, Young EP, Shon F: Adult onset supranuclear ophthalmoplegia, cerebellar ataxia, and neurogenic proximal muscle weakness in a brother and sister: Another hexosaminidase A deficiency syndrome. *J Neuro/Neurosurg Psychiatr* 50:687–690, 1987.

Two unrelated adults of Ashkenazi Jewish ancestry presented with a slowly progressive ataxia and muscle weakness since early age and with supranuclear ophthalmoplegia in their 40s and 50s. Hex A was severely deficient.

Pampiglione G, Harden A: Neurophysiological investigations in GM_1 and GM_2 gangliosidosis. *Neuropediatrics* 15(suppl):74–84, 1984.

Neurophysiologic investigations, especially when repeated at appropriate intervals during the evolution of the disease, allow assessment of the effect of the disease process on brain function.

Sewell AC: Urinary oligosaccharide excretion in disorders of glycolipid, glycoprotein and glycogen metabolism. A review of screening for differential diagnosis. *Eur J Pediatr* 134:183–194, 1980.

In Sandhoff's disease, oligosacchariduria can be demonstrated.

Raghavan SS, Krussell A, Krussel J, Lyerla TA, Kolodny EH: GM$_2$ ganglioside metabolism in hexosaminidase A deficiency status: Determination in situ using labeled GM$_2$ added to fibroblast cultures. *Am J Hum Genet* 37:1071–1082, 1985.

Feeding experiments with radiolabeled GM$_2$ gangliosides to mutant cells identified the presence of a block in the metabolism of GM$_2$ ganglioside.

Goebel HH: Morphology of the gangliosidoses. *Neuropediatrics* 15(suppl):97–106, 1984.

Neuropathologic features of the various gangliosidoses are reviewed.

MUCOPOLYSACCHARIDOSES

The mucopolysaccharidoses are a heterogeneous group of lysosomal storage disorders characterized by the intralysosomal accumulation of mucopolysaccharide in various tissues and by excessive urinary excretion of mucopolysaccharides. The mucopolysaccharide molecule consists of a protein core from which polysaccharide side chains arise. Degradation of mucopolysaccharides is primarily sequential and is catalyzed by specific exoenzymes (glycosidases or sulfatases). Deficiency of 10 specific lysosomal enzymes has been identified in various mucopolysaccharidoses. Deficiency of any one of these enzymes interrupts the sequence of degradation, resulting in the accumulation of mucopolysaccharides resistant to further cleavage by exoenzymes.

Based on mucopolysaccharides excreted in urine, one can distinguish four types of mucopolysaccharidoses (see Table 13-2). An excess of dermatan sulfate and heparan sulfate in urine in varying ratios may be produced by a defect in any one of the three specific enzymes responsible for the degradation of both dermatan sulfate and heparan sulfate (α-L-iduronidase, iduronate sulfatase, and β-glucuronidase). The clinical entities caused by alpha-L-iduronidase deficiency are grouped under the heading mucopolysaccharidoses I (MPS I): Hurler's syndrome,

Hurler-Scheie syndrome, and Scheie's syndrome. A same-enzyme defect results in a variable clinical picture. The clinical entity resulting from iduronate sulfatase deficiency is mucopolysaccharidosis II (MSP II): Hunter's syndrome. The clinical entity caused β-glucuronidase deficiency is mucopolysaccharidosis VII: Sly's syndrome.

Heparan sulfaturia characterizes Sanfilippo's syndrome (MPS III). This syndrome may be produced by the absence of any one of the four specific enzymes responsible for the degradation of heparan sulfate (heparan sulfate sulfatase, N-acetyl-α-D-glucosaminidase, acetyl CoA:alpha-glucosaminide-N-acetyl transferase, N-acetyglucosamine-6-sulfate sulfatase). The four forms of Sanfilippo's syndrome are not clinically distinguishable.

Keratan sulfaturia characterizes mucopolysaccharidoses IV (MPS IV) or the Morquio syndromes. The enzyme defect in classic Morquio's syndrome (type A) is a deficiency of N-acetyl-galactosamine-6-sulfate sulfatase, a special sulfatase for 6-sulfate linked to galactase. The deficient enzyme in type B Morquio syndrome is β-galactosidase (the same enzyme is deficient in GM$_1$ gangliosidosis).

Dermatan sulfaturia characterizes mucopolysaccharidosis VI (MPS VI) or Maroteaux-Lamy syndrome. This syndrome results from a defect in arylsulfatase B.

Clinically, mucopolysaccharidoses can be divided into two major groups. A first group characterized by a progressive mental and physical deterioration includes Hurler's syndrome, Hurler-Scheie syndrome, Hunter's syndrome, Sly's syndrome, and Sanfilippo's syndrome. A second group characterized by a normal or minimally reduced intelligence includes Scheie's syndrome, both Morquio syndromes, and Maroteaux-Lamy syndrome.

In the first group, Hurler's syndrome, the most severe form of mucopolysaccharidosis I (MPS I-H), is characterized by early onset in infancy. Infants with this syndrome may present at birth with inguinal and um-

TABLE 13-2. THE FOUR MUCOPOLYSACCHARIDOSES

Urinary Mucopolysaccharides	Enzyme Defects	Clinical Syndromes
Dermatan sulfate and heparan sulfate	α-L-Iduronidase	MPS I: Hurler (*) Hurler-Scheie (*) Scheie (−)
	Iduronate sulfatase	MPS II: Hunter (*)
	β-Glucuronidase	MPS VII: Sly (*)
Heparan sulfate	Heparan sulfate sulfatase	MPS III: Sanfilippo (*)
	N-acetyl-α-D-glucosaminidase	
	acetyl CoA:alpha glucosaminide-N-acetyltransferase	
	N-acetyl-glucosamine-6-sulfate sulfatase	
Keratan sulfate	Galactosamine-6-sulfate sulfatase	MPS IV-A: Morquio A (−)
	β-Galactosidase	MPS IV-B: Morquio B (−)
Dermatan sulfate	Arylsulfatase B	MPS VI: Maroteaux-Lamy (−)

(*) = with neurologic features; (−) = with few neurologic features.

FEATURE TABLE 13-4. MUCOPOLYSACCHARIDOSES

Discriminating Feature	Consistent Features	Variable Features
1. Specific deficiency in one enzyme involved in muco-polysaccharide catabolism in fibroblasts, serum, or leukocytes	1. Skeletal defects 2. Urine mucopolysaccharides 3. Lucent vacuoles and zebra bodies in bone marrow	1. Corneal clouding 2. Glaucoma 3. Retinitis pigmentosa 4. Mental retardation 5. Hydrocephalus, large head 6. Entrapment neuropathies 7. Hearing loss 8. Spinal cord compression 9. Coarse facial features 10. Joint stiffness 11. Hepatosplenomegaly 12. Abdominal hernia 13. Valvular cardiac disease 14. Recurrent infection

bilical hernias. Diagnosis is suggested during infancy by the deceleration of growth, the progressive mental deterioration, the appearance of hepatosplenomegaly associated with a protuberant abdomen, hernias, flexion contractures of the elbows and knees, lumbar lordosis, thoracic kyphosis, short neck, and coarse facial features (full lips, flared nostrils, low nasal bridge, hypertelorism, epicanthal folds, prominent forehead, bushy eyebrows, and large tongue). Teeth are widely and irregularly spaced and gums are hypertrophic. Most children have a history of recurrent upper respiratory tract infections and patients suffer from chronic nasal discharge. Hearing loss is progressive and language skills are limited. Communicating hydrocephalus is commonly present after the age of 2 or 3 years. Progressive clouding of the cornea, retinal pigmentation, and sometimes glaucoma are seen during the same period. Optic atrophy may occur. Death usually occurs in childhood secondary to respiratory tract infections or cardiac complications. Survival past the first decade is unusual.

Hurler-Scheie syndrome, the intermediate form of mucopolysaccharidosis I (MPS I-H/S), is characterized by gradual onset of symptoms during the first few years of life, with mild mental deficiency, growth failure, mild dysostosis multiplex without gibbus, and moderate joint limitations. A receding chin (micrognathism) is consistently found. Other facial features are a low nasal bridge, prominent lips, and corneal clouding. This constellation of findings is characteristic of Hurler-Scheie syndrome. Hepatomegaly, cardiac involvement, and hernias are variable. Survival past the second decade is common.

In Hunter's syndrome (MPS II), an appreciable variability in severity has been reported. Even within the same sibship variability makes prognostication difficult. A severe form has features similar to those of Hurler's syndrome, except for slower progression of somatic and CNS

deterioration and the lack of corneal clouding. Communicating hydrocephalus is frequent. Most patients die before the age of 15 years. A mild form is somewhat analogous to Hurler-Scheie syndrome except for the absence of corneal clouding and a prominent chin. The occurrence of pebbly ivory-colored skin lesions over the back, upper arms, and lateral aspects of the thigh is distinctive of Hunter's syndrome. The presence of the skin lesions does not correlate with the severity of the disease.

Patients with Sanfilippo's syndrome (MPS III) are characterized by severe CNS involvement and by only minimal somatic disease. After 3 years of seemingly normal development, hyperactivity, destructive tendencies, sleep disorders, and other behavioral aberrations are the most common presenting symptoms. There is a progressive deterioration in all mental and fine motor skills. Hypertrichosis and coarsening of facial features are progressive. Dwarfism is only moderate in degree, and skeletal abnormalities are minimal (very thick calvarium and persistent biconvex vertebral bodies). Motion of the joints usually is not restricted. The head may be enlarged. Corneal opacities are rare and discrete. Hepatosplenomegaly is mild. Involvement of the heart may occur. Usually by the age of 8 to 10 years these patients are severely retarded. Some patients may survive past the third decade.

Sly's syndrome (MPS VII) is an extremely rare disorder with considerable phenotypic variations. Mental retardation, coarse facies, and growth retardation are common features. Most patients lack corneal clouding. The clinical course is variable, with either an early fatal course or prolonged survival.

In the second group, Morquio's syndrome (MPS IV) is characterized by spondyloepiphyseal dysplasia, a severe form of skeletal dysplasia not found in other mucopolysaccharidoses. The intelligence is preserved or minimally reduced. In the classic form of Morquio's syndrome (type A), during the second year of life slowing of linear growth and progressive skeletal deformities may bring the patient to the attention of a physician. Genu valgum and short neck and trunk with prominence of the sternum (pectus carinatum) become striking. The head appears to lie directly on the shoulders. Many of the joints tend to be excessively loose, contributing to their instability. Usually the mouth is wide, the nose short, and the teeth widely spaced. Dental enamel is abnormally thin and pitted. Corneal opacities are present. Hepatomegaly and cardiac lesions may occur. Neurologic complications are cervical myelopathy secondary to atlantoaxial joint subluxation, and neurosensory hearing loss. Similar symptoms and complications are seen in type B Morquio's syndrome, a milder form that can be distinguished clinically from the classic form by the absence of enamel abnormality. Patients with the classic (type A) form of Morquio's syndrome may not survive beyond their 20s or 30s.

Maroteaux-Lamy syndrome (MPS VI) is characterized by clinically striking osseous and corneal changes without intellectual impairment. As in other lysosomal storage disorders, mild, intermediate, and severe forms are observed. The classic form has severe physical changes. Growth retardation usually brings the patient first to medical attention at the age of 2 or 3 years. Genu valgum, lumbar kyphosis, protrusion of the sternum, coarsening of the face (large nose, thickened lips, and low nasal bridge), joint stiffness with the development of claw hands, and corneal opacities are progressive. Associated neurologic complications include cervical myelopathy (secondary to atlantoaxial joint subluxation), communicating hydrocephalus, pachymeningitis, and nerve entrapment. Macrocephaly occurs. Hepatomegaly is frequently present. Involvement of the heart may occur. The longest survival of a patient with the severe form is probably into the late 20s. The mild and intermediate forms of Maroteaux-Lamy syndrome are characterized by a short stature. Vertebral subluxation does not occur in these forms.

Scheie's syndrome, the mild form of mucopolysaccharidosis I (MPS I-S), is characterized by joint stiffness, early clouding of the cornea, aortic valvular defects, and few other somatic defects. The onset of significant symptoms is usually after 5 years of age. The facies is characteristically coarse, with a broad mouth. Intelligence and stature are usually normal, although mental deterioration and psychosis may occur. Glaucoma and pigmentary degeneration of the retina may contribute to visual impairment. Carpal tunnel syndrome is a common complication. Most patients have a normal lifespan.

Radiologically, the constellation of skeletal abnormalities found in most mucopolysaccharidoses is referred to as dysostosis multiplex. The most consistent skeletal abnormality revealed by x rays is widening of the medial end of the clavicle and hypoplasia of the lateral end. The ribs have been described as oar-shaped: narrowed at their vertebral ends and flat and broad at their sternal ends. Vertebral bodies appear rounded and immature, and anterior vertebral wedging is responsible for kyphosis and thoracolumbar gibbus. The pelvis shows excessive flaring of the iliac wing with tapering of the distal iliac and the characteristic bilateral constriction superior to the acetabula. The acetabulae are shallow with an oblique roof. The long bones usually show thickening and sclerosis. The upper extremities are usually more affected than the lower. Skull x rays demonstrate thickened calvarium, premature closure of sutures, shallow orbits, and an enlarged J-shaped sella (i.e., a shallow elongated sella with a long anterior recess extending under the anterior clinoid processes). The mandible is broad with abnormal spacing of the teeth and dentigerous cysts. CT scan of the head may show hydrocephalus and thickened calvarium (Figure 13-1). Characteristic radiologic findings distinguishing Morquio's syndrome from other muco-

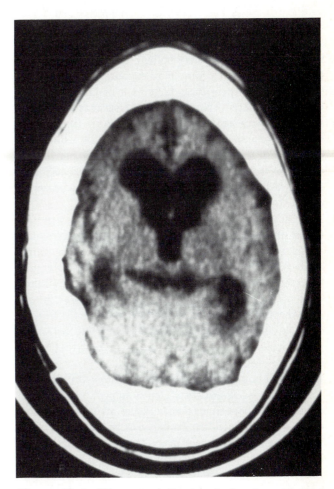

Figure 13-1. CT scan of the head showing arrested hydrocephalus and thickened calvarium in a 4-year-old black with iduronate sulfatase deficiency (Hunter's syndrome), presenting clinically with seizures, progressive mental retardation, hoarseness of voice, large head, hepatosplenomegaly, coarse facies, bushy eyebrows, low hairline, large tongue, and joint stiffness.

polysaccharidoses are, in the spine, the absence or severe hypoplasia of the odontoid process and the universal vertebra plana (spondyloepiphyseal) and, in the jaw, the absence of dentigerous cysts.

Slit lamp examination may reveal corneal opacities. Electroretinography has proved to be an effective technique for quantitative assessment of retinal involvement in mucopolysaccharidosis. Visual evoked potentials have been reported to be normal. Audiologic assessment shows virtually all patients to have some degree of peripheral sensory deficit. The EEG is frequently abnormal in patients with mental deterioration. CT scan of the head may reveal some degree of hydrocephalus in MPS I, II, and III, and IV (type A). Carpal tunnel syndrome may be demonstrated, when present, by slowing of sensory conduction of the median nerve across the wrist.

Marked mucopolysacchariduria is generally detectable by urinary screening tests. However, some patients with Sanfilippo's syndrome (MPS III), Morquio's syndrome (MPS IV), Maroteaux-Lamy syndrome (MPS VI), and Sly's syndrome (MPS VII) will be missed by certain screening tests. A quantative determination of urinary mucopolysaccharides may be helpful. However, adults with Morquio's syndrome may excrete normal keratan sulfate levels in their urine. Enzymatic diagnosis is possible for the different types of mucopolysaccharidoses. The specific enzyme activity can be measured in fibroblasts, leukocytes, amniotic cells, or chorionic villi using adequate substrates. Enzyme assays can also be performed on serum from patients with MPS I, MPS II, MPS VII, and MPS III, owing to a defect of N-acetylglucosaminidase.

Pathologically, mucopolysaccharidoses are generalized storage disorders. In the bone marrow, vacuoles with a dark basophilic granulation in their centers are found in circulating lymphocytes, bone marrow reticulocytes (Glasser cells), and bone marrow plasma cells (Buhot cells). Circulating lymphocytes may also contain metachromatic vacuoles without granulation (Mittwoch cells). Azurophilic granulations are very inconstant in polymorphonuclear leukocytes and lymphocytes (Alder-Reilly bodies). Ultrastructural studies have shown membrane-bound fibrillogranular vacuoles in all types of mucopolysaccharidoses. Dense amorphous granular material may be seen in some vacuoles. In Morquio's syndrome, the vacuoles are similar, except that myelin-like figures are frequently seen in the center of the inclusions. Storage of mucopolysaccharides in various tissues may result in collagen overproduction. The presence of ballooned cells surrounded by lakes of densely metachromatic material is characteristic of the mucopolysaccharidoses. Such findings are frequent in arterial walls (arteriosclerosis), joints, tendons, meninges, and cornea. In the viscera and CNS deposition of gangliosides besides mucopolysaccharides is a secondary phenomenon. Ultrastructural studies reveal, aside from reticulogranular vacuoles, lamellar inclusions reminiscent of zebra bodies

Pearls and Perils: Mucopolysaccharidoses

1. Dysostosis multiplex is common to mucopolysaccharidoses and mucolipidoses (except Morquio's syndrome, which is characterized by spondyloepiphyseal dysplasia).

2. Short stature is common to all mucopolysaccharidoses except MPS I-S (Scheie's syndrome) and some patients with MPS VII (Sly's syndrome).

3. Corneal clouding is common to all mucopolysaccharidoses except MPS II (Hunter's syndrome), MPS III (Sanfilippo's syndrome), and some patients with MPS IV (Sly's syndrome).

4. Joints are stiff in all mucopolysaccharidoses except MPS IV (Morquio A and B syndromes).

5. Dentigerous cysts occur in all mucopolysaccharidoses except mucopolysaccharidosis IV (Morquio's syndrome). Thin enamel allows differential diagnosis clinically between Morquio type A and type B.

6. Pebbly skin lesions over the scapula suggest MPS II (Hunter's syndrome).

7. A normal intelligence is suggestive of MPS I-S (Scheie's syndrome), MPS IV-B (Morquio B syndrome), or MPS VI (Maroteaux-Lamy syndrome). Mental retardation is most severe in MPS I-H (Hurler's syndrome) and MPS III (Sanfilippo's syndrome). Communicating hydrocephalus may develop in the severe forms of MPS associated with mental retardation.

8. Hypoplasia or aplasia of the odontoid with atlantoaxial joint subluxation is common in MPS IV (Morquio's syndrome) and severe forms of MPS VI (Maroteaux-Lamy syndrome). Compression of the spinal cord at the craniocervical junction may result. Spinal cord compression in the cervical region has also been described in Maroteaux-Lamy syndrome, in which it results from meningeal hypertrophy. Spinal cord compression in the dorsolumbar area is usually caused by gibbus deformity.

9. Mucopolysacchariduria may be missed by screens in MPS III (Sanfilippo's syndrome) and MPS VII (Sly's syndrome). Keratan sulfaturia is not unique to Morquio's syndrome and can also be found in GM_1 gangliosidosis.

10. Enzymatic diagnosis should be performed in all patients suspected to have mucopolysaccharidosis. Lysosomal enzymes are routinely assayed in serum, leukoycytes, and/or fibroblasts.

11. All reported cases of Hunter's syndrome are male.

12. The presence of lucent vacuoles and zebra bodies in various tissues is characteristic of mucopolysaccharidoses. The ultrastructural appearance of these inclusions does not permit differentiation among the different forms of mucopolysaccharidoses.

(GM₂ gangliosidosis). The neuronal storage of gangliosides may result in mental retardation.

The incidence of all mucopolysaccharidoses has been estimated at 1 in 16,000 to 30,000 live births. The three most common mucopolysaccharidoses are MPS I, MPS II, and MPS III. Mucopolysaccharidoses are panethnic diseases, with the exception of an increased incidence of Hunter's syndrome in the Jewish population in Israel and of Morquio's syndrome in French Canadians. The mucopolysaccharidoses are inherited as autosomal recessive traits with the exception of Hunter's syndrome, which is an X-linked recessive. The genes for α-L-iduronidase (deficient in MPS I), of arysulfatase B (deficient in MPS VI), and β-glucuronidase (deficient in MPS VII) have been assigned to chromosomes 22, 5, and 7, respectively. Cell hybridization studies demonstrate that Morquio type B syndrome (MPS IV-B) and GM₁ gangliosidosis belong to the same complementation group. Heterozygote identification is not routinely available.

Enzyme replacement and bone marrow transplantation are still experimental therapies. Management of mucopolysaccharidosis patients is limited to supportive care and treatment of complications. Some acute improvement in clinical function has been found after shunting. Hearing aids may be beneficial. Range of motion exercises appear to offer some benefit in preserving joint function. Physical and occupational therapy are indicated. Cardiac evaluation at regular intervals should be a part of management. Prevention of each type of mucopolysaccharidoses is possible by genetic counseling and prenatal detection.

ANNOTATED BIBLIOGRAPHY

Longdon K, Pennock CA: Abnormal keratan sulfate excretion. *Ann Clin Biochem* 16:152–154, 1979.

Finding of keratan sulfate in the urine is strong evidence for Morquio's syndrome, but mucopolysacchariduria may be missed in certain screening tests or in some older patients.

Lorincz AE, Hurst RE, Kolodny EH: The early laboratory diagnosis of mucopolysaccharidoses. *Ann Clin Lab Sci* 12:258–266, 1982.

Knowledge of the granulation nature of the urinary glycosaminoglycans coupled with their clinical manifestations can permit selection of the most appropriate enzymatic assay to establish the specific diagnosis.

Muenzer J: Mucopolysaccharidosis *Adv Pediatr* 33:269–302, 1986.

Each type of mucopolysaccharidosis has a specific lysosomal enzyme deficiency with a characteristic degree of organ involvement and rate of deterioration.

McKusick VA, Neufeld EF: The mucopolysaccharide storage disease, in Stanbury JB, Wyngaarden JB, Fredrickson DS, et al (eds): *The Metabolic Basis of Inherited Diseases*, 5th ed. New York, McGraw-Hill, 1983, p 751–777.

These authors review various aspects of mucopolysaccharidosis.

Murata F, Wohltman H, Spicer SS, Nagata T: Fine structural and ultracytochemical studies on the lymphocytes in three types of genetic mucopolysaccharidosis. *Virchows Arch B* 25:61–73, 1977.

In Morquio's syndrome the lymphocytic vacuoles contain, besides the granular material, myelin-like figures.

Mossman J, Blunt S, Stephens R, Jones EE, Pembrey M: Hunter's disease in a girl: Association with X:5 chromosomal translocation disrupting the Hunter gene. *Arch Dis Child* 58:911–915, 1983.

These authors describe a 3-year-old girl with typical Hunter's syndrome. She had an apparently balanced translocation between chromosomes X and 5 with the break in the former being between q26 and q27. This was a new mutation.

GAUCHER'S DISEASE

Gaucher's disease or glucosylceramide lipidosis is a group of lysosomal disorders characterized by the accumulation of a sphingolipid, glucosylceramide, in various tissues. Glucosylceramide is derived from the degradation of larger glycosphingolipids, such as gangliosides, in the brain and viscera, lactosylceramide in the white blood cells, and glycosphingolipids and globotetrasylceramide in red blood cells.

Gaucher's disease has been divided into three clinical subgroups, according to the presence and the severity of neurologic symptoms. Type I disease (adult type), the most common subgroup, is a nonneuronopathic chronic disorder characterized by splenomegaly with hypersplenism, pulmonary involvement, and skeletal changes. Those with early symptoms show massive splenomegaly. Episodes of bone pain and pathologic fractures of long bones or vertebrae are a feature in older children and adolescents. Pulmonary involvement may lead to pulmonary hypertension, cor pulmonale, or recurrent pneumonia. Skin hyperpigmentation and yellow-brown, wedge-shaped thickenings of the inner cornea called pinguiculae are seen in older patients. Typically, patients with type I disease rarely develop neurologic complications.

Type II disease (infantile type), much more rare, is an acute neuronopathic disorder, characterized by hepatosplenomegaly, CNS involvement, and death during infancy. Hepatosplenomegaly is invariably the first presenting sign and may be noticeable in the newborn period. Within a few months, neurologic complications develop and are almost always present by 6 months of age. Cranial nerve and brainstem abnormalities are responsible for strabismus, trismus, difficulty in swallowing, and retroflexion of the head without hyperextension of the spine, which are characteristic for this disorder. Severe and progressive spasticity, hyperreflexia, and pathologic reflexes develop. The psychomotor retardation is severe. Other difficulties include laryngeal spasm and seizures (rarely). Late in the course of the illness, the child becomes hypotonic and apathetic. Manifestations of hypersplenism may occur. Long bone x rays may show erosion with cyst-like cavities. Lung infiltrates composed of Gaucher cells may exist. Death invariably occurs before 2 years of age, usually from pulmonary infection.

Type III disease (juvenile type) is a rare subacute neuropathic disorder characterized by hepatosplenomegaly, hypersplenism, and, frequently, strabismus early in life. Other neurologic signs appear in childhood, adolescence, or adulthood. The most common neurologic symptoms are seizures and mental deterioration. Certain cases most closely resemble the acute neuronopathic variety, whereas in others the clinical course is similar in many respects to the chronic nonneuronopathic variety of the disease. Psychomotor and generalized seizures are more commonly reported than in type II disease. Myoclonus and myoclonic epilepsy may be profound and interfere with all activities. Intellectual deterioration is usually evident by about 5 years of age but may be delayed until adulthood. Mental deterioration may range from mild memory deficits to a severe global dementia of slow progression. Cranial nerves and brainstem abnormalities may occur. Other neurologic abnormalities may include spasticity, hyperreflexia, pathologic reflexes, and cerebellar ataxia. Skeletal involvement and other systemic symptoms are similar to those found in type I disease. Death may occur between the second and fourth decades.

Anemia, leukopenia, and thrombocytopenia are common. Lymphocytes are not vacuolated. The typical Gaucher cells have been found infrequently in the blood, but their detection requires careful examination of buffy coat preparations. Gaucher cells are most easily detected in marrow aspirates. The typical Gaucher cell is a large macrophage measuring 20 to 100 μm in diameter and containing one or multiple central or eccentric small nuclei. The cytoplasm is filled with fibrillary material, which gives an appearance of a "wrinkled tissue paper." The stored substance is invariably PAS positive, hematin negative, and weakly sudanophilic (even in frozen sections). On electron microscopy, membrane-bound inclusions (Gaucher bodies), ranging from 0.6 to 4 μm in diameter, are filled with "tubules" twisted around each other. These "tubules" are formed by the accumulation of polar glucosylceramide molecules. Gaucher cells are found in most tissues (e.g., spleen, liver, lymph nodes, lungs, adrenals) but not in the skin. Hepatocytes are not involved in storage of glucocerebroside. No evidence of neuronal storage is present in neurons of the gastrointestinal tract. The most characteristic CNS change is the proliferation of histiocytes in the perivascular spaces and the transformation of a few of these into Gaucher cells. The quantity of Gaucher cells increases in an anterior-posterior fashion, with the occipital lobes being the most severely affected. Solitary Gaucher cells are also found intermingled with neurons in the cerebral cortex and thalamus. The number of Gaucher cells in the CNS does not strictly correlate with the clinical severity. Loss of neurons and myelin may be noted in the vicinity of Gaucher cells in most advanced cases. Neurons are never distended by storage material. Membranous cytoplasmic bodies, less than 1 μm in diameter, containing bilayered membranous or tubular structures are occasionally found by electron microscopy in neurons of the cerebrum and cerebellum. The storage material in the neurons consists of polar glucosylceramide and psychosine (glucosylsphingosine). In those cases with the most advanced nerve cell loss, the highest levels of psychosine are found in the brain, suggesting a possible causality between intraneuronal accumulation of psychosine and neuronal degeneration.

The infiltration process seen in lung x rays of other storage diseases is infrequent in type I and type III disease, but skeletal x rays reveal characteristic findings. Such findings include flask-shaped enlargement of the distal femur with thickening and flaring of the cortexes and/or bony erosion with cyst-like cavities of various sizes. Aseptic necrosis of the femoral head and vertebral collapse may occur. CT scan of the head may reveal mild signs of atrophy in type II and type III disease. EEG may show abnormalities in all three types of Gaucher's disease. The common EEG findings are nonfocal spikes, sharp waves, and slow waves bilaterally, with photomyoclonus and

FEATURE TABLE 13–5. GAUCHER'S DISEASE

Discriminating Features	Consistent Feature	Variable Features
1. Gaucher cells in bone marrow and other tissues, except skin 2. Glucocerebroside deficiency in leukocytes, serum, and skin	1. Hepatosplenomegaly	1. Anemia 2. Fractures 3. Cirrhosis 4. Pinguicula 5. Spasticity 6. Opisthotonos 7. Horizontal oculomotor apraxia 8. Myoclonic seizures 9. Ataxia 10. Mental retardation 11. Cranial nerve involvement

photoconvulsive paroxysmal activity. EEG changes are more common in advanced stages and among splenectomized patients. Electromyography and nerve conduction velocities are normal. CSF is usually normal except when severe kyphosis leads to an elevated protein level, indicating a spinal block. Ancillary laboratory findings in the serum may include an elevation in activities of non–tartrate-inhibitable acid phosphatase and angiotensin-converting enzyme. The confirmation of the diagnosis may be obtained by measuring the quantity of glucocerebroside in tissues and serum. Although reliable procedures are available to quantify glucocerebroside, the preferred method of making the diagnosis is by direct assay of glucocerebrosidase activity in the leukocytes, skin fibroblasts, or amniocytes. The determination of enzyme activity is most reliably achieved with natural substrates. Because glucocerebrosidase is tightly bound to subcellular components, measuring β-glucosidase activity in particles may improve the diagnostic accuracy over that obtained by the assay of whole homogenates. However, these tests do not give an accurate prediction as to whether neurologic symptoms will appear. The severity of the enzyme defect, as measured by quantitative assay, is unrelated to the severity of the clinical course or type of clinical manifestations. Discrimination between the three clinical subtypes based on heat stability, or immunoblotting, has been achieved to some extent, although no single test can reliably predict the clinical course in a given patient. Recently, this biochemical characterization has been brought to the molecular level with the description of a specific mutation in the glucocerebrosidase gene. The high frequency of this mutation in patients with neuronopathic Gaucher's disease appears promising for the identification of patients who will have the neurologic sequelae of Gaucher's disease.

All three types of Gaucher's disease are inherited as autosomal recessive traits. In general, if one sibling has one clinical type of Gaucher disease, another affected sibling will have the same form, although the symptoms may differ significantly. Ethnic predilection only exists for type I disease, with an incidence in Ashkenazi Jews of about 1 in 2500 births. The absence of functional complementation between phenotypes in somatic cell hybridization studies suggests that the phenotypes of these disorders are a result of allelic mutations in the structural gene for glucocerebrosidase. The glucocerebrosidase gene is encoded on chromosome 1. The cDNA sequence predicts a primary polypeptide of 516 aminoacids. A leader peptide is removed from the precursor and the addition of a carbohydrate (mannose-6-phosphate) occurs as part of the posttranslational processing and lysosomal targeting. A single base change in the glucocerebrosidase gene results in the synthesis of catalytically defective glucocerebrosidases that are abnormally processed or improperly compartmentalized. Prenatal diagnosis has long been available for families at risk for additional children

---

Pearls and Perils:
Gaucher's Disease

1. The neurologic triad—strabismus, trismus, and retroflexion of the head—and its association with hepatosplenomegaly are suggestive of type II Gaucher's disease. Strabismus as an isolated neurologic symptom does not allow differentiation between type II and type III disease.
2. Patients with type II or type III disease have no clinical or neurophysiologic signs of peripheral nerve involvement.
3. Gaucher cells from bone marrow aspirate must be differentiated from foam cells seen in Niemann-Pick disease. Gaucher cells are commonly multinucleated and their cytoplasm has a "wrinkled tissue paper" appearance. Gaucher cells are not found in the skin.
4. Gaucher-like cells are found in patients with unusually rapid turnover in the marrow, i.e., those with leukemia, thalassemia, or multiple myeloma.
5. Gaucher bodies are only occasionally seen in neurons.
6. Caution is advised in recommending splenectomy.

---

with type II Gaucher's disease. Heterozygote detection is possible but the process has not come into widespread use.

Supportive therapy in Gaucher's disease is difficult. Splenectomy is advisable when hypersplenism develops. However, total splenectomy is followed by a high mortality from sepsis, an increase in bone involvement with osteolytic changes within a few months of surgery, and rapid deterioration of the neurologic status in patients with type II or type III diseases. Therefore, it has been suggested that splenectomy be postponed or avoided if at all possible. Partial splenectomy has been advocated with the dual goals of avoiding postsplenectomy sepsis and minimizing the deleterious effects of glucosylceramide on bones, liver, and the CNS. Specific enzyme replacement has been attempted with variable success. Delivery of exogenous enzyme by infusion of purified glucocerebrosidase has been of limited value. Organ grafts as a source of enzymes have largely been unsuccessful. Bone marrow transplants have been shown to normalize leukocyte glucocerebrosidase activity and improve bone involvement. No evidence exists at present to demonstrate that bone marrow transplants will increase glucocerebrosidase activity in the CNS, and their usefulness might be limited to nonneuronopathic cases of Gaucher's disease. More recently, somatic gene therapy has been suggested. A functional cDNA for the human enzyme has been introduced into a retroviral vector. It is possible that retroviral infection of bone marrow stem cells will prove to be as effective as bone marrow transplants and with less risk. The advantages of somatic gene therapy in neuronopathic cases of Gaucher's disease remain very speculative.

ANNOTATED BIBLIOGRAPHY

Brady, RO, Barranger JA: Glucosylceramide lipidosis: Gaucher's disease, in Stanbury JB, Wyngaarden JB, Fredrickson DS, Goldstein JL, Brown MS (eds): *The Metabolic Basis of Inherited Disease*, 5th ed. New York, McGraw-Hill, 1983, p 842–856.

Patients with type II disease (acute neuronopathic) have cranial nerve and brainstem abnormalities, in addition to hepatosplenomegaly. Patients with type III disease (chronic neuronopathic) have systemic symptoms similar to those of type I, but neurologic signs appear during childhood or adolescence.

Gravel RA, Leung A: Complementation analysis in Gaucher disease using single cell microassay techniques. Evidence for a single "Gaucher gene." *Hum Genet* 65:112–116, 1983.

The absence of functional complementation between phenotypes in somatic cell hybridization studies suggests that the phenotypes of this disorder are each a result of different allelic mutations.

Nishimura R, Omos-Lau N, Ajmone-Marsan C, Barranger JA: Electroencephalographic findings in Gaucher disease. *Neurology* 30:152–159, 1980.

Patients who appear to have the type I form of the disease but actually have type III may be distinguished by EEG. These patients are more likely to have EEG abnormalities and eventually may develop characteristic 6- to 10-Hz multiple spikes and rhythmic sharp waves diffusely but most prominently over the occipital region. Spike-wave complex discharges are also seen.

Bar-Maor JA, Govrin-Yehudain J: Partial splenectomy in children with Gaucher's disease. *Pediatrics* 76:398–401, 1985.

Partial splenectomy is preferred to total splenectomy. The immune status following the procedure is far better and the remaining spleen can be a future reservoir for storage of glucosylceramide.

Blom S, Erikson A: Gaucher disease—Norrbottnian type. Neurodevelopment, neurological, and neurophysiological aspects. *Eur J Pediatr* 140:316–322, 1983.

Neurologic abnormalities were mainly found in splenectomized patients after the first decade of life.

Nilson O, Svennerholm L: Accumulation of glucosylceramide and glucosylsphingosine (psychosine) in cerebrum and cerebellum in infantile and juvenile Gaucher disease. *J Neurol Chem* 39:709–726, 1982.

This study suggests that glucosphingonine within type II and type III Gaucher brains causes neuronal cell death.

Svennerholm L, Mansson JE, Rosengreen B: Cerebroside-beta-glucosidase activity in Gaucher brain. *Clin Genet* 30:131–135, 1986.

Cerebroside β-glucosidase activity in the brain is lower in type II disease than in type III disease.

Tsuji S, Choudary PV, Martin BM, et al: A mutation in the human glucocerebrosidase gene in neuronopathic Gaucher's disease. *N Engl J Med* 316:570–575, 1987.

In neuronopathic Gaucher's disease a specific mutation in the glucocerebrosidase gene is described.

NIEMANN-PICK DISEASE

Niemann-Pick disease or sphingomyelin lipidosis is a heterogeneous group of lysosomal disorders characterized by the accumulation of varying degrees of the phosphosphingolipid sphingomyelin in certain tissues. Sphingomyelin is a normal component of all cell membranes. The amount of sphingomyelin in each tissue and the rate of its accumulation determine the clinical course of the disease. Sphingomyelin is hydrolyzed by several specific phosphodiesterases called sphingomyelinases. In Niemann-Pick disease, the acid sphingomyelinase, a lysosomal enzyme, is deficient when the neutral nonlysosomal sphingomyelinase is not. One can distinguish two groups of Niemann-Pick disease. A first group (type A and B disease) is characterized by a severe and generalized sphingomyelinase deficiency. A second group (type C disease) is characterized by a partial and frequently less severe sphingomyelinase deficiency.

Type A disease, an acute neurovisceral form, is the most common form of Niemann-Pick disease. Type A is characterized by hepatosplenomegaly and severe early neurologic involvement. Cholestatic jaundice may appear immediately after birth or during the neonatal period, but usually disappears after 3 or 4 months. Hepatosplenomegaly may be present at birth but almost certainly becomes evident by 6 months of life. The organomegaly is responsible for feeding difficulties and failure to thrive. The infants typically become emanciated and have a protuberant abdomen. In spite of the extensive involvement of the liver and the spleen, only moderate hematologic changes occur, and liver function tests are generally normal. Delayed development and progressive loss of already acquired motor skills soon occur. By the age of 1 year, mental retardation is usually evident. Diffuse floppiness with hyporeflexic extremities is observed. No fasciculations are present. Peripheral neuropathy is demonstrated by neurophysiologic studies, nerve biopsy, or both. Patients may have an atypical "cherry-red spot" abnormality at the fovea. Mild corneal clouding and lens opacification may occur. Mild adenopathies and a fine xanthomatous rash appear during the second year. The child slowly becomes apathetic, blind, and deaf. Pupils become areflexic to light. Seizures are present occasionally, but they are not as common as in Tay-Sachs disease. Death usually occurs before the fourth year of life.

Type B disease, a chronic visceral form, is a rare disorder, characterized by organomegaly and diffuse infiltration of the lungs. Enlargement of the spleen is usually the first manifestation of the disorder and may develop as early as in type A disease, although a slightly later onset is more typical. Hepatomegaly becomes evident later. There is little, if any, impairment of liver function. During the first decade of life, no functional neurologic difficulty is apparent, although a subtle type of cherry-red spot, termed a "macular halo," and reduced peripheral nerve conduction velocity may be detected. Not infrequently, these patients are in the lowest percentile for growth and height. Sexual immaturity has been reported. Raised macular skin rash may be noted on extremities, face, and neck. Susceptibility to respiratory infections and dyspnea on exertion are common complaints. The clinical course is usually chronic with patients surviving into late adulthood; less frequently, they may succumb in the first few years of life from overwhelming infections.

Type C disease is a clinically pleomorphic chronic neurovisceral form, characterized by a variable degree of visceromegaly and a slow progression of the neurologic symptoms. Hepatosplenomegaly is less striking than in type A and type B Niemann-Pick disease. The liver is frequently normal in size and the splenomegaly may improve with age. Transient cholestasis and altered liver function tests are noted in 25% of the patients for the first several months of life. Neurologic development is normal during the first year of life. In most patients, onset of neurologic signs occurs between the ages of 2 and 10 years. The earliest neurologic changes are delayed motor development and poor school performance. In some patients with a protracted course, neurologic abnormalities may only begin between the second and fourth decades (Nova Scotia variant). Signs of dementia and ataxia are insidious in onset. Dystonia or choreoathetosis may be a presenting complaint. Emotional lability, slurred speech, and dysphagia slowly become prominent. Major motor seizures and a variety of minor motor seizures characterized by akinetic, myoclonic absence attacks (as well as gelastic seizures) may appear early. Most patients demonstrate increased myotactic reflexes. Spranuclear ophthalmoplegia (normal vertical oculocephalic response and abnormal vertical optokinetic nystagmus) is the most consistent neurologic finding. Funduscopic exam is normal. The clinical course is variable, with some patients dying during childhood and others surviving into adulthood.

In type A and type B Niemann-Pick disease, assessment of nerve conduction velocities may provide evidence of peripheral nerve involvement. ERG may show marked reduction of the wave when visual evoked potentials are only slightly abnormal. In type A disease, slit lamp examination may reveal corneal and lenticular opacifications. In both type A and B disease, chest radiography frequently shows diffuse bilateral interstitial infiltrates. CT scan of the head may be consistent with cerebral atrophy. Blood chemistry may reveal some degree of liver disease. Serum lipids usually are normal, but in some patients cholesterol is increased. An accurate diagnosis of type A or type B Niemann-Pick disease is achieved by demonstrating a profound deficiency of the sphingomyelinase activity in peripheral leukocytes, cultured fibroblasts, or cultured amniotic fluid cells. An in vitro assay of the enzyme is sensitive enough. For diagnosis of type C Niemann-Pick disease, in vivo metabolic studies in cultured fibroblasts are more reliable to demonstrate a partial sphingomyelinase deficiency.

Hematologic investigations may reveal neutropenia and thrombocytopenia on peripheral smear. Patients with Niemann-Pick disease may show discrete vacuoles in the cytoplasm of lymphocytes. These vacuoles stain negative with PAS and Sudan stains. Bone marrow aspirates show collections of Niemann-Pick cells in type A disease and in younger patients with type B disease. These cells are large macrophages 20 to 90 µm in diameter, smaller than Gaucher cells, with one or two but rarely many nuclei. The abundant pale cytoplasm is filled with lipid droplets, fairly uniform in size and highly refractable, which give a honeycombed or foamy appearance to the cells. In frozen preparations, the stored substance is invariably sudanophilic and stains unspecifically for unsaturated fatty acids and phospholipids. Under polarization microscopy many granules are birefringent. The presence of lipopigment is indicated by the appearance of a greenish-yellow autofluorescence under ultraviolet light. It is possible to demonstrate sphingomyelin histochemically with the ferric-hematoxylin method. The Schultz reaction is positive for cholesterol. The PAS reaction and the stain test for acid phosphatase may be weakly positive.

FEATURE TABLE 13-6. NIEMANN-PICK DISEASE

Discriminating Feature	Consistent Feature	Variable Features
1. Sphingomyelinase deficiency in fibroblasts and leukocytes	1. Hepatosplenomegaly	1. Failure to thrive 2. Psychomotor delay 3. Peripheral neuropathy 4. Atypical cherry-red spot 5. Vertical oculomotor apraxia 6. Seizures 7. Ataxia 8. Dystonia 9. Spasticity

In older patients with type B disease, the most prominent cells in the bone marrow are sea-blue histiocytes. These macrophages are overfilled with ceroid and stain green-blue with Wright or Giemsa stain. In type C disease, foam cells of the bone marrow have nonuniform vacuoles. They stain diffusely with PAS, suggesting glycolipid storage. In older patients, sea-blue histiocytes containing ceroid are found. On electron microscopy, the cytoplasmic vacuoles are resolved as polymorphic membrane-bound inclusions ranging from 1 to 5 μm in diameter that often contain concentrically laminated myelin-like figures with a periodicity of about 5 nm. Sometimes, the lysosomal configurations take the form of parallel palisaded lamellae, creating so-called "zebra bodies." There are occasional foci of electron-dense granular nodules, either on the surface or incorporated into these inclusions, which represent ceroid deposition. Besides the bone marrow, Niemann-Pick cells and sea-blue histiocytes are found in most organs (e.g., liver, spleen, lymph nodes, thymus, tonsils, adrenal medulla, lungs). Deposits of sphingomyelin are also found in other areas (e.g., hepatocytes, capillaries).

In both type A and type B disease, peripheral nerve involvement may be demonstrated by nerve biopsy. It has been shown that axonal degeneration is not a feature of this neuropathy. The brain in patients with type A and type C Niemann-Pick disease shows deep and cortical atrophy. The cortex is softer than usual and the underlying white matter is indurated. The cerebellum is sclerotic. Examination with the light microscope reveals vacuolization and ballooning of the large neurons, which in time leads to cell death and loss of brain substance. Neuronal loss is often accompanied by glial proliferation. This neuronal involvement is diffuse through the cerebrum, cerebellum, brainstem, and spinal cord, and extends to the ganglion cells in the peripheral plexuses as well. Ganglion cells of the retina are also swollen. Foam cells are frequently observed in the meninges. In frozen sections, neurons are sudanophilic and give a positive acid hematin reaction in type A disease. In type C disease, neurons are only weakly sudanophilic and give a negative acid hematin reaction. In type C disease, particularly in younger patients, a strong similarity to neuroaxonal dystrophy is suggested by the abundance of axonal spheroids found in the white matter. On electron microscopy, the ballooned neurons in type A Niemann-Pick disease contain membranous cytoplasmic bodies similar to those observed in Tay-Sachs disease. In type C disease, neuronal inclusions are polymorphous and smaller than in type A. They contain less numerous and more irregular membranes, and have a large dark or light membrane-free core. Contrary to the relatively uniform axonal spheroids of Seitelberger disease, axonal spheroids in Niemann-Pick type C have a pleormorphic ultrastructure, reflecting the participation of a variety of organelles, including neurofilaments.

Biochemical analysis of the tissues reveals striking

Pearls and Perils:
Niemann-Pick Disease

1. Niemann-Pick cells can very easily be distinguished from Gaucher's cells. Foam cells resembling those seen in Niemann-Pick disease are also observed in Wolman's disease, Tay-Sachs disease, Batten disease, sea-blue histiocyte syndrome, generalized gangliosidosis (infantile GM_1 gangliosidosis type I), and chronic granulomatous syndrome of childhood.
2. Peripheral neuropathy may be demonstrated by neurophysiologic studies and/or nerve biopsy in type A and type B Niemann-Pick disease.
3. Infants with type A Niemann-Pick disease are typically emaciated with a protuberant abdomen. Finding of a macular cherry-red spot excludes the diagnosis of Wolman's disease.
4. Type C Niemann-Pick disease should be suspected in patients with supranuclear ophthalmoplegia, dystonia, and splenomegaly. No funduscopic abnormality is found in those patients.
5. Splenomegaly is never severe enough to require splenectomy.

---

differences between group I and group II disease. In group I (type A and B) disease, a striking increase in sphingomyelin content is found in most organs, including the brain. Bis (monoglyceryl) phosphate, although a minor component, is regularly detected in tissues. In group II (type C) disease, there is great regional variability of sphingomyelin storage. No excess of sphingomyelin is found in the brain. The accumulated material in the neurons is a glycolipid. Storage of glycolipids in all cells affected (hepatocytes, neurons, foam cells) may be explained by a partial glucocerebrosidase deficiency found in addition to the partial sphingomyelinase deficiency. The original case of lactosylceramidosis may be reclassified as type C disease.

Niemann-Pick disease is panethnic, but the majority of patients with the classic infantile form (type A) have an Ashkenazi Jewish ancestry. No racial predilection is found in other types of Niemann-Pick disease. The disease is transmitted as an autosomal recessive trait. The gene frequency is not well established, although type A has been estimated to occur in about 1 in 100 Ashkenazi Jews. The affected siblings in a single family always manifest the same type of disorder. On the basis of somatic cell hybridization studies, type A and type B Niemann-Pick disease have been shown to be allelic disorders. Type C appears to be under a separate genetic control. Heterozygotes for type A and type B disease may be identified by determining sphingomyelinase activity in fresh peripheral leukocyte preparations or extracts of cultured skin fibroblasts. Heterozygotes for type C may be identified by the direct ultrastructural examination of skin biopsy material. It has been shown that the primary mutation in type C disease is associated with a defect in cholesterol esterification, after internalization and lysosomal processing of lipoprotein cholesterol and before the intervention of acyl CoA-cholesterol acyltransferase. A partial expression of the cholesterol esterification defect is expected in human heterozygotes.

No curative therapy is available and supportive therapy should be provided to improve the quality of survival. Preventive therapy includes genetic counseling and prenatal diagnosis. In type A and type B disease prenatal diagnosis has been achieved by demonstrating sphingomyelinase deficiency on cultured amniotic fluid cells and chorionic villi. Decreased sphingomyelinase activity has been reported in amniotic fluid and cultured amniotic cells of a fetus with autopsy-proven type C disease.

ANNOTATED BIBLIOGRAPHY

Elleder M, Cihula J: Niemann-Pick disease (variation in the sphingomyelinase deficient group). *Eur J Pediatr* 140:323–328, 1983.

These authors report a variant of the neurovisceral (type A) phenotype of Niemann-Pick disease characterized by an abnormal protracted clinical course and variable expression of neurologic symptomatology in two siblings. Sphingomyelinase activity was profoundly deficient in peripheral leukocytes and in the liver tissue (when examined). The dominant neurologic symptoms in three cases included extrapyramidal involvement (rigidity, hypokinesia) and progressive dementia. A cherry-red spot was found in all the patients.

Elleder M, Nevoral J, Spicakova V, et al: A new variant of sphingomyelinase deficiency (Niemann-Pick): Visceromegaly, minimal neurological lesions and low in vivo degradation rate of sphingomyelin. *J Inher Metab Dis* 9:357–366, 1986.

Three patients with phenotype consistent with type B disease showed low values of in vivo sphingomyelinase activity consistent with those usually found in type A disease.

Elleder M, Jirasek A, Smid F, Ledvinova J, Besley GTN, Stopekova M: Niemann-Pick disease type C with enhanced glycolipid storage. Report on further case of so-called lactosylceramidosis. *Virchows Arch A* 402:307–317, 1984.

The so-called lactosylceramidosis may well be explained as Niemann-Pick type C disease with enhanced visceral storage of the glycolipid lactosylceramide.

Gilbert EF, Callahan J, Viseskul C, Opitz JM: Niemann-Pick disease type C: Pathological, histochemical, ultrastructural and biochemical studies. *Eur J Pediatr* 136:263–274, 1981.

Two sisters who died at ages 8 and 7 years after a progressive CNS degeneration were shown to have normal total sphingomyelinase activity in the liver and spleen. However, by isoelectric focusing, sphingomyelinase activity in the range of pI 4.6 to 5.2 was markedly reduced, whereas normal amounts of more acidic components were found.

Federico A, Palmeri S, Van Diggelen O, Ferrari E, Guazzi GC: Juvenile dystonia without vertical gaze paralysis: Niemann-

Pick type C disease. *J Inher Metab Dis* 9(suppl 2):314–316, 1986.

Niemann-Pick disease type C has to be suspected in subjects presenting only with mild dystonia and rare myoclonus, even in the absence of organomegaly or vertical supranuclear ophthalmoplegia.

Wenger DA, Barth G, Githens JH: Nine cases of sphingomyelin lipidosis, a new variant in Spanish-American children. *Am J Dis Child* 131:955–961, 1977.

Clinical and enzymatic findings in juvenile variant of Niemann-Pick disease (type C) are discussed. Foamy and sea-blue histiocytes were found in bone marrow.

Levade T, Salvayre R, Douste-Blazy L: Sphingomyelinase and Niemann-Pick disease. *J Clin Chem Clin Biochem* 24:205–220, 1986.

The potential sources of error in sphingomyelinase assays are reviewed.

Vanier MT, Rousson R, Garcia I, et al: Biochemical studies in Niemann-Pick disease. III. In vitro and in vivo assays of sphingomyelin degradation in skin fibroblasts and amniotic fluid cells for the diagnosis of the various forms of the disease. *Clin Genet* 27:20–32, 1985.

For the diagnosis of type C Niemann-Pick disease, the in vivo test gives more reproducible results than the in vitro assay.

Landrieu P, Said G: Peripheral neuropathy in type A Niemann-Pick disease. A morphological study. *Acta Neuropathol* 63:66–71, 1984.

These authors demonstrate that axonal degeneration is not a feature in the peripheral neuropathy of type A and B disease.

Landas S, Foucar K, Sando GN, Ellefson R, Hamilton HE: Adult Niemann-Pick disease masquerading as sea-blue histiocytes syndrome: Report of a case confirmed by lipid analysis and enzyme assays. *Am J Hematol* 20:391–400, 1985.

In one adult, hypercholesterolemia and coronary artery diseases were associated with type B Niemann-Pick disease.

Matthews JD, Weiter JJ, Kolodny IH: Macular halos associated with Niemann-Pick type B disease. *J Ophthalmol* 93:933–937, 1986.

Macular halos are elevated, doughnut-shaped, white rings around the fovea that are pathognomonic of Niemann-Pick type B disease.

Walton DS, Robb RM, Crocker AC: Ocular manifestations of group A Niemann-Pick disease. *Am J Opthalmol* 85:174–180, 1978.

Besides the cherry-red spot abnormality of the fovea, brown granular lens abnormality and mild diffuse corneal opacification are observed.

ALPER'S DISEASE

Alper's disease, or poliodystrophia cerebri progressiva, is probably a heterogeneous group of diffuse progressive degenerative diseases of the gray matter of the cerebrum, with characteristic clinical and pathologic features. No neuronal storage is found. Some cases may result from a disturbance in neuronal pyruvate metabolism.

Clinically, the illness usually starts in the first weeks of life or late in childhood with seizures or myoclonus, which may be stimulus sensitive. Microcephaly may be

FEATURE TABLE 13-7. ALPER'S DISEASE

Discriminating Feature	Consistent Features	Variable Features
1. Spongiosis, neuronal loss, and astrocytosis, which progresses down through the brain cortex	1. Intractable seizures 2. Liver dysfunction	1. Clinical evidence of liver disease 2. Failure to thrive 3. Developmental delay 4. Ataxia 5. Hypotonia 6. Myoclonus 7. Progressive spasticity 8. Deafness 9. Blindness with optic atrophy 10. Microcephaly (late)

present at birth. Psychomotor retardation is prominent in early infancy. Other infants present with failure to thrive and feeding difficulties. The disorder is steadily progressive and characterized by spasticity, flexion contracture, hyperreflexia, dementia, seizures, blindness, and deafness. Infantile spasms may occur. Dysphagia appears late in the illness. Some instances of terminal jaundice have been described. Most patients die before 3 years of age in a decerebrate state.

EEG is variable yet often shows diffuse abnormalities with low-voltage background and numerous multifocal paroxysmal discharges. Visual evoked potentials are frequently abnormal. Nerve conduction studies and electromyogram are usually normal. CT scan of the head may show severe cortical atrophy as suggested by widened sulci and distended subarachnoid spaces. CSF proteins are usually normal. An elevated blood lactate and lactate/pyruvate ratio may be found intermittently in some patients. Biochemic evidence of liver disease may precede the onset of seizures. Diagnosis of Menkes's disease should be excluded.

In Alper's disease the brain is small with a striking cerebral cortical atrophy, giving it a "walnut" appearance. The cerebellum and brainstem are relatively spared. One cerebral hemisphere may be affected more than the other. In most cases, striate calcarine cortex is more severely involved. On coronal sections, the cortex is thin, granular, and discolored. The white matter of the centrum semiovale is symmetrically narrowed, but is of a normal white appearance. Involvement of basal ganglia is variable.

Histologic examination shows extensive pseudolaminar destruction of the nerve cells in the cerebral cortex, usually most severe and accompanied by status spongiosus in the third and often the fifth layer. There is marked astrocytic gliosis, involving both the cortex and the greatly reduced white matter. Alzheimer type II astrocytes are often present in the basal ganglia. Status spongiosus of the cortex is due to vacuolation of neuronal

processes and hydrotic swelling of astroglia. Minor developmental abnormalities in the form of ectopic neurons in the white matter and immature ganglionic cells in the cerebral cortex may be found. Electron microscopy may reveal enlarged mitochondria in the neuronal processes.

Liver biopsy may show disorganized hepatic architecture with regenerative nodules, dense fibrosis, bile duct proliferation, fatty changes, hepatocyte loss, and often cirrhosis. Acute pancreatitis with fat necrosis may also occur.

The frequency of Alper's disease is not known. Several families with multiple affected siblings have been reported. The mode of inheritance in these families is autosomal recessive. Various defects in mitochondrial metabolism have been found. Many authors have drawn attention to the morphologic similarities between Alper's disease and adult transmissible spongiform encephalopathies, such as Creutzfeldt-Jakob disease. A transmissible spongiform encephalopathy was recently reported by Manuelidis and Rorke in a 2½-year-old girl with Alper's disease.

There is no effective therapy.

Pearls and Perils: Alper's Disease

1. Convulsions and progressive microcephaly in early life distinguish Alper's disease from Canavan's disease.
2. Signs of liver disease should be sought. The liver is usually not enlarged.
3. Diagnosis of Alper's disease is established on the basis of characteristic clinical and pathologic features.
4. Alper's disease must be differentiated from Menkes's syndrome and the congenital form of neuronal ceroid lipofuscinosis.

ANNOTATED BIBLIOGRAPHY

Sandbank V, Lerman P: Progressive cerebral poliodystrophy—Alper's disease: Disorganized giant neuronal mitochondria on electron microscopy. *J Neurol Neurosurg Psychiatr* 35:749–755, 1972.

In a case of Alper's disease with elevated blood lactate level and elevated lactate/pyruvate ratio, a brain biopsy specimen was obtained and abnormal mitochrondria were found in neurons.

Jellinger K, Seitelberger F: Spongy encephalopathies in infancy: Spongy degeneration of CNS and progressive infantile poliodystrophy, in Goldensohn ES, Apple SH (eds): *Scientific Approaches to Clinical Neurology*, Vol 1. Philadelphia, Lea & Febiger, 1977, p 363–386.

A positive family history is found in 26 cases of Alper's disease. The mode of inheritance in these families is autosomal recessive.

Blackwood W, Buxton PH, Cumings JN, Robertson DJ, Tucker SM: Diffuse cerebral degeneration in infancy (Alper's disease). *Arch Dis Child* 38:193–204, 1963.

The progressive nature of the pathologic process is demonstrated by comparing biopsies taken early in the course of the disease with postmortem findings.

Gabreels FJM, Prick MJJ, Trijbels JMF, et al: Defects in citric acid cycle and the electron transport chain in progressive poliodystrophy. *Acta Neurol Scand* 70:145–154, 1984.

In five children with progressive infantile poliodystrophy, a disturbance of pyruvate metabolism was found in muscle and liver tissues, except for one case in which the defect was restricted to the brain tissue.

Harding BN: Progressive neuronal degeneration of childhood with liver disease (Alpers-Huttenlocher syndrome): A personal review. *J Child Neurol* 5:273–387, 1990.

Thirty-two autopsied cases of progressive neuronal degeneration of childhood with liver disease are reviewed.

Manuelidis EE, Rorke LB: Transmission of Alper's disease (chronic progressive encephalopathy) produces experimental Cruetzfeldt-Jakob disease in hamsters. *Neurology* 39:615–621, 1989.

A 2½-year-old girl with Alper's disease is shown to have a transmissible spongiform encephalopathy.

Leukoencephalopathies

METACHROMATIC LEUKODYSTROPHY

Metachromatic leukodystrophy or sulfatide lipidosis is a heterogeneous group of lysosomal storage disorders. The biochemic defect has been localized in the catabolism of a sphingolipid sulfatide, which is a normal constituent of myelin and cellular membranes. Sulfatide is stored in the lysosomes of the CNS, chiefly in the white matter, as well as in many somatic tissues. The metachromasia, for which the disorder is named, results from a shift of the absorption spectrum of certain cationic aniline blue stains (i.e., cresyl violet at an acid pH) toward red in the presence of the highly polar anionic sulfatide.

Clinically, at least four forms of metachromatic leukodystrophy can be distinguished. The late infantile form is the most common. The first clinical symptoms begin insidiously between the first and second years of life. The clinical picture is characterized by progressive motor losses and dysfunctions. Motor symptoms characteristically occur early and are more prominent than seizures and mental deterioration. A frequent early problem is a gait disorder, with unsteadiness. This leads within months to the loss of the ability to walk and stand. An increase in myotatic reflexes may occur in the early stage, to be replaced later by decreased reflexes. Bilateral extensor toe responses occur early and persist. Speech deteriorates as a result of dysarthria and aphasia. Ataxia and truncal titubation become obvious. Intermittent pain is a manifestation of peripheral neuropathy. Nystagmus is present. Optic atrophy and a grayish discoloration of the macula are occasionally observed. The

Hypotonia is progressively replaced by rigidity and spasticity. Megalencephaly is frequently noted. Most children are bedridden by age 3. All meaningful contact with the surroundings is progressively lost. An opisthotonic posture with flexion of the arms and equinovarus posture and scissoring of the legs are present in later stages of the illness. The final stage may last for a few months to several years.

The juvenile form has its onset between 4 and 10 years. The majority of cases develop during the first years of school with bradykinesia and poor school performance. Daydreaming, confusion, or emotional lability may be seen early. Unsteadiness of the gait, usually owing to pyramidal system involvement, may occur. Extrapyramidal dysfunction—as suggested by postural abormalities, rigidity, and tremor—may also develop. Frank cerebral signs are less common. Myotactic reflexes are usually increased. The rate of deterioration is usually slower and more variable than in the late infantile form. Patients often are not bedridden 5 to 10 years after symptoms begin.

The adult form has its onset any time after puberty. Initial symptoms consist of personality and mental changes. Such symptoms are often misdiagnosed as schizophrenia or manic-depressive illness. Disorders of movements and posture appear later. There are usually no clinical signs of peripheral neuropathy.

A rare variant of metachromatic leukodystrophy combines features of the mucopolysaccharidosis and X-linked ichthyosis with those of metachromatic leukodystrophy. It is frequently called mucosulfatidosis. The

FEATURE TABLE 13-8. METACHROMATIC LEUKODYSTROPHY

Discriminating Features	Consistent Features	Variable Features
1. Metachromasia of peripheral nerves 2. Large amount of sulfatides in urine	1. Mental deterioration 2. Ataxia 3. Extensor toe signs 4. Reduced or absent sensory action potential 5. Arylsufatase deficiency in fibroblasts or white blood cells (most cases)	1. Hypotonia (early) or spasticity (late) 2. Myotactic reflexes increased (early) or decreased (late) 3. Strabismus 4. Visual impairment 5. Psychiatric symptoms 6. Extrapyramidal dysfunction 7. Seizures (rarely) 8. Elevated CSF proteins 9. Slow motor conduction velocity 10. Mucopolysaccharidosis-like symptoms (rarely)

mucopolysacharidosis-like features include a mild gargoylism (facial changes with depressed bridge of the nose), growth retardation, limitation in extension of the elbows, radiologic changes of dysostosis multiplex, hepatosplenomegaly, and deafness. Corneal opacities do not occur. Ichthyosis, when present, develops at an early age. In general, presymptomatic development is less advanced than that of late infantile metachromatic leukodystrophy. Most children never achieve normal gait or speech. Neurologic regression follows the pattern of late infantile metachromatic leukodystrophy. By 4 to 5 years, the child is profoundly retarded, with quadriplegia, pseudobulbar paralysis, and optic atrophy.

A number of laboratory tests may reinforce a clinical suspicion of metachromatic leukodystrophy. CSF studies may show an elevated protein concentration. Nerve conduction studies may demonstrate slow nerve conduction velocities or an increase in duration and number of potential components. In the adult form, nerve conduction studies and CSF proteins may be normal. EEG abnormalities are diffuse and nonspecific. Multimodality evoked potentials may reveal a latency prolongation or loss of evoked potential components that is dependent on the type of metachromatic leukodystrophy (late infantile, juvenile, or mucosulfatidosis) and on the duration of the disease. MRI is more sensitive than CT scan of the head, and allows earlier recognition and more precise characterization of areas of demyelination (Figure 13-2). When mucosulfatidosis is suspected, additional clinical laboratory tests should include skeletal x ray series and examination of the peripheral blood smear for Alder-Reilly granules.

The diagnosis of metachromatic leukodystrophy is confirmed by demonstrating excess excretion of sulfatide

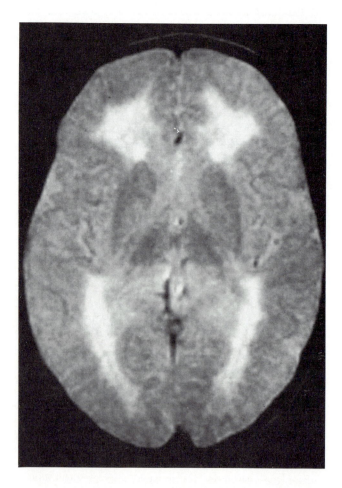

Figure 13-2. MRI of the head (SE 2100/100) showing symmetric homogeneous and diffuse elevation of signal intensity throughout the deep hemisphere white matter (sparing U fibers) in a 3-year-old white female with metachromatic leukodystrophy.

in urine and by assay of arylsulfatase-A in leukocytes or skin fibroblasts. All patients with metachromatic leukodystrophy excrete large amounts of sulfatide in the urine. Most patients with metachromatic leukodystrophy have, on cell-free preparations, a profound deficiency of arylsulfatase-A regardless of the age of onset. However, intact cells in culture are able to express subtle variations in their ability to clear sulfatide, giving a biochemic basis for varying ages of onset in metachromatic leukodystrophy. Low arylsulfatase-A activity in the cell homogenates of asymptomatic patients does not always indicate a diagnosis of metachromatic leukodystrophy. Healthy individuals with pseudo-arylsulfatase-A deficiency excrete normal amounts of urinary sulfatide. Excessive amounts of sulfatide are only found in the urine of presymptomatic cases of metachromatic leukodystrophy. In a rare variant, arylsulfatase-A activity in all homogenates is normal whereas large amounts of sulfatide are found in the urine. The molecular basis for this variant is a deficiency of the sphingolipid activator protein 1 (SAP-1) required for in vivo sulfatide catabolism. Diagnosis may be suggested by urine spot tests and mucopolysaccharide electrophoresis and proved by demonstrating decreased hydrolysis of sulfatide by intact cultured cells. In mucosulfatidosis multiple sulfatases are deficient. Not only are arylsulfatases -A, -B, and -C deficient in all homogenates, but at least three more polysaccharide sulfatases and steroid sulfateses are also deficient. Final-

ly, prenatal diagnosis of different forms of metachromatic leukodystrophy has been accomplished successfully by assays of cultured amniotic fluid cells.

Common to all forms of metachromatic leukodystrophy are a diffuse demyelination of the CNS white matter, with relative sparing of arcuated U fibers, and massive deposition of metachromatic material intracellularly and extracellularly. Although the axons are usually relatively preserved, some are fragmented. Oligodendroglial loss and astrocytosis occur in advanced cases. Swollen neurons occur in the cerebrum, thalamus, pallidum, dentate nucleus, brainstem, and spinal cord. In the peripheral nervous system, segmented demyelination occurs. Metachromatic inclusions are observed in Schwann cells and free macrophages. Metachromatic material may be found in cutaneous nerves, intramuscular nerve fibers, and myenteric plexuses (but not in the neurons of these plexuses). In some cases of the adult form, the accumulation of metachromatic material in the peripheral nerves is minimal. Visceral organs are also involved. Renal tubular epithelium is affected most severely, but considerable storage also occurs in the gallbladder. The pancreas, adrenals, liver, testes, and ovaries may be involved. The reticuloendothelial system is never affected severely. Ultrastructural analysis of the metachromatic granules by electron microscopy suggests that they are composed of several types of inclusions, among which the most characteristic are "prismatic inclusions" and "tuffstone bodies." The prismatic inclusions are formed by little disks stacked in parallel prisms with a periodicity of approximately 5.8 nm. The cross section of these prisms assumes a hexagonal honeycomb pattern. The name *tuffstone bodies* derives from the fact that these inclusions (which are membrane-bound aggregates of lamellar, granular, and vesicular structures in a mosaic-like pattern) resemble volcanic limestone.

The four forms of metachromatic leukodystrophy (late infantile, juvenile, adult, and mucosulfatidosis) are genetically distinct, with the same form recurring in the affected families. Hybridizing cell lines from patients with late infantile and adult metachromatic leukodystrophy does not restore arylsulfatase-A activity. Thus the two mutations are allelic. The locus determining the expression of arylsulfatase-A has been assigned to the long arm of chromosome 22 (22q13). Hybridizing cell lines from patients with late infantile metachromatic leukodystrophy and those from patients with mucosulfatidosis or SAP-1 deficiency restores arylsulfatase-A activity. Therefore, at least three alleles may result in metachromatic leukodystrophy. The locus determining the expression of SAP-1 has been assigned to chromosome 10. The locus determining expression of mucosulfatidosis has not yet been found. All varieties of metachromatic leukodystrophy are transmitted through an autosomal recessive pattern of inheritance. In the United States, the incidence of all forms of metachromatic leukodystrophy is

Pearls and Perils:
Metachromatic Leukodystrophy

1. Detection of large amounts of urinary sulfatides is essential for diagnosis. Urine should be kept at 4°C during collection. A urine negative for sulfatides is therefore meaningless in symptomatic patients.
2. Low arylsulfatase-A in asymptomatic patients does not always indicate diagnosis of metachromatic leukodystrophy. Presymptomatic cases of metachromatic leukodystrophy excrete excessive amounts of urinary sulfatide. Normal amounts of sulfatide are found with pseudo-arylsulfatase A deficiency.
3. Arylsulfatase-A is not always low in metachromatic leukodystrophy. Assay of arylsulfatase-A in intact cells and detection of large amounts of sulfatide in the urine allow diagnosis of SAP-1 deficiency.
4. CT scan and MRI of the head typically demonstrate mild enlargement of the ventricles and white matter changes bilaterally, maximum at the anterior and posterior poles of the central ventricles.

estimated to be 1 in 100,000 births, although the true incidence may be higher because many cases remain undiagnosed. The frequency of the trait is unknown.

Most treatments have been unsuccessful in correcting the progression of metachromatic leukodystrophy. An apparent alteration of the rate of progression of the CNS abnormality after bone marrow transplantation has been reported in several cases of late infantile metachromatic leukodystrophy. Further clinical evaluation is needed to confirm those promising results.

ANNOTATED BIBLIOGRAPHY

Hagberg B: Clinical symptoms, signs and tests in metachromatic leukodystrophy, in Folch-Pi J, Baver H (eds): *Brain Lipids and Lipoprotein and the Leukodystrophies.* Amsterdam, Elsevier, 1963, p 134–146.

The clinical features and clinical progression of the late infantile form of metachromatic leukodystrophy are described.
Bharucha BA, Naik G, Savliwala AS, Joshi RM, Kumta NB: Siblings with the Austin variant of metachromatic leukodystrophy multiple sulfatidosis. *Ind J Pediatr* 51:477–480, 1984.

The clinical features, biochemical findings, and histopathology of multiple sulfatidosis (or mucosulfatidosis) are reviewed.
Kolodny EH, Moser HW: Sulfatide lipidosis: Metachromatic leukodystrophy, in Stanbury JB, Wyngarrden JB, Fredrickson DS, Goldstein JL, Brown MS (eds): *The Metabolic Basis of Inherited Diseases.* New York, McGraw-Hill, 1983, p 881–905.

An excellent review of clinical biochemic and pathologic changes characterizing metachromatic leukodystrophy is provided.
Lutschg J: Pathophysiological aspects of central and peripheral myelin lesions. *Neuropediatrics* 15(suppl):24–27, 1984.

Neurophysiologic abnormalities in leukodystrophies are reviewed and discussed.
Kihara H, Ho CK, Fluharity AL, Tsay KK, Hartlage PL: Prenatal diagnosis of metachromatic leukodystrophy in a family with pseudo arylsulfatase-A deficiency by the cerebroside sulfate loading test. *Pediatr Res* 14:224–227, 1980.

In families that carry both the metachromatic leukodystrophy allele and the pseudo-arylsulfatase-A deficiency allele, prenatal diagnosis cannot be achieved by demonstrating low arysulfatase-A activity in cell-free homogenates. A sphingoidolipid sulfate loading test on the growing amniotic fluid cells is necessary.
Zlotogora J, Bach G: The deficiency of lysosomal hydrolases in apparently healthy individuals. *Am J Med Genet* 14:73–80, 1983.

These authors point out that lysosomal hydrolases deficient in cases of metachromatic leukodystrophy, Tay-Sachs disease, Fabry disease, and Krabbe disease are also found to be deficient in healthy persons. They introduce the concept of pseudodeficiency.
Shapiro LJ, Aleck KA, Kaback MM, et al: Metachromatic leukodystrophy without arylsulfatase-A deficiency. *Pediatr Res* 13:1179–1180, 1979.

The authors describe two siblings presenting with a variant form of metachromatic leukodystrophy caused by SAP-1 deficiency.

ADRENOLEUKODYSTROPHY

Adrenoleukodystrophy is a heterogeneous group of disorders of lipid metabolism characterized by the association of adrenal atrophy or hypoplasia with a progressive demyelination. Adrenal involvement is a constant feature, although clinical signs of adrenal insufficiency may be absent. At least two genetically distinct forms of adrenoleukodystrophy must be distinguished.

The X-linked form, the most common, has its onset in childhood or adulthood. The classic childhood X-linked adrenoleukodystrophy is characterized by behavioral, intellectual, and motor changes. Hyperactivity, withdrawal, aggressive outbursts, dementia, learning difficulties, poor memory, and gait disturbances are common signs of onset between 4 and 10 years of age. Other less common presenting symptoms include sei-

FEATURE TABLE 13-9. X-LINKED ADRENOLEUKODYSTROPHY (CHILDHOOD)

Discriminating Features	Consistent Features	Variable Features
1. Peroxisomal lignoceroyl-CoA ligase deficiency 2. Electron microscopy of brain or adrenal cortex	1. Male 2. Adrenal insufficiency (clinical or subclinical) 3. Behavioral changes 4. Visual impairment with optic atrophy 5. Abnormal gait with pyramidal tract signs 6. Elevation of very-long-chain fatty acids in plasma and cultured fibroblasts 7. CT scan of head shows cerebral white matter disease	1. CSF pleocytosis and focal production of γ-globulins 2. Elevated CSF protein 3. Skin hyperpigmentation 4. Seizures 5. Perilesional enhancement on CT scan of the head

FEATURE TABLE 13-10. X-LINKED ADRENOMYELONEUROPATHY (ADULTHOOD)

Discriminating Features	Consistent Features	Variable Features
1. Peroxisomal lignoceroyl-CoA ligase deficiency 2. Electron microscopy of brain or adrenal cortex	1. Male 2. Spastic paraparesis 3. Distal polyneuropathy 4. Adrenal insufficiency 5. Elevation of very-long-chain fatty acids in plasma and cultured fibroblasts	1. Skin hyperpigmentation 2. Hypogonadism 3. Sphincter disturbances 4. Behavior changes 5. Dementia 6. Cerebellar dysfunction 7. Focal central syndromes 8. Schizophrenia

zures, hearing and visual disturbances, and primary adrenal cortical insufficiency, leading to skin hyperpigmentation and symptoms of hypoadrenalism. In most cases, neurologic and psychologic symptoms precede clinical and laboratory signs of adrenal insufficiency. The disease runs a relentlessly progressive course lasting between 1 and 9 years. The motor examination shows signs of upper motor unit involvement with continuing progression to quadriparesis. Signs of peripheral nerve dysfunction are never prominent. Visual disturbances include homonymous hemianopsia, visual agnosia, and loss of visual acuity. Optic atrophy eventually occurs in all patients. Seizures, when present, are focal or multifocal. Duration of the illness is short. Death frequently occurs within the first 15 years of life.

Two other phenotypes of X-linked adrenoleukodystrophy are observed in the adult. Those phenotypes and childhood adrenoleukodystrophy occur in the same kindred, and are considered variant forms of the same illness. One phenotype observed in males is adrenomyeloneuropathy. This is the second most common form of adrenoleukodystrophy. Adrenal insufficiency may begin in childhood. Some patients have hypogonadism with azoospermia and hypotestosteronemia. Predominant neurologic manifestations reflect progressive myelopathy, beginning in the third decade, with resulting progressive spastic paraparesis, sensory loss for all modalities in the lower limbs, sphincter disturbances, and sexual impotence. Clinical signs of peripheral neuropathy are discrete (dysesthesia, decreased ankle jerks, and, in the early stages, spinocerebellar degeneration). Peripheral neuropathy is demonstrated by electrophysiologic studies and nerve biopsy (laminar inclusion may be demonstrated in the cytoplasm of Schwann cells). Visual symptoms are absent. Late manifestations include cerebellar ataxia, behavioral changes, or intellectual deterioration. Adrenomyeloneuropathy patients usually do not have a shortened survival. The other phenotype, observed in 10% of female heterozygotes, is characterized by the onset of a myeloneuropathy, usually less severe than that observed in adult males, without adrenal insufficiency. Survival is not shortened.

The autosomal recessive form, or neonatal adrenoleukodystrophy, shows some similarities to the cerebrohepatorenal syndrome of Zellwager. However, its clinical course is generally less severe. Presenting signs in neonates are hypotonia and seizure (paradoxically, the hallmark of gray matter degeneration). Some infants with neonatal adrenoleukodystrophy have facial characteristics reminiscent of those in Zellweger's syndrome (epicanthal folds, hypoplastic midface, ptosis). The liver is often enlarged. Cataracts, optic dysplasia or atrophy, and pigmentary retinopathy are common. Hearing and vision become severly impaired after some months. Cystic changes in the kidneys and skeletal changes (very large anterior fontanelle and stippling of the patellar) seen in the Zellweger's syndrome have not been found in neonatal adrenoleukodystrophy. Most patients with

FEATURE TABLE 13-11. AUTOSOMAL RECESSIVE ADRENOLEUKODYSTROPHY (NEONATAL)

Discriminating Feature	Consistent Features	Variable Features
1. Decreased number and size of liver peroxisomes	1. Hypotonia and hyporeflexia 2. Seizures 3. Psychomotor retardation 4. Dysmorphic features less severe than in Zellweger's syndrome 5. Metabolic abnormalities suggestive of Zellweger's syndrome	1. Enlarged liver and impaired liver function 2. Adrenal insufficiency 3. Pigmentary retinal disturbances 4. Cataracts 5. Nystagmus

neonatal adrenoleukodystrophy show some initial psychomotor development. Progression to spasticity and death occurs within the first several years of life. Clinical signs of adrenal insufficiency, although uncommon in neonatal adrenoleukodystrophy, may occur late in the clinical course. Neonatal adrenoleukodystrophy has never been observed in the same kindred as childhood adrenoleukodystrophy or adrenomyeloneuropathy. No neurologic or endocrine abnormalities have been noted in persons heterozygous for adrenoleukodystrophy.

Routine x rays of the skull are normal in adrenoleukodystrophy. In the classic childhood adrenoleukodystrophy, CT scanning of the head is often pathognomonic, demonstrating symmetric areas of decreased attenuation surrounding the ventricular trigones with perilesional contrast enhancement. At an early phase of the disease, the CT scan may be misleading, showing a unilateral lesion or lesions without the perilesional enhanced rim. Perilesional contrast enhancement diminishes or disappears as the disease progresses. The CT scan in adrenomyeloneuropathy is normal or nonspecifically abnormal, consistent with the predominant spinal and peripheral white matter involvement. In neonatal adrenoleukodystrophy, the CT scan shows evidence of cerebral white matter disease without perilesional contrast enhancement. MRI may prove useful in childhood adrenoleukodystrophy, showing a prolonged T_2 signal in deep parietal white matter and adjacent midbrain when the CT scan is still normal. The EEG demonstrates symmetric frequency in childhood adrenoleukodystrophy, showing an amplitude reduction that is maximal in the parieto-occipital region. Focal epileptiform discharges are uncommon. In contrast, in neonatal adrenoleukodystrophy the EEG frequently reveals widespread epileptiform activity. In adrenomyeloneuropathy the EEG is normal in the early stages.

Evoked potential responses are normal early in the course of childhood adrenoleukodystrophy and fail to correlate with early visual and auditory symptoms. Visual evoked responses remain normal in adrenomyeloneuropathy and heterozygotes. Brainstem auditory evoked responses may be abnormal in adrenomyeloneuropathy without auditory complaints and in heterozygotes. Abnormalities of somatosensory evoked responses have been found in adrenoleukodystrophy and in most heterozygotes. In childhood and neonatal adrenoleukodystrophies, nerve conduction velocities may be normal and fail to parallel the pathologic evidence of peripheral nerve involvement.

Except during addisonian crises, serum electrolyte levels and plasma cortisol values are normal in the neonatal and X-linked types of adrenoleukodystrophy. Baseline ACTH values may be elevated. A provocative adrenal stimulation is required in most cases to demonstrate the diminished adrenal reserve. Liver dysfunction is only seen in neonatal adrenoleukodystrophy. CSF proteins are frequently elevated in childhood adrenoleuko-

---

Pearls and Perils:
Adrenoleukodystrophy

1. Clinical and laboratory signs of adrenal insufficiency are uncommon at the onset of childhood X-linked adrenoleukodystrophy.
2. There are no clinical signs of peripheral neuropathy in childhood X-linked adrenoleukodystrophy, and nerve conduction velocities may be normal despite pathologic involvement.
3. There is no visual impairment in adult X-linked adrenoleukodystrophy.
4. Very-long-chain fatty acids in plasma and cultured fibroblasts are elevated in all forms of adrenoleukodystrophy and in Zellweger's syndrome. Patients on a ketogenic diet may show elevated very-long-chain fatty acids in plasma but not cultured fibroblasts.
5. Metabolic changes similar to those found in Zellweger's syndrome may occur in neonatal adrenoleukodystrophy.
6. CT scanning of the head is often pathognomonic in childhood adrenoleukodystrophy. The finding of a unilateral lesion or lesions without a perilesional enhanced rim does not exclude childhood adrenoleukodystrophy.
7. Except during addisonian crisis, plasma cortisol values are normal. A provocative adrenal stimulation with ACTH is usually required to demonstrate the diminished adrenal reserve.
8. In X-linked adrenoleukodystrophy, the CSF may show pleocytosis and local production of immunoglobulin G can be demonstrated. Diagnosis of multiple sclerosis (or Schilder's disease) can be excluded by analysis of the fatty acids of plasma cholesterol esters or electron microscopic examination of brain or adrenal cortex.

---

dystrophy. Diagnosis of the neonatal and X-linked types of adrenoleukodystrophy may be suggested by assays of very-long-chain fatty acids in plasma, cultured skin fibroblasts, or both. The concentration of the very-long-chain fatty acid hexacosanoic acid (C_{26}) and its ratio to docosanoic acid (C_{22}) are increased in plasma and cultured fibroblasts from patients with either form of adrenoleukodystrophy. Elevated levels of the monounsaturated $C_{26:1}$ very-long-chain fatty acid are common, suggesting a defect confined to the saturated very-long-chain fatty acids (in Zellweger's syndrome both monounsaturated and saturated very-long-chain fatty acids are elevated). It has been suggested that both forms of adrenoleukodystrophy result from a very-long-chain fatty acid oxidation defect. Carnitine-dependent very-long-chain fatty acid oxidation (mitochondrial oxidation) in fibroblasts from both forms of adrenoleukodystrophy is normal, suggesting a defect localized to peroxisomes. Metabolic abnormalities similar to those found in Zellweger's syndrome (elevation of serum pipecolic, phytanic, and di- and trihydroxicoprostanic acid levels and diminution of serum plasmalogen levels) may be found in neonatal adrenoleukodystrophy (but not in X-linked adrenoleukodystrophy). Assay of very-long-chain fatty acids on cultured amniotic cells allows prenatal diagnosis. The enzyme (or enzyme group) defect responsible for the neonatal form of adrenoleukodystrophy is still unknown. A peroxisomal lignoceroyl-CoA ligase deficiency has been found in X-linked adrenoleukodystrophy.

Characteristic pathologic changes of adrenoleukodystrophy are found in the adrenal glands and nervous system. The adrenal cortex is usually atrophic or hypotrophic. The adrenal medulla in all cases is normal. Microscopic studies of adrenal cortex reveal a preserved outer zone, or zona glomerulosa, with more significant disruption of the fascicularis and reticularis zones, which are infiltrated with enlarged cells containing a granular or hyaline eosinophilic cytoplasm. Striated PAS-positive macrophages are found in the adrenal cortex. The major neuropathologic features include a widespread peripheral and central demyelination sparing the arcuated U fibers and scattered PAS-positive and sudanophilic macrophages prominent in the areas of demyelination. On electron microscopy, the cytoplasm of macrophages in the adrenals and nervous system is packed with straight or curvilinear bilayered lamellar inclusions. The individual lamellae show a trilaminar structure consisting of paired electron-dense leaflets separated by an electron-lucent space. Recent works suggest that these lamellar inclusions are the morphologic counterparts of the accumulated cholesterol-esterified very-long-chain fatty acids.

There are striking differences in the neuropathologic features of neonatal and childhood adrenoleukodystrophy. In childhood adrenoleukodystrophy, centripetal spreading of demyelination produces characteristic zonated lesions: (1) the inner zone, with dense gliosis; (2) the peripheral zone, containing scattered macrophages and axons in various stages of demyelination; and (3) at the leading edge of the demyelination, a large rim containing perivascular inflammatory infiltrates. This inflammatory reaction is probably a secondary response to the primary breakdown of myelin, but the possible participation of accumulated IgG in the pathogenesis of these lesions has also been discussed. The inflammatory reaction with perivascular infiltrates is characteristic of childhood adrenoleukodystrophy. In both adult forms, neuropathology shows only minimal changes in the brain. In neonatal adrenoleukodystrophy, no perivascular inflammatory reaction is seen in the white matter; demyelination is more diffuse; lipid-laden macrophages can be found within the gray matter. As in Zellweger's syndrome, pachymicrogyria and mild degenerative changes are found within the gray matter, but those changes are less severe. Neonatal adrenoleukodystrophy can be distinguisned from Zellweger's syndrome by the absence of sudanophilic lipid in astrocytes (it is found in Zellweger's syndrome) and the accumulation of saturated very-long-chain fatty acids in the cholesterol esters and sphingolipids of the brain (unsaturated very-long-chain fatty acids are found in Zellweger's syndrome).

There are striking differences in the size and configuration of hepatocellular peroxisomes in both forms of adrenoleukodystrophy. In X-linked adrenoleukodystrophy, peroxisomes are normal in number and configuration. In patients with neonatal adrenoleukodystrophy, liver peroxisomes are diminished in number and size (but are not absent, differentiating this condition from Zellweger's syndrome). Finally, in neonatal adrenoleukodystrophy macrophages with membrane-bound lipid profiles are present in tissues where there is no obvious degeneration and, in particular, within the reticuloendothelial and lymphoid systems. In X-linked adrenoleukodystrophy lamellar lipid profiles are found unbound in the cytoplasm of the fibroblasts, Leydig cells of the testes, and adrenocortical cells. To date, no carrier has been studied pathologically.

The X-linked adrenoleukodystrophy gene has been mapped to the terminal segment of the long arm of the X chromosome (Xq28 locus). Clinical manifestations of the disease are thought to occur in heterozygotes because of possible selection favoring clones of cells expressing the mutant gene. Most women heterozygous for X-linked adrenoleukodystrophy can be detected by studying very-long-chain fatty acids. Plasma assay, followed by fibroblast assay when plasma is normal, identifies a total of 93% of obligate heterozygotes. The locus of the gene responsible for neonatal adrenoleukodystrophy has not been identified. Because 40 enzymes have been localized to the peroxisomes, there is adequate opportunity for genetic heterogeneity among patients with neonatal adrenoleukodystrophy. It has been shown that, if Zellweger's syndrome cells are fused with neonatal adrenoleukodystrophy cells, complementation occurs, suggesting that those conditions represent different genetic entities.

Hormonal substitution may be necessary to correct the adrenal cortical insufficiency, but this therapeutic approach does not influence the progression of the neurologic symptoms. Therapeutic intervention by dietary restriction of exogenous very-long-chain fatty acids, administration of clofibrate or carnitine, plasmapheresis, and immunosuppression have been unsuccessful in treating X-linked adrenoleukodystrophy. Allogenic bone marrow transplantation did not prove beneficial in one child with rapidly progressive X-linked adrenoleukodystrophy. Current treatment strategies involve an approach that restricts dietary intake of $C_{26:0}$ fatty acids and calls for the administration of a glyceryl trioleate oil to maintain total fat content. Preliminary evidence suggests a consistent decline in very-long-chain fatty acids on this diet. Clinical studies are under way to assess clinical response to such a treatment.

ANNOTATED BIBLIOGRAPHY

Walsh PJ: Adrenoleukodystrophy: Report of two cases with relapsing and remitting courses. *Arch Neurol* 37:448–450, 1980.

A fluctuating course more consistent with a diagnosis of multiple sclerosis is described as a childhood adrenoleukodystrophy variant that conforms to an X-linked inheritance pattern.

Moser HW, Moser AE, Singh I, O'Neill BP: Adrenoleukodystrophy: Survey of 303 cases: Biochemistry, diagnosis and therapy. *Ann Neurol* 16:628–641, 1984.

Presymptomatic and asymptomatic forms of adrenoleukodystrophy exist. Bone marrow transplant fails to arrest neurologic progression.

Powers JM, Schaumburg HH, Gaffney, CL: Kluver-Bucy syndrome caused by adrenoleukodystrophy. *Neurology* 30:1131–1132, 1980.

CT scanning may show bilateral white matter disease in cases that have a focal onset.

Aubourg P, Diebler C: Adrenoleukodystrophy—Its diverse CT appearances and an evolutive or phenotypic variant. *Neuroradiology* 24:33–42, 1982.

Atypical CT presentation is most often observed at an early phase of the disease.

Marsden CD, Obesco JA, Lang AE: Adrenomyeloneuropathy presenting as spinocerebellar degeneration. *Neurology* 32:1031–1032, 1982.

A variant form of adrenomyeloneuropathy, associated with spinocerebellar degeneration, presented on CT scan with areas of frontal lobe demyelination with an enhanced rim that proceeded posteriorly.

Garg BP, Markand ON, DeMyer WE, Warren C: Evoked response studies in patients with adrenoleukodystrophy and heterozygous relatives. *Arch Neurol* 70:356–359, 1983.

Abnormal somatosensory evoked responses were found in childhood adrenoleukodystrophy and in heterozygotes.

Johnson AB, Schaumburg HH, Powers JM: Histochemical characteristics of the striated inclusions of adrenoleukodystrophy. *J Histochem Cytochem* 24:725–730, 1976.

This work suggests that lamellar inclusions found in adrenoleukodystrophy are the morphologic counterparts of the accumulated cholesterol-esterified very-long-chain fatty acids.

Moser HW, Moser AE, Trojak JE, Supplee SW: Identification of female carriers of adrenoleukodystrophy. *J Pediatr* 103:54–59, 1983.

Of the women who are obligate heterozygote for X-linked adrenoleukodystrophy, 93% are identified by biochemic assays of very-long-chain fatty acids in both plasma and fibroblasts.

Yeager AM, Moser HW, Tutscko PJ, et al: Allogenic bone marrow transplantation in adrenoleukodystrophy: Clinical, pathologic, and biochemical studies. *Birth Defects* 22:79–100, 1986.

The selection criteria for bone marrow transplants in patients with adrenoleukodystrophy are discussed.

Kelley RI, Datta NS, Dobyns WB, et al: Neonatal adrenoleukodystrophy: New cases, biochemical studies and differentiation from Zellweger and related peroxisomal polydystrophy syndromes. *Am J Med Genet* 23:869–901, 1986.

Patients with neonatal adrenoleukodystrophy demonstrate adrenal atrophy, systemic infiltration by abnormal lipid-laden macrophages, and elevation of saturated very-long-chain fatty acids.

Nakazoto T, Sato T, Nakamura T, et al: Adrenoleukodystrophy presenting as spinocerebellar degeneration. *Eur Neurol* 29:229–234, 1989.

In early stages adrenoleukodystrophy in adults may present as spinocerebellar degeneration.

Lazo OM, Contreras A, Bhushan W, et al: Adrenoleukodystrophy: Impaired oxidation of fatty acids due to peroxisomal lignoceroyl-CoA ligase deficiency. *Arch Biochem Biophys* 270:722–728, 1989.

The activation of lignoceric acid by lignoceroyl-CoA ligase is the first and obligatory step in the peroxisomal β-oxidation of this very-long-chain fatty acid. This enzyme activity is deficient in X-linked adrenoleukodystrophy.

KRABBE'S GLOBOID CELL LEUKODYSTROPHY

Krabbe's globoid cell leukodystrophy or galactosylceramide lipidosis is a lysosomal storage disease resulting from a defect in the catabolism of a sphingolipid, galactocerebroside (or galactosylceramide). This lipid is exclusively a constituent of myelin. The characteristic metabolic defect in various forms of Krabbe's disease is a deficiency in galactocerebroside-β-galactosidase, a specific β-galactosidase involved in the catabolism of galactocerebroside.

Krabbe's disease has been divided into two clinical subgroups, according to the age of onset of neurologic symptoms. Most cases are of the infantile form. The clinical onset of the disease usually occurs between 3 and 6 months of life, although a few cases with earlier (neonatal variant) or later onset have been reported. Usually, during the first months of life, the infants have a normal development. From the onset, the course of the disease is steadily progressive and can be divided into three stages. Stage I is characterized by intermittent fever, hyperirritability, feeding difficulties, and stimulus-sensitive, tonic extensor spasms. At the same time, stagnation in motor and mental development is noted. Seizures may occur. In stage II, rapid and severe motor and mental deterioration develops. There is marked hypertonicity, with opisthotonos, scissoring of the legs, flexion of the arms, and clenching of the fists. Myotatic reflexes are hyperactive. Optic atrophy is common, and pupillary response to light may be compromised. The child remains small and may display macrocephaly. There is no visceromegaly. Various seizures (irregular myoclonic seizures, infantile spasms, major tonic-clonic seizures) frequently occur. Stage III is the "burn-out" stage. The infant is decerebrate and has no contact with the surroundings. Myotatic reflexes are depressed. Most patients die from an intercurrent infection or bulbar paralysis before 2 years of age, although a protracted course has been observed in rare cases.

The second clinical subgroup is late-onset Krabbe's

NEUROLOGIC DEGENERATIVE DISEASES

disease. In most patients, the clinical manifestations appear between the ages of 2 and 6 years, although later onset has been described. The clinical symptomatology is quite variable at the onset. The most common presenting complaint is rapidly failing vision, together with gait difficulties. The failure of vision is due to cortical blindness with optic atrophy. Gait difficulties may be due to hemiparesis, paraparesis, progressive cerebellar ataxia, or acute polyneuropathy. Rare individuals may first present at school age with dementia or psychotic traits. Despite the dissimilar presentation in the initial stage of the disease, the clinical picture progressively becomes more uniform and is dominated by demetia, cortical blindness with optic atrophy, and spastic quadriparesis. Death usually occurs 1 to 3 years from the first onset of symptoms, although a protracted course also occurs.

CT scan of the head early in the course of infantile Krabbe's disease may be normal. A later nonenhanced CT scan may show increased densities in the thalami, body of caudate nuclei, corona radiata, and cerebellum. Low attenuation in the periventricular white matter appears in the intermediate stage and in the third stage cerebral atrophy involves both gray matter and white matter. Hydrocephalus may be an additional finding. In late-onset Krabbe's disease, CT of the head shows nonspecific enlargement of the lateral ventricles and low attenuation around the frontal horns. An enhancing rim may be observed between the demyelinated white matter and the unaffected arcuate fibers. MRI in infantile Krabbe's disease may show, on T_2-weighted images, symmetric high-signal lesions in the white matter of the centrum semiovale and low-signal lesions in the thalamus and brainstem. At later stages, hydrocephalus ex vacuo can be seen (Figure 13–3). In late-onset Krabbe's disease, symmetric confluent hyperintense lesions in the peritrigonal region are associated with atrophy of the splenium of the corpus callosum. Small hyperintensity lesions can also be seen in the posterior limb of the internal capsule. There is no rim enhancement with gadolinium DTPA in late-onset Krabbe's disease.

In the early stage of infantile Krabbe's disease, the EEG abnormalities are characterized by an excess of irregular slow activity with an amplitude of between 50 and 200 μV. No EEG changes precede or accompany the episodes of screaming and hyperextension. In later stages, occasional multifocal spikes and sharp wave discharges and peculiar runs of fast activity are observed. In late-onset Krabbe's disease, the EEG shows only slight deterioration with the lapse of time. ERG is normal in all cases of Krabbe's disease. Visual evoked potential responses are markedly delayed or absent in advanced cases. Brainstem auditory evoked responses may suggest lesions involving the central and peripheral nervous systems. In the infantile form of Krabbe's disease, motor conduction velocities and distal sensory latencies are markedly delayed, whereas the amplitudes of the evoked muscle and nerve action potentials are relatively normal.

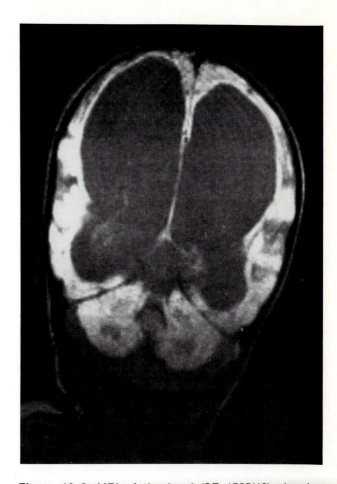

Figure 13–3. MRI of the head (SE 1585/40) showing hydrocephalus ex vacuo in a 6-year-old white male with stage III Krabbe's disease.

In late-onset Krabbe's disease, peripheral neuropathy may or may not be present.

In the first stage of infantile Krabbe's disease, the CSF protein is already elevated. The electrophoretic pattern may be diagnostically helpful in that albumin and α_2-globulin levels are elevated and β_1- and γ-globulin levels are decreased. This pattern persists throughout the course of the disease. In late-onset Krabbe's disease, CSF protein level is normal or only slightly raised, and the electrophoretic changes are nonspecific. Assays of galactocerebroside-β-galactosidase in white cells, serum, or cultured fibroblasts with the use of appropriate natural glycolipid substrates provide the means for antemortem diagnosis. When the enzyme β-galactosidase is assayed with synthetic substrates, no deficiency is found. This differentiates Krabbe's disease from GM$_1$ gangliosidosis, in which galactocerebroside-β-galactosidase activity is normal, but β-galactosidase assayed with synthetic substrates is deficient. Deficiency of galactocerebroside-β-galactosidase may be equally severe in both infantile and late-onset cases, although considerable residual activity is sometimes found in the late-onset form. Prenatal diagnosis of Krabbe's disease may be achieved by

FEATURE TABLE 13–12. KRABBE'S GLOBOID CELL LEUKODYSTROPHY

Discriminating Features	Consistent Features	Variable Features
1. Galactocerebroside-β-galactosidase deficiency in leukocytes and fibroblasts 2. Globoid cells in white matter (brain biopsy)	1. Increased CSF proteins 2. Abnormal electrophoretic pattern of CSF proteins 3. Extensor toe signs	1. Spasticity 2. Psychomotor retardation 3. Irritability 4. Spasticity, hyperextension 5. Hyperreflexia (early) and hyporeflexia (late) 6. Blindness (with optic atrophy) 7. Deafness 8. Failure to thrive 9. Macrocephaly 10. Ataxia 11. Focal motor deficits

galactocerebroside-β-galactosidase assays performed on amniotic or chorionic cells. In heterozygotes, intermediate levels of galactocerebroside-β-galactosidase are found in serum, white cells, and culture fibroblasts.

Pathologically, the brain is small with external evidence of cerebral and cerebellar atrophy. The ventricular system is dilated. The white matter is rubbery firm with sparing of subcortical arcuate fibers. Microscopically, the most important abnormality is the presence of epitheloid and globoid cells in areas of recent demyelination. Epitheloid cells are mononuclear cells that, as the demyelination proceeds, form clusters around blood vessels. Epitheloid cells, when they become multinucleated and distended with storage material, are called globoid cells. Their large cytoplasm stains strongly with PAS and faintly with Sudan dyes. As the demyelination becomes more severe, the oligodendroglial cells are progressively destroyed and axonal degeneration occurs. The white matter is progressively replaced by a dense fibrous astrocyte proliferation. Finally, the number of globoid cells decreases. On electron microscopy, globoid cells are seen to possess many pseudopods and two types of abnormal inclusions, both free in the cytoplasm and confined to membrane-bounded vacuoles. The first inclusions, characteristic for Krabbe's disease, are moderately electron-dense and appear straight or curved with hollow tubular profiles in longitudinal sections and irregularly polygonal or crystalloid in cross section. The second inclusions appear as right-handed twisted tubules in longitudinal section and irregularly round in cross section. These inclusions are reminiscent of those found in Gaucher's disease. Lipid analysis of the brain shows severe loss of myelin lipids, most severe for sulfatides. The total brain content of galactosylceramide (and its metabolites) is not elevated. This is a unique feature of Krabbe's disease among the sphingolipidoses. A high concentration of galactocerebroside is found in enriched globoid cell fractions. The morphologic abnormalities of the CNS may be detected in fetuses of as early as 20 weeks of gestation. Outside the CNS, globoid cells are rarely found in lungs, lymph nodes, and spleen. No changes are seen in peripheral blood cells or bone marrow. No globoid cells are found in peripheral nerves. Segmental demyelination is a constant finding in infantile Krabbe's disease.

Krabbe's disease is inherited as an autosomal recessive trait. In Sweden, the incidence is about 2 cases per 100,000 births. In a large Druze isolate in Israel, incidence has been found to be as high as 6 in 1,000 births. The structural gene responsible for synthesis of galactocerebroside-β-galactosidase has been localized on chromosome 12. It has been shown by somatic cell hybridization studies that the classic and late-onset forms of Krabbe's disease are allelic. There is no specific therapy for affected patients. Supportive care may improve survival. Preventive measures are available through genetic counseling and intrauterine diagnosis of affected fetuses.

Pearls and Perils: Krabbe's Globoid Cell Leukodystrophy

1. The head is usually normal in Krabbe's disease, although hydrocephalus may occur.
2. There is no visceromegaly or abnormality on x-ray films.
3. Peripheral neuropathy and elevation of CSF protein are constant findings in infantile Krabbe's disease. Those finding need not be present for the diagnosis of late-onset Krabbe's disease.
4. Galactosylceramid-β-galactosidase should always be assayed with natural substrates.

ANNOTATED BIBLIOGRAPHY

Hagberg B: Krabbe's disease: Clinical presentation of neurological variants. *Neuropediatrics* 15(suppl):11–15, 1984.

The classic irritative hypertonic presentation at between 3 and 5 months of age represents more than 90% of cases. Rare infants will present with a neonatal variant, hemiplegia variant, prolonged floppy infant variant, or infantile spasm variant. Late-onset Krabbe's disease shows considerable variation in clinical presentation.

Loonen MCB, Van Diggelen OP, Janse HC, Kleijer WJ, Arts WFM: Late-onset globoid cell leucodystrophy (Krabbe's disease): Clinical and genetic delineation of two forms and their relation to the early infantile form. *Neuropediatrics* 16:137–142, 1985.

The early infantile and late-onset forms of Krabbe's disease are allelic as shown by somatic cell hybridization.

Kliemann FAD, Harden A, Pampiglione G: Some EEG observations in patients with Krabbe's disease. *Dev Med Child Neurol* 11:475–484, 1969.

Although the EEG features in patients with infantile Krabbe's disease are in no way specific, they appear different in their time course from those seen in other inborn errors of metabolism.

Darras BT, Kwan ES, Gilmore HE, Ehrenberg BL, Rabe EF: Globoid cell leukodystrophy: Cranial computed tomography and evoked potentials. *J Child Neurol* 1:126–130, 1986.

The brainstem auditory evoked responses and the flash visual evoked potentials are abnormal in early infantile Krabbe's disease.

Wenger DA, Sattler M, Markey SP: Deficiency of monogalactosyl diglyceride β-galactosidase activity in Krabbe's disease. *Biochem Biophys Res Commun* 53:680–685, 1973.

In Krabbe's disease β-galactosidase activity is deficient toward galactosylcerebroside, psychosine, and monogalactosyl diglyceride.

Yunis EJ, Lee RE: The ultrastructure of globoid (Krabbe) leukodystrophy. *Lab Invest* 21:415–493, 1969.

By electron microscopy, two types of inclusions are found in Krabbe's disease.

Demaerel P, Wilms G, Verdru P, Carton M, Baert AL: MR findings in globoid cell leukodystrophy. *Neuroradiology* 32:520–522, 1990.

MRI of the head with gadolinium DTPA shows no rim enhancement in late-onset Krabbe's disease, although rim enhancement is seen in the early-onset form.

Corencephalopathies

WILSON'S DISEASE

Wilson's disease or familial hepatolenticular degeneration is a disorder of copper metabolism resulting in progressive degenerative changes in the brain, liver, kidneys, and cornea. The primary defects are found in the liver, resulting in an abnormal excretion of copper via the bile.

Clinically, the mean age of presentation is 15 years (range 4 to 40 years). The presentation is highly variable. A classic childhood form (also called the hepatolenticular degeneration of Wilson) can be distinguished from a juvenile or adult form (or pseudosclerosis of Westphal and Strumpell). The childhood form has its onset before puberty. The most common early symptoms are related to the liver, and include lethargy, anorexia, jaundice, and abdominal pain. Other symptoms include edema, ascites, and bleeding tendencies. In some patients, hepatosplenomegaly may remain asymptomatic. The neurologic mode of presentation in children or young adolescents may include rapidly deteriorating school performance, bizarre behavior, impulsiveness, uncontrollable agitation, dystonic postures, choreoathetoid movements, and dysarthria. Other modes of presentation are failure to thrive and hemolytic anemia. A Kayser-Fleischer ring is not often seen in the childhood form, as opposed to the adult form. The outcome of the childhood form is rapidly fatal if the patient is left untreated.

The juvenile or adult form has its onset after puberty. Presenting symptoms are predominantly related to the CNS. These symptoms are more insidious in onset than those occurring before puberty. In young adults, the first neurologic symptoms are most commonly a speech defect, tremor at rest that intensifies with voluntary movement or emotional stress, painful spasms, difficulty with fine motor tasks, and dysphagia. Facial expression may be characteristic, with a fixed, open-mouth, silly smile, the so-called Wilsonian risus. Neurologic signs and symptoms are rapidly progressive if left untreated. In older patients, flapping tremor of one arm may be the first sign before the characteristic, more generalized muscular rigidity develops. Facies tends to be expressionless. The disease is slowly progressive. As it advances, bradykinesia, rigidity, irregular tremor, and micrographia may suggest a diagnosis of Parkinson's disease. The most common psychiatric symptom is depression, followed by emotional lability, personality changes, and slow mentation. The most diagnostic clinical feature of Wilson's disease is the Kayser-Fleischer ring: a mass of golden brown pigment at the periphery of the cornea that is characteristically broad superiorly and may only form a crescent. The ring is more frequent in neurologic or psychiatric forms of the disease. It may only be detected on slit lamp examination. However, the absence of a Kayser-Fleischer ring does not rule out the diagnosis. Patients with neurologic disease become bedridden and demented. They exhibit involuntary movements, ataxia,

FEATURE TABLE 13-13. WILSON'S DISEASE

Discriminating Feature	Consistent Features	Variable Features
1. Increased copper content in the liver	1. Increased urinary excretion of copper 2. Decreased biliary excretion of copper 3. Low serum ceruloplasmin levels 4. Kayser-Fleischer ring (in neurologic form)	1. Liver failure 2. Hepatosplenomegaly 3. Abnormal behavior 4. Impaired intellect 5. Dysarthria 6. Dysphagia 7. Parkinsonism, dystonia, choreoathetosis, flapping tremor 8. Psychiatric symptoms (explosive anger and labile mood) 9. Aminoaciduria, glycosuria, phosphaturia, renal tubular acidosis 10. Hemolytic anemia 11. Rickets

and disorders of tone and posture. Pseudobulbar palsy precedes death in untreated cases.

EEG changes in patients with Wilson's disease are encountered not only in cases of neurologic symptomatology but also in predominantly hepatic forms. Only a portion of the individuals affected present with EEG changes. Those changes are usually nonspecific in nature and of mild to moderate degree. More pronounced EEG changes are likely in the juvenile form of the disease. Multimodality evoked potentials may be normal in the early stage of neurologic involvement. As the neurologic symptoms progress, somatosensory evoked potentials, brainstem auditory evoked potentials, and pattern reversal visual evoked potentials become abnormal in the majority of patients. CT scan of the head may be normal in the early stage of neurologic involvement. The most prominent CT findings include ventricular dilatation, cortical atrophy, brainstem atrophy, and cerebellar atrophy. Areas of hypodensity in the lenticular nuclei, thalami, cerebellar nuclei, and cerebral hemisphere white matter are also frequently present. Enhancement following intravenous administration of contrast material is generally not seen. Increased density in basal ganglia from copper deposition has not been described. In general T_2-weighted MRI demonstrates focal areas of increased signal in both gray and white matter. Gray matter lesions are more common. They are always bilateral and symmetric, in contrast to white matter lesions, which are generally asymmetric. Gray matter lesions are found in the lenticular nuclei, caudate nuclei, thalami, dentate nuclei, and midbrain.

Asymptomatic and symptomatic patients with Wilson's disease exhibit four abnormalities of copper metabolism: (1) a persistent deficiency or absence of serum ceruloplasmin (less than 20 mg/100 mL); (2) an increased concentration of loosely bound, nonceruloplasmin copper in the serum; (3) an increased excretion of copper in the urine; and (4) an increased copper content in the liver (more than 250 µg/g dry weight). Serum ceruloplasmin values may be in the low normal range (between 20 and 30 mg/100 mL) in up to 5% of patients with Wilson's disease. Conversely, about one fifth of heterozygotes display low serum ceruloplasmin values in the same range as in homozygotes. Low serum ceruloplasmin values may also be found in patients with acute liver failure. There may be difficulty in obtaining a complete and uncontaminated 24-hour urine specimen in a young child, and therefore results of urinary copper studies should be interpreted cautiously. The estimation of nonceruloplasmin copper in the serum may be essential for diagnosis of symptomatic or presymptomatic patients. The quantitative determination of hepatic copper content in a histologically compatible biopsy is the single most reliable diagnostic procedure. This requires that a part of the biopsy be preserved unfixed. Histochemic demonstration of copper in the liver is not reliable for diagnosis.

Other laboratory tests show the effects of damage to various organs. Liver function test abnormalities have no specificity. Aminoaciduria, glycosuria, phosphaturia, and defective urinary acidification reflect proximal renal tubular damage. The combination of renal tubular absorption defects and rickets may suggest Fanconi's syndrome. Hemolytic anemia is not common but may be severe. Thrombocytopenia and neutropenia are more frequent. Finally, in untreated patients, the blood pyruvate level is increased and pyruvate tolerance after glucose ingestion is abnormal; these findings lend support to the concept of copper toxicity to the pyruvate dehydrogenase complex.

The major pathologic changes are seen in the liver and the brain. In the early stages of the disease, hepatomegaly may occur. Abnormal fat and glycogen deposits are shown by light microscopy. Copper may be dispersed in the cytoplasm and not routinely demonstrable by histochemistry. With electron microscopy, large and grossly abnormal mitochondria are observed. Later, the liver becomes shrunken and firm. Microscopically, the characteristic appearances of macronodular cirrhosis are seen. Fibrous septa may contain perivascular collections of lymphocytes and numerous small bile ducts. Kupffer cells do not seem to take part in the reaction. Histochemic demonstration of copper may be highly variable from lobule to lobule. There is no correlation between grade of staining and liver copper content (contrary to findings in intrahepatic cholestasis of childhood, in which copper content correlates with stainable copper). Electron microscopy may demonstrate the presence of pigment granules, possibly copper, in the lysosomes of liver cells.

Neuropathologic findings vary depending on the rate of progression of the disease. In the rapidly progressive form, the pathologic changes involve primarily the striatum. Cavitation is often found in the putamen and may include part of the caudate nucleus in more severe cases. In the more chronic form, widespread degeneration of the brain is the rule, although the basal ganglia are usually more severely affected. The corpus striatum and sometimes the thalamus are shrunken and discolored. Involvement of the cerebral and cerebellar cortexes and white matter invariably occurs, but to a variable degree. The most commonly involved cerebral cortical structures are the superior and middle frontal gyri, in which softening and sometimes spongiosis in the convolutional white matter are associated with thinning of the overlying cortex. Frank degeneration of the dentate nucleus and generalized folial atrophy may occur. The spinal cord is almost always spared. The histologic findings are maximal in the putamen. Neuronal loss, proliferation of astrocytes, and vascular proliferation are frequently seen. Mononuclear Alzheimer type II astrocytes are abundant, and large multinucleate cells (Alzheimer type I astrocytes) have also been described. The reactive astrocytes do not form glial fibers. Some astrocytes are considerably enlarged (up to 15 μm in diameter) and contain yellow-brown cytoplasmic granules staining heavily for copper. Later, Opalski cells are found in the thalamus, globus pallidus, and zona reticularis of the substantia nigra but very rarely in the striatum. Such cells measure up to 35 μm in diameter and are characterized by a rounded outline without processes and by a small central nucleus. The cytoplasm is firmly granular or slightly foamy, staining a light rose color by Nissl's method and a bright orange-brown color by van Gieson's counterstain. Perivascular concretions of copper are found. Histochemic demonstration of copper is more prominent in glial cells than in nerve cells.

Wilson's disease has been reported all over the world without racial or geographic predilection. The incidence of the disease is believed to be in the range of 1 in 40,000 to 1 in 100,000 live births. Wilson's disease is an autosomal recessive disorder. Homozygotes for the same allele may present at various ages, some with neurologic and some with hepatic symptoms. Heterozygotes do not have clinical manifestations. Approximately 20% of heterozygotes have reduced ceruloplasmin (and serum copper) values. It is essential that the parents be studied, because they give an indication of the expected concentration of ceruloplasmin in the heterozygote and against this value the findings in the siblings can be interpreted. The basic biochemic defect of Wilson's disease has not yet been identified. A first step in this direction was the discovery of linkage between the locus for Wilson's disease and that for the red cell enzyme esterase D on chromosome 13. Prenatal diagnosis, although possible, has not been achieved, perhaps because of the effectiveness of available treatments.

Treatment with penicillamine is life saving in most patients with Wilson's disease, although beneficial clinical effect may take months to years. Psychiatric or neurologic deficit almost always responds to penicillamine, and many patients are able to resume a normal life. L-Dopa

Pearls and Perils: Wilson's Disease

1. Wilson's disease is not a cause of slowly progressive mental retardation. In children or young adults, behavioral and intellectual alterations, when present, are usually rapidly progressive.
2. Seizures and sensory abnormalities are lacking in Wilson's disease.
3. Because of pleomorphic presentation and severity of the untreated disease, diagnosis should always be suspected when neurologic, psychiatric, or hepatic signs and symptoms are progressing in a patient over 4 years of age.
4. A golden brown Kayser-Fleischer ring near the limbus of the eye may only be seen by slit lamp examination. Kayser-Fleischer rings are more frequent in neurologic or psychiatric forms of the disease.
5. Most patients with Wilson's disease have a low serum ceruloplasmin level. Low serum ceruloplasmin in asymptomatic siblings may represent either presymptomatic Wilson's disease or heterozygosity.
6. Although ceruloplasmin and serum copper are usually low in Menkes's syndrome and Wilson's disease, clinically these two conditions are easily distinguished.

therapy may be useful in the control of neurologic symptoms while awaiting response to penicillamine. Corresponding with the recovery in the brain, there is also recovery of hepatic and renal tubular function. Treatment with penicillamine should never be withdrawn except in the presence of life-threatening complications. The majority of these are immunologically or chemically induced. It is wise to watch the blood count, sedimentation rate, and urine for protein. Pyridoxine deficiency can be prevented by giving the appropriate vitamin. When absolute penicillamine intolerance develops, the alternative chelating agent triethylene tetramine can be used. Some patients with irreversible liver damage will benefit from liver transplantation as a last resort. As liver grafting cures the underlying biochemic defect, chelation therapy is no longer necessary, although lifelong immunosuppresion will be required.

ANNOTATED BIBLIOGRAPHY

Walshe JM: Hudson Memorial Lecture: Wilson's disease: Genetics and biochemistry. Their relevance to therapy. *J Inher Metab Dis* 6(suppl 1):51–58, 1983.

   The primary genetic defect is not known but the disease appears to result from a failure by the hepatocytes to excrete copper via the bile.

Dastur DK, Manighani DK: Wilson's disease: Inherited cuprogenic disorder of liver, brain, kidney, in Goldensohn ES, Appel SH (eds): *Scientific Approaches to Clinical Neurology.* Philadelphia, Lea & Febiger, 1977, p. 1033–1051.

   The clinical, pathologic, and laboratory features of Wilson's disease are reviewed. The estimation of serum ceruloplasmin copper level is shown to be a reliable indicator of the presence of Wilson's disease.

Goldfischer S, Sternlieb I: Changes in the distribution of hepatic copper in relation to the progress of Wilson's disease (hepatolenticular degeneration). *Am J Pathol* 53:883–901, 1968.

   Early in the disease when hepatocellular damage is prominent, the excess copper is diffusely present in the cytosol and there is little or no copper-associated protein demonstrated by histochemic techniques. Late in the disease, when liver damage is less obvious, the cytosol has been cleared of the metal, which appears to be stored in electron-dense lysosomes.

Popoff N, Budzilovich G, Goodgold A, Feigin I: Hepatocerebral degeneration. Its occurrence in the presence and in the absence of abnormal copper metabolism. *Neurology* 15:919–930, 1965.

   These authors consider that Wilson's disease is a highly distinctive histologic entity.

Starosta-Rubinstein S, Young AB, Kluin K, et al: Clinical assessment of 31 patients with Wilson's disease. Correlations with structural damages on magnetic resonance imaging. *Arch Neurol* 44:365–370, 1987.

   Dystonia and bradykinesia correlate with putamen lesions. Dysarthria correlates with lesions of both putamen and caudate. Subcortical matter, midbrain, and pontine lesions are also seen frequently. Generalized brain atrophy is common.

Chu NS: Sensory evoked potentials in Wilson's disease. *Brain* 109:491–507, 1986.

   The majority of patients with neurologic manifestations have subclinical dysfunction in three major sensory pathways.

Nevsjimalova S, Marecek Z, Roth B: An EEG study of Wilson's disease. Findings in patients and heterozygous relatives. *Electroencephalog Clin Neurophysiol* 64:191–198, 1986.

   EEG does not allow one to distinguish heterozygous from homozygous in the preclinical stage.

Frommer DJ: Urinary copper excretion and hepatic copper concentration in liver disease. *Digestion* 21:169–178, 1981.

   The administration of 10 mg/kg of penicillamine may be used diagnostically. Normal adults excrete less than 600 µg of copper in 24 hours with penicillamine, versus 1500–3000 µg in those with Wilson's disease.

MENKES'S KINKY HAIR SYNDROME

Menkes's kinky hair syndrome or trichopoliodystrophy is a progressive neurodegenerative disorder characterized by seizures, psychomotor deterioration, failure to thrive, temperature instability, and strikingly peculiar hair. The diagnostic features of Menkes's syndrome at birth may be quite subtle. Birth weight is usually normal. Hypothermia and hypotonia may develop in the first days of life. The characteristic alterations in the hair have been reported in the first week, but often develop as late as 3 or 4 months of age. The hair is short, sparse, lightly pigmented, and lusterless with a steely texture. The skin is pale and slightly hyperextensible. A mild seborrheic dermatitis may involve face and scalp. Pudgy cheeks, sparse eyebrows, and depressed nasal bridge with moderate micrognathia give these patients a similar cherubic expression. Despite an adequate intake of food, an early failure to thrive frequently precedes the onset of neurologic symptoms. Inguinal hernias and diastasis recti may be present at birth. Development may proceed normally for some weeks. Psychomotor deterioration begins before head control is achieved. Hypotonia, somnolence, and feeding difficulties soon become apparent. Focal or generalized convulsions are commonly observed early and become progressively persistent. The myotatic reflexes are hyperactive. At times, irritability and spastic quadriparesis with clenched fists, opisthotonos, and leg scissoring become prominent. Blindness has been observed in several patients. Most patients expire in a vegetative state under 3 years of age.

   Radiologic studies may reveal wormian bones in the posterior and lambdoidal sutures shortly after birth. Other radiographic signs of Menkes's syndrome develop progressively after about 2 months of age. Skeletal studies show progressive metaphyseal spurring of ribs and femur, and sometimes subperiosteal calcifications along the shaft. Bladder diverticuli can be demonstrated in most cases. Angiography may disclose tortuosity and irregularity of the lumen of the visceral, cerebral, and limb arteries. CT scan of the head shows progressive deep and cortical atrophy of the entire brain (Figure 13–4). Sub-

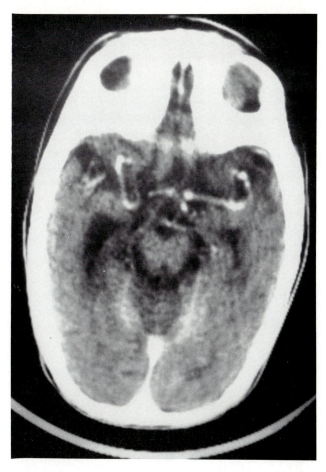

Figure 13–4. CT scan of the head showing brain atrophy with enlargement of the ambient cistern and tortuous middle cerebral arteries in a 2-year-old white male with Menkes's syndrome, who presented at 1 month of age with inguinoscrotal hernia and at 6 weeks of age with seizures, failure to thrive, and unusual hair.

skin biopsy may be preferred to obtain evidence in favor of the diagnosis. An increased uptake and an impaired efflux of copper in cultured skin fibroblasts are characteristic of the disease. Similarly, prenatal diagnosis is carried out on cultured amniotic fluid cells by showing an increased uptake of copper into the cells of affected male fetuses. After 18 weeks of gestation, the risk of a false negative is significant, however.

Neuropathologic findings in Menkes's syndrome reveal a small brain with tortuosity and dilatation of the brain vessels. Neuronal loss with marked gliosis is widespread throughout the CNS. Heterotopic neurons in the white matter suggest an early disturbance in the migration of neuroblasts. The cerebellar cortex is the more severely affected area. In the cerebellum, besides the loss of granular cells, the Purkinje cells undergo degeneration and show somatic sprouts and bizarre dendritic arborization, suggesting a state of retarded development. Electron microscopy discloses profound mitochondrial abnormalities in the various structures of the brain. Quantitative lipid analysis of fresh brain tissue shows a diminished level of docosahexanoic acid, an unsaturated fatty acid. The histologic examination of the eye reveals microcysts in the pigmented epithelium of the iris, a marked decrease in retinal ganglion cells, and partial atrophy of the optic nerve. The earliest change in the arterial wall appears in the internal elastic lamina, which undergoes disruption, fragmentation, and reduplication. Microscopically, the hair is characteristically twisted around its axis (pili torti) and brittle, as suggested by a variety of breaks and fractures, including trichoclasis, trichorrhexis nodosa, and trichoptilosis (Figure 13–5).

dural hematoma may result from tearing of bridging cortical veins as the brain recedes from the dura. In most patients, the EEG becomes abnormal before 3 months of age and shows diffuse abnormalities with multifocal sharp waves. A progressive decrease in the amptitude of the ERG and visually evoked response has been associated with the clinical deterioration.

Laboratory studies may reveal an elevated alkaline phosphatase, hypertriglyceridemia, and lactic acidosis with elevation of the lactate to pyruvate ratio. In the CSF, a similar elevation of lactate and lactate to pyruvate ratio may be found. Serum copper and ceruloplasmin are characteristically decreased. It is important to realize, however, that these levels may be within the normal range in the very early neonatal period. Copper and ceruloplasmin levels drop progressively after birth, secondary to the increased urinary copper excretion and the decreased copper absorption in the gastrointestinal tract. Liver biopsy in neonates already demonstrates decreased hepatic copper levels and may allow early diagnosis. A

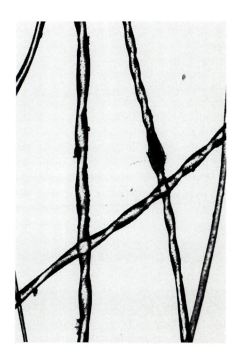

Figure 13–5. Pili torti and trichorrhexis nodosa in a patient with Menkes's syndrome.

FEATURE TABLE 13–14. MENKES'S KINKY HAIR SYNDROME

Discriminating Features	Consistent Features	Variable Features
1. Decreased copper absorption from the gastrointestinal tract 2. Increased uptake and decreased efflux of copper in cultured fibroblasts	1. Male 2. Failure to thrive 3. Psychomotor retardation 4. Hyperreflexia 5. Pili torti and trichorrhexis nodosa 6. Decreased serum ceruloplasmin 7. Increased urinary copper, decreased plasma and serum copper, decreased CSF copper, low hair copper, and decreased copper content in the liver 8. Lactic acidosis and cytochrome oxidase deficiency 9. Decreased CSF MHPG 10. Multiple Wormian bones in the lambdoid and petrosal sutures	1. Hypothermia 2. Seizures 3. Hypotonia or spasticity 4. Hernia and diathesis recti 5. Bladder diverticuli 6. Metaphyseal spurring and subperiosteal calcification 7. Tortuosity and elongation of vessels 8. Skin hyperlaxity 9. Fullness of cheeks 10. Blindness 11. Anemia 12. Recurrent bladder and respiratory infections 13. Pectus excavatum 14. Delayed eruption of teeth

The incidence of Menkes's syndrome may be as high as 1 in 35,000 live births. The syndrome is inherited as an X-linked recessive trait. The location of the Menkes gene has been proposed to be close to the centromere on the long arm of the X chromosome, near band q13. Carrier status can usually be determined by examination of multiple hairs from scattered scalp sites for pili torti. Carrier status can, of course, never be completely excluded by negative findings of such scrutiny. By measuring copper uptake into cultured skin fibroblasts from suspected carriers, it is sometimes possible to demonstrate their status, but the range of values for obligate carriers considerably overlaps those for the normal controls. The Menkes mutation is not well understood. It may result from an abnormal regulation of copper uptake. Furthermore, retention of copper is deficient in selective tissues (e.g., hair, liver, brain). The consequence is reduced activity of copper-containing enzymes (e.g., cytochrome *c* oxidase, lysyl oxidase, dopamine β-hydroxylase, ascorbic acid oxidase, tyrosinase, superoxide dismutase). The profound copper deficiency of Menkes's syndrome patients can be corrected by parenteral therapy with copper salts or oral therapy with copper nitriloacetic acid or copper histidine. This treatment improves the function of some copper-dependent oxidative enzymes. Ceruloplasmin returns to normal in the serum. CSF copper is increased but the concentration in the brain remains low. Copper therapy has not, however, demonstrated beneficial effect on the progresssive neurologic deterioration. Vitamin C therapy has been shown to prevent bone changes. Documentation of norepinephrine deficiency and absence of dopamine β-hydroxylase activity suggests a neurotransmitter deficiency as a possible etiologic factor in the neurologic impairment. For this reason, treatment with dihydroxyphenylserine, an unnatural precursor of norepinephrine, has been attempted and has resulted in a significant increase of CSF norepinephrine without improvement of neurlogic function.

Pearls and Perils: Menkes's Kinky Hair Syndrome

1. The bone changes in Menkes's syndrome are easily confused with those seen in maltreated babies and the tendency for subdural hematoma to occur in this disorder adds to the risk of confusion of the two entities. Wormian bones are present in early life.
2. Early diagnosis may be difficult because bony changes, hair abnormalities, and serum copper and ceruloplasmin may be normal in the very early neonatal period. In neonates with a positive family history, demonstration of an increased uptake of copper in skin fibroblasts may allow early diagnosis. Similarly, diagnosis may be achieved by demonstrating an increased uptake of copper into amniotic fluid cells in fetuses.
3. Menkes's disease is an X-linked autosomal recessive disorder.

ANNOTATED BIBLIOGRAPHY

Yoshimura N, Kudo H: Mitochondrial abnormalities in Menkes' kinky hair disease (MKHD): Electron-microscopy study of the brain from an autopsy case. *Acta Neuropathol* 59:295–303, 1983.

This study suggests that the mitochondrial disease is an essential abnormality and may be responsible for the progressive degeneration of the CNS in MKHD.

Horn N: Menkes' X-linked disease: Prenatal diagnosis and carrier detection. *J Inher Metab Dis* 6(suppl 1):58–62, 1983.

Horn demonstrated increased copper intake in cultured fibroblasts from amniotic fluid in at-risk pregnancies.

Gunn T, MacFarlane S, Phillips LI: Difficulties in the neonatal diagnosis of Menkes' kinky hair syndrome—trichopoliodystrophy. *Clin Pediatr* 23:514–516, 1983.

These authors show that recognition of Menkes's disease may present problems in the early neonatal period.

Menkes JH, Alter M, Steigleder G, Weakley D, Sung JH: A sex-linked recessive disorder with retardation of growth, peculiar hair, and focal cerebral and cerebellar degeneration. *Pediatrics* 29:764–779, 1962.

This article describes the major clinical and pathologic characteristics of this syndrome.

Troost D, van Rossum A, Straks W, Willemse J: Menkes' kinky hair disease II. A clinicopathological report of three cases. *Brain Devel* 4:115–126, 1982.

These authors give a detailed review of neuropathologic changes in Menkes' disease.

Grover WD, Johnson WC, Henkin RI: Clinical and biochemical aspects of trichopoliodystrophy. *Ann Neurol* 5:65–71, 1979.

Grover demonstrated normal copper levels with oral administration of large doses of copper chelated to nitriloacetic acid. The elevation of serum copper did not prevent neurologic deterioration.

Grover WD, Henkin RI, Schwartz M, et al: A defect in catecholamine metabolism in kinky-hair disease. *Ann Neurol* 12:263–266, 1982.

Grover documented abnormal catecholamine levels in blood and CSF and decreased activity of dopamine β-hydroxylase before copper therapy. The response of dopaminergic systems to copper therapy was heterogeneous.

Holdell EF, Grover WD: Catecholamine metabolism in steely-hair disease. *J Neurosci Nurs* 18:146–149, 1986.

The authors present preliminary results of dihydroxyphenylserine therapy in an attempt to correct endogenous norepinephrine deficiency.

SUBACUTE NECROTIZING ENCEPHALOPATHY OF LEIGH

Subacute necrotizing encephalopathy (SNE) of Leigh is a progressive CNS disease with cranial nerve signs, disorders of respiration, ataxia, and variable pyramidal, extrapyramidal, and visual impairment. Neuropathologic findings showing characteristic necrosis of cellular groups in the diencephalon, midbrain, and pons are diagnostic. Several biochemic abnormalities suggesting defects of mitrochondrial metabolism have been documented, supporting the genetic heterogeneity of the syndrome.

The age of onset is variable. Most cases are of the characteristic infantile form, which presents at an age of less than 2 years and often less than 1. Early psychomotor development is usually normal. The early course is usually rapid. Symptoms are made worse by intercurrent infection or a carbohydrate-rich diet. Presenting complaints may include progressive psychomotor slowing, weakness, staggering, feeding and swallowing difficulties, vomiting, poor weight gain, decreased alertness, poor visual fixation, myoclonic jerks, or generalized convulsions. On examination, clinical features that lead to the diagnosis are respiratory involvement, eye findings, and other cranial

FEATURE TABLE 13-15. SUBACUTE NECROTIZING ENCEPHALOPATHY OF LEIGH

Discriminating Feature	Consistent Features	Variable Features
1. Symmetric foci of partial necrosis with associated capillary proliferation and relative sparing of neurons in putamen, brainstem, and posterior columns of spinal cord	1. Elevated plasma and CSF lactate and pyruvate during exacerbation 2. Symmetric hyperintense lesions of putamen and brainstem on MRI 3. Ataxia 4. Signs of brainstem dysfunction (respiratory, ocular motility, or swallowing disturbances) disturbances) 5. Movement disorder (dystonia, choreoathetosis, parkinsonism) 6. Specific mitochondrial enzyme deficiency in fibroblasts and striated muscles	1. Hypo- or hyperreflexia 2. Fulminant (intermittent) or slowly progressive chronic course 3. Hypotonia or spasticity 4. Delayed neurologic development 5. Failure to thrive 6. Spasmus nutans 7. Seizures 8. Peripheral neuropathy with elevated CSF proteins 9. Visual impairment 10. Cardiac and renal involvement 11. Absence of ragged red fibers in striated muscles

nerve signs. Respiratory irregularities, a central hyper/hypoventilation syndrome, or central apnea are very remarkable. Eye findings may include nystagmus, strabismus, profound saccadic slowing, ptosis, ophthalmoplegia, optic atrophy, and atypical pigmentary degeneration of the retina. Other cranial nerve signs may include deafness, dysphagia, and facial weakness. Less specific neurologic signs may include axial hypotonia, spasticity, dystonia, choreoathetoid movements, and varying degrees of ataxia. Myotactic reflexes may be increased or decreased. Some patients are unusually hirsute. Other occasional features include cardiomyopathy and the renal de Toni-Fanconi-Debre syndrome of tubular renal acidosis. Death is the final outcome, coming often rapidly with the course of a few weeks or months. However, remissions followed by further exacerbations are sometimes seen and the child may live several years.

A rare juvenile form of the disease has also been described. The course of the illness is often characterized by an insidious onset in childhood, leading to neurologic defects, such as mild spastic paraparesis, ataxia, exercise intolerance, nystagmus, visual impairment, and Parkinson-like features. After a long quiescent period, the illness terminates acutely or subacutely during the second decade. The terminal stage is characterized by a rapid deterioration to coma and marked respiratory depression.

The results of electrophysiologic studies change with time and may vary from patient to patient. In some cases, the presence of slowed motor nerve conduction velocities is evidence of peripheral neuropathy. Needle electromyography is usually normal, but in a few cases signs of denervation have been found.

EEG may show a generalized slowing of background activity, sometimes with superimposed epileptogenic features. Brainstem auditory evoked potentials may be abnormal. Visual evoked responses may be absent. The ERG may suggest diffuse inner retinal dysfunction. CT scan of the head may show symmetric lucencies in the putamen, thalamus, and tegmentum of the brainstem. These lesions typically vary with time. Early CT scan obtained after the onset of clinical symptoms may be normal. MRI is more sensitive than CT scanning in detecting lesions (Figure 13–6). In some patients, electrocardiogram and echocardiogram abnormalities suggest a cardiomyopathy.

The main biochemic findings are intermittent metabolic acidosis with elevation of lactate/pyruvate ratios in the blood and CSF. An increase in blood alanine is also frequent. Normal biochemic findings between acute episodes do not exclude the diagnosis of SNE. The de Toni-Fanconi-Debre syndrome, with a generalized aminoaciduria, glycosuria, and phosphaturia, has been reported in some patients. Protein in the CSF may be elevated. Creatine phosphokinase is usually normal in the serum. Several biochemic abnormalities of oxidative metabolism have been documented. An inhibitor of the enzyme that forms thiamine triphosphate by

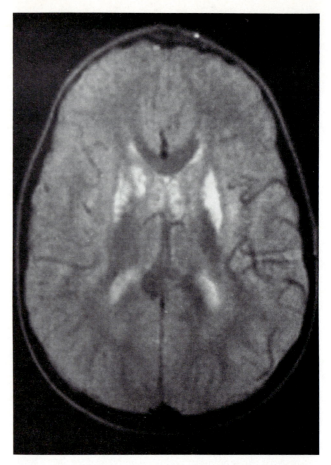

Figure 13–6. MRI of the head (SE 2100/100) showing increased signal in the putamen, caudate nucleus, and thalamus bilaterally in a 5-year-old white male with autopsy-proven Leigh's syndrome and cytochrome *c* oxidase deficiency.

phosphorylating thiamine pyrophosphate (thiamine pyrophosphate–ATP phosphotransferase) may be found in the urine of patients with SNE. This test is frequently negative in proven cases of SNE, and false positives may be found in other conditions. The urine test appears useful, but cannot be used as the only test to rule out SNE. The finding of low blood and CSF thiamine levels in patients with suspected SNE may suggest the diagnosis of beriberi as it occurs in infants.

A variety of disorders of oxidative metabolism have been associated with SNE. Biochemic testing of mitochondrial oxidative metabolism has been accomplished in various tissues (liver, muscle, heart, kidney, fibroblasts, brain, and platelets). In practice, cultured fibroblasts and skeletal muscle have been the tissues of choice for such studies, although this practice can lead to misleading sampling errors, because mitochondrial enzyme deficiency may only involve selected tissues. Defects affecting the pyruvate dehydrogenase complex, cytochrome *c* oxidase complex, and NADH-coenzyme Q oxidoreductase complex have been described in autopsy-proven cases identified as SNE. The association of isolated pyruvate carboxylase deficiency with Leigh's syndrome remains speculative. Hepatic pyruvate carboxylase deficiency has been reported in pathologically proven SNE. The estimates of pyruvate carboxylase in liver are notoriously unreliable. When pyruvate carboxylase activity is measured in cultured fibroblasts or leukocytes, no deficiency is found. It seems safe to conclude that pyruvate carboxylase deficiency is rarely, if ever, associated with the Leigh syndrome.

Characteristic pathologic findings are found in the CNS. The autopsy demonstrates symmetric foci of partial necrosis with associated capillary proliferation, and remaining intact neurons against a background of reactive glial elements in various portions of the thalamus, the putamen, the substantia nigra, the red nuclei, the periaqueductal area, the corpora quadrigemina, the dentate nucleus of the cerebellum, the inferior olives, and the tegmentum of the pons and the medulla. Sparing of the mamillary bodies and lesions of the substantia nigra differentiate Leigh's syndrome from Wernicke's disease. Demyelination may be found in the optic nerves and tracts and in the dorsal columns of the cord. Ultrastructural studies have shown abnormal brain mitochondria.

Although mitochondria are probably proliferating in Leigh's syndrome, ragged red fibers are almost never identified by light microscopy of striated muscles. In pyruvate dehydrogenase complex deficiency, histologic examination of muscle shows lipid droplets adjacent to mitochondria and an excess of primitive type II C fibers, suggesting an arrest in muscle development. Ultrastructural examination frequently shows discrete mitochondrial changes, such as increased size, bizarre shape, osmiophilic inclusions, and disoriented cristae. Hyper-

trophic cardiomyopathy and tubulopathy may be associated with SNE.

Leigh's syndrome frequently appears sporadically, but there have been cases of multiple affected siblings born to unaffected parents. These genetic observations, as well as an association with consanguinity in other kindreds, suggest that some of the biochemic abnormalities giving rise to the Leigh phenotype are inherited as autosomal recessive disorders. When several children are affected in the same sibship, age of onset, duration of the disease, and pattern of organ involvement may vary among affected siblings. Phenotypic variability within the same sibship is also seen in other mitochondrial encephalopathies.

Recognition and treatment of associated organ involvement (e.g., heart, kidney) is essential. Calories should preferably be provided as lipid. Rational use of specific therapies requires identification of the precise biochemic lesion in a given patient. Initial studies by a number of independent investigators give reason to hope that at least some oxidative disorders may be amenable to treatment. Therapy with thiamine or thiamine derivatives, such as thiamine propyldisulfide, thiamine tetrafurfuryldisulfide, and thiamine pyrophosphate (more lipid soluble), may improve clinical status in selected patients with pyruvate dehydrogenase complex deficiency. Lipoic acid therapy may also be attempted. Riboflavin therapy may be beneficial in other patients with NADH-coenzyme Q oxidoreductase complex deficiency.

ANNOTATED BIBLIOGRAPHY

Leigh D: Subacute necrotizing encephalomyelopathy in an infant. *J Neurol Neurosurg Psychiatr* 14:216–221, 1951.

Leigh describes a 7-month-old infant who died shortly after the onset of a neurologic disorder characterized by somnolence, blindness, deafness, and spasticity. The autopsy demonstrated CNS lesions similar to those of Wernicke's disease except for the sparing of the mamillary bodies and the damage to the substantia nigra.

Pincus JH: Subacute necrotizing encephalomyelopathy (Leigh's disease): A consideration of clinical features and etiology. *Dev Med Child Neurol* 14:87–101, 1972.

Eighty-six cases of SNE are reviewed in order to establish the symptomatology and natural history of the disease. The urine of affected patients may contain an inhibitor of the enzyme that catalyzes thiamine triphosphate formation.

DiMauro S, Servidei S, Zeviani M, et al: Cytochrome c oxidase deficiency in Leigh's syndrome. *Ann Neurol* 22:498–506, 1987.

Five children with pathologically proven SNE were found to have a partial defect of cytochrome c oxidase. Residual cytochrome c oxidase activity varied from tissue to tissue. One child was floppy at birth and developed hypertrophic cardiomyopathy. Two patients were unusually hirsute.

Sedwick LA, Burde RM, Hodges FJ: Leigh's subacute necrotizing encephalomyelopathy manifesting as spasmus nutans. *Arch Ophthalmol* 102:1046–1048, 1984.

Pearls and Perils: Subacute Necrotizing Encephalopathy of Leigh

1. The clinical feature that usually leads to the diagnosis of SNE is the severe and rapid onset in infancy of variable neurologic signs, among which respiratory involvement, eye findings, and cranial nerve signs are most diagnostic.
2. Radiolucencies in the thalamus, basal ganglia, and tegmentum of the brainstem are frequently seen in SNE. A normal CT scan does not exclude the diagnosis of SNE.
3. Leigh's syndrome can only be diagnosed positively by finding a characteristic pattern of brain lesions at autopsy.
4. Leigh's syndrome has clinical, biochemic, and pathologic features in common with mitochondrial encephalomyopathies.

Spasmus nutans, a clinical triad of head tilt, head nod, and nystagmus, was a presenting sign in a child with autopsy-proven SNE.

Van Erven PMM, Gabreels, FJM, Ruitenbeek W, et al: Subacute necrotizing encephalomyelopathy (Leigh syndrome) associated with disturbed oxidation of pyruvate, malate and 2-oxoglutarate in muscle and liver. *Acta Neurol Scand* 72:36–42; 1985.

A defect of NADH dehydrogenase is demonstrated in the skeletal muscle of a patient with the juvenile form of SNE.

Adams RD, Lyon G: *Neurology of Hereditary Metabolic Disease of the Child.* New York, McGraw-Hill, 1982, p 73–82.

An inhibitor of the enzyme thiamine pyrophosphate-ATP phosphoryltransferase has been found in the urine of many patients with proven SNE, but also in patients suffering from pathologically different conditions.

Walter GV, Brucher JM, Martin JJ, Ceuterick C, Pilz P, Freund M: Leigh's disease—Several nosological entities with an identical histopathological complex? *Neuropathol Appl Neurobiol* 12:95–107, 1986.

Ultrastructural examination of the brain in four autopsy-proven cases of SNE showed abnormal mitochondria in nerve cells, suggesting a mitochondriopathy.

Miyabayashi S, Ito T, Narisawa K, Iinuma K, Tada K: Biochemical study in 28 children with lactic acidosis, in relation to Leigh's encephalomyelopathy. *Eur J Pediatr* 143:278–283, 1985.

Pyruvate dehydrogenase complex deficiency was found in cultured skin fibroblasts from two patients with autopsy-proven SNE. A deficiency of cytochrome *c* oxidase was found in fibroblasts, brain, and liver of another patient with autopsy-proven disease.

Murphy JV, Isohashi F, Weinberg MB, Utter MF: Pyruvate carboxylase deficiency: An alleged biochemical cause of Leigh's disease. *Pediatrics* 68:401–404, 1981.

The estimation of pyruvate carboxylase in liver is notoriously unreliable. Pyruvate carboxylase deficiency is never documented in patients with Leigh's syndrome.

Hommes FA, Polman HA, Reenick JD: Leigh's encephalopathy: An inborn error of gluconeogenesis. *Arch Dis Child* 43:423–426, 1966.

Deficiency of pyruvate carboxylase was demonstrated in the liver of a patient with autopsy from Leigh's disease.

Paltiel HJ, O'Gorman AM, Meagher-Villemure K, Rosenblate B, Silver K, Walters GV: Subacute necrotizing encephalomyelopathy (Leigh's disease): CT study. *Radiology* 162:115–118, 1987.

CT scan of the head obtained in three patients with histologically confirmed SNE showed variable features, suggesting that the absence of radiologically detectable abnormalities in the basal ganglia does not exclude the diagnosis of SNE.

Wyatt DT, Noetzel MJ, Hilman RE: Infantile beri-beri presenting as subacute necrotizing encephalomyopathy. *J Pediatr* 100:888–892, 1987.

Infantile beri beri may present with clinical radiologic and biochemic findings indistinguishable from those of the acute form of SNE.

Medina L, Chi TL, DeVivo DC, Hilal SK: MRI findings in patients with subacute necrotizing encephalomyelopathy (Leigh's syndrome): Correlation with biochemical defect. *AJNR* 11:379–384, 1990.

In patients who present with lactic acidosis, the diagnosis of Leigh's syndrome is unlikely if the MRI shows symmetric abnormalities in the brain with sparing of the putamen.

Lombes A, Makase H, Tritschler MJ, et al: Biochemical and molecular analysis of cytochrome *c* oxidase deficiency in Leigh's syndrome. *Neurology* 41:491–498, 1991.

Cytochrome *c* oxidase deficiency in Leigh's syndrome is generalized but partial and appears to be related to a decreased amount of otherwise normal cytochrome oxidase holoenzyme.

Spinocerebellophathies

FRIEDREICH'S ATAXIA

Friedreich's ataxia is a degenerative disorder comprising progressive spinocerebellar ataxia and cardiomyopathy. The etiology of this disease remains unknown. Some patients have been found to have a primary defect in pyruvate oxidation.

Clinically, the disease usually appears before the age of 20. The peak age of onset is 11 years. The usual presenting symptoms are gait instability and difficulty with running. Cramps and aching in the legs are occasionally reported. If the patient is examined at this stage, ataxia is found to be worse in the legs than in the arms. Vibration sense and position sense are faulty in the lower limbs, but sensation is otherwise intact. The Romberg sign is usually present. Myotatic reflexes are decreased or absent. The plantar responses are extensor. As the child grows older, the gait ataxia progresses without remission. Weakness and extremity atrophy are frequently observed. Pes cavus deformities, hammer toes, and kyphoscoliosis may develop. The hands become clumsy. Speech is invariably dysarthric in the later stage of the disease. Truncal ataxia may be profound. Head titubation is sometimes observed. Patients are finally unable to walk without assistance. By the end of the third decade of life, they are reduced to a wheelchair-bound existence or are bedridden. Ocular movements remain full and pupillary reflexes are normal. Horizontal nystagmus may be present in the primary position and is increased on lateral gaze. Rotatory and vertical nystagmus is rare. Optic atrophy is infrequent, but may appear late in the course of the disease. Neurosensory hearing loss may occur. Although dementia is not a prominent feature, minor intellectual difficulties, slowing of mental processes, and emotional

FEATURE TABLE 13-16. FRIEDREICH'S ATAXIA

Discriminating Feature	Consistent Features	Variable Features
1. None	1. Ataxia of limbs 2. Decreased or absent vibratory sense 3. Absent myotatic reflexes in lower extremities (distal first) 4. Extensor plantar responses 5. Normal or mildly slow motor nerve conduction velocity 6. Absent or reduced sensory nerve potentials 7. Impaired somatosensory evoked potentials	1. Muscle atrophy and weakness (distal) 2. Truncal ataxia 3. Dysarthria 4. Loss of position sense 5. Cramp and aching in legs 6. Pes cavus and kyphoscoliosis 7. Claw hands 8. Optic atrophy 9. Nystagmus 10. Cranial nerve palsies, neurosensory hearing loss 11. Intellectual difficulties, dementia 12. Seizures 13. Abnormal echocardiogram and EKG 14. Diabetes mellitus

lability are not uncommon. Cardiac arrhythmia or congestive failure are major complications, which may begin before or after the onset of ataxia. Diabetes mellitus has been reported in less than 10% of patients.

The EEG is most often normal in Friedreich's ataxia. Visual evoked potentials may be increased in latency and reduced in amplitude, without temporal dispersion. These changes can already be seen in individuals without visual symptoms and are thought to reflect the axonal degeneration found in this condition. The ERG is usually normal. Auditory evoked potentials recorded from the cortex are usually normal whereas those recorded from mastoid electrodes are either absent or impossible to recognize. Such findings are frequently detected in patients without symptomatic hearing difficulties and are attributed to degeneration of the spiral ganglion. Somatosensory evoked potentials are impaired in all patients regardless of the duration or the severity of the illness. The motor conduction velocity of peripheral nerves is usually normal. Sensory nerve conduction, however, is practically absent in the lower limbs, and considerably slowed in the upper. On electromyography, fasciculations and an impaired interference pattern indicate denervation. Patients with Friedreich's ataxia have no or only minor abnormalities on cranial CT scan. MRI of the spine may be helpful in assessing spinal cord atrophy. The CSF is usually normal. Cardiac conduction defects as recorded by the electrocardiogram and cardiomegaly on the chest x ray, when present, may be of diagnostic value. Echocardiogram and cardiac catheter studies show left ventricular dysfunction in most patients. Attempts to localize the metabolic basis for this defect

have been unsuccessful, even though many abnormalities of enzymatic activities and substrate levels have been detected.

Nerve biopsy shows a loss of myelinated fibers, particularly the large ones, and axonal degenerative changes. Teased fiber studies show paranodal myelin enlargements, segmental demyelination, shortening, and/or variability of internodal length. In the spinal cord, atrophy and sclerosis of the posterior columns is prominent in fasciculi gracilis. Clarke's columns and the spinocerebellar tracts also degenerate. There is a "dying back" process of the pyramidal tracts, which is maximal in the lumbosacral region and diminished upwards. In the early stages of the illness, only rare neurons of the anterior horn show signs of degeneration. In the bulb, the gracile and cuneate nuclei may undergo transneuronal degeneration. Lesions in the cerebrum and cerebellum are more variable. Histologic examination of the hearts of patient's with Friedreich's ataxia show severe interstitial fibrosis without myocardial fiber disarray.

Friedreich's ataxia is one of the most common hereditary ataxias. Its prevalence is estimated as 1 to 2 cases per 100,000 births. Males and females are equally affected. The mode of inheritance is autosomal recessive. No biochemic test or electrophysiologic finding has been of value in the detection of heterozygotes. Prenatal diagnosis is not available. No treatment halts the progression of the disease. Congestive heart failure secondary to cardiomyopathy is generally treated with digitalis and diuretics. Increased taurine intake and administration of calcium channel blockers have been suggested to prevent the progression of cardiomyopathy. Scoliosis

Pearls and Perils: Friedreich's Ataxia

1. Hyporeflexia, Romberg sign, extensor plantar response, cerebellar ataxia, and loss of position and vibration sense in the first decade are the hallmarks of Friedreich's ataxia. A clinical syndrome similar to Friedreich's ataxia is seen in vitamin E deficiency. This condition is associated with pigmentary retinal degeneration, which is absent in Friedreich's ataxia. In ataxia-telangiectasia, peripheral sensory degeneration is a secondary factor that exacerbates the ataxia of cerebellar origins during the second decade.

2. In Refsum's disease, there is no extensor plantar response, and pigmentary degeneration of the retina is a prominent feature.

3. In Tabes dorsalis, there is no peripheral neuropathy.

4. In Dejerine-Sottas disease, cerebellar ataxia and extensor toe signs are not found.

5. Clinical features of B_{12}-deficient polyneuropathy are somewhat similar to those of Friedreich's ataxia. A megaloblastosis and methylmalonic aciduria are typical of B_{12} deficiency.

6. An atypical form of NCL with juvenile ataxia predominating can be distinguished by hyperreflexia in NCL and hyporeflexia in Friedreich's ataxia. An atypical spinocerebellar degeneration with hyperreflexia is also found in juvenile GM_2 gangliosidosis.

7. Adrenomyeloneuropathy may present as a spinocerebellar syndrome.

8. Leigh's syndrome may present as a spinocerebellar syndrome that can be distinguished from Friedreich's ataxia if its course is intermittently progressive and if eye involvement is present.

9. CT scan of the head is usually normal in Friedreich's ataxia (cerebellar atrophy is demonstrated in Marinesco-Sjögren-Garland syndrome and ataxia-telangiectasia).

10. An echocardiogram permits recognition of heart disease in Friedreich's ataxia before the onset of cardiac symptoms or the development of clinical signs of heart disease.

should be observed for a few years in order to assess the rate of progression of the deformity before deciding on surgical intervention, because in some patients the deformity may remain mild throughout the course of the illness.

ANNOTATED BIBLIOGRAPHY

Dijkstra U, Gabreels F, Joosten E, et al: Friedreich's ataxia: Intravenous pyruvate load to demonstrate a defect in pyruvate metabolism. *Neurology* 34:1493–1497, 1984.

In Friedreich's ataxia, disturbance in pyruvate metabolism is most directly demonstrated by the pyruvate loading test.

Diener HC, Muller A, Thron A, Poremba A, Dichgans J, Rapp H: Correlation of clinical signs with CT findings in patients with cerebellar ataxia. *J Neurol* 233:5–12, 1986.

In patients with Friedreich's ataxia, no or minor abnormalities of the cerebellum are demonstrated by CT.

St John Sutton MG, Olukotun AY, Tajik AJ, Lovett JL, Giuliani ER: Left ventricular function in Friedreich's ataxia. *Br Heart J* 44:309–316, 1980.

Echocardiography permits recognition of heart disease in Friedreich's ataxia before the onset of cardiac symptoms or development of clinical signs of heart disease.

Staya-Murti S, Cacace A, Hanson P: Auditory dysfunction in Friedreich ataxia: Result of spinal ganglion degeneration. *Neurology* 30:1047–1053, 1980.

Brainstem auditory evoked potentials obtained using a mastoid-vertex electrode derivation are useful to detect early signs of spinal ganglion degeneration.

Carroll WM, Kriss A, Baraitser M, Barrett G, Halliday AM: The incidence and nature of visual pathway involvement in Friedreich's ataxia. *Brain* 103:413–434, 1980.

Of Friedreich's ataxia patients, 64% have a generalized reduction in amplitude and prolongation of the visual evoked potential latency. Temporal dispersion and waveform are normal.

Said G, Marion MH, Selva J, Jamet C: Hypotrophic and dying-back nerve fibers in Friedreich's ataxia. *Neurology* 36:1292–1299, 1986.

Loss of large myelinated fibers in young patients and evidence of dying-back axons isolated in rare specimens fit the concept of a defect in maturation and maintenance of specific neurons.

Stumpf DA, Parks JK, Parker WD: Friedreich's disease IV. Reduced mitochondrial malic enzyme activity in heterozygotes. *Neurology* 33:780–783, 1983.

Mitochondrial malic enzyme is markedly reduced in cultured fibroblasts from Friedreich's ataxia patients. Obligate heterozygotes show 20% of the enzyme activity of controls, rather than the expected 50%. These unexpectedly low levels of enzyme activity in heterozygotes may result from negative interaction of the mutant and normal subunits in the tetrameric enzyme.

Gray RGF, Kumar D: Mitochondrial malic enzyme in Friedreich's ataxia: Failure to demonstrate reduced activity in cultured fibroblasts. *J Neurol Neurosurg Psychiatr* 48:70–74, 1985.

No abnormality of either cytosolic or mitochondrial malic enzyme in cultured fibroblasts could be detected in six patients with Friedreich's ataxia.

BASSEN-KORNZWEIG SYNDROME AND ACQUIRED VITAMIN E DEFICIENCY

Bassen-Kornzweig syndrome (BKS) or abetalipoproteinemia is a rare inborn error of lipoprotein metabolism characterized by steatorrhea, hypocholesterolemia, hematologic changes, and a progressive neurodegenerative disorder. Biochemically, the disorder is characterized by absence of all apoprotein-B–containing

FEATURE TABLE 13-17. BASSEN-KORNZWEIG SYNDROME

Discriminating Feature	Consistent Features	Variable Features
1. Absence of apolipoprotein-B in plasma	1. Diarrhea and fat malabsorption 2. Intestinal mucosa appear yellow on endoscopy 3. Acanthocytosis 4. Increased RBC sphingomyelin 5. Nearly absent plasma triglycerides 6. Decreased plasma cholesterol and phospholipids 7. Absent plasma low-density, lipoproteins, very-low-density lipoproteins, and chylomicrons	1. Mild to severe anemia 2. Retinitis pigmentosa 3. Progressive ataxia 4. Areflexia and proprioceptive changes 5. Weakness and muscle atrophy 6. Extensor plantar responses 7. Abnormal eye movements 8. Pes cavus, scoliosis 9. Vitamin E deficiency (if neurologic symptoms) 10. Vitamin A or D deficiency (rare)

lipoproteins from plasma. This apoprotein is essential for synthesis of both chylomicrons in the intestinal mucosa and very-low-density lipoproteins in the liver.

The infant with BKS is usually normal at birth. Failure to thrive and abdominal distention along with steatorrhea are the first symptoms in infancy. The diagnoses of cystic fibrosis and celiac diseases typically are entertained and later excluded by laboratory tests and failure to respond to appropriate therapy. Endoscopy reveals a yellow discoloration of the duodenum and jejunal biopsy is generally pathognomonic, showing extensively vacuolated mucosal cells packed with lipid droplets. The earliest neurologic finding is the loss of myotatic reflexes at an early age. Neurologic symptoms typically develop toward the end of the first decade of life and suggest a spinocerebellar degenerative disorder. Position and vibratory sensation are lost, and a positive Romberg sign typical of sensory ataxia can be elicited. Clinical evidence of pyramidal tract lesions usually appears later. Weakness and muscle atrophy may rapidly progress. Most subjects are unable to walk by their mid-20s. Pes cavus and scoliosis are common findings. Athetosis has been observed. Some degree of mental retardation may become apparent in 20% of the patients. Behavioral and cognitive changes may occur. Degeneration of the retina may develop during infancy but more often later. Pigmentary retinopathy is a constant finding. Reduced electroretinographic amplitudes precede visual decline. Oscillating, vertical, horizontal, and disassociated nystagmus is concomitant with the progressive loss of vision. Ophthalmoplegia may result from both supranuclear and nuclear involvement.

Chronic fat malabsorption secondary to causes other than abetalipoproteinemia (e.g., mucoviscidosis, celiac disease, intestinal lymphangiectasia, biliary atresia) may result in variable neurologic symptoms, including spinocerebellar degeneration, proprioceptive loss, areflexia, weakness, delayed motor and cognitive development,

opthalmoplegia, and retinal pigmentation. The clinical progression of neurologic symptoms is variable and depends on the etiology. In biliary atresia progression of neurologic symptoms may be more rapid than in abetalipoproteinemia. Vitamin E deficiency is thought to be responsible for the neurologic symptoms, for an isolated vitamin E deficiency without lipid malabsorption produces a similar clinical picture.

Laboratory findings suggestive of abetalipoproteinemia include a very low plasma concentration of cholesterol (less than 100 mg/mL) and triglycerides (less than 30 mg/mL) and acanthocytosis of the peripheral erythrocytes. (Acanthocytes are crenated red cells of normal size exhibiting spiny processes of various sizes. Their formation is attributed to changes in the lipid composition of erythrocyte membranes.) Severe anemia may occur. Vitamin E is undetectable in the serum of symptomatic patients. The diagnosis of abetalipoproteinemia depends on confirmation of the absence of apolipoprotein-B. Other causes of chronic fat malabsorption may result in little change in plasma, cholesterol, and triglyceride levels. In cholestatic liver disease, plasma cholesterol is elevated. In isolated vitamin E deficiency, laboratory findings are normal except for a low blood vitamin E level, elevated H_2O_2-induced hemolysis, and large amounts of thiobarbituric acid–reactive substances (lipoperoxides) in the serum.

Neuropathologic studies in abetalipoproteinemia and other causes of vitamin E deficiency show lesions of muscles, peripheral nerves, and the CNS. Muscle abnormalities include fiber type grouping suggestive of chronic denervation and abundant distinct lysosomal inclusions of ceroid lipopigment between the myofibrils, suggesting a primary insult to the muscles. Peripheral nerve studies show that demyelination is not a primary disorder but results mainly from large fiber axonal degeneration. In the CNS, the most characteristic pathologic change is the widespread presence of swollen, dystrophic axons (spheroids), most prominent in the sensory and oculomotor nuclei and absent in the cerebral and cerebellar hemispheres. Moderate to marked degrees of neuronal loss and gliosis are prominent in these areas. Neuronal lipofuscinosis is more severe in the large nerve cells, such as Betz cells. The severity of neuronal lipofuscinosis is not correlated with the neuronal disintegration. In the retina, extreme disruption of photoreceptor cells and hypertrophy of the retinal pigment epithelium with lysosomal lipopigment accumulation is the rule.

Abetalipoproteinemia is inherited as an autosomal recessive trait. Heterozygotes have normal clinical and biochemical findings. Abetalipoproteinemia results from a defective *APO B* secretion. Hypobetalipoproteinemia is another autosomal recessive condition, which can only be distinguished from abetalipoproteinemia by studying the family history. Homozygotes in hypobetalipoproteinemia have clinical and biochemic findings identical to those of abetalipoproteinemia. Heterozygotes, however, have hypocholesterolemia secondary to low levels of low-density lipoproteins and may have clinical abnormalities. Hypobetalipoproteinemia results from a defective *APO B* gene. Isolated vitamin E deficiency appears to be inherited as an autosomal recessive trait. Low normal serum vitamin E levels are found in heterozygotes. The neurologic symptoms of abetalipoproteinemia or vitamin E deficiency can be prevented or improved by large doses of vitamin E. A fat-soluable or water-miscible form of oral vitamin E is first initiated at a large dose of about 100 mg/kg per day. Serum levels of vitamin E should be carefully monitored. In abetalipoproteinemia and biliary atresia, parenteral administration is frequently necessary to obtain normal serum levels. Supplementation of other fat-soluble vitamins must be provided in cases of fat malabsorption.

Pearls and Perils:
Bassen-Kornzweig Syndrome

1. In a child showing signs of retinopathy and neurologic findings similar to those in Friedreich's ataxia, a marked hypocholesterolemia and hypotriglyceridemia should suggest abetalipoproteinemia.
2. In primary vitamin E deficiency, laboratory findings are unremarkable except for a low serum vitamin E level, elevated H_2O_2-induced hemolysis, and large amounts of thiobarbituric acid-reactive substances (lipoperoxides) in the serum.
3. Acanthocytosis is not specific for abetalipoproteinemia.
4. Homozygotes for hypobetalipoproteinemia can only be distinguished from patients with abetalipoproteinemia by studying heterozygotes.

ANNOTATED BIBLIOGRAPHY

Harding AE, Matthews S, Jones S, Ellis CJK, Booth IW, Muller DRP: Spinocerebellar degeneration associated with a selective defect of vitamin E absorption. *N Engl J Med* 313:32–35, 1985.
  A progressive neurologic disorder comprising ataxia, areflexia, and marked loss of proprioception developed at age 13. Vitamin E deficiency did not result from lipid malabsorption.
Bassen FA, Kornzweig AL: Malformation of the erythrocytes in a case of atypical retinitis pigmentosa. *Blood* 5:381–387, 1950.
  The clinical picture and hematologic changes of BKS were first described in this paper. Abetalipoproteinemia was only discovered later.
Herbert PN, Assmann G, Gotto AM, Fredrickson DS: Familial lipoprotein deficiency, in Stanbury JB, Wyngaarden JB, Fredrickson DS, Goldstein JL, Brown MS (eds): *The Metabolic Basis of Inherited Diseases*. New York, McGraw-HIll, 1983, p 589–642.
  The authors give a detailed review of abetalipoproteinemia and hypobetalipoproteinemia.
Saito R, Yokoyama T, Okaniwa M, Kamoshita S: Neuropathology of chronic vitamin E deficiency in fatal familial intrahepatic cholestasis. *Acta Neuropathol* 58:187–192, 1982.
  The neuropathology of human vitamin E deficiency is reviewed carefully.
Muller DPR, Lloyd JK, Wolff OH: The role of vitamin E in the treatment of the neurological features of abetalipoproteinemia and other disorders of fat absorption. *J Inher Metab Dis* 8(suppl):88–91, 1985.
  A therapeutic approach with vitamin E is discussed.
Ross RS, Gregg RE, Law SW, et al: Homozygous hypobetalipoproteinemia: A disease distinct from abetalipoproteinemia at the molecular level. *J Clin Invest* 81:590–595, 1988.
  Homozygous abetalipoproteinemia and homozygous hypobetalipoproteinemia can only be distinguished by plasma analysis of *ADO B*- and *APO B*-containing lipoproteins in obligate heterozygoes.

REFSUM'S DISEASE

Refsum's disease (heredopathia atactica polyneuritiformis) is a rare disorder of the mitochondrial oxidation of phytanic acid. This disorder of lipid metabolism is characterized by the tetrad of retinitis pigmentosa, cerebellar ataxia, chronic polyneuropathy, and an increased level of CSF protein with normal cell count. Additional findings may include sensorineural hearing loss, anosmia, cataracts, small myotic pupils, cardiac conduction defects, skeletal deformities, renal tubular involvement, and skin changes resembling ichthyosis.

The onset is insidious in early childhood or young adulthood. Congenital skeletal changes in the hands (symmetric hypo- or hyperplasia of fingers or metacarpals) and feet (hammer toe deformity, pes cavus, shortening or overdevelopment of metatarsals or toes) occur in up to 75% of all cases. Symmetric epiphyseal dysplasia

FEATURE TABLE 13-18. REFSUM'S DISEASE

Discriminating Features	Consistent Features	Variable Features
1. Phytanic oxidase deficiency in fibroblasts 2. Normal peroxisomal function, number, and morphology	1. Pigmentary degeneration of the retina 2. Chronic progressive sensorimotor polyneuropathy 3. Decreased motor and sensory nerve conduction 4. Hyporeflexia (ankle) 5. Distal muscular dystrophy 6. Hypertrophic demyelinating neuropathy with onion bulb formation 7. Elevated CSF proteins 8. Normal intelligence 9. No pyramidal tract signs 10. Elevated phytanic acid level in the blood	1. Ataxia (sensory and cerebellar) 2. Neural hearing loss 3. Anosmia 4. Cataracts 5. Cardiomyopathy 6. Ichthyosis 7. Bony changes 8. Pes cavus 9. Renal tubular involvement 10. Enlarged palpable peripheral nerves

of the shoulders, elbows, and knees is less frequently found. Night blindness is often the earliest manifestation. Without night blindness or pigmentary degeneration of the retina, a diagnosis of Refsum's disease should not be made. The pigmentary degeneration of the retina is often of a granular appearance, rather than the classic "bony spicule" type. It is accompanied by concentric constriction of the visual fields. Symptoms such as pigmentary degeneration of the retina, cataracts, small pupils, hyposmia, and deafness are insidious and may commence many years before a sudden deterioration. The rapid onset of ataxia, polyneuropathy (peripheral and cranial nerves), cardiac arrhythmia, or ichthyosis is usually associated with a decreased caloric intake, resulting in a weight loss. Improvement may occur when caloric intake is increased. An early onset of the disease does not necessarily indicate a particularly poor prognosis. In the early stages of sensorimotor polyneuropathy, a fairly typical syndrome of peroneal muscular atrophy develops starting distally. Myotatic reflexes become depressed and are finally lost. Sensory changes most commonly involve vibratory and proprioceptive sensation. Cerebellar signs of ataxia, dysarthria, and intension tremor may be superimposed on the sensory ataxia. Extensor toe signs do not occur, excluding Friedreich's ataxia. In some patients, the nerves may be enlarged on palpation. Skin changes, when present, may vary from dry skin or palmar hyperkeratosis to florid ichthyosis.

In Refsum's disease, nonspecific electrocardiographic changes are found. Electrophysiologic studies may reveal reduced motor and sensory nerve conduction velocity. Electromyography may show evidence of denervation. The ERG shows reduction or complete absence of rod and cone responses. The EEG is normal in most cases.

Laboratory findings suggestive of classic Refsum's disease are the isolated increase of the protein content of the CSF without a corresponding increase in the number of cells (albuminocytologic dissociation), and the increased plasma phytanic acid level (normally less than 0.3 mg/100 mL). Phytanic acid is a fatty acid derived from phytol, a component of the chlorophyll molecule. It cannot be synthesized endogenously; therefore, the only source is the diet. In Refsum's disease, phytanic acid normally present in the diet cannot be metabolized owing to a defect of the α-oxidative pathways, the initial step in catabolism of phytanic acid. In some patients with a typical clinical picture of Refsum's disease, a diet low in phytanic acid will normalize the pattern of fatty acid in the serum. In such patients, measurement of the phytanic acid oxidase activity in skin fibroblasts is necessary and proves the metabolic defect. Accumulation of phytanic acid cannot be considered diagnostic for Refsum's disease, as this acid has also been found in patients with peroxisomal disorders, such as neonatal adrenoleukodystrophy, Zellweger's syndrome, and chondrodysplasia punctata (rhizomelic type). Furthermore, measurement of the phytanic acid oxidase activity is not helpful in differentiating Refsum's disease from peroxisomal disorders. The distinction between Refsum's disease and the peroxisomal disorders can easily be made on a clinical basis. Furthermore, in Refsum's disease, contrary to peroxisomal disorders, the defect of the α-oxidative pathway is the only metabolic defect known and peroxisomes are normal in function, number, and morphology.

Pathologic changes characteristic of Refsum's disease are found in the nervous system and skin. The lesions of the nervous system are neither constant nor specific. Considerable amounts of fat may be noted in the leptomeninges, ependymal cells, and epithelium of the choroid plexus. Degeneration of the Purkinje cells, dentate neurons, inferior olives, red nucleus, and vestibular cochlear nuclei may occur. The cerebral hemispheres are well preserved in all instances. Refsum's disease may show atrophy with loss of cones and rods, loss of ganglion cells in both the inner and outer molecular layers, and damage to the pigmentary epithelium. Hypertrophic polyneuropathy is the basis of the neural lesions. Onion bulb formation affects particularly the proximal nerve trunks. It is associated with neural muscular atrophy, retrograde atrophy of the ventral horns, and secondary atrophy of the fasciculi gracili. Crystalline-like inclusions in Schwann cells seen on electron microscopy are thought to originate from mitochondria. Ultrastructural examination of the skin clearly differentiates Refsum's disease from autosomal dominant ichthyosis vulgaris and X-linked recessive ichthyosis. In the lower epidermal strata, lipid droplets (liposomes) are associated with the endoplasmic reticulum and abnormal or giant mitochondria. The epidermal liposomes have been shown to be the morphologic substrate for the cellular accumulation of phytanic acid.

Pearls and Perils: Refsum's Disease

1. Phytanic acid is characteristically elevated in Refsum's disease. It may also be elevated in peroxisomal disorders. Patients with Refsum's disease do not accumulate bile acids and very-long-chain fatty acids; synthesis of plasmalogen is normal; pipecolic acid is not found in the urine.
2. The clinical course of Refsum's disease may be improved by dietary restriction of phytanic acid.
3. Phytanic oxidase assay in skin fibroblasts is only necessary for diagnosis if phytanic acid is normal in a patient with characteristic phenotypic features of Refsum's disease.
4. Mental retardation and epileptic seizures are not part of the typical clinical picture. Patients with Refsum's disease may present with a clinical picture resembling that of relapsing or chronic polyneuropathy, or Guillain-Barré syndrome. Other patients may present with a neurologic disorder resembling other hypertrophic neuropathies (e.g., Charcot-Marie-Tooth disease or Dejerine-Sottas disease). A pigmentary degeneration of the retina distinguishes Refsum's disease.
5. Abetalipoproteinemia and other vitamin deficiency states can be readily distinguished by biochemic tests.
6. Some cases of KSS are clinically similar to Refsum's disease. Ophthalmoplegia is exceptional in Refsum's disease. Biochemic and histopathologic criteria differentiate the conditions. Skin biopsy may allow differential diagnosis between Refsum's disease and true ichthyosis.

Refsum's disease is inherited as an autosomal recessive trait. Phytanic acid oxidase activity is reduced in skin fibroblasts from obligate heterozygotes. However, the method is not sensitive enough to separate heterozygotes from homozygotic patients. As soon as the diagnosis of Refsum's disease is made, a restricted dietary intake of phytanic acid is achieved by avoiding fats obtained from herbivores (e.g., milk, beef, rabbit), fish, pork, and green vegetables. It is important to maintain sufficient caloric intake to avoid release of phytanic acid from body stores. Vitamin and mineral supplementation is required. Carefully supervised dietary restriction can lower the plasma phytanic acid levels in a few weeks, with a concomitant improvement in peripheral nerve conduction, muscle strength, and skin abnormalities. In patients with severe exacerbations of symptoms, plasmapheresis reduces plasma phytanic acid levels rapidly, reversing most clinical symptoms. Central neurologic damage, however, is permanent.

ANNOTATED BIBLIOGRAPHY

Steinberg D, Mize CE, Fales HM, Vroom FQ: Phytanic acid in patients with Refsum's syndrome and response to dietary treatment. *Arch Intern Med* 125:75–87, 1970.
　　The dietary treatment changes the natural course of the disease.
Davies MG, Reynolds DJ, Marks R, et al: The epidermis in Refsum's disease (heredopathia atactica polyneuritiformis), in Marks R, Dykes PJ (eds): *The Ichthyoses.* Lancaster, England, MTP, 1978, p 51–64.
　　The dermatologic changes in Refsum's disease are reviewed.
MacBrinn MC, O'Brien JS: Lipid composition of the nervous system in Refsum's disease. *J Lipid Res* 9:552–561, 1968.
　　Large amounts of phytanic acid are found in the central and peripheral nervous systems.
Watkins PA, Mihalik SJ: Mitochondrial oxidation of phytanic acid in human and monkey liver: Implication that Refsum's disease is not a peroxisomal disorder. *Biochem Biophys Res Commun* 167:580–586, 1980.
　　Refsum's disease is a mitochondrial disorder.

POMPE'S DISEASE

Pompe's disease or the infantile form of generalized glycogenosis (infantile type II glycogenosis) is a lysosomal glycogen storage disease resulting in early onset of cardiomegaly, hypotonia, cerebral dysfunction, failure to thrive, and early death. Lysosomal glycogen storage affects practically all the tissues in the body and results from a defect of acid α-1,4-glucosidase (or acid maltase).

Clinically, the symptoms of Pompe's disease may be apparent at birth, and usually become manifest during the first months of life. The usual presenting symptoms are feeding difficulties, dyspnea, cyanosis, poor motor activity, or sometimes febrile episodes from recurrent

FEATURE TABLE 13-19. POMPE'S DISEASE

Discriminating Feature	Consistent Features	Variable Features
1. Acid maltase deficiency in fibroblasts or other tissues	1. Hypotonia and weakness 2. Large vacuoles containing glycogen in muscle fibers 3. Hyporeflexia	1. Macroglossia 2. Hepatomegaly (mild) 3. Failure to thrive 4. Cardiomegaly (absent in childhood or adult forms) 5. Bulbar signs 6. No muscle atrophy (early) 7. Hypoglycemia or acidosis

respiratory infections. Physical examination typically reveals a severe flaccid quadriparesis with minimal spontaneous motion and frog leg position. Muscle mass appears adequate. Myotactic reflexes are decreased or absent. The mouth is kept open and the tongue is large and protruding. There are no muscular fasciculations. The infants appear alert. Umbilical and inguinal hernias are frequently reported. Dyspnea and cyanosis are the most obvious functional consequences of the cardiac dysfunction. A cardiomegaly is easily detected by percussion, whereas auscultation sometimes discloses an apical systolic murmur. The liver is typically only moderately enlarged. Failure to thrive is frequently severe. Gradually, a variable degree of muscular hypotrophy may occur. Bulbar signs, mostly difficulty in swallowing, may appear. Respiration becomes shallow. Pompe's disease is always fatal, usually within 2 years after birth. Death may be due to failure of respiratory muscles or cardiac failure.

Liver enzymes are usually elevated. However, in contrast to other glycogenoses, there are no abnormalities of glucose homeostasis. Blood lactate, uric acid, and lipid levels are normal. Cardiac and muscle enzyme levels are frequently elevated. The chest x ray shows a large, globular, cardiac silhouette. The electrocardiogram may show diffuse gigantic QRS complexes and a short PR interval. Cardiac catheterization may reveal biventricular hypertrophy sometimes with a secondary subaortic stenosis. The electromyogram displays a myopathic pattern, with normal motor and sensory conduction velocities. In some cases, characteristic changes in the electromyogram consist of postcontraction or insertional myotonic discharges, spontaneous high-frequency positive waves, and spontaneous fibrillations. CT scan of the head is normal. The diagnosis of Pompe's disease rests on the demonstration of a complete deficiency of acid α-1,4-glucosidase (acid maltase) in liver, muscle, and cultured fibroblasts. Leukocytes can be assayed after electric precipitation of a renal isoenzyme that is present in varying amounts in the leukocytes and may interfere with assays owing to its broad pH optimum. Besides Pompe's disease, a deficiency in acid α-1,4-glucosidase is found in milder forms of type II glycogenosis, which are

characterized by later onset and preferential involvement of skeletal muscles (mimicking the symptoms of slowly progressive limb girdle muscular dystrophy in children or adults).

Screening of peripherael blood may be useful in demonstrating disease-specific lysosomal inclusions in lymphocytes. PAS reaction or staining with Best's Carmine reveals small discrete cytoplasmic vacuoles. On ultrastructural studies, a few membrane-bound vacuoles are filled with round granules measuring 1 to 2 μm in diameter. Electron microscopic studies of the skin and skin fibroblast cultures demonstrate similar intracellular inclusions. Liver biopsy reveals vacuolar localization of glycogen in both hepatocytes and Kupffer cells. Ultrastructurally, membrane-bound bodies containing glycogen are larger in the hepatocytes and may reach 8 μm in diameter. Light microscopy of biopsied muscle shows a severe vacuolar myopathy with marked enlargement of muscle fibers owing to cytoplasmic vacuolization. Vacuoles are PAS positive and contain basophilic and metachromatic material. Ultrastructurally there is a severe disruption of intrinsic cytoplasmic architecture. A great deal of the sarcoplasmic glycogen is contained within vacuoles. These frequently contain dense osmiophilic remnants generally devoid of any structure. Ultrastructural studies of peripheral nerves demonstrate free and membrane-bound glycogen in Schwann cells, axons, perineural and endothelial cells, pericytes, and fibroblasts. Few ultrastructural alterations occur in the myelin sheaths. Schwann cells of unmyelinated axons may harbor a mixture of glycogen and granular lipopigments within the same lysosome. Several axons are slightly enlarged and display a proliferation of tubules, filaments, and vesicular profiles, occasionally forming clefts. These axonal lesions resemble those seen in neuroaxonal dystrophy. Neuronal glycogen storage can be demonstrated by rectal biopsy. Within the CNS neuronal glycogen storage is most prominent in the anterior horn cells of the spinal cord, dorsal root ganglias, motor cranial nerve nuclei, and parts of the basal ganglia, brainstem, and cerebellum. Free and membrane-bound glycogen is found in perikaryon, dendrites, axons, and presynaptic endings. Glycogen deposition is prominent

---

Pearls and Perils: Pompe's Disease

1. An enlarged heart in a floppy infant without tongue fasciculation is typical of Pompe's disease.
2. In contrast to symptoms of other glycogenoses, the liver is normal in size or only moderately enlarged and there are no abnormalities of glucose homeostasis in Pompe's disease.
3. Ethanolaminosis is a rare generalized storage disease resembling Pompe's disease clinically. There is widespread deposition of PAS-positive material in the tissues. Distinguishing features are the absence of glycogen abnormality and the deposition of ethanolamine in the tissues owing to a deficiency of ethanolamine kinase.
4. The localization of glycogen within lysosomal membranes is of diagnostic significance but does not allow differentiation of Pompe's disease from other later-onset acid α-1,4-glucosidase deficiencies.

---

in the white matter. The glial cells, particularly astrocytes, accumulate greatly distended glycogen-containing lysosomes. No abnormalities are seen in the myelin sheaths. In almost every cell type of the retina deposits of lysosomal glycogen are abundant.

The prevalence of Pompe's disease has been estimated to be at least equal to 1 in 150,000 live births. Pompe's disease is inherited as an autosomal recessive trait. There is a preponderance (60%) of affected males over females. Heterozygotes are detected by reduced fibroblast acid α-1,4-glucosidase activity. Only one family with both Pompe's disease and an adult form of α-glucosidase deficiency has been reported. Complementation studies by fusion of fibroblasts from patients with Pompe's disease and less severe childhood and adult forms of α-glucosidase deficiency yield no sign of nonallelism of the several forms. By study of somatic cell hybrids, the acid α-1,4-glucosidase locus has been assigned to chromosome 17 and more specifically to 17q23.

Previous therapeutic strategies including enzyme substitution and stimulation, have been ineffective in the treatment of Pompe's disease. Recently, high-protein therapy has resulted in improvement of muscle function in one case of childhood acid maltase deficiency. Whether this type of therapy has a place in the treatment of Pompe's disease is unknown. Efforts should focus on symptomatic treatment and genetic counseling. Infants with respiratory failure are artificially ventilated. Respiratory infections are treated with antibiotics. Infants with heart failure receive digitalis and diuretics. Prenatal diagnosis can be achieved by using cultured amniotic cells or chorionic villi biopsy specimens.

ANNOTATED BIBLIOGRAPHY

Broadhead DM, Butterworth J: α-Glucosidase in Pompe's disease. *J Inher Metab Dis* 1:153–154, 1978.

Leukocyte acid maltase is not always deficient in Pompe's disease owing to the presence in the leukoycytes of varying amounts of a renal α-1,4-glucosidase, which has a broad pH optimum that overlaps that of the lysosomal enzyme. This interfering activity can be removed by isoelectric precipitation at pH 5.0, allowing the unambiguous use of leukocytes for diagnosis.

Koster JF, Busch HFM, Slee RG, van Weerden TW: Glycogenosis type II: The infantile and late-onset acid maltase deficiency observed in one family. *Clin Chim Acta* 87:451–453, 1978.

A grandfather with difficulty climbing stairs after age 52 and a granddaughter with typical Pompe's disease leading to death at 16 weeks were both found deficient in acid α-1,4-glucosidase.

Bordink JM, Legato MJ, Lovelace RE, Blumenthal S: Pompe's disease. Electromyographic, electron microscopic and cardiovascular aspects. *Arch Neurol* 23:113–119, 1970.

Electromyography in Pompe's disease displays a myopathic pattern and, in some cases, a more complicated pattern, with myotonic discharges, bizarre high-frequency positive waves, and fibrillations.

Goebel HH, Lenard HG, Kohlschutter A, Pilz H: The ultrastructure of the sural nerve in Pompe's disease. *Ann Neurol* 2:111–115, 1977.

Glycogen is combined with lipopigment in lysosomes of nonmyelinating Schwann cells. Proliferation of axonal constituents indicates mild damage to axons.

Hug G, Schubert WK, Soukup S: Ultrastructure and enzymatic deficiency of fibroblast cultures in type II glycogenosis. *Pediatr Res* 5:107–112, 1971.

Fibroblasts contain numerous vacuoles that are packed with glycogen-like particles.

Hers HG, de Barsy T: Type II glycogenosis (acid maltase deficiency) in Hers HG, Van Hoof F (eds): *Lysosomes and Storage Diseases*. New York, Academic Press, 1973, p 197–216.

Clinical, pathologic, biochemic, and genetic features of type II glycogenosis are reviewed.

Slonim AE, Coleman RA, McElligot MA, et al: Improvement of muscle function in acid maltase deficiency by high-protein therapy. *Neurology* 33:34–38, 1983.

High-protein therapy was effective in one case of childhood-onset acid maltase deficiency. Whether such therapy has a place in the treatment of Pompe's disease is unknown.

Vietor KW, Havsteen B, Harms D, Busse H, Heyne K: Ethanolaminosis. A newly recognized, generalized storage disease with cardiomegaly, cerebral dysfunction and early death. *Eur J Pediatr* 126:61–75, 1977.

Ethanolaminosis is similar in several aspects to the type II glycogenosis described by Pompe.

Diffuse Encephalopathies

CEREBROHEPATORENAL SYNDROME OF ZELLWEGER

The cerebrohepatorenal syndrome of Zellweger (Zellweger's syndrome) is a peroxisomal disorder responsible for a distinct combination of congenital abnormalities and an unusual variety of profound metabolic disturbances. Congenital abnormalities characteristic of Zellweger's syndrome include typical craniofacial dysmorphism, profound generalized hypotonia, hepatomegaly, and cortical renal cysts. The appearance of the newborn with Zellweger's syndrome is characteristic: the forehead is high; the supraorbital ridges and bridge of nose are flat; the infant generally shows micrognathia, a high arched palate, and full cheeks; the anterior fontanelle and sutures (including the metopic suture) are widely patent; the eyes may show bilateral glaucoma with cloudy corneas and cataracts; and the mouth is triangular with the upper lip shaped like an inverted V (Figure 13–7). Cliteromegaly or undescended testes are common features. Limb anomalies, such as talipes equinovarus and camptodactyly, may occur. Congenital heart lesions are rare, yet septal defects and delayed closure of the ductus arteriosus and foramen ovale occur. There may be a

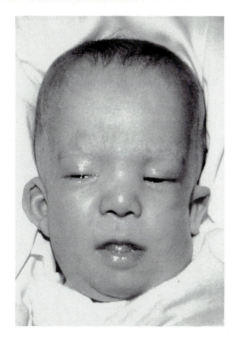

Figure 13–7. Characteristic facial features—such as flat supraorbital ridges, high forehead, ptosis, epicanthal folds, depressed nasal bridge, short anteverted nose, low-set ears, and micrognathia—in a 3-month-old white male who showed biochemic, pathologic, and radiologic evidence of Zellweger's syndrome.

history of polyhydramnios or paucity of intrauterine movements. At birth, respiration is spontaneous, but apneic episodes may occur. Sucking and swallowing difficulties necessitate gavage feedings. Postnatal weight gain is poor. The child is paretic and severely hypotonic. Moro and tendon reflexes are difficult to elicit. Psychomotor development is very limited. The infant fails to develop the ability to fix, focus vision, or follow objects, and appears unresponsive to most external stimuli. Seizures of various types are frequent. Marked variations in body temperature without evidence of localized infection or sepsis develop. Hepatomegaly is nearly a constant finding. Jaundice may develop before death. Most patients die within the first 3 months of life.

The most striking pathologic changes in Zellweger's syndrome occur in the liver, the kidney, and the nervous system. The liver is regularly increased in size and shows cirrhotic changes, hemosiderosis, and intrahepatic biliary dysgenesis. The kidneys show dysgenetic renal parenchyma and multiple small subcapsular cysts. Abnormal structure and function of mitochondria have been described in the liver and kidneys of patients with Zellweger's syndrome, but such findings do not seem obligate. More remarkable is the fact that no peroxisomes can be recognized in the liver and kidneys of Zellweger's syndrome patients. Neuropathologic studies reveal macrogyria, polymicrogyria, hypoplasia of the corpus callosum, bilateral subependymal cysts in the area of the head of the caudate nuclei, and olivary dysplasia. Lissencephaly is rarely encountered.

In the CNS, microscopic alterations characteristic of Zellweger's syndrome include a heterotopic cortex in the white matter and diffuse dysmyelination extending to the gray matter, with sudanophilic lipid deposits in the cytoplasm of astrocytes and macrophages. Those lipid deposits are made of monounsaturated and saturated very-long-chain fatty acids in the cholesterol esters and sphingolipids of the white matter.

Small subcapsular renal cysts are a constant finding and can be detected by abdominal ultrasound. Skeletal x rays show, in most cases, scattered calcified stippling in the patellar area, acetabular synchondrosis, and proximal epiphyses of femur and humerus. The epiphyses are generally spared but may be retarded in development. These findings are quite different from those in chondrodystrophia punctata congenita, in which the calcific stippling most often occurs in the epiphyses of the long bones (limbs are shortened), and no subcapsular renal cysts are found.

Laboratory studies in Zellweger's syndrome usually show evidence of liver involvement. Serum cholesterol may be low secondary to a decrease in β-lipoprotein. High serum iron levels with low iron-binding capacities are due

FEATURE TABLE 13-20. CEREBROHEPATORENAL SYNDROME OF ZELLWEGER

Discriminating Features	Consistent Features	Variable Features
1. No peroxisomes in liver and renal tubular epithelia 2. Dihydroxyacetone phosphate acyltransferase deficiency in fibroblasts	1. Seizures 2. Hypotonia 3. Characteristic facies with flat supraorbital ridges 4. Widely patent fontanelles and sutures 5. Hepatomegaly 6. Failure to thrive 7. Subcapsular renal cysts 8. Nonspecific aminoaciduria 9. Pipecolic aciduria and acidemia 10. Elevated very-long-chain fatty acids in serum and plasma 11. Abnormal bile acid metabolism	1. Cataracts, retinitis pigmentosa, glaucoma, cloudy cornea 2. Congenital heart lesions 3. Cryptorchidism or cliteromegaly 4. Limb abnormalities 5. Calcific stippling of epiphysis and patellae 6. Redundant skin on the neck 7. Fullness at the cheeks 8. Jaundice 9. Gastrointestinal bleeding 10. Elevated serum iron and total iron-binding capacity 11. Hypoglycemia 12. Vitamin E, A, D, and K deficiency

to a derangement in the reduction and delivery of ferric iron in transferrin to the ferrous iron in heme. Microcytic nonhemolytic anemia is common. An unspecific amnioaciduria may be found. A functional deficiency of the adrenal cortex may be evidenced by ACTH stimulation. Laboratory studies characteristic of Zellweger's syndrome are suggestive of a generalized impairment of peroxisomal oxidation. These characteristic findings include (1) elevated levels of pipecolic acid, an intermediary product in the catabolic pathway of lysin, in serum, urine, and CSF; (2) elevated levels of saturated ($C_{26:0}$) and monounsaturated ($C_{26:1}$) very long-chain fatty acids in the plasma, body fluids, and tissues with an elevation of the $C_{26:0}/C_{22:0}$ ratio; and (3) elevated levels of C_{27} bile acid intermediates (trihydroxycoprostanic acid and dehydroxycoprostanic acid), precursors of cholic acid in plasma and urine. In addition, the level of phytanic acid in plasma and other body fluids is sometimes elevated, resulting from a phytanic acid oxidase deficiency, but this finding is nonspecific.

Tissues of patients with Zellweger's syndrome contain less than 10% of the normal level of phosphatidylethanolamine plasmalogen, a phospholipid constituent of myelin and platelet-activating factor. The first enzyme in the pathway for plasmalogen synthesis, dihydroxyacetone phosphate acyltransferase, is located at the inner aspect of the peroxisomal membrane. This enzyme is deficient in the tissues of Zellweger's syndrome patients. Assay of this enzyme, detectable in amniotic fluid cells and chorionic villi, may be used and appears reliable for prenatal diagnosis.

Zellweger's syndrome is transmitted as an autosomal recessive trait. The assumed frequency is between 1 and 50,000 and 1 in 100,000 live births, suggesting a gene frequency of between 1 in 150 and 1 in 110. Determination of heterozygosity is still unsatisfactory. Treatment with clofibrate with the goal of stimulating production of peroxisomes has been unsuccessful. Attempts to treat the syndrome with oral plasmalogen normalize erythrocyte plasmalogen levels and may result in a clinical improvement. Bile acid (chenodeoxycholic and cholic acid)

**Pearls and Perils:
Cerebrohepatorenal Syndrome
of Zellweger**

1. Zellweger's syndrome should be suspected in newborns with craniofacial dysmorphism, seizures, and hypotonia. Cataracts and hepatomegaly may not be present at birth.
2. Renal cysts and subependymal cysts may be demonstrated by ultrasound.
3. X rays of the lower extremities may demonstrate chondral calcifications, most marked in the patellas.
4. Laboratory findings typical of Zellweger's syndrome include hyperpipecolicacidemia, elevated levels of C_{26} very-long-chain fatty acids and the $C_{26:0}/C_{22:0}$ ratio, elevated levels of C_{27} bile acid intermediates, and sometimes elevated levels of phytanic acid.
5. Dihydroxyacetone phosphate acyltransferase defects and absence of peroxisomes in the liver prove the diagnosis.

therapy may reduce hepatic sterol synthesis and prevent progression of liver and CNS damage. Dietary restriction of long-chain fatty acids has also been suggested. Replacement of adrenal steroids should be considered, particularly during stress.

ANNOTATED BIBLIOGRAPHY

Mathis RK, Watkins JB, Szczepanik-Van Leevween P, Lott IT: Liver in the cerebro-hepato-renal syndrome: Defective bile acid synthesis and abnormal mitochondria. *Gastroenterology* 79:1311–1317, 1980.

   The authors suggest that liver damage may be secondary to the accumulation of trihydroxycoprostanic acid and that bile acid therapy may decrease progression of the liver disease.

Wanders RJA, Schrakamp G, van den Bosch H, et al: Pre- and postnatal diagnosis of the cerebrohepatorenal (Zellweger) syndrome via a simple method directly demonstrating the presence or absence of peroxisomes in cultured skin fibroblasts, amniocytes, or chorionic villi fibroblasts. *J Inher Metab Dis* 9(suppl 2):317–320, 1986.

   The authors suggest a reliable method that can be used to study plasmalogen synthesis for early diagnosis of Zellweger's syndrome.

Wilson GN, Holmes RG, Custer J, et al: Zellweger syndrome: Diagnostic assays, syndrome delineation and potential therapy. *Am J Med Genet* 24:69–82, 1986.

   Therapeutic intervention is suggested for this disorder.

MITOCHONDRIAL ENCEPHALOMYOPATHIES

The mitochondrial encephalomyopathies are hereditary neurodegenerative disorders characterized by multiple features indicating dysfunction of mitochondrial aerobic oxidative metabolism: elevated levels of lactate pyruvate in the blood and/or CSF, alterations of mitochondrial morphology in various tissues, and diminished activity of oxidative mitochondrial enzymes.

   The mitochondrial encephalomyopathies are clinically, biochemically, and genetically heterogeneous. The clinical syndromes sharing features of mitochondrial encephalomyopathies are listed in Table 13–3. In this chapter, we will limit our discussion to mitochondrial encephalomyopathy, lactic acidosis, and stroke-like episode (MELAS) syndrome; myoclonic epilepsy/ragged red fiber (MERRF) syndrome; congenital mitochondrial encephalomyopathies (CMEs); and Kearns-Sayre syndrome (KSS). These syndromes differ in pattern of organ involvement and in degree of severity. The same clinical syndrome can be caused by various biochemic lesions. It appears likely that the nature of a given clinical syndrome depends not so much on the exact oxidative enzyme that is defective, but rather on the degree to which flux through oxidative pathways is impaired. Furthermore, each mitochondrial enzyme defect may lead to various clinical syndromes. Therefore, affected individuals within a single kindred may display different clinical syndromes.

TABLE 13-3. MITOCHONDRIAL ENCEPHALOMYOPATHIES

Clinical Syndrome	Enzyme Deficiency
Congenital mitochondrial encephalomyopathy	Pyruvate dehydrogenase complex Pyruvate carboxylase NADH-CoQ reductase complex Cytochrome *c* oxidase complex
Leigh's syndrome	Pyruvate dehydrogenase complex NADH-CoQ reductase complex Cytochrome *c* oxidase complex Inhibitor of thiamine pyrophosphate–ATP phosphoryltransferase
Mitochondrial encephalomyopathy, lactic acidosis, and stroke-like episode syndrome	Cytochrome *c* oxidase complex NADH-CoQ reductase complex
Myoclonic epilepsy/ragged red fiber syndrome	Cytochrome *c* oxidase complex Cytochrome *b* Succinate CoQ reductase NADH-CoQ reductase complex (?)
Kearns-Sayre syndrome	NADH-CoQ reductase complex Succinate dehydrogenase Cytochrome *c* oxidase complex Cytochrome *b* Coenzyme Q
Alper's disease	Cytochrome *c* oxidase complex NADH-CoQ reductase complex
Menkes's syndrome	Cytochrome *c* oxidase complex
Zellweger's syndrome	Succinate-CoQ reductase complex Phytanic oxidase
Refsum's disease	Phytanic oxidase

FEATURE TABLE 13-21. MITOCHONDRIAL ENCEPHALOMYOPATHIES

Discriminating Feature	Consistent Feature	Variable Features
1. Defect of mitochondrial oxidative metabolism	1. Pathologic increase in blood lactate and pyruvate after exercise or glucose loading test	1. Ragged-red fibers in striated muscles 2. Elevated CSF lactate and pyruvate

CMEs are characterized clinically by prenatal onset, as evidenced by intrauterine growth retardation, microcephaly, decreased fetal movements, or dysmorphic features. Patients with pyruvate dehydrogenase complex deficiency may show recognizable facial features, with a narrowed head, frontal bossing, a depressed nasal bridge, wide separation of the eyebrows, a small nose with anteverted nostrils and large ears. Hips may be dislocated. CT scan of the head may reveal agenesis of the corpus callosum. Micropenis and hypospadias have been found in patients with NADH-coenzyme Q (CoQ) oxidoreductase or cytochrome oxidase complex deficiency. Most infants are difficult to feed, lethargic, and floppy. The clinical course is usually characterized by recurrent episodes of lactic acidosis causing tachypnea. Seizures frequently occur. Respiratory insufficiency may be acute, causing apneic episodes. Occasional features include cardiomyopathy and the de Toni-Fanconi-Debre syndrome of tubular renal dysfunction. Most patients die within the first 3 months of life from overwhelming lactic acidosis. Those who survive after months of heroic life support are severely retarded. At autopsy, the brain shows spongy degeneration of the white matter and dysmyelination. Status spongiosus, loss of neurons, and vascular proliferation may be widespread in the CNS gray matter. Symmetric subependymal periventricular cysts near the lateral and fourth ventricles are consistently found in pyruvate dehydrogenase complex deficiency.

Patients with MELAS syndrome are usually asymptomatic in infancy and have normal early development. Symptoms begin between 2 years of age and young adulthood. Most patients are short and have recurrent epileptic seizures, which are partial or generalized. Attacks of prolonged migrainous headaches with vomiting are prominent in some patients. In the wake of migrainous headaches or focal seizures, patients may abruptly develop stroke-like episodes. The course of the disease is variable, with periods of clinical improvement without therapy. Episodes of cerebral infarction lead to a gradual decline in cognitive function, alternating hemiparesis with bilateral corticospinal signs, cortical deafness, and visual impairment with hemianopia or cortical blindness. Some patients with MELAS syndrome lack muscle symptoms, while others have muscle weakness and atrophy before the development of the CNS symptoms. In addition, some patients may have smooth muscle involvement, as suggested by recurrent abdominal pain and ileus. Most patients with MELAS syndrome do not have significant cerebellar dysfunction, interictal myoclonus, heart block, ophthalmoplegia, and retinal degeneration. CT scan of the head reveals shifting focal low-density areas, leading to diffuse cortical atrophy and ventricular dilatation. Focal lucencies may not always correspond to a vascular distribution. Cerebral angiography usually shows no abnormalities. Calcification of the basal ganglia is found in some patients in the absence of hypoparathyroidism or pseudohypothyroidism. Hypertrophic cardiomyopathy and renal dysfunction may be associated with MELAS syndrome. Pathologically multiple solitary or confluent foci of necrosis, varying in size and stage, involve predominantly the bilateral cerebral cortexes from frontal to occipital lobes and, to a lesser degree, the subcortical white matter, basal ganglia, brainstem, and cerebellum. Ultrastructural studies have suggested that brain lesions may result from a mitochondrial angiopathy, which affects the pial arterioles and small arteries most severely. Most reported cases have been sporadic, but a few familial groupings have been observed. Intrafamilial differences in disease phenotype and maternal inheritance suggest that a mutation of the mitochondrial genome may give rise to some forms of MELAS syndrome.

Typical cases of MERRF syndrome have normal early development with symptoms beginning between the ages of 5 and 42 years. The cardinal four symptoms are myoclonus, seizures, cerebellar ataxia, and mitochondrial

FEATURE TABLE 13-22. CONGENITAL MITOCHONDRIAL ENCEPHALOMYOPATHY

Discriminating Feature	Consistent Features	Variable Features
1. Mitochondrial myopathy with defects of mitochondrial oxidative metabolism	1. Short stature 2. Dysmorphic features 3. Microcephaly 4. Hypotonia 5. Lactic acidosis (recurrent)	1. Seizures 2. Cardiomyopathy 3. Renal tubular acidosis 4. Mental retardation 5. Hirsutism

FEATURE TABLE 13-23. MELAS SYNDROME

Discriminating Feature	Consistent Features	Variable Features
1. Mitochondrial myopathy with defects of mitochondrial oxidative metabolism (point mutation of mitochondrial DNA)	1. Lactic acidosis 2. Cortical blindness, hemiparesis, or hemianopsia 3. Epilepsy	1. Short stature 2. Hearing loss 3. Headaches (migraine) 4. Gastrointestinal symptoms 5. Dementia 6. Muscular atrophy and weakness (proximal) 7. Hypertrophic cardiopathy 8. Renal dysfunction 9. Ragged red fibers

myopathy. Myoclonic jerks involving the neck, trunk, and proximal portions of the limbs are triggered by attempted actions and postures, emotional reactions, or photic or auditory stimulation, and disappear at rest and during sleep. Scars of burns and traumas are related to involuntary movements and falls. Myoclonic jerks are not associated with loss of consciousness. Myoclonic epilepsy and other forms of seizures are frequently reported. Associated signs of cerebellar dysfunction include cerebellar dysarthria, intention tremor, dysmetria, and dysdiadochokinesia. This clinical presentation may suggest the diagnosis of myoclonic epilepsy or dyssynergia cerebellaris myoclonica of Ramsey-Hunt. As the disease progresses, muscle weakness and wasting increase progressively. Besides the cardinal four symptoms, other associated abnormalities may include small stature, hypothalamic dysfunction, mental deterioration, hearing loss, peripheral neuropathy with marked loss of myelinated fibers, and such symptoms reminiscent of Friedreich's ataxia as pes cavus, areflexia, and posterior column signs. Typical patients with MERRF syndrome do not have significant stroke-like episodes, ophthalmoplegia, retinal pigmentary degeneration, or heart block. CT scan of the head may not distinguish MERRF from MELAS, because basal ganglia calcifications and focal cerebellar and cerebral lucencies can be found in both syndromes. Few cases have been examined postmortem.

They presented with diffuse spongy degeneration and neuronal loss of the cerebral cortex; neuronal loss in the dentate, gracile, and cuneate nuclei; and degeneration in the posterior columns and anterior and posterior spinocerebellar tracts of the spinal cord. Maternal inheritance has been found in several kindreds, suggesting transmission of a mutation affecting the mitochondrial genome. Within a given pedigree, there is some phenotypic variation among affected individuals.

KSS is a multisystem mitochondrial disorder characterized clinically by onset before age 20, slowly progressive paralysis of extraocular muscles, atypical pigmentary degeneration of the retina, and various signs of nervous system and other organ (e.g., heart) involvement. Ptosis of the eyelids almost always precedes chronic progressive external ophthalmoplegia. Blepharoptosis may be initially asymmetrical. Ophthalmoplegia is insidious and progressive, frequently beginning with slowing of saccadic eye movements. Diplopia is not mentioned in any case report, and ophthalmoparesis usually does not cause symptoms until it is nearly total. Atypical pigmentary degeneration of the retina is usually preceded by ophthalmoplegia. Only 40% of the patients have symptoms, such as diminished visual acuity or night blindness. Pupillary responses remain normal in all patients. Other areas of the nervous system may be involved. Most often one observes cerebellar ataxia (70%

FEATURE TABLE 13-24. MERRF SYNDROME

Discriminating Feature	Consistent Features	Variable Features
1. Mitochondrial myopathy with defects of mitochondrial oxidative metabolism (point mutation of mitochondrial DNA)	1. Myoclonus 2. Cerebellar ataxia 3. Epilepsy 4. Ragged red fibers	1. Short stature 2. Dementia 3. Hearing loss 4. Peripheral neuropathy (proprioceptor) 5. Pes cavus 6. Optic atrophy 7. Hypothalamic dysfunction 8. Elevated CSF proteins (rare)

FEATURE TABLE 13-25. KEARNS-SAYRE SYNDROME

Discriminating Feature	Consistent Features	Variable Features
1. Large deletion of mitochondrial DNA and duplication of mitochondrial DNA	1. Ptosis 2. Progressive external ophthalmoplegia 3. Onset before age 15 years 4. Pigmentary retinopathy 5. Cerebellar syndrome, heart block, or CSF protein $\geq$ 100 mg/dL 6. Ragged red fibers in striated muscles	1. Short stature 2. Endocrine disorder 3. Mental retardation 4. Episodic coma 5. Hearing loss 6. Extensor toe signs 7. Renal tubular involvement

of all cases), sensorineural hearing loss (55%), and mental retardation (40%). In the advanced stage of the disease, a moderate weakness involving facial, palate, neck, or proximal limb muscles frequently appears. Pyramidal, extrapyramidal, and peripheral nerve dysfunction may also develop. Seizures occurred only in three patients with concomitant hypoparathyroidism. Patients with KSS are at risk to develop syncopal episodes and sudden cardiac arrest. Periodic electrocardiographic examination is therefore mandatory. Cardiac conduction defects range from simple prolonged intraventricular conduction time to complete atrioventricular block. Renal dysfunction (mainly tubular defects) and hepatic dysfunction may also develop. Short stature and delayed puberty are common features. CT scan of the head may show focal lucencies, cerebral and cerebellar atrophy, and basal ganglia calcifications. High CSF protein is found in most patients. Few cases have been examined postmortem. They presented diffuse neuronal loss and spongy degeneration in the Purkinje cell layer, oculomotor nuclei, cerebral cortex, basal ganglia, and cervical spine. Many cases of KSS appear to be sporadic. Within a given pedigree, there is frequently phenotypic variation among affected individuals. Maternal inheritance has been found in several kindreds, suggesting transmission of a mutation affecting the mitochondrial genome.

Important, though nonspecific, laboratory abnormalities exist in the CMEs. These often appear as elevations of lactate and pyruvate in the blood and CSF. They do not occur in all cases and the level of elevation varies considerably in severity in different patients. Patients with severe impairment of electron transport will have elevations of lactate and pyruvate even after an overnight rest. Milder deficits may become apparent after exercise or glucose tolerance tests. The blood lactate/pyruvate ratio is usually normal in pyruvate dehydrogenase complex deficiency and substantially increased in defects of the mitochondrial respiratory chain. In all lactate and pyruvate tests, it is important to chill and deproteinize specimens promptly. Blood specimens should be

drawn without the use of a tourniquet, to avoid spurious elevations from stasis. Quantative measurements of amino acids in the serum and the CSF may reveal elevation of the alanine concentration. Occasionally, the urinary findings of de Toni-Franconi-Debre syndrome (renal glycosuria, hyperphosphaturia, and generalized aminoaciduria) suggest a renal dysfunction. Increased levels of CSF protein are found in KSS and occasionally in patients with MELAS or MERRF syndrome. Recent reports of relative deficiency of CoQ in certain patients with KSS suggest that this measurement may prove useful. Occasionally, one finds elevations of creatine kinase or electromyographic changes indicative of myopathy, but usually such signs are mild or absent, even when the subsequent muscle biopsy is positive. Perhaps the most promising noninvasive test of energy metabolism involves assessment of the ratio of phosphocreatine to inorganic phosphate (Pcr/P_i) by nuclear magnetic resonance spectroscopy of skeletal muscle before, during, and after exercise. Patients with a defect in oxidative metabolism may have a reduced Pcr/P_i ratio at rest and, more dependably, for prolonged periods of time after exercise.

Although biochemic and morphologic abnormalities have been demonstrated in a variety of tissues, skeletal muscle continues to be the tissue of choice for such studies, even in patients without muscular weakness. Morphologic studies should include histochemical and enzymatic staining of frozen muscle and electron microscopy of fixed specimens. Paraffin sections are not very helpful. Specimens viewed under light microscopy should be prepared with the Gomori trichrome stain: succinic dehydrogenase, NADH, and cytochrome oxidase stains. When processed with the Gomori trichrome stain, a few of the type I, oxidative muscle fibers may show intense subsarcolemmal red-staining membranes. This appearance prompted the popular designation "ragged red fibers." Histochemic staining with oxidative stains as well as electron microscopy demonstrates these ragged red accumulations to be mitochondria. In certain enzymopathies, there is absence of reaction product for one

Pearls and Perils: Mitochondrial Encephalomyopathies

1. CME is characterized by a floppy infant syndrome associated with congenital lactic acidosis and dysmorphic or dystrophic features, suggesting prenatal onset. Specific laboratory tests can differentiate Menkes's syndrome and Zellweger's syndrome from CME.

2. MELAS syndrome is characterized by recurrent attacks of prolonged migrainous headaches, recurrent partial epileptic seizures, and repeated cerebral infarctions, ultimately leading to dementia, cortical blindness, and cortical deafness. Vascular or embolic disease may simulate MELAS syndrome.

3. Calcifications of the basal ganglia may be seen in MERRF syndrome, KSS, CME, MELAS syndrome, hypoparathyroidism, pseudohypoparathyroidism, osteopetrosis with renal tubular acidosis, Hallervorden-Spatz syndrome, and the syndrome of idiopathic cerebral calcification often referred to as Fahr's disease.

4. MERRF is a syndrome characterized by ataxia, seizures, myoclonus, and eventually dementia. This syndrome must be differentiated from NCL (late infantile, juvenile, or adult form), cherry-red spot myoclonus syndrome (sialidosis), GM_2 gangliosidosis, juvenile Gaucher's disease, juvenile Huntington's disease, and dyssynergia cerebellaris myoclonica of Ramsey-Hunt. The distinctive feature is the presence of a myopathy with ragged red fibers.

5. KSS is characterized clinically by the tetrad of onset before age 20, chronic progressive external ophthalmoplegia, atypical pigmentary degeneration of the retina, and one of the following: heart block, cerebellar syndrome, or high CSF protein (over 100 mg/dL). Chronic progressive external ophthalmoplegia should be differentiated from Wilson's disease, Huntington's disease, BKS, ataxia telangiectasia, Faxio-Londe disease, Möbius's syndrome, myasthenia gravis, myotonic muscular dystrophy, endocrine ophthalmoplegia, and various other muscular and neural ophthalmoplegias.

oxidative enzyme in fibers that show intense staining for the other enzymes in serial sections. Electron microscopy not only confirms the presence of supernumerary mitochondria, but also demonstrates that some mitochondria are enlarged, the cristae of their inner membranes are disordered or simplified, and occasionally paracrystalline "parking lot" inclusions in the matrix are seen. Biochemic testing of mitochondrial function in biopsied muscle is best accomplished on isolated mitochondria by spectrophotometric assessment of specific enxymatic reactions in the electron transport chain. Experience with evaluation of oxidative metabolism in more convenient fibroblast assays is limited to some cases of CME.

Most of the components of the electron transport chain are encoded on nuclear genes, synthesized on cytoplasmic ribosomes, and then translocated into mitochondria. Genetic errors affecting any of these steps could result in enzyme deficiency. Those disorders are segregated as Mendelian traits. Autosomal dominant or recessive inheritance has been described. However, at least 13 of the peptides that make up the different respiratory enzyme complexes (seven subunits of complex I, apocytochrome *b* of complex III, the three catalytic subunits of complex IV, and two subunits of complex V) are encoded exclusively on mitochondrial DNA. Each human cell contains about 1000 mitochondrial chromosomes, about 2 to 12 per individual mitochondrion. All the mitochondria in a zygote derive from the mother. Human sperm contains only few mitochondria, which do not penetrate into the egg. Therefore, transmission of a mutation in the mitochondrial genome is exclusively maternal. During the first few cleavage divisions, there is no replication of mitochondria. As nuclear and cell division takes place, a fixed number of mitochondria are randomly partitioned into individual cells. This explains why, within a given pedigree, there is some phenotypic variation among affected individuals when mitochondrial inheritance is involved.

At least some oxidative disorders may be amendable to treatment, by providing either vitamin cofactors (thiamine, lipoic acid, or riboflavin), artificial stimulants of defective enzymes (dichloroacetate, which stimulates pyruvate dehydrogenase complex activity), or electron-shuttling agents (CoQ, menadione, ascorbate). Generalizations about treatment should be avoided. It is best to delineate the specific biochemic defect in each individual patient or kindred, and to monitor response to any specific therapies suggested by the biochemic analysis. Other considerations include the recognition and treatment of cardiac conduction defects, seizures, migraines, and endocrine abnormalities in affected patients.

ANNOTATED BIBLIOGRAPHY

Congenital Mitochondrial Encephalomyopathy

Nyhan WL, Sakati NA: *Diagnostic Recognition of Genetic Disease*. Philadelphia, Lea & Febiger, 1987, p 221–235.

Patients with disorders of the pyruvate dehydrogenase complex may show characteristic dysmorphic features and present acutely in neonatal life with severe acidosis and rapidly progressive, fatal illness. Other patients present later in infancy with features of Leigh's encephalomyelopathy.

Moreadith RW, Batshaw ML, Ohnishi T, et al: Deficiency of the iron-sulfur clusters of mitochondrial reduced nicotinamide adenine dinucleotide-ubiquinone oxidoreductase (complex I) in an infant with congenital lactic acidosis. *J Clin Invest* 74:685–697, 1984.

After a pregnancy complicated by decreased fetal activity, a premature neonate with micropenis and hypospadias developed a progressive lactic acidosis, respiratory difficulties, hypotonia, decreased responsiveness, and hypertrophic cardiomyopathy. Neuroimaging demonstrated ventriculomegaly and white matter changes. The infant died at 16 weeks of age. The enzyme defect was centered in one of the iron-sulfur proteins in the NADH-CoQ reductase complex.

Robinson BH, Ward J, Goodyer P, Baudet A: Respiratory chain defects in the mitochondria of cultured skin fibroblasts from three patients with lactic acidemia. *J Clin Invest* 77:1422–1427, 1986.

Cytochrome oxidase deficiency was found in an infant with hypospadias, micropenis, and narrow forehead who presented recurrent episodes of lactic acidosis and development delay. NADH-cytochrome *c* reductase deficiency was demonstrated in a small-for-gestational age infant who fed poorly, developed recurrent episodes of lactic acidosis, and died on day 13. Another infant with NADH-cytochrome *c* reductase deficiency had a rapidly progressive diffuse encephalopathy, causing dysmyelination and white matter necrosis.

Seitz RJ, Langes K, Frenzel H, Kluitmann G, Wechsler W: Congenital Leigh's disease: Panencephalomyelopathy and peripheral neuropathy. *Acat Neuropathol* 64:167–171, 1984.

A dystrophic newborn presented as a floppy infant with respiratory difficulties and hypertrophic cardiomyopathy. A panencephalomyelopathy with severe white matter changes was found at autopsy.

Melas Syndrome

Hurko D, Reynafarje B, Kuncl R, Feldman E, Stern B: Familial mitochondrial encephalomyopathy, lactic acidosis, and stroke (MELAS) associated with cytochrome oxidase deficiency. *Am J Hum Genet* 25:716–717, 1986.

In one pedigree, cytochrome oxidase deficiency has resulted in severe congenital lactic acidosis in one sibling and the MELAS syndrome in her less severely affected brother.

Pollock MA, Cumberbatch M, Bennett MJ, et al: Pyruvate carboxylase deficiency in twins. *J Inher Metab Dis* 9:29–30, 1986.

Pyruvate carboxylase deficiency was found in skin fibroblasts cultured from twins presenting at birth with hypotrophy, enlarged ventricles, and severe metabolic acidosis.

Pavlakis SG, Phillips PC, DiMauro S, De Vivo DC, Rowland LP: Mitochondrial myopathy, encephalopathy, lactic acidosis, and stroke-like episodes: A distinctive clinical syndrome. *Ann Neurol* 16:481–488, 1984.

MELAS represents a distinctive syndrome well differentiated from MERRF and chronic progressive external ophthalmoplegia.

Kobayashi M, Morishita H, Sugiyama N, et al: Two cases of NADH-coenzyme Q reductase deficiency: Relationship to MELAS syndrome. *J Pediatr* 110:223–227, 1987.

NADH-CoQ reductase deficiency was found in muscle mitochondria from two patients with MELAS syndrome.

Yamamoto M, Sato T, Anno M, Ujike H, Takemoto M: Mitochondrial myopathy, encephalopathy, lactic acidosis, and stroke-like episodes with recurrent abdominal symptoms and

coenzyme Q_{10} administration. *J Neurol Neurosurg Psychiatr* 50:1475–1481, 1987.

Episodes of abdominal pain and ileus occurred in one patient with MELAS syndrome owing to an NADH-cytochrome *c* reductase deficiency.

Ohoma E, Ohara S, Ikuta F, Tanaka K, Nishizawa M, Miyatake T: Mitochondrial angiopathy in cerebral blood vessels of mitochondrial encephalomyopathy. *Acta Neuropathol* 74:226–233, 1987.

A mitochondrial angiopathy affecting the pial arterioles and small arteries of the brain was found in two autopsied patients with MELAS syndrome. Both patients also had a hypertrophic cardiomyopathy.

MERRF Syndrome

Fukuhara N, Tokiguchi S, Shirakawa K, Tusbaki T: Myoclonus epilepsy associated with ragged red fibers (mitochondrial abnormalities): Disease entity or a syndrome? *J Neurol Sci* 47:117–133, 1980.

The original case of MERRF syndrome was at first thought to have degenerative-type myoclonic epilepsy, until muscle biopsy disclosed mitochondrial pathology.

Riggs JE, Schochet SS, Fakadej AV, et al: Mitochondrial encephalomyopathy with decreased succinate cytochrome *c* reductase activity. *Neurology* 34:48–53, 1984.

A succinate-CoQ reductase deficiency is found in two siblings who developed features of MERRF syndrome at 5 years of age.

Rosing HS, Hopkins LC, Wallace DC, Epstein CM, Weidenheim K: Maternally inherited mitochondrial myopathy and myoclonic epilepsy. *Ann Neurol* 17:228–237, 1985.

Maternal inheritance and variability of clinical expression are emphasized in a three-generation pedigree containing nine patients affected with mitochondrial myelopathy. At least two patients had MERRF syndrome.

Fitzsimons RB, Clifton-Bligh P, Wolfenden WH: Mitochondrial myopathy and lactic acidemia with myoclonic epilepsy, ataxia, and hypothalamic infertility: A variant of Ramsey-Hunt syndrome? *J Neurol Neurosurg Psychiatr* 44:79–82, 1981.

Small stature and hypothalamic infertility were found in a patient with MERRF syndrome.

Mukoyama M, Kazui H, Sunohara N, Yoshida M, Nonaka I, Satoyoshi E: Mitochondrial myopathy, encephalopathy, lactic acidosis, and stroke-like episodes with acanthocytosis: A clinicopathological study of a unique case. *J Neurol* 233:228–232, 1986.

A teenager with MELAS syndrome later developed features of MERRF syndrome, suggesting overlap between the two. Acanthocytosis was found in this patient.

Kearns-Sayre Syndrome

Berenberg RA, Pellock JM, DiMauro S, et al: Lumping or splitting? "Ophthalmoplegia-plus" or Kearns-Sayre syndrome. *Ann Neurol* 1:37–54, 1977.

Thirty-six patients with complete Kearns-Sayre syndrome are reviewed. Most patients had cerebellar signs, hearing loss, vestibular dysfunction, or mental retardation.

Ishitsu T, Miike T, Kitano A, et al: Heterogeneous phenotypes of mitochondrial encephalomyopathy in a single kindred. *Neurology* 37:1867–1869, 1987.

Five patients in a single family had a CME. One patient with nephrotic diabetes insipidus had KSS.

Rivner MH, Shamsnia M, Swift TR, et al: Kearns-Sayre syndrome (mitochondrial encephalomyopathy) and a complex II deficiency. *Neurology* 38(suppl 1):188, 1988.

Succinate dehydrogenase deficiency was found in a patient with KSS.

Byrne E, Marzuki S, Sattayasai N, Dennett X, Trounce I: Mitochondrial studies in Kearns-Sayre syndrome: Normal respiratory chain function with absence of a mitochondrial translation product. *Neurology* 37:1530–1534, 1987.

In mitochondria isolated from two patients with KSS, mitochondrial protein synthesis was increased but one mitochondrial translation product was absent. This is the most direct biochemic evidence of a pathogenic mutation in mitochondrial DNA.

Schnitzle ER, Robertson WC: Familial Kearns-Sayre syndrome. *Neurology* 29:1172–1174, 1974.

Siblings with KSS are reported.

Ogasahara S, Yorifuji S, Nishikawa Y, et al: Improvement of abnormal pyruvate metabolism and cardiac conduction defect with coenzyme Q_{10} in Kearns-Sayre syndrome. *Neurology* 35:372–377, 1985.

A defect of coenzyme Q_{10} was found in serum and in muscle mitochondria from one patient with KSS.

Yorifuji S, Ogasahara S, Takahashi M, Tarui S: Decreased activities on mitochondrial inner membrane transport system from patients with Kearns-Sayre syndrome. *J Neurol Sci* 71:65–75, 1985.

Components of the inner membrane electron transport system are deficient in KSS.

GALACTOSEMIA

Classic galactosemia is a disorder of galactose metabolism characterized by hepatomegaly, cataracts, failure to thrive, and mental retardation. Most cases of classic galactosemia result from a generalized hereditary deficiency of galactose-1-phosphate uridyltransferase, the enzyme that catalyzes the conversion of galactose-1-phosphate into galactose uridine diphosphate. Signs and symptoms of classic galactosemia may also result from a generalized hereditary deficiency of uridine diphosphate galactose-4-epimerase, the enzyme that catalyzes the conversion of galactose uridine diphosphate into glucose uridine diphosphate. Galactose-1-phosphate has been incriminated as the toxic agent causing most of the pathology in classic galactosemia. Deficiency of galactokinase, the first enzyme of galactose metabolism, results in decreased production of galactose-1-phosphate and has never been associated with the picture of classic galactosemia. However, galactose is still converted into galactitol, which is responsible for cataract formation.

Most infants with classic galactosemia appear normal at birth, although a few may already have cataracts, low birth weight, and signs of cirrhosis. Signs of toxicity usually occur after the initiation of milk feedings. The presenting symptoms vary with age. Patients affected in the neonatal period often develop feeding difficulties, diarrhea, vomiting, and failure to thrive. Jaundice appears within a few days. Infants become increasingly lethargic and hypotonic. Myotactic reflexes and primitive reflexes are severely depressed. The anterior fontanelle is frequently bulging in the acute phase of the illness. Seizures are uncommon. Septicemia caused by *Escherichia coli* occurs with high frequency and is responsible for the majority of deaths during the neonatal period. By 2 weeks of age, hepatosplenomegaly is easily detectable. Ascites and edema are usually found in those infants who succumb to liver failure. Nuclear or cortical cataracts appear early but may go unnoticed for months. Lenticular opacities may be found only on slit lamp examination. In some infants, the disease is less severe and does not manifest itself until 3 to 6 months of age, when the presenting symptoms are delayed physical and mental development. There may be other patients who do not present as a failure to thrive syndrome and are seen several years after birth for evaluation of mental retardation and cataracts. These children frequently have a history of partial treatment with mild restriction. Galactokinase deficiency is generally not associated with jaundice, gastrointestinal dysfunction, and inanition in the newborn period. Cataracts may be the first and only abnormalities in children kept on an unrestricted diet. Pseudotumor cerebri has been reported in one patient.

The CT scan of the head may demonstrate cerebral edema in the acute stage of the disease. With appropriate treatment, attenuation of the white matter in the periventricular regions and moderate ventricular enlargement may be residual findings. The EEG is nonspecifically abnormal, showing excessive generalized slowing and sometimes paroxysmal features. Brainstem auditory evoked responses are frequently abnormal because of poorly formed wave IV/V complexes. Visual evoked responses are usually normal.

In classic galactosemia, renal tubular dysfunction leads to proteinuria, generalized renal aminoaciduria, and distal renal tubular acidosis with defective acidification of the urine. Usually, the urine contains a reducing substance that does not react in a glucose oxidase test. The reducing substance is identified as galactose by enzymatic or chromatographic assays. The galactosuria may disappear if food intake has been poor. Many normal infants, especially premature infants, have a physiologic galactosuria soon after introduction of milk feedings. Blood chemistry may show hypochloremic acidosis, hypoglycemia, and signs of liver dysfunction. Many babies with classic galactosemia have raised blood phenylalanine or tyrosine concentrations by the sixth day of life.

Increased concentration of galactose and galactose-1-phosphate in blood can be detected in filter paper disks. Cord blood can be used for screening as high galactose-1-

FEATURE TABLE 13–26. GALACTOSEMIA

Discriminating Features	Consistent Features	Variable Features
1. Galactose-1-phosphate 2. Uridyltransferase deficiency in blood or generalized epimerase deficiency in fibroblasts	1. Lenticular opacities 2. Increased galactose and galactose-1-phosphate in blood	1. Increased intracranial pressure 2. Failure to thrive 3. Gastrointestinal symptoms 4. Hepatomegaly 5. Jaundice 6. Lethargy 7. Psychomotor delay 8. Mental retardation 9. Cerebellar dysfunction 10. Short attention span 11. Renal tubular acidosis 12. Galactosuria

phosphate levels are already found in newborns with classic galactosemia. Microbiologic assay systems and enzymatic assays have been developed for newborn screening. Enzymatic assays offer several advantages over microbiologic assay systems. Microbiologic assay systems require overnight incubation, whereas enzymatic assays can be completed within 6 hours. Microbiologic assays are affected by antibiotic therapy. Thin-layer chromatography should be performed to confirm positive screening results and identify the specific metabolites of galactose that are elevated. The presence of galactose and galactose-1-phosphate in blood does not in itself establish the diagnosis of classic galactosemia. Severely impaired liver function owing to neonatal hepatitis, hereditary tyrosinemia, and other disorders may be accompanied by galactosemia and galactosuria.

Diagnosis of classic galactosemia must be confirmed by documenting the enzyme defect. Screening for galactose-1-phosphate uridyltransferase deficiency is easily achieved on filter paper blood specimens by the method of Beutler and Baluda. Transfused red blood cells with normal transferase activity produce false negative results. If the Beutler and Baluda test is used on cord blood, extreme caution is mandatory to prevent contamination with the mother's blood. Furthermore, transferase activity cannot be reliably measured in filter paper blood specimens after only a few weeks of storage. Therefore, negligence in mailing samples and delays in postal delivery may interfere with the reliability of results. Most patients with classic galactosemia have a complete red cell transferase deficiency. Heterozygotes for classic galactosemia have approximately 50% of normal erythrocytic transferase activity. Starch gel electrophoresis reveals a transferase with no mobility in homozygotes and one with normal mobility in heterozygotes. Some patients with a clinical picture resembling classic galactosemia have residual red cell transferase activity (7% to 40% of normal) and a different elec-

trophoretic mobility (Rennes, Indiana, Chicago, and Münster variants). Asymptomatic homozygotes for the Duarte variant have erythrocyte transferase activity equal to that of heterozygotes for classic galactosemia but with a rapid electrophoretic mobility. The deficiency of galactose-1-phosphate uridyltransferase can also be demonstrated in the white blood cells, skin fibroblasts, intestinal mucosa, and liver. In a variant confined to blacks (Negro variant), hepatic and intestinal transferase activities are 10% of normal, in spite of the absence of transferase in the red cells. Homozygotes for the Negro variant have symptoms only in infancy, when galactose intake is at its peak.

Screening for the missing enzyme is not possible for galactokinase or epimerase. Homozygotes for generalized epimerase deficiency are indistinguishable clinically from those for classic galactosemia. Their epimerase activity is less than 10% of normal in hemolysates of red blood cells, in lymphocytes cultured for 72 hours with phytohemagglutinin, and in skin fibroblasts. Heterozygotes have about 50% of normal activity in their fibroblasts. If the enzyme deficiency is limited to leukocytes and not red blood cells, affected persons show no clinical abnormality. Homozygotes for galactokinase deficiency have no detectable activity in their erythrocytes and skin fibroblasts, whereas heterozygotes have about 50% of the normal activity.

The main pathologic lesions are found in the liver and the brain. In the liver, several stages are recognized. Initially, one sees a diffuse fatty metamorphosis. If the disease remains untreated, liver cell cords are transformed into pseudoglandular structures around bile canaliculi. The final stage is pseudolobular cirrhosis. These changes are consistent with a metabolic disease, but do not indicate the precise enzymatic defect. The primary neuropathologic feature at autopsy in infants who have died in the acute phase of the disease is cerebral edema. If the condition is left untreated, diffuse Purkinje cell degeneration in the cerebellar cortex and heavy astrocytic fibrosis in the dentate nuclei are seen. Cerebral cortical neuronal degeneration is evident by depletion of the neuronal population in the entire cortex. Atrophy and fibrous gliosis of the cerebral white matter are prominent. An Alzheimer type II neuroglial reaction occurs in many areas of the cerebral gray matter, brainstem, and cerebellum. None of these neuropathologic changes is pathognomonic.

The mode of inheritance of various forms of galactosemia is autosomal recessive. The overall birth incidence for complete transferase deficiency is approximately 1 in 60,000. Geographic variation of birth incidence is considerable. Population studies have indicated that from 0.9% to 1.25% are heterozygotes for the galactosemia gene and that from 8% to 13% carry the Duarte gene. The gene for transferase activity has been localized on chromosome 9 at locus 9p13. Considerable isoallelic heterogenity exists, causing variant forms of the disorder. The estimated frequency of galactokinase deficiency is 1 in 40,000 live births with a frequency of 1 in 107 for the heterozygote carrier state. The incidence of generalized epimerase deficiency is still unknown.

Treatment of classic galactosemia or galactokinase deficiency consists of the exclusion of all galactose and lactose from the diet until after puberty. In infants, this is done by providing a formula such as Pregestimil or Nutramigen, that does not contain galactose in an absorbable form. Intermittent measurement of erythrocyte galactose-1-phosphate levels has been suggested for monitoring of diet adherence in children with transferase deficiency. Even well-controlled galactosemic children have elevated galactose-1-phosphate levels owing to endogenous formation of galactose-1-phosphate from glucose-1-phosphate. Levels appear to be fairly consistent in individuals and usually range between 30 and 45 mcg/mL RBC (normal 5 to 10 mcg/mL RBC). Treatment with a diet free of galactose results in rapid resolution of gastrointestinal symptoms. Subsequent growth is usually normal. Galactosuria, proteinuria, and aminoaciduria disappear. Cataracts regress only when dietary treatment is begun in the early weeks of life. Brain damage and hepatic cirrhosis may be permanent. Patients with classic galactosemia who receive dietary treatment from birth exhibit better intellectual progress than those treated later. Children with early treated galactosemia are still at risk for mental retardation, speech and language difficulties, cerebellar dysfunction, and shortened attention span. Prenatal exposure of galactosemic infants to galactose may lead to organic brain damage. By restricting the galactose intake during pregnancy of women who have borne galactosemic children, the incidence of physical and mental handicaps can be reduced in subsequently born homozygotes.

ANNOTATED BIBLIOGRAPHY

Pollitt RJ, Worthy E, Green A: Galactosemia detection as a bonus from screening for phenylketonuria. *J Inher Metab Dis* 5(suppl 1):51–52, 1982.

Whenever galactosemia screening is not available, galactosemia detection based on raised phenylalanine levels is a sensible precaution.

Paigen K, Pacholec F, Levy HL: A new method of screening for inherited disorders of galactose metabolism. *J Lab Clin Med* 99:895–907, 1982.

This paper reports a new microbiologic assay for blood galactose and galactose-1-phosphate using an *Escherichia coli* mutant lacking the enzyme UDP-galactose-UDP-glucose-4-epimerase and the bacteriophage C2₁.

Beutler E, Baluda MC: A simple spot screening test for galactosemia. *J Lab Clin Med* 68:137–141, 1966.

A simple spot screening test for transferase activity is devised in which blood hemolysate is incubated at 37°C with UDP-glucose and galactose-1-phosphate. After the reaction is stopped, the amount of reduced NADPH produced is determined fluorometrically. No fluorescence develops when galactosemic samples are examined.

Bowlin FG, Brown ARD: Development of a protocol for newborn screening for disorders of the galactose metabolic pathway. *J Inher Metab Dis* 9:99–104, 1986.

Enzymatic assay of galactose metabolites, thin-layer chromatography, and assay of galactose-1-phosphate uridyltransferase can be performed routinely on a single sample of blood collected on filter paper.

Kaufmann FR, Kogut MD, Donnel GN, Goebelsmann V, March C, Koch R: Hypergonadotrophic hypogonadism in female patients with galactosemia. *N Engl J Med* 304:994–998, 1981.

Pearls and Perils: Galactosemia

1. Diagnosis of galactosemia should be considered in newborn infants, older infants, or children with jaundice, hepatosplenomegaly, vomiting, feeding difficulties, poor weight gain, hepatic cirrhosis, irritability, lethargy, seizures, mental retardation, or cataract.

2. The presence of galactose in the blood or urine does not in itself establish the diagnosis of classic galactosemia. Galactosemia is not uncommon in premature infants. Galactokinase deficiency and severe liver dysfunction may be accompanied by galactosemia and galactosuria. Generalized epimerase deficiency should be suspected in infants with symptoms and signs of classic galactosemia who have normal transferase activity.

3. Mothers known to be at risk for giving birth to galactosemic infants should have their galactose intake restricted to prevent congenital cataracts and neurologic sequelae in their offspring.

4. Heterozygotes for transferase deficiency and homozygotes for the Duarte variant can be distinguished by the electrophoretic mobility of the transferase.

Girls with galactosemia are at risk for hypergonadotropic hypogonadism if dietary treatment is not initiated promptly after birth.

Garibaldi LR, Canini S, Superti-Furga A, et al: Galactosemia caused by generalized uridine diphosphate galactose-4-epimerase deficiency. *J Pediatr* 103:927–930, 1983.

Infants with positive screening tests for galactose-1-phosphate and clinical findings suggestive of classic galactosemia should be tested for generalized epimerase deficiency if transferase screening is negative.

Litman N, Kanter AI, Finberg L: Galactokinase deficiency presenting as pseudotumor cerebri. *J Pediatr* 86:410–412, 1975.

Galactokinase deficiency must be considered in patients with cataracts with or without pseudotumor cerebri.

Belman AL, Moshe SL, Zimmerman RD: Computed tomographic demonstration of cerebral edema in a child with galactosemia. *Pediatrics* 78:606–609, 1986.

In the acute phase, a CT scan of the head may demonstrate the presence of diffuse cerebral edema.

Lo W, Parkman S, Nash S, et al: Curious neurologic sequelae in galactosemia. *Pediatrics* 73:309–312, 1984.

Despite well-documented and adequate dietary management since birth, two siblings were mentally retarded, and both had tremor and prominent cerebellar signs.

Inborn Errors of Metabolism II
Lesch-Nyhan Disease and Related Disorders of Purine Metabolism

William L. Nyhan

LESCH-NYHAN DISEASE

Lesch-Nyhan disease is due to an inborn error in the metabolism of purines, leading to substantial interference with central nervous system (CNS) function and bizarre, compulsive, and aggressive behavior.

Affected children appear normal at birth and usually develop normally for the first 6 to 8 months. They almost always have impressive quantities of urate crystals, which look like orange or yellow sand, in their diapers, and they may have hematuria, urinary tract stones, or infections early in life. However, in most instances the first signs of disease are neurologic. Patients who have been sitting well begin to lose this ability. They develop opisthotonic posturing, which persists intermittently as a regular feature of the disease. Muscle tone gradually increases and in the established phenotype the child is spastic; deep tendon reflexes are increased and the plantar response is extensor. Involuntary movements are characteristic; they may be choreic, athetoid, or dystonic. Most patients are mentally retarded, but the degree of motor disability is usually greater than the degree of intellectual impairment. For instance none of these patients is able to walk or even to sit unsupported, but virtually all learn to talk, and they all appear to comprehend much of what is said to them.

The most striking feature of the behavior is self-mutilation through biting. A hallmark feature is loss of tissue about the lips. There may be partial amputations of the tongue or fingers, and most patients have had some self-induced injury to the fingers. However, the self-mutilating activity is not limited to biting; it is limited only by the patient's disability. Patients will also injure others, or try to. There is no abnormality in sensation.

Some children have convulsions. The electroencephalogram (EEG) is usually normal. The computed tomographic (CT) or magnetic resonance imaging (MRI) scan may be normal, or there may be some cerebral atrophy.

Hyperuricemia is a regular feature of the disease. Its clinical consequences of gouty arthritis, urate nephropathy, urinary tract calculi, and tophaceous deposits may be prevented by treatment with allopurinol. However, most untreated patients have died of renal failure by 10 years of age.

The concentration of uric acid in the blood is usually from 6 to 10 mg/dL, but lower levels are occasionally encountered. The urinary content of uric acid is usually 2 to 4 mg/mg creatinine, whereas in normal individuals over 1 year of age it is less than 1 mg/mg creatinine. The diagnosis depends on the demonstration of virtually absent activity of the enzyme hypoxanthine guanine phosphoribosyltransferase (HPRT). The assay can be done on erythrocytes, and the normal enzyme is quite stable during shipment at ambient temperatures. The blood should not be frozen. The companion enzyme, adenine phosphoribosyltransferase (APRT) is often run as a control on conditions of shipment. In patients with Lesch-Nyhan disease the activity of this enzyme is increased, usually to 150% of normal.

The gene for Lesch-Nyhan disease is on the long arm of the X chromosome and is fully recessive. Clinical illness is expressed only in the male. In fact, following the random inactivation of an X chromosome specified by the Lyon hypothesis, there appears to be selection against cells expressing the abnormal gene in many tissues. This makes heterozygote detection difficult, because carriers of this gene do not have two demonstrable populations of erythrocytes or of leukocytes. Hair roots are to a large extent clonal, and therefore heterozygosity can be determined by the assay of enzyme activity on a substantial number (30) of individual hair follicles. The enzyme is

FEATURE TABLE 14-1. LESCH-NYHAN DISEASE

Discriminating Feature	Consistent Features	Variable Features
1. Complete deficiency of HPRT	1. Hyperuricemia 2. Uricosuria 3. Mental retardation 4. Spastic cerebral palsy 5. Choreoathetosis 6. Self-mutilation	1. Convulsions 2. Hematuria 3. Urinary tract stones 4. Urinary tract infections 5. Tophi 6. Urate nephropathy 7. Vomiting

expressed in cultured amniocytes and chorionic villus samples. Prenatal diagnosis has been accomplished using both materials. The human gene for HPRT has been cloned and complementary (cDNA) probes have been employed with restriction endonucleases in the search for restriction fragment length patterns that might characterize the abnormal gene in individual patients. Among patients with HPRT deficiency, some have been found to have specific deletions, and so far each one defined has been different, consistent with a high rate of individual mutation in the creation of the abnormal genes. However, the majority of Lesch-Nyhan patients cannot be distinguished from normal in this way, signifying point mutations in which the base substitutions are not recognized by the restriction enzymes available. These studies have, however, shown a high degree of restriction fragment length polymorphism; in a family at risk, in which the mother is suitably heterozygous for a linked polymorphism, these methods can be used for carrier detection and successful prenatal diagnosis.

The differential diagnosis includes an enlarging spectrum of disorders caused by variants of the HPRT enzyme that are deficient in activity, but not as deficient as the Lesch-Nyhan enzyme. At one end of the spectrum are patients with hyperuricemia and gout or renal stone disease and no abnormalities of the CNS. There are others, however, in whom the degree of deficiency is so severe that they look neurologically like Lesch-Nyhan patients; but these patients have normal, or nearly normal, intelligence and their behavior is normal. The recognition of this neurologic syndrome of HPRT deficiency makes it important to screen more broadly among patients diagnosed as having cerebral palsy, rather than solely among patients demonstrating self-mutilation. The deficiency can readily be detected by the assay of erythrocytes. On the other hand the reliable distinction of these patients from classic Lesch-Nyhan patients—which may be very important for prognosis in a patient diagnosed sufficiently early that he may be either premutilative or nonmutilative—requires the assay of cultured fibroblasts.

Some patients with hyperuricemia and uricosuria and normal HPRT have abnormal phosphoribosylpyrophosphate (PRPP) synthetase levels. One of our patients also had severe deafness, some developmental retardation, and absent lacrymal glands.

Treatment of any of the overproduction hyperuricemias of childhood is with allopurinol. Patients often require larger doses than adults with gout. We aim to keep the serum uric acid level at less than 3 mg/dL. Therefore it may be useful to monitor the excretion of xanthine, hypoxanthine, and uric acid in order optimally to avoid urinary tract calculi. Many patients are less stiff, especially in the morning, if treated with valium. Operative or other orthopedic treatment directed at dislocation of the hips is not effective. The only treatment effective for the self-mutilative behavior is physical restraint.

Pearls and Perils:
Lesch-Nyhan Disease

1. If he can walk it is not Lesch-Nyhan disease.
2. If the patient is a girl it is probably not Lesch-Nyhan disease.
3. Reports on hyperuricemic patients from the routine clinical laboratory may be misleading because the accepted normal ranges given are for populations of adult males in whom hyperuricemia is common. A child with a serum uric acid level of 5 mg/dL is hyperuricemic, but the laboratory will not flag the sample as such. There may also be perils in the assay of urinary urate because it is a favorite food for contaminating microorganisms. Therefore, it is best to conduct this assay on fresh or freshly frozen urine in a local laboratory.

ANNOTATED BIBLIOGRAPHY

Nyhan WL, Sakati NA (ed): Lesch-Nyhan disease, in *Diagnostic Recognition of Genetic Disease*, Philadelphia, Lea & Febiger, 1986, p 1–8.
  A more complete, illustrated treatment of the subject.
Lesch M, Nyhan WL: A familial disorder of uric acid metabolism and central nervous system function. *Am J Med* 36:561–570, 1964.

This is the original, classic description of the syndrome.

Christie R, Bay C, Kaufman IA, Bakay B, Borden M, Nyhan WL: Lesch-Nyhan disease: Clinical experience with nineteen patients. *Dev Med Child Neurol* 24:293–306, 1982.

A compilation of the clinical phenotype in 19 patients observed as inpatients in the Clinical Research Center.

Bakay B, Nissinen E, Sweetman L, Francke U, Nyhan WL: Utilization of purine by an HPRT variant in an intelligent, nonmutilative patient with features of the Lesch-Nyhan syndrome. *Pediatr Res* 13:1365–1370, 1979.

The first example of a patient with a variant enzyme whose neurologic examination was just like that of classic Lesch-Nyhan disease, but who differed in that mental retardation and abnormal behavior were absent. He was shown to have an enzyme with some activity using an intact cell assay.

Nyhan WL: Behavior in the Lesch-Nyhan syndrome. *J Autism Child Schizophr* 6:235–252, 1976.

Practical approaches to the management of self-injurious behavior.

Nyhan WL, James JA, Teberg AJ, Sweetman L, Nelson LG: A new disorder of purine metabolism with behavioral manifestations. *J Pediatr* 74:20–27, 1969.

The initial description of a patient with a PRPP synthetase abnormality, hyperuricemia, deafness, and developmental delay.

BIBLIOGRAPHY

Becker MA, Raivio KO, Bakay B, Adams WB, Nyhan WL: Variant human phosphoribosylpyrophosphate synthetase altered in regulatory and catalytic functions. *J Clin Invest* 65:109–120, 1980.

Gottlieb RP, Koppel MM, Nyhan WL, et al: Hyperuricaemia and choreoathetosis in a child without mental retardation or self-mutilation—A new HPRT variant. *J Inher Metab Dis* 5:183–186, 1982.

Jolly DJ, Esty AC, Bernard HU, Friedmann T: Isolation of a genomic clone partially encoding human hypoxanthine phosphoribosyltransferase. *Proc Natl Acad Sci USA* 79:5038–5041, 1981.

Jolly DJ, Okayama H, Berg P, et al: Isolation and characterization of a full-length expressible cDNA for human hypoxanthine phosphoribosyltransferase. *Proc Natl Acad Sci USA* 80:477–481, 1982.

Lloyd KG, Hornykiewicz O, Davidson L, et al: Biochemical evidence of dysfunction of brain neurotransmitters in the Lesch-Nyhan syndrome. *N Engl J Med* 305:1106–1111, 1981.

Page T, Bakay B, Nyhan WL: An improved procedure for the detection of hypoxanthine-guanine phosphoribosyltransferase heterozygotes. *Clin Chem* 28:1181–1184, 1982.

Nyhan WL: The Lesch-Nyhan syndrome. *Dev Med Child Neurol* 20:376–380, 1978.

Wilson JM, Stout JT, Pallela TD, Davidson BL, Kelley WN, Caskey CT: A molecular survey of hypoxanthine-guanine phosphoribosyltransferase deficiency in man. *J Clin Invest* 77:188–195, 1986.

PURINE NUCLEOSIDE PHOSPHORYLASE DEFICIENCY

Deficiency of purine nucleoside phosphorylase (PNP), like deficiency of adenosine deaminase, leads to severe combined immunodeficiency. In this disorder T-cell function is always impaired, while B-cell function may be normal or somewhat impaired. There is an associated lymphopenia and deficiency of thymic function. Autopsies have revealed hypoplasia of the thymus and cortical depletion. Tonsils and lymph nodes may be hard to find. T-lymphocyte-mediated immunity is markedly deficient. Skin tests for delayed hypersensitivity are negative and lymphocytes do not respond to phytohemagglutinin. As a consequence affected patients have frequent life-threatening infections. Most have died of infection. One patient developed vaccinia gangrenosa following vaccination against smallpox. Malignant neoplasms have also been observed, as has autoimmune hemolytic anemia.

Two of the earliest patients described had mild mental retardation and spastic tetraparesis. Another patient had a mild intention tremor. It has only recently been recognized that surviving patients with virtually complete deficiency of PNP may have more severe neurologic features. Five siblings from two families had severe developmental retardation and spastic tetraparesis. Spastic diplegia and behavioral abnormalities were reported in another patient. Patients with PNP deficiency may be suspected in the laboratory by the presence of hypouricemia, and an associated low level of excretion of uric acid in the urine. Nevertheless, they overproduce purines and excrete large amounts of inosine and guanosine in the urine. Concentrations of guanosine triphosphate (GTP) and other guanine nucleotides in erythrocytes are low. Levels of PRPP are increased.

The molecular defect in PNP can be demonstrated in erythrocytes and leukoyctes, as well as other cells; most

FEATURE TABLE 14-2. PURINE NUCLEOSIDE PHOSPHORYLASE DEFICIENCY

Discriminating Feature	Consistent Features	Variable Feature
1. Deficiency of PNP	1. Immunodeficiencies 2. T-cell depletion 3. Infections 4. Hypouricemia 5. Nucleoside accumulation	1. Neurologic abnormalities

---

Pearls and Perils: Purine Nucleoside Phosphorylase Deficiency

1. The importance of early diagnosis cannot be overemphasized; in the presence of a suitable sibling donor this otherwise fatal disease is curable by bone marrow transplantation.

---

severely affected patients have essentially no detectable activity.

PNP deficiency is inherited in an autosomal recessive fashion. Heterozygotes display activity of PNP that is intermediate between the activities of patients and controls. Prenatal diagnosis should be possible.

The disease can be cured by bone marrow transplantation. Improvement has been reported using repeated erythrocyte transfusions.

ANNOTATED BIBLIOGRAPHY

Giblett ER, Ammann AJ, Wara DW, Sandman R, Diamond LK: Nucleoside phosphorylase deficiency in a child with severely defective T-cell immunity. *Lancet* 1:1010–1013, 1975.

The first description of the entity.

Stoop JW, Zegers BJM, Hendrick GFM, et al: Purine nucleoside phosphorylase deficiency associated with selective cellular immunodeficiency. *N Engl J Med* 296:651–655, 1977.

Documentation of impaired T-cell function in a patient with no tonsils. Two siblings in this family had PNP deficiency along with mild mental retardation and spastic tetraparesis.

Simmonds HA, Fairbanks LD, Timms P: Erythrocyte GPT depletion in PNP deficiency presenting with haemolytic anaemia and hypouricaemia. *Pediatr Res* 19:776, 1985.

The first report on severe neurologic abnormalities in PNP deficiency.

BIBLIOGRAPHY

Nyhan WL, Sakati NA: Purine nucleoside phosphorylase deficiency, in *Diagnostic Recognition of Genetic Disease*, Philadelphia, Lea & Febiger, 1986, p 23–26.

Polmar SH, Stern RC, Schwartz AL, Wetzler EM, Chase PA, Hirschhorn R: Enzyme replacement therapy for adenosine deaminase deficiency and severe combined immunodeficiency. *N Engl J Med* 295:1337–1343, 1976.

Rich KC, Mejias E, Fox IH: Purine nucleoside phosphorylase deficiency: Improved metabolic and immunologic function with erythrocyte transfusions. *N Engl J Med* 303:973–977, 1980.

Staal GEJ, Stoop JW, Zegers BJM, et al: Erythrocyte metabolism in purine nucleoside phosphorylase deficiency after enzyme replacement therapy by infusion of erythrocytes. *J Clin Invest* 65:103–108, 1980.

PHENYLKETONURIA

Phenylketonuria (PKU) is due to an inborn error in the metabolism of phenylalanine that causes severe mental retardation. The metabolic defect also interferes with pigment development. Affected individuals are always less deeply pigmented than their relatives and they are often blonde and blue eyed. However, the only significant effect of the disease is that on the brain. Untreated patients usually have IQ levels of less than 30. Early symptoms include irritability and vomiting severe enough to have led to surgery for pyloric stenosis. An eczematoid rash may occur on the face, but this is not commonly seen. A characteristic odor, which is that of phenylacetic acid, has been variously described as mousey, wolflike, musty, or barny.

Neurologic findings other than severe mental retardation are found in about two thirds of patients. About half of these have subtle findings, such as some hypertonicity or an upgoing toe, but some patients may have severe spastic cerebral palsy. There may be purposeless hand posturing, rhythmic rocking, and tremors of the hands. Hyperkinetic activity, uncontrollable temper, and other behavioral problems are common. Seizures occur in about one fourth of the patients, predominantly in those most severely retarded. EEG abnormalities have been described in approximately 80% of patients. The CT or MRI scan may reveal cortical atrophy.

The neuropathology of PKU consists of a delay in myelination in the CNS. Thus autopsies carried out in childhood have revealed dysmelination in the subcortical white matter. These findings are absent in patients studied after 21 years of age. Thus the formation of myelin is delayed by the chemical abnormality.

Patients with PKU accumulate large amounts of

FEATURE TABLE 14-3. PHENYLKETONURIA

Discriminating Features	Consistent Features	Variable Features
1. Deficient hepatic phenylalanine hydroxylase	1. Mental retardation	1. Vomiting
2. Elevated plasma phenylalanine	2. Diminished pigment	2. Eczematoid rash
3. Depressed plasma tyrosine	3. Phenylpyruvic aciduria	3. Odd odor
	4. Phenyllactic aciduria	4. Restriction fragment length polymorphism
	5. Phenylacetylglutamic aciduria	

Pearls and Perils: Phenylketonuria

1. Mental retardation caused by PKU should be preventable in developed countries by programs of routine neonatal screening, definitive diagnosis, and the early institution of dietary therapy.
2. Infants now go home from the hospital so soon after birth that patients with PKU may be missed because the patient has not been receiving protein long enough to experience a diagnostic rise in the concentration of phenylalanine.
3. Physicians can avoid this problem by the routine determination of phenylalanine in blood at the first office visit after neonatal discharge from the hospital.

phenylalanine in body fluids and convert some of this phenylalanine to intermediates, such as phenylpyruvic acid, phenyllactic acid, phenylacetic acid, and phenylacetylglutamine. All of these compounds have been tested to detect the disease. In fact, the disease was first discovered because of the green color that results from the reaction of ferric chloride with phenylpyruvic acid. The optimal method for the detection of PKU is the analysis of the blood for phenylalanine. This technique has been adapted to the assay of spots of dried blood on filter paper, and has permitted the development of universal neonatal screening programs that now are the rule in all the developed countries of the world. In this way patients are detected before the development of brain damage and treated with diets restricted in phenylalanine.

The enzymatic defect in PKU is in the enzyme phenylalanine hydroxylase, which catalyzes the conversion of phenylalanine to tyrosine. It is expressed only in liver. Its activity in classic PKU is undetectable and immunochemical studies have revealed no cross-reacting material. The messenger RNA coding for phenylalanine hydroxylase has been purified and its cDNA prepared, and the structural gene has been cloned in rat and in man. Studies using this cDNA as a probe and a variety of restriction endonucleases have revealed considerable polymorphism, but the cells of patients have not been differentiated from controls in this way. The probe has been used to define the locus of the PKU gene on chromosome 12. This new methodology permitted the development of a method for prenatal diagnosis. Analysis by means of a panel of restriction enzymes revealed a considerable polymorphism linked tightly to the phenylalanine hydroxylase, and this polymorphism has been employed in informative families* for heterozygote detection and for prenatal diagnosis. PKU is transmitted as an autosomal recessive characteristic. The involved

*An informative family is one in which the carrier parents are heterozygous for polymorphic bands detectable with the cDNA probe.

child is homozygous for one of the two bands and an unaffected sibling may be homozygous for the other band. A child found to be heterozygous for the two bands will be a carrier for PKU. In prenatal diagnosis cells from a fetus that is homozygous for the same band as the patient will signify an affected fetus. In two families at risk monitored prenatally, one fetus was diagnosed as having PKU and the other was a heterozygote.

Treatment of PKU is accomplished by restriction of dietary intake of phenylalanine. This strategy has been successful in the prevention of the clinical manifestations of the disease when instituted in the neonatal period as a result of case finding in siblings of previous patients or through a program of routine neonatal screening. Preparations such as Lofenalac and Milupa make long-term treatment economically feasible and palatable. Dietary therapy readily lowers levels of phenylalanine in the blood, and phenylpyruvic acid and its metabolic products disappear.

The management of infants on a low-phenylalanine diet is demanding. All infants require a certain amount of phenylalanine, including those with PKU, for whom the minimal requirements are similar to those of normal infants. Patients with PKU often vomit or refuse feedings, and infections may complicate the altered metabolic state. Management should be directed by a clinician with experience with the problem and access to facilities for accurate determination of serum concentrations of phenylalanine. If phenylalanine is restricted below levels required for growth, catabolism results and levels of phenylalanine increase. Hypoglycemic convulsions and death can occur. The optimal time for termination of dietary therapy is unclear. It was once customary to stop the diet at 5 years of age, but recent experience has indicated that discontinuation of dietary treatment at 6 years of age may lead to a reduction in IQ. Nevertheless, the rigidity of dietary restriction is usually relaxed after 6 years of age.

ANNOTATED BIBLIOGRAPHY

Nyhan WL: *Abnormalities in Amino Acid Metabolism in Clinical Medicine*, East Norwalk, CT, Appleton-Century-Crofts, 1984, p 129–148, 393–400.

  A more comprehensive treatment of this disease, which is a model for the understanding of inborn errors of amino acid metabolism. It includes a chapter on neonatal screening programs.

Jervis GA: Phenylpyruvic oligophrenia. *Assoc Res Nerv Ment Dis Proc* 33:259–282, 1954.

  A classic description of untreated PKU from a time before the development of treatment regimens.

Partington MW: The early symptoms of phenylketonuria. *Pediatrics* 27:465–473, 1961.

  A description of the earliest signs of PKU, emphasizing that vomiting is the most prominent.

Woo SLC, Lidsky AS, Güttler F, Thirumalachary C, Robson

KJ: Prenatal diagnosis of classical phenylketonuria by gene mapping. *JAMA* 251:1998–2002, 1984.

Modern molecular biology and the cloning of the gene for phenylalanine hydroxylase permit prenatal diagnosis and heterozygote detection.

BIBLIOGRAPHY

Bickel H, Guthrie R, Hammersen G (eds): *Neonatal Screening for Inborn Errors of Metabolism,* Berlin, Springer-Verlag, 1980.

Ledley FD, Grenett HE, DiLella AG, Kwok SC, Woo SL: Gene transfer and expression of human phenylalanine hydroxylase. *Science* 228:77–79, 1985.

Smith I, Lobascher ME, Stevenson JE, et al: Effect of stopping low-phenylalanine diet on intellectual progress of children with phenylketonuria. *Br Med J* 2:723–726, 1978.

ABNORMALITIES IN THE METABOLISM OF BIOPTERIN

A group of disorders, which have variously been referred to as malignant hyperphenylalaninemia or atypical phenylketonuria, result from abnormalities in the synthesis of tetrahydrobiopterin, the cofactor for the phenylalanine hydroxylase reaction, or from defective recycling of the cofactor.

Initially most children were identified because of progressive neurologic degeneration in those thought to have PKU because of a positive neonatal screening test; previous management included good dietary control of the blood levels of phenylalanine. Now children are being detected earlier by testing for biopterin defects in those with hyperphenylalaninemia detected by screening programs.

In the fully developed phenotype the patient is hypertonic or even rigid and has extensor posturing or episodic opisthotonus. Convulsions may occur as early as 3 months of age. Myoclonic seizures are common. Deep tendon reflexes are exaggerated, the Babinski sign is positive, and clonus is often elicited. Patients are difficult to feed. They have problems with their secretions and commonly drool. The patient appears expressionless or drowsy, and may have tremors or dystonic movements. The intelligence deteriorates progressively to the range of profound retardation. CT or MRI scan reveals cerebral atrophy, and ultimately the patient is microcephalic. Death usually supervenes in childhood.

Concentrations of phenylalanine in the blood are elevated. The levels are usually more like those in atypical hyperphenylalaninemia than in classical PKU. Worrisome is the fact that these disorders can occur, at least in infancy, without elevation of the serum concentration of phenylalanine, as documented in one patient diagnosed early because of an affected sibling.

Ultimately, of course, levels of phenylalanine should rise, because tetrahydrobiopterin is the cofactor required for activity of phenylalanine hydroxylase. Defects have been noted in the synthesis of biopterin at the initial GTP cyclohydrolase step and later in the formation of the reduced biopterin itself. The syndrome also results when there is a deficiency of dihydropteridine reductase, which catalyzes the recycling of tetrahydrobiopterin from the inactive quinonoid oxidation product of the phenylalanine hydroxylase reaction. Tetrahydrobiopterin is also the cofactor for the hydroxylation of tryptophan and tyrosine. Deficiency in this compound interferes with the synthesis of serotonin, dopamine, and norepinephrine.

The diagnosis of these disorders is readily made by the administration of tetrahydrobiopterin. This leads to a prompt decrease to normal of serum concentrations of phenylalanine in patients with defects in synthesis or the reductase, whereas there is no change in the patient with PKU. The test must be done while the patient is receiving a normal diet. The usual dose is 2 mg/kg. It has been recommended that the test be given to every infant identified in the screening for PKU.

The definitive diagnosis in dihydropteridine reductase deficiency is made by assay of the enzyme in biopsied liver or cultured fibroblasts or lymphoblasts, or in freshly isolated lymphocytes. Patients with defective biosynthesis of tetrahydrobiopterin can be diagnosed by assay of the pattern of excretion of pterins in the urine or by quantitative assay of tetrahydrobiopterin in plasma, especially after the administration of a phenylalanine load.

These disorders are all thought to be autosomal recessive. Heterozygote detection is possible in dihydropteridine reductase deficiency by assay of the enzyme. Prenatal diagnosis should be possible.

Treatment is by the administration of tetrahydro-

FEATURE TABLE 14-4. ABNORMALITIES IN THE METABOLISM OF BIOPTERIN

Discriminating Features	Consistent Features	Variable Features
1. Defective activity of dihydropteridine reductase 2. Evidence of deficient synthesis of tetrahydrobiopterin	1. Hyperphenylalaninemia 2. Degenerative neurologic disease 3. Convulsions 4. Spasticity	1. Rigidity 2. Tremors 3. Dystonic movements

Pearls and Perils: Abnormalities in the Metabolism of Biopterin

1. Everyone with a positive neonatal screen for phenylalanine does not have PKU. Some have benign hyperphenylalaninemia. A few have defects in biopterin metabolism. In the absence of early recognition and effective therapy, the effects of defective biopterin metabolism on the nervous system are profound.

biopterin. It has been recommended that these patients also be treated with the precursors of the biogenic amines 5-hydroxytryptophan and DOPA.

ANNOTATED BIBLIOGRAPHY

Danks DM, Schlesinger P, Firgaira F, et al: Malignant hyperphenylalaninemia—Clinical features, biochemical findings, and experience with administration of biopterins. *Pediatr Res* 13:1150–1155, 1979.

A clinical description of the phenotype and the use of tetrahydrobiopterin in diagnosis.
Bartholomé K, Byrd DJ: L-Dopa and 5-hydroxytryptophan therapy in phenylketonuria with normal phenylalanine hydroxylase. *Lancet* 2:1042–1043, 1975.

This paper discusses the role of biogenic amine precursors in therapy.

BIBLIOGRAPHY

Brewster TG, Moskowitz HA, Kaufman S, Breslow JL, Milstein S, Abroms IF: Dihydropteridine reductase deficiency associated with severe neurologic disease and mild hyperphenylalaninemia. *Pediatrics* 63:94–99, 1979.
Endres W, Niederwieser A, Curtus H-Ch, et al: Atypical phenylketonuria due to biopterin deficiency. *Helv Paediatr Acta* 37:489–498, 1982.
Kaufman S, Holtzman NA, Milstein S, Butler IJ, Krumholz A: Phenylketonuria due to a deficiency of dihydropteridine reductase. *N Engl J Med* 293:785–790, 1975.
Kaufman S, Berlow S, Summer GK, et al: Hyperphenylalaninemia due to a deficiency of biopterin. *N Engl J Med* 299:673–679, 1978.
Narisawa K, Arai N, Ishizawa S, et al: Dihydropteridine reductase deficiency: Diagnosis by leukocyte enzyme assay. *Clin Chim Acta* 105:335–342, 1980.
Niederwieser A, Blau N, Wang M, Joller P, Ataré S, Cardesa-Garcia J: GTP cyclohydrolase I deficiency, a new enzyme defect causing hyperphenylalaninemia with neopterin, biopterin, dopamine, and serotonin deficiencies and muscular hypotonia. *Eur J Pediatr* 141:208–214, 1984.
Smith I: Atypical phenylketonuria accompanied by a severe progressive neurological illness unresponsive to dietary treatment. *Arch Dis Child* 49:245, 1974.

MAPLE SYRUP URINE DISEASE

Maple syrup urine disease (MSUD) is an inborn error in the metabolism of the branched-chain amino acids that is fatal in the neonatal period in a majority of patients. Even those diagnosed promptly and treated carefully may die in infancy. The survivors are often retarded in mental development. The metabolic abnormality is so devastating that, even in those states in which there are neonatal screening programs for MSUD, it is not uncommon to find a patient in extremis by the time the initial positive result becomes known.

In MSUD leucine, isoleucine, and valine are not effectively catabolized because of a defect in their common branched-chain ketoacid decarboxylase. The activity of this enzyme and its deficiency in MSUD are readily demonstrable in leukocytes and in cultured fibroblasts by assay of the conversion of $[^{14}]CO_2$ to $^{14}CO_2$.

Infants with MSUD appear well at birth but symptoms begin within 24 hours to 5 days of life with feeding difficulty or irregular respirations. There is progressive loss of vigor and the Moro reflex. Severe hypoglycemia may occur. Characteristically these patients develop convulsions, opisthotonos, and generalized muscular rigidity with or without intermittent flaccidity. Coma may be profound. Death usually occurs following the development of decerebrate rigidity. On CT or MRI scan cortical atrophy may be seen along with hypodense myelin. This finding is consistent with the defective myelinization that has been observed at autopsy.

FEATURE TABLE 14-5. MAPLE SYRUP URINE DISEASE

Discriminating Feature	Consistent Features	Variable Features
1. Complete deficiency of branched-chain ketoacid decarboxylase	1. Elevated concentrations of leucine, isoleucine, and valine 2. Positive dinitrophenyl-hydrazine test of urine 3. Branched-chain ketoaciduria	1. Maple syrup odor of urine 2. Mental retardation 3. Spasticity 4. Opisthotonos 5. Coma 6. Convulsions 7. Hypodense cerebral myelin

The name of the disease derives from the odor of the urine, which is reminiscent of maple syrup. The branched-chain amino acids are present in high concentration in the blood and urine, and the ketoacid analogues are found in the urine. Diagnosis is best made by the quantitation of the amino acids of the blood plasma. Ketoacids may be recognized in the urine by the yellow precipitate that forms on the addition of 2,4-dinitrophenylhydrazine.

Milder forms of the disorder occur, representing less complete deficiencies of the decarboxylase enzyme. Patients with some of these enzyme variants have been referred to as having intermittent branched-chain ketoaciduria because of the intermittent occurrence of the symptoms. The enzyme abnormality is always present, just as in classic MSUD. Ataxia and repeated episodes of lethargy may progress to coma in patients with or without mental retardation. The episodes may be precipitated by infection, surgery, or anesthesia. A variant form of the disease has been described that is responsive to the administration of thiamine.

All of the forms of branched-chain ketoaciduria are transmitted as autosomal recessive traits.

The enzyme is expressed in cultured amniocytes. The disorder has been detected prenatally in a number of affected fetuses. In addition methods have been developed for rapid, accurate diagnosis in very small numbers of cells on microtiter plates. This methodology should be applicable to chorionic villus samples.

Any patient shown to be responsive to thiamine should be treated accordingly. The mainstay of treatment for the majority of patients is dietary regulation. The intakes of leucine, isoleucine, and valine are maintained at levels at which the concentrations of the branched-chain amino acids in plasma are kept within normal limits. This therapy may be difficult. However, in patients in whom diagnosis is made very early a normal IQ may be achieved. Commercial products are available that are useful in management.

Pearls and Perils: Maple Syrup Urine Disease

1. The characteristic maple syrup, or caramel, odor can be detected in urine, skin, or hair and may be very striking. However, the odor may not be detected at all, especially in very ill patients who may not have ingested protein for days. Freezing the urine intensifies the odor in an oil that forms at the top of the specimen.

2. A pitfall was reported in an infant in whom prenatal assay of the enzyme was normal but who went on to develop typical elevations of amino acids in the blood. It has not been possible to detect MSUD prenatally by analysis of the amino acids of amniotic fluid.

ANNOTATED BIBLIOGRAPHY

Menkes JH, Hurst PL, Craig JM: A new syndrome: Progressive familial infantile cerebral dysfunction associated with an unusual urinary substance. *Pediatrics* 14:462–466, 1954.

This is the classic paper: an example of the value of careful clinical observation—and a good nose—in the definition of a new disease.

Snyderman SE: Maple syrup urine disease, in Nyhan WL (ed): *Heritable Disorders of Amino Acid Metabolism.* New York, John Wiley & Sons, 1974, p 17–31.

The definitive work on the dietary management of MSUD.

Scriver CR, MacKenzie S, Claw CL, Delvin E: Thiamine-responsive maple syrup urine disease. *Lancet* 1:310–312, 1971.

Not many patients with MSUD will respond to thiamine, but they all should be tested. If the patient is responsive, management is enormously simplified and the prognosis should be very good.

BIBLIOGRAPHY

Clow CL, Reade TM, Scriver CR: Outcome of early and long-term management of classicial maple syrup urine disease. *Pediatrics* 68:856–862, 1981.

Cox RP, Hutzler J, Dancis J: Antenatal diagnosis of maple-syrup-urine disease. *Lancet* 2:212, 1978.

Dancis J, Hutzler J, Rokkones T: Intermittent branched chain ketoaciduria: Variant of maple syrup urine disease. *N Engl J Med* 276:84–89, 1967.

Danner DJ, Armstrong N, Heffelfinger SC, Sewell ET, Priest JH, Elsas LJ: Absence of branched chain acyl-transferase as a cause of maple syrup urine disease. *J Clin Invest* 75:858–860, 1985.

Fensom AH, Benson PF, Baker JE: A rapid method for assay of branched-chain keto acid decarboxylation in cultured cells and its application to prenatal diagnosis of maple syrup urine disease. *Clin Chim Acta* 87:169–174, 1978.

Litwer S, Danner DJ: Identification of a cDNA clone in λgtll for the transacylase component of branched chain ketoacid dehydrogenase. *Biochem Biophys Res Commun* 131:961–967, 1985.

Mantovani JF, Naidich TP, Prensky AL, Dodson WE: Presentation with pseudotumor cerebri and CT abnormalities. *J Pediatr* 96:279–281, 1980.

Wendel U, Rüdiger HW, Passarge E, Mikkelsen M: Maple syrup urine disease: Rapid prenatal diagnosis by enzyme assay. *Humangenetik* 19:127–128, 1973.

PROPIONIC ACIDEMIA AND DISORDERS OF PROPIONATE METABOLISM

Propionic acidemia is the protypic organic acidemia. In this disorder and in methylmalonic acidemia and multiple carboxylase deficiency, the patient presents in early infancy with life-threatening acidotic illness, characterized clinically by vomiting and dehydration and progressing to deep coma. It is characterized metabolically by massive ketosis, a low serum concentration of bicarbonate, and a low pH. There may be an elevated blood concentration of ammonia. Concentrations of glycine in blood and urine are elevated.

There are recurrent episodes of metabolic acidosis associated with the ketosis, similar to those observed in diabetic coma. Patients usually have neutropenia and thrombocytopenia, and may be anemic. Osteoporosis may be severe enough to lead to pathologic fractures. Mental retardation may occur, but this appears to be a consequence more of the complications of overwhelming illness in a young infant (such as shock and diminished cerebral perfusion) or of complicating hyperammonemia, than of the metabolic defect itself.

Symptoms usually begin with vomiting and patients have been diagnosed as having pyloric stenosis. Convulsions and EEG abnormalities may be present. The disease is transmitted as an autosomal recessive trait.

The diagnosis of propionic acidemia is most readily made by organic acid analysis of the urine, in which the diagnostic compound is methylcitrate. It may be suspected by finding elevated quantities of glycine. Other distinctive metabolites found in the urine are hydroxypropionate, tiglate, tiglylglycine, and propionylglycine.

The molecular defect is in the activity of propionyl CoA carboxylase, an enzyme on the catabolic pathway for isoleucine, valine, threonine, and methionine, which catalyzes the conversion of propionyl CoA to methylmalonyl CoA. The enzyme may be assayed in leukocytes or cultured fibroblasts. Prenatal diagnosis has been carried out by assay of this enzyme in cultured amniocytes. However, an index of the difficulties inherent in this approach is the fact that the first pregnancy in which the prenatal diagnosis was reported was already so far advanced that termination was not feasible; a baby with

FEATURE TABLE 14-6. DISORDERS OF PROPIONATE METABOLISM

Discriminating Features	Consistent Features	Variable Features
Propionic Acidemia 1. Deficiency of propionyl CoA carboxylase	1. Methylcitraturia 2. Hydroxypropionaturia 3. Propionic acidemia 4. Recurrent episodes of ketosis and acidosis leading to coma and potentially fatal illness 5. Osteoporosis 6. Vomiting 7. Hypotonia 8. Anorexia 9. Moniliasis	1. Hyperammonemia 2. Anemia 3. Hyperglycinemia, hyperglycinuria 4. Pathologic fractures 5. Mental retardation 6. Immunodeficiency
Methylmalonic Acidemia 1. Deficiency of methylmalonyl CoA mutase	As in propionic acidemia, plus: 10. Failure to thrive	As in propionic acidemia
Multiple Carboxylase Deficiency 1. Deficiency of holocarboxylase synthetase	As in propionic acidemia, plus: 10. Alopecia 11. Dermatosis 12. Lactic acidemia, lactic aciduria 13. Deficient leukocyte carboxylases	As in propionic acidemia
2. Deficiency of biotinidase	As in propionic acidemia, plus: 10. Sensorineural deafness and visual defects 11. Ataxia	As in propionic acidemia

propionic acidemia was born who died in infancy. This type of experience has been a stimulus for the development of more rapid methods of prenatal diagnosis. Among them has been the incorporation of [^{14}C]propionate into macromolecules, a technique that requires only two to four passages to obtain a sufficient number of amniocytes. It can be applied also to the diagnosis of methylmalonic acidemia. Propionyl CoA carboxylase can also be assayed in chorionic villus samples. The direct chemical prenatal diagnosis of propionic acidemia can be accomplished by the demonstration of methylcitric acid in the amniotic fluid. Stable isotope dilution and selected ion monitoring gas chromatography-mass spectrometry (GCMS) have made for rapid, highly sensitive prenatal diagnosis of the fetus with propionic acidemia. Patients with methylmalonic acidemia and multiple carboxylase deficiency can also be diagnosed in this way.

Prenatal diagnosis permits the institution of prenatal treatment. This has been accomplished with excellent results in B$_{12}$-responsive methylmalonic acidemia and in biotin-responsive multiple carboxylase deficiency. Prenatal therapy of a pregnant woman carrying a fetus with methylmalonic acidemia or multiple carboxylase deficiency with pharmacologic doses of cobalamin or biotin has been highly successful. This approach permits the avoidance of the initial catabolic episode, which can occur within hours of birth and can be fatal.

Methylmalonic acidemia and multiple carboxylase deficiency also present with an identical picture of overwhelming illness that is usually fatal in the neonatal period. These infants have episodes of acidosis with massive ketosis, dehydration, and hyperammonemia, progressive to deep coma. Infants with multiple carboxylase deficiency have in addition generalized erythematous cutaneous lesions and alopecia totalis. Each has a characteristic pattern of organic acid excretion. The first is characterized by the excretion of large amounts of methylmalonic acid, but 3-hydroxypropionic acid and methylcitric acid are also found in the urine. In multiple carboxylase deficiency 3-hydroxypropionic acid and methylcitric acid are found, along with 3-methylcrotonylglycine and large amounts of 3-hydroxyisovaleric acid and lactic acid.

Patients with methylmalonic acidemia have defective activity of methylmalonyl CoA mutase. In a B$_{12}$-responsive subset of patients, the fundamental defect is in the conversion of hydroxycobalamin to deoxyadenosylcobalamin, the cofactor for the mutase enzyme. Similarly patients with multiple carboxylase deficiency have abnormal activity of propionyl CoA carboxylase, 3-methylcrotonyl CoA carboxylase, and pyruvate carboxylase, but the fundamental defect in the infantile form is in the enzyme holocarboxylase synthetase. A second form of multiple carboxylase deficiency is due to deficiency of biotinidase.

Therapy in propionic acidemia and methylmalonic acidemia requires profound restriction of the dietary in-

---

Pearls and Perils: Disorders of Propionate Metabolism

1. Quantitative assay of the organic acids is essential for the unraveling of these conditions. Hydroxyisovalerate occurs nonspecifically in ketosis and therefore may be found along with methylcitrate and hydroxypropionate in propionic acidemia. In the absence of quantitation this could suggest a diagnosis of multiple carboxylase deficiency, and the reduction of levels of metabolites induced by fasting and parenteral fluids may be mistaken for a response to biotin. This could be a fatal mistake if the patient is sent home consuming the usual quantities of protein. Quantitation resolves these issues because hydroxyisovalerate is a major metabolite in multiple carboxylase deficiency, whereas in the ketotic infant with propionic acidemia it is a minor one.

2. In a ketotic infant who appears to have an organic aciduria, repeat the analyses after resolution of ketosis. Methylcitrate, and even methylmalonate, may disappear at times of ketosis.

3. Loading tests with the offending amino acids are not recommended under these conditions.

---

take of protein. In B$_{12}$-responsive methylmalonic acidemia treated with B$_{12}$, dietary restriction may be less severe, and in multiple carboxylase deficiency treatment with biotin, usually in doses as small as 10 mg/day, is all that is required for effective therapy.

Dietary therapy in propionic acidemia and methylmalonic acidemia requires the amounts of protein to be individually determined. For most patients the requirements are less than 1.0 g/kg per day. Infants diagnosed early and treated with good dietary management may have normal intelligence. Episodes of intercurrent acidosis must be treated vigorously with large amounts of parenteral fluid and electrolytes containing sodium bicarbonate.

ANNOTATED BIBLIOGRAPHY

Childs B, Nyhan WL, Borden M, Bard L, Cooke RE: Idiopathic hyperglycinemia and hyperglycinuria, a new disorder of amino acid metabolism. *Pediatrics* 27:522–538, 1961.

This is the initial description of this order.

Wolf B, Hsia YE, Sweetman L, Gravel R, Harris DJ, Nyhan WL: Propionic acidemia: A clinical update. *J Pediatr* 99:835–846, 1981.

A clinical compilation of experience in multiple centers.

Naylor G, Sweetman L, Nyhan WL, et al: Isotope dilution analysis of methylcitric acid in amniotic fluid for the prenatal diagnosis of propionic and methylmalonic acidemia. *Clin Chim Acta* 107:175–183, 1980.

The method for direct prenatal diagnosis by GCMS of the amniotic fluid.

Nyhan WL: Disorders of propionate metabolism, in Bickel H, Wachtel U (eds): in *Inherited Diseases of Amino Acid Metabolism: Recent Progress in Understanding, Recognition and Management.* Stuttgart, Georg Thieme, 1985, p 363–382.

This chapter summarizes the most up-to-date approach to dietary treatment of these disorders.

BIBLIOGRAPHY

Ampola MG, Mahoney MJ, Nakamura E, Tanaka K: Prenatal therapy of a patient with vitamin B_{12} responsive methylmalonic acidemia.

Buchanan PD, Kahler SG, Sweetman L, Nyhan WL: Pitfalls in the prenatal diagnosis of propionic acidemia. *Clin Genet* 18:177–183, 1980.

Burri BJ, Sweetman L, Nyhan WL: Heterogeneity of holocarboxylase synthetase in patients with biotin-responsive multiple carboxylase deficiency. *Am J Hum Genet* 37:326–337, 1985.

Cathelineau L, Briand P, Ogier H, Charpentier C, Coude F-X, Saudubray J-M: Occurrence of hyperammonemia in the course of 17 cases of methylmalonic acidemia. *J Pediatr* 99:279–280, 1981.

Cowan MJ, Wara DW, Packman S, et al: Multiple biotin-dependent carboxylase deficiencies associated with defects in T-cell and B-cell immunity. *Lancet* 2:115–118, 1979.

Fenton WA, Rosenberg LE: The defect in the *cbl B* class of human methylmalonic acidemia: Deficiency of cob(1)alamin adenosyltransferase activity in extracts of cultured fibroblasts. *Biochem Biophys Res Commun* 98:283–289, 1981.

Ney DN, Bay C, Saudubray J-M, et al: An evaluation of protein requirements in methylmalonic acidaemia. *J Inher Metab Dis* 8:132–142, 1985.

Packman W, Cowan MJ, Golbus MS, et al: Prenatal treatment of biotin-responsive multiple carboxylase deficiency. *Lancet* 1:1435–1438, 1982.

Roth K, Yang W, Foremen J, Rothmar R, Segal S: Holocarboxylase synthetase deficiency: A biotin-responsive organic aciduria. *J Pediatr* 96:845–849, 1980.

Sweetman L: Prenatal diagnosis of the organic acidurias. *J Inher Metab Dis* 7:18–22, 1984.

Sweetman L, Bates SP, Hull D, Nyhan WL: Propionyl-CoA carboxylase deficiency in a patient with biotin-responsive 3-methylcrotonylglycinuria. *Pediatr Res* 11:1144–1147, 1977.

Willard HF, Ambani LM, Hart AC, Mahoney MJ, Rosenberg LE: Rapid prenatal and postnatal detection of inborn errors of propionate, methylmalonate, and cobalamin metabolism. *Hum Genet* 34:277–283, 1976.

Willard HF, Rosenberg LE: Inherited methylmalonyl CoA mutase apoenzyme deficiency in human fibroblasts: Evidence for allelic heterogeneity, genetic compounds, and codominant expression. *J Clin Invest* 65:690–698. 1980.

Wolf B, Grier RE, Allen RJ, et al: Phenotypic variation in biotinidase deficiency. *J Pediatr* 103:233–237, 1983.

ISOVALERIC ACIDEMIA

Isovaleric acidemia is a disorder of the catabolism of leucine that is remembered as the "sweaty foot syndrome" because of the characteristic pungent odor of isovaleric acid. Patients usually present with severe illness in early life, much like that of propionic acidemia; onset may occur with vomiting. Neurologic abnormalities include tremors and convulsions. The course is progressive to deep coma. Laboratory assessment reveals prominent acidosis and ketosis. Some patients have hyperammonemia. Patients with isovaleric acidemia may also have leukopenia, thrombocytopenia, and anemia. Death may occur within a few days or weeks of birth.

Infants who survive the initial episode of illness are subject to recurrent attacks of vomiting, acidosis, and ataxia, progressive to coma. Such episodes may follow infections or surgery. The odor is more likely to be appreciated during an episode of acute illness, but it may be absent. Mental retardation may be a sequela.

The diagnosis is best based on the detection of isovalerylglycine in the urine. This compound is excreted in amounts up to 3 g/day. It is quite stable, and can also be employed to monitor the success of therapeutic measures, and especially to fine tune dietary management. Isovaleric acid itself may be detected in the serum, but its volatility makes assay more difficult. During acute episodes concentrations in the serum may be as high as 10 mM.

3-Hydroxyisovaleric acid is also found in the urine. Levels of glycine may be elevated. The molecular defect is in the activity of isovaleryl CoA dehydrogenase, through which isovaleryl CoA is converted into 3-methylcrotonyl CoA. Enzyme assay is not easy and is not generally available.

Treatment of the acute episode requires the vigorous

FEATURE TABLE 14-7. ISOVALERIC ACIDEMIA

Discriminating Features	Consistent Features	Variable Features
1. Isovalerylglycinuria 2. Deficiency of isovaleryl CoA dehydrogenase	1. Episodes of acute illness 2. Ketoacidosis 3. Neutropenia, thrombocytopenia	1. Acrid "sweaty foot" odor 2. Mental retardation 3. Hyperammonemia 4. Anemia 5. Ataxia 6. Convulsions

Pearls and Perils:
Isovaleric Acidemia

1. The excretion of hydroxyisovalerate may engender confusion because it is a regular concomitant of this disease and of multiple carboxylase deficiency. It also occurs in any infant with ketosis. The diagnosis of isovaleric acidemia requires a demonstration of the presence of isovalerylglycine.
2. In the acutely hyperammonemic infant whose condition is improved by means of dialysis or exchange, resist the urge to begin protein feedings until levels of ammonia are normal and stable, and then begin with very small quantities.

use of parenteral fluids containing glucose and electrolytes, as outlined for the management of propionic acidemia. Hemodialysis, exchange transfusion, or peritoneal dialysis may be useful, especially in the hyperammonemic neonate. Supplemental glycine and its conjugation with isovaleric acid may be useful in acute management. Doses employed have been 250 mg/kg.

Glycine has also been employed in doses of 800 mg/day in chronic management, where the mainstay of the treatment is the restriction of the dietary intake of leucine by lowering the intake of protein until the amounts of leucine ingested are those just necessary for growth.

ANNOTATED BIBLIOGRAPHY

Tanaka K, Budd MA, Efron ML, Isselbacher KJ: Isovaleric acidemia: A new genetic defect of leucine metabolism. *Proc Natl Acad Sci USA* 56:236–242, 1966.

This is the classic initial description of the disease.

Ando T, Nyhan WL, Bachmann C, Rasmussen K, Scott R, Smith EK: Isovaleric acidemia: Identification of isovalerate, isovalerylglycine, and 3-hydroxyisovalerate in urine of a patient previously reported as having butyric and hexanoic acidemia. *J Pediatr* 82:243–248, 1973.

An index of the problems with specific diagnosis in organic acidemia is the fact that these patients were originally described as having a different entity.

BIBLIOGRAPHY

Dubiel B, Wetts R, Tanaka K: Heterogenity in diseases of leucine metabolism: Complementation studies using cultured skin fibroblasts. *Pediatr Res* 14:521, 1980.

Hine DG, Tanaka K: The identification and the excretion pattern of isovaleryl glucuronide in the urine of patients with isovaleric acidemia. *Pediatr Res* 18:508–512, 1984.

Jakobs C, Sweetman L, Nyhan WL, Packman S: Stable isotope dilution analysis of 3-hydroxyisovaleric acid in amniotic fluid: Contribution to the prenatal diagnosis of inherited disorders of leucine catabolism. *J Inher Metab Dis* 7:15–20, 1984.

Kelleher J, Yudkof M, Hutchinson R, August CS, Cohn RM: The pancytopenia of isovaleric acidemia. *Pediatrics* 65:1023–1027, 1980.

Lehnert W, Niederhof H: 4-Hydroxyisovaleric acid: A new metabolite in isovaleric acidemia. *Eur J Pediatr* 136:281–283, 1981.

Rhead WJ, Hall CL, Tanaka K: Novel tritium release assays for isovaleryl CoA dehydrogenases. *J Biol Chem* 256:1616–1624, 1981.

Rhead WR, Tanaka K: Demonstration of a specific mitochondrial isovaleryl CoA dehydrogenase deficiency in fibroblasts from patients with isovaleric acidemia. *Proc Natl Acad Sci USA* 77:580–583, 1980.

Truscott RJW, Malegan D, McCairns E, et al: New metabolites in isovaleric acidemia. *Clin Chim Acta* 110:187–203, 1981.

Williams KM, Peden VH, Hillman RE: Isovalericacidemia appearing as diabetic ketoacidosis. *Am J Dis Child* 135:1068–1069, 1981.

GLUTARIC ACIDURIA

Glutaric aciduria type I is a neurodegenerative disorder first described in two siblings, one of whom also had a tendency to a compensated metabolic acidosis. There is a progressive neurologic deterioration. Patients have convulsions, spasticity, and involuntary movements. The cardinal characteristic is massive excretion of glutaric acid. This increases after lysine loading and decreases after the restriction of the dietary intake of protein. This pattern distinguishes this disease from glutaric aciduria type II, in which several organic acids are excreted in the urine, along with glutaric acid. These include a number of other dicarboxylic acids and hydroxy acids, especially ethylmalonic adipic, suberic, and sebacic acids, as well as unsaturated suberic acids. Among the latter are α-hydroxybutyric, p-hydroxyphenyllactic, and

FEATURE TABLE 14–8. GLUTARIC ACIDURIA

Discriminating Feature	Consistent Features	Variable Feature
1. Glutaric aciduria	1. Spasticity 2. Convulsions 3. Cerebral degeneration 4. Involuntary movements	1. Metabolic acidosis

Pearls and Perils: Glutaric Aciduria

1. This condition raises the importance of screening for organic aciduria in a sizable population of patients with seizures and neurologic deterioration.

α-hydroxyglutaric acids. Lactic acid is also present in massive amounts, and concentrations of the amino acids citrulline, lysine, ornithine, and proline are elevated in plasma and urine.

In glutaric aciduria type I the molecular defect is in glutaryl CoA dehydrogenase. Glutaryl CoA is an intermediate in the catabolism of lysine, tryptophan, and hydroxylysine. α-Ketoadipic acid is a common product of each of these three amino acids, which is decarboxylated to form glutaryl CoA. Glutaryl CoA dehydrogenase converts glutaryl CoA to glutaconyl CoA. It is a mitochondrial FAD-dependent enzyme found in liver and kidney.

Treatment of glutaric aciduria type I has been reported to be modestly effective. Treatment with a diet specifically low in tryptophan and lysine was followed by a decrease in the excretion of glutaric acid in the urine to about one third of the usual level. A low-protein diet and treatment with riboflavin, the coenzyme for glutaryl CoA dehydrogenase, were also followed by substantial reduction in glutaric aciduria. Slight clinical improvement was reported. In treatment of patients diagnosed early, the use of diet, riboflavin, and the GABA agonist Lioresal has been recommended.

No successful treatment has been reported for classic glutaric aciduria type II. It has proven uniformly fatal. Exchange transfusion or peritoneal dialysis might be useful in acute management, but subsequent therapy is not available. However, patients with milder forms of multiple acyl CoA dehydrogenase deficiency, some referred to as having ethylmalonic aciduria, have responded well to restriction in fat intake. A trial of riboflavin is reasonable.

ANNOTATED BIBLIOGRAPHY

Goodman SI, Markey SP, Moe PG, Miles BS, Teng CC: Glutaric aciduria: A "new" disorder of amino acid metabolism. *Biochem Med* 12:386–391, 1975.
This is the classic description of the disease.
Kyllerman M, Steen G: Intermittently progressive dyskinetic syndrome in glutaric aciduria. *Neuropediatrics* 8:397–404, 1977.
A good clinical description of the progressive disease.
Sweetman L, Nyhan WL, Trauner DA, Merritt TA, Singh M: Glutaric aciduria type II. *J Pediatr* 96:1020–1026, 1980.
A description of the dysmorphic form of glutaric aciduria type II, in which there are polycystic kidneys.

BIBLIOGRAPHY

Brandt NJ, Gregersen N, Christensen E, Grøn IH, Rasmussen K: Treatment of glutaryl-CoA dehydrogenase deficiency (glutaric aciduria). *J Pediatr* 94:669–673, 1979.
Christensen E, Brandt NJ: Studies on glutaryl-CoA dehydrogenase in leucocytes, fibroblasts and amniotic fluid cells. The normal enzyme and the mutant form in patients with glutaric aciduria. *Clin Chim Acta* 88:267–276, 1978.
Goodman SI, Norenberg MD, Shikes RH, Breslich DJ, Moe PG: Glutaric aciduria: Biochemical and morphologic considerations. *J Pediatr* 90:746–756, 1977.
Goodman SI, Stene DO, McCabe ER, et al: Glutaric acidemia type II: Clinical, biochemical, and morphologic considerations. *J Pediatr* 100:946–950, 1982.
Przyrembel H, Wendel U, Becker K, et al: Glutaric aciduria type II: Report of a previously undescribed metabolic disorder. *Clin Chim Acta* 66:227–239, 1976.
Rhead W, Mantagos S, Tanaka K: Glutaric aciduria type II: In vitro studies on substrate oxidation, acyl CoA dehydrogenases and electron transferring flavoprotein in cultured skin fibroblasts. *Pediatr Res* 14:1339–1342, 1980.
Stokke O, Goodman SI, Thompson JA, Miles BS: Glutaric aciduria: Presence of glutaconic and β-hydroxyglutaric acids in urine. *Biochem Med* 12:386–391, 1975.
Tanaka K, Rosenberg LE: Disorders of branched chain amino acid and organic acid metabolism, in Stanbury JB, Wyngaarden JB (eds): *The Metabolic Basis of Inherited Disease*, 5th ed. New York, McGraw-Hill, 1982, p 440–473.

3-HYDROXY-3-METHYLGLUTARIC ACIDURIA

3-Hydroxy-3-methylglutaric aciduria differs from the other organic acidemias in that it presents as hypoketotic hypoglycemia. Thus it must be considered in the differential diagnosis of disorders of fatty acid oxidation. However, it also presents with metabolic acidosis and hyperammonemia, so that the major problem in diagnosis is its distinction from Reye's syndrome. It should always be considered in children with "recurrent" attacks of Reye's syndrome. Episodes of the illness are, like those of Reye's syndrome, likely to follow an acute infectious illness.

Acute episodes of life-threatening illness occur in early infancy and lead to coma. Persistent vomiting may be the first symptom. Apnea and death may ensue unless vigorous measures of resuscitation, including mechanical ventilation, are employed. Some patients have had convulsions. Most have had hepatomegaly. One patient presented with acute pancreatitis. Chronic features may include mental retardation, neurologic abnormalities, and cerebral atrophy. Death and permanent neurologic disability have been reported.

Serum concentrations of glucose may be very low. Levels less than 10 mg/dL were recorded in the first three patients. The absence of ketonuria distinguishes these patients from all of the others with organic acidemia. Nevertheless, there may be a prominent metabolic acidosis and

FEATURE TABLE 14-9. 3-HYDROXY-3-METHYLGLUTARIC ACIDURIA

Discriminating Features	Consistent Features	Variable Features
1. 3-Hydroxy-3-methylglutaric aciduria 2. 3-Hydroxy-3-methylglutaryl CoA lyase deficiency	1. 3-Methylglutaconic aciduria 2. 3-Methylglutaric aciduria 3. Hypoketotic hypoglycemia 4. Acute overwhelming illness 5. Metabolic acidosis 6. Lethargy or coma	1. Lactic aciduria 2. Lactic acidemia 3. Hyperammonemia 4. Hypotonia 5. Hepatomegaly 6. Vomiting 7. Elevated liver function tests 8. Convulsions 9. Cerebral atrophy

reduction in the serum bicarbonate. Neonatal hyperammonemia is common. Liver function tests may be abnormal.

The organic aciduria is characteristic. The index feature is the excretion of large quantities of 3-hydroxy-3-methylglutaric acid. In addition, 3-methylglutaconic acid and 3-methylglutaric acid are found in the urine. These compounds represent successive steps in the catabolism of leucine, as well as the reduction of 3-methylglutaconic acid. At times of acute illness the urine also contains large amounts of lactic acid. The molecular defect is in 3-hydroxy-3-methylglutaryl CoA lyase, which catalyzes the conversion of 3-hydroxy-3-methylglutaryl CoA to acetyl CoA and acetoacetate. The activity of the lyase can be assayed in fibroblasts, leukocytes, and cultured amniocytes. The disorder is transmitted as an autosomal recessive trait. Heterozygotes may be detected by enzyme assay of leukocytes or fibroblasts.

Management of the acute crisis requires large amounts of water, electrolytes, and glucose. Long-term management depends on the avoidance of fasting and attendant hypoglycemia. Parents should bring the patient in early when the oral route is compromised by fasting or anorexia. A high-carbohydrate diet is useful, and the intake of both fat and protein should be limited. Glucose polymers may be useful.

ANNOTATED BIBLIOGRAPHY

Faull K, Bolton P, Halpern B, et al: Patient with defect in leucine metabolism. *N Engl J Med* 294:1013, 1976.
   This is the original description of the entity.
Wilson WG, Cass MB, Søvik O, Gibson KM, Sweetman L: 3-Hydroxy-3-methylglutaryl-CoA lyase deficiency in a child with acute pancreatitis and recurrent hypoglycemia. *Eur J Pediatr* 142:289–291, 1984.
   This paper describes a case that presented with vomiting and abdominal pain, leading to a diagnosis of pancreatitis.
Gibson KM, Sweetman L, Nyhan WL, Page TM, Greene C, Cann HM: 4-Hydroxy-3-methylglutaric aciduria: A new assay of 3-hydroxy-3-methylglutaryl-CoA lyase using high-performance liquid chromatography. *Clin Chim Acta* 126:171–181, 1982.
   This article describes the definitive enzyme assay in which the products of the reaction are isolated and quantified.

Pearls and Perils:
3-Hydroxy-3-Methylglutaric Aciduria

1. The urine of every patient with Reye's syndrome should be subjected to an organic acid analysis. In a patient who has had more than one attack, or in an infant under 2 years of age thought to have Reye's syndrome, organic acid analysis is mandatory.
2. Hypoketotic hypoglycemia is an unusual syndrome. 3-Hydroxy-3-methylglutaric aciduria is a well-defined cause of the syndrome. Look for carnitine deficiency or deficiency of carnitine palmitoyl transferase as another.

BIBLIOGRAPHY

Greene CL, Cann HM, Robinson BB, et al: 3-Hydroxy-3-methylglutaric aciduria. *J Neurogenet* 1:165–173, 1984.
Leonard JV, Seakins JWT, Griffin NK: β-Hydroxy-β-methylglutaricaciduria presenting as Reye's syndrome. *Lancet* 1:680, 1979.
Robinson BH, Oei J, Sherwood WG, Slyper AH, Heininger J, Mamer OA: Hydroxymethylglutaryl CoA lyase deficiency: Features resembling Reye syndrome. *Neurology* 30:714–718, 1980.
Schutgens RBH, Heymans H, Ketel A, et al: Lethal hypoglycemia in a child with a deficiency of 3-hydroxy-3-methylglutaryl-coenzyme A lyase. *J Pediatr* 94:89–91, 1979.

FEATURE TABLE 14-10. γ-HYDROXYBUTYRIC ACIDURIA

Discriminating Feature	Consistent Features	Variable Features
1. Succinic semialdehyde dehydrogenase deficiency	1. γ-Hydroxybutyric aciduria 2. Convulsions 3. Ataxia 4. Mental retardation	1. Hyperactivity 2. Somnolence

γ-HYDROXYBUTYRIC ACIDURIA

γ-Hydroxybutyric aciduria is an inborn error of GABA metabolism that is unusual in that the compound that accumulates is of known neuropharmacologic activity. γ-Hydroxybutyric acid was once developed by the pharmaceutical industry as an intravenous anesthetic. It was designed as a GABA analogue that could cross the blood-brain barrier, but it was abandoned when it was found to produce convulsions in animals.

Affected patients have had seizures as well as mental retardation and ataxia. Ataxia has been nonprogressive. Marked hypotonia has been observed regularly. Psychomotor delay may be mild. In one patient ocular mobility was that of a mild apraxia. Language development has usually been retarded. In one patient speech was dysarthric. Pyramidal tract signs are not observed, and there is no sensory deficit.

The hallmark feature is the accumulation of γ-hydroxybutyric acid in urine, serum, and cerebrospinal fluid (CSF). Acidosis is characteristically absent.

The molecular defect is in the enzyme succinic semialdehyde dehydrogenase. The succinic semialdehyde that accumulates is reduced to γ-hydroxybutyric acid. The enzyme is not expressed in fibroblasts, but it is active in lymphocytes and cultured lymphoblasts and the molecular diagnosis has been established in these cells. It is also active in chorionic villus samples. Therefore, the disease should be diagnosable prenatally by chorionic villus biopsy. Heterozygous carriers are detectable by assay of the enzyme in lymphocyte or lymphoblast lysates. An effective treatment regimen has not been developed.

ANNOTATED BIBLIOGRAPHY

Jakobs C, Bojasch M, Monch E, Rating D, Siemes H, Hanefeld F: Urinary excretion of gamma-hydroxybutyric acid in a patient with neurological abnormalities. The probability of a new inborn error of metabolism. *Clin Chim Acta* 111: 169–178, 1981.
   The original description of the disease.
Gibson KM, Nyhan WL, Jaeken J: Inborn errors of GABA metabolism. *Bioessays* 4:24–27, 1986.
   A good review of the chemical and clinical features.

BIBLIOGRAPHY

Divry P, Baltassat P, Rolland MO, et al: A new patient with 4-hydroxybutyric aciduria, a possible defect of 4-aminobutyrate metabolism. *Clin Chim Acta* 129:303–309, 1983.
Gibson KM, Sweetman L, Nyhan WL, et al: Succinic semialdehyde dehydrogenase deficiency: An inborn error of gamma-aminobutyric acid metabolism. *Clin Chim Acta* 133:33–42, 1983.
Gibson KM, Sweetman L, Nyhan WL, Lenoir G, Divry P: Defective succinic semialdehyde dehydrogenase activity in 4-hydroxybutyric aciduria. *Eur J Pediatr* 142:257–259, 1984.
Gibson KM, Kansen I, Sweetman L, et al: 4-Hydroxybutyric aciduria: A new inborn error of metabolism. III. Enzymology and inheritance. *J Inher Metab Dis* 7(suppl 1):95–96, 1984.
Gibson KM, Sweetman L, Nyhan WL, Rating D: Succinic semialdehyde dehydrogenase in cultured human lymphoblasts. *J Neurogenet* 1:213–218, 1984.
Gibson KM, Sweetman L, Nyhan WL, Jansen I: Demonstration of 4-aminobutyric acid aminotransferase deficiency in lymphocytes and lymphoblasts. *J Inher Metab Dis* 8:204–208, 1985.
Rating D, Hanefeld F, Siemes H, et al: 4-Hydroxybutyric aciduria: A new inborn error of metabolism. I. Clinical review. *J Inher Metab Dis* 7(suppl 1):90–92, 1984.

Pearls and Perils:
γ-Hydroxybutyric Aciduria

1. This disorder presents another good reason for screening the urine for organic acids in the presence of rather nonspecific neurologic disease, such as convulsions, mental retardation, and ataxia.
2. γ-Hydroxybutyric acid may be missed in some systems of organic acid analysis.

NONKETOTIC HYPERGLYCINEMIA

Nonketotic hyperglycinemia is an inborn error of metabolism in which large amounts of glycine are found

FEATURE TABLE 14-11. NONKETOTIC HYPERGLYCINEMIA

Discriminating Features	Consistent Features	Variable Features
1. Elevated CSF/plasma glycine ratio 2. Defective hepatic glycine cleavage enzyme	1. Hyperglycinemia 2. Hyperglycinuria 3. Neonatal coma and apnea 4. Myoclonic seizures 5. EEG burst suppression pattern 6. Cerebral atrophy	1. Hypertonia 2. Hypotonia 3. Increased deep tendon reflexes 4. Hiccuping

in body fluids, and there is no detectable accumulation of organic acids.

The currently accepted diagnostic feature is the elevated concentration of glycine in the CSF. The child generally presents with severe illness within a few days of birth. Death usually occurs in the first year. Most patients develop apnea and, if admitted to a neonatal intensive care unit, usually require ventilator support. Children who survive usually have severe mental retardation in which there is little evidence of functional cortical activity. These infants have severe seizure disorders—many have virtually continuous seizures. Hiccuping and myoclonic seizures are the rule.

Microcephaly, hypertonicity, and hypotonicity may be found. Deep tendon reflexes are exaggerated. Cerebral atrophy is found on CT or MRI scan. The EEG displays a distinctive burst suppression pattern.

Heterogeneity has also been described in this condition and there are some patients with milder clinical pictures. Such patients may have only a modest developmental delay, but this presentation is rare. Glycine concentrations in plasma are elevated; levels usually approximate 6 to 12 mg/dL. Glycine excretion in the urine may be enormous. Concentrations in the CSF of patients with nonketotic hyperglycinemia average at least eight times the control level of 0.1 mg/dL. The ratio of the CSF concentration of glycine to that in the plasma is very useful in delineating the diagnosis. The ratio is substantially higher in patients with nonketotic hyperglycinemia than in hyperglycinemic patients with organic

acidemia. Normally the ratio is only 0.02. In nonketotic hyperglycinemia the mean ratio was 0.17 ± 0.09. Patients with milder versions of the disorder than the classic phenotype tend to have lower ratios. The molecular defect is in the glycine cleavage enzyme, which catalyzes the conversion of glycine to CO_2 and hydroxymethyltetrahydrofolic acid. This is a multienzyme system, with four distinct protein components designated P, H, T, and L. Among the few patients with nonketotic hyperglycinemia studied definitively by assay of the system in autopsied liver or brain, individual defects have been described in the H protein, the P protein, and the T protein.

Treatment is generally unsatisfactory. Heroic measures are probably not justified. Treatment with strychnine has been reported but it is clear that it is not useful in the classic phenotype. A concerted effort to lower the CSF concentration as much as possible within the limits of the toxicity of benzoate may ameliorate seizures in a surviving patient.

ANNOTATED BIBLIOGRAPHY

Gerritsen T, Kaveggia E, Waisman HA: A new type of idiopathic hyperglycinemia with hypo-oxaluria. *Pediatrics* 36:882–891, 1965.
    The original description of the disease.
Nyhan WL, Sakati NA: *Diagnostic Recognition of Genetic Disease.* Philadelphia, Lea & Febiger, 1986, p 85–95.
    A thorough summary of the clinical phenotype.
Hayasaka K, Tada K, Kikuchi G, Winter S, Nyhan WL: Nonketotic hyperglycinemia: Two patients with primary defects of P-protein and T-protein, respectively, in the glycine cleavage system. *Pediatr Res* 17:967–970, 1983.
    A report on the enzyme defect.
Wolff JA, Kulovich S, Yu A, Qiao CN, Nyhan WL: The effectiveness of benzoate in the management of seizures in nonketotic hyperglycinemia. *Am J Dis Child* 140:596–602, 1986.
    A concerted attack on the CSF glycine level using sodium benzoate may ameliorate seizures.

BIBLIOGRAPHY

Ando T, Nyhan WL, Gerritsen T, Gong L, Heiner DC, Bray PF: Metabolism of glycine in the nonketotic form of hyperglycinemia. *Pediatr Res* 2:254–263, 1968.

Pearls and Perils: Nonketotic Hyperglycinemia

1. In the workup of an infant in metabolic coma, routine clinical laboratory tests are very helpful. First hypoglycemia must be ruled out. Metabolic acidosis and reduction of the serum bicarbonate lead one to the diagnosis of an organic acidemia. Hyperammonemia in the absence of acidosis signifies a urea cycle defect. Most other patients will have nonketotic hyperglycinemia.

Ando T, Nyhan WL, Bicknell J, Harris R, Stern J: Nonketotic hyperglycinaemia in a family with an unusual phenotype. *J Inher Metab Dis* 1:79–83, 1978.

Baumgartner R, Ando T, Nyhan WL: Nonketotic hyperglycinemia. *J Pediatr* 75:1022–1030, 1969.

Frazier DM, Summer GK, Chamberlin HR: Hyperglycinuria and hyperglycinemia in two siblings with mild developmental delays. *Am J Dis Child* 132:777–781.

Hiraga K, Kochi H, Hayasaka K, Kikuchi G, Nyhan WL: Defective glycine cleavage system in nonketotic hyperglycinemia. Occurrence of a less active glycine decarboxylase and an abnormal aminomethyl carrier protein. *J Clin Invest* 68:525–534, 1981.

Matalon R, Michals K, Naidu S, Hughes J: Treatment of nonketotic hyperglycinaemia with diazepam, choline and folic acid. *J Inher Metab Dis* 5:3–5, 1982.

Rampini S, Vischer D, Curtius HC, et al: Hereditäre Hyperglycinämie: Klinisches Bild und Bestimmung von Glyoxylsäure und Oxalsäure im Urin bei je einem Patienten mit der acidotischen und der nichtacidotischen Form. *Helv Paediatr Acta* 22:135–159, 1967.

Shuman RM, Leech RW, Scott CR: The neuropathology of the nonketotic and ketotic hyperglycinemias: Three cases. *Neurology* 28:139–145, 1978.

Simila S, Viskorpi JK: Clinical findings in three patients with nonketotic hyperglycinaemia. *Ann Clin Res* 2:151–156, 1970.

Trauner D, Page T, Greco C, Sweetman L, Kulovich S, Nyhan WL: Progressive neurodengenerative disorder in a patient with nonketotic hyperglycinemia. *J Pediatr* 81:272–275, 1981.

VonWendt L: Nonketotic hyperglycinaemia. A clinical and experimental study. *Acta Univ Ouluen Ser D* 53 (8):53–64, 1980.

HOMOCYSTINURIA

Homocystinuria is an inborn error of metabolism of a sulfur-containing amino acid in which there is defective activity of the enzyme cystathionine synthetase. This enzyme catalyzes the conversion of homocysteine and serine to cystathionine. Homocystinuria is a disorder of connective tissue with similarities to Marfan's syndrome. It is also characterized by thromboembolic disease, and therefore the resultant clinical picture is often a consequence of which vessel or vessels become involved. In homocystinuria clinical manifestations tend to be progressive, because many of its clinical manifestations result from thrombotic complications.

Patients with homocystinuria generally appear normal at birth. However, typical clinical features have been observed as early as 1 month of age. An early manifestation may be failure to thrive. Death may occur prior to 1 year of age but less severely affected documented patients have been asymptomatic. The most characteristic feature of this disorder is subluxation of the ocular lens. In some patients this is the only manifestation of disease. Iridodonesis may alert one to the presence of the detached lens. Myopia, cataracts, glaucoma, and other ocular manifestations may occur.

Among the other connective tissue abnormalities are changes in the bones. Genu valgum is the most characteristic, but there may be valgus at the ankle as well as pes cavus, or pectus excavatum or carinatum. The gait is peculiar or shuffling and "Charlie Chaplin–like." The joints tend to be limited in mobility.

The hair is usually fair, fine, and sparse. The complexion is usually fair and the eyes are blue. A malar flush is striking and many patients have had livido reticularis.

Thromboembolic phenomena are both arterial and venous, and are frequently the cause of death. Pulmonary emboli, renal artery thrombosis, and cerebral thrombosis have been common, as well as carotid or coronary thrombosis. Classic tests of clotting function are normal, but platelets from these patients show unusual adhesiveness. Furthermore, the addition of homocystine to normal blood causes the platelets to become sticky. Mental retardation is a common but by no means invariable feature of the disease. Among retarded patients the IQ has been 30 to 75. There may be acute signs of a stroke, or the insidious development of hemiplegia. Some patients have a spastic cerebral palsy. Many have seizures, and even more have abnormalities of the EEG.

The most prominent metabolic characteristic is the excretion of homocystine in the urine. Homocysteine is an intermediate in the metabolism of methionine. Free homocysteine condenses with itself to form the disulfide homocystine, as cysteine does to form cystine. The diagnosis is made by the demonstration of homocystine in the urine. Levels of methionine in blood and urine are usually elevated. Mixed disulfide of cysteine and homocysteine is also present in the urine.

Homocystine is unstable. Therefore testing should be done only on fresh urine. For the analysis of plasma,

FEATURE TABLE 14-12. HOMOCYSTINURIA

Discriminating Features	Consistent Feature	Variable Features
1. Homocystinuria 2. Cystathionine synthase deficiency	1. Mixed disulfide of cysteine and homocysteine in urine	1. Hypermethioninemia 2. Ectopia lentis 3. Mental retardation 4. Thromboembolic phenomena 5. Failure to thrive 6. Genu valgum 7. Osteoporosis

Pearls and Perils: Homocystinuria

1. Ectopia lentis or a thrombotic event in a pediatric patient warrants a search for homocystinuria.
2. Homocystine is unstable. Never be satisfied with less than fresh urine.
3. In order to assay for homocystine in the plasma, proteins must be precipitated with acid at the bedside. Otherwise the homocystine links with the proteins and is absent when further analysis is performed.

it is important to precipitate the protein immediately, or homocystine will attach to the proteins and be removed prior to analysis. Screening of urine can be carried out by the cyanide-nitroprusside test.

The enzymatic defect in the most usual form of homocystinuria is in cystathionine synthase, which catalyzes the conversion of homocysteine and serine to cystathionine. The enzyme defect can be demonstrated in biopsied liver or in cultured fibroblasts or amniotic fluid cells. The disorder is transmitted as an autosomal recessive trait, and heterozygotes have reduced cystathionine synthase activity.

Some patients respond to the administration of pyridoxine with an impressive reduction in the accumulation of homocystine. The usual doses are 100 to 500 mg/day, but up to 1000 mg/day may be necessary. Those who respond are effectively managed by treatment with pyridoxine. Folate deficiency is avoided by concomitant administration of 1 to 15 mg/day of folate.

In patients unresponsive to pyridoxine, betaine has been used successfully to provide a methyl donor, reducing concentrations of homocysteine by converting it to methionine. Dietary therapy has also been recommended: methionine is restricted and supplemental cystine is provided.

ANNOTATED BIBLIOGRAPHY

Carson NAJ, Cusworth DC, Dent CE, Field CMB, Neill DW, Westall RG: Homocystinuria: A new inborn error of metabolism associated with mental deficiency. *Arch Dis Child* 38:425–436, 1963.
   This classic description of the disease clearly lays out its clinical manifestations.
Barber GW, Spaeth GE: The successful treatment of homocystinuria with pyridoxine. *J Pediatr* 76:463–478, 1969.
   This demonstration that some patients respond to vitamin B₆ established genetic heterogeneity in homocystinuria. It also provided a means of highly effective therapy in responsive patients.

BIBLIOGRAPHY

Dunn HG, Perry TL, Dolman CL: Homocystinuria: A recently discovered cause of mental defect and cerebrovascular thrombosis. *Neurology* 16:407–420, 1966.
Fleischer LD, Longhi RC, Tallan HH, Beratis NG, Hirschhorn K, Gaull GE: Homocystinuria: Investigations of cystathionine synthase in cultured fetal cells and the prenatal determination of genetic status. *J Pediatr* 85:677–680, 1974.
Francois J: Ocular manifestations in aminoacidopathies. *Adv Ophthalmol* 25:28–103, 1972.
Komrower GM, Wilson VK: Homocystinuria. *Proc R Soc Med* 56:996–997, 1963.
Mudd SH, Finkelstein JD, Irreverre F, Laster L: Homocystinuria: An enzymatic defect. *Science* 143:1443–1445, 1964.
Mudd SH, Skovby F, Levy HL, et al: The natural history of homocystinuria due to cystathione β-synthase deficiency. *Am J Hum Genet* 37:1–31, 1985.
Nyhan WL, Sakati NA: *Diagnostic Recognition of Genetic Disease.* Philadelphia, Lea & Febiger, 1986, p 140–150.
Valle D, Pai GS, Thomas GH, Pyeritz RE: Homocystinuria due to cystathionine β-synthase deficiency: Clinical manifestations and therapy. *Johns Hopkins Med J* 146:110–117, 1980.
Wilcken DEL, Wilcken B, Dudman NPB, Tyrrell PA: Homocystinuria—The effects of betaine in the treatment of patients not responsive to pyridoxine. *N Engl J Med* 309:448–453, 1983.

UREA CYCLE DISORDERS

The prototypic disorders of the urea cycle include carbamyl phosphate synthetase (CPS) deficiency, ornithine transcarbamylase (OTC) deficiency, citrullinemia, and argininosuccinic aciduria. Each presents classically with massive neonatal hyperammonemia. This picture may also be produced by transient hyperammonemia of the newborn. The classic disorder of urea cycle function is uniformly fatal in the first days of life. Transient hyperammonemia of the newborn, on the other hand—although lethal if untreated—resolves within 5 days with proper care, and its long-term prognosis is excellent. Most of the urea cycle disorders are autosomal recessive, but OTC deficiency, the most common single disorder of the urea cycle, is determined by a gene on the X chromosome. The disease is expressed in both males and females. Affected male infants have the classic phenotype, in which the disease is fatal in the first days of life. In affected females there is variable expression, owing probably to the variable inactivation of the X chromosome carrying the normal gene or its counterpart carrying the abnormal one.

The infant with a defect of the urea cycle is normal at birth and may do well for some time, usually until 12 to 48 hours after feedings begin. Refusal of feedings and lethargy develop, followed by grunting or rapid respirations. There may be hypotonia or hypertonia. Some infants have convulsions. Progression is rapid to apnea and hypothermia. The appearance is that of surgical anesthesia. The patient survives only if intubated and provided with mechanical ventilation. The family history may include siblings who died very early in life.

Children with less complete deficiency of a urea cycle enzyme may present with neurologic abnormalities or mental retardation. Some have had recurrent episodes of vomiting, headaches, or ataxia. Even these patients may be at risk of death in hyperammonemic coma. Children with later-onset argininosuccinic aciduria have also had trichorrhexis nodosa, in which scalp hair is brittle and breaks off, leaving such short hair that the child may appear to be bald.

The hallmark feature in children with disorders of the urea cycle is the presence of hyperammonemia. Plasma concentrations of ammonia may vary with protein intake and the presence of a catabolic stimulus. In neonatal hyperammonemic coma, ammonia concentrations of 600 to 2600 $\mu g/dL$ have been observed.

In hyperammonemic patients, the concentrations of glutamine and alanine, and occasionally aspartate, increase as nonspecific responses the increased ammonia levels. Similarly, when carbamylphosphate accumulates, orotic acid excretion is increased. Orotic aciduria is characteristic of OTC deficiency. It also occurs in citrullinemia, and in argininosuccinic aciduria. It may be used to distinguish patients with these abnormalities from those with CPS deficiency or transient hyperammonemia of the newborn. Hepatomegaly and increased serum activities of serum glutamic oxaloacetic transaminase and serum glutamic pyruvate transaminase occur at times when ammonia concentration is increased, and may be confused with hepatic coma.

In the workup of a patient with hyperammonemia the first step is the quantitative analysis of the amino acids of the plasma and urine. Citrulline is found in large amounts in both plasma and urine in citrullinemia; argininosuccinic acid in the urine in argininosuccinic aciduria. In patients without elevation of an amino acid of the urea cycle, orotic aciduria is used to distinguish those with OTC deficiency from those with deficiency of CPS. To distinguish patients with transient hyperammonemia of the newborn from those with CPS deficiency, one looks carefully for the peaks of citrulline and arginine. They should be absent in a newborn with massive hyperammonemia because of a complete defect in CPS, whereas some of each is usually present in transient hyperammonemia of the newborn.

The molecular defect in CPS deficiency is in the first step of the urea cycle. The enzyme catalyzes the formation of carbamyl phosphate from ammonium and bicarbonate and thus provides a branch point to pyrimidine biosynthesis as well as urea synthesis. Assay of the enzyme requires liver biopsy. Biopsy is ideally postponed until the patient has been shown to be stable and able successfully to survive catabolic states such as infection.

Carbamyl phosphate reacts with ornithine in the presence of OTC to form citrulline. The OTC enzyme is exclusively present in the liver. Prenatal diagnosis has not been possible in the usual ways. It has been attempted by biopsy of the fetal liver and assay of the enzyme in liver tissue, but OTC activity in the liver does not develop until the second trimester. Therefore this rather heroic type of prenatal diagnosis has had to be delayed until 18 to 20 weeks of gestation.

The cloning of the OTC gene has permitted the early prenatal diagnosis of amniocytes and chorionic villus tissue. It also permits heterozygote detection. The cDNA probe does not usually detect the mutation in the gene directly, but in informative families restriction fragment length polymorphisms linked to the gene permit the diagnosis of the affected fetus. Among 15 affected males

FEATURE TABLE 14-13. UREA CYCLE DISORDERS

Discriminating Features	Consistent Features	Variable Features
1. OTC deficiency	1. Orotic aciduria	1. Hyperalaninemia
	2. Hyperammonemia	2. Hyperaspartic acidemia
	3. Hyperglutaminemia	3. Convulsions
	4. Coma	4. Mental retardation
2. CPS deficiency	As in OTC, except for orotic aciduria	As in OTC deficency
3. Argininosuccinic synthase deficiency	As in OTC deficiency, plus: 5. Citrullinemia 6. Citrullinuria	As in OTC deficiency
4. Argininosuccinase deficiency	As in OTC deficiency, plus: 5. Increased concentrations of argininosuccinate in urine and CSF	As in OTC deficiency, plus: 5. Trichorrhexis nodosa

Pearls and Perils: Urea Cycle Disorders

1. Neonatal hyperammonemic coma is harmful to the brain. Most male infants with OTC deficiency rescued with benzoate or phenylacetate treatment are retarded, and they tend to worsen with each subsequent episode. Best results are obtained in infants diagnosed prenatally who are prevented from ever having serious hyperammonemia. This may be easier done in CPS deficiency or argininosuccinic aciduria, or in the female with OTC deficiency, possibly in citrullinemia.
2. Patients undergoing this type of therapy should be followed with repeated MRI scans.

studied with the cDNA probe, 14 were indistinguishable from normal, while 1 was found to have a deletion. In two pregnancies at risk a hemizygous normal male was detected in one and a heterozygous female in the other.

In citrullinemia the molecular defect is in argininosuccinate synthase, which catalyzes the formation of argininosuccinic acid from citrulline. Argininosuccinic acid synthase has been found to be deficient in liver and in cultured fibroblasts. Heterozygotes may be detected by assay of fibroblasts, and prenatal diagnosis has been accomplished.

Argininosuccinic acid is an intermediate in the urea cycle that is formed from citrulline and aspartic acid. It is not normally found in body fluids. In argininosuccinic aciduria there is very efficient renal clearance of the compound, so that plasma concentrations are low and urinary concentrations very high. High concentrations of argininosuccinic acid are also found in the CSF. Argininosuccinic aciduria represents a failure in the cleavage of this compound to arginine and fumaric acid, which is catalyzed by argininosuccinase. The defective enzyme may be demonstrated in erythrocytes and cultured fibroblasts as well as in liver. The disease has been diagnosed prenatally.

The treatment of disorders of the urea cycle has been altered dramatically by the advent of alternative approaches to the elimination of waste nitrogen. Thus benzoate is given in order to tie up glycine as hippurate and phenylacetate or phenylbutyrate are given to tie up glutamine as phenylacetylglutamine. Both compounds are efficiently excreted in the urine. In addition arginine is provided as an essential amino acid in case of a complete block and as a source of ornithine to keep the cycle moving. This approach is especially useful in citrullinemia and argininosuccinic aciduria. In the management of the acute episode of coma, hemodialysis is more efficient than exchange transfusion or peritoneal dialysis.

ANNOTATED BIBLIOGRAPHY

Campbell AGM, Rosenberg LE, Snodgrass PJ, Nuzum CT: Ornithine transcarbamylase deficiency: A cause of lethal neonatal hyperammonemia in males. *N Engl J Med* 288:1–6, 1973.

A classic description of the lethal nature of neonatal hyperammonemic coma in urea cycle defects.

Leibowitz J, Thoene J, Spector E, Nyhan WL: Citrullinemia. *Virchows Arch A* 377:249–258, 1978.

Citrullinema, too, when presenting in the neonatal period, was once uniformly fatal.

Brusilow SW, Batshaw ML, Waber L: Neonatal hyperammonemic coma. *Adv Pediatr* 29:69–103, 1982.

This paper sets out the newer approaches to the management of hyperammonemia and of patients with defects of the urea cycle.

Rozen R, Fox J, Fenton WA, Horwich AL, Rosenberg LE: Gene deletion and restriction fragment length polymorphisms at the human ornithine transcarbamylase locus. *Nature* 313:815–817, 1985.

A discussion of the use of molecular biology in the assessment of OTC deficiency.

Ballard RA, Vinocur B, Reynolds JW, et al: Transient hyperammonemia of the preterm infant. *N Engl J Med* 299:920–925, 1978.

The initial description of this syndrome.

BIBLIOGRAPHY

Batshaw ML, Brusilow SW: Treatment of hyperammonemic coma caused by inborn errors of urea synthesis. *J Pediatr* 97:893–900, 1980.

Davies KE, Briand P, Ionasecu V, et al: Gene for OTC: Characterisation and linkage to Duchenne muscular dystrophy. *Nucleic Acids Res* 13:155–165, 1985.

Horwich AL, Fenton WA, Williams KR, et al: Structure and expression of a complementary DNA for the nuclear coded precursor of human mitochondrial ornithine transcarbamylase. *Science* 224:1068–1074, 1984.

Pembrey ME, Old JM, Leonard JV, Rodeck CH, Warren R, Davies KE: Prenatal diagnosis of ornithine carbamoyl transferase deficiency using a gene specific probe. *J Med Genet* 22:462–465, 1985.

ARGININEMIA

Argininemia is a disorder of the urea cycle in which the clinical picture is very different from that of the other disorders of the cycle. The picture is that of a spastic diplegia or tetraplegia. The clinical onset of the disease may be with convulsions in the neonatal period or with signs of cerebral palsy first noted in the early months or years of life. Developmental delay may be the first evidence of abnormality. In the established phenotype the patient is very spastic and opisthotonic. Scissoring of the lower extremities is common. Muscle tone is hypertonic and the deep tendon reflexes are accentuated. There

FEATURE TABLE 14-14. ARGININEMIA

Discriminating Features	Consistent Features	Variable Features
1. Arginase deficiency 2. Argininemia	1. Spastic diplegia 2. Developmental delay 3. Hypertonia 4. Opisthotonus 5. Involuntary movements	1. Hyperammonemia 2. Hepatomegaly 3. Abnormal liver function tests 4. Convulsions 5. EEG abnormalities

may be involuntary movement, which may be choreic or athetoid. Some patients have tremors. Drooling and dysphagia are common. Along with convulsions there are abnormalities of the EEG. Psychomotor retardation is usually severe. Ultimately there is microcephaly and cerebral atrophy on CT or MRI scan.

Concentrations of ammonia are elevated only intermittently in argininemia, and hyperammonemia, when it occurs, tends to be moderate. The diagnosis is made by the analysis of the amino acids of the blood or urine.

Plasma concentrations of arginine are 4 to 20 times normal. Concentrations in CSF are also markedly elevated. The concentration of arginine in the urine is elevated, but the urine also contains increased quantities of lysine, cystine, and ornithine because of competition for reabsorption by the large amounts of arginine in tubular urine. Patients with argininemia also have massive orotic aciduria. This feature of the disease is not a consequence of hyperammonemia as it is in other urea cycle defects, but rather a consequence of the stimulation by accumulated arginine of N-acetylglutamate synthesis, which leads to increased synthesis of carbamylphosphate. In the presence of limiting quantities of ornithine this leads preferentially to pyrimidine biosynthesis.

The molecular defect is in the activity of arginase, which is readily measured in erythrocytes. The defect has also been demonstrated in liver, but the enzyme is not expressed in cultured fibroblasts.

Heterozygosity may be demonstrated by assay of arginase in erythrocytes. Prenatal diagnosis is not available.

Nutritional therapy designed to keep levels of arginine within normal limits has been known to lead to normal neurologic development. Sodium benzoate may be employed in those patients who develop hyperammonemia.

ANNOTATED BIBLIOGRAPHY

Terheggen HG, Schwenk A, Lowenthal A, VanSande M, Colombo JP: Hyperargininämie mit Arginasedefkt: Eine neue familiäre Stoffwechselstorung. *Z Kinderheilkd* 107:298–312, 1970.
   The original description of the disease.
Terheggen HG, Lavinha F, Colombo JP, VanSande M, Lowenthal A: Familial hyperargininemia. *J Hum Genet* 20:69–84, 1972.
   A description for those who do not read German.
Yoshino M, Kubota K, Yoshida I, Murakami T, Yamashita F: Argininemia: Report of a new case and mechanisms of orotic aciduria and hyperammonemia, in Lowenthal A, Mori A, Marescau B (eds): *Urea Cycle Diseases.* New York, Plenum Press, 1982, p 121–125.
   A classic phenotype, and some critical observations on the orotic aciduria.

BIBLIOGRAPHY

Bachman C, Colombo JP: Diagnostic value of orotic acid excretion in heritable disorders of the urea cycle and in hyperammonemia due to organic acidurias. *Eur J Pediatr* 134:109–113, 1980.
Cederbaum SD, Shaw KNF, Spector EB, Verity MA, Snodgrass PJ, Sugarman GI: Hyperargininemia with arginase deficiency. *Pediatr Res* 13:827–833, 1979.
Michels VV, Beaudet AL: Arginase deficiency in multiple tissues in argininemia. *Clin Genet* 13:61–67, 1978.
Qureshi IA, Letarte J, Ouellet R, Batshaw ML, Brusilow S: Treatment of hyperargininemia with sodium benzoate and arginine-restricted diet. *J Pediatr* 104:473–476, 1984.
Serrano AP: Argininuria, convulsiones y oligofrenia: Un nuevo error innato del metabolismo? *Rev Clin Esp* 97: 76–183, 1965.
Snyderman SE, Sansaricq CC, Cheu WJ, Norton PM, Phansalkar SW: Argininemia. *J Pediatr* 90:563–568, 1977.

Pearls and Perils: Argininemia

1. The diagnosis of argininemia may be missed on the basis of a screening pattern of amino acids in the urine because the pattern may appear to be that of cystinuria. The question is readily resolved by the quantitative analysis of the amino acids of the plasma.

GALACTOSEMIA

Please see pages 359 through 362 for a complete discussion.

Neoplastic Diseases

Michael E. Cohen
Patricia K. Duffner

Intracranial tumors represent the second most common neoplasm in childhood, exceeded only by leukemia. The incidence of central nervous system (CNS) neoplasia for children under 15 years of age is approximately 2.4 in 100,000 births. Based on a United States population of 50 to 70 million children under 15 years of age, there are approximately 1200 to 1500 newly diagnosed cases each year.

Unfortunately, advances in treatment have lagged behind those of other forms of childhood cancer. Several factors unique to brain tumors account for the poor results. These include the inability to debulk CNS tumors safely; the presence of a blood-brain barrier that restricts access of chemotherapeutic agents to the CNS; the low mitotic grade of many CNS tumors; and the often unacceptable toxicity associated with current treatment modalities.

The diagnosis of a brain tumor depends on clinical suspicion and the diagnostic acumen of the physician. Diagnosis is confirmed by neuroimaging procedures and surgical exploration. Signs and symptoms of brain tumors vary, depending upon the age of the child, the location of the tumor, and the amount of neurologic tissue compromised. This chapter will be confined to a discussion of tumors relative to location in the nervous system, regardless of the various histopathologies. In particular, the chapter will discuss tumors of the posterior fossa, including tumors of the brainstem and cerebellum; midline tumors, including visual pathway tumors; tumors of the thalamus, hypothalamus, and pineal region and craniopharyngiomas; and supratentorial tumors.

SIGNS AND SYMPTOMS

Children with brain tumors present with signs and symptoms of both a localizing and a nonlocalizing nature.

Nonlocalizing Symptoms

The nonlocalizing signs and symptoms usually reflect increased intracranial pressure. These symptoms occur early in patients with tumors located in the posterior fossa, as masses in this area can readily occlude the aqueduct of Sylvius or the fourth ventricle, leading to obstructive hydrocephalus. In contrast, a tumor located in the cerebral hemispheres must be of relatively greater size before it significantly compresses the lateral ventricles or foramen of Monro or has enough mass effect to cause increased intracranial pressure. Tumors located in the midline tend to cause increased intracranial pressure by compression of the third ventricle.

Headache

Headache is an important symptom of increased intracranial pressure. Although most headaches in children do not reflect mass lesions, certain symptoms strongly suggest increased intracranial pressure. The location of the headache is of variable significance. Persistently focal headaches must be evaluated to exclude underlying structural disease. In general, however, headaches tend to occur in the frontotemporal regions as a result of referred pain. Consequently, a frontal location is common in patients with migraine and anxiety-related headaches, as well as brain tumors. Similarly, although headaches in the occiput and neck suggest disease in the posterior fossa, tension headaches may also be associated with neck pain resulting from contraction of the neck musculature. The presence of neck pain in a patient with increased intracranial pressure may be a warning of impending herniation created by the downward extension of the cerebellar tonsils, with resulting irritation of cervical roots.

Another important symptom in analyzing a headache history is the time of day at which the headache occurs. Headaches that wake a child from sleep or occur early in the morning strongly suggest organic disease. In contrast, headaches that occur as the day progresses are much less likely to be due to mass lesion.

The tempo and progression of headaches associated with a mass lesion are different from those identified with either tension- or migraine-related headaches (Figure 15-1). Headaches resulting from brain tumors typically increase in intensity over time. The exception to this rule is the headache occurring in the very young child with tumor in which there may be a biphasic course. For example, a 2-year-old child may awaken each morning for several weeks with headaches and vomiting. After several hours, the headache will abate and the child will play normally. Each morning, however, the symptoms may reappear. After a few weeks, these symptoms may disappear entirely and the child will appear perfectly normal. Unfortunately, the cycle will recur in the near future. The symptoms resolve because the child is able to accommodate the increased intracranial pressure by separating his cranial sutures. The cycle recurs when the ability to compensate for the pressure is lost.

Headaches that increase with Valsalva maneuvers also suggest increased intracranial pressure. Thus, a child who complains that the headache increases with coughing, sneezing, or straining while having a bowel movement must be investigated for increased intracranial pressure. This symptom almost never occurs in anxiety-related headaches.

Headaches may be the sole early symptom of patients with brain tumor. By the time the child has had 8 to 12 weeks of headache symptoms, however, he or she will usually have clinical signs detectable on ophthalmologic exam. Thus, the index of suspicion must be highest in those children with the shortest duration of symptoms.

Diplopia

Diplopia is another important nonlocalizing symptom of increased intracranial pressure. Although young children rarely verbalize this complaint, double vision can be recognized by observation of the child. The youngster may turn the head to the side or tilt it. The head turning either allows the child's nose to occlude vision from one eye or places the head in a plane of gaze that eliminates the double image. At other times, children may close one eye voluntarily. Benign "strabismus" does not present initially in a 6-year-old child. Furthermore, children with nonparalytic squints do not "see double." Consequently, children presenting with either an acquired strabismus or complaint of diplopia should be investigated for oculomotor palsies, particularly of the sixth nerve. The diplopia is usually due to involvement of the sixth cranial nerve, which, because of its long free intracranial course, is readily compressed against bony structures with increased intracranial pressure. Third-nerve palsy is less

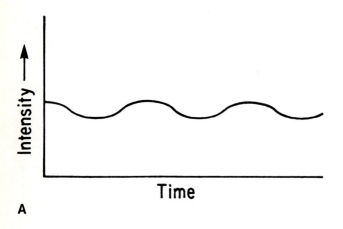

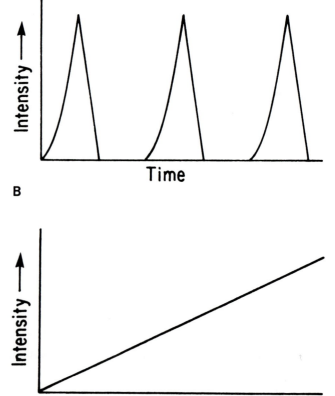

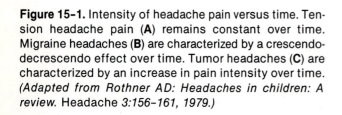

Figure 15-1. Intensity of headache pain versus time. Tension headache pain (**A**) remains constant over time. Migraine headaches (**B**) are characterized by a crescendo-decrescendo effect over time. Tumor headaches (**C**) are characterized by an increase in pain intensity over time. *(Adapted from Rothner AD: Headaches in children: A review.* Headache *3:156–161, 1979.)*

common, but, because of the nerve's anatomical proximity to the temporal lobe, it may be compressed secondary to a herniating mass in the region.

Personality Change

Personality change can be an important sign of brain tumor and/or increased intracranial pressure. Unfortunately, the combination of personality change and headache, especially in adolescents, commonly raises the question of emotional problems rather than a mass lesion. The association of personality change with deteriorating school performance also suggests an organic rather that a psychogenic etiology.

Vomiting

Vomiting is a characteristic symptom of increased intracranial pressure. The symptom may be nonlocalizing, owing to increased intracranial pressure, or may reflect tumor invasion of the vomiting center in the floor of the fourth ventricle. Vomiting is rarely seen in nonneoplastic hydrocephalus. The vomiting associated with increased intracranial pressure is generally not projectile in nature.

Nonlocalizing Signs

The physical signs of increased intracranial pressure are expanding head circumference, papilledema, and sixth-nerve palsy. These signs are not unique to tumors, as papilledema and sixth-nerve palsies commonly occur with all causes of increased intracranial pressure. The value of head circumference in the evaluation of possible increased intracranial pressure decreases with age. However, it is of prime importance in the young. Head circumferences should be monitored in all children because the absolute head circumference is less important than a change in percentiles.

Papilledema is an important sign of increased intracranial pressure. Unfortunately, examination of the fundus in the young child may be extremely difficult. Persistence on the part of the examiner is vital. In cases in which the examiner is not certain whether or not the child has papilledema or pseudopapilledema, assessment of the blind spot may be helpful. Although visual acuity is normal in the presence of early papilledema, children may complain of vision that tends to be clouded at times (obfuscation of vision). Papilledema may not occur in patients who have developed optic atrophy. Thus, other signs of increased intracranial pressure must be sought.

Most cases of sixth-nerve palsy are apparent, as the child is unable to fill the lateral canthus. Ways of differentiating functional from organic diplopia include observation of the complaint that there is increased separation of the double image as the patient looks in the direction of function of the paretic eye, or elimination of diplopia with closure of one eye.

FEATURE TABLE 15-1. SIGNS AND SYMPTOMS

Discriminating Features	Consistent Features	Variable Features
Nonlocalizing Signs and Symptoms		
Signs of ICP		
1. Papilledema	1. Enlarged blind spot	1. Headache
	2. Irritability	2. Diplopia
	3. Vomiting	3. Personality change
Localizing Signs and Symptoms		
Posterior Fossa		
1. Truncal ataxia	1. Papilledema	1. Headache
2. Appendicular ataxia	2. Vomiting	2. Diplopia
3. Ipsilateral cranial nerve signs, contralateral long tract signs		
Midline		
1. Visual field loss	1. Papilledema	1. Personality change
2. Decreased visual acuity	2. No lateralizing signs	2. Optic atrophy
3. Endocrinopathies		3. Headache
4. Precocious puberty		
Supratentorial		
1. Lateralizing long tract and sensory signs	1. Progressive neurologic deficit	1. Seizures
2. Seizures	2. Papilledema	2. Mass effect
	3. Abnormal CT or MRI	3. Vomiting
		4. Personality change

Localizing Signs

In addition to the signs and symptoms of increased intracranial pressure that are essentially nonlocalizing in nature, there are also signs that are quite specific to the location of the tumor. These localizing signs can be separated by location, for example, in the posterior fossa above the tentorium, supratentorial, or in the midline.

Posterior Fossa

Most children with tumors located in the posterior fossa, especially in the cerebellum and sixth ventricle, tend to present early with increased intracranial pressure. In addition to the nonlocalizing signs discussed previously, clinical signs will reflect the location of the tumor. Children whose tumors are located in the midline of the cerebellum tend to present with truncal ataxia. These children have difficulty walking and crawling. Those children whose tumors are located in the hemisphere of the cerebellum are more likely to have appendicular dysmetria. These children will have particular difficulty with finger-to-nose or heel-to-shin maneuvers. Other signs referable to cerebellar involvement include pendular reflexes, cerebellar speech, hypotonia, and nystagmus. The nystagmus, if present, generally is coarser toward the side of the lesion.

Tumor located in the brainstem is heralded by the combination of cranial neuropathies, motor signs, and cerebellar signs. Typically, the cranial neuropathies are ipsilateral to the site of the tumor, motor signs are contralateral, and cerebellar signs are generally ipsilateral. The presence of a sixth-nerve palsy in a child with a brainstem glioma is localizing when it is associated with other cranial neuropathies on one side and a contralateral hemiparesis. Children whose tumors are located in the brainstem, unlike those with cerebellar masses, usually develop increased intracranial pressure much later in their course. Although multiple cranial nerves may be involved, patients typically have difficulty with swallowing and associated nasopharyngeal regurgitation. Speech abnormalities include dysarthria and hypernasality.

Midline Tumors

Tumors located in the midline of the brain tend to interrupt visual pathways as well as the hypothalamic-pituitary axis. Thus, children with such tumors may present with decreased visual acuity, visual field abnormalities, or nystagmus. Tumors directly involving the optic nerve are more likely to present as either exophthalmos or decreased vision. Those tumors located in the chiasm are more commonly associated with either bilateral visual field abnormalities or nystagmus. In the latter case, they are easily confused in the young child with congenital nystagmus or spasmus nutans.

Tumors located within or near the hypothalamic-pituitary axis are commonly associated with a variety of endocrinopathies. These may manifest themselves as either weight gain or loss, precocious or delayed puberty, abnormalities of growth, or diabetes insipidus.

Supratentorial Lesions

Children whose tumors are located in the supratentorial region will also present with signs and symptoms referable to the location of the tumor. Thus, a child whose tumor is located in the motor strip is likely to present with a contralateral hemiparesis. Subtle weakness suggests compressive rather than destructive disease of the motor pathways. The child with a tumor located in the parietal region is more likely to present with visual field or sensory abnormalities.

Patients with supratentorial lesions commonly pre-

Pearls and Perils:
Signs and Symptoms

1. Signs of increased intracranial pressure occur early in children with posterior fossa tumors.
2. Headache that awakens a child from sleep, occurs in the morning with vomiting, and increases with Valsalva maneuvers suggests structural disease.
3. Focal headache should be investigated.
4. Headache in patients with brain tumors that is present for more than 8 weeks is usually associated with oculomotor signs.
5. Children with sixth-nerve palsy tend to turn their heads or obscure one eye to prevent diplopia.
6. Vomiting associated with increased intracranial pressure need not be projectile.
7. The blind spot increases in papilledema but visual acuity is usually normal.
8. Obfuscation of vision is typical of papilledema.
9. Nystagmus associated with chiasmatic tumors may mimic congenital nystagmus or spasmus nutans.
10. Neck pain in the presence of increased intracranial pressure may be a warning of impending herniation.
11. Children with nonparalytic squints do not complain of double vision.
12. Patients with optic atrophy may not develop papilledema, even in the presence of increased intracranial pressure.
13. Clues to the development of tumor in a population of long-term epileptics include personality change, change in school performance, change in neurologic exam, change in quantity or quality of seizures, and abnormal neuroradiologic studies.
14. Sixth-nerve palsy may be nonlocalizing, secondary to increased intracranial pressure, or localizing as a result of direct involvement of the brainstem.

sent with deteriorating school performance and personality change. In addition, seizures are an important symptom of patients with hemispheric lesions. Although most seizures in children are not due to tumors, the incidence of seizures in patients with hemispheric tumors ranges from 30% to 60%. The most epileptogenic areas are those in the sensorimotor regions of the brain and the temporal lobes. In general, seizures are more commonly associated with slowly growing than rapidly evolving tumors. At times, a child will be followed for many years for what is presumed to be an idiopathic seizure disorder only to be diagnosed years later as having a tumor. Such cases have led some workers to suggest the value of a magnetic resonance imaging (MRI) scan in newly diagnosed partial (focal) epilepsies. Clues to the development of tumor in this population of epileptics include change in personality or school performance, change in neurologic examination, slow wave focus on the electroencephalogram (EEG), increase in frequency of seizures, change in quality of seizures, and abnormalities on skull films.

POSTERIOR FOSSA TUMORS

The posterior fossa is bounded anteriorly by the tentorium of the cerebellum and posteriorly by the foramen magnum. This area traditionally includes the cerebellum, lower mesencephalon, pons, and medulla, i.e., those structures traversed by the aqueduct of Sylvius and the fourth ventricle. Excluded from consideration as posterior fossa structures are the hypothalamus, thalamus, and anterior visual pathway anteriorly, and the cervical spinal cord inferiorly and posteriorly. The most common posterior fossa tumors in childhood are cerebellar astrocytomas, medulloblastomas, brainstem gliomas, and ependymomas.

Cerebellar Astrocytomas

The cerebellar astrocytoma has the most favorite prognosis of any childhood neoplasm. It represents approximately 11% of brain tumors in children under 18 years of age. The peak incidence of this tumor is from 5 to 14 years of age. Although the location of the cerebellar astrocytoma is primarily hemispheric, the vermis may also be involved. Typical signs of a hemispheric lesion are appendicular dysmetria with cerebellar dysfunction lateralized to one side. Vermal symptoms typically consist of truncal ataxia. Infrequently, skewed deviation with coarse nystagmus increasing on fixation is also identified. As previously indicated, because of early occlusion of the fourth ventricle, these patients are likely to present with papilledema and signs of increased intracranial pressure.

The tumor usually consists of a single large cyst with a solid mural nodule or, less commonly, is solid with smaller cysts seen throughout the substance of the tumor. In 1930, Cushing recognized that the mural nodule repre-

sented the neoplastic element of the tumor. Until this time, failure to remove the nodule had been associated with regrowth of the tumor.

The 25-year survival rate for cystic cerebellar astrocytoma or juvenile cerebellar astrocytoma is 94%, compared with a 38% 25-year survival rate for patients with a diffuse type of cerebellar astrocytoma.

Surgery is the primary treatment for tumors of this type. When total surgical removal is possible, 5-year survival rates approach 90% to 95%. Reoperation following recurrence is also associated with long-term survival. Chemotherapy and radiotherapy are limited to those patients in whom there has been partial resection, recurrence of the tumor, or possibly diffuse pathology. In these situations, local radiation to the tumor bed is recommended. Because of the benign nature of cerebellar astrocytomas, experience with chemotherapy has been limited.

Medulloblastomas

Of all tumors of childhood, the greatest advances in treatment have been made in children with medulloblastomas. In 1930, Cushing reported a series of 61 children with medulloblastomas. Only 1.6% were alive at the end of 3 years. In contrast, during the last few decades, several large studies have reported 5-year survival rates of 30% to 60%. Certain subsets of patients do better than others. These include children who are greater than 3 to 4 years of age at the time of diagnosis and those who have had gross surgical removal. Those who do the worst are young children treated with biopsy alone, whose tumor involves the brainstem, or who show evidence of tumor spread throughout the subarachnoid space or extraneural metastases.

In 1925, Bailey and Cushing coined the term *medulloblastoma* because of the tumor's biologic nature and histopathologic features. The tumor was called a medulloblast because it was thought to be composed of embryonal stem cells with a pleuripotential ability. However, the medulloblast as a naturally occurring cell capable of differentiating along either neuronal or glial cell lines has not been satisfactorily identified. Histopathologically, the medulloblastoma is thought to derive from remnants of the fetal external granular layer of the cerebellum or from cell rests in either the posterior medullary or anterior medullary velum of the cerebellum. Because of this location, the medulloblastoma tends to occur in the vermis of the cerebellum. Macroscopically, it is soft, fleshy, and well demarcated. Hemorrhagic cyst formation and calcification are common. As with cerebellar astrocytomas, the tumor tends to rapidly obstruct or fill the cavity of the fourth ventricle. Thus, early in its course, signs of increased intracranial pressure and papilledema are recognized. The tumor consists of small round cells that may harbor evidence of glial differentiation. Ependymal differentiation of the tumor may occur either independently or in association with astrocytic differentiation.

Perhaps more than any other histologic subtype, the medulloblastoma is characterized by its tendency to seed the subarachnoid space both locally and distally. However, 70% to 80% of recurrences occur in the posterior fossa. Following diagnosis, the patient should have myelograms to determine if there has been seeding to the spinal cord as well as cerebrospinal fluid (CSF) cytology for evidence of subarachnoid spread. Extraneural metastases are well documented and, in some series, occur in 5% to 30% of patients. Placement of a ventricular shunt to circumvent an obstructed fourth ventricular outlet, as well as the primary surgery, may allow the tumor to spread beyond the confines of the CNS. Remote metastases may be seen in bone, bone marrow, and lymph nodes. Occasionally, other viscera may be involved.

Following clinical consideration, the diagnosis is confirmed with either computed tomographic (CT) or MRI scanning. Both forms of neuroimaging usually show a homogeneous midline mass with secondary hydrocephalus. Most recently, polyamines have been used to assess the possible recurrence of medulloblastoma. Polyamines are elevated in biologic tissue characterized by high growth and rapid turnover. A good correlation has been found between the presence of polyamine and the recurrence of medulloblastoma. This raises the possibility of making the diagnosis of recurrence of medulloblastoma prior to finding evidence of tumor on CT or MRI.

Treatment of medulloblastoma begins with operative removal of the tumor. Aggressive surgery without compromising neurologic function provides definitive pathologic diagnosis, opens CSF pathways, and eliminates in most cases the need for postoperative or intraoperative shunting, thus obliterating a possible portal for extraneural metastasis.

Total removal is unlikely. However, attempts to debulk as much tumor as possible are necessary because both radiation and chemotherapy destroy by a log kill hypothesis. Following surgery, there is overwhelming consensus supporting the role of radiotherapy in extending survival. The development of a high-energy source of radiation and increasing doses of radiation to the posterior fossa and craniospinal areas account for the major changes in radiotherapy in the last several decades. Since the late 1960s and early 1970s, there has been good documentation of the value of craniospinal radiation as well as high-dose radiation to the tumor bed. Survival of those treated with whole-CNS radiation is significantly better than that of those in whom the CNS is partially irradiated. Radiation doses over this period of time have continually changed. In the late 1960s, less than 40 Gy was considered adequate radiation to the posterior fossa and 30 Gy adequate for the spinal cord. Currently,

FEATURE TABLE 15-2. DIAGNOSTIC FEATURES OF POSTERIOR FOSSA TUMORS

Discriminating Features	Consistent Features	Variable Features
Cerebellar Astrocytoma		
1. Pathologic examination of surgical specimen	1. Ataxia (usually appendicular, may be truncal) 2. Papilledema 3. CT or MRI shows cystic lesion with mural nodule	1. Headache 2. Diplopia 3. Vomiting
Medulloblastoma		
1. Pathologic examination	1. Truncal ataxia 2. Short course 3. Papilledema 4. Neuroimaging shows noncystic midline lesion	1. Headache that resolves after 3 to 4 weeks 2. Diplopia 3. Neck pain 4. Vomiting
Brainstem Tumor		
1. Fusiform swelling of brainstem on MRI or CT	1. Ataxia 2. Long tract signs 3. Cranial nerve signs 4. Short course	1. Papilledema (late) 2. Feeding and swallowing abnormalities
Ependymoma		
1. Pathologic examination	1. Ataxia 2. Obliteration of fourth ventricle on CT or MRI 3. Papilledema	1. Headache 2. Vomiting

recommended radiation doses are 40 to 55 Gy to the posterior fossa, 40 to 45 Gy to the whole head, and 35 to 40 Gy to the spinal cord. In specific subsets of patients using these doses, 5-year survival rates are greater than 50% to 60%. In planning radiation, care should be taken to include underdosed areas of the neuroaxis such as the retroorbital and subfrontal regions.

Although 5-year survival rates have improved dramatically, 10-year survival tends to be limited and recurrence is invariably followed by death. Furthermore, high-dose radiation has been associated with unacceptable long-term treatment effects. Because most treatment failures present as either recurrent or metastatic disease unresponsive to surgery, the use of chemotherapy either as a primary adjuvant or as a treatment for recurrent disease is a logical consideration. Reports began to appear as early as the 1960s suggesting a role for chemotherapy in the treatment of medulloblastoma. These tumors are theoretically well suited for treatment with chemotherapy because of their rapid growth rate, high mitotic index, and location in close proximity to the ventricular cavity and subarachnoid space. Initially, chemotherapy reports were limited to single agents. But now combination chemotherapy has replaced the use of most single agents. Currently, most of the phase III trials for medulloblastoma in the Pediatric Cancer Consortium Groups consist of multiple agents. Although the results are not definitive, there are some trends suggesting that chemotherapy may be effective in those children under 4 years of age who have residual tumor at the time of surgery and whose tumor invades the lateral recesses and the brainstem.

Increasingly, in an effort to eliminate the synergistic effects of chemotherapy and radiotherapy, preradiotherapy protocols have been suggested. These protocols are developed in an attempt to eliminate the leukoencephalopathy associated with the combination of methotrexate and radiotherapy given together. Because the dose of radiotherapy appears to be at the upper limits of tolerance, it appears unlikely that an increase in survival will result from a change in radiotherapy protocols. Chemotherapy will continue to play a role in the treatment of extraneural metastasis as well as local recurrences. In an effort to decrease long-term treatment effects and increase the quality of life associated with recurrent treatment modalities, new and different approaches of chemotherapy are being considered in the hope that radiation doses can be reduced and in turn that the side effects can be diminished. Despite these caveats, of all malignant brain tumors, results with medulloblastomas continue to be the most encouraging. Today, the child over 3 to 4 years of age treated with total resection and appropriate doses of radiotherapy can expect a 5-year survival rate above 50%.

Brainstem Tumors

Brainstem tumors, occupy the region of the brain traversed by the aqueduct of Sylvius and the fourth ventricle. This includes the mesencephalic, pontine, and medullary regions. As a group, the presentation and prognosis of tumors in this area are quite different from those of tumors presenting in the spinal cord or in the diencephalon. Tumors in the brainstem are either fibrillary or pilocytic. However, malignant glioblastomas also occur. Cysts may be found in both malignant and slow-growing varieties.

The prognosis for brainstem tumors has never been directly related to histology. In part, this relates to the small tissue size obtained at biopsy or the failure to obtain pathologic confirmation at the time of diagnosis. There has been some suggestion that the more histologically aggressive tumors are found in the pons and medulla and that those arising in the upper brainstem tend to be less aggressive. On occasion, a slowly growing tumor with exophytic features is recognized. These tumors present in the region of the fourth ventricle, occupy the cerebellar-pontine angles, or extend into the lateral recesses. Exophytic features permit reasonable surgical access. Furthermore, it has been postulated that, because the tumor tends to grow into areas of least resistance, the bulk of these tumors may present exophytically and be surgically removed.

The usual tendency of gliomas of this area to distort and expand the brainstem produces diffuse enlargement of the pons, leading to the use in the older literature of the term *pontine hypertrophy*. The growth of tumor between nerve fiber tracts gives a pilocytic rather than a fibrillary appearance to the astrocyte. Thus, the pilocytic characteristic of the tumor may represent an epiphenomenon resulting from specific patterns of growth.

These tumors represent somewhat less than 11% of all brain tumors in childhood. They most commonly are seen in children 5 to 14 years of age but may occur in any age group. The consideration of a brainstem mass begins with a typical triad of clinical findings, consisting of cranial nerve signs, cerebellar signs, and long tract signs. Ataxia coupled with hyperreflexia, extensor plantar responses, and cranial neuropathies suggest involvement of tracts passing to and from the cerebellum and the pons and the corticospinal tracts descending from the cortex.

Multiple types of nystagmus are associated with intrinsic abnormalities of the brainstem. Vertical nystagmus on upward gaze, bilateral nystagmus on lateral gaze, primary position nystagmus on horizontal gaze, and nonfatigable position nystagmus should suggest brainstem pathology. Conversion retraction nystagmus suggests involvement of the median longitudinal fasciculus. Signs of difficulty with swallowing, eating, and respiration reflect medullary involvement, as do asymmetry of the palate, absent gag reflexes, atrophy of the tongue, and nasal regurgitation of food. Since most of these tumors present on the ventral surface of the brainstem, obstructive hydrocephalus, when it occurs, is seen late in the course of the disease.

The clinical suspicion of a pontine mass is confirmed

FEATURE TABLE 15-3. PATHOLOGY AND COURSE OF POSTERIOR FOSSA TUMORS

Discriminating Features	Consistent Features	Variable Features
Cerebellar Astrocytoma		
1. Cerebellar hemisphere or midline 2. Cystic with mural nodule 3. Less frequently diffuse 4. Seldom spreads	1. Papilledema secondary to obstructive hydrocephalus 2. Greater than 95% survival for cystic type, somewhat less for diffuse 3. Cured with surgery alone if mural nodule removed	1. On recurrence may require radiotherapy 2. Malignant glioma unusual
Medulloblastoma		
1. Mostly midline of cerebellum 2. Papilledema 3. Obstructive hydrocephalus 4. Truncal ataxia 5. Short course 6. Seeds subarachnoid space early in course	1. Responds to radiotherapy 2. Midline mass without cyst on CT 3. Rapidly progressive 4. Short duration of symptoms	1. 50% to 70% survival, depending on age, location, and degree of removal at surgery 2. Certain subsets respond to chemotherapy
Ependymoma		
1. Fourth ventricle 2. Papilledema 3. Secondary obstructive hydrocephalus 4. Seeds subarachnold space	1. Requires adjuvant therapy following surgery 2. Homogeneous fourth-ventricular mass on CT 3. Variable course	1. Metastasis to CSF late in course 2. Response to radiotherapy and chemotherapy variable 3. 39% 5-year survival depending on location and ?histology
Brainstem		
1. Papilledema late in course 2. Triad of ataxia, cranial neuropathy, and long tract signs suggests brainstem pathology	1. Astrocytomas most common tumor 2. Hypodense lesion on CT suggests malignant course 3. Rapid course to death	1. Response to therapy limited 2. 15% to 30% 5-year survival; most die within 12 months of diagnosis 3. A small subset may be long-term survivors 4. Histopathology, when obtained, is of questionable prognostic help

by either CT or MRI. Since MRI does not image bone, the posterior fossa is better seen with this modality rather than with CT. Furthermore, MRI readily provides images in multiple planes, that is, sagittal, coronal, and axial. Using MRI alone, the existence of a tumor cyst may be misinterpreted as edema. By obtaining both CT and MRI, one can determine the anatomic extent of the tumor, whether a cyst is present, and whether, following contrast enhancement, there is alteration of the blood-brain barrier.

Although most physicians continue to recommend against surgical exploration, obtaining tissue prior to treatment may provide a clearer picture of the natural history of the tumor and help clarify the controversy concerning the prognostic role of histology in making a diagnosis. Additionally, surgical exploration provides a means of evacuating a cyst, amputating an exophytic

tumor, and permit identification of pathology. The latter step will eliminate such mistaken diagnoses as brainstem encephalitis, abscess, arteriovenous malformation, and tuberculoma. Identification of the pathology helps to avoid the possibility of committing the child to potentially damaging treatment in the absence of a specific diagnosis. Differences in clinical presentation, the availability of diagnostic studies, and a voidability in natural history suggest that tumors of the brainstem cannot be treated as a homogeneous entity.

Following confirmation of the diagnosis, by either direct or indirect means, the mainstay of treatment is radiotherapy. Unfortunately, there is no consensus regarding response curves for radiation of the brainstem. Additionally, survival statistics have not improved appreciably with increasing doses of radiation. Today, the generally accepted dose of radiation is 50 to 55 Gy given directly to the tumor bed over a 5- to 6-week period. In an effort to avoid radiation necrosis, the radiation dose should not exceed 1.50 to 1.80 Gy/day. Response to radiation occurs early in the course of treatment followed by a plateau effect. As a generalization, long-term survival is seen in patients with a long history of symptoms prior to diagnosis. Although most tumors of the brainstem are considered to be relentlessly progressive with an inexorable course to death, there is a small subset of patients who have a slowly nonprogressive course. The overall 5-year survival rates in most series are less than 20%, although rates as high as 30% have been reported in the literature.

Because of the poor prognosis for brainstem tumors, cooperative groups have considered newer methods of increasing radiation dose. At present, there is an ongoing study evaluating the use of hyperfractionated radiation. Rather than once a day, children are radiated twice a day in doses of 1.1 to 1.7 Gy. By this method, radiation is increased by 10% to 20%, without, one hopes, increasing concomitant side effects.

Results of chemotherapeutic trials in the treatment of brainstem tumors have been even more difficult to assess than those with radiotherapy. Comparison of differing chemotherapy protocols is compicated by the multiplicity of drugs, varying dose schedules, short-lived effects, multiple delivery systems, and lack of uniformity

in approach. Results, when positive, are invariably short-term or tempered by previous treatment with radiotherapy. Beneficial effects in most reports are achieved in small numbers of patients using either single-agent or combination chemotherapy. Most responses are measured in weeks rather than months. No one treatment regimen has been found to be effective.

Overall, results of treatment of tumors of the brainstem with either surgery, radiation, or chemotherapy alone or in combination have been disappointing. Of all tumors of childhood, treatment has been least helpful in this group. Short-term results have been seen with both radiation and chemotherapy but long-term results are poor. Radiation response is usually early, followed by a plateau effect. The margin of error for treatment of tumors in this region is extremely limited. The compactness of vital structures and limited room for expansion continue to dampen the enthusiasm for debulking surgery other than biopsy. These anatomic considerations have influenced the decision to treat aggressively with either radiation or chemotherapy without initial surgery. Unfortunately, although brainstem tumors are bathed by spinal fluid, administration of chemotherapy via the subarachnoid route has not had measurable benefit. Because of these poor outcomes, there is a continuing effort by cooperative groups to consider alternative approaches to treatment. These include hyperfractionated radiation and novel systems of drug delivery.

Ependymomas

The fourth most common tumor of the posterior fossa presenting with signs of increased pressure and obstructive hydrocephalus is the ependymoma. Ependymomas represent approximately 9% of intracranial tumors in childhood. The majority occur in children in the first half decade of life. Although the tumors arise in relation to any part of the ventricular system, they are twice as common in the posterior fossa than in the supratentorial areas. As with medulloblastomas, spinal cord seeding is common and is found in approximately 11% of intracranial ependymomas. The incidence of seeding may vary with the location and histologic aggressiveness of the tumor. The more aggressive tumors and those located in the fourth ventricle are associated with a higher risk of subarachnoid spread than ependymomas of a more benign histologic nature or those located supratentorially.

Ependymomas initially present as well-defined, homogeneous masses that are partially encapsulated. Like other posterior fossa tumors, they may be cystic. Gross calcification may be found regardless of location or degree of malignancy. Ependymal rosettes characterize the histologic nature of the tumor. These usually are rosettes of cells grouped around a central lumen. When the tumor coats the surface of the ventricle, cilia and blepharoplasts can be recognized. Additionally, perivascular pseudorosettes are identified. These consist of radiating and

Pearls and Perils: Posterior Fossa Tumors

1. Children with posterior fossa masses are more likely to have signs of increased intracranial pressure than focal neurologic signs.
2. Papilledema occurs late in patients with brainstem tumors.
3. Histopathology, even with brainstem gliomas, is helpful prior to initiating therapy.
4. Of all posterior fossa tumors, the greatest change in prognosis has been seen with medulloblastomas. In certain subsets, survival approaches 70%, which is a marked change from the 1.6% 3-year survival reported in 1930.
5. Irradiation of the tumor bed and craniospinal axis is mandatory in patients with medulloblastoma. Craniospinal radiation is indicated in some patients with ependymoma and not required in those patients with cerebellar astrocytomas or brainstem gliomas.
6. Treatment of patients with radiotherapy may be associated with intellectual decline, endocrinopathies, and second primaries.
7. Surgery of the brainstem may cause severe neurologic sequelae.
8. Nonspecific short-term headache, with and without vomiting, may be the only sign of a posterior fossa mass.

tapering processes of tumor oriented toward a blood vessel. The ependymoma tends to be graded either as benign or malignant. Malignant ependymomas are characterized by mitosis, pleomorphism, and hyperchromasia. Some pathologists characterize a more intermediate form of ependymoma consisting primarily of a benign histologic appearance with infrequent features of focal pleomorphism and mitosis. The myxopapillary ependymoma is more commonly found in the spinal cord. This variety is associated with a much more benign course than the ependymomas identified above the foramen magnum.

The duration of symptoms prior to diagnosis may vary between 18 and 36 months, with the majority presenting around 12 months of age. Supratentorial tumors have an average duration of symptoms prior to diagnosis of 7 months, whereas posterior fossa tumors have an average duration of symptoms prior to diagnosis of 9 months. Duration of symptoms prior to diagnosis is longer in patients with calcified versus noncalcified supratentorial ependymomas. This difference is not found in the posterior fossa.

As with most neoplasms, treatment begins with debulking surgery. Unfortunately, owing to their frequent attachment to the floor of the fourth ventricle, there may be a high degree of morbidity associated with aggressive removal. Because surgery, regardless of grade or location, is not curative, operation is followed by radiation. Controversies involving radiation concern the volume of radiation administered to the brain, spinal cord, and tumor bed. Variability in treatment reflects the tumor's tendency to involve the CSF pathways. Most radiotherapists recommend treatment of low-grade supratentorial ependymomas with local radiation and high-grade supratentorial tumors and posterior fossa tumors with craniospinal irradiation. Presently, there is an active Pediatric Oncology Group protocol to assess the optional volume of radiation for patients with ependymomas. Patients with high-grade supratentorial tumors receive craniospinal radiation, whereas those with low-grade posterior fossa tumors receive local radiation with margins including the upper cervical cord. In those patients who have tumors that are both high grade and occur in the posterior fossa, there is general consensus that craniospinal radiation is appropriate.

As with most tumors of the CNS, the value of chemotherapy and the ideal type are still not clear. Many centers have used both single and combination chemotherapy in patients with ependymomas. Unfortunately, results of chemotherapy are available in only a limited number of patients. Differences in response by location and grade are not available in the literature. Theoretically, high-grade tumors adjacent to the fourth ventricle should be most receptive to chemotherapy.

As with medulloblastomas, extraneural metastases do occur. There have been reports of metastasis in liver, bone marrow, scalp, diaphragm, lymph nodes, and lung.

The overall survival rate of children with ependymomas is approximately 30%. Prognosis varies with age of the patient and location and grade of tumor. Long-term survival rates are worse in children under 2 years of age. Despite combination treatments with surgery, radiation, and chemotherapy, the diagnosis of ependymoma in most children portends a poor prognosis.

MIDLINE TUMORS

Midline tumors consist of tumors involving the thalamus, hypothalamus, pineal region, and visual pathways. The most common histologies identified in this area are astrocytomas, craniopharyngiomas, optic gliomas, pinealomas, germinomas, and teratomas. This section will discuss craniopharyngiomas, visual pathway tumors, tumors of the thalamus and hypothalamus, and pineal region tumors.

Craniopharyngiomas

Since the initial description by Erdheim in 1904, there has been universal agreement that the craniopharyngioma arises from retained elements of Rathke's pouch. This tissue is the embryologic forerunner of the anterior pituitary gland. The tumor is thought to arise from embryonic squamous cell rests occurring along the involuted tract of the hypophysiopharyngeal duct. Others have suggested that the tumor results from embryonic cell rests arising from metaplasia in cells of the adenohypophysis. Because of its putative origins, the tumor was named a craniopharyngioma by Cushing in 1932.

Craniopharyngiomas account for 3% of all tumors in adults and 6% to 10% of all tumors in children. Diagnosis peaks in the latter half of the first decade and the early part of the second decade. There is no clear sexual preference. The tumor is quite variable in location, size, texture, and adherence to surrounding structures. The majority are suprasellar in location, although on occasion an intrasellar location is recognized. They can fill the cavity of the third ventricle and extend either posteriorly to involve the clivus, anteriorly and superiorly to involve the visual pathways, or posteriorly to involve much of the hypothalamus.

Grossly, craniopharyngiomas are largely cystic or partially solid with a firm capsule. The tumor is grayish red in color and of varying size with a smooth, nodular surface. It has a firm structure associated with the inherent calcification. Cystic contents are thick, brownish yellow, or green, with machine oil–like fluid rich in cholesterol crystals. At surgery, the cystic content may erupt into the subarachnoid space, causing a symptomatic chemical arachnoiditis.

Histologically, the tumor presents as an epithelial microcystic mass. Cells are found arranged in cords or angulated columnar cells resting on a collagen basement membrane. Keratin and pearls may be found among the squamous epithelium. The keratin may become confluent and undergo calcification and even new bone formation.

As expected, signs and symptoms depend on the extent and location of the tumor. Because of its tendency to occupy the anterior hypothalamus and obstruct the foramen of Monro, nonspecific signs of increased intracranial pressure are not infrequent. Visual defects, depending of the location of the tumor above, below, or behind the visual axis, result from compression of either the optic nerve chiasm or tracts. Because of the asymmetric nature of these tumors, visual field defects are more likely to be asymmetric or unilateral rather than presenting as a more classic bitemporal hemianopsia. As with any optic pathway tumor that is slowly progressive in nature, the child is not likely to complain of visual loss until late in the course of the disease. Involvement of the optic pathway is more likely to be suspected during a school visual examination or on findings of optic atrophy or papilledema on routine funduscopic examination. Despite the existence of increased intracranial pressure, compression of the visual pathway may lead to funduscopic findings of optic atrophy rather than papilledema.

Endocrine abnormalities are common but variable. The most usual endocrine abnormalities in children are short stature, hypothyroidism, or diabetes insipidus. Children with growth retardation present with bone delay and deceleration of linear growth. Hypothyroidism is suggested by increased weight gain, easy fatigability, lethargy, and declining school performance. Excessive thirst, frequent urination, or abnormalities of specific gravity raise the question of diabetes insipidus.

Diagnosis is confirmed by CT scanning, with or without plain skull films. Calcification is either patchy, diffuse, or linear and is seen in up to 80% of children with craniopharyngioma. Intrasellar masses are suggested by downward displacement of the floor of the sella, erosion of the dorsum, and changes in the clinoid processes. CT scanning, especially coronal views, can readily identify extent, location, and degree of calcification. CT features consist of calcification, low density, cyst formation, and contrast enhancement. MRI, although not able to portray graphically the calcification present in patients with craniopharyngioma, more readily identifies the anatomic extent of the lesion.

There is universal agreement on the need for surgery, although the ideal type and extent of surgery has not yet been fully determined. Complete removal of craniopharyngiomas is advocated by some, whereas others suggest partial removal followed by local radiation. With the advent of steriod replacement pre- and postoperatively, operative mortality has declined. However, most neurosurgeons note that the tumor does not present with an adequate cleavage plane, dooming to failure attempts at total removal. Skilled endocrine management removes the fear of intraoperative and postoperative hypopituitarism and has led some to a more aggressive surgical approach.

FEATURE TABLE 15-4. DIAGNOSTIC FEATURES OF MIDLINE TUMORS

Discriminating Features	Consistent Features	Variable Features
Craniopharyngioma		
1. Suprasellar mass	1. Papilledema	1. Suprasellar calcification
2. Pathologic examination	2. Endocrinopathies	2. Visual loss
		3. Visual field abnormalities
Visual Pathway Tumor		
1. Visual loss	1. Optic atrophy	1. Headache
2. Nystagmus	2. Asymmetric visual field loss	2. Papilledema
	3. Abnormal visual evoked response	3. Endocrinopathies
Tumors of Thalamus and Hypothalamus (Diencephalic Syndrome)		
1. Pathologic examination	1. Nystagmus	1. Visual loss
2. Failure to thrive	2. Normal intelligence	2. Euphoria
	3. CT or MRI shows diencephalic mass	
	4. Lack of focal neurologic signs	
Pineal Region Tumor		
1. Papilledema	1. Lack of focal neurologic signs	1. Precocious puberty
2. CT or MRI shows pineal region mass	2. Spread throughout the CSF pathways	2. Elevated α-fetoprotein
3. Pathologic examination	3. More common in males	3. Elevated chorionic gonadotropin

Radiation therapy following surgery was first used in 1937. However, only since the 1960s has there been increasing acceptance of the use of radiotherapy in combination with subtotal excision for the treatment of craniopharyngioma. Results of radiation therapy following subtotal surgical removal suggest that recurrences are strikingly decreased in the irradiated group. Even in those reports in which there has been total excision, the rate of recurrence approaches that of patients treated with radiotherapy. Following either surgery or radiotherapy, most children develop significant diabetes insipidus, which is likely to be permanent. This disorder can readily be treated with appropriate forms of vasopressin. There have also been several observations of normal growth after surgery and radiation despite growth hormone deficiency. Growth spurts after surgery have been documented in many children. Hyperphagia with obesity is greatest immediately following surgery. Weight gain may or may not parallel gains in growth.

In general, craniopharyngiomas present with a complex set of medical and surgical problems. Total surgical removal with limited morbidity depends on the skill of the surgeon, the location and size of the tumor, the presence of a well-defined surgical plane, and the age of the patient. Surgery is invariably associated with endocrine complications, usually consisting of diabetes insipidus with or without other abnormalities of anterior pituitary lobe function. Although total surgical removal has its advocates, approximately 50% of removed tumors will recur and thus may require radiotherapy. Overall survival is excellent although significant morbidity is to be expected.

Visual Pathway Tumors

The optic pathway tumor is one of the most common neuroglial tumors found in the midline. Such tumors represent approximately 3% of all childhood intracranial tumors. The association of optic nerve tumors with neurofibromatosis has been recognized for years. The incidence of optic gliomas in children 2 to 9 years of age may approach 3% to 10%. Conversely, of all children with optic gliomas, approximately 50% have neurofibromatosis. The natural history of this tumor is determined by its location in either the orbit or chiasm and by its association with neurofibromatosis. Because of the variability in natural history, approaches to treatment are confused and complicated. Most tumors of the anterior visual pathways are histologically benign and are generally classified as pilocytic astrocytomas. Anaplastic tumors and glioblastomas are much less common. Tumors of the optic pathway may be limited to a single optic nerve, occur bilaterally, invade the optic chiasm anteriorly, or involve the entire chiasm. Fusiform enlargement of the nerves may be seen intraorbitally or may be limited to one side of the chiasm. Tumors that involve the chiasm may extend anteriorly to obstruct the foramen of Monro or posteriorly to invade the interpeduncular fossa. Oc-

casionally, these tumors may extend along anatomic pathways as far posteriorly as the lateral geniculate body or even the visual cortex. Extension of these tumors beyond the anatomic limits of the visual apparatus is well recognized.

The most common presenting sign is diminished visual acuity. Decreased vision may be brought to the attention of an unsuspecting parent after a routine eye examination. A reducible and nonpulsatile proptosis suggests the presence of an intraorbital mass. The presence of nystagmus should suggest chiasmatic involvement. Nystagmus usually takes the form of constant short arcs and rapid oscillations with scanning or searching slow wide arcs. A spasmus nutans–like picture and congenital nystagmus have been incorrectly diagnosed in children with optic chiasm tumors.

As expected with any infiltrative lesion, visual fields are variable and consist of variations of central, centrosecal, and eccentric field cuts. Bilateral field cuts, either congruous or incongruous, should suggest involvement of the optic chiasm or tract while a unilateral field loss should suggest disease limited to the orbit. Signs of papilledema and intracranial pressure reflect involvement of the anterior hypothalamus with obstruction of the foramen of Monro. Even in the absence of visual disturbances, the findings in an asymptomatic child 2 to 10 years of age of axillary freckling, a large head, and cafe au lait spots should raise the possibility of neurofibromatosis and initiate a search for an unsuspected optic glioma.

The diagnostic study of choice is either CT or MRI scanning. Appropriate views in both the axial and coronal sections allow definition of an enlarged intraorbital nerve or optic chiasm. These modes of neuroimaging have essentially eliminated other diagnostic modalities from consideration. However, enlargement of the optic nerve on CT scan may occur as a result of papilledema rather than a glioma. Furthermore, tortuousity of the optic nerve may be mistaken for intraorbital enlargement. In order to assure an artifact-free picture, a CT scan should be obtained with the nerve on stretch, a status that can be achieved by having the eye look straight ahead and neither up nor down.

Although modern neuroimaging techniques provide unparalleled ability to identify the anatomy of the visual pathway, these modalities provide little information regarding the functional integrity of the optic nerve. Visual evoked responses offer the possibility of identifying functional abnormalities of the system. In one of our patients, an initial CT scan was misleading because of a tortuous optic nerve. The failure of the visual evoked response to correlate with the CT abnormality led to repeat scanning and reinterpretation. Repeat scan revealed that the nerve, which initially had been reported as abnormal, was scanned in the wrong plane. Thus, the presence of an equivocal CT scan and normal visual evoked response suggested that long-term evaluation and a conservative approach were warranted.

Despite the fact that there are many series reported

in the literature of patients with visual pathway tumors, there is no universal approach to treatment. The decision to remove surgically a tumor that has not extended into the optic chiasm in a sighted eye presumes that intraorbital tumors are malignant and, if not treated, will progress. This may not be the case, because many of these neoplasms are pilocytic with slow growth potential. Furthermore, there is some evidence that the bulk of an optic glioma may be composed of hyperplastic arachnoid cells rather than frank neoplastic elements.

Surgery, when considered, consists of biopsy or excision of the nerve. With complete excision, the nerve should be flush with the optic chiasm. When there is profound loss of vision, total rather than partial amputation is advocated. In a patient who has slowly progressive loss of vision, biopsy offers the advantage of histologic confirmation while preserving the possibility of vision. When chiasmatic tumors are associated with obstructive hydrocephalus, a shunt procedure may be necessary.

Radiation, like surgery, is also controversial. Radiation may preserve vision although complications include vasculopathy, cataracts, and endocrinopathies. Some have suggested that radiation does not provide significant benefit whereas others unequivocally point to improved long-term results. The dose of radiation to the tumor varies between 30 and 50 Gy.

By and large, the prognosis of patients with tumor limited to the optic nerve is better than that for those with chiasmatic extension. It is our current belief that, in patients with visual pathway tumors, there should be continuous ongoing assessment with neuroimaging, visual evoked response studies, and testing of visual acuity and visual fields. These procedures allow documentation of the progression of the lesion. Visual evoked response studies in selected cases may identify abnormalities prior to the identification of a field defect. As with so many other tumors of the nervous system, newer neuroimaging techniques are altering our concept of the natural history and long-term prognosis of visual pathway tumors. At present, it is generally recommended that those children with chiasmatic extension be subject to intervention on diagnosis, whereas those in whom tumor is limited to the orbits be followed expectantly until there is evidence of visual loss or posterior extension into the optic canal. If there is evidence of progression on visual assessment and the tumor is shown to extend posteriorly into the optic canal, then surgical amputation of the nerve at the junction of the nerve with the chiasm is recommended. In those patients who have chiasmatic tumors, surgical biopsy followed by radiotherapy is the preferred treatment. Chemotherapeutic results in these patients are limited and reports are based mainly on small numbers of patients.

Tumors of the Thalamus and Hypothalamus

Tumors of the diencephalon occupy that region normally surrounding the third ventricle. These include tumors of the thalamus, hypothalamus, and pineal region. Thalamic tumors are rare, accounting for less than 1% of brain tumors in childhood. Age of onset is usually under 20 years. Thalamic region tumors are aggressive and have a truncated course, unlike hypothalamic tumors. Duration of symptoms prior to diagnosis is usually less than 1 year. Most of these tumors are of the astrocytic series and vary in malignancy from benign to highly aggressive. Long-term survival without treatment is well documented with low-grade astrocytomas. Other tumors occurring in the lateral midline are ganglioneuromas, oligodendrogliomas, and ependymomas.

Symptoms of thalamic tumors are nonspecific and consist of confusion, memory loss, and emotional lability. Increased intracranial pressure, when it occurs, is usually secondary to obstruction of the foramen of Monro. Mental symptoms are thought to reflect involvement of the medial thalamic nuclei and their projection to the frontal cortex. Lateralizing signs reflect involvement of fibers either entering or leaving the thalamus. Motor abnormalities such as tremor and dysmetria may be confused with cerebellar lesions, whereas dystonic movements and unilateral chorea imply abnormalities of the basal ganglia or the subthalamus.

A 30% incidence of seizures has been reported in at least one series of thalamic tumors. Nonspecific EEG findings consisting of symmetric, high-voltage delta and theta occurring in the waking state may reflect increased intracranial pressure. Specific EEG correlates include ipsilateral depression of normal background rhythms, presence of lateralized polymorphic delta activity, or the finding of sleep spindles during the waking state. Thus the emerging profile of thalamic tumors is characterized by signs and symptoms that suggest functional derangement not specifically related to the anatomic site of involvement.

Confirmation of a thalamic mass is obtained by neuroimaging. The density of the mass, depending on the degree of malignancy, may be greater than, equal to, or less than that of the surrounding tissue. Treatment of tumors of the thalamus, in general, is unsatisfactory. Debulking surgery is usually contraindicated because of the fear of significant neurologic residua. Radiotherapy is considered the treatment of choice; however, overall results have been discouraging, with reported 5-year survival rates of 20% to 30%. On the other hand, low-grade tumors may be associated with long-term survival. Because large treatment series comparing treatment modalities are not available, it is difficult to assess the potential role of either chemotherapy or radiotherapy.

Midline gliomas of childhood, occupying the region of the third ventricle, have a different biology than those occurring in the thalamus. These tumors may blend histologically imperceptibly into neoplasms originating in the optic chiasm. Thus distinction between these two types of tumors may be arbitrary. Gliomas of the hypothalamus are generally classified as juvenile pilocytic astrocytomas. Unlike tumors found more laterally, they are not graded histologically according to degree of

FEATURE TABLE 15–5. PATHOLOGY AND COURSE OF MIDLINE TUMORS

Discriminating Features	Consistent Features	Variable Features
Craniopharyngioma 1. Endocrinopathy 2. Suprasellar location 3. Papilledema secondary to obstruction of foramen of Monro 4. Calcified cystic mass 5. Visual field abnormalities	1. Diabetes insipidus following surgery 2. Long-term survival is the rule 3. Must be followed and treated for panhypopituitarism	1. Over 50% recur despite putative total removal 2. Radiation indicated in those patients who do not have total removal and in those who recur 3. Growth acceleration may occur following removal
Visual pathway tumor 1. Optic astrophy 2. Visual loss 3. 50% associated with neurofibromatosis 4. Proptosis 5. Neuroimaging localizing	1. Tumor either intraorbital or chiasmatic 2. Long-term survival is the rule 3. Do not require treatment unless there is visual loss or evidence of growth	1. May be confused with spasmus nutans or congenital nystagmus 2. Pathology either low-grade astrocytomas or hamartoma 3. Longterm survivals reported regardless of form of treatment, i.e., no treatment surgery, or radiation
Diencephalic Syndrome 1. May occur in thalamus or hypothalamus 2. Failure to thrive associated with midline tumor 3. Usually pilocytic low-grade astrocytoma	1. Failure to thrive seen in young child with hypothalamic tumors 2. "Diencephalic syndrome?" 3. Long tract signs seen in thalamic tumors 4. Hypothalamic tumors are more commonly associated with endocrinopathies	1. Prognosis better in hypothalamic tumors, worse in thalamic tumors 2. Response to radiation is variable 3. Midline tumors likely to be juvenile "pilocytic astrocytomas"
Pineal Region 1. Teratomas, germinomas, and pinealomas found in midline area 2. Suprasellar germinomas found in girls and pineal region pinealomas found in boys 3. Precocious puberty seen in boys	1. Germinomas are highly radiosensitive 2. Teratomas do not respond to radiation 3. Presence of α-fetoprotein or chorionic gonadotropin suggests malignant behavior	1. Prognosis depends on histologic grade and evidence of seeding 2. Germinoma may resemble a primitive neuroectodermal tumor 3. Vascularity of region may limit attempts at total surgical removal

malignancy. Necrosis and hemorrhage do not necessarily imply an aggressive nature. Rosenthal fibers and lack of vascular reaction are the usual histologic features. Signs and symptoms of a hypothalamic mass include endocrinopathies as well as midline neurologic abnormalities. Prior to surery, differentiation from other parasellar masses, such as craniopharyngiomas, may be difficult.

Since it was first reported in 1951, the diencephalic syndrome, consisting of failure to thrive and inanition, has suggested an astrocytoma of the anterior hypothalamus or optic chiasm. This syndrome is usually seen in children between 18 months and 3½ years of age. Its failure to occur in older children is unexplained. Hypoglycemia may or may not be present. Anorexia or excessive appetite may be the predominant features. Long bone growth continues or may even be accelerated. Despite these features, emaciation with profound loss of subcutaneous tissue (the "concentration camp syndrome") is the hallmark of the diencephalic syndrome. Some have suggested that the emaciation implies that the mass is limited to a small proportion of the anterior hypothalamus. When the subsequent growth of the tumor extends into other portions of the hypothalamus, cachexia may be replaced by obesity, vegetative states, and delayed puberty. The diencephalic syndrome is usually seen in children under 3 years of age. Above this age, obesity, diabetes insipidus, and hypogonadism or precocious puberty are more common.

Treatment of hypothalamic tumors consists of surgical biopsy followed by radiotherapy. The results of this therapy in patients with hypothalamic tumors may be quite striking. Radiation doses of 50 to 60 Gy to this area may be associated with reversal of symptoms and long-term cures. Five-year survival rates of 71% and 10-year survival rates of 56% have been recognized. Again, the role of chemotherapy is problematic. Currently, our present policy is to limit the treatment of patients with hypothalamic tumors to high-dose radiation. Combination chemotherapy is considered when there is evidence of progression or recurrence of disease.

Pineal Region Tumors

Pineal region tumors represent 0.4% to 4.2% of brain tumors. They are more common in Oriental than in Western countries. Tumors are classified into three different histologic groups: (1) germ cell tumors, including germinomas, teratomas, choriocarcinomas, and embryonal carcinomas; (2) pineal parenchymal tumors, including pineocytomas and pineoblastomas; and (3) other histologic types, such as gangliogliomas, pineal area cysts, and meningiomas.

The germinoma represents 50% of all tumors occurring in this region. Its morphology is similar to that of the testicular seminoma. Tumors that occur in the pineal region are more commonly found in boys and are likely to be more radioresponsive than suprasellar germinomas. Those masses that occur in the posterior region of the third ventricle can spread anteriorly to involve the cavity of the third ventricle, superiorly to involve the corpus callosum and roof of the third ventricle, and posteriorly to involve the cerebellar vermis and brainstem. Suprasellar germinomas are more common in adolescent girls. They may be multilobular and encompass the region of the anterior third ventricle, pituitary stalk, or optic chiasm.

Microscopically, germinomas consist of large, vesicular cells that are mixed with small cells resembling lymphocytes. Mitosis is usually confined to the larger cell type.

The presence of dermoids, teratomas, and epidermoids in the pineal area reflects the potential of growth from the three primordial germ cell layers. Grossly, this tumor may be lobulated with multicystic areas. The literature is confusing and suggests an uneasy separation of teratomas from germinomas because both may have elements of one or the other. Choriocarcinoma, on the other hand, is highly malignant, grows rapidly, and is known to metastasize extracranially.

Assay of human chorionic gonadotrophin and α-fetoprotein may be of some use in assessing intracranial tumors. These markers are abnormally elevated in the serum and CSF in patients with embryonal carcinomas and choriocarcinomas. The finding of increased oncofetoproteins in the presence of an avascular cystic suprasellar pineal region tumor should suggest a teratoma rather than a germinoma. CSF cytology and cell markers may yield important prognostic information. These markers may

---

Pearls and Perils: Midline Tumors

1. The most common intracranial tumor in young children with neurofibromatosis is a tumor of the visual pathway.
2. The pilocytic astrocytoma is most commonly seen in childhood and most commonly found in the hypothalamus.
3. Tumors of the thalamus are more likely to be fibrillary astrocytomas or glioblastomas.
4. Although craniopharyngiomas may present with growth hormone deficiency, paradoxically there is likely to be catch-up growth after removal of the tumor.
5. Diabetes insipidus and hypersatiation syndrome with pathologic obesity are the common endocrinopathies following treatment for craniopharyngiomas.
6. Pineal region germinomas may be exquisitely sensitive to radiation, whereas teratomas of this region are less responsive.
7. Headaches of short duration, with or without vomiting, and CT findings of obstructive hydrocephalus may be the only signs and symptoms of a midline intracranial mass. Midline tumors characteristically are unassociated with focal neurologic findings.
8. Because most young children do not complain of visual loss, visual pathway tumors may not be identified until late in their course.
9. The diagnosis of congenital nystagmus and spasmus nutans should not be made until visual pathway tumors are excluded.
10. The treatment of craniopharyngioma is invariably associated with endocrinopathies. Ruptured craniopharyngioma cysts may produce severe chemical arachnoiditis.
11. Extensive surgery for a hypothalamic or thalamic mass may be associated with significant neurologic residual, including apathy, lethargy, and focal neurologic deficits.
12. Of all tumors presenting in the midline, pineal region tumors are the most likely to seed the cranial subarachnoid space.
13. Intracranial tumors should be considered in the workup of patients with failure to thrive, precocious puberty, and acute onset of headache with and without pernicious vomiting.

provide a means by which to measure the success of chemotherapy following recurrence of the tremor.

The treatment for pineal region tumors depends on whether the tumor is of germ cell or neuroectodermal origin. Operative mortality rates for subtotal resection or biopsy have been reported to be as high as 33% to 50%. Ventricular cisternostomy is the most common diverting procedure for those patients in whom the tumor occupies the cavity of the third ventricle. Direct approaches are difficult because of large venous channels present in the area of the tumor. Lack of direct surgical access at times does not allow debulking or even surgical biopsy. However, in the last decade, the use of the operating microscope has permitted a more aggressive surgical approach. Once hemostasis is obtained, the tumor can be removed by either aspiration or piecemeal dissection.

All authors agree that after surgery the patient should receive radiation. Although radiation is the procedure of choice for germinomas, there is no universal agreement on the dose or volume of radiation. Most radiotherapists suggest 50 Gy to the tumor bed and 35 to 40 Gy rads to the craniospinal axis. After radiation 5-year survival rates may be as high as 50–80%. Survival rates tend to be age-dependent. Rates for patients under 25 years of age are better than those for older patients. Because pineal germinomas are analogous to those occurring in the gonads, histologic verification theoretically should permit radiation schedules similar to those for seminomas. Doses of 25 Gy to the gonads in 1-Gy fractions have produced impressive results, with relapse rates of less than 10%. A similar response might be expected with intracranial germinomas. If, in the future, operative approaches to biopsy consistently yield pathologic material without undue mortality, dose-response curves to radiation based on pathology may be forthcoming.

Recurrence, when seen, may occur anywhere from 6 months to many years after initial treatment. There is a suggestion that suprasellar germinomas are more likely to metastasize through the craniospinal subarachnoid than pineal germinomas. Also, patients with suprasellar germinomas have worse survival rates than those with pineal region tumors.

As with other tumors, results of chemotherapy trials are limited. There has been some suggestion that those agents used for treatment of disseminated seminomas may also be helpful for patients with intracranial germinomas. These drug regimens include a varying combination of vincristine, cis-platinum, procarbazine, and VP-16. The Einhorn regimen used in the treatment of extraneural seminoma consists of bleomycin, vinblastine, and cis-platinum. Successful results with this combination treatment have been reported.

In conclusion, the approach to the treatment of pineal area tumors continues to be variable. The germinoma is highly radiosensitive and may also respond to chemotherapy, whereas parenchymatous tumors are less responsive. Surgery in this area remains difficult and, despite successful reports, an operative tour de force. Overall 50% to 80% survival rates have been reported.

HEMISPHERIC TUMORS

Approximately 30% to 50% of brain tumors in children are located in the supratentorial region. The majority of these tumors are astrocytomas, although oligodendrogliomas, primitive neuroectodermal tumors, and ependymomas may also be present. Low-grade astrocytomas are the most common tumor type in children regardless of age. Other supratentorial tumors occur with relatively less frequency. High-grade astrocytomas and glioblastoma multiforme range in incidence from 2% to 10%.

Astrocytomas are generally diffuse and ill-defined, with infiltration of white matter, cortex, and basal ganglia. There are a variety of pathologic types. The most common is the fibrillary astrocytoma, which tends to occur in tumors of the cerebellum and brainstem. The tumors are firm with occasional cellular pleomorphism. Mitoses are absent and endothelial proliferation is not recognized. Pilocytic astrocytomas of the cerebrum are often microcystic or have a single large cyst. In these cases, they resemble the cystic astrocytomas of the cerebellum. Gemistocytic astrocytomas tend to have a worse prognosis and may dedifferentiate over time into glioblastoma multiforme. The tumors are well circumscribed and may be cystic. Cell bodies are typically globoid with short fibrillated processes and cytoplasm is eosinophilic and homogeneous.

Anaplastic astrocytomas have increased cellularity, cellular pleomorphism, and mitoses as well as features typical of astrocytomas. Glioblastoma multiforme is usually quite diffuse, with necrosis, fatty degeneration, and hemorrhage. The most common microscopic features include pleomorphism, necrosis, endothelial proliferation, and multinucleated giant cells. Mitoses and hemorrhages are common.

The signs and symptoms of hemispheric supratentorial astrocytomas relate to the area of involvement. Headache and vomiting are common. Persistent focal headache correlates strongly with site of tumor. Seizures occur most often with tumors located in the sensorimotor regions of the brain. Seizures are more common with slowly growing tumors than with glioblastoma multiforme, and as such tend to be associated with a better prognosis. In general, prolonged duration of symptoms prior to diagnosis is a good prognostic sign. Physical findings present with hemispheric tumors include hemiparesis, hemisensory loss, and visual field abnormalities.

CT and, more recently, MRI scans have allowed rapid diagnosis of hemispheric supratentorial astrocytomas. Low-grade astrocytomas tend to be better

FEATURE TABLE 15-6. DIAGNOSTIC FEATURES OF HEMISPHERIC TUMORS

Discriminating Features	Consistent Features	Variable Features
Low-Grade Astrocytoma		
1. Pathologic examination	1. Lateralizing signs	1. Seizures
	2. Slow progression	2. Nonenhancing CT
	3. Long duration of symptoms	3. Headache
High-Grade Astrocytoma		
1. Pathologic examination	1. Rapid progression	1. Papilledema
	2. Short duration of symptoms	2. Headache
	3. Enhancing mass on CT	3. Seizures
	4. Lateralizing signs	4. Subarachnoid spread
Primitive Neuroectodermal Tumors		
1. Pathologic examination	1. Large mass on CT or MRI	1. Calcification
	2. Papilledema	2. Cranial neuropathy associated with subarachnoid seeding
	3. Subtle signs	3. Seizures
Oligodendroglioma		
1. Pathologic examination	1. Long duration of symptoms	1. Seizures
	2. Low-density lesion on CT with calcification	2. Lateralizing signs
	3. Minimal mass effect	

delineated and regular in shape than high-grade astrocytomas.

Mass effect is a reliable sign of malignancy but contrast enhancement on CT is not. Although glioblastoma multiforme typically enhances, low-grade astrocytoma may also enhance at times. Ring-like enhancement is characteristic of glioblastoma multiforme.

The approach to the treatment of children with low-grade supratentorial astrocytomas is undergoing reexamination. At the present time, most neurooncologists recommend biopsy and attempts at removal of the tumor. Unfortunately, only with cystic cerebral astrocytomas is complete surgical resection a possibility. Results of radiation appear to improve the prognosis in the short term but have limited effect on long-term prognosis. Consequently, there has been increasing interest in surgical removal with longitudinal followup before deciding on a course of cranial radiation. Although dedifferentiation to more malignant pathology occurs in adult astrocytomas, it appears to be less common in childhood tumors. Thus, at least in grade I astrocytomas, a conservative approach may be warranted, especially since 5-year survival rates of children with low-grade supratentorial astrocytomas in the SEER Registry approach 70%.

The approach to the child with glioblastoma multiforme is quite different. Here, the outcome is uniformly poor. The surgeon should attempt to maximally remove tumor, although complete resection is impossible. Following this procedure, radiation to the whole brain should be given. Glioblastoma multiforme may metastasize throughout the CSF axis, particularly in the very young child. Baseline evaluation must include myelography and CSF cytology. If results suggest CSF spread, radiation to the entire CSF axis is indicated. Despite radiation therapy, the long-term survival rates of patients with glioblastoma are very limited. It is of interest, however, that survival rates in adults are far worse than those in children. Whereas adults with glioblastoma multiforme have survivals measured in months, the survivals in children have been measured in years. Indeed, in the SEER Registry data, children with high-grade astrocytomas and glioblastoma multiforme had approximately a 30% 5-year survival rate.

There may be a role for chemotherapy in the treatment of high-grade astrocytomas. A recent report from the Children's Cancer Study Group has suggested that a combination of vincristine and 1, 3-bis-(2-chloroethyl)-1-nitrosourea (BCNU) has offered a significant advantage in survival over treatment with radiation alone following surgery. In adult studies the results with chemotherapy have been far less impressive. Although BCNU does appear to improve outcome, survival is still measured in months.

Primitive Neuroectodermal Tumors

Primitive neuroectodermal tumors (PNETs) are a group of tumors occurring in the cerebrum of children and young adults. PNETs represent a considerable proportion of tumors in infancy. They are highly malignant with a rapid course from diagnosis to death. The tumors are 90% to 95% undifferentiated and consist of highly

FEATURE TABLE 15-7. PATHOLOGY AND COURSE OF HEMISPHERIC TUMORS

Discriminating Features	Consistent Features	Variable Features
Low-grade astrocytoma		
1. Supratentorial hemispheric mass with pilocytic, fibrillary, or gemistocytic appearance	1. Slow progression 2. Long duration of symptoms 3. Up to 70% 5-year survival	1. Possibly contrast enhancement on CT 2. Slow wave focus on EEG 3. Seizures, headache, focal motor/sensory signs, visual field abnormalities
High-grade astrocytoma		
1. Supratentorial hemispheric mass with mitoses, necrosis, hemorrhage, endothelial proliferation, and multinucleated giant cells	1. Possibly ring enhancement, mass effect, edema on CT 2. Rapid progression 3. Short-duration symptoms 4. Increased intracranial pressure 5. Focal signs 6. Rapid downhill course, limited survival	1. Seizures, subarachnoid spread, extraneural metastases
Primitive neuroectodermal tumors		
1. 90% to 95% undifferentiated, mitoses, necrosis, endothelial hyperplasia 2. Focal areas of differentiation (possibly)	1. Increased intracranial pressure, mass effect, focal signs 2. Cysts, hemorrhage, and enhancement on CT 3. Rapid downhill course	1. Seizures, personality change, subarachnoid metastases, extraneural metastases
Oligodendrogliomas		
1. Honeycomb appearance, microcalcification	1. Calcium, decreased density, mass lesions on CT 2. Slow wave focus on EEG 3. May be cured with surgery, with or without radiation	1. Subarachnoid metastases (uncommon), seizures, focal motor signs

primitive cells. Grossly, the tumors often have areas of necrosis, cyst formation, and calcification. On microscopic examination, they consist of small, undifferentiated cells without observable cytoplasm and dark, oval to irregular nuclei. They have frequent mitotic figures, endothelial hyperplasia, and necrosis. Although the tumors are largely undifferentiated, there may be focal areas of differentiation toward neuronal or glial lines.

These tumors are often extremely large on presentation and consequently, patients have signs and symptoms of increased intracranial pressure. It has been the experience of many investigators that, although these children generally present with increased intracranial pressure and long tract signs, they function remarkably well despite the large mass of tumor. There is generally a short duration from onset of symptoms until diagnosis.

CT scans reveal large tumors with mass effect, cyst formation, hemorrhage, and contrast enhancement. MRI or myelography may reveal subarachnoid seeding with positive cytology. The EEG may demonstrate focal slowing.

Treatment has had limited success. The tumors seed the subarachnoid space and therapy must be directed to the entire neuroaxis. In addition, the tumors occasionally metastasize extraneurally. Initial treatment includes surgical resection followed by craniospinal radiation. In addition, a variety of centers have used chemotherapy. Unfortunately, responses to chemotherapy, although initially impressive, are short lived.

Oligodendrogliomas

Oligodendrogliomas, another supratentorial tumor of childhood, represent only about 1% of brain tumors in children 0 to 14 years of age. The tumor is more common in older children than in infants and young children.

The tumors are usually mixed gliomas. They have a characteristic honeycomb appearance of uniform cells with clear cytoplasm and pale perinuclear halos. The cytoplasm often stains for mucin. Mitotic figures may be identified. There is frequent microcalcification. In general, there is a lack of correlation between histology and

Pearls and Perils: Hemispheric Tumors

1. The most common brain tumor in children is the low-grade supratentorial astrocytoma.
2. Treatment for PNETs includes surgery, craniospinal radiation, and/or chemotherapy. Survival rates are very poor.
3. Patients with oligodendrogliomas often present with seizures.
4. Patients followed for seizures for many years may have a low-grade brain tumor. MRI should be done in all children with new onset complex partial seizures to rule out temporal lobe tumor.
5. Glioblastoma multiforme and PNETs are associated with CSF seeding. Evaluation should include myelography and examination of CSF cytology.

biologic behavior. Although oligodendrogliomas are generally considered benign, they occasionally disseminate through the CSF pathways.

As with all tumors, signs and symptoms relate to the tumor's location. Oligodendrogliomas are classically associated with seizures. The incidence of patients with oligodendrogliomas presenting with seizures may approach 50% to 70%. Other prominent symptoms include vomiting, headache, and focal motor dysfunction.

CT scans reveal low-density masses, usually with calcification. Cystic components are common and approximately 50% have contrast enhancement. EEGs typically reveal a slow wave focus.

The prognosis for oligodendrogliomas is generally good and prolonged survivals are well known. In one study, a 10-year survival rate of 58% was recognized, with no advantage to postoperative radiation compared to surgery alone. However, because these tumors are relatively unusual in children, the data are necessarily limited. Most observers suggest that radiation should be delayed following surgery until there is evidence of recurrence. Tumor may recur many years later and so patients must be continuously reassessed.

LONG-TERM CLINICAL EFFECTS

The physician taking care of a child with a brain tumor should be aware of the potential adverse effects of radiation and chemotherapy. It is the pediatrician, in particular, who provides the ongoing long-term care after the child has recovered from initial treatment of the tumor. Therefore, although we will briefly describe some of the early effects of radiation therapy on the CNS, it is the long-term effects that have the most bearing on the quality of life and the associated role of the pediatrician in providing continuity of care.

Effects of Radiation

Early Delayed Effects

One of the first delayed effects commonly seen in children following irradiation of the CNS is the somnolence syndrome. These children develop somnolence, anorexia, apathy and headaches 6 to 8 weeks following radiation. They may last from 4 to 14 days and usually respond well to prednisone. The symptoms resolve completely without physical or mental sequelae. Recognition of the benign nature of this clinical syndrome can allay fears of recurrence.

Unlike the somnolence syndrome, there is a more severe early delayed effect of radiation associated with rapidly progressive clinical deterioration. This syndrome is quite unusual and generally reflects demyelination within the field of radiation.

The most serious late delayed effect of radiation is radiation necrosis. This condition mimics a recurrent tumor. The peak incidence of radiation necrosis is between 1 and 3 years following completion of treatment. The symptoms are similar to those of a recurrent intracranial mass lesion, with focal motor signs, seizures, dementia, and increased intracranial pressure. Differentiation of radiation necrosis from recurrent tumor is difficult, since these two conditions may have similar CT, brain scan, EEG, and lumbar puncture findings. Even pathologic examination is sometimes confusing. It is, however, necessary to diagnose the condition correctly, because treatment for radiation necrosis will be entirely different from the recurrent tumor.

Beyond these early and late delayed effects of radiation, concern has developed over the possible long-term effects of radiation on the child's quality of life. These remote effects include dementia, endocrinopathies, and the possible development of secondary malignancies.

Intellectual Function

In recent years there has been increasing concern over the long-term effects of radiation on learning. Previously, the survivals of most children with brain tumors were so limited that concerns over long-term effects of therapy were unnecessary. However, with survival rates approaching 70% in some cases, quality of life issues are becoming of increasing importance.

The adverse effects of radiation on intelligence were first identified in children with acute lymphoblastic leukemia who received CNS radiation as part of CNS prophylaxis. Studies demonstrated that children who received radiation had significantly lower IQs than children treated with chemotherapy alone. However, the general functioning of the children was within the normal range. The children were in regular classes and seemed to be performing age-appropriate work. Unfortunately, this has not been the case in children with brain tumors. The dose of radiation to the brain in a child with a CNS malignancy is 50 to 60 Gy compared to 18 to 24 Gy for a child with leukemia. Thus, the effects on the CNS are much

Pearls and Perils: Long-term Clinical Effects

1. The somnolence syndrome is benign and self limited, occurring 6 to 8 weeks following cranial irradiation.
2. Following cranial irradiation, children may have slowly progressive dementia as well as learning problems.
3. Growth hormone deficiency and associated growth failure are common following cranial irradiation for brain tumor. Replacement therapy is effective if given prior to epiphyseal fusion at puberty.
4. Radiation to the cervical spine may be associated with primary hypothyroidism (decreased levels of T_4) and thyroid cancer.
5. Radiation to the hypothalamic-pituitary axis may be associated with secondary or tertiary hypothyroidism (decreased thyroid-stimulating hormone and T_4 levels).
6. Radiation to the spine may adversely affect spinal growth.
7. Second malignancies have been reported following CNS prophylaxis with radiation for acute lymphoblastic leukemia and radiation treatment for primary brain tumors.
8. Radiation to the cervical spine may be associated with the development of thyroid cancer.
9. Children younger than 3 are at greatest risk for long-term treatment effects from radiation therapy.
10. Growth failure may be secondary to growth hormone deficiency, spinal shortening, or hypothyroidism.
11. Late effects of radiation therapy are progressive over many years and require constant monitoring.
12. Leukoencephalopathy may develop in children treated with chemotherapy alone as well as combined with cranial radiation.
13. Radiation necrosis mimics recurrent tumor.
14. Tumor "recurrence" in an unusual location or at an unusual time should be evaluated to exclude a secondary malignancy.

more severe. Multiple studies have now demonstrated that irradiated children develop progressive intellectual deterioration. Retrospective studies reported that 30% to 40% of children with brain tumors had IQs in the retarded range. These effects were found to be worse in children younger than 2 years of age at the time of treatment. Not only were a large number of children functioning in the retarded range, but only 10% to 20% had IQs above 90. A variety of explanations have been suggested for the learning problems. One theory is that the demetia is secondary to either the child's increased intracranial pressure or the tumor itself, rather than adverse effects

of radiation therapy. In response to this hypothesis, a study was done in which children who had been operated on for cerebellar astrocytomas were compared with children who had received surgery, radiation, and chemotherapy for medulloblastoma. In both groups, the site of the tumor was similar and all patients had increased intracranial pressure. The major difference between the two groups was treatment with radiation and chemotherapy. Children treated with radiation in this study had significantly worse IQs than children treated with surgery alone, implicating the therapy rather than the tumor or its location.

Prospective studies of children with brain tumors have revealed much less severe effects on intellect. These studies have noted a slow but steady decrease in IQ over time in some patients. However, in the majority of studies children are functioning within the wide range of normal. Unfortunately, there has been a high incidence of neuropsychologically based learning disorders. Most of the children have required special classes and have had difficulty with attention and impulse control.

It is of prime importance that these children receive yearly psychoeducational evaluations. The effects on intelligence are progressive over time and a single evaluation at the conclusion of therapy is not adequate. When indicated, the children should have access to resource services or self-contained classes for cognitively impaired children. Unfortunately, children with brain tumors may be considered terminally ill by school personnel, leading to falsely elevated grades in the face of less stringent academic demands. These well-intentioned acts are inappropriate for those children who may be cured of their tumors. Specific educational approaches directed at their deficiencies are far more helpful.

Endocrine Dysfunction

Initial endocrine studies performed on children with leukemia who had received cranial irradiation for CNS prophylaxis showed biochemic evidence of growth hormone deficiency in the face of normal linear growth. Unfortunately, when children with brain tumors were similarly evaluated, it was found that they had clinical growth failure. As many as 80% of children treated with cranial irradiation for brain tumors will show growth hormone deficiency as early as 1 year following completion of radiation. Fortunately, these children do respond to growth hormone replacement therapy. Treatment must be instituted prior to puberty and fusion of epiphyseal centers. If the rate of growth is less than 4 cm/year, investigative studies and replacement therapy should be considered.

Other children may develop hypothyroidism on either a primary, secondary, or tertiary basis. Children who have had radiation to the cervical spine have their thyroid gland included within the port. Consequently, these children may develop low T_4 levels, suggesting primary hypothyroidism. Those children who have received high-dose radiation to the whole brain may develop evidence of low thyroid-stimulating hormone levels in the face of low T_4 levels, suggesting either secondary or tertiary hypothyroidism. Hypothyroidism may contribute to the child's difficulty in learning as well as to growth failure. Appropriate replacement therapy potentially should eliminate these effects.

In general, children who have had cranial irradiation have not been gonadotrophin deficient unless the tumors are located in the hypothalamic-pituitary axis. Similarly, abnormalities of adrenocorticotropic hormone have also been uncommon in children whose tumors are remote from the hypothalamic-pituitary axis.

An additional problem associated with radiation to the spine has been adverse effects on longitudinal vertebral growth. This effect on spinal growth has been most severe in very young children treated with spinal radiation.

In summary, endocrine dysfunction following cranial irradiation is a serious but treatable long-term complication. Unfortunately, although many children with brain tumors are operated on and irradiated, the importance of close pediatric follow-up may be overlooked. Pediatricians should make every effort to monitor growth and other endocrine functions and institute replacement therapy, when necessary.

Oncogenesis

The most devastating long-term effect of radiation is oncogenesis. It has recently been recognized that children treated with CNS prophylaxis for leukemia may develop brain tumors several years later. As with other adverse effects of radiation, the significance of this complication becomes of increasing importance as children survive their primary tumors. Thus, they may be cured of their initial cancer only to die of a second tumor. Children treated for primary brain tumors have also been noted to have a variety of secondary brain tumors, which develop 5 to 25 years following initial treatment. These second malignancies have been meningiomas, astrocytomas of all grades, and medulloblastomas. In addition, non-CNS malignancies have developed in children who have received radiation to the cervical spine. Thus, thyroid neoplasia is now becoming of major clinical import as children have survived tumors requiring craniospinal irradiation. Thyroid carcinoma tends to develop between 7 and 18 years following original treatment. Children with cervical spine irradiation will require lifelong monitoring.

Effects of Chemotherapy

In addition to those of radiotherapy, chemotherapy presents a variety of long-term complications. Methotrexate has been associated with the development of leukoencephalopathy characterized by seizures, dementia, and focal motor signs. BCNU has caused pulmonary fibrosis. Long-term use of cytoxan has been associated with hemorrhagic cystitis as well as sterility. Procarbazine has been noted to cause secondary tumors, particularly in young children. By and large, however, the adverse effects of chemotherapy are seen acutely and relate to hematologic, renal, and hepatic toxicity. Long-term effects of chemotherapy appear to be much less severe than those of radiation.

Conclusion

Many of the adverse effects of radiation and chemotherapy are amenable to therapy, particularly in the area of endocrine dysfunction. Appropriate class placement will improve the educational life of the child, but will not reverse the persistent neuropsychologic effects on cognition. Until newer forms of treatment become available, it is incumbent on the pediatrician to follow closely patients who have been treated for malignancies to improve their quality of life.

ANNOTATED BIBLIOGRAPHY

Cohen ME, and Duffner PK: *Brain Tumors in Children: Principles of Diagnosis and Treatment*, Raven Press, New York, 1984.

The initial chapters of this book review the principles of diagnosis, epidemiology, radiation therapy, chemotherapy, and neurosurgery. The remainder is devoted to diagnosis and management of common intracranial tumors of childhood. The book has over 1500 references and is a compendium of treatment issues of the various tumors discussed. It is the only book available dealing solely with brain tumors in children.

Plum F, Posner JB: *Diagnosis of Stupor and Coma*, 3rd ed. Philadelphia, FA Davis, 1980.

This book discusses the clinical approach to coma. It is especially valuable in separating the clinical signs and symptoms of intracranial disease from those of extracranial abnormalities causing coma.

Harisiadis L, Chang CH: Medulloblastoma in children: A correlation between staging and results of treatment. *Int J Radiat Oncol Biol Phys* 2:833–841, 1977.

The staging of tumors recommended in this article is used in formulating the prognosis for patients with medulloblastomas. Specifically, the authors emphasize the excellent prognosis in those children who fit into the best categories.

Gjerris F, Klinken L: Long-term prognosis in children with benign cerebellar astrocytoma. *J Neurosurg* 49:179–184, 1978.

This paper reviews the long-term prognosis for children with benign cerebellar astrocytomas. In particular, the authors differentiate those children with cystic astrocytomas, who have an excellent prognosis, from those with the more diffuse type of astrocytoma, in whom the prognosis is less favorable.

Bloom, HJG: Intracranial tumors: Response and resistance to therapeutic endeavors, 1970–1980. *Int J Radiat Oncol Biol Phys* 8:1083–1113, 1982.

This reference, by one of the most respected radiation oncologists in the United Kingdom, describes the results of treatment of patients with intracranial tumors, with an emphasis on posterior fossa tumors.

American Cancer Society Workshop Conference on Pediatric Brain Tumors. Niagara-on-the-Lake, Ontario, Canada, June 18–20, 1984. *Cancer* 56:1743–1904, 1985.

This article reviews the results of the symposium on intracranial brain tumors held in Canada in 1985. It is an excellent resource for the current treatment preferences and thinking of a body of experts concerned with the treatment of children with intracranial tumors.

Cohen ME, Duffner PK, Heffner RR, Lacey DJ, Brecher MK: Prognostic factors in brainstem gliomas. *Neurology* 36:602–605, 1986.

This article reviews the prognosis in patients with brainstem gliomas and points out the existence of two populations of children with these tumors: those who have a poor prognosis and those who are likely to be long-term survivors. A rationale for considering biopsy of tumors in this very strategic area is presented.

Imes RK, Hoyt WF: Childhood chiasmal gliomas: Update on the fate of patients in the 1969 San Francisco Study. *Br J Ophthalmol* 70:179–182, 1986.

This article describes the experience of a leading neuroophthalmologist's treatment of children with optic pathway tumors. The controversies in the approach to these tumors are reviewed.

Bloom HJG: Recent concepts in the conservative treatment of intracranial tumors in children. *Acta Neurochir* 50:103–116.

This article from the major treatment center in the United Kingdom reviews the results of radiotherapy and conservative treatment in patients with hypothalamic and thalamic gliomas.

Fazekas JT: Treatment of grades I & II brain astrocytomas. The role of radiotherapy. *Int J Radiat Oncol Biol Phys* 2:661–666, 1977.

This is a retrospective analysis of 68 patients with grade I or II astrocytomas. The authors suggest that radiation does not improve on the 5-year survival rate when tumor resection is grossly complete. In incompletely excised cases, adjuvant radiotherapy does improve survival. However, by 10 years, there does not appear to be any difference in cumulative survival rate regardless of treatment and prognostic parameters.

Hart MN, Earle KM: Primitive neuroectodermal tumors of the brain in children. *Cancer* 32:890–897, 1973.

This is the original article describing PNETs in children. The authors describe the pathologic entity and clinical course. The biologic behavior of these tumors, first described in 1973, has unfortunately been relatively static over these years and still carries a very poor prognosis.

Duffner PK, Cohen ME, Freeman AI: Pediatric brain tumors: An overview. *CA* 35:287–301, 1985.

This is a widely disseminated review article on the causes of and approaches to children with intracranial tumors. In addition to reviewing the clinical presentation of patients with brain tumors, the article deals with the wide range of side effects, their diagnosis, and approaches to remediation.

Chapter Sixteen

16

Neuromuscular Diseases

Shawke Soueidan

This chapter addresses the rather common complaint of weakness in infancy and childhood. Clearly, neuromuscular diseases represent a significant proportion of pediatric neurologic disorders, either as primary pathologic entities involving anterior horn cells, peripheral nerves, muscle fibers, and neuromuscular junctions, or as a prominent manifestation of a systemic disorder. The chapter will be divided into two principal sections, one dealing with the general approach to neuromuscular diseases and the other with specific entities. The first section will highlight the approach to the hypotonic infant and then consider the differential diagnosis of new-onset or progressive weakness. The second section will concentrate on the main clinical and diagnostic features of four main categories of neuromuscular diseases: motor neuron diseases, primary diseases of muscle, neuromuscular junction defects, and diseases of peripheral nerves.

General Approach to Neuromuscular Diseases

HYPOTONIC CHILDREN

Hypotonia is the decrease of tonic muscle resistance or contraction. The normal tone is the product of complex central nervous system (CNS) interactions involving the cortex, cerebellum, and basal ganglia, with effects on the corticospinal tract and ultimately the peripheral nerves and muscles. This tone allows maintenance of body posture, be it sitting, standing, or lying; dysfunction in any of these systems will cause abnormalities in certain or all of the postures. As postures are developmental milestones, knowledge of which posture is affected or not attained is a prospective clue to when the child was afflicted with a disease. The resulting hypotonia can be broken into neonatal and infantile causes, with some overlap. Implied in the diagnosis of hypotonia is potential involvement of nonpostural muscle systems, such as those involved with sucking, swallowing, and breathing.

GENERAL CHARACTERISTICS OF HYPOTONIA

The hypotonic neonate and infant have characteristic general features, such as abducted thighs (the frog leg posture) with a decrease in spontaneous movement. This lack of movement will cause the child to rub a bald spot on the scalp and may cause flattening of the occiput. The cry may be weak and often the parents will complain of poor feeding, with difficulty swallowing and subsequent regurgitation and aspiration. Severe hypotonia can result in respiratory failure, necessitating ventilatory support. Other signs of respiratory weakness are diaphragmatic or paradoxical breathing and pectus excavatum.

Infants will not attain the ability to sit erect by 6 months, and, if an infant is placed in this position, the head will fall forward with the arms dangling at the sides. Only if there are focal findings of differential affliction of the limbs and head can a localization of the cause be quickly ascertained; otherwise all infants appear the same irrespective of the lesion's locale. Those with cerebral causes of hypotonia will have fisting of their hands and adduction of the thighs (scissoring) when the child is suspended vertically.

The physical examination uses several different maneuvers to confirm the presence and extent of the hypotonia. Limbs should be moved through range of motion and resistance compared to normal. Maneuvers such as the traction response and vertical and horizontal suspension should be done. Tendon reflexes should always be elicited. Those with normal or brisk reflexes probably have an upper motor neuron lesion. Unsustained clonus is a normal finding in infants but sustained clonus is not. Decrease in tendon reflexes implies muscle or nerve disease or an acute CNS lesion, usually spinal. Those with cerebral lesions may have abnormal postural reflexes, such as the Moro reflex, that are exaggerated or maintained past the age at which they are usually lost.

In neonates, only when there are limb deformities can the etiology be assumed to have begun in utero. Such infants will present with arthrogryposis, the most common and least disabling being club foot. The most devastating deformity would be severe flexion contraction of all limbs. Another common deformity is dislocation of the hips, because muscle contractions are needed to maintain hip joint integrity. Subjective clues to intrauterine difficulties include reports from the mother of decreased movement of the child during pregnancy. The presence of dysmorphic features or other organ abnormalities usually indicates a developmental etiology for the hypotonia.

It should be noted that certain diseases, especially the metabolic diseases, can affect more than one aspect of the nervous system. Thus, if cerebrum, peripheral nerve, and muscle are affected, combined or conflicting signs may result. Hypotonia also has gradations, even in cases of systemic disease, and one region of muscles or function may be more severely affected than others (e.g., an infant may be squirming about relatively well but have a significant swallowing problem).

CENTRAL CAUSES OF HYPOTONIA

It is useful to break the CNS down into two distinct areas, the brain and the spinal cord, because their respective signs and symptoms, as well as pathologies, are often distinctive.

The hallmark of cerebral dysfunction is decreased level of arousal and seizures. These symptoms plus the previously discussed findings should allow one to make the diagnosis. Dysmorphic features and other organ maldevelopment also speak for cerebral dysfunction. Birthing complications are the most common cause of cerebral lesions. These lesions are secondary to hypoxia or ischemia from a myriad number of problems. Premature neonates also suffer from intraventricular hemorrhage (IVH), that can cause significant hypotonia. Intrauterine infections such as the TORCH syndrome can severely damage the cerebrum. Neonatal infections such as meningitis can cause hypotonia but differ from the above etiologies in that the affected neonate is normal initially and then develops hypotonia, whereas the TORCH neonate is born hypotonic and remains so. Other causes, such as cerebral palsies, are idiopathic.

Another large category is neural tube closure defects. Some, such as the grossly deformed cyclops or anencephalics, are easily diagnosed. These neonates are usually born dead, but one does not need much brainstem to live and some have survived for months. Other more subtle neural tube defects, such as lobar holoprosenceph-

aly, or neural migration defects, such as lissencephaly, may vary greatly in severity. All the above maladies should be evaluated with computed tomographic (CT) scans and/or cranial ultrasound. Treatment is mostly supportive. Those with IVH may require an intraventricular shunt for hydrocephalus.

SPINAL LESIONS

Spinal malformations include myelomeningocele, which can occur anywhere along the spine but is most common in the lumbosacral area. Affected children will have differential affliction of legs compared to arms and head depending on the site of the defect. Those with high cervical lesions will have quadraparesis but retain sucking and eye movements. Any cord lesion will cause bladder distension with overflow incontinence, decreased rectal tone, and a segmental sensory loss.

Birth trauma can also cause spinal lesions secondary to breech or cervical presentations. These traction injuries occur during difficult deliveries and may be added to the hypoxia and cerebral trauma from birthing. High cervical lesions cause approximately 25% of the traction lesions and are due to a midforceps rotation, in which the head is twisted and the trunk does not follow. The cord may have variable amounts of damage, from partial shearing and intraparenchymal hemorrhage to complete severing. Lower cervical and upper thoracic regions are the most common sites, accounting for 75% of the traction injuries. These occur in breech deliveries when the head is hyperextended, which causes compression of the spinal arteries. This results in infarction, which can later become hemorrhagic. The compression can also cause upward herniation of the cord through the foramen magnum.

Evaluation of suspected spinal lesions requires an x ray of the spine to determine bone formation. If the bones are normal and cord traction is then suspected, a myelogram or magnetic resonance imaging (MRI) scan will usually show if the cord is swollen or has been severed. Those with high lesions will require ventilator assistance and will often die after several weeks. The severe edema of the cord may extend into the brainstem, leading to unconsciousness. In those with myelomeningocele, the defect must be closed to protect the cord; otherwise supportive care is the mainstay.

CHROMOSOMAL, GENETIC, AND METABOLIC DEFECTS

Certain chromosomal abnormalities such as trisomies, as well as hereditary diseases, such as Riley-Day syndrome, cause hypotonia. The pathology is present throughout the CNS and peripheral nerves, and children fail to thrive secondary to decreased swallowing. Metabolic disease such as adrenoleukodystrophy (ALD) cause hypotonia.

ALD is characterized by an increase in long-chain fatty acids (C_{26}) with CNS white matter dysfunction and peripheral nerve demyelination. Patients may have hyporeflexia or hyperreflexia depending on which part has greater pathology. Other metabolic diseases, such as Tay-Sachs disease and acid maltase deficiency, also cause multiple lesions. A history of other afflicted family members along with appropriate serum and tissue testing is needed for diagnosis. Treatment is symptomatic and supportive. Other neuromuscular causes of hypotonia will be discussed later.

WEAKNESS IN CHILDHOOD

Weakness in children is usually brought to medical attention by family or teachers who notice that the child either waddles, has difficulty running or going up steps, or (less often) shows changes in facial expression or voice. In younger children and infants, one usually notes delay in motor development. In addition to this chronic or subacute presentation, acute weakness also deserves special attention.

When approaching diseases of the peripheral nervous system causing weakness, it is helpful to try to make a mental classification of the particular signs and symptoms in a given patient. Specifically, one should ask oneself is the weakness acute or chronic, is it proximal or distal, were the reflexes absent or present, and is there sensory involvement. It is important to arrive at these conclusions at the time the history is taken and the physical examination performed. Obtaining a detailed family history and occasionally examining family members can be quite informative.

Using inspection, one should comment on muscle bulk. More commonly, atrophic muscles will imply denervation from either anterior horn cell diseases or axonal diseases. It must be remembered, however, that chronic dystrophies will ultimately lead to atrophy. On the other hand, hypertrophy or pseudohypertrophy of certain muscle groups can lead one to suspect certain muscle dystrophies, such as enlargement of the gastrocnemius muscle in Duchenne's muscular dystrophy. One should look carefully for the presence or absence of fasciculation, a finding that usually implies denervation. This is seen as rippling under the skin best noted on the long muscles of the legs, the deltoids, and the pectoralis muscles. However, one should inspect all groups. Palpation and percussion while paying attention to texture and tenderness can be helpful. Duchenne's patients have a rubbery, flabby muscle consistency, whereas inflamed muscles may be tender. In myotonic dystrophy percussion can often make the diagnosis.

One should examine the tone and passive range of motion of all joints. Patients with proximal weakness who have a lordotic waddling gait overcompensate with toe walking usually associated with shortening of the Achilles tendons. Such a gait may be secondary to either a myopathic process or even CNS disease and the tone is often helpful in differentiating the two. Evaluation of strength can be best achieved by combining observation of functional abilities and direct examination of various muscle groups. This will help categorize the weakness as proximal, distal, or both. Testing the infant depends more on observation, whereas in older subjects one should comment on ability to rise from the floor, looking for a tripod sign and trying to elicit a Gower's sign. Other helpful maneuvers include arising from a chair, stepping on a stool, heel walking, toe hopping, and raising the arms above the head. One should also assess strength by testing movements across joints using the standard rating system. One should comment on facial strength and ocular mobility, as they are crucial in myotonic dystrophy and myasthenia gravis. Both these diseases may present with ptosis and facial weakness, but only myasthenia affects ocular mobility.

Examinations of reflexes and sensation are helpful in differentiating upper motor from lower motor, and peripheral nerve from muscular causes of weakness. It is obvious that hyperreflexic weakness is likely to be due to a central disease of the upper motor neurons, whereas hyporeflexic or areflexic weakness is more difficult to classify. In general, lower motor neuron or neuropathic causes of areflexia are usually associated with atrophy, and loss of reflexes is proportional to the degree of weakness and atrophy. On the other hand, myopathic processes would result in a loss of reflexes earlier, even before any evidence of atrophy or with only mild weakness observed. In peripheral neuropathies with significant sensory involvement, reflexes are lost early even in the absence of any demonstrable weakness.

Three patterns of weakness are commonly observed in childhood: progressive proximal weakness, progressive distal weakness, and acute weakness.

- *Progressive proximal weakness* in childhood is most commonly due to a myopathy. Less common causes are the juvenile muscular atrophies and certain forms of myasthenia gravis. The myopathies include dystrophies, inflammatory and metabolic myopathies, and endocrine myopathies. Rarely, certain acquired neuropathies will be more proximal but should have distal involvement as well; one such neuropathy is chronic inflammatory demyelinating neuropathy.

- *Progressive distal weakness*, on the other hand, is more commonly caused by a neuropathy. Such neuropathies are mixed sensory and motor and usually are hereditary. However, spinal muscular atrophy can present with predominantly distal weakness. Two myopathies that should be thought of in this setting are myotonic dystrophy and hereditary distal myopathy.

- *Acute weakness* deserves special attention, as

there are few situations in which disorders must be considered and a diagnosis established quickly, because prompt institution of appropriate therapy can be lifesaving (see Table 16–1).

The differentiatial diagnosis usually comprises myasthenia gravis, Guillain-Barré syndrome, poliomyelitis, and transverse myelitis. Early on, all these can present with flaccid paralysis. Clearly transverse myelitis should not involve bulbar muscles. If the patient in question has no bulbar weakness, then early bladder involvement favors a diagnosis of myelitis.

The differentiation ultimately rests on a combination of clinical, electrophysiologic, and cerebrospinal fluid (CSF) findings. Later evaluation of the patient should show a typical progression for the various disease entities mentioned. The myelitis patient will develop an increased tone and spasticity; the electromyogram (EMG) in poliomyelitis will show evidence of denervation (with

TABLE 16–1. CAUSES OF ACUTE WEAKNESS

Spinal cord diseases
    Transverse myelitis
Motor neuron diseases
    Poliomyelitis
Peripheral nerve diseases
    Guillain-Barré syndrome
    Tick paralysis
Neuromuscular junction diseases
    Myasthenia gravis crisis
    Botulism
Muscle diseases
    Inflammatory myopathy
    Periodic paralysis

fibrillation and other findings); and nerve conduction velocities are ultimately slowed in Guillain-Barré syndrome. These entities will be discussed individually in later sections.

Specific Neuromuscular Diseases

MOTOR NEURON DISEASES: SPINAL MUSCULAR ATROPHIES

Diseases affecting the motor neurons include a number of disorders. Some are limited to the lower motor neurons, others involve both upper and lower motor neurons, and in some, disease of the motor neurons is only a part of a systemic illness. In this chapter discussion will be limited to the spinal muscular atrophies (SMAs).

The SMAs are similar in clinical presentation and pathology except for age of onset. All present with weakness secondary to loss of the alpha motor neuron. No etiologic cause or genetic marker has been identified, and for the most part they are all recessively transmitted. There is no sensory loss nor are there upper motor neuron signs, and the reflexes are usually lost. The SMAs are classified according to age of onset and rate of progression. There is little variability among affected members of the same pedigree.

Signs and Symptoms. Type I SMA (Severe SMA, Werdnig-Hoffman Disease, Acute SMA). Type I SMA runs a very stereotyped course in affected children. The onset is between the second and sixth months of life. Progression is rapid, with death occurring in the second year owing to pulmonary complications. Many infants are identified from birth or in the first few weeks of life. They are hypotonic and have a characteristic posture with the legs in the frog leg position. The cry is weak and there

is constant drooling secondary to swallowing difficulties. Proximal muscles are affected first and early on there is some distal extremity movement. Most infants have a lively expression with no involvement of extraocular or facial muscles. Fasciculations are seen in the tongue in about half the patients, but are seldom seen in the limbs. It is uncommon for contractures to be present at birth.

Type II SMA (Intermediate or Chronic Werdnig-Hoffman Disease). Type II SMA is a little more variable than type I. Onset is between the sixth and twelfth months of life. The child may ultimately be able to sit, but only for a short period, and most children are wheelchair bound by the third year. In addition to generalized weakness, which is worse proximally, patients may have mild facial weakness. Children seldom have difficulty chewing or swallowing. Fasciculations are common, as is a fine tremor of the hands. Skeletal deformities, particularly kyphoscoliosis, develop with time. After an initial progressive course, patients stabilize and ultimately succumb to respiratory insufficiency.

Type III SMA (Kugelberg-Welander Disease or Late-Onset Juvenile SMA). The onset of weakness in type III SMA occurs between 5 and 15 years of age, and the disease pursues a slowly progressive course. The weakness is predominantly proximal and may resemble limb girdle dystrophy. Toe walking and early contractures are uncommon. Patients are usually wheelchair bound by their mid-30s and weakness of the hands occurs last. Involvement of cranial muscles is rare, and fasciculations are seen in about half the cases.

FEATURE TABLE 16–1. MOTOR NEURON DISEASES

Disease	Discriminating Features	Consistent Features	Variable Features
Type I SMA	1. A combination of severe weakness and Type 1 fiber hypertrophy on muscle biopsy	1. Severe progressive weakness, sparing the face 2. Autosomal recessive 3. Absent reflexes 4. Neurogenic EMG	1. Skeletal deformities 2. Death within 2 to 3 years
Type II SMA	1. A combination of later age of onset and slow progression	1. Nonprogressive or slowly progressive course 2. Hand tremor 3. Autosomal recessive 4. Neurogenic EMG	1. Fasciculations 2. CK elevation
Type III SMA	1. A combination of later onset, slow progression, and proximal weakness and neurogenic muscle biopsy	1. Proximal weakness 2. Delayed motor milestones	1. Tongue fasciculations 2. CK elevation

Pearls and Perils: Spinal Muscular Atrophies

1. In contrast to infantile myotonic dystrophy, patients with type I SMA do not have facial weakness.
2. Patients with type II SMA develop skeletal deformities as the disease progresses. Kyphoscoliosis is particularly common and more severe than that seen in Duchenne's muscular dystrophy.
3. Patients with SMAs have elevated CK levels. However, in contrast to Duchenne's dystrophy, as the disease progresses the CK level rises.
4. Gastrocnemius enlargement is common in juvenile SMA. Unlike Duchenne's dystrophy, there is no early toe walking or shortening of the heel cords.
5. The typical patient with type I SMA usually dies within the first 2 years of life. If there is any doubt that this is the correct diagnosis, or a suspicion that the child's disorder is of the more chronic variety, it is worthwhile being aggressive with surgical intervention to correct contractures, scoliosis, and joint deformities.
6. Patients with juvenile SMA should not be simply managed with supportive rehabilitation and passive exercises. Rather, active exercises should be performed to strengthen available muscles.
7. There are a few SMA lookalikes that should not be forgotten. The most important to remember is Tay-Sachs disease. The importance lies in our ability to detect the infants prenatally.

Investigation and Diagnosis. The investigation of any progressive weakness usually includes serum creatine kinase (CK) measurement, EMG, and commonly a muscle biopsy. In the SMAs, CK levels are abnormally elevated, but not to the same degree as in Duchenne's dystrophy. The EMG shows neuropathic features with fibrillations and increased insertional activity. The muscle biopsy shows neurogenic changes with grouped atrophy and fiber type grouping. In type I SMA the grouped atrophy usually involves large fascicles, and there are large hypertrophic fibers that are characteristically type I fibers. The diagnosis is usually established on clinical grounds and supported by the ancillary tests.

Treatment. There is no specific therapy for the SMAs. Physical therapy and surgical intervention to correct deformities may be needed.

PRIMARY MUSCLE DISEASES

CONGENITAL MYOPATHIES

The congenital myopathies include the following disorders: central core disease, nemalin (rod body) myopathy, centronuclear (myotubular) myopathy, congenital fiber type disproportion, and congenital muscular dystrophy.

All of these disorders can present in the neonatal period with various degrees of severity of joint deformities and hypotonia. Most, however, present with delay of motor milestones or an unsteady gait. Rarely, these disorders can cause severe neonatal weakness or a severe progressive myopathy that leads to respiratory compromise and death. The two myopathies with greater incidence of the severe form are centronuclear myopathy and congenital muscular dystrophy, which also have an autosomal recessive pattern of inheritance. The rest of the congenital myopathies are inherited as autosomal dominant traits.

Signs and Symptoms. As already mentioned, this group of dystrophies usually runs a benign course. Presenting early in infancy with motor developmental delays, affected infants are noted to have various forms of skeletal deformities, usually kyphoscoliosis, congenital hip dislocation, and foot deformities. Most of these patients have either a very slowly progressive myopathy or even a static one; some are even felt to improve.

Facial and pharyngeal muscle weakness is more commonly encountered in the severe forms and it is these forms that also demonstrate diminished or absent reflexes. Atrophy of muscles may be present and correlates with the severity of the disease. Intelligence is not affected except in the Fukuyama variant of congenital muscular dystrophy.

Investigation and Diagnosis. As with all patients with hypotonia, proximal weakness, and delayed motor development, the workup should include serum CK measurement, EMG, and nerve conduction studies. If these are indicative of a myopathic process, a muscle biopsy with histochemic analysis is warranted. In these

---

Pearls and Perils:
Congenital Myopathies

1. All of these myopathies present with hypotonia. With the exception of myotubular myopathy, there is rarely involvement of extraocular muscles.
2. Both congenital muscular dystrophy and fiber type disproportion myopathy usually present with marked skeletal deformities. All of the congenital myopathies have a high incidence of congenital dislocation of the hips.
3. Patients with central core disease have a high tendency to develop malignant hyperthermia when under general anesthesia.

---

disorders, the CK is usually normal; it is only elevated in the two severe forms. EMG shows a myopathic pattern in all forms, with small short-duration polyphasic potentials and early recruitment.

Pathology. The pathology in these disorders is interesting in that, except for congenital muscular dystrophy, all show a relative predominance of type I fibers, which are also atrophied. This had led some authors to suggest that these disorders should be classified as congenital fiber type disproportion myopathies, with each one having a characteristic feature of its own. Central core disease shows areas of absent oxidative staining in the center of the fibers, which represent absent mitochondria. Nemalin

---

FEATURE TABLE 16-2. CONGENITAL MYOPATHIES

Disease	Discriminating Features	Consistent Features	Variable Features
Central core disease	1. Presence of central cores on biopsy	1. Autosomal dominant 2. Benign course 3. Type 1 fiber predominance	1. Skeletal deformities
Nemalin (rod body) myopathy	1. Rod bodies originating from Z bands	1. Autosomal dominant 2. Type 1 fiber predominance 3. Moderate atrophy	1. Skeletal deformities 2. Bulbar weakness
Centronuclear (myotubular) myopathy	1. Chains of central nuclei	1. Type 1 fiber predominance 2. CK elevation 3. Absent reflexes	1. Autosomal recessive 2. Extraocular muscle involvement
Congenital fiber type disproportion	1. A combination of clinical features and type 1 fiber predominance	1. Autosomal dominant 2. Contractures and skeletal deformities 3. Short stature	1. Myopathic EMG
Congenital muscular dystrophy	1. A combination of clinical features and myopathic muscle biopsy	1. Autosomal recessive 2. Elevated CK 3. Contractures and skeletal deformities	1. Benign and severe forms

myopathy shows rod bodies originating from the Z lines; however, these are not pathognomonic for this disease. Centronuclear or myotubular myopathy shows chains of central nuclei with a normal-looking peripheral myofibrillar pattern. Congenital fiber type disproportion shows only the predominance of the smaller type I fibers. Finally, congenital muscular dystrophy shows nonspecific fiber size variation and degenerating fibers, although these findings are compatible with any dystrophy.

Treatment. There is no available treatment for these myopathies. However, providing orthosis for correction of skeletal deformities or even surgical correction often leads to improvement of functional disabilities as these myopathies are usually nonprogressive.

MUSCULAR DYSTROPHIES

The muscular dystrophies are a group of inherited muscle diseases characterized primarily by their clinical presentation and pattern of muscle involvement. The group includes Duchenne's muscular dystrophy (DMD), Becker's muscular dystrophy (BMD), facioscapulohumeral (FSH) dystrophy, Emery-Dreifuss muscular dystrophy, limb girdle muscular dystrophy, and such other less common disorders as scapuloperoneal, oculopharyngeal, and distal muscular atrophy. With the exception of DMD all present later in childhood or

adolescence; however, in each category one can find case reports of patients with earlier onset or a more severe progression.

Duchenne's Muscular Dystrophy

DMD is an X-linked recessive disorder affecting about 20 to 30 of every 100,000 boys. It is a progressive dystrophy with a rather stereotyped and grim prognosis. Recent work has identified the genetic defect and the gene product, dystrophin.

Signs and Symptoms. As with other muscle dystrophies, the earlier the onset the less specific the clinical presentation is, and patients may only present with delay in motor development and hypotonia. Boys with DMD are first noted to be late in walking. They have an accentuated lordosis while walking on their toes, and the calves are hypertrophied. By 3 to 4 years of age the child is unable keep up with his peers and running is never well established. Between 3 and 6 years the child looks as though he is improving; however, there are more frequent falls and the tightening of the heel cords forces him to have a perched posture. By now the child has more difficulty with climbing stairs and independent walking. By 12 years essentially all patients are wheelchair bound. As the child is further immobilized pulmonary compromise ensues. This is the usual cause of death, which occurs by the second to third decade. It is important to note that about 15% of patients with DMD may remain am-

FEATURE TABLE 16-3. MUSCULAR DYSTROPHIES

Disease	Discriminating Features	Consistent Features	Variable Features
Duchenne's muscular dystrophy	1. Xp21.2 gene deletion with very low or absent dystrophin	1. Steadily progressive contractures 2. Pseudohypertrophy 3. Age of onset within first 5 years 4. CK grossly elevated	1. Cardiomyopathy 2. Mental retardation
Becker's muscular dystrophy	1. Xp21.2 gene deletion with abnormal dystrophin	1. Slowly progressive ambulation beyond 16 years 2. CK grossly elevated 3. Pseudohypertrophy 4. Normal intelligence	1. Age of onset 2. Cardiomyopathy
Facioscapulohumeral dystrophy	1. A combination of clinical findings and myopathic biopsy	1. Autosomal dominant 2. Facial and scapuloperoneal weakness 3. Sparing of deltoids	1. Age of onset 2. Deafness 3. Coats's syndrome 4. CK elevation
Emery-Dreifuss muscular dystrophy	1. Xq28 lows in addition to clinical features	1. Rigid neck or spine 2. Humeroperoneal weakness 3. Slowly progressive course	1. Degree of weakness 2. Cardiac arrhythmia 3. CK elevation
Limb girdle muscular dystrophy	None	1. Shoulder and pelvic girdle weakness 2. Myopathic EMG	1. Autosomal recessive 2. CK elevation

bulatory for a slightly longer time; such patients are considered outliers.

On examination the child initially manifests the waddling lordotic gait so characteristic of the disease. The calves are enlarged and the muscles feel compact and rubbery. Deep tendon reflexes are lost early in the illness, and as the disease progresses all muscles are affected, beginning proximally and ending distally. Interestingly, the facial musculature is only mildly affected and extraocular muscles are completely spared. Another hallmark of the disease is the early development of contractures involving the heel cords, hip flexors, and ilio-tibial bands. Ultimately all joints are involved. In addition to the muscular difficulties, boys with DMD tend to have an overall IQ below that of age-matched controls.

Investigation and Diagnosis. The investigation should include measurement of CK levels (which are grossly elevated), EMG to help differentiate between neurogenic and myopathic weakness, and a muscle biopsy. The electrocardiagram (EKG) is abnormal in about 75% of cases. Patients with DMD may have arrhythmias but they rarely become symptomatic from cardiac disease. The EMG shows the typical myopathic findings of short-duration polyphasic units with early recruitment. The diagnosis is established by a muscle biopsy, which shows fiber size variation, endomesial thickening, and many foci of necrosis and phagocytosis. Most of the fibers are small circular fibers with internal nuclei. There is no fiber type predominance.

Researchers have now identified the DMD/BMD gene in the Xp21.2 region. This gene is one of the largest known genes, and its size may explain the high incidence of this disease, because there may be greater chance for mutations or deletions. Not only can one now screen for such deletions, but the gene product dystrophin can also be assayed. This protein is a structural muscle protein that is essentially absent in DMD, and has an altered molecular weight in BMD. Thus carriers and patients alike can be tested for the deletion and have their dystrophin assayed. This allows definitive establishment of the diagnosis, detection of carriers, and prenatal diagnosis of affected fetuses.

Treatment and Prognosis. The prognosis remains grim for patients with DMD. Treatment is limited at present to supportive care. This is not to say that one should give up. Physical therapy and appropriate surgery to lengthen various tendons and so prevent contractures, and early rodding to prevent or correct scoliosis, can provide the patient with significant ambulatory and functional time.

Becker's Muscular Dystrophy
BMD was considered for a long time to be at the more benign end of the spectrum of DMD. This is not the case. Although it is an X-linked recessive disorder and shares the same genetic marker and the same gene product with DMD, BMD probably represents a separate, more functional deletion or mutation with preservation of dystrophin. Total dystrophin level may be reduced or the molecule may have a lower molecular weight. Pedigrees of BMD or DMD do not usually show phenotypic variation among affected members.

Signs and Symptoms. Patients with BMD have a more benign course than patients with DMD. The initial presentation is very similar but more delayed (until the fifth year of life), and ambulation is not lost until the late teens, with prolonged survival to the middle of adult life. As in most myopathies, proximal muscles are affected first and the disease could be confused with limb girdle dystrophy were it not for the X-linked inheritance. The examination is very similar to that of patients with DMD except for showing milder deficits and normal intelligence.

Investigation and Diagnosis. The same tests apply here as in DMD. The CK levels are elevated and the EMG demonstrates myopathic activity. The EKG is not as frequently abnormal. The muscle biopsy shows similar findings but these are not as severe. Carrier detection and prenatal diagnosis are the same.

Treatment. Supportive care follows the same principles as that in DMD.

Facioscapulohumeral Muscular Dystrophy
FSH, as the name implies, is a dystrophy involving the facial, shoulder girdle, and lower limb muscles. The disease is dominantly inherited with a marked variability within the same pedigree. The weakness is usually slowly progressive.

Signs and Symptoms. Most cases become symptomatic in the second to third decade, but presentations as early as 5 years of age and as late as the fifth decade have been reported. The first symptoms are related to lower limb proximal weakness. The patients may then recall that they have never been able to whistle or suck through a straw and examination shows the facial and shoulder girdle weakness. There is usually a strong family history or at least evidence of facial weakness and a pectoral fold in clinically unsuspecting members. The patients have a characteristic appearance, with facial weakness, winging of the scapulae, and thin arms with well-developed "Popeye" forearms. There is no extraocular muscle involvement and the deltoids are usually spared. Progression is slow and patients die of other complications. There is an infantile form with a rapidly progressive severe myopathy. It is important to recognize in the juvenile cases the co-occurence of sensorineural hearing loss in a subgroup of patients. Others may also have Coats's syn-

---

Pearls and Perils:
Muscular Dystrophies

1. Children with DMD often complain of leg pains early in the course of their illness.
2. A normal CK level excludes the diagnosis of DMD, and typically the CK falls as the disease progresses.
3. Some patients will remain ambulatory for longer periods of time than expected. Some of these patients may be identified by having relative sparing of neck flexors.
4. In severe cases of FSH the distal muscles become involved late in the course. Interestingly, wrist extensors are affected to a much greater degree than flexors.
5. Boys with DMD often appear to be improving between the ages of 4 and 6 years. The diagnosis should be established with confidence so as not to give the parents false hopes.
6. Malignant hyperthermia may be seen in patients with DMD.
7. The muscle weakness in Emery-Dreifuss muscular dystrophy is very slowly progressive. These patients die from cardiac arrhythmias. It is very important to place pacemakers in some individuals early in the course of their illness.

---

drome, that is, retinal exudative telangiectasia; these patients can have their abnormal retinal vessels photocoagulated to prevent blindness.

Investigation and Diagnosis. The CK level is moderately elevated in about half the cases. The EMG is myopathic and the muscle biopsy shows a nonspecific myopathy with occasional neurogenic changes. The diagnosis is based on the strong family history and clinical presentation with confirmation by the EMG and biopsy. Audiometry and careful funduscopy should be performed.

Treatment. As with other dystrophies therapy is aimed at prevention and correction of contractures and scoliosis. Certain patients benefit from scapular fixation to assist them in raising their arms.

Emery-Dreifuss Muscular Dystrophy
The Emery-Dreifuss form is an interesting dystrophy with very peculiar clinical findings. The inheritance is X-linked recessive with great variability within the same pedigree. Linkage analysis has shown that the gene is located in the Xq28 region but it has not yet been identified. Cardiac involvement can be life threatening.

Signs and Symptoms. The onset is in childhood or adolescence and begins with mild walking difficulties. The patients typically are toe walking because of peroneal distribution weakness and they have thin and weak biceps. (This distribution gives the disease its alternate name of humeroperoneal dystrophy.) Most patients will have the characteristic contractures at the time of presentation even in the absence of significant weakness. Posterior neck ligaments, biceps, and Achilles tendons are most commonly involved. Cardiac involvement is in the form of conduction defects and atrial arrhythmias. The disease is very slowly progressive and patients can live long if cardiac catastrophes are prevented.

Investigation and Diagnosis. The clinical picture with its strong family history usually provides the diagnosis. CK levels may be mildly elevated and the EMG is myopathic. EKG and Holter monitoring are very important to detect abnormalities. The biopsy is also myopathic. A probe is available to look for the gene in potential carriers or presymptomatic individuals.

Treatment. The same principles apply as in the other myopathies. It is important to detect cardiac abnormalities early on, because pacemaker insertion can be lifesaving.

Limb Girdle Muscular Dystrophy
The limb girdle dystrophies constitute a heterogeneous group of proximal dystrophies with variable clinical presentations and modes of inheritance, the most common being autosomal recessive. This entity must be differentiated from inflammatory myopathies, juvenile spinal muscular atrophy, and FSH with only mild facial involvement. There is no specific clinical sign for limb girdle dystrophy; however, one feature that distinguishes it from FSH is the sparing of the deltoids in the latter.

Diagnosis is based on clinical and electrophysiologic findings and the biopsy confirms the presence of a myopathy. The biopsy is important in order to exclude the SMAs and detect a potentially treatable inflammatory myopathy. There is no specific treatment.

MYOTONIC DYSTROPHIES

Myotonia is the failure of the muscle to relax after contraction. Myotonia can be produced by voluntary activity of the muscle, percussion or other mechanical stimulation, and, in some disorders, cold temperature. Multiple drugs are known to cause myotonia but they will not be discussed here.

Myotonia is probably due to membrane abnormalities that may also be present in other tissues, although membrane defects have not been characterized for all the diseases with myotonia.

In this section three diseases will be described: myotonic dystrophy, myotonia congenita (Thomsen's disease), and paramyotonia congenita.

Myotonic Dystrophy

Myotonic dystrophy is inherited as an autosomal dominant condition. There is extreme variability in the clinical presentation of patients within the same pedigree. The membrane defect has not been fully characterized but seems to involve other tissues as well. Patients with myotonic dystrophy often have other abnormalities, such as gonadal atrophy, gallbladder dysfunction, cataracts, mental retardation, early baldness, and cardiac conduction defects. It is one of the commoner dystrophies, with a prevalence of 3 to 5 in 100,000 births. The gene is probably located on chromosome 19, but it has not been identified yet.

Signs and Symptoms. Often patients with myotonic dystrophy do not seek medical attention until late adolescence or occasionally early childhood. The presenting symptoms are invariably related to weakness, which is strikingly distal. Thus they present with foot drop and hand weakness. Patients do not usually complain of myotonia; however, they may recall having unusual stiffness or cramping. The patients rarely complain about their facial weakness. Their appearance is so characteristic that one can sometimes make the diagnosis based solely on their slender facies, tapered mouths with the upper lip inverted like a V, and atrophy of temporal, jaw, and neck muscles. The patients usually have a nasal voice and ultimately develop severe dysarthria and swallowing difficulties. In the final stages of the disease, wasting of all muscle groups develops along with contractures. Patients die from cardiorespiratory complications.

The myotonia can be elicited easily with percussion or activation of muscles but disappears with repeated exercise. One should examine muscles that are not wasted in order not to miss the myotonia. Rarely the myotonic phenomena are significantly disabling.

Neonates and infants with myotonic dystrophy present with the characteristic appearance of the mouth and face and extreme floppiness. At presentation they do not display the myotonic phenomena; these tend to appear by the fourth to fifth year of life. They have various degrees of joint deformities, most commonly club feet. The diagnosis is made by examining the mother, who usually displays some features of myotonic dystrophy, namely the facial weakness. Interestingly, it is the mothers and not the fathers of the majority of infants with myotonic dystrophy who are affected.

Investigation and Diagnosis. The usual tests for all dystrophies are supportive but not necessary to make the diagnosis. The CK levels are mildly to moderately elevated, and the EMG shows the characteristic rapid firing during delayed relaxation with waxing and waning. The sound this electric activity makes has been likened to that of dive bombers. The EKG shows conduction abnormalities, usually a first degree atrioventricular block. The muscle biopsy has the typical myopathic features of fibrosis, internal nuclei, and small rounded fibers. There is a striking type I fiber atrophy with a large number of internal nuclei.

Treatment. Supportive care follows the same lines as that outlined for other neuromuscular diseases. Myotonia can be alleviated with Diamox, Dilantin, procainamide, or quinine. However, patients rarely are sufficiently disabled by their myotonia to warrant therapy. Counseling of parents is of paramount importance because techniques for prenatal diagnosis are not well established.

FEATURE TABLE 16-4. MYOTONIC DYSTROPHIES

Disease	Discriminating Features	Consistent Features	Variable Features
Myotonic dystrophy	1. Myotonia plus clinical features	1. Autosomal dominant 2. Muscle weakness and wasting 3. Facial weakness 4. Percussion myotonia	1. Cataracts 2. Premature balding 3. Cardiomyopathy 4. Gonadal atrophy 5. Intellectual deficit
Myotonia congenita	1. Myotonia is the only symptom	1. No weakness 2. Muscle hypertrophy 3. Percussion myotonia 4. Activity relieves myotonia	1. Autosomal dominant and recessive 2. Tends to improve with time
Paramyotonia congenita	1. Combination of cold-induced stiffness and spontaneous muscle activity on EMG	1. Autosomal dominant 2. Increasing weakness with repeated activity	1. Cold-induced paramyotonia and paralysis

Myotonia Congenita

Myotonia congenita is also a disease with a membrane defect producing myotonia. The defect has been characterized as reduced chloride conductance. The myotonic phenomena are the major symptoms and the disease seems to be inherited in two forms. The autosomal dominant form presents earlier in childhood but has only mild (if any) progression. The autosomal recessive variety is noticed in the middle of the first decade and is the more severe form. Patients do not have the other associated features affecting other organ systems, as in myotonic dystrophy.

Signs and Symptoms. The patient presents with the complaint of stiffness and weakness that begins immediately after resting from exercise. As the patient tries to ambulate or exercise again, he or she is unable to move freely and feels stiff. As the patient moves about mobility increases and eventually returns to normal. Although patients complain of weakness this is not usually demonstrable on examination. The patients may have marked muscular hypertrophy.

Investigation and Diagnosis. The EMG can be helpful in establishing the diagnosis. Usually the muscle biopsy is normal or has few nonspecific findings.

Treatment. Because the main symptoms are related to the myotonic phenomena, a trial of Dilantin or procainamide

---

Pearls and Perils: Myotonic Dystrophies

1. Patients with myotonic dystrophy have such a characteristic appearance that one should make the diagnosis based on their nasal voice, thin faces, and withered sternocleidomastoids.
2. It seems that with each succeeding generation of families with myotonic dystrophy, the illness appears earlier and earlier.
3. Myotonia should not be confused with the normal contraction produced by percussion of a muscle.
4. One should be careful when prescribing procainamide or quinine for patients with myotonic dystrophy. These drugs prolong the PR interval on the EKG, and these patients already have conduction defects. Furthermore, seldom are these patients bothered by the myotonic phenomena.
5. If a patient with suspected myotonia congenita develops muscle weakness, then most likely this is not the correct diagnosis and further studies are warranted.

---

is worthwhile. Unfortunately the beneficial effects are short lived.

Paramyotonia Congenita

Signs and Symptoms. Paramyotonia congenita is a dominantly inherited disorder in which the main symptoms are muscular stiffness and relaxation difficulty. The symptoms are worsened by cold and exercise. Unlike myotonia, the failure to relax is accentuated with repeated exercise and may occur spontaneously in cold temperature. These symptoms are probably present from childhood and do not improve with time. Exposure to cold can cause true weakness even after the paramyotonia disappears, and the weakness may last longer than the exposure to cold.

Investigation and Diagnosis. The EMG is able to document electrical myotonia produced by percussion. Characteristically the EMG shows spontaneous activity with exposure to cold. Unlike myotonia there is little muscle activity during the phase of delayed relaxation, which may indicate a contracture rather than abnormal contraction.

Treatment. Therapy with Tocainide has been tried and seems to have promising results.

INFLAMMATORY MYOPATHIES: DERMATOMYOSITIS

In this section only dermatomyositis (DM) will be discussed because polymyositis is predominantly a disease of adults. Most investigators feel that childhood DM differs from adult DM. Other causes of inflammatory myopathies include infectious etiologies, but they are beyond the scope of this text.

Signs and Symptoms. The disease follows a subacute course with the weakness developing over a period of weeks. There are, however, less common, more acute presentations. Childhood DM is so typical that the history and physical examination alone are often sufficient to make the diagnosis. The child becomes irritable and initially has a nonspecific illness that includes respiratory or gastrointestinal symptoms. Commonly there is generalized malaise and fever. A rash may precede, accompany, or follow the onset of the weakness. The rash is violaceous in color and is present on the face, around the eyelids, and on the extensor surfaces of the hands and other limbs. There is an associated edema of the affected areas. The weakness typically involves proximal muscles, but later may involve all groups.

Characteristically neck flexors are weak, in contrast to myasthenia, in which extensors are involved. Less com-

FEATURE TABLE 16–5. INFLAMMATORY MYOPATHIES: DERMATOMYOSITIS

Discriminating Feature	Consistent Features	Variable Features
1. A combination of the characteristic rash and typical muscle biopsy	1. Violaceous rash 2. Proximal weakness 3. Perifascicular atrophy on muscle biopsy 4. Elevated CK 5. Miserable child	1. Bulbar and respiratory weakness 2. GI symptoms 3. Myocarditis and pericarditis 4. Arthralgias

monly bulbar and respiratory muscles are affected, but dysphagia is a common complaint.

Children with DM are often miserable and appear ill. They have other symptoms of gastrointestinal ulceration, pericarditis or myocarditis, and respiratory involvement.

Investigation and Diagnosis. The serum muscle enzymes are markedly elevated in the active phase of the disease, and the EMG shows myopathic features with marked muscle irritability, usually indicative of necrosis. The pathology in DM is quite characteristic and shows marked necrosis and inflammation. The atrophy and necrosis are typically perifascicular and are probably due to vascular infarction secondary to vasculitis.

Treatment. Treatment should be reserved for patients with progressive acute or subacute weakness that is also disabling, because many patients go into spontaneous remission. (Some clinicians believe all patients should be treated.) The mainstay of therapy is prednisone, which may be supplemented with plasma exchange during relapses or other forms of immunosuppression if there is no response to steroids.

Prognosis. The disease can run a monophasic course with spontaneous remission or can follow a relapsing remitting pattern. With therapy prognosis is good. In chronic cases calcinosis may develop.

Pearls and Perils:
Inflammatory Myopathies

1. The rash in patients with DM may accompany, precede, or follow the onset of weakness.
2. Muscle pains are not always present in patients with DM.
3. It is important to recognize that patients with DM can occasionally have severe bulbar and respiratory weakness.
4. Childhood DM is probably a systemic vasculitis and patients may develop severe gastrointestinal ulcerations.

METABOLIC MYOPATHIES

Metabolic myopathies derive from defects in energy production, which include abnormalities in glycogen/glucose and lipid metabolism and respiratory chain dysfunction. These diseases have a spectrum of clinical manifestations. At one end the patients suffer from exercise intolerance and little permanent or progressive weakness. At the other there is profound weakness and systemic abnormalities with little exercise intolerance. Only the prototype diseases in each category will be discussed.

Disorders of Glycogen Metabolism

Glycogen Storage Diseases

The classic glycogen storage disease with exercise intolerance is myophosphorylase deficiency (McArdle's disease or glycogenosis type 5). The enzyme breaks down glycogen to provide glucose for immediate utilization.

Signs and Symptoms. The disease is transmitted as an autosomal recessive trait. The cardinal symptom, exercise intolerance, is manifested as fatigue, muscle pains, and contractures. These signs are associated with necrosis, CK level elevation, and myoglobinuria. Symptoms begin before 10 years of age, and with time the exercise-induced fatigue and pain become increasingly severe and require less exertion. Episodes are relatively stereotyped. Immediately after heavy exercise the patient starts having cramps in the muscle and may develop a contracture. The muscle cannot be stretched passively and feels swollen and tender. This condition may last for hours and is usually associated with myoglobinuria. Thigh and other proximal muscles are commonly affected. The muscle strength is initially normal; however, with repeated episodes permanent weakness develops.

Another interesting phenomenon is the so-called second wind phenomenon. As patients get fatigued they learn to rest or slow down, and after a brief period they are able to resume their activities without limitations. Because the enzyme is limited to muscle other organs are spared. The preceding clinical description holds essentially true for a number of glycogen/glucose metabolism defects, which include: phosphofructokinase deficiency (glycogenosis type 7), phosphoglycerate mutase deficiency (glycogenosis type 10), phosphoglycerate kinase deficiency (glycogenosis type 9), and lactate dehydrogenase deficiency.

Investigation and Diagnosis. The CK level is elevated during bouts of pain, and the EMG is usually normal except in later stages of the disease, when it becomes myopathic. The muscle biopsy may show vacuoles and electron microscopy demonstrates subsarcolemmal deposits of glycogen. An accurate diagnosis is made with histochemic staining showing absence of myophosphorylase activity. The other disorders are diagnosed by assaying the specific enzyme activity in the muscle.

The clinical picture is rather stereotyped, and the forearm ischemic exercise test will confirm or exclude the diagnosis of a glycogen metabolism defect. Because the enzymatic defects occur before the formation of lac-

tate in the glycolysis pathway, under ischemic conditions failure to produce lactate essentially rules in one of the above disorders.

Treatment. Despite our understanding of the biochemic defect, therapy has been less rewarding than one would hope. Oral administration of glucose and adrenergic stimulation with isoproterenol is usually recommended. One should also remember that frank rhabdomyolysis can occur during bouts of pain and can lead to renal dysfunction; thus appropriate recognition and management can be lifesaving.

Acid Maltase Deficiency (glycogenosis type 2)

Acid maltase deficiency affects muscles as well as other tissues. There are at least two forms. The infantile form presents with generalized weakness resembling that

FEATURE TABLE 16-6. METABOLIC MYOPATHIES

Disease	Discriminating Features	Consistent Features	Variable Features
Glycogen Metabolism Disorders			
Glycogen storage disease types 5, 7, 9, and 10	1. Assays for specific enzymes	1. Exercise intolerance 2. Positive forearm ischemic exercise test 3. Autosomal recessive 4. Myoglobinuria 5. Muscle pain and cramps 6. Fatigue	1. Permanent weakness 2. Myopathic EMG and muscle biopsy
Acid maltase deficiency	1. Absent enzyme activity in all forms	1. Severe myopathy in the infantile form with organomegaly and cardiomyopathy 2. Autosomal recessive 3. Vacuolar myopathy 4. CK elevation	1. Slower rate of progression in the mild form with variable organomegaly
Lipid Metabolism Disorders			
CPT deficiency	1. Low CPT activity in muscles	1. Exercise intolerance 2. Muscle pain and tenderness 3. No weakness 4. Increased lipid in muscles 5. Normal EMG 6. Precipitated by fasting 7. Myoglobinuria	1. Cramps and contractures
Mitochondrial Disorders			
Mitochondrial myopathies	1. Respiratory chain component assays or ?DNA analysis	1. Exercise intolerance 2 Lactic acidosis or acidemia 3. Ragged red fibers	1. Variable degrees of myopathy, encephalopathy 2. Deafness 3. Ophthalmoplegia 4. Cardiomyopathy 5. Pigmentary retinal degeneration

observed in the SMAs and involves other tissues as well. Infants have hepatosplenomegaly and cardiomyopathy. The inheritance is autosomal recessive and the infants die before 1 year of age.

A milder form exists that presents in infancy and childhood; however, the rate of progression is much slower. The patients usually do not survive beyond the second decade.

CK levels in this disorder are usually elevated and the EMG is myopathic. The biopsy shows a striking vacuolar myopathy that is characteristic of the disease. Assays for acid maltase show absence of enzyme activity in all forms. There is no available treatment yet.

Disorders of Lipid Metabolism

Free fatty acids are oxidized in the mitochondria. The acids are mobilized into the mitochondria by several enzymes and carrier proteins, of which the clinically important ones are carnitine palmityl transferase (CPT) and carnitine.

Carnitine Palmityl Transferase Deficiency

Signs and Symptoms. Patients with CPT deficiency suffer from symptoms similar to those of patients with glycogenoses. They complain of fatigue, muscle pain and cramps, and repeated bouts of myoglobinuria. They do not have any demonstrable weakness. The pains are milder and the muscles are tender, but contractures do not occur. The episodes are triggered by prolonged exertion and not by short bouts of heavy exercise. They are also precipitated by fasting.

Investigation and Diagnosis. CK levels are usually elevated during attacks only. The EMG is normal and so is the muscle biopsy. Special stains for fats demonstrate increased lipid content in the muscle. The forearm ischemic exercise test shows a normal rise in lactate as expected. Enzymatic assays for CPT show the enzyme deficiency. Patients are advised not to fast and informed about the complications of prolonged exercise.

Carnitine Deficiency

Several clinical syndromes are associated with carnitine deficiency; some are limited to muscle and others are more systemic. Muscle carnitine deficiency usually manifests in adulthood as progressive myopathy. The diagnosis is established by muscle biopsy and by demonstrating low muscle carnitine content.

Mitochondrial Disorders

As we learn more about mitochondrial physiology and genetics it has become increasingly difficult to classify mitochondrial disorders. The earlier classifications used constellations of signs and symptoms as the basis for differentiation. Newer schemes use the enzymatic abnor-

malities as the basis. Now some researchers are suggesting that the genetic abnormalities should be the focal point. Rather than going into controversial details about the new genetic and enzymatic discoveries, this section will focus on the main symptoms of mitochondrial defects and how to recognize them and make the diagnosis.

Signs and Symptoms. These are a heterogeneous group of disorders. They all are characterized by defects in energy production; thus exercise intolerance is a salient feature. There is less muscle pain and cramping and minimal myoglobinuria.

Some patients have a progressive myopathy involving the extraocular muscles, the syndrome of progressive external ophthalmoplegia. Some have additional pigmentary retinal degeneration, cerebellar and other CNS symptoms, and a generalized myopathy. This constitutes the Kearns-Sayre syndrome. Others have sensorineural hearing loss and seizures, and some have stroke-like episodes, encephalopathy, and lactic acidosis, giving rise to the syndromes of MERRF (myoclonic epilepsy/ragged red fiber) or MELAS (mitochondrial encephalopathy, lactic acidosis, and stroke-like episodes), respectively. The onset of symptoms is usually in childhood but can vary somewhat. The severity is quite variable. Inheritance is com-

---

Pearls and Perils:
Metabolic Myopathies

1. Patients with McArdle's disease show a peculiar fluctuation in their symptoms. Although at times they are incapacitated by the mildest exercise, at other times they lead normal lives.
2. Patients with CPT deficiency can sustain heavy activity in abnormal fashion. However, significantly milder exercise, if sustained for longer periods, can be devastating.
3. The family history is extremely important when trying to establish the diagnosis of mitochondrial diseases. It should be remembered that these disorders can affect multiple systems. Therefore, one must inquire about those systems as well in taking the family history.
4. It is important to remember that, although the ischemic forearm exercise test establishes the diagnosis in glycogen storage myopathies, it causes muscle contractures and necrosis in affected patients. The test should not be routinely repeated for demonstration purposes, and, as soon as contractures begin, the test should be terminated.
5. One cannot overemphasize the need to recognize rhabdomyolysis. In certain cases the myoglobinuria reaches magnitudes that can cause acute renal failure.

plex because some mitochondrial enzymes are coded for by nuclear DNA and others by mitochondrial DNA, which is maternally transmitted. Some of the patients have a relatively benign course, others have respiratory insufficiency requiring assisted ventilation, and others have cardiac conduction defects and arrhythmias.

Investigation and Diagnosis. Usually baseline serum lactate and pyruvate are elevated, along with certain CSF amino acids and proteins. The EMG is nonspecific and the muscle biopsy shows a mild myopathy with the characteristic ragged red fibers using the modified Gomori trichrome stain. Electron microscopy shows subsarcolemmal collections of abnormally large mitochondria. A definitive diagnosis is made by enzymatic assay of the oxidative function of the mitochondria, and determining the site of dysfunction along the respiratory chain. Currently DNA analysis is not readily available. EKG and Holter monitoring are useful in detecting early cardiac abnormalities.

Treatment. Some patients respond to certain vitamins that can act as electron transporters along the respiratory chain and thus bypass the defects; however, there are few case reports indicating success with such trials. The vitamins include CoQ_{10}, ascorbic acid, and vitamin K. Succinate has also been used. Otherwise, treatment is aimed toward controlling seizures and managing cardiac abnormalities.

NEUROMUSCULAR JUNCTION DEFECTS

Neuromuscular junction defects are characterized by abnormal acetylcholine transmission. The defect may be at the presynaptic or at the receptor end. The most common disorders are the myasthenic syndromes and botulism.

MYASTHENIC SYNDROMES

In the myasthenic category one encounters several disorders of neuromuscular transmission that can be separated clinically and electrophysiologically. These include transient neonatal myasthenia, congenital myasthenia, juvenile myasthenia gravis, and the Lambert-Easton syndrome. The latter is extremely rare in children and will not be discussed here.

Transient Neonatal Myasthenia

Signs and Symptoms. Neonates with transient neonatal myasthenia are born to mothers with myasthenia gravis (MG) and present immediately or soon after birth with hypotonia. They have variable degrees of weakness proximally more than distally. Characteristically sucking and occasionally swallowing are impaired. The neonates may

FEATURE TABLE 16-7. NEUROMUSCULAR JUNCTION DEFECTS

Disease	Discriminating Features	Consistent Features	Variable Features
Transient neonatal myasthenia	1. A combination of an affected mother and a transiently weak infant	1. Hypotonia 2. Affected mother 3. Course less than 12 weeks 4. Positive Tensilon test	1. Degree of weakness 2. Antibodies to AchR
Congenital or infantile myasthenia	1. A combination of clinical findings and absent antibodies to AchR	1. Fixed ophthalmoparesis 2. Nonaffected mother 3. No antibodies to AchR 4. Fatigable muscles	1. Response to Tensilon
Juvenile myasthenia gravis	1. Antibodies to AchR	1. Fatigable weakness 2. Autoimmune nature 3. Antibodies to AchR 4. Neck extensor weakness more than flexors	1. Bulbar weakness 2. Response to thymectomy
Botulism	1. Presence of *Botulinum* toxin	1. Pupillary nonreactivity 2. Bulbar weakness 3. Posttetanic facilitation 4. Presence of toxin 5. Areflexia	1. Fatigable weakness 2. Response to Tensilon

also have breathing difficulties, but the condition lasts no more than 3 months. Interestingly, the presence of this condition cannot be predicted from the clinical status of the mother nor from her antibody titer. Nonetheless, it is felt to be due to passive transfer of maternal antibodies to the fetus. These antibodies are directed at the acetylcholine receptor (AchR).

Investigation and Diagnosis. The edrophonium (Tensilon) or Neostigmine tests should support the diagnosis. Levels of circulating antibodies to AchR are helpful, but they have been seen in unaffected babies of myasthenic mothers as well.

Treatment. Pyridostigmine can be used if weakness is significant. One can usually reassure the parents that the condition is temporary, and that the prognosis is good.

Congenital Myasthenia

Signs and Symptoms. Congenital myasthenia is a much less common disorder, which is present from birth. Boys are more frequently affected and usually have ptosis and extraocular and bulbar muscle weakness. They also have the other symptoms of fatigable proximal muscle weakness. The disease does not seem to progress significantly and the extraocular motility dysfunction remains fixed. Patients do respond to Tensilon and other acetylcholinesterase inhibitors, albeit not dramatically. There is usually a positive family history but not necessarily one affecting the mother.

Investigation and Diagnosis. The Tensilon test usually supports the diagnosis, but antibodies to AchR are absent. Repetitive stimulation usually demonstrates a typical decrement, which confirms the diagnosis. Single-fiber EMG shows increased jitter, which is an indication

of defective neuromuscular transmission; however, this test is difficult to perform on children. Some researchers have found cases with acetylcholinesterase deficiency, abnormal acetylcholine, and slow ion channel defects.

Treatment. Treatment is limited to administration of acetylcholinesterase inhibitors.

Juvenile Myasthenia Gravis

Signs and Symptoms. Juvenile MG is essentially the same as the adult form of MG. The patients present with fatigable weakness of the extraocular and bulbar muscles, and they later develop generalized weakness. In about 15% of cases the disease is limited to the eyes, and about half of them never develop generalized symptoms. As in the adult form, patients are subject to fluctuations of symptoms, which include the myasthenic crisis. A certain percentage will have a spontaneous remission.

Investigation and Diagnosis. The Tensilon test and repetitive stimulation usually establish the diagnosis. There is usually an elevation of antibody titers.

Treatment. Most physicians believe that generalized autoimmune MG should be treated with immune suppression. The same strategy is recommended for juvenile MG. Along with steroids, plasma exchange is beneficial during the acute crisis. If patients do not respond to steroids other forms of immune suppression can be used. Most patients with generalized symptoms should undergo thymectomy as this increases the likelihood of remission.

BOTULISM

Botulism is caused by the exotoxin of *Clostridium botulinum*. The toxin is extremely potent in its ability to block neuromuscular transmission. It impairs the ability of nerve terminals to release acetylcholine.

Signs and Symptoms. Patients present with bulbar symptoms, diplopia, dysphagia, and occasionally nausea and vomiting. The weakness spreads rapidly; respiratory paralysis is almost inevitable and usually is the cause of death. Symptoms usually begin 2 hours to 7 days after ingestion of contaminated food. Cases have been seen secondary to wound infection. The patients are usually areflexic and the pupils are unreactive. There is no sensory involvement and fatigability is not as prominent as in MG. However, patients may have a positive response to Tensilon.

Infants may become irritable and weak and usually are constipated. As in older patients, bulbar and respiratory weakness is common. The disease is due to ingestion of the bacterium itself and elaboration of the toxin in the gut.

Pearls and Perils: Neuromuscular Junction Defects

1. Of patients with ocular myasthenia who will develop generalized symptoms, 90% will do so in the first year.
2. Patients who do not show a response to Tensilon should be tested further with intramuscular neostigmine. This is particularly important in patients with ocular myasthenia.
3. Hot temperatures worsen the transmission defect.
4. Patients with myasthenia can have crises precipitated by mild systemic illnesses.
5. A number of drugs should be avoided in patients with MG. The most notorious are the aminoglycoside antibiotics.

Investigation and Diagnosis. The Tensilon test is somewhat positive. These patients may be confused with those with Guillain-Barré syndrome, but when spinal taps are done the CSF is normal. Electrophysiology supports the diagnosis. There is a decrement to repetitive stimulation as in MG. However, the compound muscle action potential is diminished and there is a posttetanic facilitation similar to that seen in the Lambert-Eaton Syndrome. Sensory evoked responses and nerve conduction velocities are normal. The diagnosis is established by detecting and typing the toxin in the serum. The test is an antibody neutralization test usually performed at the Centers for Disease Control. Gastric contents and a stool specimen should also be sent.

Treatment. Generally supportive measures to manage respiratory failure are all that is needed. Patients may require a tracheostomy, because recovery may take several months. The mortality rate is 25%. One can administer botulinum antitoxin, but the side effects are frequent and the efficacy is not proven.

DISEASES OF PERIPHERAL NERVES

Although peripheral neuropathies are not common in childhood and infancy, two topics should be discussed: these are the hereditary motor sensory neuropathies (HMSNs) and acute acquired inflammatory demyelinating polyradiculoneuropathy or the Guillain-Barré syndrome (GBS).

HEREDITARY MOTOR SENSORY NEUROPATHIES

The HMSNs are a group of inherited neuropathies classified on the basis of the pathophysiologic process involved. These processes can be demyelinating, axonal, or both.

FEATURE TABLE 16–8. PERIPHERAL NEUROPATHIES

Disease	Discriminating Features	Consistent Features	Variable Features
Charcot-Marie-Tooth Neuropathy			
HMSN-1	1. Demyelinating neuropathy and dominant inheritance	1. Onion bulb formation 2. Hypertrophic nerves 3. Pes cavus and hammer toes 4. Linkage to Duffy locus 5. Slow conduction velocities	1. Degree of weakness
HMSN-2	1. Axonal neuropathy and dominant inheritance	1. Nerves are not palpable 2. Pes cavus and hammer toes 3. Axonal degeneration	1. Degree of weakness
Dejerine-Sottas Neuropathy			
HMSN-3	1. A combination of clinical features and pattern of inheritance	1. Infantile onset 2. Hypertrophic nerves 3. Autosomal recessive 4. Demyelinating and axonal neuropathy 5. Marked onion bulb formation 6. Severe hypotonia 7. Elevated CSF protein	1. Degree of weakness
Guillain-Barré Syndrome			
	1. Albuminocytologic dissociation in CSF (CSF protein elevation without pleocytosis)	1. Demyelination 2. Early muscle pains 3. Facial weakness 4. Depressed reflexes 5. Slow conduction velocities with blocks	1. Axonal degeneration 2. Respiratory involvement 3. Autonomic involvement

Charcot-Marie-Tooth Neuropathy (HMSN-1)

Signs and Symptoms. HMSN-1 is a dominantly inherited hypertrophic neuropathy. The disease is linked to the Duffy locus on the long arm of chromosome 1. The motor system is predominantly affected with variable degrees of sensory and autonomic involvement. There is a marked heterogeneity within the same pedigree. The weakness begins with the anterior tibial compartment muscles, and patients develop pes cavus and hammer toes. In severe cases generalized weakness ensues, involving both upper and lower extremities, distally more than proximally; patients may be wheelchair bound by their 40s. In the mildest forms only pes cavus is noted and the diagnosis is based on electrophysiologic tests. There is marked atrophy of the lower leg muscles when affected; initially this spares the posterior compartment. Reflexes are absent diffusely and a variable degree of predominantly proprioceptive sensory loss is found. The nerves are easily palpated.

Investigation and Diagnosis. The diagnosis is suspected clinically. Nerve conduction velocities are markedly and uniformly slowed in all extremities. There are usually no conduction blocks and the reduced velocities are present in minimally affected members as well. The pathology shows marked reduction of myelinated fiber density, increased number of fibers undergoing demyelination, and onion bulb formation.

HMSN-2

Signs and Symptoms. This is a predominantly axonal neuropathy with a dominant inheritance. The clinical course is very similar to that of HMSN-1 except for the absence of palpable hypertrophic nerves. There is also less sensory involvement.

Investigation and Diagnosis. No genetic linkage has been identified. The diagnosis is made based on clinical signs and symptoms and nerve conduction velocities, which support an axonal neuropathy. There is a diminished compound muscle action potential with preserved conduction velocities. The EMG shows evidence of denervation. The pathology typically shows axonal degeneration with little demyelination or onion bulb formation.

Dejerine-Sottas Neuropathy (HMSN-3)

HMSN-3 is a recessively inherited variant of the hypertrophic form, HMSN-1. The onset occurs in infancy and the children are severely affected. The nerve conduction velocities are extremely slow and there is typically an elevation of CSF protein. The nerves are hypertrophied with striking onion bulb formation. These patients are usually confined to a wheelchair by their second decade.

Treatment

No specific therapy is available for any of the HMSNs. No prenatal diagnosis can be made, nor can one accurately predict the prognosis. Supportive care in the form of physical therapy, splints, and surgical intervention is of paramount importance to improve functional abilities.

ACUTE ACQUIRED INFLAMMATORY DEMYELINATING POLYRADICULONEUROPATHY (GUILLAIN-BARRÉ SYNDROME)

GBS is much less common among children than adults, although it can affect all age groups. It is believed to be an autoimmune disorder that may be provoked by an antecedent viral infection, surgery, or immunization. Several viruses have been suspected to induce GBS. These include, among others, cytomegalovirus and Epstein-Barr, human immunodeficiency, or hepatitis viruses.

Signs and Symptoms. A history of a viral illness preceding the onset of the weakness by about 1 to 3 weeks is commonly obtained. The illness tends to be an upper respiratory tract or gastrointestinal infection. Patients present with a rapidly progressive ascending paralysis. The symptoms peak in about a week, but may progress for 3 weeks or more. Proximal muscles are weaker occasionally and there is a variable degree of sensory loss. Tendon reflexes are lost early in the course and sometimes never return. Cranial nerve involvement is com-

---

Pearls and Perils: Diseases of Peripheral Nerves

1. Among families with type 1 HMSN, the earlier the disease appears, the faster the progression seems to be.
2. Although patients with HMSN-1 rarely complain of sensory loss, they are often unable to walk at night. This probably represents proprioceptive loss that can be demonstrated clinically.
3. Patients with GBS almost always have weakness of their hamstring muscles even when other thigh muscles are minimally involved.
4. Patients with GBS succumb to two major complications aside from respiratory weakness: infections and autonomic dysfunction. This autonomic instability, if unrecognized, can be the cause of death.
5. Fewer than 10% of patients with GBS have an early relapse. Recent studies have shown that this may be related to inadequate plasma exchange.

mon and at times is the presenting symptom. In severe cases respiratory muscles are involved, necessitating mechanical ventilation. There is usually an element of bladder dysfunction and autonomic instability, which may be severe. Pain and muscle cramps are early and common symptoms and persist until the patient starts to recover. In most patients, recovery is incomplete and may take months. Few, however, recover fully.

Investigation and Diagnosis. The differential diagnosis of acute weakness has been discussed earlier. Establishing a diagnosis will depend on finding CSF protein elevation without pleocytosis, and supportive electrophysiologic tests. Initially both the CSF and nerve conduction velocities may be normal. Ultimately the nerve conduction velocities show conduction blocks, slow velocities, and prolonged F waves. Variable degrees of axonal damage may be evident on EMG and nerve conduction velocities. The pathology is of segmental demyelination with an inflammatory infiltrate.

Treatment. Early plasma exchange seems to hasten recovery. It should be instituted before the patient's weakness plateaus. Because most cases recover spontaneously, therapy is reserved for those with a rapidly progressive weakness with loss of ambulation or early bulbar involvement. Steroids have not been clearly beneficial. Prognosis is related to the degree of axonal loss and whether respiratory weakness was present.

ANNOTATED BIBLIOGRAPHY

Dubowitz V: *A Color Atlas of Muscle Disorders in Childhood.* Chicago, Wolf, 1989.

This is probably the most illustrative text in its category. It combines excellent pathologic specimens with representative case reports. The disease description is in tabular form; however, it is complete and concise.

Brooke M: *A Clinician's View of Neuromuscular Diseases,* 2nd ed. Baltimore, Md, Williams & Wilkins, 1986.

Brooke's clinical descriptions and anecdotes are by far the most pleasurable to read. They are complete, informative, and coupled with the recent pathophysiologic understanding of the individual disorders.

BIBLIOGRAPHY

Carpenter S, Karpati G: *Pathology of Skeletal Muscle.* Edinburgh, Churchill Livingstone, 1984.

Dalakas M: *Polymyositis and Dermatomyositis.* Boston, Butterworths, 1988.

Dyck PJ, Thomas PK, Lambert EH, Bunge R: *Peripheral neuropathy,* 2nd ed. Philadelphia, WB Saunders, 1984.

Engel AG, Banker B: *Myology.* New York, McGraw-Hill, 1986.

Fenichel G: *Clinical Pediatric Neurology: A Signs and Symptoms Approach.* Philadelphia, WB Saunders, 1988.

Hausmanowa-Petrusewicz I, Karwanska A: Electromyographic findings in different forms of infantile and juvenile spinal muscular atrophy. *Muscle and Nerve* 9:37–46, 1986.

Hausmanowa-Petrusewicz I, Zaremba J, Borkowska J: Chronic proximal spinal muscular atrophy of childhood and adolescence: Problems of classification and genetic counselling. *J Med Genet* 22:350–353, 1985.

McKhann GM, Griffin JW, Cornblath DR, Mellits ED, Fisher RS, Quaskey SA: Plasmapheresis and Guillain-Barré syndrome: Analysis of prognostic factors and the effect of plasmapheresis. *Ann Neurol* 23:347–353, 1988.

Riggs JE (ed): *Muscle Diseases.* Philadelphia, WB Saunders, 1988.

Walton JN: *Disorders of Voluntary Muscle,* 5th ed. Edinburgh, Churchill Livingstone, 1988.

Malformations of the Central Nervous System I

Neurocutaneous Syndromes of the Dermal Pigmentary Unit

Daniel W. Stowens

Neurocutaneous syndromes are disorders in which the dermal and neurologic signs and symptoms are believed to arise from the same mechanism, or at least from synchronous mechanisms. Most of the disorders are genetic diseases, and, as is emphasized in this chapter, important aspects of the clinical syndrome are thought to be based on the common embryology of skin and brain. More specifically, the disorders are expressions of the abnormal function or structure of cells formed before or during the stage of differentiation of the central nervous system (CNS) from the (neuro)ectodermal layer of the embryo.

With our ever-increasing knowledge of the biologic pathology of human disease, the disparities among the various disorders included in a chapter such as this one have become more evident. The list of disorders to be discussed in detail is arbitrary—if not capricious or idiosyncratic. The most satisfactory plan would be to organize the discussion to correspond with basic pathologic principles. With understanding of the molecular biology of growth, development, maintenance of cellular integrity, and the like, the classification of these disorders would be much easier than it now is. A successful classification scheme based on embryologic principles alone has not yet been developed, and its creation will not be attempted here.

There are many diseases, disorders, and syndromes that have been labeled *neurocutaneous*. An incomplete list includes the following:

Neurofibromatosis
Tuberous sclerosis
Incontinentia pigmenti

Hypomelanosis of Ito
Primary meningocutaneous melanosis
Albinism
Waardenburg's syndrome
Lentiginosis-deafness-cardiomyopathy

Linear sebaceous nevus
Epidermal nevus
Basal cell nevus syndrome
Focal dermal hypoplasia

Sjögren-Larsson syndrome
Neuroichthyosis

Sturge-Weber syndrome
Ataxia-telangiectasia
Cutaneomeningospinal
    angiomatosis
Hereditary hemorrhagic
    telangiectasia (Osler-Rendu-Weber disease)
Klippel-Trenauney-Weber syndrome

Neurocutaneous lipomatosis
Phenylketonuria
Homocystinuria
Argininosuccinic aciduria
Citrullinemia
Fabry's disease
Menkes's kinky hair disease
Fabry's disease
Refsum's syndrome
Fucosidosis
Biotin-responsive multiple
    carboxylase deficiency

Chediak-Higashi syndrome

von Hippel-Lindau disease
Xeroderma pigmentosum
Cockayne's syndrome

Poikiloderma congenitale
Progeria
Albright's syndrome
Familial dysautonomia

Many of the historical entries on this list are discussed in other chapters. For example, several of the syndromes are now commonly classified with the lysosomal enzyme defects, organic acidemias, and other known metabolic diseases. Future lists of neurocutaneous syndromes will be even shorter than this one, as familial tumor syndromes, DNA repair defects, and angioplastic disorders are similarly reclassified.

In lieu of convincing embryologic explanations for the syndromes, a grouping of the disorders by skin pathology will be used in this discussion. Furthermore, several of the more common syndromes involve a specific component of skin, the pigmentary unit, and they will be discussed together. The other disorders will be reviewed in chapter 18 as examples of more specifically neurologic malformations. For many of the diseases the embryologic features are not well understood. In others the combined nervous system and cutaneous involvement is the result of those organs reflecting a systemic process. I have tried to include disorders not discussed elsewhere in this volume. It is hoped that some clinical parallel exists between the syndromes discussed and others omitted or only mentioned in passing.

NEUROFIBROMATOSIS AND TUBEROUS SCLEROSIS

The archetypical neurocutaneous syndromes are characterized by prominent dysfunction of the pigmented cells of the epidermis. Besides abnormalities of the melanocytes and their innervated keratinocytes, the disease complexes manifest other dermal abnormalities. The physically evident pigmentary changes are important diagnostic and pathogenic clues. The two most common autosomal dominant diseases are neurofibromatosis and tuberous sclerosis.

Neurofibromatosis

Neurofibromatosis includes at least two distinct syndromes: type I, von Recklinghausen's disease, and type II, bilateral acoustic neuroma. Both have recently been linked to specific chromosomal regions: the long arm of chromosome 17 (17q11.2) for type I, and the long arm of chromosome 22 (between 22 q11 and 22q12) for type II. Given the appropriate family setting, accurate determination of carrier status and prenatal diagnosis is possible. Rapid improvement in the precision of the genetic assignment is anticipated, with much more clinically useful capabilities eagerly awaited.

The neurofibromatoses are archetypical neurocristopathies; most manifestations of the diseases are linked to, if not explained by, putative dysfunction of the ubiquitous cells of that lineage. In both disorders the clinical manifestations of the diseases are variable enough in intensity and anatomic distribution to weaken the hypothesis of an overabundance of a systemic hormone, growth factor, or similar substance. There are abnormalities of growth factors in the neurofibromatoses; for example, cerebrospinal nerve growth factor concentrations are elevated in the type II syndrome. However, an aberration of a cell surface receptor or cytoskeletal structure, or other such "end-organ" mechanism in cells of the neuroectoderm, would be a more inclusive theory of pathogenesis.

A possibly distinct form, segmental neurofibromatosis, reveals signs similar to those of type I disorder in only a segment of the body that received cells from one portion of the neural crest. Presumably, the type I genetic abnormality has arisen by somatic mutation and is expressed in only the clonal neuroectodermal derivatives. This form has been classified as a separate type of neurofibromatosis because of the obvious differences in the clinical and genetic implications of this diagnosis and that of type I. The cellular biologic disorder may be identical. Combinations of signs and symptoms have been recognized that suggest neurofibromatosis with significantly different anatomic localization (for example, palmar neurofibromata); variant time course (for example, late onset); or limited expression (for example, only numerous cafe au lait spots). Thus naming of at least one more type of neurofibromatosis is warranted—variant neurofibromatosis. The clues to the pathogenesis of the neurofibromatoses are certainly present in the variant forms—histologic, genetic, anatomic, physiologic. To date an elegant synthesis of concepts and observations has eluded even the most persistent and enthusiastic students of the disorders. In practical terms, for those of us struggling to deal with today's patients despite our relative ignorance, it is probably useful to assign each patient a diagnosis of typical type I, typical type II, segmental, or other (variant) type. A discussion of the typical presentations follows.

Neurofibromatosis Type I (von Recklinghausen's Disease, Peripheral Neurofibromatosis)

Neurofibromatosis type I is the newest designation of the most common disorder in the group of neurofibromatoses. This autosomal dominant disease, the result of a derangement of a gene near the centromere on the long arm of chromosome 17, has been estimated to occur in anywhere from 1 in 2500 or 3300 to 1 in 8000 individuals. The true prevalence is most likely somewhere in between. As the molecular genetic diagnosis becomes easier, more accurate determinations will be made and genetic features will be refined or confirmed. The penetrance of the neurofibromatosis I gene is very near 100%, based on the examination of obligate heterozygotes and other defined genetic populations. An intimately related feature is a very high rate of spontaneous mutation. Even with the genetic tools at hand, some large population studies are needed to generate the necessary data for accurate genetic epidemiologic measurements. In neurofibromatosis I the gene has been altered by virtually every form of chromosomal derangement possible—deletion, point mutation, translocation, and insertion. The exact product of the very large, possibly compound, gene is as yet unknown.

The pathogenesis of the disorder remains a mystery. That the cells of neural crest derivation express the abnormal gene is clear. That expression can occur before birth, perhaps as the result of decreased responsiveness to normal growth control factors, has also been established. However, a variety of abnormalities in the CNS has been reported. Accordingly, disordered growth of tissues other than the neural crest may be involved. Alternatively, the pluripotent neural crest cells may demonstrate the genetic pathology as another form of abnormal response to growth suppression and promotion factors, lack of restriction of differentiation. The peculiar features of the CNS in neurofibromatosis I may be the manifestations of neural crest cells usually only derived from the caudal portion of the crest. The generation of a protein like guanosine-diphosphatase activating protein in part by the gene for neurofibromatosis I, presumably interacting with oncogene functions, is a plausible route for such disordered embryologic functions. Although future editions of this chapter may be able to give a detailed description of the molecular biology of the disorder, for now a clinical overview will have to suffice.

The diagnosis of neurofibromatosis I rests on the occurrence of several features that can be combined, in any one patient, in different ways. According to a National Institutes of Health consensus conference (July 1987), the diagnosis is confirmed in people with two of the following features: cafe au lait spots, neurofibromas, axillary or inguinal freckling, optic glioma, iris (Lisch) nodules, one of the distinctive osseous lesions (thoracic scoliosis, anterolateral bowing of the tibias, pseudoarthrosis, sphenoid wing dysplasia), or a family history of neurofibromatosis I. The criteria are thought to be stringent enough to ensure a very high likelihood of correct positive diagnosis. Conversely, it is now known that people who do not have neurofibromas, cafe au lait spots, or Lisch nodules do not have neurofibromatosis I. The caveats and exceptions to the rules have to do with the age of the subject. Whereas virtually all afflicted individuals have Lisch nodules at age 20 years or older, some younger ones do not. Cafe au lait spots may not be recognized until after the first birthday. Neurofibromas develop or, at least increase in size, with age as well. The diagnosis may thus be suspected in infants and young children and not confirmed until the patient has aged sufficiently. Because of the extraordinarily high penetrance of the gene, a child's parents can be said not to have the gene (disease) if they meet the exclusionary criteria and are older than 20 years.

Dermatology. The skin manifestations of neurofibromatosis I are multiple. The most readily recognized sign is the cafe au lait spot. Typically oval, larger than 10 mm in diameter, and sharply demarcated with smooth borders, cafe au lait spots in neurofibromatosis may nevertheless be atypical in any of those features. The number of spots needed to suggest or confirm the diagnosis increases slightly with age: six spots larger than 15 mm in diameter after puberty, five spots larger than 5 mm before. A person with neurofibromatosis I with no cafe au lait spots is almost never seen, and this sign is virtually pathognomonic for the disease in itself. Histologically, the cafe au lait spots of neurofibromatosis are nearly

FEATURE TABLE 17–1. NEUROFIBROMATOSIS TYPE I

Discriminating Features	Consistent Features	Variable Features
1. Multiple cafe au lait spots	1. Diffuse pigmentary changes	1. Megalencephaly
2. Lisch nodules	2. Migraine	2. Specific orthopedic deformities
3. Multiple neurofibromas		3. Learning disability
		4. Generalized pruritis
		5. Brain tumors
		6. Epilepsy
		7. Mental retardation
		8. Meningocele
		9. Megacolon
		10. Hypertrophic neuropathy

identical to the cafe au lait spots of normal skin. The
neural crest–derived melanocytes of the cafe au lait spot
produce more pigment to be transmitted to the overlying keratinocytes than those of the surrounding skin.
The melanocytes of neurofibromatosis I have more giant
pigmented granules (fused melanosome with lysosome,
secondary megalomelanosome, melanin macroglobule
[MMG]) than those of any other disorder, including
other forms of neurofibromatosis. It is not only the melanocytes of the cafe au lait spots that have more MMGs.
The melanocytes of type I are a consistent, diffuse neural crest manifestation of the genetic abnormality. Col-
lectively, skin cells of neuroectodermal origin may be abnormally numerous. Alternatively, a larger than normal
proportion of them may develop into the pigmented
cells of the cafe au lait spots.

Other pigmentary abnormalities are present in
neurofibromatosis I. The spots of so-called axillary freckling are not true freckles but very small, diffuse cafe au
lait spots. The diagnostic features of the freckling are the
location (sun-shy areas, such as the axillae, groin, and
popliteal fossae) and the inducing factors (minor trauma
such as intertrigo or abrasion of tight clothing, such as
brassieres and collars). The sign is pathognomonic for
neurofibromatosis I.

A diffuse hyperpigmentation, perhaps the macroscopic manifestation of the melanin MMGs, can often
allow relatives to differentiate affected family members
from nonaffected individuals. With experience, clinicians can recognize the sallow, very slightly grayish skin
tone as different from the normal variation in Caucasian
coloration. A similar, subtle aberration of coloration may
be present in dark-complected races, but my experience
and perceptive sensitivity have been insufficient to detect it.

Dermal tumors in neurofibromatosis I have been
classified primarily by location, as cutaneous, subcutaneous, or proximal (plexiform) neurofibromas. The peripheral nerve tumors in general are of four histologic
varieties: schwannoma, neurofibroma, plexiform neurofibroma, and neurofibrosarcoma. The schwannomas,
in which the tumor cell is clearly the Schwann cell, arise
proximally in major nerve roots and trunks. These tumors are rare in type I; they are the predominant nerve
tumor in type II. Distal tumors—cutaneous, subcutaneous, and plexiform—are all neurofibromas. The tumor
cells in these lesions are of neural crest origin with cell
surface markers and the intracellular chemistry of
Schwann cells, the perineural cells. Neurofibromas involve nerves diffusely, unlike schwannomas, which
arise from better-differentiated precursors and expand
to the periphery of the nerve. Cutaneous neurofibromas
involve the distal branches of the cutaneous nerves.
More proximal cutaneous nerves yield the subcutaneous
form. With tumorous expansion of larger, even more
proximal nerves, the plexiform neurofibromas arise. It

is these larger tumors that produce a clinical neuropathy. It is also only from the plexiform neurofibromas
that the malignant neurofibrosarcoma develops.

Neurology. The neurologic problems of people with
neurofibromatosis I can be subdivided into those of the
central and peripheral nervous systems. The clinical
problems in the latter group include pain, dysfunction,
secondary orthopedic reactions, disfigurement, and
neoplastic development. The signs and symptoms arising from the effects of neurofibromatosis on the brain
and spinal cord include headaches, developmental delays, mental retardation, other deficits of higher cortical
function, seizures, loss of vision, and secondary orthopedic reactions.

In a general overview, the usual presenting neurologic problems are developmental delays or frank
mental retardation and seizures. Much more common neurologic symptoms are headaches, pruritus, and
neuropathic and tumoral pain.

Formal mental retardation is more common in neurofibromatosis than in the general population, but less
severe deficits of higher cortical function are even more
prevalent. More precise estimates of the number of neurofibromatosis children with speech delay, motor developmental delays, and deficits of specific learning functions are being developed in multispecialty clinics for
neurofibromatosis. The prevalence of these disorders, in
some cases rather subjectively defined, in the general
pediatric population of the United States is unknown.
Comparison between groups of children may be difficult.

The most common expression of developmental
delay in neurofibromatosis I is a lag in the development
of speech. As only a very small percentage of older
people with the disorder have a developmental language disorder, the symptom must truly reflect a delay
in cortical maturation of function rather than a malformative lesion of the dominant cerebral hemisphere. Delays in motor development are seen less frequently. Occasional associations between neurologic deficits and
abnormalities of brain on magnetic resonance imaging
(MRI) or computed tomography (CT) are recognized.
One 3-year-old boy showed delays in development of
ambulation; stereotaxic biopsy of a T_2-bright brainstem
lesion revealed only a subtle disproportion between
neural structures and cerebral microvasculature. Usually the relationship between patches of high-intensity
tissue on T_2 MRI and cerebral dysfunction is not clear.
In the majority of patients such "brain spots" are associated with no specific deficit. A consensus is developing
that the more spots are present, the more likely there
is to be a deficit of higher cortical function. Attentional
deficits, distractibility, dyslexia, deficits of short-term
memory, and other learning disorders are well represented in children with the disorder.

Somewhat surprisingly, seizures in patients with neurofibromatosis I are generalized in some patients and focal in others. The electroencephalographic and clinical features of the seizures are no different from those of most other epilepsies. Both major subtypes of generalized seizures are seen, absence and major motor, perhaps reflecting more the age of the patient than the formal pathophysiologic basis of the epilepsy. Focal seizures seem to originate slightly less often in the temporal lobe than in other epileptics. This observation may be heavily biased by my predominant exposure to children with the disease. True temporal lobe foci dominate much less often in children than in adults.

Migraine headaches—and the panoply of other paroxysmal autonomic symptoms, including recurrent abdominal pains, paroxysmal vertigo, syncope, motion sickness, recurrent limb pains (''growing pains''), and the parasomnias—occur in at least 80% of children with neurofibromatosis I.

Pain arising from neurofibromas, usually plexiform, is the most common indication for surgery on the tumors. Statistical data are not available on the responsiveness of the neuropathic pain to medical management.

The neuropathology of neurofibromatosis I has revealed a diversity of abnormalities. The peripheral nerve tumors were mentioned in the discussion of the dermatology of the disorder. The schwannoma is seen frequently in neurofibromatosis, but recent reviews of the neuropathology by type of disorder strongly suggest that the true Schwann cell tumor is the predominant extra-axial tumor in neurofibromatosis II and is distinctly rare in type I. Acoustic neuromas almost never arise in type I; soon confirmatory data from intensive monitoring will be available.

More proximal neuropathologic features include meningiomas, arising in both the cranial and the spinal compartments. The tumors are always multiple in neurofibromatosis and show an unusual predilection for the choroid plexus. The type of neurofibromatosis in which meningiomas occur has not yet been clarified, but they are very frequent in type II. A clinically more prominent meningeal abnormality, dural ectasia, is definitely common in type I. The pathologically extended and expanded investment of cranial and spinal nerves by the dura gives rise to radiographic features very easily confounded with nerve involvement by tumor. Dural ectasia of the optic nerves can be important; very-high-resolution studies are needed to rule out the presence of an optic glioma. Dural ectasia of the acoustic nerves may suggest acoustic neuroma, leading to individual clinical confusion as well as causing academic controversy about the type distribution of the tumor. Clinical symptoms can arise from spinal dural ectasia if the structural integrity of vertebrae is compromised. Meningoceles are found in neurofibromatosis patients as well.

Often occurring in the nearly pathognomonic thoracic region, those defects are rarely symptomatic.

More central manifestations of type I have only recently been carefully discriminated from those of type II, ''central'' neurofibromatosis. Macrocephaly with or without infrequently symptomatic hydrocephalus is common enough to be part of the minor diagnostic criteria of type I. T_2-bright patches or spots on the MRI of the brain, or hypodense CT areas, are seen in about one-third of the patients undergoing those studies. Histology is limited, but gliosis, focal or more diffuse, in the subependymal and molecular layers was discovered in about half the cases of type I that were studied. Whether the glial proliferation is a hamartomatous process or a reactive state has not been clarified.

The foci of abnormal glia are strongly reminiscent of low-grade neoplasms. A high incidence of astrocytoma and malignant glioma in later years has been reported. Certain tumors are relatively common in children with neurofibromatosis I, including optic pathway and brainstem gliomas. The prognosis for CNS tumors is significantly better if they are associated with neurofibromatosis I than if they are not. Perhaps some of the neoplasms are hamartomas, or the gliomas actually reactive gliosis.

Vascular abnormalities have been discovered in the CNS in neurofibromatosis I. Cellular hyperplasia in small vessels is said to be similar to that seen in visceral organs. The exact cell type involved is not known. Endothelial cells, smooth muscle cells, or perineural cells of the vascular wall are candidates. Large vessel disease produces progressive occlusion of the carotid termini, perhaps by a related mechanism. Although rare, the vascular disorder with secondary moyamoya (collateralization) is more frequent in afflicted children than in the general population.

Syringomyelia, hydromyelia, and secondary myelopathic involvement from orthopedic spinal disease round out the CNS effects of neurofibromatosis I.

Nonneurocutaneous Manifestations. The skeleton is the other organ system frequently and significantly affected by the disease. Several malformative lesions are so highly linked to the diagnosis that they form part of the diagnostic criteria: dysplasia of the sphenoid wing, tibial or radial pseudoarthrosis, and thoracic vertebral anomalies with sharply angulated scoliosis or meningocele. The pathogenesis of the bony abnormalities is unknown. Clinically, the lesions respond poorly to surgical correction, suggesting a primary role for juxta- or periosteal soft tissue influences on bone.

There is no correlation between extent of involvement and severity of disease in the various organ systems: skin, nervous system, and bone. Also independent of the degree of expression in the primarily affected tissues are the infrequent pheochromocytomas, Wilms's

Pearls and Perils:
Neurofibromatosis Type I

1. Hyperpigmented patches over the midline of the back indicate an underlying neurofibroma involving the spinal cord or adjacent roots.

2. The characteristic bony lesions —sphenoid wing hypoplasia, tibial or radial pseudoarthroses, and thoracic vertebral anomalies— should be considered diagnostic for neurofibromatosis in children.

3. Probably the most common "false positive" diagnostic sign is multiple cafe au lait spots. Very, very few patients with neurofibromatosis have only these markers of the disorder.

4. The subcutaneous nerves in the neck are quite easily seen on clinical examination. They are often the nerves first recognized as involved by neurofibromatosis.

5. Slit-lamp ophthalmologic examination of parents is a rapid, quite accurate screen for the presence of the gene. Pigmentary features are more useful in prepubertal siblings.

tumors, rhabdomyosarcomas, leukemias, and short stature.

Clinical Management. The optimal management of the variety of problems in neurofibromatosis requires the coordinated attention of several concerned specialists. In the setting of a multispecialty clinic, now increasingly common in the United States, the management of orthopedic, neurologic, dermatologic, and genetic problems is made more efficient. In this chapter, the discussion of treatment will be limited to neurologic concerns, with acknowledgment of the importance of the other specialties and of general pediatric care.

Developmental delays and mental retardation respond to medical, behavioral, and educational therapies without significant concern for the specific etiology. Psychological evaluation, determination of visual and auditory acuity, and delineation of any overt neurologic deficits with the appropriate laboratory tests should be carried out at an early age. Support of the child and family can most easily be provided when expectations and prognosis are accurately developed.

The treatment of seizures should be no different from that of those in other epilepsies—valproate in the generalized epilepsies, carbamazepine in the focal epilepsies. I have avoided using phenytoin out of concern for the combined effects on subcutaneous tissues of both the disease and the drug. Other hydantoins (mephenytoin or ethotoin), valproate, chlorazepate, primidone, and oxcarbazepine are useful alternatives to carbamazepine. If valproate cannot be used, or is ineffective in

the generalized epilepsies, the barbiturates, hydantoins, carbamazepine, and benzodiazepines should be tried. Seizures in neurofibromatosis I do not require special consideration save for the cutaneous, partly cosmetic concerns noted earlier. Surgical treatment of focal seizures can be dramatically effective and should not be avoided on the basis of a diagnosis of neurofibromatosis I. Many neurofibromatosis patients have multifocal seizures, but the likelihood of successful surgery can be determined by the obligatory preoperative evaluation.

Common forms of prophylactic antimigraine therapy may be as effective in the children with the disorder as in those without it. Cyproheptadine works to reduce pruritus as well; amitriptyline is often helpful in reducing the intensity of pain in neurofibromas.

Medical management of pain can use carbamazepine, phenytoin, or the tricyclic antidepressants, as well as analgesics. Anecdotal experience speaks to the efficacy of this approach in some patients. Attempts to modify the growth, and thus dysfunction, of the tumors have been carried out using a variety of agents. Hormonal therapy, following the observation of tumor growth (and hyperpigmentation) during pregnancy, has been unsuccessful. An anti–mastcell antihistamine, ketotifen, has been used effectively for generalized pruritus; measurements of tumor number, size, and distribution are still being collected.

Neurofibromatosis Type II (Bilateral Acoustic Neuroma, Central Neurofibromatosis)

Neurofibromatosis II is now the preferred designation for a disorder that occasionally has clinical manifestations of cafe au lait spots and cutaneous neurofibromas. Intraaxial tumors, most frequently multiple (bilateral) schwannomas of the vestibular portion of the acoustic nerves, are always present. Although the cutaneous manifestations are always less prominent than in type I, the disorder was classified as neurofibromatosis in the early 19th century. Bilateral acoustic neuroma has gradually been recognized, characterized, and then proven to be a separate type. It is now known that it is genetically distinct, clinically separate, and pathogenetically different from type I neurofibromatosis.

Diagnostic criteria for the diagnosis are a little more broad than simply the presence of bilateral acoustic neuromas. The disorder is manifest through the status of Schwann cells, pigmented cells of the meninges, and glial cells. Multiple tumors of any of these cells, particularly in a patient younger than 30 years, may be sufficient criteria for the diagnosis. Cutaneous neurofibromas and cafe au lait spots may raise suspicion of the disease, or lend support to the diagnosis. The absence of Lisch nodules and presence of posterior capsule lens opacities clinically confirms the diagnosis. As the disorder is an autosomal dominant disease with high penetrance, the presence of an affected family member defines the genetic risk in any patient and confirms the clinical diagnosis. The responsible gene is on chromosome 22, with flanking markers available. It is possible, in many families, to detect a linkage pattern and assign a diagnosis of affected, carrier state, or not at risk. It is currently estimated that the disorder has a prevalence of about 0.1 case per 100,000 individuals; no ethnic, regional, or racial prominence is known.

The gene product causing neurofibromatosis II, and in fact the gene itself, are unknown. However, the linkage to abnormalities of the long arm of chromosome 22 has been found in sporadic (nongenetic) tumors of the same type found in the familial disorder. It is to be expected that research on the two varieties of tumors will be mutually supportive and thus speed the acquisition of clinically useful information.

Dermatology. The cafe au lait spots of type II neurofibromatosis do not have the MMGs of type I. The cutaneous neurofibromas are probably the same, although careful analysis of the dominant cell in the tumors of type II has not yet been published. No additional cutaneous involvement associated with type II has been described.

Neurology. The tumors of type II appear to arise from a different population of neuroectodermal cells than give rise to the tumors of type I. Acoustic neuromas rarely, perhaps never, arise in type I. Other schwannomas occur much more frequently in type II neurofibromatosis than in type I. Meningiomas occur more frequently, and primary glial tumors, except optic gliomas, may be seen significantly more frequently in type II than type I. The clinical symptoms of the disorder are exclusively those produced by the tumors. Higher cortical dysfunction, seizures, macrocephaly, and short stature have specifically not been reported more frequently in type II than in the general population.

Pathologically, in addition to the neoplastic lesions of the CNS, a variety of hamartomatous abnormalities have been seen in type II. The predominant form of malformation is diffuse rests of ectopic cells—Schwann cells in the dorsal horn and perivascular regions of the spinal cord, meningeal cells in the deep cerebral nuclei and perivascular spaces, ependymal cells in the spinal cord in proximity to ependymomas. Proliferation of cortical microvascular structures may represent a type of malfor-

---

Pearls and Perils: Neurofibromatosis Type II

1. A careful family history should be taken from all patients with acoustic neuromas. The younger the patient, the more likely the diagnosis of neurofibromatosis.
2. The tumors of type II do not seem to respond to hormonal changes as do those of type I.

---

mation as well. Syringomyelia and hydromyelia occur more frequently in type II neurofibromatosis than in the general population. Rarely do the ancillary neuropathologic abnormalities produce any clinical signs or symptoms, but they will be detected by the increasingly higher/resolution studies of the nervous system that are becoming available for routine use. It is predicted that confusion about the significance of an individual lesion on the MRI of a patient with type II disease will arise—is the area a tumor or a malformation? With experience one may be able to predict the clinical nature and implications of the spot on the scan. Histologically the patterns in the malformations are identical to those, more widespread or extensive, in the tumors of the disease.

Clinical Management. The natural history or evolution of the disorder will undoubtedly determine management in the future, as it does now. Presently, loss of vestibular function, tinnitus, deafness, headaches, hydrocephalus, and more extensive brainstem dysfunction outline the evolution of the acoustic neuromas. Because hearing can be preserved if surgery can be performed when the tumor is small, it is now recommended that every attempt be made to detect the presence of such tumors as early as possible. Imaging studies of the acoustic nerves, electrophysiologic studies of hearing and balance, and indications of clinical signs and symptoms referable to the cranial nerve VIII must be obtained periodically in affected individuals. Similar attention should be given to those at high risk for the disease (family members) who cannot be proven to be free of the gene by genetic studies. All other tumors and their associated manifestations should be treated symptomatically. The progression of the problems varies quite

---

FEATURE TABLE 17-2. NEUROFIBROMATOSIS TYPE II

Discriminating Features	Consistent Features	Variable Features
1. Bilateral acoustic neuromas	1. Bilateral deafness	1. Tinnitus
2. Multiple schwannomas	2. Fewer than five cafe au lait spots	2. Headaches
3. Multiple meningiomas	3. Optic gliomas never seen	3. Cranial nerve palsies
	4. Autosomal dominant transmission	4. Elevated cross-reacting nerve growth factor titers in cerebrospinal fluid

widely from person to person, even within families. Nonneurologic manifestations of type II neurofibromatosis are secondary to the tumor growth of the disease, such as spinal disease around an intraforaminal schwannoma, or a myelopathy from an ependymoma. Nonsurgical management of CNS tumors is identical to the treatment of the same diseases without neurofibromatosis.

ANNOTATED BIBLIOGRAPHY

Riccardi VM, Eichner JE: *Neurofibromatosis: Phenotype, Natural History, and Pathogenesis.* Johns Hopkins Series in Contemporary Medicine and Public Health. Baltimore, Md, Johns Hopkins University Press, 1986.

This book describes the findings from a huge clinic population, the Baylor neurofibromatosis program study. The bibliography is exhaustive. Chapter 16 touches on a wide range of treatment issues.

Riccardi VM, Mulvihill JJ (eds): *Advances in Neurology,* vol 29: *Neurofibromatosis (von Recklinghausen Disease): Genetics, Cell Biology, and Biochemistry.* New York, Raven Press, 1981.

The reviews of the clinical problems, neuropathology, and associated malignancies complement the other more recent references. A practical summary of neurofibromatosis type II can be found in the fifth paper. The history of the study of the disorder(s) is included, with a partial translation of von Recklinghausen's original paper of 1882.

Riccardi VM: Neurofibromatosis: Past, Present, and Future [editorial]. *N Engl J Med* 324(18) 1283–1285, 1991.

An expression of the state of the art in neurofibromatosis type I.

Rubenstein AE, Bunge RP, Housman DE (eds): *Neurofibromatosis: Results of a Conference, May 22–24, 1985. Ann NY Acad Sci,* 1986.

This volume includes discussions of a large variety of topics in neurofibromatosis. Many of the papers deal with basic embryologic, pathologic, and biochemical studies of the disease. The second section of the book is devoted to the neural crest.

Wallace MR, Marchuk DA, Andersen LB, et al: Type 1 neurofibromatosis gene: Identification of a large transcript disrupted in three NF1 patients. *Science* 249(4965): 181–186, 1990.

The discovery of the gene for neurofibromatosis 1 is reported in this paper.

Tuberous Sclerosis

The next most prevalent neurocutaneous syndrome, after neurofibromatosis type I, is tuberous sclerosis. The disease is an autosomal dominant disorder, with high penetrance and a presumed high spontaneous mutation rate. It consists of disordered development of neural structures, many of which are directly derived from neural crest progenitor cells. Other pathologic structures are probably influenced by components of crest origin. The lesions of tuberous sclerosis are either malformations (hamartias, tumors), hamartomas, or neoplasms (hamartoblastomas). The first group of lesions is made up of malformed, bizarre cells apparently of neuronal lineage. The second form includes clear hyperplasia of the same type of cells, and the third form is probably a neoplastic transformation of a tumorous lesion. The cancers are only seen, inexplicably, in the kidney. The brain (and its ocular extension, the retina), skin, kidney, heart, and lungs can all be affected by the disordered growths. Clinical symptoms vary across a wide spectrum of distribution and severity between patients both within and between families.

The genetic disorder is estimated to be prevalent at a rate of 10 to 14 cases per 100,000 individuals. Certain aspects of the epidemiology of tuberous sclerosis have been observed in all studies to date: the prevalence is high in children, highest in those under 5 years old. The number of cases with no detectable family members is high: 50% to 70%! The association between symptoms of the disease and the objective, diagnostic signs is very close. The most recent data suggest a prevalence of about 6.5 per 100,000 at birth and 2.9 per 100,000 overall. How the other 3.6 disappear is unclear; little has been written about the natural history of the disease. There is evidently a major early childhood mortality with a lesser, but still significant, decrease in adult expected life span.

Because many patients have no diagnosed family members, it is presumed that a very high spontaneous mutation rate accounts for the high prevalence. Recent molecular genetic studies have linked the disease to two separate regions in several different families—the distal long arm of chromosome 9 (9q34), and the distal long arm of chromosome 11 (11q21–23). Apparently, about 35% of families carry the chromosome 9 genetic disease. A recent report suggests another family with possible linkage to chromosome 14. The genetic heterogeneity has no clinical counterpart. This finding has led to the speculation that the lesions of tuberous sclerosis require dysfunction of at least two genes—a situation parallel to that of another familial tumor syndrome, retinoblastoma. It is possible that genetic transmission supplies the miscoding in one gene, with spontaneous mutation providing the other. Either genetic event could occur postconception, or even postnatally. If the rate of spontaneous mutation were high enough, then an extremely broad, random variability in symptoms would be predicted.

The diagnosis currently rests on clinical grounds. The classical triad of mental retardation, epilepsy, and adenoma sebaceum is too exclusive. Many affected patients do not demonstrate both or, occasionally, either of the cerebral symptoms. The diagnosis thus rests on the detection of one of the distinctive malformations—cerebral cortical focal dysplastic island (tuber), subependymal nodule (candle-guttering), giant cell astrocytoma, retinal astrocytic hamartoma, facial angiofibroma, or ungual fibroma—or multiple less specific lesions—cardiac rhabdomyomas, renal angioleimyolipomas, pulmonary angiomyolipomas, or rectal polyps. Hypopigmented skin macules, the ashleaf spots, are suggestive and can support the diagnosis when another feature is detected. Similarly, angiomyolipomas of liver, gonads, or adrenals; adenoma of the thyroid; and osteomatous lesions of the bones suggest the diagnosis. Of course, a family history of tuberous sclerosis adds strong confirmatory pressure, requiring much less extensive demonstration of the characteristic or even nonspecific lesions. Imaging studies of various types can be used to detect the expressions of the tuberous sclerosis complex in a variety of organs. The vast majority of patients with tuberous sclerosis have more than one manifestation of the disorder. Suspicion of the disorder will often thus be rewarded by clinical confirmation. Pursuing the diagnosis in close family members is also likely to prove successful. Given the current assumption of very high penetrance, negative examinations (and images) can be used to confirm or support the diagnosis of unaffected or noncarrier. However, there are well documented, but very rare, cases of "skipped" generations and otherwise irrefutable evidence of nonpenetrance. An absolute assurance of noncarrier status must await perfection of molecular genetic testing methods.

Dermatology. There are several dermal abnormalities in tuberous sclerosis. The most obvious skin lesions are the facial angiofibromas. Clinically the misnamed adenoma sebaceum are pink to reddish nodules less than 0.5 cm in diameter with bilaterally symmetric distribution in the nasolabial folds, on the cheeks, and occasionally on the chin, forehead, and scalp. There is often faint telangiectasia associated with the nodular lesions, adding to the ruborous coloration. Histologically the lesions are localized hamartomas composed of fibrous and vascular tissue. Larger flat tumors of fibrous more than vascular tissue on the forehead and scalp of patients are pathognomonic signs. A distinctive clustering of fibrous hamartomas, fused into a relatively large patch, the shagreen patch, is seen on the trunk of about 25% of patients with tuberous sclerosis. Because the fibrous hamartomas of all three varieties develop after a variable period of life, the signs are not as useful diagnostically as the pigmentary lesions. The characteristic abnormality of pigmentation is hypomelanosis, but many of the tuberous sclerosis patients have multiple cafe au lait spots as well. The decreased pigmentation is evident as numerous scattered macules, predominantly on the abdomen, back, and anterior and lateral aspects of the limbs. The macules come in three distinct shapes. The least diagnostically specific, but most common, version is the polygonal macule (thumbprint) that varies in size from 0.5 to 2 cm in diameter. The lance-ovate, or ash leaf–shaped, spot is much more specific, ranges in size from 1 to 12 cm in diameter, and occurs in about one-fifth of the tuberous sclerosis population. The confetti type of hypopigmented macule (1 to 3 mm in diameter) is pathognomonic for tuberous sclerosis. Because the hypopigmented spots are evident soon after birth, they have more diagnostic power than the more specific dermal hamartomas. The detection of the spots is enhanced by ultraviolet illumination. Histologically, the hypopigmented macules contain normal numbers of melanocytes (distinctively unlike the decreased numbers in vitiligo) that produce smaller and less pigmented melanosomes. The pathogenesis of the undermelanization has not yet been elucidated.

Additional dermal abnormalities include the pathognomonic ungual or periungual fibromas, which again are hamartomas of the dermal connective tissues.

Neurology. From a list of symptoms of cerebral dysfunction—migraine, seizures, mental retardation, specific cognitive deficits, higher motor deficits (apraxias, movement disorders), developmental language disorders, autism, formal thought disorders, behavioral disorders—only the first has not been emphasized as an important, common feature in tuberous sclerosis. There is a rough correlation between the extent to which the cerebrum is abnormal and the severity of symptoms. The recognition of more specific anatomic-symptomatic connections awaits more extensive use of imaging studies and neurophysiologic measures of sufficiently sophisticated resolution.

The neuropathology of tuberous sclerosis has revealed characteristic lesions almost exclusively in the cerebral hemispheres. Disordered growth of isolated germinal cells in the periventricular matrix is produced by abnormal differentiation. Abnormal neuronal, astrocytic, and bizarrely hybrid cells suggest that the affected

FEATURE TABLE 17-3. TUBEROUS SCLEROSIS

Discriminating Features	Consistent Features	Variable Features
1. CNS and retinal hamartomas (clinical or radiographic) 2. Dermal (angio) fibromas 3. Multiple renal angiomyolipomas	1. Hypomelanotic macules 2. Rectal polyps	1. Epilepsy, including infantile spasms 2. Mental retardation 3. Cardiac rhabdomyomas 4. Thyroid adenoma 5. Gingival fibromas

cells are quite primitive. The effects on differentiation also produce abnormal migration, by either disordered growth of radial glia, neuronal interaction with the glia, or both. The resultant migration defects are expressed very early in the development of the cortex. Most of the foci of abnormal cells are in the subependymal region, representing no migration from the bed of the germinal matrix at all. Lesions in the molecular layer demonstrate the earliest and shortest migration. The subependymal nodules, candle-gutterings, and tubers are the macroscopic descriptions of these lesions.

In the foci, abnormal neurons, abnormal astroglia, and peculiar-looking cells that have histologic and immunocytologic characteristics of both neurons and astrocytes are dispersed in a network of denser than normal astrocytic fibers and diminished myelinated bundles. Some of the glia are giant multinucleated astrocytes that are nearly pathognomonic for tuberous sclerosis.

The disordered migration is expressed later in gestation as well. The other major neuropathologic finding is diffusely deranged radial columns of the same abnormal cells spanning the entire width of the cortex. Some indistinct layers can be recognized in the transcortical foci. It bears emphasizing that the abnormalities appear to affect only a few of the early neuroblasts. The tubers, subependymal nodules, and radial rests are dispersed through and within otherwise completely normal cortex.

A variety of cell adhesion molecules, growth factors, and neurotrophic factors have offered a rich field for research into the molecular biology of the disease. Undoubtedly, the definition of the gene and its product will play a pivotal role in the advancement of knowledge in these areas.

The clinical manifestations of tuberous sclerosis arise from dysfunction of the cerebral cortex. Seizures are a very common symptom of tuberous sclerosis. The first description by Bourneville in 1880 included epilepsy. Only with modern imaging techniques has it been possible to detect more than an occasional patient with the disease who does not have seizures. Approximately 8% of the total diagnosed population does not have seizures, but a current study of extended families has found about 20% of their members to be nonepileptic. Although a variety of seizure types have been reported in the disorder, it is very likely that all seizures in tuberous sclerosis are focal at onset, with the possible exception of infantile spasms. The age of the patient with the seizures seems to determine the clinical expression more than differences in pathophysiology. Infantile spasms are seen in children less than 1 year old, posterior focal (partial) seizures before 2 years, and frontal and temporal seizures later. In a majority of children with apparently generalized seizures, electroencephalographic (EEG) and monitoring data have demonstrated focal or multifocal seizure onset. Secondary bilateral EEG synchrony is seen almost exclusively with exten-

sive bilateral frontal involvement. It has been possible to correlate EEG foci with cortical malformations (tubers) in a very high percentage of epileptic patients. In the few patients with EEG foci not correlated with imaged lesions it is assumed that the anatomic abnormality is subtle or otherwise invisible to the techniques available. It is expected that some of these patients will eventually undergo surgical treatment of their epilepsy and reveal clinical-pathologic correlations.

Occasional cerebellar lesions destructive, not malformative, in nature, have been discovered on pathologic examination. As the atrophic, often heavily calcified, folia have been seen in the brains of patients with the most severe problems with seizures, the lesions probably represent secondary pathologic effects. To date, no clinical manifestations of the cerebellar disease have been reported.

Mental retardation is common in the disorder, the percentage of occurrence varying between studies. Children with tuberous sclerosis referred for medical attention demonstrate the deficit of intellect about two-thirds of the time. Their otherwise asymptomatic siblings and parents are much less frequently retarded. Careful large clinical studies with precision in diagnosis are only now feasible. More precise definition of the genetic defect will allow more reliable data to be gathered. A current study has detected mental retardation in about half of the patients of all ages. Interestingly, 80% of patients had seizures; all retarded patients had seizures. Thus, one-third had seizures but no retardation. The cerebral dysfunction must produce seizures and, if more extensive or intense, also mental retardation. In small studies of less extensive defects in higher cortical function all the patients with autism, developmental language disorders, and specific behavioral disorders also had seizures. Only the mentally normal tuberous sclerosis patients had not had seizures.

Nonneurocutaneous Manifestations. After the CNS, the kidneys are the most frequently affected organs in tuberous sclerosis. There are two dominant pathologic features: renal cysts and renal angiomyolipomas. The cysts are lined by distinctive cells, probably related to the epithelial cells of Bowman's capsule. All portions of the nephron are involved, glomerulus, tubules, and ducts. The extent of involvement and severity of the cystic disease vary remarkably among patients. Probably more than one-third of patients have renal cysts, but a much smaller fraction have clinically significant signs or symptoms of renal disease. There is a rough correlation between the extent of cystic disease and renal insufficiency and hypertension.

Renal angiomyolipomas are very frequent in tuberous sclerosis; about two-thirds of adult patients have detectable tumors. Although there is a small but significant risk of malignancy associated with the angiomyolipomas, they are much less clinically symptomatic than the renal cysts. The tumors very rarely compress renal arteries, causing hypertension, infrequently are associated with flank pain and the risk of bleeding, and sometimes are associated with renal insufficiency.

Cardiac involvement is also quite common, but usually asymptomatic. About half of all patients, children and adults, have been found to harbor rhabdomyomas. The benign tumors can be found in any of the heart chambers but show a predilection for the ventricles, and the left side in general. Rarely do the tumors cause cardiac symptoms, but younger patients more frequently have symptomatic heart disease. There is an early cardiac mortality in tuberous sclerosis. Many different arrhythmias have been reported in cardiac tuberous sclerosis. There is a distinctive association between Wolff-Parkinson-White syndrome and tuberous sclerosis, independent of the presence of cardiac tumors.

A very high percentage of patients have rectal polyps, but these are never symptomatic and are not prone to malignant transformation. Pulmonary cystic disease is rare in tuberous sclerosis, but carries a high mortality. Cystic, sclerotic, and other bony lesions are seen, but are rarely symptomatic. Vascular lesions, particularly hemangiomas, small vessel dysplasias, are common. Medium and large vessel disease, aneurysmal malformation of the intracranial great vessels and aorta, is very rare.

Clinical Management. The proper treatment of tuberous sclerosis requires not only management of acute symptoms, but also anticipation of certain specific problems. CNS malformations, renal cysts, and angiolipomas are susceptible to growth as well as malignant tumor development. It is not known how best to anticipate the appearance of the important changes in pathology. Therefore, periodic imaging of the afflicted organs is needed. Contrast enhancement in the CT brain scan is presumptive evidence of the development of a giant cell astrocytoma. Most surgical treatment is postponed until symptoms from the growing tumors appear, but the true risk of metastatic renal cell carcinoma has yet to be defined.

The management of acute symptoms of tuberous sclerosis is more straightforward. The treatment of seizures in the disorder is independent of the etiology. Adrenocorticotropic hormone (ACTH) or other steroids are used in infantile spasms. Carbamazepine, phenytoin, primidone, and other drugs are used for focal seizures. Surgical treatment of well-defined focal epilepsies is an important consideration for many patients. Aggressive management of the various epileptic syndromes of tuberous sclerosis should always be attempted. Attention must be paid to the relationship between poorly controlled seizures and mental retardation, and to the more important converse: no seizures, no mental retardation.

The presence of mental retardation must be documented and defined. Educational and behavioral therapies are as likely to be successful in tuberous sclerosis as in the general retarded population. Less global deficits in higher cortical functioning, for example, developmental language disorders, need to be treated much more specifically with appropriate educational, physical, and speech therapies. Movement disorders respond to the same medical treatments as in other diseases. Autism and other behavioral-psychiatric symptoms often yield to the appropriate medical and nonmedical treatments. Interactions between medicines for these disorders and anticonvulsants are always a concern. Occasionally a single medicine can be found for several symptoms—such as carbamazepine for seizures and behavioral problems, or amitriptyline for attentional deficits, sleep disorder, and the affective component of autism.

A variety of medical, surgical, and nonmedical treatments are used for the renal and cardiac complications of tuberous sclerosis.

A common concern in the treatment of all problems of tuberous sclerosis is the ultimate prognosis for the disease. Generally, the severity of the various symptoms changes little over the years. A severely delayed infant with infantile spasms, spastic quadriparesis, and renal disease will not recover with maturity. On the other hand, a child with easily controlled seizures and normal development will be, at worst, only mildly neurologically impaired in the future. For the large group of patients whose status and prognosis are unknown I would prefer to treat vigorously and expect the best. It is more humane, albeit more expensive, to treat some

---

Pearls and Perils: Tuberous Sclerosis

1. About 25% of children with infantile spasms have tuberous sclerosis.

2. Abdominal (renal) ultrasound and echocardiograms should be considered in screening parents of tuberous sclerosis patients for manifestations of the disease.

3. Surgical decompression, possibly percutaneous, may ameliorate clinical symptoms of renal cysts.

4. Retinal hamartomas are not symptomatic and do not change significantly with age.

5. Pulmonary lymphangiomyomatosis, although very rarely seen in tuberous sclerosis, is pathognomic for the disorder.

6. The fat content of hepatic angiomyolipomas is diagnostic on ultrasound or CT.

7. Dental enamel pitting can be easily demonstrated with plaque disclosing solution and dye. The diffuse small pits have been seen in 100% of adults with tuberous sclerosis.

severely impaired children too much than to treat some ultimately near normal children too little.

ANNOTATED BIBLIOGRAPHY

Gomez MR (ed): *Tuberous Sclerosis: Neurologic and Psychiatric Features,* 2nd ed. New York, Raven Press, 1988.
   Complete discussions of major clinical concerns. Detailed descriptions of findings in specific organs. Extensive bibliographies.

Johnson WG, Gomez MR (eds): *Tuberous Sclerosis and Allied Disorders: Clinical, Cellular, and Molecular Studies. Ann NY Acad Sci,* 1991.
   A series of papers on tuberous sclerosis that covers the wide range of clinical, genetic, pathologic, and biochemic aspects of the disorder.

INCONTINENTIAS

Incontinentia Pigmenti (Bloch-Sulzberger Syndrome)

Incontinentia pigmenti is seen almost exclusively in girls. A dominant, possibly X-linked, transmission, prenatally fatal to the affected hemizygote, has been proposed. The ratio of females to males with the diagnosis has remained about 20:1 in the years since the first description of the syndrome in the late 1930s.

Dermatology. The pigmentary disturbance of the skin develops after an acute inflammatory process. The vesicles and bullae on the trunk and extremities are seen in the first 6 months of life and, in about one-quarter of the children, in the first few days of life. The swirling, splashed distribution of the hyperpigmented residua becomes apparent afterwards. The initial inflammatory vesicles and bullae develop in crops and may persist for months, but are never associated with fever. During this phase of the cutaneous development marked eosinophilia can usually be detected. The epidermal vesicles are filled with eosinophils, and the upper dermal, perivascular, inflammatory infiltrates include numerous eosinophils. As the vesicular phase resolves, a verrucous phase develops with hyperkeratosis, acanthosis, and occasional dyskeratotic cells on histologic examination. The third phase of the pigmentary changes follows, with overlap of the other two stages: phagocytosis of the otherwise unremarkable melanin occurs in the

dermis (the dermal-epidermal junction is incontinent) resulting in the deep blue or gray coloration. The pigmentary patterns—cobweb, chinese-character, streaks, swirls, splatters—do not always have complete 1:1 correspondence to the preceding inflammatory lesions. Many of the children have hypopigmented streaks, often on the calves but otherwise on the trunk and extremities without correlation with the other cutaneous components of the disorder. As the hyperpigmented lesions frequently fade or completely disappear in adolescence, the streaks of underpigmented skin may be the only residual cutaneous manifestation in the women of the family. Anhydrosis, alopecia, and dystrophy of hair, teeth, and nails represent additional cutaneous abnormalities in the disorder.

Neurology. The neurologic manifestations are predominantly cortical in clinical localization—mental retardation, developmental delays, seizures. Microcephaly, hydrocephalus, and slowly developing flaccid paralysis have been reported. Involvement of more extensive regions of the CNS must occur in those cases. The developmental delays and mental retardation are seen in about one-third of affected patients, and seizures are seen independently of the cognitive deficits. Although always stated as an important component of the disorder, the seizures are actually reported in less than 5% of cases. They are of both focal and generalized pathogenesis, but very little specific information about the epilepsy has been published. Girls are most frequently referred to a neurologist for evaluation of their slowed development.

   Weakness of the limbs has been reported as both flaccid and spastic. A few cases have been studied at autopsy. Degeneration of anterior horn cells in a pattern indistinguishable from that of motor neuron disease, type I, was seen in one case. In two other children, a destructive encephalopathy was radiologically demonstrated. In several girls stepwise deterioration has accompanied systemic signs of an inflammatory disease. Some have had documented viral or fungal infections of the CNS. Most of the brains studied postmortem showed encephaloclastic lesions. Several have shown malformations of cortical development owing to early embryologic insults. Global abnormalities of the brain have been noted, including microcephaly and hydrocephalus, neither of which has been explained in pathologic or physiologic terms.

   Ocular abnormalities occur as frequently as do

FEATURE TABLE 17–4. INCONTINENTIA PIGMENTI

Discriminating Feature	Consistent Feature	Variable Features
1. Characteristic swirled hyperpigmented lesion(s)	1. Female sex	1. Mental retardation 2. Epilepsy 3. Hemihypertrophy

Pearls and Perils:
Incontinentia Pigmenti

1. Boys with the disorder have been diagnosed (14 out of 255 cases). Some have had polyploidy of the X chromosome, notably Klinefelter's syndrome.

2. Children with incontinentia pigmenti are small-for-gestational-age infants more frequently than would be predicted in the general population.

3. Retrolental fibroplasia in an infant not exposed to high concentrations of oxygen should suggest the diagnosis of incontinentia pigmenti.

CNS problems. Avascularity of the peripheral retina, retinal dysplasia, and fibrovascular proliferation are the abnormalities reported.

Linkage to a particular region of the X chromosome, Xq28, has been discovered in a few families. Several reports of X chromosome fragility raise the possibility of a primary defect in DNA maintenance or repair. Secondary defects then could account for the pronounced variability in distribution, timing, extent, and severity of neurocutaneous involvement.

Clinical Management. The dermatologic manifestations of the disease are usually self-limited and do not produce clinical distress. If needed, antiinflammatory treatment helps. A careful examination of female relatives is required for genetic counseling. Treatment of infantile seizures with ACTH or other steroids is usually successful. Aggressive antiinflammatory treatment in cases of progressive CNS disease may be warranted, but infectious complications must be considered. No general recommendations can be given. Early detection of ocular lesions should preclude unnecessarily aggressive treatment for suspected retinal glioma or retinoblastoma. Serial examinations can document the rate of change and refine the differential diagnosis. Finally, supportive treatment of mental retardation and specific deficits of higher cortical function, to be optimally effective, should be offered early in development.

ANNOTATED BIBLIOGRAPHY

Catalano RA: Incontinentia pigmenti, *Am J Ophthalmol* 110 (6): 696–700, 1990.
This paper discusses the ocular findings in the disorder. A very interesting hypothetical pathogenesis is proposed to explain genetic, pathologic, and clinical findings.

O'Doherty N: Bloch-Sulzberger syndrome, incontinentia pigmenti, in (ed): *The Phakomatoses. Handbook of Clinical*

Neurology, Vol 14. Amsterdam, North-Holland, 1972, p 213–222.
Although an older reference, this chapter in the encyclopedic *Handbook* still is a useful practical description of the clinical manifestations of the disorder.

Hypomelanosis of Ito

The genetics of the pigmentary disorder that has been called incontinentia pigmenti achromians is unknown. The alternative name was applied because the skin lesion resembles, in reverse, that of incontinentia pigmenti. Swirled, reticular, splotchy, or splashed areas of decreased rather than increased coloration are present on the trunk and limbs. There is no incontinence of pigment and the disorder is distinctly different from incontinentia pigmenti in most respects. The name hypomelanosis of Ito is more appropriate. The associated signs and symptoms include neurologic, ocular, and skeletal abnormalities.

There is considerable controversy about the genetics of the disorder. In isolated families, autosomal dominant, autosomal recessive, and X-linked modes of inheritance have been proposed. In all series such inherited cases represent a tiny percentage. It is likely that the disorder is heterogenous, both genetically and phenotypically. Any theory of pathogenesis must explain the predominance of female cases seen in all reported series. The female to male ratio has varied from 1.5:1 to 3.3:1.

Dermatology. The hypopigmented areas have normal numbers of melanocytes, and the distribution of innervated keratinocytes is normal. There is a decreased amount of pigment in both cell types in comparison to the adjacent more deeply colored skin. In the most intensively studied cases two distinct populations of melanocytes are described. Highly arborized dendritic cells with less than normal numbers of melanosomes are interspersed with blunted cells with sparse cytoplasm and little pigment. The melanocytes in the darker adjacent skin have normal morphology and stronger melanization. Most modern studies postulate cellular mosaicism. Two populations of pigmented, neural crest-derived cells migrate from the dorsal aspect of the embryo along the dermal lines of Blaschko, giving rise to the distinctive pattern. Older reports demonstrate some concern that the lesion is actually a diffuse hyperpigmentation with only an apparent loss of coloration by comparison. Reflectance measurements have shown, in some cases, increased pigmentation on average, similar to the results of such measurements in incontinentia pigmenti.

Neurology. More than half of the patients with the skin manifestation of hypomelanosis of Ito have neurologic problems. Series that are drawn from patients seen by neurologists or pediatricians rather than dermatologists show neurologic manifestations in 75% to 95%. Delayed

FEATURE TABLE 17–5. HYPOMELANOSIS OF ITO

Discriminating Feature	Consistent Feature	Variable Features
1. Characteristic hypomelanotic skin lesion(s)	1. None.	1. Mental retardation 2. Epilepsy 3. CNS migration defects 4. Other pigmented skin lesions 5. Hemihypertrophy, macrocephaly, microcephaly 6. Syndactyly and other acrosketetal anomalies 7. Megacolon

development, mental retardation, seizures, nystagmus, macrocephaly, weakness, and hypotonicity have been reported. Sensorineural hearing loss and deafness are seen in a small percent of cases, but much more frequently than in the general pediatric population.

The neuropathology is poorly defined. Autopsy findings in two children demonstrated migration defects, with ulegyria, neuronal heterotopias, lamination defects, and both pachygyria and polymicrogyria. The distribution of the cerebral lesions was extensive. MRI in many more children has revealed regional, patchy, or focal areas of presumed migration defects. Destructive lesions, porencephaly, ventricular dilatation with cortical atrophy, and focal encephalomalacia are also radiographically demonstrated in the disorder.

Nonneurocutaneous Features. Ocular and skeletal abnormalities occur only slightly less frequently than neurologic problems. In a grand compilation of several series, about half the published cases had those extraneurocutaneous signs. It is not clear, however, how severe the ocular findings had to be to be included in the general category. Microphthalmia, iris nevi, heterochromia, colobomas, corneal and lenticular opacities, choroidal atrophy, and optic atrophy are well documented. Strabismus, myopia, epicanthic folds, hyperopia, slow pupillary reactions, nystagmus, ptosis, and astigmatism are much less so. Although it is reported that these latter symptoms and signs are much more frequent in children with hypomelanosis of Ito than in the general population, accurate statistics are not available.

Scoliosis, leg length discrepancy, hemihypertrophy, macrocrania, cervical ribs, and facial anomalies or dysmorphisms are the skeletal abnormalities of the disorder. About half of 34 children referred for neurologic abnormalities had orthopedic problems.

Clinical Management. Of the neurologic problems in hypomelanosis of Ito, developmental delays and mental retardation are the most common. The retardation can be severe, requiring institutional care when the patients are adults or older children. The disorder is never progressive, so early testing is predictive. Educational, be-

havioral, and rarely medical therapies are as effective in these children as in other disorders. No published data are available on the prevalence of specific cognitive, language, or learning disorders in this syndrome. Autism has been reported, presumably as responsive to intensive behavior modification therapy as in other etiologies. Affective, attentional, behavioral, and other psychiatric disorders have not been described but have been present in anecdotal, personal cases. Treatment with stimulants, tricyclic antidepressants, and major antipsychotic medications as indicated by the clinical symptoms was successful. The static encephalopathy has shown no specific complications to any of the medical therapies.

Treatment of the seizures can be difficult. Particularly in infancy, intractable seizures may be unresponsive to all nonanesthetic doses of anticonvulsants including ACTH and other steroids. No published reports of surgical seizure treatment are available. An occasional patient with focal seizures of hypomelanosis of Ito will qualify for operative therapy. However, most of the epi-

---

**Pearls and Perils:
Hypomelanosis of Ito**

1. Genetic mosaicism has been discovered in children with the disorder. Circulating lymphocytes do not demonstrate the chromosomal variations; skin fibroblasts are needed.

2. If a clear family history is present, the possibility of the wrong diagnosis exists. Patients with incontinentia pigmenti may have similar–appearing skin signs, distinguishable by biopsy.

3. Although half the children with hypomelanosis of Ito have clear "hard" neurologic abnormalities, the prevalence of less severe problems (e.g., migraine, attentional deficits, learning disabilities, and behavioral abnormalities) may be higher than expected in the other half of the population.

lepsy in the disorder has been described as generalized, with various subtypes well represented. There is no specific contraindication to, or clinical concern with, the use of any of the available anticonvulsants.

ANNOTATED BIBLIOGRAPHY

Glover MT, Brett EM, Atherton DJ: Hypomelanosis of Ito: Spectrum of the disease. *J Pediatr* 115(1): 75–80, 1989.

Discussion generated by clinical review of 19 cases. Chromosomal/genetic mosaicism is offered as a hypothesis for the distribution of the cutaneous lesions.

Pascual-Castroviejo I, López-Rodriguez L, de la Cruz Medina M, Salamanca-Maesso C, Herrero CR: Hypomelanosis of Ito. Neurological complications in 34 cases. *Can J Neurol Sci* 15(2): 124–129, 1988.

Review of a fairly large population of neurologically affected children. Distribution of various neurologic signs and symptoms is clinically helpful. Additional mention is made of numerous nonneurocutaneous abnormalities.

Sybert VP: Hypomelanosis of Ito (commentary). *Pediatr Dermatol* 7(1), 74–76, 1990.

A refreshing, isolated opinion about the lack of usefulness of the syndromic diagnosis. This is a plea for careful evaluation and description of patients' problems and findings.

OTHER PIGMENTARY DISORDERS

Primary Meningocutaneous Melanosis

The skin signs of this disorder are pigmented nevi. Meningeal and intracerebral melanin is visibly present. The pathogenesis of the hydrocephalus seen in this autosomal dominant disorder is unknown.

Albinism

The hypopigmentation of this group of disorders is a result of inadequate formation of melanin granules within otherwise normal melanocytes. The disease complex is subdivided into oculocutaneous and ocular albinism. Both have marked deficits in retinal pigments as well as absent coloration of the iris. Specific abnormalities of the lateral geniculate nuclei and more central visual structures of the brain are present in humans, as well as a large number of other species. Clinical manifestations of the CNS problems are nystagmus, head nodding, and decreased visual acuity. The ocular form is an X-linked recessive disorder, the oculocutaneous an autosomal recessive disease.

Waardenburg's Syndrome

The hypopigmentation of this autosomal dominant disease is strictly patterned: a white forelock. Another dermal abnormality is synophrys or unfused, excessive eyebrows. Dysmorphic facial features, lateral displacement of the medial canthi, hypoplasia of the ala nasi, cleft lip, cleft palate, prognathism, and broad nasal root are, to variable degrees, common in the syndrome. Neurologic manifestations include high-tone sensorineural hearing loss and heterochromia of the iridites.

Lentiginosis-Deafness-Cardiomyopathy

This disorder has also been called "leopard syndrome" as an acronym for lentigines, electrocardiographic conduction defects, ocular hypertelorism, pulmonary stenosis, abnormal genitalia, retarded growth, deafness. The skin lesions are small, rather darkly pigmented lesions with numerous melanocytes and excessively melanized basal keratinocytes. They are present at birth and increase in number, darkness, and size with age. The 1- to 5-mm spots are usually prominent on the upper trunk with decreasing concentration centrifugally. The conduction defects are secondary to ventricular hypertrophy and may be fatal. The cardiomyopathy is often progressive: hypertrophy worsening in the face of pulmonic or subaortic stenosis. Skeletal abnormalities besides the hypertelorism and growth retardation include pectus deformities, kyphosis, and prognathism. More overt endocrine abnormalities include cryptorchism, hypoplastic testes or ovaries, hypospadias, and delayed puberty. Sensorineural hearing loss, slowed peripheral nerve conduction velocities, intellectual deficits, and abnormal EEGs make up the neurologic component of the syndrome. The disorder is transmitted in an autosomal dominant pattern.

Management centers primarily on the cardiac disease. Patients vary in their need for medical and surgical therapy of the arrhythmias and stenoses. Treatment of the hearing deficits with aids and special education programs is usually needed. Surgical treatment of hypospadias and cryptorchism should be undertaken as needed. Specific endocrine therapy has not been emphasized in the literature. It is anticipated that formal hormonal deficits can now be corrected.

BIBLIOGRAPHY

Neurofibromatoses

Arkhipov BA, Sadovskaia IuE: Epileptic paroxysms in Recklinghausen's neurofibromatosis. *Zh Nevropatol Psikhiatr* 90(3):20–23, 1990 [in Russian].

Barson AJ, Cole FM: Neurofibromatosis with congenital malformation of the spinal cord. *J Neurol Neurosurg Psychiatr* 30:71–74, 1967.

Bognanno JR, Edwards MK, Lee TA, et al: Cranial MR imaging in neurofibromatosis. *AJR* 151(2):381–388, 1988.

Bolande RP: Neurofibromatosis—The quintessential neurocristopathy: Pathogenic concepts and relationships, in Riccardi VM, Mulvihill, JJ (eds): *Advances in Neurology, Vol 29: Neurofibromatosis (von Recklinghausen Disease)* New York, Raven Press, 1981, p 67-75.

Burke AP, Sobin LH, Shekitka KM, Federspiel BH, Helwig EB: Somatostatin-producing duodenal carcinoids in patients with von Recklinghausen's neurofibromatosis. A predilection for black patients. *Cancer* 65(7):1591-1595, 1990.

Cammarata CA, Deveikis JR, Schellinger D, Patronas NJ, Stull MA: Neuroradiology case of the day. Neurofibromatosis 2. *AJR* 154(6):1337-1338, 1990.

Carey JC: Von Recklinghausen neurofibromatosis: General, historical, and overview. *Abstracts, NIH Consensus Development Conference.* 1987, p 21-24.

Clementi M, Barbujani G, Turolla L, Tenconi R: Neurofibromatosis-1: A maximum likelihood estimation of mutation rate. *Hum Genet* 84(2):116-118, 1990.

Crawford AH: Neurofibromatosis in the pediatric patient. *Orthop Clin North Am* 9: 11-23, 1978.

Crawford AH Jr, Bagamery N: Osseous manifestations of neurofibromatosis in childhood. *J Pediatr Orthop* 6(1):72-88, 1986.

Denckla MB: Von Recklinghausen's neurofibromatosis: Neurological and cognitive assessment with sibling controls. *Am J Dis Child* 143(7):833-837, 1989.

DiPrete DA, Abuelo JG, Abuelo DN, Cronan JJ: Acute renal insufficiency due to renal infarctions in a patient with neurofibromatosis. *Am J Kidney Dis* 15(4):357-360, 1990.

Dunn DW, Purvin V: Optic pathway gliomas in neurofibromatosis. *Dev Med Child Neurol* 32(9):820-824, 1990.

Eldridge R: Bilateral acoustic neurofibromatosis: Genetic basis, natural history, and counseling. *Abstracts, NIH Consensus Development Conference.* 1987, p 25-31.

Fontaine B, Hanson MP, VonSattel JP, Martuza RL, Gusella JF: Loss of chromosome 22 alleles in human sporadic spinal schwannomas. *Ann Neurol* 29:183-186, 1991.

Gardner WJ, Frazier CH: Bilateral acoustic neurofibromas: A clinical study and field survey of a family of five generations with bilateral deafness in thirty-eight members. *Arch Neurol Psychiatr* 23:266-302, 1930.

Glasscock ME 3d: Neurofibromatosis type II: Diagnosis and decision making. *Am J Otol* 11(3):212-213, 1990.

Grobman LR, Fisch U, Pollack A: Central neurofibromatosis: A clinical-pathological correlation. *Am J Otol* 11(2):108-112, 1990.

Harkens K, Dolan KD: Correlative imaging of sphenoid dysplasia accompanying neurofibromatosis. *Ann Otol Rhinol Laryngol* 99(2 Pt 1):137-141, 1990.

Hegg CA, Flint A: Neurofibroma of the ovary. *Gynecol Oncol* 37(3):437-438, 1990.

Hochstrasser H, Boltshauser E, Valavanis A: Brain tumors in children with von Recklinghausen neurofibromatosis. *Neurofibromatosis* 1(4):233-239, 1988.

Holt GR: E.N.T. manifestations of von Recklinghausen's disease. *Laryngoscope* 88(10):1617-1632, 1978.

Hurst RW, Newman SA, Cail WS: Multifocal intracranial MR abnormalities in neurofibromatosis. *AJNR* 9(2):293-296, 1988.

Huson SM, Compston DA, Harper PS: A genetic study of von Recklinghausen neurofibromatosis in south east Wales. II. Guidelines for genetic counselling. *J Med Genet* 26(11):712-721, 1989.

Ilgren EB, Kinnier-Wilson LM, Stiller CA: Gliomas in neurofibromatosis: A series of 89 cases with evidence for enhanced malignancy in associated cerebellar astrocytomas. *Pathol Ann* 20(Pt 1):331-358, 1985.

Jaakkola S, Muona P, James WD, et al: Segmental neurofibromatosis: Immunocytochemical analysis of cutaneous lesions. *J Am Acad Dermatol* 22(4):617-621, 1990.

Jadayel D, Fain P, Upadhyaya M, et al: Paternal origin of new mutations in von Recklinghausen neurofibromatosis. *Nature* 343(6258):558-559, 1990.

Kamerer DB: Gamma knife for neurofibromatosis type II [letter]. *Am J Otol* 11(3):213-214, 1990.

Kameyama O, Ogawa R: Pseudarthrosis of the radius associated with neurofibromatosis: Report of a case and review of the literature. *J Pediatr Orthop* 10(1):128-131, 1990.

Kantor W, Eldridge R, Fabricant R, Allen J, Koerber T: Central neurofibromatosis: Genetic, clinical, and biochemical distinctions from peripheral neurofibromatosis. *Neurology* 30(8): 851-859, 1980.

Kiwit JC, Nicola N, Roosen N, et al: The influence of magnetic resonance tomography on diagnosis and therapy in patients with intracranial manifestation of neurofibromatosis (Recklinghausen disease). *Neurosurg Rev* 10(4):283-286, 1987.

Kousseff BG: The phakomatoses as paracrine growth disorders (paracinopathies). *Clin Genet* 37(2):97-105, 1990.

Landau K, Dossetor FM, Hoyt WF, Muci-Mendoza R: Retinal hamartoma in neurofibromatosis 2. *Arch Ophthalmol* 108(3):328-329, 1990.

Lewis RA, Gerson LP, Axelson KA, Riccardi VM, Whitford RP: Von Recklinghausen neurofibromatosis. II. Incidence of optic gliomata. *Ophthalmology* 91(8):929-935, 1984.

Lisch K: Ueber Beteiligung der Augen, insbesondere das Vorkommen von frisknötchen bei der Neurofibromatose (Recklinghausen). *Z Augenheilkd* 93:137-143, 1937.

Listernick R, Charrow J: Neurofibromatosis type 1 in childhood. *J Pediatr* 116(6):845-853, 1990.

Listernick R, Charrow J, Greenwald MJ, Esterly NB: Optic gliomas in children with neurofibromatosis type 1. *J Pediatr* 114(5): 788-792, 1989.

Lott IT, Richardson EP Jr: Neuropathological findings and the biology of neurofibromatosis, in Riccardi VM, Mulvihill JJ (eds): *Advances in Neurology, Vol 29: Neurofibromatosis (von Recklinghausen Disease): Genetics, Cell Biology, and Biochemistry.* New York, Raven Press, 1981, p 23-32.

Lubs M-LE, Bauer MS, Formas ME, Djokic B: Lisch nodules in neurofibromatosis type I. *N Engl J Med* 324:1264-1266, 1991.

Martuza R, Eldridge R: Neurofibromatosis 2 (bilateral acoustic neurofibromatosis). *N Engl J Med* 318(11):684-688, 1988.

Mayfrank L, Mohadjer M, Wullich B: Intracranial calcified deposits in neurofibromatosis type 2. A CT study of 11 cases. *Neuroradiology* 32(1):33-37, 1990.

Menon AG, Anderson KM, Riccardi VM, et al: Chromosome 17p deletions and p53 gene mutations associated with the formation of malignant neurofibromatosis in von Recklinghausen neurofibromatosis. *Proc Natl Acad Sci USA* 87:5435-5439, 1990.

Milstein JM, Geyer JR, Berger MS, Bleyer WA: Favorable prognosis for brainstem gliomas in neurofibromatosis. *J Neurooncol* 7(4):367-371, 1989.

Mirowitz SA, Sartor K, Gado M: High-intensity basal ganglia

lesions on T_1-weighted MR images in neurofibromatosis. *AJR* 154(2):369–373, 1990.

Morier P, Merot Y, Paccaud D, Beck D, Frenk E: Juvenile chronic granulocytic leukemia, juvenile xanthogranulomas, and neurofibromatosis. Case report and review of the literature. *J Am Acad Dermatol* 22(5 Pt 2):962–965, 1990.

Mulvihill JJ, Parry DM, Sherman JL, Pikus A, Kaiser-Kupfer MI, Eldridge R: NIH conference. Neurofibromatosis 1 (Recklinghausen disease) and neurofibromatosis 2 (bilateral acoustic neurofibromatosis). An update. *Ann Intern Med* 1 113(1):39–52, 1990.

Murray MR, Stout AP: Schwann cell versus fibroblast as the origin of the specific nerve sheath tumor. Observations of normal nerve sheaths and neurilemomas in vitro. *Am J Pathol* 16:41–60, 1940.

Penfield W, Young AW: The nature of von Recklinghausen's disease and the tumors associated with it. *Arch Neurol Psychiatr* 23:320–344, 1930.

Pierce SM, Barnes PD, Loeffler JS, McGinn C, Tarbell NJ: Definitive radiation therapy in the management of symptomatic patients with optic glioma. Survival and long-term effects. *Cancer* 65(1):45–52, 1990.

Pou-Serradell A, Ugarte-Elola AC, Llorens-Terol J: Optic pathway gliomas in neurofibromatosis. *Neurofibromatosis* 2(4):227–232, 1989.

Raffel C, McComb JG, Bodner S, Gilles FE: Benign brain stem lesions in pediatric patients with neurofibromatosis: Case reports. *Neurosurgery* 25(6):959–964, 1989.

Ratner N, Lieberman MA, Riccardi VM, Hong DM: Mitogen accumulation in von Recklinghausen neurofibromatosis. *Ann Neurol* 27(3)298–303, 1990.

Riccardi VM: Neurofibromatosis and Albright's syndrome. *Dermatol Clin* 5(1):193–203, 1987.

Riccardi VM: Neurofibromatosis: Past, present, and future [editorial]. *N Engl J Med* 324 (18):1283–1285, 1991.

Riccardi VM, Eichner JE: *Neurofibromatosis: Phenotype, Natural History, and Pathogenesis.* Johns Hopkins Series in Contemporary Medicine and Public Health. Baltimore, Md, Johns Hopkins University Press, 1986.

Robinson RG: Intrathoracic meningocele and neurofibromatosis. *Br J Surg* 51:432–437, 1964.

Rosner J: Clinical review of neurofibromatosis. *J Am Optom Assoc* 61(8):613–618, 1990.

Rouleau G, Wertelecki W: Genetic linkage of bilateral acoustic neurofibromatosis to a DNA marker on chromosome 22. *Nature* 329:246–248, 1987.

Rouleau GA, Seizinger BR, Wertelecki W, et al: Flanking markers bracket the neurofibromatosis type 2 (NF2) gene on chromosome 22. *Am J Hum Genet* 46(2):323–328, 1990.

Rubenstein AE, Bunge RP, Housman DE (eds): *Neurofibromatosis: Results of a Conference, May 22–24, 1985. Ann NY Acad Sci,* 1986.

Samuelsson B: *Neurofibromatosis (v. Recklinghausen disease): A clinical-psychiatric and genetic study.* Gothenburg, Sweden, University of Gothenburg, 1981.

Schreiber D, Quade B: CNS involvement in neurofibromatosis. A postmortem study. *Zentralbl Allg Pathol* 136(1–2):67–76, 1990 [in German].

Seizinger B, De La Monte : Molecular approach to human meningioma: Loss of genes on chromosome 22. *Proc Natl Acad Sci USA* 84:5414–5423, 1987.

Seizinger B, Martuza RL: Loss of genes on chromosome 22 in tumorigenesis of human acoustic neuroma. *Nature* 322:644–647, 1986.

Seizinger B, Rouleau GA: Common pathogenetic mechanism for three tumor types in bilateral acoustic neurofibromatosis. *Science* 236:317–319, 1987.

Shapeero LG, Vordermark JS: Bladder neurofibromatosis in childhood. Noninvasive imaging. *J Ultrasound Med* 9(3):177–180, 1990.

Shields JA, Shields CL, Lieb WE, Eagle RC: Multiple orbital neurofibromas unassociated with von Recklinghausen's disease. *Arch Ophthalmol* 108(1):80–83, 1990.

Shul WJ, Crowe FW: Neurocutaneous syndromes in the M kindred. A case of simultaneous occurrence of tuberous sclerosis and neurofibromatosis. *Neurology* 3:904–909, 1953.

Sirois JL 3d, Drennan JC: Dystrophic spinal deformity in neurofibromatosis. *J Pediatr Orthop* 10(4):522–526, 1990.

Sloan JB, Fretzin DF, Bovenmyer DA: Genetic counseling in segmental neurofibromatosis. *J Am Acad Dermatol* 22(3): 461–467, 1990.

Sorensen SA, Mulvihill JJ, Nielsen A: Long-term follow-up of von Recklinghausen neurofibromatosis. Survival and malignant neoplasms. *N Engl J Med* 314:1010–1015, 1986.

Strauss S, Pansky M, Lewinsohn G: Hemorrhagic pheochromocytoma in a pregnant patient with neurofibromatosis. Sonographic appearance. *J Ultrasound Med* 9(3):165–167, 1990.

Summers CG, MacDonald JT: Paroxysmal facial itch: A presenting sign of childhood brainstem glioma. *J Child Neurol* 3(3):189–192, 1988.

Tarlov IM: Origin of the perineural fibroblastoma. *Am J Pathol* 16:33–40, 1940.

Thomas PK, King RH, Chiang TR, Scaravilli F, Sharma AK, Downie AW: Neurofibromatous neuropathy. *Muscle Nerve* 13(2):93–101, 1990.

Turek M, Raistrick ER, Hart CD: Retinal tumors in neurofibromatosis. *Can J Ophthalmol* 12:68–70, 1977.

Unger PD, Taff ML, Song S, Schwartz IS: Sudden death in a patient with von Recklinghausen's neurofibromatosis. *Am J Forensic Med Pathol* 5(2):175–179, 1984.

Von Recklinghausen F: Ein Herz von einem Neugeborenen, Welches mehrere theils nach aussen, theils nach den Hohlen prominirenden Tumoren (Myomen) trug. *Monatsschr Geburtsk Frauenkr* 20:1–2, 1862.

Walker AE: "Astrocytosis arachnoidal cerebelli (a rare manifestation of von Recklinghousen's neurofibromatosis)," *Archives of Neurologic Psychiatry,* Vol. 45 (1951): 520–532.

Wallace MR, Marchuk DA, Andersen LB, et al: Type 1 neurofibromatosis gene: Identification of a large transcript disrupted in three NF1 patients. *Science* 249(4965):181–186, 1990.

Walsh NM, Bodurtha A: Auerbach's myenteric plexus. A possible site of origin for gastrointestinal stromal tumors in von Recklinghausen's neurofibromatosis. *Arch Pathol Lab Med* 114(5):522–525, 1990.

Wander JV, Das Gupta TK: Neurofibromatosis. *Curr Probl Surg* 14(2):1–81, 1977.

Ward K, O'Connell P, Carey JC, et al: Diagnosis of neurofibromatosis I by using tightly linked, flanking DNA markers. *Am J Hum Genet* 46(5):943–949, 1990.

Wertelecki W, Rouleau G, Superneau D, et al: Neurofibromatosis 2: Clinical and DNA linkage studies of a large kindred. *N Engl J Med* 319(5):278–283, 1988.

Weston JA: The regulation of normal and abnormal neural crest cell development, in Riccardi VM, Mulvihill JJ (eds): *Advances in Neurology,* Vol 29: *Neurofibromatosis (von Recklinghausen Disease): Genetics, Cell Biology, and Biochemistry.* New York, Raven Press, 1981, p 77–95.

Xu G, O'Connell P, Viskochil D, et al: The neurofibromatosis type 1 gene encodes a protein related to GAP. *Cell* 62:599–608, 1990.

Young DF, Eldridge R, Nager GT, Deland FH, McNew J: Hereditary bilateral acoustic neuroma (central neurofibromatosis), *Birth Defects* 7(4):73–86, 1971.

Tuberous Sclerosis

Arseni C, Alexianu M, Horvat L, et al: Fine structure of atypical cells in tuberous sclerosis. *Acta Neuropathol (Berlin)* 21:185–193, 1972.

Awan KJ: Leaf-shaped lesions of ocular fundus and white eyelashes in tuberous sclerosis. *South Med J* 75:227–228, 1982.

Barsky D, Wolter JR: The retinal lesions of tuberous sclerosis: An angiomatous hamartoma? *J Pediatr Ophthalmol* 8:261–265, 1971.

Bender BL, Yunis EJ: Central nervous system pathology in tuberous sclerosis in children. *Ultrastruct Pathol* 1:287–299, 1980.

Bender BL, Yunis EJ: The pathology of tuberous sclerosis. *Pathol Ann:* 17(Pt 1):339–382, 1982.

Berg G, Zacharisson CG: Cystic lungs of rare origin: Tuberous sclerosis. *Acta Radiol* 22:425–436, 1941.

Bernstein J, Robbins TO, Kissane JM: The renal lesions of tuberous sclerosis. *Semin Diagn Pathol* 3:97–105, 1986.

Blume WT, Pillay N: Electrographic and clinical correlates of secondary bilateral synchrony. *Epilepsia* 26:636–641, 1985.

Bonnin JM, Rubinstein LJ, et al: Subependymal giant cell astrocytoma: Significance and possible cytogenetic implications of an immunohistochemical study. *Acta Neuropathol (Berlin)* 62:185–193, 1984.

Borberg, A: Clinical and genetic investigations into tuberous sclerosis and Recklinghausen's neurofibromastosis. Contribution to elucidation of interrelationship and eugenics of the syndrome. *Acta Psychiatr et Neurol Scand* (Suppl 71):3–239, 1951.

Bourneville DM: Contribution à l'étude de l'idiotie. Sclérose tubéreuse des circonvolutions cérébrales: Idiotie et epilepsie hémiplégique. *Arch Neurol* 1:81–90, 1880.

Braffman BH, Bilaniuk LT, Zimmerman RA: The central nervous system manifestations of the phakomatoses on MR [review]. *Radiol Clin N Am* 26(4):773–800, 1988.

Brown J: Tuberous sclerosis with malignant astrocytoma. *Med J Aust* 1:811–814, 1975.

Bye AM, Matheson JM, Tobias VH, MacKenzie RA: Selective epilepsy surgery in tuberous sclerosis. *Aust Paediatr* 25(4):243–245, 1989.

Caviness VS Jr, Williams RS: Cellular patterns in developmental malformations of neocortex: Neuron-glial interactions, in Arima M, Suzuki Y, Yabuuchi H (eds): *The Developing Brain and Its Disorders.* Tokyo, University of Tokyo Press, 1984, p 43–67.

Caviness VS, Misson J-P, Gadisseux J-F: Abnormal neuronal patterns and disorders of neocortical development, in Galaburda A (ed): *From Reading to Neurons.* Boston, MIT Press, 1989, p 405–439.

Charmley P, Foroud T, Wei S, et al: A primary linkage map of the human chromosome 11q22-23 region. *Genomics* 6:316–323, 1990.

Chow CW, Klug GL, Lewis EA: Subependymal giant cell astrocytoma in children. *J Neurosurg* 68:880–883, 1988.

Christophe C, Bartholome J, Blum D, et al: Neonatal tuberous sclerosis. US, CT and MR diagnosis of brain and cardiac lesions. *Pediatr Radiol* 19:446–448, 1989.

Connor JM, Stephenson JBP, Hadley MDH: Non-penetrance in tuberous sclerosis. *Lancet* 1:1275, 1986.

Curatolo P, Cusmai R: Autism and infantile spasms in children with tuberous sclerosis. *Dev Med Child Neurol* 29:550–551, 1987.

Davidson S: Tuberous sclerosis with fusiform aneurysms of both internal carotid arteries manifested by unilateral visual loss and papilledema. *Bull Los Angeles Neurol Soc* 39:128–132, 1974.

Dawson J: Pulmonary tuberous sclerosis and its relation to other forms of the disease. *Q J Med* 23:113–145, 1954.

De Sevilla TF, Muniz R, Palou J, et al: Renal leiomyosarcoma in a patient with tuberous sclerosis. *Urol Int* 43:62–64, 1988.

Devroede G, Lemineux B, Masse S, et al: Colonic hamartomas in tuberous sclerosis. *Gastroenterology* 94:182–188, 1988.

Dulac O, LeMaitre A, Plouin P: Maladie de Bourneville: Aspects cliniques et électroencéphalographiques de l'épilepsie dans la première année, *Boll Lega It Epil* 45–46:39–42, 1984.

Farrow GM, Harrison EG Jr, Utz DC, Jones DR: Renal angiomyolipoma: A clinicopathologic study of 32 cases. *Cancer* 22:564–570, 1968.

Fenoglio JJ, McAllister HA, Ferrans VJ: Cardiac rhabdomyoma: A clinicopathologic and electron microscopic study. *Am J Cardiol* 38:241–251, 1976.

Fitzpatrick TB: History and significance of white macules, earliest visible sign of tuberous sclerosis. *Ann NY Acad Sci* 615:26–35, 1991.

Fitzpatrick TB, Szabo G, Hori Y, et al: White leaf-shaped macules: Earliest sign of tuberous sclerosis, *Arch Dermatol* 98:1–6, 1968.

Fleury P, deGroot WP, Delleman JW, et al: Tuberous sclerosis: The incidence of sporadic versus familial cases. *Brain Dev* 2:107–117, 1980.

Fryer AE, Chalmers A, Connor JM, et al: Evidence that the gene for tuberous sclerosis is on chromosome 9. *Lancet* 1:659–661, 1987.

Fujiwara S, Kakaki T, Hikita T, Nishio S: Subependymal nodules and giant-cell astrocytomas associated with tuberous sclerosis. Do subependymal nodules grow? *Child Nerv Syst* 5:43–44, 1989.

Gold AP, Freeman JM: Depigmented nevi: The earliest sign of tuberous sclerosis. *Pediatrics* 335:1003–1005, 1965.

Gomez MR (ed): *Tuberous Sclerosis: Neurologic and Psychiatric Features,* 2nd ed. New York, Raven Press, 1988.

Gomez MR: Strokes in tuberous sclerosis: Are rhabdomyomas a cause? *Brain Dev* 11:14–19, 1989.

Gomez MR: Phenotypes of the tuberous sclerosis complex with a revision of diagnostic criteria. *Ann NY Acad Sci* 615:1–7, 1991.

Gomez MR, Kuntz NL, Westmoreland BF: Tuberous sclerosis, early onset of seizures, and mental subnormality: Study of discordant homozygous twins. *Neurology* 32:604–611, 1982.

Gonzalez-Angulo A, Alford BR, Greenberg SD: Tuberous sclerosis: An otolaryngic diagnosis. *Arch Otolaryngol* 80:193–199, 1964.

Good CH, Garb J: Systemic nevi of the face, tuberous sclerosis, epilepsy and fibromatous growth on scalp. *Arch Dermatol Syphilol* 47:197–215, 1943.

Gould SR, Stewart JB, Temple LN: Rectal polyposis in tuberous sclerosis. *J Ment Defic Res* 34:465–473, 1990.

Grover WD, Harley RD: Early recognition of tuberous sclerosis by funduscopic examination. *J Pediatr* 75:991–995, 1969.

Gunther M, Penrose LS: Genetics of epiloia. *J Genet* 31:413–430, 1935.

Hajdu SI, Foote FW Jr: Angiomyolipoma of the kidney: Report of 27 cases and review of the literature. *J Urol* 102:396–401, 1969.

Harley WD, Grover RD: Tuberous sclerosis: Description and report of 12 cases. *Ann Ophthalmol* 1:477–481, 1970.

Hirano A: Neuronal and glial processes in neuropathology. *J Neuropathol Exp Neurol* 37:365–374, 1978.

Hirano A, Tuazon R, Zimmerman HM: Neurofibrillary changes, granulovacuolar bodies and argentophilic globules observed in tuberous sclerosis. *Acta Neuropathol (Berlin)* 11:257–261, 1968.

Hockfiel S, McKay RDG: Identification of major cell classes in the developing mammalian nervous system. *J Neurosci* 5:3310–3328, 1985.

Hogood CO, Garvin DD, Lactina FM, et al: Abdominal aortic aneurysm and renal hamartoma in an infant with tuberous sclerosis. *Surgery* 79:713–715, 1976.

Hunt A: Tuberous sclerosis: A survey of 97 cases. III. Family aspects. *Dev Med Child Neurol* 25:353–357, 1983.

Hunt A, Dennis J: Psychiatric disorder among children with tuberous sclerosis. *Dev Med Child Neurol* 29:190–198, 1987.

Hunt A, Lindenbaum RH: Tuberous sclerosis: A new estimate of prevalence within the Oxford region. *J Med Genet* 21:272–277, 1984.

Huttenlocher PR, Wollman RL: Cellular neuropathology of tuberous sclerosis. *Ann NY Acad Sci* 615:140–148, 1991.

Imaizumi M, Nukada T, Yoneda S, et al: Tuberous sclerosis with moyamoya disease: Case report. *Med J Osaka* 28:345–353, 1978.

Inoue Y, Nakajima S, Fukuda T, et al: Magnetic resonance images of tuberous sclerosis. Further observations and clinical correlations. *Neuroradiology* 30(5):379–384, 1988.

Janssen LAJ, Sandkuyl LA, Merkens EC, et al: Genetic heterogeneity in tuberous sclerosis. *Genomics* 8(2):237–242, 1990.

Janssen LAJ, Povey S, Attwood J, et al: A comparative study on genetic heterogeneity in tuberous sclerosis: Evidence for one gene on 9q34 and a second gene on 11q22–23. *Ann NY Acad Sci*, 615:306–315, 1991.

Jimbow K, Fitzpatrick TB, Szabo G, Hori Y: Congenital circumscribed hypomelanosis: Characterization based on electron microscopic study of tuberous sclerosis, nevus depigmentosus and piebaldism. *J Invest Dermatol* 64:50–62, 1977.

Johnson WG, Gomez MR (eds): Tuberous sclerosis and allied disorders: Clinical, cellular, and molecular studies. *Ann NY Acad Sci* 615, 1991.

Journel H, Roussey M, Plais MH, et al: Prenatal diagnosis of familial tuberous sclerosis following detection of cardiac rhabdomyoma by ultrasound. *Prenat Diagn* 6:283–289, 1986.

Kinder RSL: The ocular pathology of tuberous sclerosis. *J Pediatr Ophthalmol* 9:106–107, 1972.

Kingsley DPE, Kendall BE, Fitz CR: Tuberous sclerosis: A clinical-radiological evaluation of 110 cases with particular reference to atypical presentation. *Neuroradiology* 28:38–46, 1986.

Koprowski C, Rorke LB: Spinal cord lesions in tuberous sclerosis. *Pediatr Pathol* 1:475–480, 1983.

Lane VW, Samples JM: Tuberous sclerosis: Case study of early seizure control and subsequent normal development. *J Autism Dev Disord* 14:423–427, 1984.

Lie JT: Pulmonary manifestations, in Gomez MR (ed): *Tuberous Sclerosis: Neurologic and Psychiatric Features*, 2nd ed. New York, Raven Press, 1988, p 159–168.

McLaurin RL, Towbin RB: Tuberous sclerosis: Diagnostic and surgical considerations. *Pediatr Neurosci* 12:43–48, 1985–1986.

Messinger HC, Clarke BE: Retinal tumors in tuberous sclerosis. Review of the literature and report of a case with special attention to microscopic structure. *Arch Ophthalmol* 18:1–11, 1937.

Morimoto K, Mogami H: Sequential CT study of subependymal giant-cell astrocytoma associated with tuberous sclerosis. Case report. *J Neurosurg* 65:874–877, 1986.

Moss JG, Hendry GMA: The natural history of renal cysts in an infant with tuberous sclerosis: Evaluation with ultrasound. *Br J Radiol* 61:1074–1076, 1988.

Muller L, DeJong G, Falck V, et al: Antenatal ultrasonographic findings in tuberous sclerosis. *S Afr Med J* 69:633–638, 1986.

Pinto-Lord MC, Abroms IF, Smith TW: Hyperdense cerebral lesion in childhood tuberous sclerosis: computed tomographic demonstration and neuropathologic analysis. *Pediatr Neurol* 2:245–248, 1986.

Reagan TJ: Neuropathology, in Gomez MR (ed): *Tuberous Sclerosis: Neurologic and Psychiatric Features*, 2nd ed. New York, Raven Press, 1988, p 63–74.

Ribadeau-Dumas JL, Poirier J, Escourolle R: Etude ultrastructurale des lésions cérébrales de la sclérose tubéreuse de Bourneville. *Acta Neuropathol (Berlin)* 25:259–270, 1973.

Richardson EP Jr: Pathology of tuberous sclerosis. *Ann NY Acad Sci* 615:128–139, 1991.

Rolfes DB, Towbin R, Bove KE: Vascular dysplasia in a child with tuberous sclerosis. *Pediatr Pathol* 3:359–373, 1985.

Russell DS, Rubinstein LJ: Subependymal astrocytomas, in: *Pathology of Tumours of the Nervous System*, 5th ed. Baltimore, Md, Williams & Wilkins, 1989, 114–120.

Sampson JR, Scahill SJ, Stephenson JBP, et al: Genetic aspects of tuberous sclerosis in the West of Scotland. *J Med Genet* 26:28–31, 1989a.

Sampson JR, Yates JRW, Pirrit LA, et al: Evidence for genetic heterogeneity in tuberous sclerosis. *J Med Genet* 26:511–516, 1989b.

Sharp D, et al: Tuberous sclerosis in an infant of 28 weeks gestational age. *J Neurol Sci* 10:59–62, 1983.

Sidman RL, Rakic P: Neuronal migration, with special reference to developing human brain: A review. *Brain Res* 62:1–35, 1973.

Sinclair W, Wright JL, Churg A: Lymphangioleiomyomatosis in a postmenopausal woman. *Thorax* 40:475–476, 1985.

Smith M, Smalley S, Cantor R, et al: Mapping of a gene determining tuberous sclerosis to human chromosome 11q14–11q23. *Genomics* 6:105–114, 1990.

Stefansson K, Wollman RL: Distribution of the neuronal specific protein, 14-3-2, in central nervous system lesions of tuberous sclerosis. *Acta Neuropathol (Berlin)* 53:113–117, 1981.

Stefanson K, Wollmann RL, Huttenlocher PR: Lineages of cells in the central nervous system, in Gomez MR (ed): *Tuberous Sclerosis:* 2nd ed. New York, Raven Press, 1988, p 75–87.

Szeiles B, Herholz K, Heiss WD, et al: Hypometabolic cortical lesions in tuberous sclerosis with epilepsy: Demonstration by positron emission tomography. *J Comput Assist Tomogr* 7:946–953, 1983.

Trombley IK, Mirra SS: Ultrastructure of tuberous sclerosis: Cortical tuber and subependymal tumor. *Ann Neurol* 9:174–181, 1981.

Van Bogaert L, Paillas JE, Mme Berar-Badier Payan H: Etude sur la sclérose tubéreuse de Bourneville à forme cérébelleuse. *Rev Neurol* 98:673–689, 1958.

Van der Hoeve J: Eye symptoms in tuberous sclerosis of the brain. *Trans Ophthalmol Soc* 40:329–334, 1920.

Vogt H: Zur Diagnostik der tuberosen Sklerose. *Z Erforsch Behandl Jugendl Schwachsinns* 2:1–12, 1908.

Watson GH: Cardiac rhabdomyomas in tuberous sclerosis. *Ann NY Acad Sci* 615:50–57, 1991.

Weinblatt ME, Kahn E, Kochen J: Renal cell carcinoma in patients with tuberous sclerosis. *Pediatrics* 80:898–903, 1987.

Wiederhold WC, Gomez MR, Kurland LT, Incidence and prevalence of tuberous sclerosis in Rochester, Minnesota: 1950–1962. *Neurology* 35:600–603, 1985.

Incontinentia Pigmenti

Ashley JR, Burgdorf WH: Incontinentia pigmenti: Pigmentary changes independent of incontinence. *J Cutan Pathol* 14(4):248–250, 1987.

Bolognia JL, Pawelek JM: Biology of hypopigmentation. *J Am Acad Dermatol* 19(2 Pt 1):217–255, 1988.

Brown CA: Incontinentia pigmenti: The development of pseudoglioma. *Br J Ophthalmol* 72(6):452–455, 1988.

Brunquell PJ: Recurrent encephalomyelitis associated with incontinentia pigmenti. *Pediatr Neurol* 3(3):174–177, 1987.

Caputo R, Gianotti F, Innocenti M: Ultrastructural findings in incontinentia pigmenti. *Int J Dermatol* 14(1):46–55, 1975.

Carney RG: Incontinentia pigmenti. A world statistical analysis. *Arch Dermatol* 112(4):535–542, 1976.

Cohen BA: Incontinentia pigmenti. *Neurol Clin* 5(3):361–377, 1987.

Diamantopoulos N, Bergman I, Kaplan S: Actinomycosis meningitis in a girl with incontinentia pigmenti. *Clin Pediatr* 24(11):651–654, 1985.

El-Benhawi MO, George WM: Incontinentia pigmenti: A review. *Cutis* 41(4):259–262, 1988.

Fellner MJ, Weinstein LH: Incontinentia pigmenti in a boy. *Int J Dermatol* 17(1):67–68, 1978.

Garcia-Dorado J, de Unamuno P, Fernandez-Lopez E, Salazar VJ, Armijo M: Incontinentia pigmenti: XXY male with a family history. *Clin Genet* 38(2):128–138, 1990.

Guerrier CJ, Wong CK: Ultrastructural evolution of the skin in incontinentia pigmenti (Bloch-Sulzberger). Study of six cases. *Dermatologica* 149(1):10–22, 1974.

Honig PJ, Miller ME: Incontinentia pigmenti—A possible immunologic disorder. *J Pediatr* 80(2):334–336, 1972.

Jessen RT, Van Epps DE, Goodwin JS, Bowerman J: Incontinentia pigmenti. Evidence for both neutrophil and lymphocyte dysfunction. *Arch Dermatol* 114(8):1182–1186, 1978.

Kunze J, Frenzel UH, Huttig E, Grosse F-R, Wiedemann H-R: Klinefelter's syndrome and incontinentia pigmenti Bloch-Sulzberger. *Hum Genet* 35(2):237–240, 1977.

Larsen R, Ashwal S, Peckham N: Incontinentia pigmenti: Association with anterior horn cell degeneration. *Neurology* 37(3):446–450, 1987.

Lucky AW: Pigmentary abnormalities in genetic disorders. *Dermatol Clin* 6(2):193–203, 1988.

Martinez G, Carnazza MML, Caltabiano C: Melanosomes, melanocytes and keratinocytes in the human epidermis in incontinentia pigmenti. *Arch Ital Anat Embriol* 95(1):65–76, 1990 [in Italian].

Menni S, Piccianno R, Biolchini A, Delle Piane RM, Bardare M: Incontinentia pigmenti and Behçet's syndrome: An unusual combination. *Acta Dermatol Venereol* 66(4):351–354, 1986.

Menni S, Piccinno R, Biolchini A, Plebani A: Immunologic investigations in eight patients with incontinentia pigmenti. *Pediatr Dermatol* 7(4):275–277, 1990.

Moss C, Ince P: Anhidrotic and achromians lesions in incontinentia pigmenti. *Br J Dermatol* 116(6):839–849, 1987.

Nazzaro V, Brusasco A, Gelmetti C, Ermacora E, Caputo R: Hypochromic reticulated streaks in incontinentia pigmenti: An immunohistochemical and ultrastructural study. *Pediatr Dermatol* 7(3):174–178, 1990.

O'Brien JE, Feingold M: Incontinentia pigmenti. A longitudinal study. *Am J Dis Child* 139(7):711–712, 1985.

Pallotta R, Dalpra L: Chromosomal instability in incontinentia pigmenti: Study of four families. *Ann Genet* 31(1):27–31, 1988.

Roberts WM, Jenkins JJ, Moorhead EL 2d, Douglass EC: Incontinentia pigmenti, a chromosomal instability syndrome, is associated with childhood malignancy. *Cancer* 62(11):2370–2372, 1988.

Sasaki M, Hanaoka S, Suzuki H, Takashima S, Arima M: Cerebral white matter lesions in a case of incontinentia pigmenti with infantile spasms, mental retardation and left hemiparesis. *No To Hattatsu* 23(3):278–283, 1991 [in Japanese].

Schamburg-Lever G, Lever WF: Electron microscopy of incontinentia pigmenti. *J Invest Dermatol* 61(3):151–158, 1973.

Schmalstieg FC, Jorizzo JL, Tschen J, Subrt P: Basophils in incontinentia pigmenti. *J Am Acad Dermatol* 10(2 Pt 2):362–364, 1984.

Shuper A, Bryan RN, Singer HS: Destructive encephalopathy in incontinentia pigmenti: A primary disorder? *Pediatr Neurol* 6(2):137–140, 1990.

Siemes H, Schneider H, Dening D, Hanefeld F: Encephalitis in two members of a family with incontinentia pigmenti (Bloch/Sulzberger syndrome). The possible role of inflammation in the pathogenesis of CNS involvement. *Eur J Pediatr* 129(2):103–115, 1978.

Simonsson H: Incontinentia pigmenti, Bloch-Sulzberger's syndrome, associated with infantile spasms. *Acta Paediatr Scand* 61(5):612–614, 1972.

Takematsu H, Seiji M: The role of macrophages in incontinentia pigmenti histologica. Migration and phagocytosis of macrophages. *J Dermatol* 7(5):335–339, 1980.

Wiley HE 3d, Frias JL: Depigmented lesions in incontinentia pigmenti. A useful diagnostic sign. *Am J Dis Child* 128(4):546–547, 1974.

Worret WI, Nordquist RE, Burgdorf WH: Abnormal cutaneous nerves in incontinentia pigmenti. *Ultrastruct Pathol* 12(4):449–454, 1988.

Zillikens D, Mehringer A, Lechner W, Burg G: Hypo- and hyperpigmented areas in incontinentia pigmenti. Light and electron microscopic studies. *Am J Dermatopathol* 13(1):57–62, 1991.

Hypomelanosis of Ito

Amon M, Menapace R, Kirnbauer R: Ocular symptomatology in familial hypomelanosis Ito. Incontinentia pigmenti achromians. *Ophthalmologica* 200(1):1–6, 1990.

Donat JF, Walsworth DM, Turk LL: Focal cerebral atrophy in incontinentia pigmenti achromians. *Am J Dis Child* 134(7):709–710, 1980.

Flannery DB: Pigmentary dysplasias, hypomelanosis of Ito, and genetic mosaicism. *Am J Med Genet* 35(1):18–21, 1990.

Fleury P, Dingemans K, de Groot WP, et al: Ito's hypomelanosis (incontinentia pigmenti achromians). A review of four cases. *Clin Neurol Neurosurg* 88(1):39–44, 1986.

Glover MT, Brett EM, Atherton DJ: Hypomelanosis of Ito: Spectrum of the disease. *J Pediatr* 115(1):75–80, 1989.

Hamada K, Tanaka T, Ohdo S, et al: Incontinentia pigmenti achromians as part of a neurocutaneous syndrome: A case report. *Brain Dev* 1(4):313–317, 1979.

Hara M, Mitsuishi Y, Yajima K, et al: Ito syndrome (hypomelanosis of Ito) as a cause of intractable epilepsy. *Jpn J Psychiatr Neurol* 43(3):487–489, 1989.

Ito M: Studies on melanin. XI. Incontinentia pigmenti achromians: A singular case of nevus depigmentosus systematicus bilateralis. *Tohoku J Exp Med* 55(suppl):57–59, 1952.

Klug H, Schreiber G, Hauschild R: Incontinentia pigmenti achromians (Ito syndrome). Cell morphological aspects. *Dermatol Monatsschr* 168(10):680–685, 1982 [in German].

Morohashi M, Hashimoto K, Goodman TF Jr, Newton DE, Rist T: Ultrastructural studies of vitiligo, Vogt-Koyanagi syndrome, and incontinentia pigmenti achromians. *Arch Dermatol* 113(6):755–766, 1977.

Morohashi M, Maeda T, Takahashi S, Igarashi R: Ultrastructure of incontinentia pigmenti achromians, with special reference to melanocytes and nerve endings. *J Dermatol* 8(5):401–409, 1981.

Moss C, Burn J: Genetic counselling in hypomelanosis of Ito: Case report and review. *Clin Genet* 34(2):109–115, 1988.

Pascual-Castroviejo I, López-Rodriguez L, la Cruz Medina M, Salamanca-Maesso C, Herrero CR: Hypomelanosis of Ito. Neurological complications in 34 cases. *Can J Neurol Sci* 15(2):124–129, 1988.

Ross DL, Liwnicz BH, Chun RW, Gilbert E: Hypomelanosis of Ito (incontinentia pigmenti achromians)—A clinicopathologic study: Macrocephaly and gray matter heterotopias. *Neurology* 32(9):1013–1016, 1982.

Rott HD, Lang GE, Huk W, Pfeiffer RA: Hypomelanosis of Ito (incontinentia pigmenti achromians). Ophthalmological evidence for somatic mosaicism. *Ophthal Paediatr Genet* 11(4):273–279, 1990.

Rubin MB: Incontinentia pigmenti achromians. Multiple cases within a family. *Arch Dermatol* 105(3):424–425, 1972.

Schwartz MF Jr, Esterly NB, Fretzin DF, Pergament E, Rozenfeld IH: Hypomelanosis of Ito (incontinentia pigmenti achromians): A neurocutaneous syndrome. *J Pediatr* 90(2):236–240, 1977.

Turleau C, Taillard F, Doussau de Bazignan M, et al: Hypomelanosis of Ito (incontinentia pigmenti achromians) and mosaicism for a microdeletion of 15q1. *Hum Genet* 74(2):185–187, 1986.

Other Pigmentary Neurocutaneous Disorders

Barbieri F, Santangelo R, Indaco A, De Furio M, Buscaino GA: Neurocutaneous melanosis, neurofibromatosis and spinal meningioma: An unusual association. *Acta Neurol* 12(2):115–121, 1990.

Bussone G, La Mantia L, Vaghi MA, et al: Amelanotic leptomeningeal malanoblastosis. Case report. *Ital J Neurol Sci* 11(2):171–175, 1990.

Hoperskaya OA: Induction—The main principle of melanogenesis in early development. *Differentiation* 20(2):104–116, 1981.

Kasantikul V, Shuangshoti S, Pattanaruenglai A, Kaoroptham S: Intraspinal melanotic arachnoid cyst and lipoma in neurocutaneous melanosis. *Surg Neurol* 31(2):138–141, 1989.

Rhodes RE, Friedman HS, Hatten HP Jr, et al: Contrast-enhanced MR imaging of neurocutaneous melanosis. *AJNR* 12(2):380–382, 1991.

Van Heuzen EP, Kaiser MC, de Slegte RG: Neurocutaneous melanosis associated with intraspinal lipoma. *Neuroradiology* 31(4):349–351, 1989.

Witkop CJ Jr, Jay B, Creel D, Guillery RW: Optic and otic neurologic abnormalities in oculocutaneous and ocular albinism. *Birth Defects* 18(6):299–318, 1982.

Malformations of the Central Nervous System II

Given the complexity of embryologic development of the brain and spinal cord in gross as well as microscopic structure, malformations of the central nervous system (CNS) are hardly unexpected. Many are associated with chromosomal aberrations, whereas others may be under polygenic influence. The anomalies that follow are some of the more common that will confront a primary care physician. They are presented not so much because of their frequency but because of the variations and complications that are of practical importance when caring for affected infants and children. The interested reader is referred to the bibliography for further references.

Other Neurocutaneous Disorders

Daniel W. Stowens

This portion of the chapter presents an incomplete listing of malformative syndromes that include cutaneous features other than the prominent pigmentary components of the preceding chapter. How the CNS abnormalities are related to the skin signs is, as yet, unknown. As the dermal components are essential for the diagnoses, brief discussions of the skin pathology are included.

ABNORMALITIES OF NONPIGMENTED EPIDERMAL CELLS

The term *nevus* has somewhat diffuse or broad usage in dermatology. More precisely it is applied to circumscribed congenital abnormalities of any cell type. Through common usage, the term has been applied to benign tumors and pigmented lesions of the skin. A qualifying adjective, usually denoting the anatomic or histologic derivation, is appended to the term for more specificity, as in *epidermal nevus, junctional nevus, intradermal nevus, melanocytic nevus,* or *vascular nevus.*

Several nevus syndromes have been reported, separate because they had different nevi as the cutaneous expressions of the disorders: linear nevus sebaceous, nevus unis lateris, basal cell nevus, giant hairy nevus, and organoid nevus. Two types of disorders can be distinguished for the interested neurologist: those with cutaneous lesions including nevus cells and those without.

Congenital giant pigmented nevi, with nevus cells, have been associated with a wide variety of nervous system malformations. Epidermal nevi, a generic name for a group of cutaneous tumors without nevus cells, have been noted to occur familially in relation to several relatively specific neuropathologic findings and consistent clinical features.

Congenital (Giant) Pigmented Nevi

The giant congenital nevus syndrome is a sporadic disorder. The most important clinical feature is the risk of the development of malignant, often fatal, melanomas. The neurologic symptoms have been managed symptomatically with no reported special concerns. No histologic or embryologic correlation has been reported between the presence of the nevus cells in the skin and the malformations of neurologic structures. Skin lesions over the spine have been associated with spina bifida and meningomyelocele. Those on the scalp have been associated with brain malformations and the attendant symptoms, such as seizures, mental retardation, and central motor deficits.

The nevus cell is thought to be a slightly aberrant derivative of the neural crest. The nevus cell is capable of differentiating into melanocytic or Schwann cell–like structures, either because it is bi- or pluripotent, or because there are two subpopulations of nevus cells. One

FEATURE TABLE 18-1. GIANT CONGENITAL NEVUS

Discriminating Feature	Consistent Feature	Variable Feature
1. Congenital pigmented nevus in garmentlike distribution	1. Malformative lesions of underlying brain or spine	1. High likelihood of developing malignant melanoma

---

Pearls and Perils: Giant Congenital Nevus Syndrome

1. The topographic extent of the CNS involvement is predicted by the extent of scalp and midline dorsum skin involvement.

---

would expect the CNS histopathology in the congenital nevus syndrome to shed some light on the role and fate of these cells, but the necessary details are not yet available.

Clinical Management

Symptomatic treatment of seizures, mental retardation, and spasticity is uncomplicated in the giant pigmented nevus syndrome. The extent of the cutaneous lesions makes dermatologic management difficult. The propensity for the development of malignant melanoma is high. Prophylactic removal of the nevi is rarely practical or possible.

Epidermal Nevus Syndrome

The combination of one of the epidermal nevi (most frequently on the face, less commonly on the scalp) and anomalous development of brain, eye, skeleton, heart, or kidneys is called the epidermal nevus syndrome. Although most cases are sporadic, autosomal dominant inheritance has been reported in rare families.

Dermatology

The epidermal nevi of the syndrome are identical to the varieties noted in isolation. Histologic features are hyperkeratosis, papillomatosis, and acanthosis. Additional cutaneous findings are frequently noted: areas of hypopigmentation, cafe au lait spots, and other nevi all have the microscopic appearance of similar nonsyndromic lesions.

Neurology

A combination of neuropathologic features can be considered to define a specific neurologic variant of the syndrome. Hemimegalencephaly with neuronal migration defects and hyperplasia and hypertrophy of neurons and glia ipsilateral to the nevus produce mental retardation, seizures, and contralateral hemiparesis. Those are the major components of the neurocutaneous syndrome. Approximately half of the population with detected epidermal nevi have neurologic abnormalities. Secondary CNS manifestations include infarcts, atrophy, porencephaly, hydrocephalus, and calcifications. Those may be the result of vascular anomalies, including angiomas, arteriovenous malformations, absent dural sinuses, and systemic malformations such as coarctation of the aorta.

Clinical Management

The seizures of the epidermal nevus syndrome are readily responsive to standard anticonvulsant treatment. Mental retardation is usually mild. Specific deficits of higher cortical function and behavioral disorders may be more prevalent than has been reported.

Pearls and Perils: Epidermal Nevus Syndrome

1. All children with focal seizures must be scrutinized for an epidermal nevus. The nevus is usually near the midline on the upper face, but can be concealed by hair on the scalp.

2. Hypertrophy of the half of the body ipsilateral to the abnormal and enlarged cerebral hemisphere should suggest one of the nevus syndromes. Atrophy or hypoplasia contralateral to the abnormal hemisphere is the expected effect of a parietal lesion, not usually the manifestation of a neurocutaneous syndrome.

FEATURE TABLE 18-2. EPIDERMAL NEVUS SYNDROME

Discriminating Feature	Consistent Features	Variable Feature
1. Epidermal nexus	1. Partial seizures 2. Mental deficiency 3. Hemihypertrophy and other skeletal abnormalites	1. Hemimegalencephaly

ANNOTATED BIBLIOGRAPHY

Pavone P, Curatolo P, Rizzo R, et al: Epidermal nevus syndrome: A neurologic variant with hemimegalencephaly, gyral malformation, mental retardation, seizures, and facial hemihypertrophy. *Neurology* 41(2 Pt 1):266–271.

This paper is not only a report of firsthand observations of children with the syndrome, but also a review of reported cases. The current, eclectic approach to the diagnosis is well represented. Clinicians will recognize features of the syndrome present in various combinations and degrees in their own patients with the disorder. These patients have the syndrome itself, not a ''forme fruste.''

Basal Cell Nevus Syndrome

Also known as multiple nevoid cell carcinoma syndrome, or Gorlin's syndrome, this autosomal dominant disorder is one of the familial tumor syndromes. Multiple basal cell epitheliomas, locally invasive low-grade malignancies, can appear after the age of 2 years. They increase in number at puberty, and arise in crops thereafter. Other cutaneous lesions are commonly noted in affected individuals. Milia of the face, epidermal cysts, fibromas, lipomas, cafe au lait spots, and pigmented nevi have been reported. Skeletal abnormalities of the skull, jaw, spine, ribs, sternum, and metacarpals have been seen in about 75% of patients. Mental retardation, congenital hydrocephalus, deafness, and calcification of the dura are the dominant neurologic features. Medulloblastomas occur in a larger than expected proportion of the affected population.

DISORDERS OF OTHER EPIDERMAL CELLS

Ichthyosis is a disorder of skin characterized by dryness and scaling. Several pathophysiologic factors are now recognized as producing ichthyosis: increased transepidermal water loss, increased rate of cell arrival at the surface of the epidermis, and decreased rate of cell loss at the surface. The primary cutaneous disorders have been classified into two major groups. In lamellar ichthyosis and epidermolytic hyperkeratosis there is marked hyperkeratosis, a thickened layer of cornifying keratinocytes just under the surface cells (granular layer). There is also a marked decreased in transit time from basal cells to surface. In ichthyosis vulgaris, auto-

Pearls and Perils: Sjögren-Larsson Syndrome

1. A developmental language disorder, independent of the mental deficiency, is so common in this syndrome that it may actually be a constant feature.
2. In some families, there is a distinct correlation between the extent of the skin disease and the severity of the neurologic disease.
3. All children with congenital ichthyosis should be carefully followed for the development of spasticity and mental retardation (evident before the age of 3 years), yielding the diagnosis.
4. All children with spastic diplegia should be examined for ichthyosis, and a family history of the skin disorder should be sought.

somal dominant and X-linked recessive forms, there is decreased thickness, or even absence, of the granular layer and normal transit time.

Several syndromes have been described in which neurologic dysfunction, beyond peripheral nerve involvement, is associated with ichthyosis most closely resembling lamellar ichthyosis.

Sjögren-Larsson Syndrome

The neurologic manifestations of this autosomal recessive disease include mental retardation, spastic paralysis most prominent in the lower extremities, and degeneration of the pigment epithelium of the retina. Together with congenital ichthyosis the first two neurologic features make up the diagnostic triad. About half of the children are born prematurely, but are of appropriate weight for gestational age. They tend to have few of the severe problems of prematurity. The ichthyosis is present at birth. The spasticity is recognizable in the first year of life and does not appear to be progressive. About one-third of patients have seizures, not well characterized in the literature. Pubertal development is normal, though this may be by diagnostic definition; Rud's syndrome consists of ichthyosis, mental retardation, hypogonadism, and epilepsy. The mental retardation ranges

FEATURE TABLE 18-3. SJÖGREN-LARSSON SYNDROME

Discriminating Features	Consistent Features	Variable Features
1. Congenital ichthyosis	1. Autosomal recessive inheritance	1. Retinal pigment degeneration
2. Mental retardation	2. Dysarthria and dysphonia	2. Widely spaced teeth, enamel dysplasia
3. Spastic di- or quadriparesis	3. Hypertelorism	3. Diffuse cortical atrophy
4. Glistening dots on the optic fundi		

from severe to mild, with half of the patients' IQs falling below 50. Abnormalities in serum phospholipids were reported in 1982 but not subsequently confirmed. In the few cases examined postmortem, neuronal loss in the basal ganglia and dysmyelination of the frontal lobes were described.

ANNOTATED BIBLIOGRAPHY

Jagell S, Heijbel J: Sjögren-Larsson syndrome: Physical and neurological features. A survey of 35 patients. *Helv Paediatr Acta* 37:519–530, 1982.

This review of the findings in a large population from a small country demonstrates the consistent features that define the syndrome.

Selmanowity VJ, Porter MJ: The Sjögren-Larsson Syndrome. *Am J Med* 42:412–422, 1967.

This review of non-Swedish cases points out the associated facial and dermal dysmorphisms that may be common in the disorder, even in heterozygote carriers.

Sjögren T, Larsson T: Oligophrenia in combination with congenital ichthyosis and spastic disorders. A clinical and genetic study. *Acta Psychiatr Scand* 32:1–113, 1957.

The original report, still quite complete in clinical details.

Neuroichthyoses

Distinctions have been made between patients with ichthyosis and a variety of cutaneous and neurologic signs and symptoms. The primary reason for classifying patients with dysplastic nails, alopecia, abnormal hair, abnormal teeth, growth retardation, hypogonadism, mental retardation, epilepsy, spasticity, and deafness separately is the lack of overlap in the families. All of the disorders appear to be autosomal recessive.

Rud's syndrome. Mental retardation, seizures, and disordered statural growth and sexual development associated with lamellar-like ichthyosis are the dominant manifestations of this autosomal recessive disorder. The mental deficiency is often profound, and the seizures commonly are very difficult to control.

Keratitis, ichthyosis, and deafness (KID syndrome). Alopecia, including eyelashes and brows, dystrophy of the nails, and sensorineural deafness distinguish this syndrome from other neuroichthyoses.

Tay's syndrome. Distinctive abnormalities of hair

Pearls and Perils: Neuroichthyosis

1. Patients with ichthyosis of any sort, with neurologic involvement without spasticity, are probably best classified as having "nonspecific" neuroichthyosis.
2. Patients with more than the cardinal features of Sjögren-Larsson syndrome probably can be assigned to another named diagnostic pigeonhole.

---

formation, ichthyosis, dystrophic nails, hypogonadism, mental retardation, microcephaly, spasticity, and basal ganglia calcification are the features of this disorder.

Ichthyosis with neutral lipid storage disease. Deafness, cataracts, and myopathy, with ichthyosis, are sometimes seen in patients with prominent leukocyte lipid granules or vacuoles. The obligate heterozygotes have vacuolated eosinophils.

Other combinations of signs and symptoms have been reported in different, unrelated families. The link between the pathogenesis of the neurologic abnormalities and the epidermal disease in any of the syndromes is not understood.

VASCULAR SYNDROMES

The neurocutaneous syndromes that are produced by abnormalities of the vascular component of both dermal and neural systems fall into two broad classes. One, nongenetic, is the result of a vascular malformation that produces skin and brain dysfunction by virtue of the proximity of the two organs at the head—Sturge-Weber syndrome. The other class includes the telangiectasias. Ataxia-telangiectasia is associated with a defined molecular biologic feature: defective DNA repair. The group of disorders with similar defects includes Cockayne's syndrome, xeroderma pigmentosum, and others. The cutaneous and neurologic manifestations develop later in life and thus complicate the embryologic explanations of the disease.

FEATURE TABLE 18-4. NEUROICHTHYOSIS

Discriminating Features	Consistent Features (Specific Syndromes)	Variable Features
1. Icthyosis 2. CNS dysfunction	1. Mental retardation 2. Short stature 3. Delayed pubertal development 4. Spasticity	1. Developmental language disorders 2. Epilepsy 3. Dermal derivative abnormalities (hair, teeth, sweat glands)

FEATURE TABLE 18-5. STURGE-WEBER SYNDROME

Discriminating Features	Consistent Features	Variable Features
1. Port wine stain (nevus flammeus) in trigeminal distribution 2. Ipsilateral meningocortical venous malformation	1. Progressive cortical deficits 2. Focal (partial) epilepsy 3. Glaucoma	1. Truncal, limb cutaneous vascular malformations 2. Mental retardation 3. Hemihypertrophy, hemiatrophy

Sturge-Weber Syndrome

The vascular malformation of Sturge-Weber syndrome is a congenital dysplasia of mature capillaries, identical to nevus flammeus (port wine stain birthmark), seen anywhere on the body. If the malformation involves the skin innervated by the superior division of the trigeminal nerve, the vascular disorder very frequently is expressed in the ipsilateral leptomeninges and cerebral cortex, as Sturge-Weber syndrome. It is not clear whether the anatomic, and presumably embryologic, specificity for the ophthalmic nerve is more refined to the frontal and, possibly, lacrimal subbranches of the first trigeminal branch. Why there is such a close relationship between the distribution pattern of the vascular malformation and the innervation of the face is unknown. Review of the embryologic phases of development of the trigeminal nerve and the vasculature of the head reveals that the ophthalmic branch has reached the skin at Streeter stage XIX. The blood vessels have just separated into external, dural, and cerebral networks or strata at the same stage. The separation of the dural vascular system from the external system appears to be dependent on the formation of the membranous skull. The superior orbital fissure, the most lateral (and latest formed) extent of which carries the lacrimal and frontal branches of the ophthalmic nerve, represents a defect, albeit normal, in the skull. The cranial induction of vascular formation might be faulty. The most minimal anatomic distribution of the deficit would then be the last region of the head to undergo vascular system separation; earlier appearance of the malformation would include those areas induced afterward. How such a mechanism could explain the involvement of the skin on the neck, upper trunk, and upper extremities, as is occasionally seen, is not clear.

The pathogenesis of the neurologic symptoms is probably progressive ischemia of the adjacent cerebral cortex. Predictably, seizures, deficits of cortical motor function, specific deficits of higher cortical function, and mental retardation are seen in a very high percentage of the affected children. The neurologic manifestations of the disorder are progressive, frequently recognized in the latter half of the first year of life. The neurologic problems of Sturge-Weber syndrome are always cortical in origin and, obviously, focal in character.

Clinical Management

Recommendations for very early surgical removal of the intracranial vascular malformation, with the surrounding cerebral cortex, can no longer be accepted. Operation in infancy may avoid the inevitable deterioration in neurologic function and take advantage of the remarkable capacity of infants to ameliorate cerebral deficits. However, current understanding of the mechanism of the disorder's progression had led to medical therapy. Acetylsalicylic acid alters the natural history of the disease to such a degree that complete avoidance of important neurologic sequelae can be anticipated in the majority of cases. Additional treatment aimed at avoiding venous and capillary thrombosis should be used in those patients who are unable to tolerate aspirin. Anecdotal experience with pentoxifylline has not yielded any information. Doses small enough for infants could not be readily produced, and aspirin became recognized as effective before the experimental treatment was refined. The seizures respond to those agents effective in the focal epilepsies, carbamazepine and the hydantoins, and if necessary can be treated surgically after the appropriate preoperative evaluations are made. The seizures will not spontaneously remit, so early operative treatment is possible in the disorder if medical therapy fails.

The dermatologic management of Sturge-Weber syndrome is primarily cosmetic. Hemoglobin's absorption of light energy in the frequency band of the argon laser can be used to produce extremely restricted denaturation of the vascular malformation and marked reduc-

---

Pearls and Perils:
Sturge-Weber Syndrome

1. Hemihypertrophy, seen in the disorder, is usually associated with a vascular malformation of the affected limb(s). A similar enlargement is seen in the skull ipsilateral to the port wine stain.
2. Prilosec or other ulcer medicine may be used to allow the administration of aspirin in some otherwise intolerant children.

tion in the intensity of coloration of the nevus. Local surgical treatment of mucosal involvement is sometimes needed, and very frequently (45% of cases) glaucoma must be treated both operatively and medically.

Ataxia-Telangiectasia

Ataxia-telangiectasia is an autosomal recessive disease; the gene has been mapped to the long arm of chromosome 11 (11q22–23). Recent observations on the incidence of solid cancers in heterozygotes, notably breast cancer in women, suggest high penetrance and beg the definition of recessive. An estimate of the prevalence of the carrier state is about 1% of the North American population. Although the gene defect has not been identified yet, there is sufficient information to allow reasonable hypotheses to be developed about the pathogenesis of the disorder. One of the most intriguing is that the disorder is caused by defective regulation of the immunoglobulin gene superfamily. The manifestations explained by this theory are the well-documented immunodeficiency, the progressive neurologic disorders, and the defect in repair of radiation-induced DNA damage. Other clinical features of the syndrome include thymic dysplasia, frequent lymphoreticular malignancies, and mucocutaneous telangiectasia.

Dermatology

The characteristic dilated venules, capillaries, and arterioles that are the telangiectases develop after the age of 3 years. Initially recognized on the bulbar conjunctivae, the dermal vascular lesions become increasingly evident on the sun-exposed skin of the head, face, neck, chest, and then extremities. Other dermatologic findings include cafe au lait spots, premature graying of scalp hair (but no reports of vitiligo), eczema, and hirsutism.

Neurology

Children with ataxia-telangiectasia appear normal, although small, in infancy. After development of the ability to walk, clumsiness and slowly progressive ataxia are seen. Movement disorders of basal ganglia origin develop to a greater or lesser degree, and decreased movements of the face with abnormal eye movements suggest progressive brainstem involvement. Telangiectasia in the brainstem has been demonstrated. The clinical

---

Pearls and Perils:
Ataxia-Telangiectasia

1. Oculomotor abnormalities in ataxia-telangiectasia are a constant feature. They are distinctly more complex than the signs of pure cerebellar dysfunction. They include slow initiation of saccades and interrupted pursuit, absent optokinetic nystagmus.

2. Heterozygotes for the ataxia-telangiectasia gene are hypersensitive to ionizing radiation. It is thought that about 1.5% of the United States population carries the gene.

3. Serum α-fetoprotein and carcinoembryonic antigen levels are high in ataxia-telangiectasia.

4. Progressive death of neurons is seen, not only in the cerebellum, but also in the brainstem and spinal cord, and later in the cerebral hemispheres themselves. The clinical correlates of disorders at these locations have also been recognized—spinal muscular atrophy and early dementia.

---

symptoms, however, rarely correlate with the vascular malformations. The deterioration in neural function with paucity of demonstrable pathologic changes resembles the paraneoplastic syndromes. No recognized association exists between the development of a lymphoproliferative malignancy and the neurologic signs in ataxia-telangiectasia. However, there is such an association between lymphoma or lymphocytic leukemia and cerebellar degeneration in general. The role of immune defects in the pathogenesis of various symptoms of the disorder is being studied.

Clinical Management

The most important clinical problems relate to the immunodeficiency; a significant fraction of the patients die from respiratory infections. A recent report of treatment with intravenous immunoglobulins needs confirmation, but raises the hope of the more effective treatment than that provided by the antibiotic therapies used to date. Unfortunately, those patients who do not die as the re-

---

FEATURE TABLE 18–6. ATAXIA-TELANGIECTASIA

Discriminating Features	Consistent Features	Variable Features
1. Conjunctival and cutaneous telangiectasia	1. Thymic hypoplasia	1. Leukemia, lymphoma
2. Progressive cerebellar ataxia	2. CD3+/CD4+ lymphocyte deficiency	2. Solid tumors of breast, pancreas, stomach, bladder, and ovary
3. Increased chromosomal sensitivity to radiation-induced breakage	3. Sinopulmonary infections	3. High α-fetoprotein levels
4. Low serum IgA levels		4. Ovarian dysgenesis
		5. Endocrine disorders

sult of an infectious disease have an exceptionally high chance of developing a fatal neoplastic disease. Not only lymphosarcoma, Hodgkin's disease, and leukemia, but also recently recognized solid tumors of the breast, pancreas, stomach, bladder, and ovary occur very frequently.

Neurologic treatment of the brainstem and cerebellar deficits has been ineffective. Perhaps therapy directed at the immunologic aberrations of the disease will be more successful.

(*Ataxia-telangiectasia is further discussed on pages 273 and 274.*)

ANNOTATED BIBLIOGRAPHY

Gatti RA, Boder E, Vinters HV, Sparkes RS, Norman A, Lange K: Ataxia-telangiectasia: An interdisciplinary approach to pathogenesis. *Medicine* 70(2):99–117, 1991.

A comprehensive review of current knowledge. This article includes a notably complete description of the disease's neuropathology and a discussion of its embryologic implications. The essay ends with a detailed analysis of the genetic studies done to date.

Hereditary Hemorrhagic Telangiectasia

Osler-Rendu-Weber disease is an autosomal dominant disorder. Telangiectasia of the skin, mucosal surfaces, and lungs with marked fragility or tendency to bleed are the hallmarks of the disorder. Other organs, including the brain, can be the site of vascular malformations. Much more frequently, cerebral problems are secondary to the progressive pulmonary disease. Cerebrovascular accidents, transient ischemic attacks, and cerebral abscesses are the most common and serious neurologic complications.

Klippel-Trenauney-Weber Syndrome

A diffuse vascular malformation with cutaneous manifestations of telangiectasia (port wine stain) associated with hypertrophy of the skeletal structures underlying the lesion is the diagnostic hallmark of the disorder. If the port wine stain is in the scalp, macrocephaly occurs. The clinical distinction between Sturge-Weber syndrome with extension onto the trunk and upper extremities and the cephalic extension of this syndrome rests on the lack of cerebral involvement in the Klippel-Tren-

auney-Weber syndrome. If the skin lesion consists of multiple cavernous hemangiomas with scalp involvement and macrocephaly, the disorder is called the Riley-Smith syndrome. This autosomal dominant disorder is probably very similar to Klippel-Trenauney-Weber.

VON HIPPEL-LINDAU DISEASE

Von Hippel-Lindau disease is an autosomal dominant disease that has been traditionally included with the neurocutaneous syndromes because it commonly exhibits retinal lesions. Van der Hoeve named the lesions of the eye and skin phakomas (*phakoi*=lentil-shaped) in 1923. Von Hippel-Lindau diseases does not affect the skin. The CNS is commonly affected in the disorder. One of the hereditary cancer syndromes, von Hippel-Lindau disease is apparently genetically homogeneous. The gene responsible for the disease has been mapped to the distal short arm of chromosome 3 (3p25–p26). Additionally, it has been shown that the normal gene in heterozygotes is lost in the cancers that develop over time in the disease.

Retinal hemangiomas are the earliest ocular signs of the disorder. They can be detected in the fundi of children from about 5 years of age on. They usually progress asymptomatically. The retina can become displaced, or detached, by accumulation of an exudate from the tumor. Retinal hemangioblastomas tend to overlie the optic disk, and may be mistaken for papilledema. At least 10% of patients with retinal hemangioblastoma have an intracranial tumor as well, they have von Hippel-Lindau disease. The diagnosis can be made by detecting the intracranial (usually cerebellar) or retinal hemangioblastoma and one other characteristic lesion: a renal, pancreatic, or epididymal cyst or renal carcinoma. At least 60% of patients have cerebellar hemangioblastomas. Although the posterior fossa tumors produce signs of increased intracranial pressure and progressive brainstem dysfunction, they can be detected in the presymptomatic stage by modern imaging techniques. Hemangiomas of the brainstem, spinal cord, and cerebral hemispheres are also seen, but much less frequently. Renal carcinoma metastatic to brain also occurs in the disorder.

The renal lesions of von Hippel-Lindau disease include cysts, adenomas, hemangiomas, and the malig-

FEATURE TABLE 18-7. VON HIPPEL-LINDAU DISEASE

Discriminating Features	Consistent Features	Variable Features
1. Retinal hemangioblastoma 2. Intracranial hemangioblastoma	1. Autosomal dominant inheritance 2. Renal, pancreatic, or epididymal cysts	1. Cysts and hemangiomas of the viscera 2. Pheochromocytoma 3. Adrenal adenoma

nant hypernephromas and renal cell carcinomas. If the cancer can be detected before metastasis, it can be surgically treated. About 45% of autopsy cases show the renal cancers.

Cysts and hemangiomas of most visceral organs are seen much more frequently in von Hippel-Lindau disease than in the general population. The pancreas, adrenal glands, epididymis, liver, spleen, ovaries, lungs, bones, bladder, and skin have all manifested the vascular tumors and benign cysts and tumors of the disorder.

The principal concern in the clinical management of the disorder is the detection of the tumors at an early stage. Periodic examinations, with indirect ophthalmoscopy to examine the periphery of the fundus, should start in childhood. Imaging studies of the brain and kidneys must be repeated at intervals. The average age of onset of symptoms of cerebellar hemangioblastomas is 13 years; that of signs of renal carcinoma, 41 years. Polycythemia may be present with a cerebellar hemangioblastoma, the result of erythropoietic activity of the tumor. As the disorder is autosomal dominant with high penetrance, careful repeated examinations of the family members at risk should be carried out.

ANNOTATED BIBLIOGRAPHY

Filling-Katz MR, Chouke PL, Oldfield E, et al: Central nervous system involvement in Von Hippel-Lindau disease. *Neurology* 41(1):41–46, 1900.

This article is a nice statistical assessment of the neurologic involvement in the disorder. Suggestions for the use of modern imaging techniques and other modes of testing are well supported.

BIBLIOGRAPHY

Nevus Syndromes

Choi BH, Kudo M: Abnormal neuronal migration and gliomatosis cerebri in epidermal nevus syndrome. *Acta Neuropathol (Berl)* 53:319–325, 1981.

David P, Elia M, Garcovich A, et al. A case of epidermal nevus syndrome with carotid malformation. *Ital J Neurol Sci* 11(3):293–296, 1990.

Dobyns WB, Garg BP. Vascular abnormalities in epidermal nevus syndrome. *Neurology* 41:276–278, 1991.

Eichler C, Flowers FP, Ross J. Epidermal nevus syndrome: Case report and review of clinical manifestations. *Pediatr Dermatol* 6(4):316–320, 1989.

Ellis DL, Nanney LB, King LE Jr. Increased epidermal growth factor receptors in seborrheic keratoses and acrochordons of patients with the dysplastic nevus syndrome. *J Am Acad Dermatol* 23:1070–1077, 1990.

Feuerstein RC, Mims LC. Linear nevus sebaceous with convulsions and mental retardation. *Am J Dis Child* 104:675–679, 1962.

Hager BC, Dyme IZ, Guertin SR, et al. Linear nevus sebaceous syndrome: Megalencephaly and heterotopic gray matter. *Pediatr Neurol* 7(1):45–49, 1991.

Hodge JA, Ray MC, Flynn KJ. The epidermal nevus syndrome. *Int J Dermatol* 30(2):91–98, 1991.

Kelley RS, Wagner RF Jr, Sanchez RL, Duff RR. Complete spontaneous regression of multiple basal cell carcinomas in the basal cell nevus syndrome: The possible role of transepithelial elimination. *J Dermatol Surg Oncol* 16(11):1039–1042, 1990.

Manz HJ, Phillips TM, Rowden G, McCullough DC. Unilateral megalencephaly, cerebral cortical dysplasia, neuronal hypertrophy, and heterotopia: Cytomorphometric, fluorometric, cytochemical, and biochemical analyses. *Acta Neuropathol* 45:97–103, 1979.

Nuno K, Mihara M, Shimao S. Linear sebaceous nevus syndrome. *Dermatologica* 181(3):221–223, 1990.

Pavone L, Curatolo P, Rizzo R, et al. Epidermal nevus syndrome: A neurologic variant with hemimegalencephaly, gyral malformation, mental retardation, seizures, and facial hemihypertrophy. *Neurology* 41:266–271, 1991.

Rogers M, McCrossin I, Commens C. Epidermal nevi and the epidermal nevus syndrome. A review of 131 cases. *J Am Acad Dermatol* 20(3):476–488, 1989.

Sakuta R, Aikawa H, Takashima S, Yoza A, Ryo S. Epidermal nevus syndrome with hemimegalencephaly: A clinical report of a case with acanthosis nigricans-like nevi on the face and neck, hemimegalencephaly, and hemihypertrophy of the body. *Brain Dev* 11(3):191–194, 1989.

Solomon LM, Esterly NB. Epidermal and other congenital organoid nevi. *Curr Prob Pediatr* 6:1–56, 1975.

Zaremba J. Jadassohn's naevus phakomatosis: 2. A study based on a review of thirty-seven cases. *J Ment Defic Res* 22:103–123, 1978.

Goldberg LH, Hsu SH, Alcalay J. Effectiveness of isotretinoin in preventing the appearance of basal cell carcinomas in basal cell nevus syndrome. *J Am Acad Dermatol* 21(1):144–145, 1989.

Hasegawa K, Amagasa T, Shioda S, Kayano T. Basal cell nevus syndrome with squamous cell carcinoma of the maxilla: Report of a case. *J Oral Maxillofac Surg* 47(6):629–633, 1989.

Mustaciuolo VW, Brahney CP, Aria AA. Recurrent keratocysts in basal cell nevus syndrome: Review of the literature and report of a case. *J Oral Maxillofac Surg* 47(8):870–873, 1989.

Pearlman RL, Herzog JL. Arachnoid cyst in a patient with basal cell nevus syndrome. *J Am Acad Dermatol* 23:519–520, 1990.

Neuroichthyoses

Andria G, Ballabio A, Parenti G, Di Maio S, Piccirillo A. Steroid sulphatase deficiency is present in patients with the syndrome "ichthyosis and male hypogonadism" and with "Rud syndrome." *J Inherited Metab Dis* 7(Suppl 2):159–160, 1984.

Anibaldi A, Cieri E, Finocchi G. Sjögren-Larsson syndrome (contribution of 2 cases with familial features). *Minerva Pediatr* 19(11):483–487, 1967.

Boudouresques J, Khalil R, Vigouroux RA, Poncet M, Bille J. Complex neuro-ectodermic dysplasia associated with oligophrenia, spastic paraplegia, epilepsy, cataract and congenital ichthyosis. Nosological discussion. *Acta Neurol Belg* 69(4):241–248, 1969.

Dykes PJ, Marks R, Harper PS. Syndrome of ichthyosis, hepatosplenomegaly and cerebellar degeneration: Steroid sulphatase activity. *Br J Dermatol* 102(3):353–354, 1980.

Fivenson DP, Lucky AW, Iannoccone S. Sjögren-Larsson syndrome associated with the Dandy-Walker malformation: Report of a case. *Pediatr Dermatol* 6(4):312–315, 1989.

Gellis SS, Feingold M. Sjögren-Larsson syndrome (congenital ichthyosis with spastic paralysis and oligophrenia). *Am J Dis Child* 116(6):653–654, 1968.

Gilbert WR Jr, Smith JL, Nyhan WL. The Sjögren-Larsson syndrome. *Arch Ophthalmol* 80(3):308–316, 1968.

Giovannini M, Riva E, Besana R, Daroda C, Romeo A. A case of congenital lamellar ichthyosis, alopecia universalis and hypohidrosis with psychomotor retardation and epilepsy. Rud syndrome? *Minerva Pediatr* 31(24):1775–1779, 1979.

Guilleminault CG, Harpey JP, Lafourcade J. Sjögren-Larsson syndrome. Report of two cases in twins. *Neurology* 23(4):367–373, 1973.

Happle, R. The lines of Blaschko: A developmental pattern visualizing functional X-chromosome mosaicism. *Curr Probl Dermatol* 17:5–18, 1987.

Heijer A, Reed WB. Sjögren-Larsson syndrome. Congenital ichthyosis, spastic paralysis, and oligophrenia. *Arch Dermatol* 92(5):545–552, 1965.

Ignatowicz R, Michaowicz R, Kubicka K, Kmiec T, Jozwiak S. Clinical symptomatology and diagnostic criteria in Rud's syndrome. *Pol Tyg Lek* 40(49):1374–1375, 1985.

Larbrisseau, A, Carpenter S. Rud syndrome: Congenital ichthyosis, hypogonadism, mental retardation, retinitis pigmentosa and hypertrophic polyneuropathy. *Neuropediatrics* 13(2):95–98, 1982.

Maldonado RR, Tamayo L, Carnevale A. Neuroichthyosis with hypogonadism (Rud's syndrome). *Int J Dermatol* 14(5):347–352, 1975.

Marxmiller J, Trenkle I, Ashwal S. Rud syndrome revisited: Ichthyosis, mental retardation, epilepsy and hypogonadism. *Dev Med Child Neurol* 27(3):335–343, 1985.

McLennan JE, Gilles FH, Robb RM. Neuropathological correlation in Sjögren-Larsson syndrome. Oligophrenia, ichthyosis and spasticity. *Brain* 97(4):693–708, 1974.

Munke M, Kruse K, Goos M, Ropers HH, Tolksdorf M. Genetic heterogeneity of the ichthyosis, hypogonadism, mental retardation, and epilepsy syndrome. Clinical and biochemical investigations on two patients with Rud syndrome and review of the literature. *Eur J Pediatr* 141(1):8–13, 1983.

Nissley PS, Thomas GH. The Rud syndrome: Ichthyosis, hypogonadism, mental retardation. *Birth Defects* 7(8):246–247, 1971.

Rodriguez Sanchez, MD, Corral Carames MJ, Rodriguez Arnao MD, et al. Ichthyosis, epileptic crises and infantilism: 4 cases of Rud syndrome. *An Esp Pediatr* 25(3):201–203, 1986.

Ruiz-Maldonado R, Tamayo L. Classification of neuroichthyosis. *Mod Probl Paediatr* 17:65–70, 1975.

Stormorken H, Sjaastad O, Langslet A, et al. A new syndrome: Thrombocytopathia, muscle fatigue, asplenia, miosis, migraine, dyslexia and ichthyosis. *Clin Genet* 28(5):367–374, 1985.

Sylvester PE. Pathological findings in Sjögren-Larsson syndrome. *J Ment Defic Res* 13(4):267–275, 1969.

Theiss B. Uniovular twins with ichthyosis vulgaris, discordantly combined with multiple malformations. *Helv Paediatr Acta* 23(5):429–444, 1968.

Try K. Herdopathia atactica polyneuritiformis (Refsum's disease). The diagnostic value of phytamic acid determination in serum lipids. *Eur Neurol* 2(5):296–314, 1969.

Sturge-Weber Syndrome

Avila JO, Radvany J, Huck FR, et al. Anterior callosotomy as a substitute for hemispherectomy. *Acta Neurochir Suppl (Wien)* 30:137–143, 1980.

Bebin EM, Gomez MR. Prognosis in Sturge-Weber disease: Comparison of unihemispheric and bihemispheric involvement. *J Child Neurol* 3(3):181–184, 1988.

Chaudary RR, Brudnicki A. Sturge-Weber syndrome with extensive intracranial calcifications contralateral to the bulk of the facial nevus, normal intelligence, and absent seizure disorder. *AJNR* 8(4):736–737, 1987.

Chiron C, Raynaud C, Dulac O, et al. Study of the cerebral blood flow in partial epilepsy of childhood using the SPECT method. *J Neuroradiol* 16(4):317–324, 1989.

Chugani HT, Mazziotta JC, Phelps ME. Sturge-Weber syndrome: A study of cerebral glucose utilization with positron emission tomography. *J Pediatr* 114(2):244–253, 1989.

Cibis GW, Tripathi RC, Tripathi BJ. Glaucoma in Sturge-Weber syndrome. *Ophthalmology* 91(9):1061–1071, 1984.

Di Trapani G, Di Rocco C, Abbamondi AL, Caldarelli M, Pocchiari M. Light microscopy and ultrastructural studies of Sturge-Weber disease. *Childs Brain* 9(1):23–36, 1982.

Enjolras O, Riche MC, Merland JJ. Facial port-wine stains and Sturge-Weber syndrome. *Pediatrics* 76(1):48–51, 1985.

Fishman MA, Baram TZ. Megalencephaly due to impaired cerebral venous return in a Sturge-Weber variant syndrome. *J Child Neurol* 1(2):115–118, 1986.

Fukuyama Y, Tsuchiya S. A study on Sturge-Weber syndrome. Report of a case associated with infantile spasms and electroencephalographic evolution in five cases. *Eur Neurol* 18(3):194–204, 1979.

Furukawa T. Klippel-Trenaunay-Weber syndrome. *Nippon Rinsho* 35(Suppl 1):524–525, 1977.

Garcia JC, Roach ES, McLean WT. Recurrent thrombotic deterioration in the Sturge-Weber syndrome. *Childs Brain* 8(6):427–433, 1981.

Ito M, Sato K, Ohnuki A, Uto A. Sturge-Weber disease: Operative indications and surgical results. *Brain Dev* 12(5):473–477, 1990.

Iwach AG, Hoskins HD Jr, Hetherington J Jr, Shaffer RN. Analysis of surgical and medical management of glaucoma in Sturge-Weber syndrome. *Ophthalmology* 97(7):904–909, 1990.

Lee S. Psychopathology in Sturge-Weber syndrome. *Can J Psychiatry* 35(8):674–678, 1990.

Mancardi GL. Pathologic anatomy of cerebral arteriovenous malformations. *Minerva Med* 77(25):1157–1163, 1986.

Marini D, Bonavia L, Buzzetti I, Veraldi S. Sturge-Weber syndrome. Clinico-therapeutic study of 107 patients. *G Ital Dermatol Venereol* 123(12):661–663, 1988.

Masson C, Gallet JP, Cheron F, Masson M, Cambier J. Epilepsy with bilateral cortical calcifications. Discussion of a durable post-critical deficit. *Rev Neurol (Paris)* 144(8–9):499–502, 1988.

McNaughton FL, Rasmussen T. Criteria for selection of patients for neurosurgical treatment. *Adv Neurol* 8:37–48, 1975.

Neetens A, Martin JJ, Neetens I, Smets RM. The Klippel-Trenauney-Sturge-Weber syndrome. *Bull Soc Belge Ophtalmol* 224:123–137, 1987.

Norman MG, Schoene WC. The ultrastructure of Sturge-Weber disease. *Acta Neuropathol (Berl)* 37(3):199–205, 1977.

Phelps CD. The pathogenesis of glaucoma in Sturge-Weber syndrome. *Ophthalmology* 85(3):276–286, 1978.

Probst FP. Vascular morphology and angiographic flow patterns in Sturge-Weber angiomatosis: Facts, thoughts and suggestions. *Neuroradiology* 20(2):73–78, 1980.

Rappaport ZH. Corpus callosum section in the treatment of intractable seizures in the Sturge-Weber syndrome. *Childs Nerv Syst* 4(4):231–232, 1988.

Riela AR, Stump DA, Roach ES, McLean WT Jr, Garcia JC. Regional cerebral blood flow characteristics of the Sturge-Weber syndrome. *Pediatr Neurol* 1(2):85–90, 1985.

Sarwar M. Deep venous occlusion in the Sturge-Weber syndrome. *Rev Interam Radiol* 2(3):159–161, 1977.

Sperner J, Schmauser I, Bittner R, et al. MR-imaging findings in children with Sturge-Weber syndrome. *Neuropediatrics* 21(3):146–152, 1990.

Stimac GK, Solomon MA, Newton TH. CT and MR of angiomatous malformations of the choroid plexus in patients with Sturge-Weber disease. *AJNR* 7(4):623–627, 1986.

Taly AB, Nagaraja D, Das S, Shankar SK, Pratibha NG. Sturge-Weber-Dimitri disease without facial nevus. *Neurology* 37(6):1063–1064, 1987.

Uram M, Zubillaga C. The cutaneous manifestations of Sturge-Weber syndrome. *J Clin Neuro Ophthalmol* 2(4):245–248, 1982.

Vassella F. Epileptic manifestations of cerebrovascular origin in children. *Schweiz Rundsch Med Prax* 73(24):759–763, 1984.

Wagner RS, Caputo AR, Del Negro RG, Neigel J. Trabeculectomy with cyclocryotherapy for infantile glaucoma in the Sturge-Weber syndrome. *Ann Ophthalmol* 20(8):289–291, 1988.

Wilkins RH. Natural history of intracranial vascular malformations: A review. *Neurosurgery* 16(3):421–430, 1985.

Witschel H, Font RL. Hemangioma of the choroid. A clinicopathologic study of 71 cases and a review of the literature. *Surv Ophthalmol* 20(6):415–431, 1976.

Yoshikawa H, Fueki N, Sakuragawa N, Ito M, Iio M. Crossed cerebellar diaschisis in the Sturge-Weber syndrome. *Brain Dev* 12(5):535–537, 1990.

Telangiectasias

Bridges BA, Harnden DG. Untangling ataxia-telangiectasis (letter). *Nature* 289(5795):222–223, 1981.

Brown LR, Coulam CM, Reese DF. Ataxia-telangiectasia (Louis-Bar syndrome). *Semin Roentgenol* 11(1):67–70, 1976.

Cleaver JE. DNA repair in man. *Birth Defects* 25(2):61–82, 1989.

Cohen MM, Levy HP. Chromosome instability syndromes. *Adv Hum Genet* 18:43–149, 365–371, 1989.

Cowan MJ, Wara DW, Packman S, et al. Multiple biotin-dependent carboxylase deficiencies associated with defects in T-cell and B-cell immunity. *Lancet* 1979;2(8134):115–118, 1979.

Doi S, Saiki O, Hara T, et al. Administration of recombinant IL-2 augments the level of serum IgM in an IL-2 deficient patient. *Eur J Pediatr* 148(7):630–633, 1989.

Fischer A. Primary immunodeficiencies. *Curr Opin Immunol* 2(3):439–444, 1989–1990.

Friedberg EC, Henning K, Lambert C, et al. Microcell-mediated chromosome transfer: A strategy for studying the genetics and molecular pathology of human hereditary diseases with abnormal responses to DNA damage. *Basic Life Sci* 52:257–267, 1990.

Griscelli C. Current data on congenital lymphocytic immune deficiencies. *Brux Med* 58(10):511–523, 1978.

Hannan MA, Greer W, Smith BP, et al. Skin fibroblast cell lines derived from non-Hodgkin's–lymphoma (NHL) patients show increased sensitivity to chronic gamma irradiation. *Int J Cancer* 47(2):261–266, 1991.

Hecht F, Hecht BK. Cancer in ataxia-telangiectasia patients. *Cancer Genet Cytogenet* 46(1):9–19, 1990.

Hittelman WN. Direct measurement of chromosome repair by premature chromosome condensation. *Prog Clin Biol Res* 340B:337–346, 1990.

Houldsworth J, Cohen D, Singh S, Lavin MF. The response of ataxia-telangiectasia lymphoblastoid cells to neutron irradiation. *Radiat Res* 125(3):277–282, 1991.

Lehmann AR, Jaspers NG, Gatti RA. Fourth International Workshop on Ataxia-Telangiectasia. *Cancer Res* 49(21):6162–6163, 1989.

London WP. Gamma/delta T-cell receptors (letter). *Lancet* 337(8741):613, 1991.

Matsumoto S, Sakiyama Y, Kajii N, et al. Ataxia telangiectasia and characterization of its immunological disorders. *No To Hattatsu* 22(2):103–111, 1990.

Minegishi M, Tsuchiya S, Minegishi N, et al. Functional and molecular characteristics of acute lymphoblastic leukemia cells with a mature T-cell phenotype from a patient with ataxia telangiectasia. *Leukemia* 5(1):88–89, 1991.

Mirzayans R, Paterson MC. Lack of correlation between hypersensitivity to cell killing and impaired inhibition of DNA synthesis in ataxia telangiectasia fibroblasts treated with 4-nitroquinoline 1-oxide. *Carcinogenesis* 12(1):19–24, 1991.

Muriel WJ, Lamb JR, Lehmann AR. UV mutation spectra in cell lines from patients with Cockayne's syndrome and ataxia telangiectasia, using the shuttle vector pZ189. *Mutat Res* 254(2):119–123, 1991.

Peterson RD, Funkhouser JD. Speculations on ataxia-telangiectasia: Defective regulation of the immunoglobulin gene superfamily. *Immunol Today* 10(9):313–314, 1989.

Preud'homme JL, Hanson LA. IgG subclass deficiency. *Immunodefic Rev* 2(2):129–149, 1990.

Rosen FS. Genetic deficiencies in specific immune responses. *Semin Hematol* 27(4):333–334, 1990.

Schlesinger I. Ataxia telangiectasia: A familial multisystem disorder. *Conn Med* 53(3):135–137, 1989.

Schwartzman JS, Sole D, Naspitz CK. Ataxia-telangiectasia: A clinical and laboratory review study of 14 cases. *Allergol Immunopathol (Madr)* 18(2):105–111, 1990.

Shiraishi Y. Nature and role of high sister chromatid exchanges in Bloom syndrome cells. Some cytogenetic and immunological aspects. *Cancer Genet Cytogenet* 50(2):175–187, 1990.

Swift M. Genetic aspects of ataxia-telangiectasia. *Immunodefic Rev* 2(1):67–81, 1990.

Swift M, Chase CL, Morrell D. Cancer predisposition of ataxia-telangiectasia heterozygotes. *Cancer Genet Cytogenet* 46(1):21–27, 1990.

Taylor AM, Metcalfe JA, McConville C. Increased radiosensitivity and the basic defect in ataxia telangiectasia. *Int J Radiat Biol* 56(5):677–684, 1989.

Taylor YC, Duncan PG, Zhang X, Wright WD. Differences in the DNA supercoiling response of irradiated cell lines from ataxia-telangiectasia versus unaffected individuals. *Int J Radiat Biol* 59(2):359–371, 1991.

Thacker J. Inherited sensitivity to X-rays in man. *Bioessays* 11(2–3):58–62, 1989.

Hereditary Hemorrhagic Telangiectasia

AAssar OS, Friedman CM, White RI Jr. The natural history of epistaxis in hereditary hemorrhagic telangiectasia. *Laryngoscope* 101(9):977–980, 1991.

Adams HP Jr, Subbiah B, Bosch EP. Neurologic aspects of hereditary hemorrhagic telangiectasia. Report of two cases. *Arch Neurol* 34(2):101–104, 1977.

Bartolucci EG, Swan RH, Hurt WC. Oral manifestations of hereditary hemorrhagic telangiectasia (Osler-Weber-Rendu disease). Review and case reports. *J Periodontol* 53(3):163–167, 1982.

Bean WB. Retinal involvement in hereditary hemorrhagic telangiectasia. *Arch Ophthalmol* 86(6):726, 1971.

Bick RL. Hereditary hemorrhagic telangiectasia and disseminated intravascular coagulation: A new clinical syndrome. *Ann N Y Acad Sci* 370:851–854, 1981.

Borman JB, Schiller M. Osler's disease with multiple large vessel aneurysms. *Angiology* 20(3):113–118, 1969.

Brant AM, Schachat AP, White RI. Ocular manifestations in hereditary hemorrhagic telangiectasia (Rendu-Osler-Weber disease). *Am J Ophthalmol* 107(6):643–646, 1989.

Braverman IM, Keh A, Jacobson BS. Ultrastructure and three-dimensional organization of the telangiectases of hereditary hemorrhagic telangiectasia. *J Invest Dermatol* 95(4):422–427, 1990.

Ceccotti EL, Schuj RA, Yasnig F, Ferretti E. Hereditary hemorrhagic telangiectasia (Rendu-Osler-Weber disease). *Rev Asoc Odontol Argent* 78(3):165–166, 1990.

Conlon CL, Weinger RS, Cimo PL, Moake JL, Olson JD. Telangiectasia and von Willebrand's disease in two families. *Ann Intern Med* 89(6):921–924, 1978.

Cooke DA. Renal arteriovenous malformation demonstrated angiographically in hereditary haemorrhagic telangiectasia (Rendu-Osler-Weber disease). *J R Soc Med* 79(12):744–746, 1986.

Cos LR, Rabinowitz R, Bryson MF, Turula J, Valvo JR. Hereditary hemorrhagic telangiectasia of bladder in a child. *Urology* 20(3):302–304, 1982.

Cynamon HA, Milov DE, Andres JM. Multiple telangiectases of the colon in childhood. *J Pediatr* 112(6):928–930, 1988.

Daly JJ, Schiller AL. The liver in hereditary hemorrhagic telangiectasia (Osler-Weber-Rendu disease). *Am J Med* 60(5):723–726, 1976.

David DG, Smith JL. Retinal involvement in hereditary hemorrhagic telangiectasia. *Arch Ophthalmol* 85(5):618–621, 1971.

De Cenzo JM, Morrisseau PM, Marrocco G. Osler-Weber-Rendu syndrome. Urologist's view. *Urology* 5(4):549–552, 1975.

Flint SR, Keith O, Scully C. Hereditary hemorrhagic telangiectasia: Family study and review. *Oral Surg Oral Med Oral Pathol* 66(4):440–444, 1988.

Gammon RB, Miksa AK, Keller FS. Osler-Weber-Rendu disease and pulmonary arteriovenous fistulas. Deterioration and embolotherapy during pregnancy. *Chest* 98(6):1522–1524, 1990.

Gold MH, Eramo L, Prendiville JS. Hereditary benign telangiectasia. *Pediatr Dermatol* 6(3):194–197, 1989.

Goodman RM, Gresham GE, Roberts PL. Outcome of pregnancy in patients with hereditary hemorrhagic telangiectasia. A retrospective study of 40 patients and 80 matched controls. *Fertil Steril* 18(2):272–277, 1967.

Guillen B, Guizar J, de la Cruz J, Salamanca F. Hereditary hemorrhagic telangiectasia: Report of 15 affected cases in a Mexican family. *Clin Genet* 39(3):214–218, 1991.

Hashimoto K, Pritzker MS. Hereditary hemorrhagic telangiectasia. An electron microscopic study. *Oral Surg Oral Med Oral Pathol* 34(5):751–768, 1972.

Heffner RR Jr, Solitare GB. Hereditary haemorrhagic telangiectasia: Neuropathological observations. *J Neurol Neurosurg Psychiatry* 32(6):604–608, 1969.

Iannuzzi MC, Hidaka N, Boehnke M, et al. Analysis of the relationship of von Willebrand disease (vWD) and hereditary hemorrhagic telangiectasia and identification of a potential type IIA vWD mutation (Ile865 to Thr). *Am J Hum Genet* 48(4):757–763, 1991.

Jahnke V. Ultrastructure of hereditary telangiectasia. *Arch Otolaryngol* 91(3):262–265, 1970.

King CR, Lovrien EW, Reiss J. Central nervous system arteriovenous malformations in multiple generations of a family with hereditary hemorrhagic telangiectasia. *Clin Genet* 12(6):372–381, 1977.

Kristoffersson A, Domellof L, Kullenberg K. Gastrointestinal manifestations of hereditary haemorrhagic teleangiectasia. *Ann Chir Gynaecol* 76(2):96–98, 1987.

Kwaan HC, Silverman S. Fibrinolytic activity in lesions of hereditary hemorrhagic telangiectasia. *Arch Dermatol* 107(4):571–573, 1973.

Lande A, Bedford A, Schechter LS. The spectrum of arteriographic findings in Osler-Weber-Rendu disease. *Angiology* 27(4):223–240, 1976.

Lawrence G, Thruston C, Shultz K, Mengel M. Acanthosis nigricans, telangiectasia and diabetes mellitus. *Birth Defects* 7(8):322–323, 1971.

Livandovskii, IA, Klusova EV, Anikina EV. The lung in Osler-Rendu disease. *Klin Med (Mosk)* 67(12):68–71, 1989.

Martini GA. The liver in hereditary haemorrhagic teleangiectasia: An inborn error of vascular structure with multiple manifestations: A reappraisal. *Gut* 19(6):531–537, 1978.

Menefee MG, Flessa HC, Glueck HI, Hogg SP. Hereditary hemorrhagic telangiectasia (Osler-Weber-Rendu disease). An electron microscopic study of the vascular lesions before and after therapy with hormones. *Arch Otolaryngol* 101(4):246–251, 1975.

Merry GS, Appleton DB. Spinal arterial malformation in a child with hereditary hemorrhagic telangiectasia. Case report. *J Neurosurg* 44(5):613–616, 1976.

Moss HD. Hereditary hemorrhagic telangiectasia. *Gen Dent* 35(4):312–314, 1987.

Myles ST, Needham CW, LeBlanc FE. Alternating hemiparesis associated with hereditary hemorrhagic telangiectasia. *Can Med Assoc J* 103(5):509–511, 1970.

Nikolopoulos N, Xynos E, Vassilakis JS. Familial occurrence of hyperdynamic circulation status due to intrahepatic fistulae in hereditary hemorrhagic telangiectasia. *Hepatogastroenterology* 35(4):167–168, 1988.

Ona FV, Ahluwalia M. Endoscopic appearance of gastric angio-dysplasia in hereditary hemorrhagic telangiectasia. *Am J Gastroenterol* 73(2):148–149, 1980.

Péery WH. Clinical spectrum of hereditary hemorrhagic telangiectasia (Osler-Weber-Rendu disease). *Am J Med* 82(5):989–997, 1987.

Plauchu H, de Chadarevian JP, Bideau A, Robert JM. Age-related clinical profile of hereditary hemorrhagic telangiectasia in an epidemiologically recruited population. *Am J Med Genet* 32(3):291–297, 1989.

Reagan TJ, Bloom WH. The brain in hereditary hemorrhagic telangiectasia. *Stroke* 2(4):361–368, 1971.

Reilly PJ, Nostrant TT. Clinical manifestations of hereditary hemorrhagic telangiectasia. *Am J Gastroenterol* 79(5):363–367, 1984.

Roman G, Fisher M, Perl DP, Poser CM. Neurological manifestations of hereditary hemorrhagic telangiectasia (Rendu-Osler-Weber disease): Report of 2 cases and review of the literature. *Ann Neurol* 4(2):130–144, 1978.

Sobel D, Norman D. CNS manifestations of hereditary hemorrhagic telangiectasia. *AJNR* 5(5):569–573, 1984.

Solomon S, Kleiman AH. Hereditary hemorrhagic telangiectasia associated with polycystic disease of kidneys. *N Y State J Med* 71(13):1665–1668, 1971.

Stanley IM, Hunter KR. Neurological manifestations of hereditary haemorrhagic telangiectasis. *Br Med J* 3(724):688, 1970.

Steel D, Bovill EG, Golden E, Tindle BH. Hereditary hemorrhagic telangiectasia. A family study. *Am J Clin Pathol* 90(3):274–278, 1988.

Sureda A, Cesar J, Garcia Frade LJ, et al. Hereditary hemorrhagic telangiectasia: Analysis of platelet aggregation and fibrinolytic system in seven patients. *Acta Haematol* 85(3):119–123, 1991.

Teragaki M, Akioka K, Yasuda M, et al. Hereditary hemorrhagic telangiectasia with growing pulmonary arteriovenous fistulas followed for 24 years. *Am J Med Sci* 295(6):545–547, 1988.

Varma DG, Schoenberger SG, Kumra A, Agrawal N, Robinson AE. Osler-Weber-Rendu disease: MR findings in the liver. *J Comput Assist Tomogr* 13(1):134–135, 1989.

Vase I, Vase P, Ocular lesions in hereditary haemorrhagic telangiectasia. *Acta Ophthalmol (Copenh)* 57(6):1084–1090, 1979.

Wells, RS, Dowling GB. Hereditary benign telangiectasia. *Br J Dermatol* 84(1):93–94, 1971.

von Hippel-Lindau Disease

Atuk NO, McDonald T, Wood T, et al. Familial pheochromocytoma, hypercalcemia, and von Hippel-Lindau disease. A ten year study of a large family. *Medicine (Baltimore)* 58(3):209–218, 1979.

Boughey AM, Fletcher NA, Harding AE. Central nervous system haemangioblastoma: A clinical and genetic study of 52 cases. *J Neurol Neurosurg Psychiatry* 53(8):644–648, 1990.

Connor JM. von Hippel-Lindau disease (editorial; comment). *Q J Med* 77(283):1099–1100, 1990.

Decker HJ, Gemmill RM, Neumann HP, Walter TA, Sandberg AA. Loss of heterozygosity on 3p in a renal cell carcinoma in von Hippel-Lindau syndrome. *Cancer Genet Cytogenet* 39(2):289–293, 1989.

Filling-Katz MR, Choyke PL, Oldfield E, et al. Central nervous system involvement in Von Hippel-Lindau disease. *Neurology* 41(1):41–46, 1991.

Frank TS, Trojanowski JQ, Roberts SA, Brooks JJ. A detailed immunohistochemical analysis of cerebellar hemangioblastoma: An undifferentiated mesenchymal tumor. *Mod Pathol* 2(6):638–651, 1989.

Glenn GM, Daniel LN, Choyke P, et al. Von Hippel-Lindau (VHL) disease: Distinct phenotypes suggest more than one mutant allele at the VHL locus. *Hum Genet* 87(2):207–210, 1991.

Goodman MD, Goodman BK, Lubin MB, et al. Cytogenetic characterization of renal cell carcinoma in von Hippel-Lindau syndrome. *Cancer* 65(5):1150–1154, 1990.

Hoffman RW, Gardner DW, Mitchell FL. Intrathoracic and multiple abdominal pheochromocytomas in von Hippel-Lindau disease. *Arch Intern Med* 142(10):1962–1964, 1982.

Hubschmann OR, Vijayanathan T, Countee RW. Von Hippel-Lindau Disease with multiple manifestations: Diagnosis and management. *Neurosurgery* 8(1):92–95, 1981.

Hull MT, Warfel KA, Muller J, Higgins JT. Familial islet cell tumors in Von Hippel-Lindau's disease. *Cancer* 44(4):1523–1526, 1979.

Ismail SM, Jasani B, Cole G. Histogenesis of haemangioblastomas: An immunocytochemical and ultrastructural study in a case of von Hippel-Lindau syndrome. *J Clin Pathol* 38(4):417–421, 1985.

Jennings CM, Gaines PA. The abdominal manifestation of von Hippel-Lindau disease and a radiological screening protocol for an affected family. *Clin Radiol* 39(4):363–367, 1988.

Jennings AM, Smith C, Cole DR, et al. Von Hippel-Lindau disease in a large British family: Clinicopathological features and recommendations for screening and follow-up. *Q J Med* 66(251):233–249, 1988.

Kiechle-Schwarz M, Neumann HP, Decker HJ, et al. Cytogenetic studies on three pheochromocytomas derived from patients with von Hippel-Lindau syndrome. *Hum Genet* 82(2):127–130, 1989.

Komatsu K, Misaki T, Hisazumi H, et al. A case of von Hippel-Lindau disease associated with bilateral renal cell carcinoma. *Hinyokika Kiyo* 34(9):1621–1625, 1988.

Kragel PJ, Walther MM, Pestaner JP, Filling-Katz MR. Simple renal cysts, atypical renal cysts, and renal cell carcinoma in von Hippel-Lindau disease: A lectin and immunohistochemical study in six patients. *Mod Pathol* 4(2):210–214, 1991.

Labauge R, Campello C, Barjon P, Mery C, Pages M. Hemangioblastoma of the cerebellum, bulbo-spinal cord syringomyelia and bilateral pheochromocytoma. *Rev Neurol (Paris)* 144(3):194–201, 1988.

Lamiell JM, Salazar FG, Hsia YE. von Hippel-Lindau disease affecting 43 members of a single kindred. *Medicine (Baltimore)* 68(1):1–29, 1989.

Lee KR, Kishore PR, Wulfsberg E, Kepes JJ. Supratentorial leptomeningeal hemangioblastoma. *Neurology* 28(7):727–730, 1978.

Lozes G, Lesoin F, Fallas P, Biserte J, Jomin M. Multivisceral expression of von Hippel Lindau disease. *Rev Otoneurooph-talmol* 54(5):453–460, 1982.

Maher ER, Yates JR, Ferguson-Smith MA. Statistical analysis of the two stage mutation model in von Hippel-Lindau disease, and in sporadic cerebellar haemangioblastoma and renal cell carcinoma. *J Med Genet* 27(5):311–314, 1990.

Maher ER, Yates JR, Harries R, et al. Clinical features and natural history of von Hippel-Lindau disease. *Q J Med* 77(283):1151–1163, 1990.

Maher ER, Bentley E, Yates JR, et al. Mapping of von Hippel-Lindau disease to chromosome 3p confirmed by genetic linkage analysis. *J Neurol Sci* 100(1–2):27–30, 1991.

Maloney KE, Norman RW, Lee CL, Millard OH, Welch JP. Cytogenetic abnormalities associated with renal cell carcinoma. *J Urol* 146(3):692–696, 1991.

Michels VV. Investigative studies in von Hippel-Lindau disease. *Neurofibromatosis* 1(3):159–163, 1988.

Mottow-Lippa L, Tso MO, Peyman GA, Chejfec G. von Hippel angiomatosis. A light, electron microscopic, and immunoperoxidase characterization. *Ophthalmology* 90(7):848–855, 1983.

Nerad JA, Kersten RC, Anderson RL. Hemangioblastoma of the optic nerve. Report of a case and review of literature. *Ophthalmology* 95(3):398–402, 1988.

Neumann HP, Wiestler OD. Clustering of features of von Hippel-Lindau syndrome: Evidence for a complex genetic locus (comments). *Lancet* 337(8749):1052–1054, 1991.

Neumann HP, Dinkel E, Brambs H, et al. Pancreatic lesions in the von Hippel-Lindau syndrome. *Gastroenterology* 101(2):465–471, 1991.

Nicolaij D, Vogel-Kerebyn C, van den Bergh R, Steeno OP. Bilateral epididymal cysts as the first clinical manifestation of von Hippel-Lindau-disease. A case report. *Andrologia* 11(3):234–235, 1979.

Peterson GJ, Codd JE, Cuddihee RE, Newton WT. Renal transplantation in Lindau-von Hippel Disease. *Arch Surg* 112(7):841–842, 1977.

Pou Serradell A, Mares Segura R, Lamarca Ciuro JL. Combined medullary hemangioblastoma and syringomyelia in a patient with von Hippel-Lindau disease: Pathological study *Rev Neurol (Paris)* 144(6–7):456–458, 1988.

Reich H, Hollwich F. Von Hippel-Lindau syndrome. *Klin Monatsbl Augenheilkd* 184(6):513–519, 1984.

Schmidt D, Neumann HP, Eggert HR, Friedburg H. Neuro-ophthalmologic findings in hemangioblastoma of the cerebellum and brain stem—downbeat nystagmus as the first symptom of hemangioblastoma in Hippel-Lindau disease. *Fortschr Ophthalmol* 85(4):427–433, 1988.

Solomon D, Schwartz A. Renal pathology in von Hippel-Lindau disease. *Hum Pathol* 19(9):1072–1079, 1988.

Tory K, Brauch H, Linehan M, et al. Specific genetic change in tumors associated with von Hippel-Lindau disease. *J Natl Cancer Inst* 81(14):1097–1101, 1989.

Congenital Malformations of the Central Nervous System

Jerome S. Haller

SPINA BIFIDA

The terms *spina bifida, myelodysplasia,* and *myelomeningocele* are used interchangeably to describe infants with vertebral arch fusion defects and varying degrees of involvement of the spinal cord and its covering (Table 18–1).

Spina bifida is the failure of fusion of vertebral arches, most commonly found in the lumbosacral area and with lesser frequency in the thoracic and cervical regions. Failure of fusion of the entire spinal column, rachischisis, is very uncommon and not compatible with life. Meningocele indicates that the contents of the spinal canal are externally exposed, a meningeal sac overlying the spinal cord and interposed between the unfused dorsal arches. Nerve roots may be visible extending from the cord and following their normal course. The infant can be free of any neurologic deficit despite this anatomic abnormality. Closure of the defect is required to prevent rupture and meningitis, although in some infants the defect is small and closes naturally by overgrowth of skin. More extensive anatomic involvement of the spinal cord along with spina bifida is incorporated into the term *myelomeningocele*. The cord at the site of the defect may be intact but not covered by pia-arachnoid or it may be splayed open, giving the appearance of the embryonic state before closure of the neural tube: dorsal columns laterally and ventral columns medially with varying degrees of cover of this defect by abnormal arachnoid.

Neurologic Deficits

Deficits are determined by the level at which the cord is malformed. Joint contractures of hips, knees, and ankles may already be present at birth, the result of in utero paralysis.

Functional levels can be determined in part by observation of the infant's spontaneous muscular activity below the defect and in part by the level of the lesion itself. With a sacral defect the infant may be expected to have little, if any, impairment of muscle function. There is normal muscle strength and movement down to the feet, where plantar flexion could be weakened. Bladder and anal sphincters remain intact. A lumbar myelomeningocele produces paresis/paralysis of musculature about the ankles and knees, but generally leaves hip musculature intact. In general, a thoracolumbar defect will result in paresis/paralysis of muscles of the hip girdle and below. In both of these latter defects, bladder sphincter and musculature and anal sphincter will be affected.

TABLE 18-11. SPINA BIFIDA: A SUMMARY

Axial Anomaly	Dermal Defects	Bony Defects	Nervous System Defects
Spina bifida occulta	Hypesthetic midline thin-skinned area or hairy patch over lower lumbar spine	By x ray only: Nonfusion of arches	May have no significance or minimal distal weakness May be associated with lipoma, tethered cord syndrome Progressive lower extremity weakness and sphincter defects
Spina bifida aperta Meningocele	Cutaneous defect with cord and covering visible	Nonfusion of dorsal spines above and below visible defect	No to minimal involvement of lower extremities distally
Myelomeningocele, myelodysplasia	Fusion of dura and arachnoid with skin Cord intact or malformed	As above	Variable and level dependent: from minimal distal weakness to total paralysis of lower extremities and bladder and anal sphincter malfunction

Arnold-Chiari Type II Malformation

Arnold-Chiari type II malformation is present in nearly all of these infants. This malformation, which is associated with spina bifida, consists of elongation and herniation of the cerebellar vermis, through the foramen magnum and extending over the upper cervical cord, along with displacement and distortion of the medulla, including the fourth ventricle. The cerebellar hemispheres may be flattened around the caudal brainstem and even partially herniated. Adhesions and fibrotic meninges impede the flow of ventricular fluid and, as a consequence, hydrocephalus may develop. Aqueductal stenosis may also occur as a result of the distortion of the brainstem. However, macrocephaly need not be present at birth despite early acquired hydrocephalus. Complications of the associated Arnold-Chiari malformation and/or hydrocephalus are being recognized more frequently and include apnea, vocal cord paralysis, stridor, and other clinical signs of lower bulbar dysfunction (Paposozomenos and Roessmann, 1981; Hest and Wolraich, 1985). These have been variously attributed to (1) crowding of the medulla in the posterior fossa and

herniation into the upper cervical spinal canal, (2) progressive hydrocephalus with further herniation of the lower brainstem, (3) combinations of (1) and (2), and (4) repeated ischemic/hemorrhagic infarcts of the displaced brainstem from distortion of its vascular supply. Surgical correction has been attempted by enlarging the foramen magnum and/or shunt revision. In some children, respiratory embarrassment will require tracheostomy and permanent ventilatory support. Surgical intervention may not be effective in all cases in view of the various etiologic possibilities. The initial workup should include x rays of the entire spine to eliminate vertebral anomalies at other levels and a computed tomographic (CT) scan of the head or magnetic resonance imaging (MRI) study for visualization of the ventricular system and brainstem.

If shunting is necessary because of hydrocephalus, the infant must be followed closely for shunt malfunction. Acute failure in the infant results in a bulging anterior fontanelle and possible lethargy and vomiting. When the fontanelle has closed, lethargy, vomiting, and (with progression) a sixth-nerve palsy may develop. Acute respiratory arrest has also been reported (Tomita and McClone, 1983). In the infant chronic malfunction

FEATURE TABLE 18-8. SPINA BIFIDA OCCULTA

Discriminating Features	Consistent Features	Variable Features
1. Hypesthetic midline thin-skinned area or hairy patch over lower lumbar spine 2. By X-ray only: nonfusion of arches	1. None	1. May have no significant or minimal distal weakness 2. May be associated with lipoma, tethered cord syndrome 3. Progressive lower extremity weakness and sphincter defects

<table>
<tr><td>

Pearls and Perils: Spina Bifida

1. Many persons with low back pain are found to have spina bifida occulta without any CNS defects.
2. The bony abnormality of spina bifida aperta may be more extensive than the cutaneous defect. Other spine anomalies or nonfused arches may be found at these levels. Spine x rays should be taken from the cervical through the sacral spine.
3. The functional level of the cord defect can be inferred by observing the posture of the resting limbs and spontaneous movement as well as movement induced by painful stimulation above the cutaneous defect. Painful stimuli applied below the defect to lower limbs can produce movement but only as a reflection of isolated spinal cord reactivity.
4. Development of hyperreflexia and spasticity of the upper extremities may reflect the development of hydromyelia. In one of our own patients, spasticity of one upper extremity was produced by a bony spur impinging on the cervical cord.
5. Macrocephaly and hydrocephalus need not be present at birth. Cranial ultrasound can be used effectively to follow lateral ventricular size.

</td></tr>
</table>

results in continuing macrocephaly (over the 98th percentile). In the older child chronic shunt failure may produce gait disturbances (Torkelson et al., 1985) or more subtle effects on learning or intellect without complaints of headache, intermittent lethargy, and vomiting. Chronic shunt malfunction and the resultant normal-pressure hydrocephalus must be kept in mind for all children with shunts—not only those with spina bifida. Infants with an open anterior fontanelle can be evaluated periodically with ultrasound until the fontanelle is closed. If the ventricular size remains stable, then repeat CT scanning is not likely to be helpful. A CT scan should be done if there is any suspicion of a change in neurologic status or learning skills.

Bladder Dysfunction

Bladder dysfunction, which accompanies thoracolumbar lesions, should not be glossed over as "neurogenic bladder" because there are variations on the theme of dysfunc-

tion. The detrusor musculature may be contracted, leading to a "spastic" condition with a flaccid or spastic external sphincter, or the reverse condition may be present (Park et al., 1985). Urodynamic studies are necessary to manage properly this component of the malformation. Because these infants and children have problems involving multiple systems, long-term care is best managed in a multidisciplinary clinic.

Intellectual Outcome

Factors that may aid in predicting the intellectual capabilities of children with spina bifida include the occurrence of CNS infection (ventriculitis, meningitis) and seizures (McClone et al., 1982; Bartoshesky et al., 1985). The association of hydrocephalus and spina bifida/myelomeningocele does not significantly alter the child's testable IQ (Mapstone et al., 1984). However, complications such as ventriculitis, birth anoxia, and seizures, do. Although seizures may develop as a result of CNS infection, they can also occur in its absence. Presumably the latter course reflects abnormalities of the cortical gray matter including heterotopias and microgyria. In either case, the median IQ in children with complications of shunting, anoxia, infection, or seizures is significantly lower than that in children with uncomplicated hydrocephalus.

Spina Bifida Occulta

The frequency of spina bifida occulta is uncertain because it can exist without any deficit or manifested only by a thinned discolored area of skin in the midline lumbosacral region, by a patch of hair, or by a palpable mass or dermal sinus (Anderson, 1985). Involvement of the spinal cord or the nerve roots may be manifested by a structural asymmetry of the lower extremities with one shortened and smaller leg. Late-onset clinical features include persistent enuresis or progressive weakness of one or both legs. Pathologically there are two types of lesions: those that can compress the cord or conus (lipomata or dermal or epidermal cysts) and those that cause traction on the cord (the so-called tethered cord or diastomatomyelia, with a cartilagenous or bony spicule or spur). Radiologic investigation and surgery should be undertaken to avoid progressive and potentially irreversible injury to the cord.

FEATURE TABLE 18-9. SPINA BIFIDA APERTA MENINGOCELE

Discriminating Features	Consistent Features	Variable Feature
1. Cutaneous defect with cord and covering visible 2. Nonfusion of dorsal spines above and below visible defect	1. None	1. No to minimal involvement of lower extremities distally

FEATURE TABLE 18–10. MYELOMENINGOCELE, MYELODYSPLASIA

Discriminating Features	Consistent Feature	Variable Features
1. Fusion of dura and arachnoid with skin 2. Cord intact or malformed	1. Level dependent minimal distal weakness to total paralysis of lower extremities and bladder and anal sphincter malfunction	1. None

ENCEPHALOCELE

Statistically, encephalocele is seven times less frequent than spina bifida. It too represents a deficit in bone, in this case of the calvarial or basal skull through which nervous tissue extends (Diebler and Dulac, 1983). An occipital encephalocele with microcephaly, polydactyly, polycystic kidney and other facial anomalies makes up the Meckel-Gruber syndrome (Jones, 1988).

Encephaloceles generally occur in the midline, most commonly in the occipital area, less often in the frontal region and uncommonly in defects at the base of the skull. The protruding tissue may consist solely of dura and meninges covered by skin and easily detectable by transillumination, or it may include normal or abnormally structured cerebral tissue. An occipital encephalocele may be confined above the tentorium or may extend to involve nervous tissue of the posterior fossa with cerebellar hypoplasia or aplasia or disorganized cerebellar structure and/or brainstem disorganization. In this circumstance, bifid upper cervical vertebral arches are additional bony defects. Surgical resection of an occipital encephalocele is possible, depending on the size and extent of the cerebral lesion as determined by a CT scan (Lorber, 1967). Hydrocephalus may complicate the postoperative course. An anomaly that externally has the appearance of an occipital encephalocele is the extracranial extension of a fourth ventriculocele (Fernstermaker et al., 1984). This would, in simplistic terms, be a Dandy-Walker–like malformation with external extension of the fourth ventricle because of the absence of the suboccipital bone. A CT or MRI scan should distinguish these anomalies, because the fourth ventriculocele anomaly will not contain any of the supratentorial tissue of the occipital lobes.

FRONTAL ENCEPHALOCELES

Facial malformation and/or hypertelorism accompanies the encephaloceles in this malformation. The cerebral defect extends through the lamina cribrosa of the frontal fossa into the nose, through the ethmoid, into the orbit, or between the orbits to protrude at the glabella. An encephalocele can also develop at the distal end of the metopic suture, where a considerable portion of one or both frontal lobes may be encountered. The infranasal site may only be appreciated if respiratory difficulties result from its location.

Reconstructive surgery is possible for all these forms of frontal encephalocele.

AGENESIS OF THE CORPUS CALLOSUM AND RELATED DISORDERS

A review article on holoprosencephaly (Leech and Shuman, 1986) incorporates a number of malformations into a continuum of dysgenesis of the prosencephalon. Thus, the various forms of holoprosencephaly, complete and partial agenesis of the corpus callosum and the disorder septo-optic dysplasia, and absence of the septum pellucidum can be perceived in a unified fashion.

Agenesis of the corpus callosum is associated with several chromosomal anomalies, including trisomy 13 and 18, and with a wide assortment of non–nervous system, nonchromosomal anomalies as well. Midline facial defects accompany this malformation both with and without chromosomal abberations (Parrish et al., 1979; Lacey, 1985; Jeret et al., 1987). Clinically, other than the midline facial defects, there is nothing distinctive to predict this anomaly. The radiologic investigation of infants with infantile spasms may reveal the presence of agenesis of the corpus callosum in many (Singer et al., 1982). Aicardi's syndrome describes females with infantile spasms, severe retardation, and chorioretinal lacunae in addition to agenesis (Aicardi et al., 1965). Other seizure types can occur at any age with this malformation. In several reports of children with agenesis of the corpus callosum, ventricular dilatation has been found. A few, because of macrocephaly, have been shunted. It should be appreciated that ventricular dilatation is a commonly associated finding, particularly involving the occipital horns, and does not reflect progressive hydrocephalus. The specific enlargement of the occipital horns has been called colpocephaly.

Although retardation is commonly felt to be associated with agenesis, it should not be assumed that all those afflicted will be retarded. A number of patients reported in the literature had average intelligence (Field et al., 1978; Gott and Saul, 1978; Lynn et al., 1980). Carefully carried out neuropsychologic testing does reveal subtle differences in higher cortical function compared to normal persons of the same age and education. Early development of seizures, especially infantile spasms, is predictive of retardation.

AGENESIS OF THE SEPTUM PELLUCIDUM/SEPTO-OPTIC DYSPLASIA

"Lumpers and splitters" have described various combinations of absence of the septum pellucidum, hypoplastic optic nerves, and hypothalamic-pituitary dysfunction, thus muddling this condition (O'Dwyer et al., 1980; Acers, 1981; Arslanian et al., 1984; Izenberg et al., 1984; Costin and Murphree, 1985; Menezes et al., 1988). A recent paper associates absence of the septum pellucidum with various forms of porencephaly, including schizencephaly (O'Dwyer et al., 1980). In its purest form absence/agenesis of the septum pellucidum exists without other associations. Clinically symptomatic infants and children with septo-optic dysplasia will have nystagmus or other evidence of impaired vision and small optic nerve heads or optic nerves, and may have hypoglycemic episodes with or without seizures, short stature, or delayed growth rate. A careful funduscopic examination with pupillary dilatation should be done in the infant with early onset of nystagmus or failure to develop visual tracking. Small or pale, oval or unusually shaped optic disks are additional evidence in the diagnosis of septo-optic dysplasia.

Patients have been reported under the same rubric with a normal septum pellucidum but with hypoplastic optic nerves and hypopituitarism.

Any child with these clinical characteristics will need neuroradiologic, ophthalmologic, and endocrinologic evaluation because of the multifaceted effects of this neuroanatomic malformation.

DANDY-WALKER SYNDROME

The classic triad of hydrocephalus, cystic dilatation of the fourth ventricle, and hypoplasia of the cerebellum constitutes the signs of the Dandy-Walker syndrome (Dandy, 1921). While the latter two components of this disorder must be present at birth, hydrocephalus need not be (Hirsch et al., 1984). Although some infants will have macrocrania and hydrocephalus at birth, others develop this complication in later infancy and even into childhood. It may even turn up unexpectedly without symptoms at autopsy. In one study of 40 patients, only 5 infants had hydrocephalus at birth, though by 1 year the number had increased to 31 (Hirsch et al., 1984). Of 59 additional patients in two other reports, 7 patients did not have this complication at the time of report (Hart et al., 1972; Tal et al., 1980). In infancy, patients may present with progressive macrocephaly or, in the older child, with symptoms of increased intracranial pressure (headache, vomiting), or with signs of cerebellar dysfunction, ataxia (either axial alone or with limb involvement), and nystagmus.

While CT or MRI are definitive, skull transillumination in the young infant is predictive of this anomaly. In the suboccipital area, a triangular pattern of illumination is formed by the torcular at the peak of the triangle and the abnormal site of attachment of the tentorium, with the area of illumination corresponding to the dilatated fourth ventricle.

Of importance to the physician caring for the child is the association of the syndrome with other CNS anomalies as well as other system malformations. Of 89 patients with Dandy-Walker syndrome, 39 children had other CNS structural anomalies (other than cerebellar hypoplasia), including 12 with agenesis of the corpus callosum. Of 49 children, 10 had malformations involving other systems, for example, digit or limb abnormalities, facial clefts, and cardiac abnormalities. Of 48 children evaluated, 19 were retarded or had IQs less than 80. In contrast to some CNS malformations, retardation is not an obligatory component in the Dandy-Walker syndrome.

The authors of a report constituting a review of 21 autopsy-proven cases and 92 patients culled from the literature discuss the possible genetic factors and the likelihood of recurrence (Murray et al., 1985). Dandy-Walker syndrome may be an autosomal recessive disorder when combined with other anomalies, as in the Meckel-Gruber syndrome. Guidelines for genetic counseling are provided.

RETROCEREBELLAR CYSTS

Retrocerebellar cysts, a congenital arachnoidal malformation, can at times be confused with the Dandy-Walker syndrome (Haller et al., 1971; Gilles and Rockett, 1971).

FEATURE TABLE 18-11. DANDY-WALKER SYNDROME

Discriminating Features	Consistent Features	Variable Features
1. Hydrocephalus 2. Cystic dilitation of fourth ventricle 3. Hypoplasia of cerebellum	1. None	1. Age of onset of hydrocephalus 2. Agenesis of corpus callosum 3. Other malformations 4. Retardation

They have been associated with progressive macrocephaly and can in some cases produce obstructive hydrocephalus. Radiologic distinction can be made between the Dandy-Walker syndrome and retrocerebellar cysts by identifying the fourth ventricle. Because of the position of the retrocerebellar cyst, the fourth ventricle is normal but displaced forward and sometimes downward. Insufficient CT scan "cuts" of the posterior fossa contents can trap the unwary into identifying the cyst as an enlarged fourth ventricle.

OTHER MALFORMATIONS

Schizencephaly, lissencephaly, pachygyria, and other similar structural abnormalities are invariably accompanied by retardation and often microcephaly and seizures. There are no non-CNS anomalies specifically associated with these malformations that would cause the pediatrician to consider them. They are generally identified by CT scanning or MRI as part of an evaluation of neonatal seizures, unexplained microcephaly, or retardation.

ANNOTATED BIBLIOGRAPHY

Friede RL: *Developmental Neuropathology*, 2nd ed. New York, Springer-Verlag, 1975.
  Chapter 21 specifically addresses spina bifida and related abnormalities, and Chapter 22 contains information on the Arnold-Chiari malformation.
Lemire RJ, Loeser JD, Leech RW, Alvard ED: *Normal and Abnormal Development of the Human Nervous System*. Hagerstown, Md, Harper & Row, 1975.
  This volume contains an excellent chapter on the development (normal and abnormal) of the spinal cord.
Freeman JM: *Practical Management of Meningomyelocele*. Baltimore, Md, University Park Press, 1974.
  This is a good review of the underlying embryology and the neurologic examination, and a discussion of dysraphism.
Brocklehurst G: *Spina Bifida for the Clinican. Developmental Medicine*, No. 57. Philadelphia, JB Lippincott, 1976.
  This book discusses the evaluation and management of spina bifida aperta and occulta.
Vinken PJ, Bruyn GW, Klawans HL (eds): *Handbook of Clinical Neurology*, Vol 50: *Malformations*. Amsterdam, Elsevier 1987.
  Chapter 29 is a well-organized discussion of spina bifida, from epidemiology, to associated lesions of the brain and spinal cord, to the management and complications of this complex disorder.

REFERENCES

Acers TE: Optic nerve hypoplasia: Septo-optic-pituitary dysplasia syndrome. *Trans Am Ophthalmol Soc* 74:425–457, 1981.

Aicardi J, Lefebvre J, Lerique-Loechlin A: A new syndrome: Spasm in flexion, callosal agenesis, ocular abnormalities. *Electroencephalogr Clin Neurophysiol* 19(suppl):609–610, 1965.
Anderson FM: Occult spinal dysraphism: A series of 73 cases. *Pediatrics* 55:826–835, 1985.
Arslanian SA, Rothfus WE, Foley TP, et al: Hormonal, metabolic, and neuroradiologic abnormalities associated with septo-optic dysplasia. *Acta Endocrinologica* 107:282–288, 1984.
Bartoshesky LE, Haller J, Scott MR, et al: Seizures in children with meningomyelocele. *Am J Dis Child* 139:400–402, 1985.
Costin G, Murphree AL: Hypothalamic-pituitary function in children with optic nerve hypoplasia. *Am J Dis Child* 139:249–254, 1985.
Dandy WE: The diagnosis and treatment of hydrocephalus due to occlusions of the foramina of Magendie and Luschka. *Surg Gynecol Obstet* 32:112–124, 1921.
Diebler C, Dulac O: Cephaloceles: Clinical and neuroradiological appearances. *Neuroradiology* 25:199–216, 1983.
Fernstermaker RA, Roesmann U, Rekate HL: Fourth ventriculoceles with extracranial extension. *J Neurosurg* 61:348–350, 1984.
Field M, Ashton R, White R: Agenesis of the corpus callosum: Report of two pre-school children and review of the literature. *Dev Med Child Neurol* 20:47–61, 1978.
Gilles FH, Rockett FX: Infantile hydrocephalus: Retrocerebellar "arachnoidal" cyst. *J Pediatr* 79:436–443, 1971.
Gott PS, Saul RE: Agenesis of the corpus callosum: Limits of functional compensation. *Neurology* 28:1272–1279, 1978.
Haller JS, Wolpert SM, Rabe EF, et al: Cystic lesions of the posterior fossa in infants: A comparison of the clinical, radiological, and pathological findings in Dandy-Walker syndrome and extra-axial cysts. *Neurology* 21:493–506, 1971.
Hart MN, Malamud N, Ellis WG: The Dandy-Walker syndrome. A clinicopathological study based on 28 cases. *Neurology* 22:771–780, 1972.
Hesz N, Wolraich M: Vocal-cord paralysis and brainstem dysfunction in children with spina bifida. *Dev Med Child Neurol* 27:522–531, 1985.
Hirsch JF, Pierre-Kahn A, Renier D, et al: The Dandy-Walker malformation. *J Neurosurg* 61:515–522, 1984.
Izenberg N, Rosenblum M, Parks JS: The endocrine spectrum of septo-optic dysplasia. *Clinical Pediatrics* 23:632–636, 1984.
Jeret JS, Serur D, Wisniewski K, et al: Clinicopathological findings associated with agenesis of the corpus callosum. *Brain Dev* 9:255–264, 1987.
Jones KL (ed): Meckel-Gruber syndrome, in *Smith's Recognizable Patterns of Human Malformations*, 4th ed. Philadelphia, WB Saunders, 1982, p 152–153.
Lacey DJ: Agenesis of the corpus callosum. Clinical features in 40 children. *Am J Dis Child* 139:953–955, 1985.
Leech RW, Shuman RM: Holoprosencephaly and related midline cerebral anomalies: A review. *J Child Neurol* 1:3–18, 1986.
Lorber J: The prognosis of occipital encephalocele. *Dev Med Child Neurol* 13(suppl):75–86, 1967.
Lynn RB, Buchanan D, Fenichel GM, et al: Agenesis of the corpus callosum. *Arch Neurol* 37:444–445, 1980.
McLone DG, Czyzewski D, Raimondi AJ, et al: Central ner-

vous system infections as a limiting factor in the intelligence of children with myelomeningocele. *Pediatrics* 70:338–342, 1982.

Mapstone TB, Rekate HL, Mulsen FE, et al: Relationship of CSF shunting and IQ in children with myelomeningocele: A retrospective analysis. *Child's Brain* 11:112–118, 1984.

Menezes L, Aicardi J, Goutieres F: Absence of the septum pellucidum with porencephalia. A neuroradiologic syndrome with variable clinical expression. *Arch Neurol* 45:542–545, 1988.

Murray JC, Johnson JA, Bird TD: Dandy-Walker malformation: Etiologic heterogeneity and empiric recurrence risks. *Clin Genet* 28:272–283, 1985.

O'Dwyer JA, Newton TH, Hoyt WF: Radiologic features of septo-optic dysplasia: De Morsier syndrome. *Am J Neurol Res* 1:443–447.

Paposozomenos S, Roessmann U: Respiratory distress and Arnold-Chiari malformation. *Neurology* 31:97–100, 1981.

Park TS, Cail WS, Maggio WM, et al: Progressive spasticity and scoliosis in children with myelomeningocele. *J Neurosurg* 62:367–375, 1985.

Parrish ML, Roessmann U, Levinsohn MW: Agenesis of the corpus callosum: A study of the frequency of associated malformations. *Ann Neurol* 6:349–354, 1979.

Singer WD, Haller JS, Sullivan LR, et al: The value of neuroradiology in infantile spasms. *J Pediatr* 100:47–50, 1982.

Tal Y, Freigang B, Dunn HG, et al: Dandy-Walker syndrome: Analysis of 21 cases. *Dev Med Child Neurol* 22:189–201, 1980.

Tomita T, McLone DG: Acute respiratory arrest: A complication of malformation of the shunt in children with myelomeningocele and Arnold-Chiari malformation. *An J Dis Child* 137:142–144, 1983.

Torkelson RD, Leibrock LG, Gustavson JL, et al: Neurological and neuropsychological effects of cerebral spinal fluid shunting in children with assumed arrested "normal pressure" hydrocephalus. *J Neurol Neurosurg Psychiatr* 48:799–806, 1985.

Disorders of Motor Execution I Cerebral Palsy

Barry S. Russman

Cerebral palsy is "characterized by aberrant control of movement or posture of a patient, appearing early in life (secondary to a central nervous system lesion, damage or dysfunction), and not the result of a recognized progressive or degenerative brain disease" (Nelson and Ellenberg, 1978). In addition to motor deficits, the patient may suffer from other manifestations of cerebral dysfunction, including mental retardation, epilepsy, sensory deficits (hearing or vision loss), learning disabilities, and emotional problems. The diagnosis is established by a history of nonprogressive motor disability. Physical examination localizes the problem to the central nervous system (CNS) as opposed to the motor unit (anterior horn cell, peripheral nerve, nerve-muscle junction, muscle). Efforts to establish an etiology should be made, and these, in combination with the specific type of cerebral palsy (e.g., spastic, dyskinetic) can lead to a prognosis and a rational treatment program. *Cerebral palsy* often has been referred to as a "wastebasket" term. A complete understanding of the meaning and implication of the diagnosis will erase this attitude.

HISTORICAL REVIEW

The words *cerebral palsy* became prominent as a result of the work of Dr. George Little in the 1860s. He defined a specific type of cerebral palsy, namely spastic diplegia, which is still referred to as Little's disease (see Classification). Furthermore, he is credited with the observation that birth anoxia was causally related to cerebral palsy. Sigmund Freud, in his classic 1897 text *Infantile Cerebral Paralysis*, emphasized the existence of associated problems that required attention when analyzing the problems of a patient with this disorder.

During the early part of the twentieth century, most research related to the development of different treatment programs for cerebral palsy patients. The gamut ranged from inhibiting movement with braces to facilitating movement with various stimulation techniques (Weiss and Betts, 1867). Much of the confusion and disagreement regarding treatment related to a lack of knowledge regarding the etiology, pathology, and physiology of cerebral palsy. In addition, an acceptable classification system that would allow comparison of similar patients had not yet been developed.

In the mid- and late 1950s, a classification system was finally established (Minear, 1956). Furthermore, epidemiologic studies were launched in the United States, Western Australia, and Sweden (Nelson and Ellenberg, 1978; Dale and Stanley, 1980; Hagberg et al., 1982, 1984). The study by Nelson and Ellenberg, the National Collaborative Perinatal Project (NCPP), deserves special mention as it is the only prospective one. Twelve hospitals in the United States enrolled over 50,000 pregnant mothers the first time each presented herself for prenatal care. Labors and deliveries were monitored using a carefully designed protocol. The child was evaluated in the delivery room, at 1 day of age, at 3 days of age, at 4 months, at 8 months, at 1 year, at 2 years, at 4 years, and finally at 7 years of age. Included in these evaluations were developmental, neurologic, and psychologic examinations. Although the last patient reached the age of 7 in 1973, analyses of the data will be published for several more years. Much of the information presented in the following sections of this chapter will be summaries of the studies from the NCPP, as well as from the Swedish and Western Australian reports.

CLASSIFICATION

The classification system that is the standard today was published in 1956, the effort of a committee of the American Academy of Cerebral Palsy (Minear, 1956). The system is a clinical one based on the physiology of

TABLE 19-1. CLASSIFICATION OF CEREBRAL PALSY: MOTOR AND TOPOGRAPHIC

A. Spastic
   Diplegia—legs more than arms
   Quadriplegia—all four extremities equally involved
   Hemiplegia—one-sided involvement, usually arm more than leg
   Double Hemiplegia—arms involved more than legs
B. Dyskinetic
   Hyperkinetic or choreoathetoid
   Dystonic
C. Ataxic
D. Mixed

Reproduced from Minear (1956).

TABLE 19-3. CEREBRAL PALSY: RISK FACTORS

Prenatal
   Two or more previous abortions
   Maternal disorder
   Bleeding during pregnancy in births at term
   Preeclamptic signs
   Small-for-gestational-age baby
   Placental infarction
   Multiple births

Perinatal
   Asphyxia
   Cerebral hemorrhage
   Placental ablation
   Hypoxia
   Hyperbilirubinemia
   CNS infection

Reproduced from Hagberg et al. (1984).

the motor dysfunction and the number of limbs involved (Table 19–1). The system establishes an orderly approach to describing a patient's disability. However, it does not afford insight into the pathology or etiology of the problem.

A *complete* description of the patient's difficulties necessitates an attempt to establish the etiology or at least identify the risk factors (Tables 19–2 and 19–3), a listing of the patient's associated problems (Table 19–4), and a summary of his or her functional capacity (Table 19–5).

Physiologic (Motor) Grouping

Table 19–1 summarizes the motor and anatomic grouping. *Spasticity* is defined as increased muscle tone, determined by passively flexing and extending muscle groups across a joint. A satisfactory, reproducible system of grading muscle tone has never been developed. Therefore, in the questionable case, the most experienced examiner will usually make the determination. Associated with spasticity are enhanced deep tendon reflexes, usually with clonus and a positive Babinski response. However, the latter is sometimes difficult to elicit in the infant and even in the older child with spastic cerebral palsy.

Dyskinesias are defined as abnormal motor movements that are most obvious when the patient initiates a movement. The motor patterns and postures of patients with dyskinesias are secondary to inadequate regulation

of muscle tone and coordination (Brun and Kyllerman, 1979; Kyllerman, 1982; Kyllerman et al., 1982). When the patient is totally relaxed, usually in the supine position, a full range of motion and decreased muscle tone are found. Dyskinetic patients are subdivided into two groups: hyperkinetic or *choreoathetoid* patients show purposeless, often massive involuntary movements with motor overflow (that is, the initiation of a movement of one extremity leads to movement of other muscle groups). The *dystonic* group manifest abnormal shifts of general muscle tone induced by movement. Typically, these patients assume and retain abnormal and distorted postures in the same stereotyped patterns. The dyskinesias may occur together in the same patient or independently. Dystonia may be confused with spasticity. In many instances, it is important to distiguish the specific physiologic abnormality, as the etiology, treatment, associated problems, and prognosis are different.

Patients with *ataxias* have a disturbance of the coordination of voluntary movements owing to dyssynergia of the muscles. They commonly walk with a widely based gait and have at least mild intention tremors. A subgroup in the ataxia category is called the disequilibrium syndrome (Sanner, 1973). These patients not only have dysmetria, but also have a pronounced difficulty in maintaining posture and equilibrium. They tend to be hypotonic for the first several years of life prior to the development

TABLE 19-2. CEREBRAL PALSY: ETIOLOGIC GROUPS

Obvious postnatal
Obvious prenatal
   Simple inheritance
   Defined prenatal syndromes
   Unequivocal prenatal infections
   Cerebral malformations
Potential pre- or perinatal
   Presence of one or more risk factors
Unknown
   None of the above

TABLE 19-4. CEREBRAL PALSY: MOTOR DISABILITY AND ASSOCIATED PROBLEMS

	IQ 50	Seizure Disorder
Dyskinesia	30%	27%
Diplegia	33%	31%
Hemiplegia	39%	67%
Quadriplegia	64%	56%

Reproduced from Gibbs et al. (1963).

TABLE 19-5. SEVERITY OF CEREBRAL PALSY

	Gross Motor	Fine Motor	Cognitive	Speech	Overall
Mild	Independent walker	Unlimited function	IQ > 70	More than two words	Independent life
Moderate	Supported walk or creep	Limited function	IQ 50–70	Single words	Need of assistance
Severe	No locomotion	No function	IQ < 50	Indistinct	Total care

Based on Minear (1956) and Veelken et al. (1983).

of useful function. Retardation is almost invariable in this group. Until further studies are published, patients placed in this category should be considered to have a genetic disease.

The mildest form of ataxia might preferably be labeled as apraxia, rather than ataxic cerebral palsy (Gubbay, 1975, page 39). Patients in this category demonstrate normal coordination on a standard neurologic examination but have an impairment in the ability to carry out purposeful gross and fine motor acts. If the treatment program will *not* include orthopedic care, and if the motor limitations are minimal, it is preferable to label the child as being apraxic rather than as having cerebral palsy, recognizing that the latter term carries the implication of associated problems, including mental retardation.

The fourth category that is commonly used in the physiologic and motor classification is the *mixed* group. Patients in this category commonly have mild spasticity with dystonia. Furthermore, ataxia might also be a component of the motoric dysfunction in patients placed in this group.

Anatomic Grouping

Diplegic refers to the involvement of all four extremities, the lower extremities more than the upper. *Quadriplegia* is the term that reflects dysfunction of all four extremities,

although in some patients one upper extremity might be less involved; the term *triplegia* then would be substituted. *Hemiplegia* describes those individuals with one-sided motor dysfunction, and, in most patients, the upper extremity is more severely involved than the lower.

Finally, an unusual situation can occur in which the upper extremities are much more involved than the lower, and the term *double hemiplegia* is applied to this group of patients.

ANNOTATED BIBLIOGRAPHY

Nelson KB, Ellenberg JH: Epidemiology of cerebral palsy, in Schoenberg BS (ed): *Advances in Neurology.* New York, Raven Press, 1978, p 421–435.

This article provides an overview regarding general statistics about cerebral palsy from the NCPP.

Weiss H, Betts HB: Method of rehabilitation in children with neuromuscular disorders. *Pediatr Clin North Am* 14:1009–1016, 1967.

This paper presents a historic perspective on the various treatment programs offered to patients with cerebral palsy over the past 40 years.

Minear WL: A classification of cerebral palsy. *Pediatrics* 18: 841–852, 1956.

This article provides the best insight into the classification system.

FEATURE TABLE 19-1. CLASSIFICATION SYSTEM

Discriminating Features	Consistent Features	Variable Features
Spastic Diplegia 1. Lower extremities more involved than upper	1. Commonly associated with prematurity	1. May have other CNS deficits (cognitive, language)
Spastic Hemiplegia 1. One side of body involved 2. Upper extremity more involved than lower	1. Usually will walk independently 2. May have a parencephalic cyst on CT scan	1. Seizures 2. Learning disabilities
Spastic Quadriplegia 1. All four extremities are involved 2. Legs may be slightly worse than upper extremities	1. Retardation or learning disabilities	1. Seizures
Spastic Double Hemiplegia 1. Upper extremities more dysfunctional than lower, but all four extremities are abnormal	1. Mental retardation	1. Epilepsy

FEATURE TABLE 19-2. CEREBRAL PALSY VERSUS OTHER MOTOR DISORDERS

Discriminating Features	Consistent Features	Variable Features
1. Hyperreflexia, as a rule, establishes the motor disability to be secondary to a brain dysfunction as opposed to a spinal cord or motor unit abnormality 2. Asymmetry of motor abnormalities is not uncommon in cerebral palsy; it is the exception rather than the rule in patients with motor unit disease	1. Gross and fine motor delay 2. Physical examination, history, or imaging procedure establishes the fact that a dysfunction in the central nervous system is responsible for the motor abnormalities	1. Epilepsy 2. Mental retardation 3. Spasticity 4. Dystonia 5. Ataxia

EPIDEMIOLOGY AND ETIOLOGY

Epidemiologic studies of the cerebral palsy population are important for several reasons:

1. The prevalence of disabilities in the population at any one time allows society to plan for and develop programs and facilities.
2. The different types of cerebral palsy can be correlated with gestational age, birth weights, perinatal and postnatal complications, and presumed prenatal abnormalities. This information allows

for the development of hypotheses regarding the etiology of cerebral palsy, which then can be tested.

3. The changing statistics on children being born with cerebral palsy can shed light on the benefits of or problems created by the ability to provide sophisticated care to the very sick newborn (Nelson and Ellenberg, 1978).

Table 19–6 summarizes the incidence of cerebral palsy by physiologic and anatomic abnormalities in the NCPP study. From a population of approximately 38,000 who completed all evaluations through age 7, 202 children had cerebral palsy of at least a mild degree (5 per 1000 of those who completed the study; 3 per 1000 of those who entered the study): 32% had diplegia, 29% hemiplegia, 24% quadriplegia, and 14% either dyskinesia or ataxia (Nelson and Ellenberg, 1978). The NCPP did not separate the dyskinesias and ataxias; the Swedish and Western Australian studies did separate these entities.) More than half the children with cerebral palsy in the NCPP population were born at term. Of the children, 63% were appropriate for gestational age and 15% were small for gestational age. Although only 10% of the children with cerebral palsy weighed less than 1500 g at birth, the risk of developing cerebral palsy in this group was found to be extremely high (90 per 1000). This compared to 3 per 1000 children who were born at the appropriate age and weighed more than 2500 g. A further 12% developed cerebral palsy as a result of a postnatal event (Table 19–7).

Pearls and Perils: Classification

1. The classification system for cerebral palsy is a clinical one. It does not provide insight into etiology, treatment, or prognosis.
2. Positive Babinski responses are uncommon in cerebral palsy even though one associates Babinski responses with a central nervous system dysfunction.
3. The term *apraxia* is best used in a patient with mild hypotonic or ataxic cerebral palsy if orthopedic intervention is deemed unnecesssary. This allows one to avoid the connotations of the term *cerebral palsy.*
4. *Cerebral palsy* refers to a motor dysfunction only. Associated problems must be identified and clearly discussed with the parents and therapists.
5. In a patient with pure paraplegia (legs only), one must assure that a spinal cord lesion is not present. A careful sensory examination and possible computed tomographic (CT) or magnetic resonance imaging scan of the spine might be necessary.
6. Cerebral palsy is not the same as mental retardation. Cerebral palsy is a term that, if used correctly, helps the parents understand that the child will only get better.

TABLE 19-6. INCIDENCE OF CEREBRAL PALSY AT AGE 7 YEARS

Spastic	
Diplegia	32%
Hemiplegia	29%
Quadriplegia	24%
Dyskinetic/ataxia	14%

Reproduced from Nelson and Ellenberg (1978).

**TABLE 19–7. INCIDENCE OF CEREBRAL PALSY
BY GESTATIONAL AGE**

Term	60%–65%
Preterm	35%–40%
Postnatal	12%

Reproduced from Nelson and Ellenberg (1984).

The Swedish and Western Australian studies provide longitudinal data comparing the incidences of cerebral palsy over different periods of time, revealing some interesting trends. The Swedish studies show that the incidence from 1959 through 1968 was 1.88 per 1000 live births. The number then fell from 1967 through 1970 to 1.44 per 1000 births, and in the most recent analysis, from 1975 through 1977, the incidence rose to 1.63 per 1000 births (Hagberg et al., 1984).

The recent change has been attributed primarily to the number of cerebral palsy children who were born prematurely as well as those who develped dyskinetic cerebral palsy and were born at term.

The data from the epidemiologic studies not only provide insight into the prevalence of the disease and its changing incidence, but also provide some understanding of the causation of cerebral palsy. Just as important, the data provide information about risk factors—those prenatal or perinatal events that are correlated with a child's developing cerebral palsy. Specifically, since the initial description of cerebral palsy by Little, a belief has persisted that labor and delivery complications are causes of cerebral palsy. The NCPP was developed to study this issue in depth, with the expectation that corrective measures could be introduced that would prevent the development of cerebral palsy as a result of poor obstetric management. The conclusions were unexpected.

A multivariate analysis of the NCPP data revealed that prenatal risk factors associated with cerebral palsy include maternal mental retardation, toxemia of pregnancy, maternal bleeding, and multiple births (Nelson and Ellenberg, 1986). In a survey of 681 Swedish cases, chronic infection and diabetes in the mother, as well as multiple births, were identified as prenatal risk factors (Hagberg and Hagberg, 1984). Nonmaternal prenatal risk factors include small-for-gestational-age babies, placental infarction, and a head circumference more than three standard deviations below the mean (Ellenberg and Nelson, 1979; Nelson and Ellenberg, 1984).

On the other hand, very few identifiable prenatal events have been definitively established as *causes* of cerebral palsy. A few rare genetic diseases have been definitively determined to be causes (Fisher and Russman, 1974). Prenatal infections in the fetus, such as toxoplasmosis and rubella, as well as cerebral malformations have also been etiologically related to cerebral palsy.

The major controversy regarding the etiology of cerebral palsy relates to *perinatal* events. Little argued that asphyxia and/or obstetric "factors" were definite

causes of cerebral palsy. However, the Swedish and NCPP studies have shown only that these problems are risk factors. For example, only 20% of children with Apgar scores less than 3 at 5 minutes developed cerebral palsy in the NCPP (Nelson and Ellenberg, 1981). Furthermore, if the Apgar score at 5 minutes was more than 7, it is unlikely that obstetric "complication" caused the brain damage (Nelson and Ellenberg, 1984). Postnatally, specific causes include CNS infections and trauma. Stroke is a very uncommon cause of cerebral palsy (Blair and Stanley, 1982).

In addition to evaluating the prenatal and perinatal risk factors, the data for preterm and term births with cerebral palsy have been analyzed. In the Swedish series, 6% of the preterm babies had obvious prenatal causes, such as cerebral malformation or purely prenatal risk factors, such as maternal retardation. Twenty-three percent had combined prenatal and perinatal risk factors and 51% had purely perinatal risk factors. Of those children born at term, 24% had prenatal risk factors, 20% had both prenatal and perinatal risk factors, and 19% had perinatal risk factors alone (Hagberg et al., 1982, 1984). Specific prenatal risk factors were generally more common among the term cases. The NCPP analysis revealed that babies weighing less than 1500 g at birth had a 9% risk of developing cerebral palsy, as opposed to 0.3% for babies weighing 2500 g at birth (Table 19–8).

The Swedish studies also correlated the anatomic and physiologic abnormalities with prenatal and perinatal risk factors as well as being born preterm or at term. Children with spastic diplegia were almost universally appropriate for gestational age, 55% were born preterm. Furthermore, there was a lower proportion of prenatal risk factors among this group of infants. The diplegic children born at term had a much more complex situation, having both prenatal and perinatal risk factors in a much higher frequency. These included toxemia, placental infarction, and evidence of intrauterine asphyxia, including meconium staining (Hagberg et al., 1981, 1984).

The dyskinetic syndromes are most likely to occur with perinatal risk factors, such as asphyxia and hyperbilirubinemia. Of these patients, 37%, in addition to having perinatal risk factors, also had prenatal risk factors

**TABLE 19–8. CORRELATION OF BIRTH WEIGHT
AND GESTATIONAL AGE WITH INCIDENCE
OF CEREBRAL PALSY**

Birth Weight and Gestational Age	Incidence of Cerebral Palsy at Age 7 Years
>2500 g	3.3/1000
<1500 g	90.4/1000
1500–2500 g, SGA	22.9/1000
1500–2500 g, AGA	6.7/1000

Denominator = number of patients who completed the study, SGA = small-for-gestational-age; AGA = average-for-gestational-age.
Reproduced from Nelson and Ellenberg (1984).

TABLE 19-9. GENETIC SYNDROMES PRESENTING AS CEREBRAL PALSY

Ataxia-telangiectasia (progressive by second decade)

Behr's syndrome

Disequilibrium syndrome

Familial spastic paraplegia (progressive by second or third decade)

Hereditary microcephaly

Lesch-Nyhan disease

Marinesco-Sjögren syndrome

Phenylketonuria

Sjögren-Larsson syndrome

Reproduced from Fisher and Russman (1974).

present, such as fetal deprivation (being small for gestational age) (Kyllerman, 1982, Kyllerman et al., 1982).

Can one predict the development of cerebral palsy in a specific child? Under rare conditions this is possible, such as when the child has a disorder that has been identified as a definite genetic cause (Table 19-9), has a serious congenital malformation, or has suffered a severe in utero or perinatal infection. Otherwise, one can only talk about the presence of risk factors, whether they occurred in the mother (such as retardation), in utero (such as being small for gestational age), or perinatally (such as severe asphyxia). Other perinatal observations that should raise a concern about future cerebral palsy include decreased activity in the baby, poor feeding, apneic episodes, and hypertonia or hypotonia (Nelson and Ellenberg, 1979).

ANNOTATED BIBLIOGRAPHY

Nelson KB, Ellenberg JH: Epidemiology of cerebral palsy, in Schoenberg BS (ed): *Advances in Neurology*. New York, Raven Press, 1978, p 421-435.

   The basic epidemiologic data from the NCPP are presented in this article. It is extremely comprehensive and very help-

ful for those who want to understand the incidence of the different types of cerebral palsy.

Hagberg B, Hagberg G, Olow I: The changing panorama of cerebral palsy in Sweden. IV. Epidemiological trends, 1959-1978. *Acta Paediatr Scand* 73:433-440, 1984.

   The title of this article is self-explanatory; it provides insight into changing incidences of cerebral palsy, at least in Sweden.

Nelson K, Ellenberg JH: Antecedents of cerebral palsy. Multivariate analysis of risk. *N Engl J Med* 315:81-86, 1986.

   This is a most comprehensive paper delineating risk factors in patients who will develop cerebral palsy. The article further defines the role of asphyxia in cerebral palsy and points out that "birth trauma" is not *the* cause of cerebral palsy.

DIAGNOSIS

The child must have an *obvious motor deficit* for the diagnosis of cerebral palsy to be considered. The chief complaint usually is a concern that the child is not reaching motor milestones at the normal time. A careful history must emphasize that the child is *not losing function*, assuring that the patient does not have a progressive disease. This history, combined with a neurologic examination establishing that the patient's motor deficit can be explained by a CNS abnormality, leads to the diagnosis of cerebral palsy. (Some children with cerebral palsy will lose function, especially during the early second decade of life. This usually relates to the development of contractures, excessive weight gain, or lack of motivation. The latter is especially noted in those patients who are barely able to ambulate.) Finally, pseudoregression may occur in association with changing muscle tone or with increasing body size (such as in adolescence). The "loss" of function will be secondary to the dyskinesia.

   The physical examination establishes the motor abnormalities as being caused by a CNS abnormality. Cerebral palsy is easily diagnosed in a child who is not developing motor skills, whose muscle tone is generally increased, and who is not regressing. However, a common diagnostic problem is presented by the child who is not developing normally, and who has normal or decreased muscle tone. The presence of the developmental or primitive reflexes beyond the time that they should have been lost or the lack of development of the protective reflexes at the expected time are important findings on the neurologic examination, suggesting a CNS abnormality (Taft and Barabas, 1982). The Moro reflex should be unobtainable after 6 months of age. The asymmetric tonic neck response should never be obligatory when the child is placed in the appropriate position; that is, the infant should "break" the tonic neck posture spontaneously after 15 to 30 seconds, and it should be unobtainable after 6 months of age. The side protective reflexes should be evident after 5 months of age and the parachute reflex is typically obtained after 10 months of age. Another im-

---

Pearls and Perils: Epidemiology and Etiology

1. Cerebral palsy as an outcome of difficult labor has not been clearly established.
2. Many children who had low birth weight, breech presentation, or clinical depression at birth were perfectly normal 7 years later.
3. Risk factors or causation are established in only 35% to 40% of patients with cerebral palsy.
4. A diagnosis of cerebral palsy is based on history and physical exam, not on the presence or absence of risk factors. The lack of a history of prematurity or "birth trauma" does not preclude the diagnosis of cerebral palsy.

portant observation in the physical examination is the finding of hand preference. A child should not cross the midline when reaching for an object until after 1 year of age and should not show hand preference until 18 to 24 months of age. The development of handedness prior to this time suggests a hemiplegia.

The diagnosis of cerebral palsy in the hypotonic child can be quite difficult. To establish the diagnosis under these circumstances might necessitate serial examinations. If the infantile reflexes have disappeared at the appropriate time, and if the protective reflexes have developed as indicated, then one should suspect a motor unit disease, such as spinal muscular atrophy or a congenital myopathy. In these instances, an electromyogram, measurement of nerve conduction times, and a muscle biopsy might be necessary.

Laboratory tests, such as x rays and an electroencephalogram, are not necessary to confirm the diagnosis. However, they can be helpful to establish an etiology and prognosis. CT scans are frequently abnormal, the primary abormality being cortical atrophy. At least two separate studies have demonstrated a correlation between the severity of the abnormality, and the extent of the motor disability, cognitive deficits, and the presence of epilepsy (Cohen and Duffner, 1981; Pedersen et al., 1982). The finding of agenesis of the corpus callosum would suggest that "birth trauma" was not the etiology of the cerebral palsy. A recent personal experience was very instructive. During the course of a cerebellar stimulator study, the CT scan revealed hypotrophy of the cerebellum in a patient who subsequently was rejected as a candidate for this procedure (Gahm et

al., 1981). On being informed of the rejection, the parents expressed relief rather than disappointment. For 14 years they had felt that dropping of their child at 5 days of age, even though there was no obvious change in his behavior and no loss of consciousness, had been the etiologic explanation for his cerebral palsy.

ANNOTATED BIBLIOGRAPHY

Ellenberg JH, Nelson KB: Birth weight and gestational age in children with cerebral palsy or seizure disorder. *Am J Dis Child* 133:1044–1048, 1979.
  This paper presents the data correlating premature birth with cerebral palsy as the primary risk factor.
Hanson RA, Berenberg W, Byers RK: Changing motor patterns in cerebral palsy. *Dev Med Child Neurol* 12:309–314, 1970.
  This article discusses the changing of motor tone as the patients with cerebral palsy mature. That the motor tone changes does not obviate the diagnosis.

ASSOCIATED PROBLEMS

Optimal management of the cerebral palsy patient occurs only after an in-depth evaluation, including careful assessment of the associated disabilities. The presence of one brain dysfunction should alert the examiner to search for other CNS abnormalities. Epilepsy, mental retardation, learning disabilities, vision difficulties, strabismus, dysarthria, and hearing loss occur with higher frequency in the cerebral palsy population compared to control groups (Robinson, 1973). Table 19–4 summarizes the incidence of mental retardation and epilepsy seen in the specific types of cerebral palsy (Gibbs et al., 1963).

Hemiplegic Cerebral Palsy

Epilepsy occurs most frequently in this group of cerebral palsy patients. Usually, the seizure will develop in the first 2 years of life; only 4 of 51 patients in one series developed seizures after age 10 years (Cohen and Duffner, 1981). Furthermore, the presence of seizures and mental retardation correlated with the extent of anatomic abnormality as determined by CT scan. Data from the NCPP found mental retardation especially in patients with postnatal onset of hemiplegia.

In addition to these findings, patients in this group experience other problems that are unique. Homonymous hemianopsia is frequently found. Classroom seating is an important consideration when this associated problem is identified. For example, a patient with a right homonymous hemianopsia should sit on the right side of the room because the left peripheral vision is still intact. Many hemiplegic patients have a significant sensory loss in addition to the motor disability. The prognosis for useful function of the involved hand relates more to the sensory abnormality than to spasticity. It is important to

---

Pearls and Perils: Diagnosis

1. Handedness should not develop before 1 year of age.
2. Poor head control, present at 3 months of age, should make one suspicious of cerebral palsy. The presence of risk factors should heighten that diagnostic concern.
3. One cannot establish a precise etiology in cerebral palsy in more than 55% to 60% of the cases. Most of these are due to dysplastic brain development, though perhaps at a microscopic level. The diagnosis is established by a nonprogressive history and a physical exam that suggests that the patient's problem is in the CNS.
4. The most common diagnosis for the floppy baby is cerebral palsy. It is not uncommon for a floppy baby to develop a dyskinesia by age 2 years. This should not preclude the diagnosis of cerebral palsy.
5. Cerebral palsy does not mean mental retardation. It is important to highlight this issue in discussing the diagnosis with the parents.

Pearls and Perils: Associated Problems

1. Hemiplegic cerebral palsy patients commonly will have a very small hand and a smaller foot compared to normal sizes. This is not the result of disuse, but rather the result of the lack of a "trophic" factor. Such a hand not only will be small but also will have a significant sensory loss. One can unequivocally state that the hand will not be very useful functionally. Therapists may be unrealistically enthusiastic about making this hand "normal" with an aggressive program, but it is important to be realistic.

2. Hemiplegic patients commonly have homonymous hemiopsia. Identification of this problem is important so that one can give advice regarding appropriate seating in the classroom.

note that the asymmetry of hand growth in this group of patients is not related to disuse, but rather to the sensory loss. The involved foot is invariably smaller than the normal foot and yet the patient is ambulatory, confirming that lack of a "trophic" factor and not disuse is a more likely explanation for the size disparity.

Diplegia

Most studies have noted a higher incidence of moderate to severe retardation in term infants with diplegic cerebral palsy and a more favorable prognosis for the preterm patient (Veelken et al., 1983). The Western Australian studies challenge these statistics, presenting data indicating that the babies weighing less than 1500 g with diplegia are now showing a high incidence of moderate to severe retardation (Dale and Stanley, 1980).

Dyskinesia

Seizures are less common in this group, but mental retardation, especially in the dystonic cerebral palsies, occurs in about 50% of cases.

Ataxia

Seizures are rare or nonexistent. However, mental retardation is common, especially in the disequilibrium group.

ANNOTATED BIBLIOGRAPHY

Robinson RO: The frequency of other handicaps in children with cerebral palsy. *Dev Med Child Neurol* 15:305–312, 1973.
    This paper presents a very clear discussion of the associated problems of patients with cerebral palsy.

TREATMENT

Some general treatment principles must be established before discussing specific treatment methods and programs:

1. The goals of a treatment program for the infant and young child differ from the goals for an adolescent, which, in turn, differ from those for an adult.
2. Because the manifestations of cerebral palsy vary from patient to patient, treatment programs must be individualized.
3. The severity of the associated problems must be considered during the formulation of the treatment plans.
4. As in the treatment of a child with a motor unit disease, the treatment of a child with cerebral palsy is best accomplished by a team of knowledgeable individuals with different expertises (Russman, 1984). A typical team includes a physician trained in the evaluation and treatment of developmentally disabled children. The diagnosis must be established, progressive diseases eliminated, and, if possible, specific genetic syndromes identified. A knowledgeable orthopedist should be the second physician member of the team. Contractures, subluxed or dislocated hips, and scoliosis are the deformities that can interfere with function as well as a more comfortable lifestyle. Nonphysician members of the team usually include a physical therapist, occupational therapist, and clinical nurse specialist. Many programs have found that a psychologist, social worker, and educator can play vital roles.

Infancy and Toddler Age

The diagnosis of cerebral palsy in most patients is established during the first 2 years of life. The patient, at this time, becomes involved in a physical or occupational therapy program or both. Because cerebral palsy is not one disease, as might be anticipated, there are a variety of therapy programs. Initially, passive range of motion exercises (to prevent contractures) and bracing (to prevent the abnormal muscle from interfering with normal muscle function) were used (Weiss and Betts, 1967). In the late 1950s and early 1960s, the Bobaths developed a program now known as neurodevelopmental treatment, which was aimed at inhibiting the primitive reflexes and facilitating normal movement by active patient participation (Bobath, 1967).

Variations of this form of therapy have been advocated during the past 15 years, although attempts to validate any one treatment program have been unsuccessful (Paine, 1962; Tizzard, 1980). Early intervention pro-

Pearls and Perils: Treatment

1. None of the various occupational or physical therapy programs has ever been validated. Empirically, they seem to be extremely helpful, especially for providing emotional support for families.
2. Early intervention programs to enhance motor and cognitive development in the physically handicapped population have not been shown to be beneficial, as opposed to early intervention programs for the environmentally deprived population (e.g., Head Start). Emotional support must be considered when one is developing a program.
3. The goals of any specific treatment program must be carefully outlined. Orthopedic intervention is not necessarily intended to change function dramatically. Rather, the goal of a specific procedure might merely be better positioning.

grams, which provide not only specific, "hands-on" therapy but also psychologic support, are beneficial, although there is no evidence that they enhance the child's development (Russman, 1983).

Pre-School Age, School Age, and Adolescence

As the child with cerebral palsy approaches school age, the goals of the therapy programs begin to shift from enhancing motor develpment and minimizing contractures toward helping the child cope with the expectations of the classroom. Sitting properly and moving about the environment (including the use of a wheelchair) are gross motor needs that might require therapy. Use of the small muscles for fine motor function, such as writing and cutting, must be enhanced. Most important is a therapy program to help the child communicate, either with speech or communication devices. Dressing, feeding, use of the toilet, and activity of daily living skills are important needs that should be incorporated into the educational/"treatment" program. The occupational therapist is usually the team member who works with the patient toward these ends.

Orthopedic Surgery

During the preschool years, spastic patients especially, despite an excellent treatment program, will develop contractures (Paine, 1962). The persistent shortening of the spastic muscle coupled with bone growth is responsible for the development of this problem. Both spastic and dyskinetic patients are at risk of developing dislocated hips, a source of pain and poor sitting posture (Moreau

et al., 1979). A knowledgeable orthopedist, who preferably is an integral member of the cerebral palsy team, has much to offer. Unless fixed bony deformities develop, it is preferable for the orthopedist to remain a therapeutic nihilist until the patient's gait pattern has been well established. This does not occur until age 7 or 8 years, as opposed to the pattern in the "normal" child, who establishes an "adult" gait pattern by age 4 (Sutherland, 1980). At that time, surgical correction of the deformities, followed by an intensive physical therapy program and judicious use of orthoses, is recommended. Currently, procedures are planned depending on a subjective impression of the effect of the deformities on the patient's function. However, a recent addition to the armamentarium of the orthopedist is the gait laboratory (Gage et al., 1984). With the use of computers to integrate a videotape of a patient walking with simultaneous electromyogram recording, an analysis of the gait can be obtained. This allows a more logical approach to the surgical corrections. Scoliosis is another important deformity that requires attention. This becomes a significant problem during the growth years and even into adulthood.

Orthoses

By changing the position of the neck and truncal muscles, the muscle tone in the upper and lower extremities can be altered, allowing the patient to use these muscles more efficiently and effectively. Use of a carefully designed chair with head and trunk supports to accomplish these goals is now commonplace (Nwaobi et al., 1983). In more severely involved cases, when inoperable deformities have developed, a custom-designed seating device, molded to the patient, can be fabricated by an experienced orthotist. The orthosis can then be placed into a wheelchair and used as a car seat, allowing comfort, stability, and some functional use of the extremities. Foot and leg orthoses also continue to play a role, but to provide support and not to inhibit movement.

Neurosurgery

In the mid-1970s chronic cerebeller stimulation was proposed as a way of decreasing spasticity that, in turn, would allow functional improvement in patients with spastic cerebral palsy (Cooper et al., 1976). A subsequent paper, controlling for the placebo effect, could not confirm the initial findings (Gahm et al., 1981). A recent article suggests that this form of surgery can decrease spasticity but not necessarily improve function (Penn, 1982).

A second neurosurgical procedure is stereotaxic thalamotomy, which has been offered as a procedure to alter either tone or movement disorders (Broggi et al., 1983). To date, this has been effective in decreasing hemiparetic tremors only. Finally, neurectomies are necessary under circumstances in which the spasticity is extreme, preventing adequate perineal care, and when myotomies and medication have been unsuccessful.

Medication

Spasticity, dyskinesia, and ataxia are the three types of motor disabilities. No medication has been found to be of benefit for the latter two problems, including artane, carbamezapine, dopamine, or diazepam. Spasticity can be reduced by dantrolene sodium (Ford et al., 1976) and baclofen (Milla and Jackson, 1973). However, in the few published studies, the use of these medications has not altered function, although it has enhanced care for the severely involved patient in some instances. By decreasing spasticity, for example, peroneal care and transfers may be made easier.

ANNOTATED BIBLIOGRAPHY

Russman BS: Comprehensive management of children with muscular disorders. *Pediatr Ann* 13:103–112, 1984.

This article discusses the team approach to the management of patients with neuromuscular problems.

Bobath B: The very early treatment of cerebral palsy. *Dev Med Child Neurol* 9:373–390, 1967.

The Bobath form of treatment is very popular among physical and occupational therapists. It is important for the physican to have a working knowledge of the principles of this type of therapy.

Paine RS: On the treatment of cerebral palsy. The outcome of 177 patients, 74 totally untreated. *Pediatrics* 29:605–616, 1962.

Although this study is retrospective, it provides insight into the natural course of the disease. Unfortunately, therapists, in their enthusiasm, occasionally tend to ignore what might have occurred naturally.

Gage JR, Fabian D, Hicks R, Tashman S: Pre- and postoperative gait analysis in patients with spastic diplegia. *J Pediatr Orthop* 17:46–52, 1984.

This article presents the new innovative approach to evaluating gait with the anticipation that a more scientific approach to orthopedic intervention is forthcoming.

PROGNOSIS

When the diagnosis of cerebral palsy is first established in a nonambulator, the first question asked is "Will my child walk?" Criteria for predicting independent walking have been developed (Bleck, 1975) (Table 19–10). If, by the age of 1 year, the patient still has persistent primitive reflexes and the protective reflexes have not developed, it is unlikely that the child will ever ambulate independently. Furthermore, if the child has severe dyskinesias, or falls into the disequilibrium category, ambulation will not be achieved. Even though cerebral palsy is a result of a nonprogressive CNS lesion, the marginal ambulator, on entering the early teens, may lose walk-

TABLE 19–10. PROGNOSIS FOR INDEPENDENT WALKING

_____	1. Asymmetric tonic neck reflex
_____	2. Symmetric tonic neck reflex
_____	3. Moro reflex
_____	4. Neck-righting reflex
_____	5. Extensor thrust
_____	6. Foot placement reaction
_____	7. Parachute reaction

Legend: At age 1, give 1 point for each item, 1–5 that is found; give 1 point each if 6 and 7 are not found. 0 = good prognosis; 1 = guarded prognosis; 2 = poor prognosis.
Reproduced from Bleck (1975).

ing ability because of contractures, excess weight gain, or lack of motivation. Those involved with the care of cerebral palsy patients must be alert to these potential problems and take early preventive measures.

Because cerebral palsy is commonly associated with mental retardation, parents also express concerns about the child's cognitive development. Data from the analyses of large series help address this issue. The quadriplegic patient who has epilepsy will almost certainly be, at best, educably mentally retraded. Of patients with disequilibrium syndrome, 90% are also retarded. In most patients, a prognosis about intellectual development must be deferred pending the development of language because this skill is correlated with intellectual development. Therefore, in questionable situations, a prognosis cannot and should not be rendered until after age 2 years. Furthermore, in the athetoid patient who might have a severe dysarthria, a prognosis about intelligence should be postponed until school age is attained. An examiner experienced with the severely disabled dyskinetic population should perform the evaluation, for the patient may be a poor examinee because of motor disability and the scores might thus be misleading.

As the child matures, changes in muscle tone and function may occur, which might raise concerns about the diagnosis (Hanson et al., 1970). For example, the hypotonic infant and toddler commonly develop spasticity or athetoid movements. This is typical in the patient, who might begin to self-mutilate at age 3 years. A test for uric acid in the hypotonic infant should always be requested (to eliminate the possible existence of Lesch-Nyhan disease). Not only may the muscle tone change, but the disability may lessen or disappear entirely. An analysis of the data from the NCPP showed that 118 children diagnosed as having mild cerebral palsy at age 1 year did not show a motor disability at age 7 years (Nelson and Ellenberg, 1982). However, as a group, they had a higher incidence of learning difficulties and afebrile seizures. Obviously, even the child who improves over time is at risk for the associated problems.

Finally, the examiner must be able to discuss issues of lifestyle with the parents. Communication is the most important skill required by a human being. Without this

Pearls and Perils: Prognosis

1. Marginal ambulators, upon reaching the early teens, may stop walking because of contractures, excessive weight gain, or lack of motivation. This does not necessarily mean that the patient has a progressive disease.
2. Quadriplegic patients with epilepsy will at best be mildly retarded.
3. Muscle tone in some patients will change over the years. Hypotonic patients may eventually become ataxic or might develop dyskinesias. Hypotonic boys should always have a uric acid test to rule out Lesch-Nyhan disease.
4. Some children with the diagnosis of cerebral palsy at age 1 year will not have significant motor disabilities at age 7 years. However, such children have a higher incidence of learning disabilities.
5. Communication is much more important than ambulation or even having self-help skills.
6. Do not think that all cerebral palsy patients, who cannot speak, are retarded. This specifically applies to the patient with choreoathetosis.
7. Change for the worse in muscle tone or status does not necessarily mean that the patient has a progressive disease.

ability, even with a normal intellect, the patient is "locked in." However, the technical advances being made, and expected to be made in the future, will allow a more positive outlook for the most severely disabled patient with cerebral palsy.

ANNOTATED BIBLIOGRAPHY

Nelson KB, Ellenberg JH: Children who "outgrew" cerebral palsy. *Pediatrics* 69:529–536, 1982.

This article points out that the initial diagnosis of cerebral palsy can be altered as the patient matures. On the other hand, one must be concerned about other associated problems, including learning disability and seizures, in such patients.

CONCLUSIONS AND SUMMARY

Cerebral palsy is a term used to describe a patient who has a nonprogressive brain lesion leading to a motoric deficit. That the motor disability might change over the years does not preclude the diagnosis. Associated problems—including seizures, mental retardation, language disorder, and speech deficits, as well as a strabismus—must be evaluated and treated appropriately. There are many causes of cerebral palsy, including genetic diseases

and embryologic abnormalities. Most often, a specific cause cannot be identified. However, risk factors can be identified in about 30% to 40% of cases; risk factors alert the clinician to anticipate the presence of cerebral palsy in a patient and they should be considered separately from causative factors.

Cerebral palsy is an acceptable term as long as it is used appropriately and as long as the issues associated with this term are carefully explained to the parents. Cerebral palsy ranges in severity, from minimal limitations requiring no treatment to severe impairment requiring total care and intensive treatment. It is those who require total care whom the public commonly associates with the term *cerebral palsy*. Consequently, the diagnosis must be carefully articulated to the parents, emphasizing the various degrees of impairment. If one anticipates a treatment program including physical therapy and potential orthopedic intervention, the term is appropriate and should be used.

REFERENCES

Blair E, Stanley FJ: An epidemiological study of cerebral palsy in Western Australia, 1956–1975. III. Postnatal aetiology. *Dev Med Child Neurol* 24:575–585, 1982.

Bleck EE: Locomotor prognosis in cerebral palsy. *Dev Med Child Neurol* 17:18–25, 1975.

Bobath B: The very early treatment of cerebral palsy. *Dev Med Child Neurol* 9:373–390, 1967.

Broggi G, Angelini L, Bono R, Giorgi C, Nardocci N, Franzini A: Long-term results of stereotactic thalamotomy for cerebral palsy. *Neurosurgery* 12:195–202, 1983.

Brun A, Kyllerman M: Clinical pathogenetic and neuropathological correlation in dystonic cerebral palsy. *Eur J Pediatr* 131:93–104, 1979.

Cohen ME, Duffner PK: Prognostic indicators in hemiparetic cerebral palsy. *Am Neurol* 9:353–357, 1981.

Cooper IS, Riklan M, Amin I, Waltz JM, Cullinan T: Chronic cerebellar stimulation in cerebral palsy. *Neurology* 26:744–753, 1976.

Dale A, Stanley FJ: An epidemiological study of cerebral palsy in Western Australia, 1956–1975. Spastic cerebral palsy and perinatal factors. *Dev Med Child Neurol* 22:13–25, 1980.

Ellenberg JH, Nelson KB: Birth weight and gestational age in children with cerebral palsy or seizure disorder. *Am J Dis Child* 133:1044–1048, 1979.

Fisher RL, Russman BS: Genetic syndromes associated with cerebral palsy. *Clin Orthop* 99:2–11, 1974.

Ford F, Bleck EE, Aptekan RG, Collins FJ, Stevick D: Efficacy of dantrolene sodium in the treatment of spastic cerebral palsy. *Dev Med Child Neurol* 18:770–783, 1976.

Freud S: Infantile cerebral paralysis. Russin LA (transl). Miami, University of Miami Press, 1968 [1897],

Gage JR, Fabian D, Hicks R, Tashman S: Pre- and postoperative gait analysis in patients with spastic diplegia. *J Pediatr Orthop* 17:46–52, 1984.

Gahm NH, Russman BS, Cerciello RL, Fiorentino MR, McGrath DM: Chronic cerebellar stimulation for cerebral palsy. A double-blind study. *Neurology* 31:87–90, 1981.

Gibbs FA, Gibbs EL, Perlstein MA, Rich CL: Electroencephalographic and clinical aspects of cerebral palsy. *Pediatrics* 30:73–84, 1963.

Gubbay S: *The Clumsy Child: A Study of Developmental Apraxia and Agnostic Ataxia.* Philadelphia, WB Saunders, 1975.

Hagberg B, Hagberg G: Prenatal and perinatal risk factors in a survey of 681 Swedish cases, in Stanley F, Alberman E (eds): *The Epidemiology of the Cerebral Palsies.* Philadelphia, JB Lippincott, 1984, p 116–134.

Hagberg B, Hagberg G, Olow I: Gains and hazards of intensive neonatal care: An analysis from Swedish cerebral palsy epidemiology. *Dev Med Child Neurol* 24:13–19, 182.

Hagberg B, Hagberg G, Olow I: The changing panorama of cerebral palsy in Sweden. IV. Epidemiological trends, 1959–1978. *Acta Paediatr Scand* 73:433–440, 1984.

Hanson RA, Berenberg W, Byers RK: Changing motor patterns in cerebral palsy. *Dev Med Child Neurol* 12:309–314, 1970.

Kyllerman M: Dyskinetic cerebral palsy. II. Pathogenetic risk factors and intra-uterine growth. *Acta Paediatr Scand.* 71: 559–568, 1982.

Kyllerman M, Bager B, Bensch J, Billie B, Oslow I, Voss H: Dyskinetic cerebral palsy. I. Clinical categories, associated neurological abnormalities and incidences. *Acta Paediatr Scand* 71:543–558, 1982.

Milla JJ, Jackson ADM: A controlled trial of baclofen in children with cerebral palsy. *J Int Med Res* 5:398–404, 1973.

Minear WL: A classification of cerebral palsy. *Pediatrics* 18: 841–852, 1956.

Moreau M, Drummond DS, Rogala E, Ashworth A, Porter T: Natural history of the dislocated hip in spastic cerebral palsy. *Dev Med Child Neurol* 21:749–753, 1979.

Nelson KB, Ellenberg JH: Epidemiology of cerebral palsy, in Schoenberg BS (ed): *Advances in Neurology.* New York, Raven Press, 1978, p 421–435.

Nelson KB, Ellenberg JH: Neonatal signs as predictors of cerebral palsy. *Pediatrics* 64:225–232, 1979.

Nelson KB, Ellenberg JH: Apgar scores as predictors of chronic neurologic disability. *Pediatrics* 68:36–44, 1981.

Nelson KB, Ellenberg JH: Children who "outgrew" cerebral palsy. *Pediatrics* 69:529–536, 1982.

Nelson KB, Ellenberg JH: Obstetric complications as risk factors for cerebral palsy or seizure disorders. *JAMA* 251: 1843–1848, 1984.

Nelson KB, Ellenberg JH: Antecedents of cerebral palsy. Multivariate analysis of risk. *N Engl J Med* 315:81–86, 1986.

Nwaobi OM, Brubaker CE, Cusick B, Sussman MD: Electromyographic investigation of extensor activity in cerebral-palsied children in different seating positions. *Dev Med Child Neurol* 25:175–183, 1983.

Paine RS: On the treatment of cerebral palsy. The outcome of 177 patients, 74 totally untreated. *Pediatrics* 29:605–616, 1962.

Pedersen H, Tandorf K, Melchior JC: Computed tomography in spastic cerebral palsy. *Neuroradiology* 223:275–278, 1982.

Penn RD: Chronic cerebellar stimulation for cerebral palsy: A review. *Neurosurgery* 10:116–121, 1982.

Robinson RO: The frequency of other handicaps in children with cerebral palsy. *Dev Med Child Neurol* 15:305–312, 1973.

Russman BS: Early intervention for the biologically handicapped infant and young child: Is it of value? *Pediatr Rev* 5:51–55, 1983.

Russman BS: Comprehensive management of children with muscular disorders. *Pediatr Ann* 13:103–112, 1984.

Sanner G: The dysequilibrium syndrome. A genetic study. *Neuropaediatrie* 4:403–413, 1973.

Sutherland DH: The development of mature gait. *J Bone Joint Surg* 62A:336–353, 1980.

Taft LT, Barabas G: Infants with delayed motor performance. *Pediatr Clin North Am* 29:137–149, 1982.

Tizzard JPM: Cerebral palsies: Treatment and prevention. *J R Coll Physicians London* 14:72–80, 1980.

Veelken N, Hagberg B, Hagberg G, Olow I: Diplegia cerebral palsy in Swedish term and preterm children. Differences in reduced optimality, relations to neurology and pathogenetic factors. *Neuropaediatrie* 14:20–28, 1983.

Weiss H, Betts HB: Method of rehabilitation in children with neuromuscular disorders. *Pediatr Clin North Am* 14:1009–1016, 1967.

Disorders of Motor Execution II Higher-Order Motor Deficits

Ruthmary K. Deuel

Disorders of motor execution that accompany paralysis, spasticity, and movement disorders may be called disorders of primary motility. This chapter describes a different type of motor disorder, one that does not affect primary motility and does not result in grossly detectable alterations of strength, tone, or posture, but rather is manifest by clumsiness and inadequate performance of sequential motor acts. Children's motor development and performance may be quite severely handicapped by such higher-order motor deficits. The true incidence of such deficits is not known, but estimates range from 2% to 12% of first graders in regular schools (Prechtl and Stemmer, 1962; Brenner and Gillman, 1966; Gubbay, 1975; Iloeje, 1987; Nichols, 1987). Thus, disorders of cerebral function that result only in clumsiness and dyspraxia without paralysis or spasticity are rather common, and probably similar in incidence to "specific learning disorders," with which they are often associated (Johnson et al., 1981; Deuel and Robinson, 1987; Nichols, 1987).

Higher-order motor deficits were first clearly described less than 100 years ago in adult patients with acquired brain damage (Liepmann, 1900), and it is only recently that these disorders have received attention in the general neurologic literature (Geschwind and Damasio, 1985). They really were not recognized in children until the 1920s (Orton, 1925). The fact that they were recognized later in children than in adults probably reflects the fact that no obvious alteration in strength, tone, coordination, or sensation accompanies them (Liepmann, 1900, 1908; DeRenzi et al., 1968, 1980; Geschwind and Damasio, 1985). On examination, some higher-order motor abnormalities may be detected only if age-appropriate sequences of individual motions are performed under the examiner's surveillance. For example, in the finger to nose test of a standard pediatric neurologic exam the child is told "put this finger on the tip of your nose, and then touch my finger with it." Younger (below

about 9 years) apraxic children frequently follow only the first part of the instruction. Thereafter, instead of moving the finger from the nose, the child uses a finger from the other hand to touch the examiner's finger, or uses this second finger to touch the nose a second time. In this example the individual motions are fluidly and easily made, but the sequence is inappropriate to the command, with extra motions (parapraxis) inserted. Generally the child recognizes that his response is incorrect and yet cannot correct it even after a second instruction or sample performance by the examiner.

For children, higher-order motor execution deficits may be defined as "failure to learn or perform voluntary motor activities with an age-appropriate efficiency, despite adequate strength, sensation, attention and volition" (David et al., 1981). This general definition, of course, may be made more specific in relation to the different types of higher-order deficits (to be more fully discussed in the sections describing each deficit). The relationship of the loose category of "neurologic soft signs" (Deuel and Robinson, 1987) to the disorders of higher-order motor execution will also be taken up separately with each disorder. In general there has been an unfortunate tendency in the pediatric literature to call any manifestation of clumsiness or dyspraxia a "soft neurologic sign," and to value the finding only as a diagnostic marker for more commonly recognized neuropsychiatric disorders of childhood, such as hyperactivity or attention deficit disorder (ADD). Although the literature firmly supports a high incidence of disorders of higher-order motor execution among groups of children with cognitive disorders (Prechtl and Stemmer, 1962; Pyfer and Castelman, 1972; Denckla and Rudel, 1978), there is absolutely no support for the view that disorders of motor execution are inevitably linked to them in individual children (Deuel, 1981; Nichols, 1987).

Children with disorders of higher motor execution may have been exposed to the same sources of brain damage (infection, head trauma, intracranial vascular accident, or cerebral hypoxia) that lead to the disorders of primary motility, characterized by gross static neurologic findings, such as deficient strength, coordination, and muscle tone. Alternatively there may be no such history in the child with the higher-order motor execution deficit. Nonetheless, both in school and at home the child's higher-order deficits lead him to be "behind" or "slow" in motor performance. Regardless of the etiology then, one important reason to search out higher-order motor deficits is their propensity to cause long-term severe educational and social handicaps (Gubbay, 1975, 1985; Knuckey and Gubbay, 1983). In addition, higher-order motor deficits may be the first sign of significant underlying neurologic disease, such as subacute sclerosing panencephalitis (Jabbour, 1969; Percy et al., 1977). Rett's syndrome (Hagberg et al., 1983), or other degenerative disorders of the nervous system (Swaiman et al., 1983). In addition, cerebellar lesions (e.g., a cystic cerebellar astrocytoma, a fully curable disorder if operated on early) may lead to motor execution deficits. Medication side effects, familial paroxysmal chorea, Gilles de la Tourette syndrome, dystonia musculorum deformans, and collagen vascular disorders are some other entities that may present as a higher-order motor deficit.

Particularly because such higher-order motor deficits may not be clear to historians, or even declare themselves during a general physical examination, it is mandatory that they be specifically sought out during neurologic evaluation of the school-age child. If the child has a problem with academic achievement or if there is a question of an underlying pathologic diagnosis that may affect the cortical or subcortical gray matter, it is especially important to add particular items to the exam and establish on an objective basis whether or not the child does suffer from such a deficit (Table 20-1). When such a higher-order deficit is found and does appear to be handicapping the child (irrespective of its diagnostic significance for a disease or condition), some form of long-term remedial management is in order. Such specifically

TABLE 20-1. MOTOR EXECUTION BATTERY

Psychometric
1. Purdue Peg Board
2. Kaufman ABC
   a. Hand movements
   b. Visual spatial memory—David Roeltgen
Neurologic
1. Historic
   Gross motor milestones—walked at which month?
   When showed hand preference?
   Tie shoes, color within lines, print name
   Write name in cursive
   Button shirt or blouse
   Make bed, cook, construct models, play with Barbie
      dolls, build with Legos
   Ride bike, play baseball or soccer
2. Neurologic exam protocol, including especially apraxia
   tests (see Chapter 4)

directed management is often very helpful in restoring functional ability, even in children with cerebral palsy and other disorders of primary motility, who, as commonly happens, suffer additionally from higher-order motor dysfunction (Crothers and Paine, 1959; Frei, 1986). To analyze the deficits with the goal of determining their handicapping potential for the individual child, and to recommend specifically directed management if warranted, it is best to consider the disorders under separate headings: *dypraxia*, which is separable from *clumsiness*, and has somewhat different management programs, *material-specific dyspraxias*, (notably dysgraphia), and *adventitious movements*.

DYSPRAXIA

Dyspraxia (otherwise called apraxia or deficient motor planning) in childhood is defined as inability to perform developmentally appropriate sequences of voluntary movements in the face of preserved volition, power, coordination, sensation, and cooperation. Individual fine and gross movements are often quite dexterous and appropriate. However, depending on the type of activity required, an incorrect sequence of individual movements may be produced, sometimes with additions of unrequired movements (parapraxes) (Poeck, 1986) or with the spatial requirements of the movements poorly estimated, or both. Thus the final product of what looks like a quick, dexterous sequence may be completely ineffectual or incorrect.

The characteristic failure in the elaboration of a complex voluntary act, without even slowness of performance, may be the reason why dyspraxia is generally unrecognized as a source of "slowness." Indeed, as dyspraxic children look and act normal, a motor deficit is seldom suspected by experienced professionals. Furthermore, because primary motility (strength, coordination, and dexterity) is preserved, even a neurologic examination may not reveal the dyspraxic deficit unless it evaluates the child's performance in learning or completing such acts. Although some extended or "neurodevelopmental" exams for "soft signs" do contain items that would be affected by dyspraxia, dyspraxia per se, not contaminated by clumsiness, is not one of the commonly cited soft signs (see the section on Clumsiness). Thus an unrecognized dyspraxic motor deficit may lead the child to be labeled as lazy, naughty, or stupid, with adverse effects on self-esteem, motivation, and conduct. Any of a wide array of school and behavior problems may be the presenting complaint for the dyspraxic child. However, if a detailed account of motor developmental progress can be rendered, the history may be indicative of a motor abnormality to the examiner asking the right questions. Dyspraxic children are usually delayed in dressing and grooming themselves independently—

FEATURE TABLE 20-1. MOTOR DYSPRAXIA

Discriminating Feature	Consistent Features	Variable Features
1. Inability to perform developmentally appropriate sequences of voluntary movements in the face of preserved volition, power, coordination, and sensation	1. Abnormal outcome of movement sequences. 2. Ability to choose the correct sequence when alternatives are modeled 3. Extra or inappropriate movements (parapraxis)	1. Association with clumsiness 2. May affect facial, manual, or pedal motions separately

specifically in buttoning, snapping, zippering, donning coats and boots, tying shoes, and manipulating combs, toothbrushes, and scissors. They are often unwilling even to attempt coloring, carpentry, sewing, and cooking. This may happen despite the fact that gross motor (sitting, walking, and climbing stairs) milestones were normal.

The etiologies of dyspraxia are diverse. In ones with known pathology cerebral hemisphere gray matter is usually affected: dyspraxia is frequently seen in frank cerebral palsy (Frei, 1986); it may follow stroke in childhood (Crothers and Paine, 1959), and it may be one of the first signs of a dementing disease such as subacute sclerosing panencephalitis or metachromatic leukodystrophy of childhood or adolescent onset (Jabbour, 1969; Percy et al., 1977). Although dyspraxia is said to occur in mental retardation, perhaps if a developmental quotient of praxic ability could be reliably determined, it would be commensurate with the intelligence quotient in most mentally retarded children, as it is in normal children. In most developmental dyspraxia that is associated with learning and attention problems, the etiology is obscure, just as it is in dyslexia and dysgraphia. It seems likely that involvement of the association cortex in some fashion underlies the behavioral deficit (Deuel, 1977), but direct evidence is not available.

To test for dyspraxia it is best to do a complete neurologic examination that includes several types of subject-performed tasks, including pantomiming of actions, imitating actions of the examiner, and using actual familiar objects (DeRenzi et al., 1980) (see Chapter 4). Some possible items for pantomime testing in younger children are asking a child to blow a kiss or wave goodbye. For imitation testing, simple finger and hand movements as described in the Lincoln/Oseretsky tests (Sloan, 1948) may be used. For testing the use of actual objects, having the child fold a piece of paper to fit into an envelope or roll up the paper and use it as a pretend telescope are interesting items, although precise age- and sex-normative expectations are unclear. Ideally such tasks should demand of the child age-appropriate complex voluntary motor activity (as described in Chapter 4). To be truly deemed dyspraxic, a child should be able to pick the action he or she was unable to perform out of several alternative modeled actions. Choosing the correct one demonstrates the child's recognition of the act and under-

standing of the command. Effective completion of an act by a dyspraxic child, unlike completion by a clumsy child, does not improve appreciably with extra long periods of time allowed for the completion. This facet of the dyspraxic's performance can help differentiate

Pearls and Perils: Dyspraxia

1. The best screening test for manual dyspraxia is an accurate, detailed history of motor development and current motor learning.
2. On a general-purpose neurologic examination of young children the item most prone to be disturbed in manual dyspraxia is the finger to nose test (for the child it is a new, "nonsense" motor sequence).
3. To ascertain dyspraxia definitively, a standard manual apraxia battery may readily be administered in conjunction with the neurologic examination. Elements of such a battery are presented in Chapter 4.
4. Buccal-facial dyspraxia is generally seen in the developmental language disorder called verbal apraxia or dilapidated speech (Aram and Horwitz, 1983). The finding of buccal facial dyspraxia can help differentiate this diagnostic entity from other speech and language disorders and point the way to appropriate therapy.
5. Motor deficit is usually not the presenting complaint of a purely dyspraxic child. Parents and teachers may not recognize a motor deficit in the apraxic child.
6. Dyspraxia is not systematically ascertained on the general-purpose neurologic exam, nor is it tested specifically in most "extended" or "neurodevelopmental" exams designed to detect neurologic "soft signs."
7. The secondary developmental effects of dyspraxia—diminished self-esteem and avoidance of motor sequencing tasks—may be much more handicapping than the motor deficit per se. The secondary effects may remain long after the child has developed near-normal or normal praxis.
8. Speech pathologists may understand the term *dyspraxia* to refer only to "dyspraxia of speech."

clumsiness from dyspraxia, although some children demonstrate both difficulties.

There are no psychometric-style tests for dyspraxia that come close to providing the amount of information that a neurologic exam with an apraxia battery provides. However, the Kaufman ABC (Kaufman and Kaufman, 1983) test has a hand movement copying subtest that does at least test sequential manual abilities and has normative standards from 2½ to 12½ years. Gubbay (1975, pp. 96–103) has standardized a motor performance battery, but it fails to provide any means of differentiating apraxia from clumsiness and adventitious movements. The same problem exists with an extended version of the Purdue Peg Board.

The management of dyspraxia especially depends on its handicapping significance and the age of the child displaying it. Simple recognition of the apraxic deficit, and the counseling of the child and his parents that it is due to "mechanical problems"—and not carelessness, laziness, or other voluntary oppositional personality traits—may be very helpful in removing an inhibitory stigma from the child. Especially if the dyspraxia is the result of static brain damage or is idiopathic, further management should include a combination of practice of the required motor sequences and bypass of complex motor acts at certain junctures. Dyspraxia is most likely to be handicapping and obvious where it interacts with new situations or new demands, that is, learning a new complex motor sequence. One 10-year-old child was introduced to throwing darts when visiting at the home of friends of her parents. At each attempt she threw the dart backwards, with incremental embarrassment to her parents. The incident caused them to seek medical consultation for "mental retardation" in their child. Another dyspraxic child performing a science experiment for the first time in the third grade repeatedly attempted to measure the temperature of a fluid with a thermometer placed upside down in the container. "The more explanation, the less understanding" was the teacher's comment. These apraxic children, placed in unfamiliar situations that required unfamiliar acts, were not able to devise correct motor sequences.

Such embarrassing motor inefficiencies cannot be completely avoided by dyspraxic children, but certain amounts of deliberate rational ritual (cognitive self-cuing) can help avoid some predictable difficulties, particularly in the older child. The child can develop a system of conscious self-questioning: "How are the other kids in line ahead of me doing this? Which hand comes first, which part of the object is the front/the left/the right?" Such questions may help the older apraxic child orient himself or herself and consciously control motor sequencing. (A nondyspraxic child of course seldom uses such explicit cognitive aids.) The child should be made aware of situations in which the apraxic deficit will surface and will clearly be detrimental to self-esteem or performance of academic requirements. He or she should be taught to

actively avoid such situations. In addition, practice of a given motor sequence is sometimes very helpful, just as it is with clumsiness, although obviously every motor sequence to be encountered cannot be practiced.

Because it has not been previously evaluated separately from clumsiness and adventitious movements, both the *incidence* of pure idiopathic dyspraxia and the *prognosis* are unclear. In many instances it seems to be developmental, in that the ability to carry out effective complex motor sequencing improves with age. Idiopathic dyspraxia does occur alone, but more frequently it occurs in conjunction with clumsiness, adventitious movements, or other disorders of higher cerebral function, at least in this author's experience. Unfortunately, for the reasons cited previously, there is no published data on this point.

MATERIAL-SPECIFIC DYSPRAXIAS

Material-specific dyspraxias are the most limited type of higher-order motor deficit. They cannot be detected unless the material that causes the difficulty is presented for test manipulation. The most common material-specific dyspraxia is called dysgraphia. Dysgraphia results in poor quality of written verbal output at every stage of a child's development. Children with dysgraphia generally have difficulty with spelling, or at least legibility. Written productions are sparse, with poor grammatic construction. There may be an interaction between the difficulty of spelling a word and the quality of the writing of the constituent letters. In some types of dysgraphia the child cannot orally spell words correctly. If oral spelling is incorrect, a true material-specific kind of dysgraphia is present and may be seen with or without marked or clear dyslexia and without any other trace of language disorder. When children make written letters and words very poorly, spell incorrectly in both written and oral attempts, and truncate written assignments but read fluently and with good comprehension, they are clearly different from the dyslexics, who have the written language disorder described, plus an inability to read. Far from 100% of children with dysgraphia have severe dyslexia, whereas some form of dysgraphia does appear in 100% of severely dyslexic children (Deuel, 1981). The material specificity of the disorder is certainly best exemplified by the dyslexic child with dysgraphia, as many such dyslexic children have excellent fine and gross motor abilities when tested on other material than written expression of letters, words, and sentences. An example is seen in Figure 20–1, in which printed spelling words may be compared with the same child's drawing of a bicycle.

Children who are otherwise clumsy may also be called dysgraphic, but in them the defect is not *material*-specific, as oral spelling is normal or at least much superior to written spelling, and they show other evidence of clumsiness or maladroitness for drawing and other fine motor activities on examination and by history. Still,

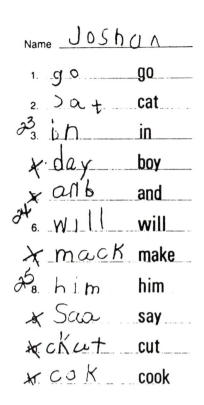

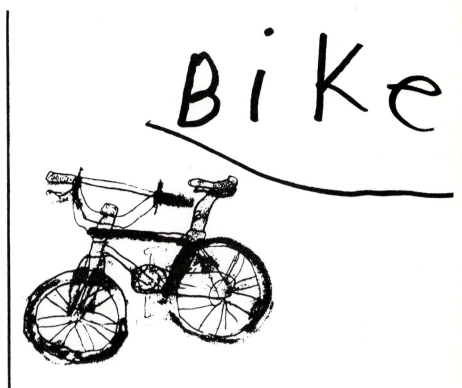

Name Joshua

1. g o .... go
2. ⊃ a t ...... cat
3. i n .... in
4. d a y ...... boy
5. a n b ...... and
6. w ı l l ...... will
7. m a c k .. make
8. h i m ...... him
9. S a a ...... say
10. c k u t .... cut
11. c ⊃ k ...... cook

Figure 20-1. Contrasting efficiency of graphomotor skills for separate types of material. The first panel shows the written spelling to dictation of an 8-year-old with normal full-scale IQ (104, WISC-R) who was referred for reading difficulties. The words that were dictated (from the Wide Range Achievement Test—Level 1) appear to the right of the patient's productions. The second panel shows a spontaneous drawing of a bicycle by the same patient.

when writing is required of them the individual letters may be poor and individual words may be elided. All written production is abbreviated, presumably because of the labor involved in setting out the words on paper. This more mechanical dysgraphia problem does occur without other evidence of clumsiness, but very rarely.

To evaluate dysgraphia, a pertinent history is important, and review of written schoolwork is helpful. A good examination can be carried out by using the Test of Written Language (Hammill and Larson, 1978). More informally, one may request an age-appropriate sample of spontaneous written composition (of words, sentences, or paragraphs, depending on the subject's educational status). Copying of an age-appropriate written sample should also be evaluated. To determine if spelling deficits are related to writing, as in the clumsy child with dysgraphia, the child should be asked to spell words aloud. All of this can take place during a neurologic examination. When giving these tasks it is important to remember that letter reversals are common in normal young children and do not presage the development of dyslexia nor proclaim it.

Constructional dyspraxia is a second kind of material-specific dyspraxia, in which the child appears

---

**Pearls and Perils:
Dysgraphia**

1. Highly abbreviated handwritten output in the verbally advanced or normal child suggests isolated dysgraphia as a cause.
2. In dysgraphia, scores on individual IQ tests, such as the WISC-R, are generally normal on all subtests with the frequent exception of the "coding" subtest.
3. Neat but very slow writing characterizes some dysgraphic children, again leading to paucity of written output.
4. The first-grade child who writes letters backwards should not be declared dyslexic or dysgraphic.
5. It is important to test writing speed in the child whose school performance is under consideration.
6. It is important to test for oral spelling in a child who always fails written spelling. Otherwise, an incorrect attribution to a linguistically based abnormality rather than a simple motor abnormality may be made.

to have poor spatial intuition and great difficulty in drawing, and most especially in putting together three-dimensional models. Testing to include the latter material-specific dyspraxia should include drawing age-appropriate shapes and figures in addition to the writing and spelling exercises. More formal tests include the Bender Gestalt test (Bender, 1946) and the Benton test of visual memory (Benton, 1974).

The management of material-specific dyspraxias is various. Dysgraphia can be severely handicapping scholastically, and its treatment with bypass methodologies (e.g., dictation of essays) is well known to most educators. Word processors with spelling checkers are very helpful, but some dysgraphics do better to avoid written compositions as completely as possible.

CLUMSINESS

A child with clumsiness, the classic "klutz," suffers from slowness in completion of very simple (single-phase) acts, such as flexing a finger or rotating the wrist and forearm. This developmental motor disability has in the past been considered together with pure apraxia (Ford, 1960, p. 197; Gubbay, 1975; Iloeje, 1987), but is in fact separable from it on empirical grounds (David et al., 1981; Poeck, 1986). The main point of differentiation of clumsiness from pure apraxia is that primary motility is affected in clumsiness, not in terms of strength or muscle tone, but rather in terms of speed and dexterity. Although purists would certainly argue that clumsiness is really a "lower-order" type of deficit, they should recall that it fulfills most of the criteria for Liepmann's (1908) "limb kinetic apraxia" or Kleist's (1934) "melokinetic" apraxia. These authors describe a decrement in dexterity and speed of movements without strength or tone changes in adult stroke victims. The purely clumsy child similarly exhibits slow and thus often ineffectual fine and/or gross motor performance in the face of an otherwise normal neurologic exam. Fortunately items such as finger tapping and wrist supination and pronation are part of the standard exam, so direct recognition of clumsiness is more likely than recognition of pure apraxia.

The incidence of pure clumsiness by itself is unknown, but Gubbay's study of Australian school children in regular schools screened for clumsiness, apraxia, and adventitious movements together, and it yielded an incidence of 5.6% of children with higher-order motor deficits. The perinatal study (Nichols, 1987) used a somewhat different data base, but also reported a high incidence of clumsiness. Of 7-year-olds with an IQ of above 80 and without gross evidence of cerebral palsy, 8.1% demonstrated "motor soft signs." These percentages probably include children with all of the types of higher-order motor deficits being discussed here. Because clumsiness seems to account for the largest proportion of these percentages, they may be considered as guidelines for the true incidence, which can only be determined when large numbers of children are examined with a battery that separates pure dyspraxia from clumsiness and adventitious movements.

To evaluate children for clumsiness, a detailed history of motor development should be the starting point. The clumsy child's problem, unlike that of a dyslexic or even a dyspraxic child, has almost invariably created difficulties and tensions at home throughout the preschool years. Before the child ever gets to school he or she has often gained a reputation as slow, lazy, or uncooperative (Annell, 1949; Ford, 1960; Gubbay, 1975). After taking a history, the most efficient way to determine specific clumsiness is with a neurologic examination. This will both rule out accompanying or underlying conditions and also positively identify the slow, ineffectual motions that constitute clumsiness. In addition, a neurologic exam allows evaluation of various body parts, such as face, upper extremities, lower extremities, trunk, and axial musculature. It allows evaluation of interdigit and interlimb coordination. Clumsiness is also usually clear to observers of both drawing and writing. In the younger child, clumsiness can be noted in simple manipulations, such as buttoning buttons, putting on clothes, tying shoes, or stringing beads. With the clumsiness disorder, bimanual coordination—such as that required for setting pegs, taking pegs from a reservoir and putting them in a board, or stringing beads on a string—is generally deficient, as is all interdigit coordination. Some children are affected not only in fine but also in gross motor activities. Other children appear to have adequate fine motor abilities but are affected only in gross motor activities, such as throwing, running, walking, riding a bicycle, and kicking. Thus, both gross and fine motor abilities must be studied for a thorough evaluation of clumsiness.

In passing, it should be pointed out that clumsiness

FEATURE TABLE 20–2. CLUMSINESS

Discriminating Feature	Consistent Features	Variable Features
1. Slow completion of single-phase movements of single joints, in the absence of weakness	1. Finger and/or foot tapping too slow for age. 2. Outcome of movement sequences improved when there are no time constraints	1. Association with dyspraxia 2. Association with adventitious movements 3. May affect facial, pedal, or axial motion separately

is not a "soft" sign in the sense that it is ephemeral or unquantifiable. It is readily measured and detectable by different observers in the same individual over several examinations (Denckla, 1973, 1974; Roach and Kephardt, 1966). It seems to have been relegated to the "soft" category because to observe it properly the patient must be watched (for quality of response) and timed (for speed) while in action, and timing the appropriate action was not part of the classic "hard" neurologic exam (Denny-Brown, 1958). Of course other types of examinations may reveal clumsiness, particularly if the examination happens to be testing the body part involved. However, the other types do not rule out primary motility disorders such as cerebral palsy as the origin of the clumsiness, nor do they allow for segregating of dyspraxia and adventitious movements from clumsiness. Most "neurodevelopmental" protocols, or exams for "soft signs," contain numerous items to evaluate for clumsiness, but as most of them grade outcome rather than the motor process, they again cannot differentiate among types of higher-order motor disability (Deuel and Robinson, 1987).

Manual clumsiness may be reliably ascertained using the Purdue Pegboard Test (Rapin et al., 1966) or the finger tapping test and quantified by using the Denckla (1973, 1974), Spreen and Gaddes (1969), or Goodenough (1935) criteria. While evaluating only a very limited aspect of motor behavior, these tests have the major advantage of sex- and age-appropriate standards.

Some tests do generally quantitate various motor behaviors but, as with the cited "neurodevelopmental" exams, the *process* of motor activity is generally not evaluated by them, only the *outcome*, so it is not possible to use them for subtyping causes of failure. Still, the tests are standardized and norms are available, so results can reliably alert one to look more specifically for clumsiness or other causes of outcome failure. Frankenberg's Denver Developmental Screening Test (Frankenberg and Dodds, 1967) and the McCarthy Scales (McCarthy, 1972) are two such tests that are widely used. The Lincoln-Oseretsky Test of Motor Behavior is also well known (Sloan, 1948) and normative data are available for children between the ages of 6 and 14 years. It is highly correlated with academic success. The Halsted-Reitan Battery was initially developed with a view to ascertainment of locus of brain damage in children. Although it is not currently used for that purpose, the motor items do have developmental norms and are useful for qualitative screening for clumsiness and other higher-order motor deficits (Reitan, 1969). The Kaufman Battery also contains hand movement evaluations (Kaufman and Kaufman, 1983).

Children with cerebral palsy and actual weakness and spasticity also always suffer from lack of dexterity, but they have telltale neurologic signs to alert the examiner to the problem. Even in the cerebral palsied, quantitative specific tests of dexterity, praxis, and manual coordination are valuable in defining the degree of impairment from clumsiness versus dyspraxia and thus guiding therapy for more successful everyday living for these children.

To help a clumsy child, the limits and influence of

Pearls and Perils: Clumsiness

1. Clumsiness is very conducive to low self-esteem, starting very early in development. This early secondary low self-esteem mediates depression, continued failure, and thus failure in areas that have no motor requirements whatsoever.

2. Clumsiness is often a primary cause of school failure in the early grades, when mechanical demands are heavy and intellectual ones light. Even though the child may have no measurable difficulty in processing ideas or in reading or calculating, his or her clumsiness may prevent proper school achievement.

3. Clumsiness is often a primary cause of "hyperactivity" or "inattention" in the young child whose motor performance is inadequate.

4. Some clumsy individuals can improve their performance with a specific modality of input guiding them. For example, the child who is a poor soccer player is not necessarily a poor dancer and may perform aerobic exercises readily and handily to music.

5. Treating clumsiness as a "soft sign" of other disorders, such as ADD, is a mistake. Although it is statistically significantly associated with ADD (Denckla and Rudel, 1978; Nichols, 1987), it is not an indicator of ADD or vice versa (in fact some would hold that it is one of several possible causes of ADD).

6. Occasionally an artistically or verbally gifted clumsy child's performance improves on specific material that falls into the child's area of talent. For instance, the musically gifted clumsy child may be a superb performer on the flute. It is important to evaluate a range of motor performances.

7. Often a simple explanation to parents and teachers of the mechanical difficulties at the root of the child's slow and labored performances will change these authorities' attitudes and demands to a great extent, allowing marked increase in the child's self-esteem and improved performance through improved motivation.

8. If clumsiness is not handicapping an individual child, investment of time and money by parents in direct remediation should be avoided. Rather, particularly in the older clumsy child, secondary effects of clumsiness (depression and low self-esteem) may be much more important to address therapeutically than the motor deficit per se.

the motor disability on the total disability must first be defined. The major effective remedy for clumsiness is practice. However, the allowance of extra time to complete fine motor tasks is also helpful to self-esteem and relieves interfering anxieties. The reduction of mechanical impediments to speedy production in required activities (a so-called "bypass" method) is often used. For example, Velcro flap shoes instead of laced shoes, zippers instead of buttons, or elastic bands rather than buckled belts may be provided. While practice generally improves the child's performance of a given act, anxiety and tension may lead to disintegration of the performance once again. Thus, under stress (as when dressing for school) certain amounts of help may be granted, but when the child is in a more relaxed situation (as when undressing for bed or dressing for a Saturday occasion), this additional help can be withdrawn. It is important to realize that machines can be very helpful to purely clumsy children, whose disorder is generally a fully mechanical one in that the motor program is appropriate to the goal of the action, and only the speed of execution is deficient.

As for prognosis, severe clumsiness (or maladroitness, as it is politely called by some of the earlier authors [Ford, 1960]) is unlikely to be completely gone by maturity (Knuckey and Gubbay, 1983). However, a sufficient degree of dexterity may be achieved that the maturing child is capable of at least the minimum dexterity that he or she must achieve in order to function in a society of people who are more adroit. A general rule is that if the child can learn to overcome or go around mechanical blocks, and thus avoid the deficit in self-esteem created by the performance deficit, the primary deficit will not be a severe handicap in the adult life of a normally intelligent individual (Ford, 1960).

ADVENTITIOUS MOVEMENTS

A type of motor abnormality, very often accompanying clumsiness (Nichols, 1987) but readily separable from it, is adventitious movements. There are two major varieties of adventitious movements. One appears whether the subject is attempting a voluntary movement or not. This type moves the limb that may be in voluntary play in an unwanted direction or in fact appears when no voluntary motions of the limb are going on. The best-known and most common adventitious movement of this sort is chorea, which manifests itself as a sudden rapid motion of the face, fingers, limbs, or even trunk that may interrupt or disturb an ongoing voluntary movement or may come about irrespective of lack of willed activities. In the neurologic literature chorea is not classified as a higher-order motor deficit, yet the literature of "soft signs" gives it much discussion (Prechtl and Stemmer, 1962; Barlow, 1974; Deuel and Robinson, 1987). Chorea is best tested by having the subject stand with the legs slightly apart, the arms extended in the prone position

---

**Pearls and Perils:
Adventitious Movements**

1. The acute or subacute appearance of chorea or emotional lability in a school-age child alerts one to look for rheumatic or collagen vascular disease. Its sudden appearance differentiates it from developmental chorea, which has often been noted throughout early childhood by parents.
2. Choreiform movements can be confused with tardive dyskinesia in mentally retarded children on neuroleptics.
3. Children with agenesis of the corpus callosum appear to have a greater propensity to mirror movements than others.
4. Chorea is sometimes an early symptom of a treatable nervous system disorder, such as rheumatic disease or Wilson's disease. Serious consideration of such diagnoses is important in its presence.
5. A cerebellar lesion must be considered in every instance in which an intention tremor is discovered.

---

with the wrists dorsiflexed and the digits abducted, and with the eyes closed, for about 20 seconds (Barlow, 1974). The examiner will observe rapid twitch-like movement of the fingers most advantageously with the subject in this position. With marked or severe chorea, flinging movements of the arms and face may appear. There are many other ways to test this symptom directly, but most effective are observation during other items (such as walking gaits) of a neurologic examination (Deuel and Robinson, 1987). There is a familial benign chorea that is recognized as nonprogressive and is also generally treated (Damasio et al., 1977). Otherwise, other chorea is treated as indicated by etiology.

Tremor is another variety of adventitious movement. Tremor, involuntary oscillations of a body part that may occur at rest or during willed action, also frequently hinders voluntary movement. Intention tremor, when the oscillation increases as the limb in motion nears its target, is known as a sign of cerebellar disease. To test for it, use the finger-to-nose and the heel-to-shin test of the neurologic examination and observe for it during the tandem gait test and during writing, drawing, and picking up small objects. In a developmental setting tremor and chorea are often accompanied in the same individual by decreased limb girdle and axial tone with near-normal or normal strength. Decreased ability to perform accurate simple movements usually occurs when tremors are plentiful. Benign familial tremor occurs in children as well as in adults and must be differentiated from tremors with more dire prognosis. Management of tremors without underlying cerebellar pathology is predicated on their handicapping significance. If the tremor causes significant functional impediment to the child, medication may be helpful.

The third variety of adventitious movement is called synkinesis. It is manifest as unwilled activity of voluntary musculature (involuntary movement) that occurs during the course of a voluntary action, and is elicited by production of the voluntary target action. Examples include involuntary opening of the eyes when a child is told to stick out his or her tongue. Involuntary opening of the mouth when the child voluntarily opens his or her eyes very wide is another commonly encountered example.

This disorder, like chorea, is best evaluated as part of a neurologic exam. One item that directly elicits this type of synkinesis is the Fog test (Fog and Fog, 1963), which requires the child to walk on the sides of the feet, either the insides or the outsides of the sole. When the child performs this maneuver, especially if a relatively narrow base is demanded, the arms and hands frequently enter distorted postures. This test has been reevaluated and is quite useful, especially using Wolff's new data (Wolff et al., 1983).

Mirror movements are a well-known form of synkinesis. These are synkineses that occur in groups of muscles directly homologous to the groups that are in voluntary play. During the performance of the finger tapping test a mirror movement commonly occurs: the hand that has not been commanded to tap nevertheless carries out the very same tapping activity, which may persist even in the face of a command to stop. The occurrence of mirror movements in the nondominant hand when the dominant hand is performing is an abnormality above the age of 6 years. On the other hand, the occurrence mirror movements in the dominant hand when the nondominant hand is performing is not an abnormality, even above the age of 8 years, unless the effort involved is very little or the adventitious movements are very copious. It has been confirmed that the amount of effort required for the voluntary (commanded) activity predicates mirror synkineses in normal children (Todor and Lazarus, 1986). Thus, when searching for true "excess" mirror synkinesis it is best to avoid tasks that require extraordinarily strenuous efforts. A patient suffering from extreme degrees of mirror movements will produce them in simple, "nonstrenuous," everyday unimanual activities, such as turning a door handle.

The incidence of mirror movements is much less (2%) in the Perinatal Project cohort of children, previously mentioned in the section on Clumsiness (Nichols, 1987), than that of higher-order motor deficits in general. The reason is not clear, but it may relate to how the mirror movements were elicited in the Perinatal Project. As clumsy children very often exhibit mirror movements, the above-mentioned finding about the interaction between degree of exertion and occurrence of mirror movements may play a role in their occurrence in clum-

sy children, who have to exert a large amount of effort to accomplish simple motor acts. Fortunately mirror movements tend to diminish with increasing age (Wolff et al., 1983). An effective treatment is not known, but it may be helpful to deliberately engage the hand not involved in the voluntary action with grasping or pressing a surface. Some children spontaneously use this maneuver.

ANNOTATED BIBLIOGRAPHY

Liepmann, H: *Drei Aufsätze aus dem Apraxiegebiet.* Berlin, Karger, 1908.

This is a thoughtful synoptic text that reviews the general concept of apraxia (or dyspraxia) as a higher-order motor deficit. It discusses various schemes of classification and mentions a number of common forms of apraxia seen after localized cerebral lesions in adults. It also gives general rules for testing for dyspraxia, and discusses parapraxis as incorrect or supernumerary movements. The book ends with a very modern concept—that there are many brain areas that initiate movement, and that whether or not these areas are used depends on the type and purpose of the movement to be performed.

Gubbay SS: Clumsiness, in Fredriks JAM (ed): *Handbook of Clinical Neurology,* Vol 46: *Neurobehavioural Disorders.* Amsterdam, Elsevier/North-Holland, 1985, p 159–167.

This chapter tells a great deal about the general dilemma of a child with higher developmental disorders of motor execution. However, it fails to differentiate various forms of these disorders.

Deuel RK, Robinson DU: Development motor signs, in Tupper DE (ed): *Soft Neurological Signs.* New York, Grune & Stratton, 1987, p 95–129.

This is a critical review of literature concerning developmental motor soft signs. It points out some common methodologic failures in the large literature on the subject, and therefore the difficulty in comparing studies. It describes many studies in detail.

Nichols PL: Minimal brain dysfunction and soft signs: The Collaborative Perinatal Project, in Tupper DE (ed): *Soft Neurological Signs.* New York, Grune & Stratton, 1987, p 179–199.

A statistical evaluation of the Perinatal Project outcome concerning soft signs in a large cohort of children, this chapter is especially pertinent to the question of motor execution deficits in relation to other developmental higher cerebral function deficits. The 30,000 subjects all received a standard battery of tests, including a WISC and a neurologic exam at age 7 years. They had all been followed since birth.

REFERENCES

Annell AL: School problems in children of average or superior intelligence. *J Mental Sci* 95:901–909, 1949.

Aram DM, Horwitz SU: Sequential and non-speech praxic abilities in developmental verbal apraxia. *Dev Med Child Neurol* 25:197–206, 1983.

Barlow C: "Soft signs" in children with learning disabilities. *Am J Dis Child* 128:605–606, 1974.

Bender LA: *Instructions for the Use of the Visual-Motor Gestalt Test and Its Clinical Use*. New York, American Orthopsychiatric Association, 1946.

Benton AL: *The Revised Visual Retention Test*. New York, Psychological Corporation, 1974.

Brenner M, Gillman S: Visuomotor ability in school children: A survey. *Dev Med Child Neurol* 8:686–712, 1966.

Crothers B, Paine RS: *The Natural History of Cerebral Palsy*. Cambridge, Mass, Harvard University Press, 1959.

Damasio H, Antunes L, Damasio A: Familial nonprogressive involuntary movements of childhood. *Ann Neurol* 1:602–603, 1977.

David R, Ferry P, Gascon G, et al: *Proposed Nosology of Disorders of Higher Cerebral Function in Children*. Minneapolis, Minn, Task Force on Nosology, Child Neurology Society, 1981.

Denckla MB: Development of speed in repetitive and successive finger-movements in normal children. *Dev Med Child Neurol* 15:635–645, 1973.

Denckla MB: Development of motor co-ordination in normal children. *Dev Med Child Neurol* 16:729–741, 1974.

Denckla MB, Rudel RG: Anomalies of motor development in hyperactive boys. *Ann Neurol* 3:231–233, 1978.

Denny-Brown D: *Handbook of Neurological Examination*. Cambridge, Mass, Harvard University Press, 1958, p 21–35.

DeRenzi E, Pieczuro A, Vignolo LA: Ideational apraxia: A quantitative study. *Neuropsychologia* 6:41–52, 1968.

DeRenzi E, Motti F, Nichelli P: Imitation gestures. A quantitative approach to ideomotor apraxia. *Arch Neurol* 37:6–10, 1980.

Deuel RK: Loss of motor habits after cortical lesions. *Neuropsychologia* 15:205–215, 1977.

Deuel RK: Minimal brain dysfunction, hyperkinesis, learning disabilities, attention deficit disorder. *J Pediatr* 98:912–915, 1981.

Deuel RK, Robinson DU: Developmental motor signs, in Tupper DE (ed): *Soft Neurological Signs*. New York, Grune & Stratton, 1987, p 95–129.

Fog E, Fog M: Cerebral inhibition examined by associated movements. *Clin Dev Med* 10, 1963.

Ford F: *Diseases of the Nervous System in Infancy, Childhood and Adolescence*. Springfield, Ill, Charles C. Thomas, 1960.

Frankenberg W, Dodds J: The Denver Developmental Screening Test. *J Pediatr* 71:181–191, 1967.

Frei H: Das "ungeschickte" Kind: Differentialdiagnose und Therapieindikationen. *Schweiz. Med Wochenschr* 116:294–299, 1986.

Geschwind N, Damasio A: Apraxia, in Fredriks JAM (ed): *Handbook of Clinical Neurology*, Vol 45: *Clinical Neuropsychology*. Amsterdam, Elsevier/North-Holland, 1985, p 7–22.

Goodenough F: A further study of tapping speed in early childhood. *J Appl Psychol* 19:309, 1935.

Gubbay S: *The Clumsy Child: A Study of Developmental Apraxia and Agnostic Ataxia*. Philadelphia, WB Saunders, 1975.

Gubbay SS: Clumsiness, in Fredriks JAM (ed): *Handbook of Clinical Neurology*, Vol. 46: *Neurobehavioural Disorders*. Amsterdam, Elsevier/North-Holland, 1985, p 159–167.

Hagberg B, Aicardi J, Dias K, Ramos D: A progressive syndrome of autism, dementia, ataxia and loss of purposeful hand use in girls: Rett's syndrome. *Ann Neurol* 14:471–479, 1983.

Hammill DD, and Larson SC: *The Test of Written Language*. Austin, Tex, Pro-Ed, 1978.

Iloeje SO: Developmental apraxia among Nigerian children in Enugu, Nigeria. *Dev Med Child Neurol* 29:502–507, 1987.

Jabbour J: Subacute sclerosing panencephalitis: A multidisciplinary study of eight cases. *JAMA* 207:2248–2254, 1969.

Johnson R, Stark R, Mellits E, Tallal P: Neurological status of language impaired and normal children. *Ann Neurol* 10:159–165, 1981.

Kaufman A, Kaufman N: *Kaufman Assessment Battery for Children (K-ABC). Administration and Scoring Manual*. Circle Pines, Minn, American Guidance Service, 1983.

Kleist K: *Gehirnpathology*. Leipzig, Barth, 1934.

Knuckey NW, Gubbay SS: Clumsy children: A prognostic study. *Aust Paediatr J* 19:9–13, 1983.

Levine M, et al: The PEEX: Studies of neurodevelopmental examination for 7 to 9 year old children. *Pediatrics* 71:894–903, 1983.

Liepmann H: Das Krankheitsbild der Apraxie. Monographie. *Monatsschr Psychiatr Neurol (Berlin)* 8:15–44, 102–132, 182–197, 1900.

Liepmann H: *Drei Aufsätze aus dem Apraxiegebiet*. Berlin, Karger, 1908.

McCarthy D: *McCarthy Scales of Children's Abilities*. New York, The Psychological Corporation, 1972.

Nichols PL: Minimal brain dysfunction and soft signs: The Collaborative Perinatal Project, in Tupper DE (ed): *Soft Neurological Signs*. New York, Grune & Stratton, 1987, p 179–199.

O'Malley PJ, Griffith JF: Perceptuo-motor dysfunction in the child with hemiplegia. *Dev Med Child Neurol* 19:172–178, 1977.

Orton ST: "Word blindness" in school children. *Arch Neurol Psychiatr* 14:581–615, 1925.

Percy A, et al: Metachromatic leukodystrophy: A comparison of early and late onset forms. *Neurology* 27:933–944, 1977.

Poeck K: The clinical examination for motor apraxia. *Neuropsychologia* 24:129–134, 1986.

Prechtl H, Stemmer C: The choreiform syndrome in children. *Dev Med Child Neurol* 4:119–127, 1962.

Pyfer JL, Castelman BR: Characteristic motor development of children with learning disabilities. *Percept Motor Skills* 35:291–296, 1972.

Rapin I, Tourk LM, Costa LD: Evaluation of the Purdue pegboard as a screening test for brain damage. *Dev Med Child Neurol* 8:45–54, 1966.

Reitan R: *Manual for Administration of Neuropsychological Test Batteries for Adults and Children*. Privately published by author, 1969.

Roach E, Kephardt N: *The Purdue Perceptual Motor Survey*. Columbia, Mo, Chas C Merrill, 1966.

Skubic V, Anderson V: The interrelationship of perceptual motor achievement, academic achievement and intelligence in fourth grade children. *J Learn Disabil* 3:413–420, 1970.

Sloan W: *The Lincoln Adaptation of the Oseretsky Tests: A Measure of Motor Proficiency*. Lincoln, Ill, Lincoln State School, 1948.

Spreen O, Gaddes W: Developmental norms for 15 neuropsychological tests ages 6-15. *Cortex* 5:170–181, 1969.

Swaiman K, Smith SR, Track GL, Siddiqui RR: Sea blue histiocytes, lymphocytic cytosomes, movement disorders and ^{59}Fe uptake in the basal ganglia. *Neurology* 33:301–305, 1983.

Todor JI, Lazarus JA: Exertion level and the intensity of associated movements. *Dev Med Child Neurol* 28:205–212, 1986.

Wolff H, Gunnoe CE, Cohen C: Associated movements as a measure of developmental age. *Dev Med Child Neurol* 25:417–429, 1983.

Disorders of Higher Cortical Function in Preschoolers

Ruth D. Nass
Diane Koch

This chapter will focus primarily on the developmental language disorders and the autistic spectrum disorders, two not uncommon developmental disorders presenting in the preschool years. Attention deficit disorder, disorders of temperament, and visuomotor and spatial difficulties will be briefly described.

DEVELOPMENTAL LANGUAGE DISORDERS

General Discussion

When presented with a child with language delay the clinician must first document that the child has the two major prerequisites for language acquisition: intact hearing and adequate intellect. Mentally retarded children may on occasion have specific language impairments. However, preschool children with IQs under 50 generally do not develop communicative language. The language disability here is nonspecific and stems from the general cognitive deficit. Although children with developmental language disorders may score in the subnormal intellectual range on measures taxing verbal skills (e.g., the Wechsler Verbal Scale), a number of measures are available to assess nonverbal intelligence in the preschooler (e.g., the Leiter Performance Scale, the Weschler Performance Scale; see Chapter 3 for discussion). The criteria used by the Child Neurology Society Higher Cortical Function Nosology Task Force to separate autistic spectrum disorder (ASD) from developmental language disorder (DLD) from nonautistic mental deficiency (NAMD) are shown in Figure 21–1.

Hearing loss should be ruled out by formal audiologic assessment in the child with language delay. The current availability of techniques for measuring brainstem evoked responses makes a gross assessment of the uncooperative young child possible. However, mild and even moderate deficits can sometimes be missed by this technique because of the high stimulus threshold. Thus behavioral audiometry should be used when possible.

Diagnosis

With so much individual variability in rate of language acquisition, it is at times difficult to distinguish DLDs from initial delay in acquisition with eventual catch-up and normal language. Morley (1965) charted language acquisition in approximately 1000 ultimately normal British children. First word acquisition occurred at anywhere from age 6 to 30 months and phrase acquisition at anywhere from 10 to 44 months. Prevalence of language impairment in the preschooler has been reported at between 1% and 25% (Stevenson and Richman, 1976). The percent with language impairment at elementary school entry is estimated around 5% (Morley, 1965). Generally, failure to develop normal expressive language by age 3 years is pathologic (Rapin and Allen, 1983). The 2-year-old without expressive language and a receptive deficit is also of concern. In addition, children with DLDs (regardless of subtype) fail to maximize the communicative use of language (pragmatics; Donahue, 1987). Question exchanges and the ability to make conversation develop excessively late in these children as compared to normal children (Rapin and Allen, 1983).

Risk factors for DLDs have been identified. The National Collaborative Perinatal Project identified low birth weight, low gestational age, and parental mental retardation. Language failures at age 3 years correlated best with failure to vocalize to social stimuli (pragmatic deficit) and failure to vocalize two syllables (babble) at the 8-month assessment (Bayley Mental and Motor Scales). These two subtests were highly predictive of language failure at age 8 years as well (Lassman et al., 1980). Historical information about these two early language milestones may thus be quite useful. Sex chromosome abnormalities characterized by an extra X chromosome, i.e., XXX and

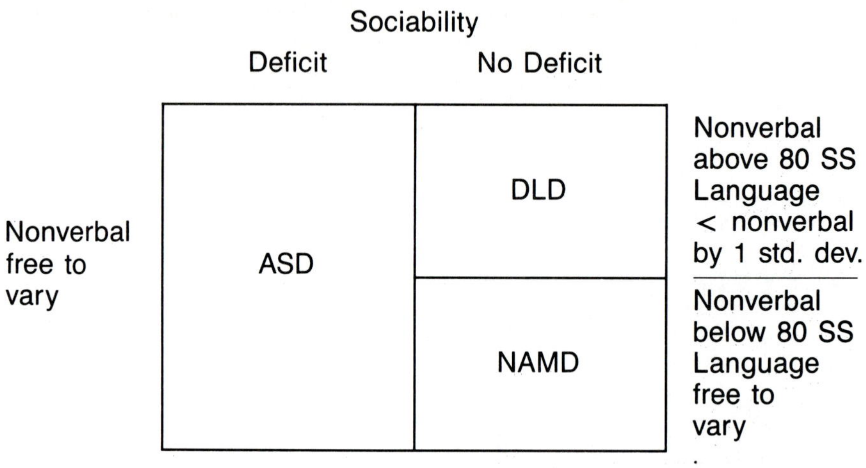

Sociability

Deficit   No Deficit

Figure 21-1. Sociability, language, and cognitive abilities are used to define three disorders: developmental language disorder (DLD), autistic spectrum disorder (ASD), and nonautistic mental deficiency (NAMD). *(Reproduced from the Child Neurology Society Higher Cortical Function Nosology Task Force with permission.)*

Nonverbal free to vary

ASD

DLD

NAMD

Nonverbal above 80 SS Language < nonverbal by 1 std. dev.

Nonverbal below 80 SS Language free to vary

XXY syndromes (Netley, 1983), also put a child at risk for specific language disorders. A negative effect of testosterone on language development is suggested by the increased incidence of DLDs and autism in males (Geschwind and Galaburda, 1985).

Signs and Symptoms

DLDs vary enormously in their characteristics; definition of etiology, prognosis, and treatment depends on subtyping (Rapin, 1982; Rapin and Allen, 1983, 1988; Allen et al., 1988). The traditional subtyping of both adult and childhood aphasia delineates them as receptive and expressive. The problem with this dichotomy, however, is that those with expressive difficulties are not wholly free of comprehension problems, and vice versa. The dichotomy of fluent versus nonfluent has therefore replaced the traditional classification with respect to expressive skills. Both in adult acquired aphasias and in studies of the DLDs, recent investigation has centered on psycholinguistic classification (Nass and Gazzaniga, 1987).

A variety of subtyping systems have been proposed.

This chapter concentrates on that of the Child Neurology Society Higher Cortical Function Nosology Task Force schema. Deficits in different linguistic processes, for example, syntax (see Glossary), differentiate subtypes. Table 21-1 shows the linguistic deficits to be anticipated in each syndrome.

Verbal Auditory Agnosia

In the verbal auditory agnosia subtype, meaningful language cannot be understood despite intact hearing. The characteristic language deficit pattern has been reported on a congenital/developmental basis (Rapin et al., 1977; Maccario et al., 1982) and has also been termed *generalized low performance* (Aram and Nation, 1982) and *global dysfunction* (Wilson and Risucci, 1986; Wolfus et al., 1980). Low-functioning autistic children often show evidence of this syndrome. However, Landau and Kleffner (1957) first described the acquired epileptic and most common form of this relatively uncommon DLD. (We will therefore concentrate on this form unless otherwise noted.) Typically, a previously normal, usually male child between the ages of 3 and 7 years develops a specific disorder of language functioning. A deterioration in the

TABLE 21-1. LINGUISTIC DEFICITS IN DEVELOPMENTAL LANGUAGE DISORDERS

	Verbal Auditory Agnosia	Verbal Apraxia	Semantic-Pragmatic Deficit Syndrome	Lexical-Syntactic Deficit Syndrome	Phonologic-Syntactic Deficit Syndrome
Comprehension					
Phonology	↓↓				
Syntax	↓↓				↓
Semantics	↓↓		↓↓	↓	
Production					
Semantics (lexical)	↓↓		↓	↓↓	
Syntax	↓↓			↓	↓↓
Phonology	↓↓	↓↓			↓
Repetition	↓↓	↓	↑↑	↓	↓
Fluency	↓↓	↑ or ↓	↑	↓	↓
Pragmatics	↑ or ↓		↓↓	↓	

Reproduced with modifications from Rapin and Allen (1988), with permission.

child's ability to comprehend language occurs over days to weeks. Often parents think that their child is becoming deaf. However, the child is able to hear, as attested to by the fact that he responds to the environmental sounds and by the fact that in the laboratory both the audiogram and brainstem auditory responses are normal. But the child cannot meaningfully process the language he hears. The loss of the ability to understand language is followed by the insidious progressive loss of the ability to speak, sometimes to the point of mutism. Poorly articulated, dysprosodic speech is the rule. Some children with this disorder are capable of accessing language in the visual modality; they can gesture, learn signs, and read and write. Except for their language impairment these children are generally intellectually normal, for example, as measured by performance IQ. Sometimes they have behavioral difficulties like hyperactivity or even frank psychosis, presumably a secondary response to their impaired ability to function in the linguistic domain. Language deficits consistent with verbal auditory agnosia and paroxysmal electroencephalographic (EEG) findings with or without seizures have recently been reported in typically developmentally autistic children (Nass and Petrucha, 1990; Payton and Minshew, 1987).

All seizure types have been reported in association with this language syndrome. EEG abnormalities have generally been bilateral: bitemporal, generalized, or multifocal. However, unilateral paroxysmal abnormalities on both right and left have been reported in about 10% of cases. Generally seizures are easy to control. Considerable controversy exists as to the extent of the parallel between the presence and severity of the EEG abnormalities and the aphasic disorder. Most investigators (e.g., Shoumaker et al., 1974; Cole et al., 1988) have demonstrated, in children with fluctuating aphasia, a similarly fluctuating EEG. Deuel and Lenn (1977) document, in a child treated early with anticonvulsants, a remarkable parallel between EEG and clinical improvement. By contrast (Sandt-Koenderman et al., 1984; Lou et al., 1977), two children followed prospectively for 3 and 10 years, respectively, evidenced no parallel between EEG and clinical status. The issue of the relationship between EEG abnormalities and clinical language deficit is further confounded by studies of children with DLDs of all linguistic subtypes, which demonstrate as many as 50% with abnormal paroxysmal EEGs (Maccario et al., 1982).

The outcome from the acquired disorder is variable. Although many suggest anticonvulsant treatment, even to the point of treating the EEG in the absence of seizures, no definite parallel between treatment course and language outcome has been demonstrated. Nonetheless, EEG assessment and a limited trial of anticonvulsants should the EEG prove paroxysmal (even in the absence of clinical seizures) appears warranted in the child presenting with an isolated developmental or acquired language disorder.

Long-term (greater than 10-year) follow-up suggests that about one third of patients have normal language, one third have mildly impaired language, and one third have severely impaired language. Younger age of onset may be associated with a worse prognosis (Bishop, 1985). Mantovani and Landau (1980) reported follow-up of nine of the original patients, 10 to 28 years after the onset of the aphasia. Four of the five with the best outcome had diminished visuoperceptual ability, while the three tested patients with moderate residual language disability had normal visuoperceptual ability as measured by the Benton Visual Retention Test.

The etiology of this disorder is unknown. Some suggest that it is a form of chronic focal encephalitis (Worster-Drought, 1971; Lou et al., 1977). Biopsy in one patient revealed lymphocytic infiltration of the meninges, gliosis, and neuronal loss (Lou et al., 1977). However, the patient was somewhat atypical for the eventual development of a bulbar palsy. McKinney and McGreal (1974) found no abnormalities on biopsy. Cole et al. (1988) reported two patients who were subject to seizure surgery, neither of whom evidenced pathology in the corticectomy specimen, a finding consistent with an encephalitic process. Reports of left temporal horn dilatation lend some favor to a destructive process as etiology.

The extent of underlying pathology, be it focal or diffuse, is also debated. Nass and Walker (1989) reported a patient with a left temporal ganglioglioma whose severe seizures and aphasia improved dramatically when the tumor was resected. Mantovani and Landau's (1980) neuropsychologic data also support a focal origin for this disorder; recovery of language, when it occurs, compromises ordinarily right hemisphere–mediated functions, a finding that suggests transfer of recovered language from the left to the right hemisphere. Teuber (Woods and Teuber, 1973) coined the term "crowding" to explain such a recovery pattern when it occurred after early structural left brain damage in the child. However, the fact that recovery from this syndrome is significantly less frequent than that from acquired aphasia owing to structural left brain injury raises questions about the putative left focal nature of this disorder. Positon emission tomographic scanning of a patient atypical for severe epilepsy revealed right temporal hypometabolism, as well as an extremely active left temporal epileptic focus (Cole et al., 1988). Magnetic resonance imaging (MRI) data analyzing volumetric parameters revealed reduced posterior temporal volumes bilaterally in two patients (Filipek et al., 1987). Xenon inhalation blood flow assessment in one patient revealed decreased posterior perisylvian flow bilaterally, and failure of verbal activation to increase flow in the left perisylvian language region (Lou et al., 1984). Finally, two patients with developmental verbal auditory agnosia without epilepsy evidenced bilateral disease. A patient of Landau and associates (1960) had bitemporal cystic changes with retrograde degeneration of the medial geniculate bodies. Congenital rubella and severe spastic quadriparesis were observed in a patient of Fuller and colleagues (1983).

Verbal Apraxia

Morley (1965) is credited with the first description of a cohort of children whose language deficit was characterized by markedly impaired articulation in the face of otherwise adequate comprehension skills. She found by history that the majority (69%) of the members of her 114-child sample were speaking intelligibly by age 2 years (55% of the boys and 82% of the girls) and that by age 3 years 84% (77% of the boys and 91% of the girls) had intelligible speech. (Note the more rapid maturation of articulation skills in girls as compared to boys.) At age 3 years, 9 months 11% had unintelligible (to strangers) speech (Figure 21–2). Minor (group I: articulation normal except for the defective use of [th] and/or [r]) and mild (group II: intelligible speech but with some consonant substitutions other than or in addition to [th] and/or [r]) defects in articulation were still present in almost 50% of the normal sample. At the age of 4 years, 9 months, one third of the normal sample continued to have minor to mild articulation defects. In 4% speech was still unintelligible. At the 6½-year assessment 3% continued to show relapsing articulation deficits (regression to a less mature pattern during times of stress). Such regression had been quite common during the preschool transition from immature to mature articulation patterns. One child still had unintelligible speech at 6½ years.

Morley also assessed 162 children with defective articulation (with or without delay in the development of speech). Males outnumbered females by 2 to 1. Overall, speech development was slower in the children with defective articulation. The average age for first word use was 15 months, almost 4 months later than the average age in the entire sample. The average age for the use of phrases was 24 months compared with 18 months. Despite the initial delay, even severe defects of articulation (44 children) were not associated with delay in the use of language at 3½ years (Figure 21–3).

Based on the findings and developmental patterns demonstrated in her study, Morley classified disorders of articulation into five types: defective articulation owing to deficient hearing, defective articulation caused by various structural abnormalities, developmental dysarthria caused by known brain damage, dyslalia, and developmental verbal apraxia. Dyslalia refers to the articulation difficulties of children whose speech intelligibility is relatively late in developing.

More recently, Ferry and associates (1975) defined verbal apraxia as a neurologically based disorder of speech wherein articulatory ability is impaired despite motor and sensory abilities sufficient to carry out purposeful articulatory movements. In generating their 60-patient cohort, aged 4 to 30 years, the authors required delay in speech of greater than 1 year; intact hearing; normal receptive language skills; inconsistent omissions, substitutions, and distortions of speech sounds; increasing problems as phonics increased in complexity; an elaborate gesture system; limited progress in articulatory skills despite prolonged therapeutic intervention; and a

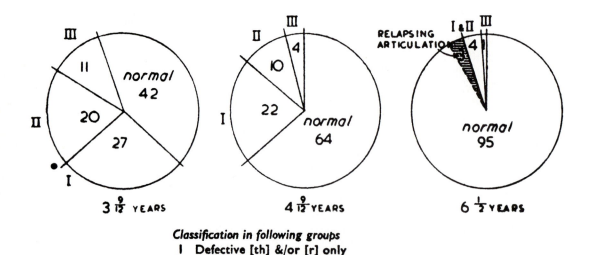

Classification in following groups
I   Defective [th] &/or [r] only
II Intelligible speech, but defects of articulation
III Unintelligible speech
% of children in group of 114 children

Figure 21–2. Classification of articulation in 114 children. Gradual and spontaneous improvement is seen with age. *(From Morley, 1965, with permission.)*

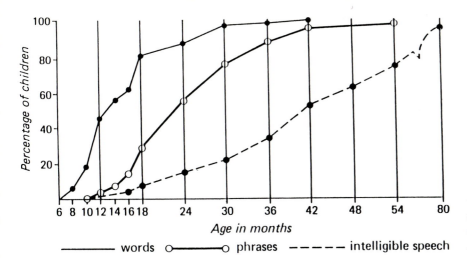

Figure 21–3. Rate of language acquisition in children with articulation defects. *(From Morley, 1965, with permission.)*

struggle to position muscles of articulation. The majority of patients in this series had associated neurologic abnormalities, including orofacial dyspraxia (36), spastic diplegia (13), mild motor delay (10), tremor (2), hemiplegia (1), and chorea (1). Ferry and colleagues concluded that if a child with this disorder does not have intelligible speech by 6 years, he is unlikely to acquire it.

There is considerable controversy as to how often nonverbal apraxic deficits—oral apraxia for nonspeech movements (the struggle to position muscles of articulation) and general motor apraxia or clumsiness—occur in this disorder. Many of these children are clumsy or have documented difficulty in learning nonspeech motor acts (Aram and Nation, 1982). The presence of a more general apraxic deficit has significant therapeutic implications, because these children are very dependent on their signing and writing skills for communication. Pearce and colleagues (1987) have demonstrated in a small cohort, aged 2 years 11 months to 5 years 10 months, that the patients had more trouble learning (but no more than controls) and recalling manual signs and Bliss symbols. Because some did better on manual signs than Bliss symbols and others did better with Bliss symbols than manual signs, the investigators suggest that a preliminary paired associate learning task might help select the best communication method for a particular child. However, there is clearly heterogeneity in this disorder because many of these children become very skilled in signing.

The etiology of this disorder is not yet known. The excess of males and familial tendency support a genetic basis. Worster-Drought (1953) reported a patient with a similar speech disorder who also manifested signs of suprabulbar palsy and was found to have hypoplasia of the motor tract running from the Rolandic region to cranial nerve nucleii X and XII. Rapin and Allen (1988) suggest that the disorder most resembles the adult aphasia-aphemia. Patients with this disorder, unlike those with Broca's aphasia, generally evidence good writing skills despite their severely reduced language corpus

(Benson, 1979). The pathology in aphemia is in or near Broca's area, in the lower sensorimotor cortex, or in the connections between the supplementary motor area or Broca's area and the orofacial region of the sensorimotor cortex (Benson, 1979; Kertesz, 1983). Lou and associates (1984) reported that patients with this disorder manifest decreased blood flow, as measured by the xenon inhalation technique, in the frontal regions. Verbal activation failed to increase perfusion in Broca's area.

Semantic-Pragmatic Syndrome

The semantic-pragmatic syndrome is among the most common and often most subtle of the developmental language disorders. Other names for it (Aram and Nation, 1982) include *repetition strength* and *comprehension deficit disorder* and *language without cognition* (Curtiss, 1988). Children with this disorder are fluent, even verbose. Phonologic and syntactic skills are generally intact. Vocabulary is often large although somewhat formal. Parents are often inappropriately encouraged by these children's sizable vocabulary, only to find later that this was not a harbinger of superior verbal skills. These children fall short in basic semantic skills required for meaningful conversation and informative exchange of ideas. They talk to talk. Comprehension is impaired. They may, for example, answer a different "wh-" question from the one being asked (Rapin and Allen, 1983). Furthermore, their pragmatic skills are lacking. They have not learned the rules that govern the use of language in context (Bates, 1976). Children with the semantic-pragmatic syndrome do not know how to make appropriate use of such conversational techniques as turn taking, topic maintenance, and varying style depending on whether or not the person being addressed is a peer. Finally, children with the semantic-pragmatic syndrome often evidence deficits in prosody. Their speech often has a singsong quality and they therefore cannot convey the additional pragmatic intentions that prosody affords.

This syndrome is sometimes seen in the higher-functioning, more verbal autistic child (Rapin and Allen, 1983). This clinical population in particular often has exceptional repetition skills, which may manifest as immediate echolalia or as delayed echoing, often of lengthy commercials, nursery rhymes, or songs. Apparently exceptional memory abilities are sometimes present (Obler and Fein, 1988).

This syndrome is also reported under the name *cocktail party syndrome* in children with hydrocephalus, particularly in the setting of myelomeningocoele. Tew and Lawrence (1979) found that at age 5 years children with the cocktail party syndrome could be distinguished from other children with spina bifida by their lower IQ, retarded social skills, and decreased visuoperceptual abilities. Despite a good score on the syntactic portion of a standardized language test, their creative language capacities were inferior. At age 7 years they performed poorly academically and had impaired attention. The frequency of the syndrome tended to diminish with age. Those children still meeting the criterion at age 10 years were mentally retarded. Poorer outcome tended to be associated with being female and having more severe spina bifida. Studying 11 shunted hydrocephalics with spina bifida (ages 2 to 9 years, IQs 65 to 106), Swisher and Pinsker (1971) found them to be more talkative, more repetitive, and more inappropriate and bizarre in their language use than age- and socioeconomically matched controls. Language was also inferior on a standardized language test. Dennis and colleagues (1988), assessing children with hydrocephalus of many etiologies including spina bifida, found relatively little evidence of cocktail party syndrome; rather they found individual and variable language impairments. Notably, left-handers were most at risk for language impairment. Darwish and Pearce (1983) reported three children with agenesis of the corpus callosum and the semantic-pragmatic syndrome.

The neuroanatomic basis of this disorder is unknown. Repetition strength in the setting of fluent speech with impaired comprehension characterizes the adult aphasia syndrome of transcortical sensory aphasia (Rapin and Allen, 1988; Rubens and Kertesz, 1983). Prognosis in adults with this acquired aphasia is generally good. Pathology in the reported cases of this relatively rare syndrome is found in the left temporo-occipital area. The primary perisylvian language region is spared. Interestingly, fluent echolalic aphasia is often seen in Alzheimer's disease, the pathology there being nonspecific diffuse atrophy. Some form of disconnection may be implied by the fact that hydrocephalics have thin corpus callosums and by the cases with agenesis of the corpus callosum. The bulk of the pathology in hydrocephalus is in the subcortical white matter, presumably sparing the classic perisylvian language region. Difficulties with prosody and pragmatics suggest right hemisphere dysfunction as well as left (Nass and Gazzaniga, 1987).

Lexical-Syntactic Syndrome

Although the lexical-syntactic syndrome has not yet received much attention as an entity, it was noted in 14% of 104 preschool subjects (Wilson and Risucci, 1986). Speech is generally dysfluent, even to the point of stuttering, because of word-finding difficulties and poor syntactic skills, with many hesitancies and false starts. Paraphasias of both the literal and semantic variety are common. Phonology, however, is spared and repetition generally exceeds spontaneous speech skills. Pragmatics may or may not be impaired, and, if it is, only to a relatively minor degree. When this syndrome is seen in autistic children, pragmatics tends to be more impaired. Comprehension is generally acceptable, although complex questions and other forms taxing higher-level syntactic skills are generally impaired (Rapin and Allen, 1983).

Lexical and syntactic deficits (see Phonologic-Syntactic Syndrome) have been frequently studied in isolation in children with DLDs. Lexical development has been well studied in the normal child. Two types of speakers have been identified during the single-word stage, and this dichotomy appears to persist throughout and probably precede the single-word stage: referential and expressive (Bates and Marchman, 1988). The former speakers tend to emphasize nouns in their early vocabulary, while the latter emphasize action words and social "phrases." Interestingly, normal referential speakers tend to acquire language faster than expressive speakers, although there is no evidence to suggest that their language skills are ultimately better. When the semantic capabilities of children falling within the general rubric of DLD are compared to mean length of utterance–matched younger normals, both similarities and differences have been noted. For example, both language styles are noted at the 50-word vocabulary level (Weiss et al., 1983). Inappropriate extensions (e.g., ball for moon) are seen in both groups (Chapman et al., 1983). Single-word conversational replies were even more varied than in the younger normal controls (Leonard, 1986).

Rapin and Allen (1988) do not consider that there is an exact counterpart for this syndrome among the adult acquired aphasias. While the lexical impairment is clearly analogous to that in anomic aphasia, the fluent nature of the latter disorder differentiates it from the lexical syntactic syndrome. The resemblance to conduction aphasia is mitigated by the absence of the poor repetition cardinal to that syndrome.

Phonologic-Syntactic Syndrome

Called by a variety of different names, the phonologic-syntactic syndrome is probably the most common DLD (Aram and Nation, 1982; Wilson and Risucci, 1986; Ingram, 1975; Wolfus et al., 1980). The phonologic disturbances consist of omissions, substitutions, and distortions of consonants and consonant clusters in all word positions. Thus, the phonologic output problem differs from purely developmental articulation difficulties, which, as discussed previously, affect specific consonants and occur primarily at the ends of words. The sounds these children produce are unpredictable as well as unrecognizable, often making the child impossible to understand. Syntactic impairment is generally evidenced by the lack of small grammatical words (e.g., *and, but*) and the absence of appropriate inflected endings (e.g., *-ed, -ing*). Again, the deficit is not just a developmental lag. While the normal young child may say "baby cry" or "a baby crying," these children will say "the baby is cry." The presence or absence of difficulties in other language areas is variable. Overall, comprehension clearly exceeds expressive abilities, although it is not wholly spared. Semantic skills tend generally to be intact. Repetition may or may not be affected in this disorder. The same is true for pragmatics and for prosody (Rapin and Allen, 1983).

Neurologic dysfunction is common in this language subtype, particularly oromotor difficulties. Some children have abnormalities on the motor exam, including increased tone and difficulties with dexterity. There is historical evidence of buccal-lingual difficulties. Feeding problems involving sucking, swallowing, and chewing are common, and drooling is often persistent. The exam may reveal signs of pseudobulbar palsy like a hyperactive jaw jerk. Oromotor apraxia is often evidenced by difficulties with movement of the tongue (clicking, side-to-side, elevating), lip (pursing), and jaw (side-to-side sequences). Although children with this syndrome without oromotor difficulties tend to have more intelligible speech, the fact that the syndrome can occur with or without neurologic buccal-lingual impairment implicates a central phonologic programming problem as a part of the syndrome (Rapin and Allen, 1983).

The question of whether syntactic skills in the child with DLDs are delayed or deviant has been much debated. Menyuk (1964) was among the first to investigate this question by comparing the grammar of 10 children with "infantile speech" to that of 10 children with normal speech aged 2 to 3 years. Those children with immature speech formulated their sentences using the most general grammatical rules, whereas those children with normal speech used increasingly differentiated rules for different structures. Moorehead and Ingram (1973)—comparing 15 language-impaired children with 15 normals matched for same stage of early grammatical acquisition—found differences in usage of less general aspects of syntax. Overall, they concluded that the children with DLDs used language less creatively. Steckol and Leonard (1979) reported that language-impaired children displayed less grammatical morpheme usage than their mean length of utterance–matched controls. However, they found no use of alternative features that had semantic import, suggesting to them that no unique patterns of acquiring language were in operation. Leonard (1979) argues in general that it is frequency of usage rather than actual deviance that distinguishes normal from developmentally language-impaired children. This controversy has yet to be resolved.

Although there is not a total overlap, this developmental syndrome most resembles Broca's aphasia. Broca's aphasia is usually associated with large lesions involving the third frontal gyrus, frontal operculum, insula, and areas of cortex superior and inferior to these regions (Mohr, 1976). Levine and Sweet (1983) suggest that the precentral gyrus is the critical area for producing Broca's aphasia. On the other hand, Mohr argues that no particular area within the above-described complex is critical; rather it is necessary that more than one region be damaged to produce a lasting deficit. As in those with Broca's aphasia, comprehension is spared overall, but the system most affected at the output level—syntax—is also affected at the receptive level when careful assessment is performed (Nass and Gazzaniga, 1987). The syndrome also resembles (although it is present there in a milder form) the language impairment in children with congenital left hemisphere damage and early hemispherectomy (Dennis and Whitaker, 1976), as well as children with "recovered" acquired aphasia of childhood (Woods and Carey, 1979). The crucial similarity may be that the left hemisphere is innately specialized to mediate syntactic function, and this function is never adequently taken over by the right hemisphere (see Nass and Gazzaniga, 1987; Witelson, 1985, for review). Lou and associates (1984) demonstrated bilateral anterior and posterior perisylvian hypoperfusion in a patient with this syndrome.

Follow-Up of Preschool Language Disorders

Despite the fact that follow-up studies of the preschooler with language disorders do not divide them into the above-delineated categories, retrospective and even some prospective data are available about the disorders as a

FEATURE TABLE 21-1. DEVELOPMENTAL LANGUAGE DISORDERS

Discriminating Feature	Consistent Feature	Variable Features
1. Language deficit	1. Problems with comprehension or production	1. Mental retardation 2. Social problems 3. Pragmatics difficulty

whole. A language disorder in the preschool years is bound to affect later educational achievement, vocational status, and social adjustment. Preschool language skills are the best single predictor of latter reading ability and disability.

Retrospective studies addressing outcome demonstrate the long-term impact of early language problems. Griffiths (1969), studying 49 graduates of the Horniman School in England, demonstrated a link between the initial language impairment and eventual language, academic achievement, and social-emotional status. In 58 children who had presented at a hospital with delayed speech, Garvey and Gordon (1973) also found that later language, academic achievement, and behavior were affected. Hall and Tomblin (1978) found that adults with an initial language problem fared less well academically than those with an initial articulation problem. Aram and Nation (1980), reporting the 5-year follow-up of children presenting as preschoolers with language difficulties, found that 40% still manifested language or articulatory disorders, as well as reading and spelling difficulties. King and colleagues (1982) found that almost half of 50 adolescents and young adults with preschool problems still had communication difficulties or had required tutoring in academic subjects.

Weiner (1974) followed a single child for a 12-year period and also (1972) reassessed seven children 2 years after presentation with the same battery originally used. In both instances the language difficulties persisted. Wolpaw and associates (1976) reassessed 30 school-age children who had been assessed 5 years previously as preschoolers in a group of 47 by Aram and Nation (1975). Two thirds were having academic difficulties. For some the language profiles were relatively constant in terms of strengths and weaknesses, while for others, although language remained a problem, the deficit pattern had shifted. Ten-year follow-up of 20 of the original 47 children (Aram et al., 1984) revealed that 15 were receiving special education, 4 in classrooms for the educably mentally retarded. The majority evidenced persistent language problems and were rated by their parents as having socioemotional problems as compared to their peers. Nonverbal intelligence as measured by the Leiter Performance Scale was the best single predictor of outcome. The Northwestern Syntax Test, expressive scale, was the best predictor of adolescent language skills. Stark and colleagues (1984) found that 80% of 29 children with developmental language disorders at 4 to 8 years still had deficits at 8 to 12 years. Most were dyslexic. In the National Collaborative Perinatal Project children with receptive and expressive language problems at age 3 years were at significantly increased risk for one of the study-defined minimal brain dysfunction syndromes—hyperkinesis, soft signs, or learning disabilities—at age 7 years (Nichols and Chen, 1981). Thus it appears that residual language and academic difficulties are the rule in DLDs.

Whether intensive early therapy ameliorates this situation to any degree has yet to be determined.

Emotional ramifications have also been reported. For example, Cantwell and Baker (1987), comparing children from ages 5 to 8 years with speech versus language disorders, found that the latter had a higher rate of psychiatric diagnoses. Of 600 children (mean age 5.7 years) selected from a community speech clinic, 50% were found to have diagnosable psychiatric disorders according to DSM-III criteria. The children carrying psychiatric diagnoses had more neurologic abnormalities on exam. The biggest differentiating factor between those with and without a psychiatric diagnosis was the degree of language deficit. Conversely, the prevalence rate of speech and language disorders was found to be 65% among 116 children referred for psychiatric services at an average age of 5 years. Thus, children presenting with speech and language difficulties are at risk for psychiatric disturbance and should be screened and followed.

Workup

The workup of the child with a DLD must include an assessment of hearing and an assessment for level of cognitive functioning. If there is any suggestion of seizures or if the deficit pattern is of the verbal auditory agnosia type, an EEG should be obtained. By and large neuroimaging is not a necessary part of management to the extent that it does not alter therapy unless focal abnormalities are suspected by history (e.g., a nonfamilial early-declaring left-hander) or on exam (see Chapter 3).

Treatment

Treatment of language-disordered preschool children varies according to the kind of language impairment as well as its degree of severity. Children with a moderate to severe language impairment who suffer associated social, cognitive, and behavioral difficulties are best treated in a therapeutic nursery environment. Mildly impaired children who can participate in formal language remediation tasks often can do well in a regular nursery program when they are also given individual speech-language therapy. Play materials are used by the speech-language therapist with the preschool child in a directive way (Green, 1976). Every activity becomes a language activity in that the child's actions are given words by the therapist. Play activities are also helpful to engage children with severe expressive difficulties. Pleasurable activities involving the mouth, such as blowing bubbles or initiating mouth movements and sounds, as well as nonvocal imitative games, such as hand clapping, have been found to foster language initiations (Allen et al., 1989). Formal language work typically begins at the phonologic level, involving repetition of sounds and sound sequences to encourage fluency. Treatment of receptive disorders often necessitates the use of visual modalities such as signs

Pearls and Perils: Developmental Language Disorders

1. If in any doubt, assess hearing. Missing a hearing loss is missing a potentially treatable cause of DLD.
2. In spite of individual variability, failure to develop normal expressive language skills by age 3 is pathologic.
3. An EEG is a useful screening procedure in the DLDs, as treatment of an underlying paroxysmal disorder may improve language function.
4. Failure to develop intelligible speech by age 6 is a poor prognostic sign in verbal apraxia.
5. DLDs often diminish, but the basic deficit affects language-related academic skills, particularly reading. Suggesting to the parents that they are merely an immaturity is generally inaccurate.
6. Regression of articulation skills during stress and excitement is common during preschool years. The articulation in the office may be less adept than is actually the case.
7. Beware of the child whose conversation is fluent but lacking in content. His parents may be the most resistant to accepting the diagnosis of a DLD.
8. The child with developmental language problems is at risk for emotional difficulties and should be monitored for possible intervention.
9. The child who appears to "talk to talk" rather than to communicate and whose head is large ought to be assessed for hydrocephalus, in view of the frequency of the cocktail party syndrome in this disorder.
10. Later reading problems are common in the child with a DLD. Expectant assessment should be performed if there is any hint of reading readiness difficulties.

and gestures. Less severe disorders of comprehension are addressed through practiced structuring of conversations with the child. Developmentally language-disordered children with receptive problems rarely progress in treatment as well as children with primary expressive disorders.

ANNOTATED BIBLIOGRAPHY

Aram D, Nation J: *Child Language Disorders.* St. Louis, CV Mosby, 1982.

Rapin I, Allen D: Developmental language disorders: Nosologic considerations, in Kirk U (ed): *Neuropsychology of Language, Reading and Spelling.* New York, Academic Press, 1983.

Rapin I, Allen D: Syndromes of developmental dysphasia and adult aphasia, in Plum F (ed): *Language, Communication and Brain.* New York, Raven Press, 1988.

These are good reviews of the general definition and nosology of the DLDs. The last relates the developmental syndromes to the acquired aphasias.

Lassman FM, Fisch RO, Vetter DK, LaBenz ES: *Early Correlates of Speech, Language and Hearing.* Littleton, Mass, PSG Publishing, 1980.

Nicholas P, Chen T: *Minimal Brain Dysfunction.* Hillsdale, NJ, Lawrence Erlbaum, 1981.

These volumes provide the data on language development and outcome from the National Collaborative Perinatal Project.

Rapin I, Mattis S, Rowan A, Golden G: Verbal auditory agnosia. *Dev Med Child Neurol* 19:192–207, 1977.

Cole AJ, Anderman F, Taylor A, et al: The Landau-Kleffner syndrome of acquired epileptic aphasia: Unusual clinical outcome, surgical experience and absence of encephalitis. *Neurology* 38:31–38, 1988.

These are key references on verbal auditory agnosia.

Morley ME: *The Development and Disorders of Speech in Childhood,* 2nd ed. Baltimore, Md, Williams & Wilkins, 1965.

Ferry P, Hall S, Hicks J: Dilapidated speech: Developmental verbal apraxia. *Dev Med Child Neurol* 17:749–756, 1975.

These are classic works on verbal apraxia.

Curtiss S: Special grammatical abilities, in Obler L, Fein D (eds): *Neuropsychology of Special Abilities.* New York, Guilford Press, 1988.

Swisher LP, Pinsker E: The language characteristics of hyperverbal hydrocephalic children. *Dev Med Child Neurol* 13:746–755, 1971.

These papers—together with Rapin and Allen (1983), mentioned earlier—review the semantic pragmatic syndrome.

Wilson B, Risucci D: A model for clinical quantitative classification. *Brain and Language* 27:281–309, 1986.

This nosologic study of the DLDs provides a specific discussion of the lexical syntactic syndrome.

Leonard L: What is deviant language? *J Speech Hear Disord* 37:427–446, 1979.

This is a good theoretic review of the syntactic deficits in the developmental language disorders.

Wolfus B, Moscovitch M, Kinsbourne M: Subgroups of developmental language disorders. *Brain and Language* 9:152–171, 1980.

The phonologic syntactic syndrome is discussed under different names in this reference, Wilson and Risucci (1986), and Aram and Nation (1982).

AUTISTIC SPECTRUM DISORDERS

General Discussion

In 1943 Kanner reported a series of patients with varyingly severe developmental impairments of social skills, verbal and nonverbal communication skills, and play skills. The DSM-III-R currently categorizes autistic disorder under the more general rubric of pervasive developmental disorders (Table 21-2). The Child Neurology Society Higher Cortical Function Nosology Task Force separates autistic spectrum disorder from developmen-

TABLE 21-2. DIAGNOSTIC CRITERIA FOR AUTISTIC DISORDER

A. Impairment in reciprocal social interaction
   1. Unaware of others' feeling or existence
   2. Failure to seek comfort in distress
   3. Impaired imitation
   4. Abnormal social play
   5. Inability to make peer friendships
B. Impairment in verbal and nonverbal communication
   1. No mode of communication
   2. Abnormal nonverbal communication like eye-to-eye gaze
   3. Absent imaginative play
   4. Abnormal speech prosody
   5. Abnormal speech content
   6. Inability to maintain a conversation
C. Restricted activities and interests
   1. Stereotyped body movements
   2. Preoccupation with object parts or attachment to unusual objects
   3. Distress over trivial changes
   4. Excess insistence on routines
   5. Restricted range of interests

Modified from DSM-III-R.

tal language disorders and nonautistic mental deficiency based on IQ and sociability criteria (see Figure 21–1).

Signs and Symptoms

A number of subtypes within the more general ASDs have been proposed in order to streamline a heterogeneous population, to define differing etiologies leading to autistic behaviors, and to clarify prognosis on a more individual basis.

Asperger's syndrome (Asperger, 1944) is the only ASD that has achieved an eponym. The patients tend to be higher functioning (Wing, 1981). Hence, concern as to the child's social interactions and communicative and play behaviors may not become apparent until after age 30 months (the outside time of presentation for the DSM-III-R criteria to be met). The criteria elaborated by Wing (1981) to define this syndrome include pedantic, aprosodic, bizarre speech; clumsy and uncoordinated nonverbal communication; withdrawn or clumsy interpersonal relatedness; defect in empathy for others; repetitive activity; resistance to change in the environment; stereotyped bodily movements; adequate to excellent rote memory; and circumscribed interest patterns.

Other subtyping systems have considered the three potentially defining aspects of ASDs: deficits of cognitive function, sociability, and language.

Cognition

By definition children with ASDs may function in the inferior, average, or superior range of intellectual ability. Fein and colleagues (1985) defined, based on neuropsychologic test results for 54 children with pervasive developmental disorder ranging in age from 5 to 17 years,

four main cognitive skill profiles. There were no age, IQ, or sex differences among the subgroups, suggesting that the subgroups did not just reflect level of intellectual functioning or extent of maturation. The subgroups did differ in patterns of verbal, perceptual, quantitative, and memory strengths and weaknesses: (I) visuospatial strength and variable receptive language skills, (II) verbal strength, (III) quantitative and verbal strength, and (IV) even profile. Motor skills and degree of manual asymmetry also differentiated the subgroups. The patterns suggested differential hemispheric involvement, i.e., right and left hemisphere–deficient subgroups. Behavioral and attentional deficit patterns were not related to cognitive subgroups, suggesting that behavioral or psychiatric features may occur independently of cognitive deficit patterns, that is, may be differently localized.

Sociability

Based on a social interaction scale and a checklist (Table 21–3), Wing (Wing and Gould, 1979; Wing and Attwood, 1987) has differentiated three different social deficits: aloof, passive, and interactive but odd. The *aloof* group is most similar to the popular notion of autism. The signs of abnormal attachment are already apparent in the first years. These children do not follow their parents around, run to greet them, or seek comfort when in pain. This subgroup tends to be rather low functioning in terms of verbal skills and nonverbal communication, and evidences very little symbolic play. The *passive* group is

TABLE 21-3. WING'S SOCIAL INTERACTION SCALE

0 Does not interact—aloof and indifferent.

1 Interacts to satisfy needs, otherwise indifferent.

2 Responds to (and may initiate) *physical* contact only, including rough-and-tumble games, chasing, and cuddling.

3 Generally does not initiate but responds to *social* (not just physical) contact, if others, including peers, make approaches. Joins in passively, e.g., as baby in game of mothers and fathers. Tries to copy, but with little understanding. Shows some pleasure in passive role (unlike Groups 0, 1, and 2, who move away once physical needs are satisfied).

4 Makes social approaches actively, but these are usually inappropriate, naive, peculiar, or bizarre—"one sided." The behavior is not modified according to the person being approached.

5 Shy, but makes social contacts appropriate for mental age with familiar people, including peers. (Also used for children who refuse to talk to adults, but interact with other children.)

6 Makes social contacts appropriate for *mental* age with children and adults. Looks up with interest and smiles when approached. Responds to the ideas and interests of people of similar mental age and contributes to the interactions. (Nonmobile people without speech can show social interest by means of eye contact and eye pointing.)

Reproduced from Wing and Attwood (1987), with permission.

somewhat higher functioning. Their speech may fit that in the semantic-pragmatic syndrome as delineated previously. Children in this group do not make social approaches, but they accept such approaches when made by others. They will join in games although they take a passive role, for example, as the baby in the game of "mothers and fathers." The *interactive but odd* group will make spontaneous social approaches to others, but they do so in a peculiar, naive, and one-sided fashion. They tend to talk *at* other people. Their approach may be so persistent as to become unwelcome. Their language lacks pragmatic constraints. For example, questions are used as conversational openers without the preceding social graces. They are capable of pretend symbolic play, but it is extremely repetitive. Asperger's syndrome patients fall into this subgroup.

Allen's (1988) subtyping system delineates autism as a spectrum disorder that has different sociability deficits as the universal classifying variable and different language and play deficits (Table 21–4) as additional subtyping variables (Figure 21–4). The language subtypes for this classification system are based on those developed by Rapin and Allen (1983, 1988) to delineate developmental language disorders: verbal auditory agnosia, semantic-pragmatic deficit syndrome, lexical-syntactic deficit syndrome, and phonologic-syntactic deficit syndrome. Four social deficit patterns are defined. *Socially unavailable* describes the most severely impaired children, who are unavailable for interpersonal contact with adults or other children. These children may appear to be oblivious to their surroundings and just wander about. When in need or in distress, they do not usually seek human contact, but rather cry or scream inconsolably. The *socially remote* category includes children who tend to engage only in solitary activity. The child may become interested in the activities of another person, but not in the person himself. If someone attempts to intrude into their solitary state, these children may respond by ignoring, moving away, or vocally protesting. Some of the children engage in simple physical activities, such as tickling or chasing, when directed by an adult. The higher-functioning children in this group may permit an adult to join them in limited areas of special interest. The *inappropriately interactive* category includes children who are easier to engage. Nonetheless, they have difficulty initiating or maintaining social interactions. Their efforts at socialization are usually inadequate, immature, or bizarre. The *pseudosocial* category includes the most verbal of the autistic spectrum children. These children are engageable, though their attempts at social interaction are immature, inadequate, or bizarre. They are mechanical, stilted, and pedantic. They may be obsessed with or preoccupied by particular topics. They do not engage with other children. Because these children are so verbal, they may appear to have more social skills than they actually have.

The importance of the sociability deficit in the overall definition of autism subtypes and in determining

TABLE 21-4. ALLEN'S PLAY RATING SCALE

Level 1 No appropriate or functional use of toys or play materials. No symbolic play. Activities restricted to repetitive stereotypic pursuits, and indiscriminate sensory use of objects (e.g., mouthing, rubbing) even when directed by an adult.

Level 2 Objects used functionally (drinks from cup), but toy play consists primarily of repetitive stereotypic pursuits (e.g., opening and closing doors) except when directed by an adult. Some capacity to imitate action-naming (brushing a doll's hair) with adult support. Beyond this, there is no symbolic play.

Level 3 Objects used functionally but range of toys is limited. Prefer cognitive activities (e.g., puzzles) but when left to their own devices, tend to use even these activities perseveratively. Activities are primarily repetitive and stereotypic, unless directed by an adult. May learn to engage in simple symbolic play (e.g., doll house scene).

Level 4 Objects used functionally and a variety of toys used appropriately. These children enjoy running, catching, and tickling games, with adults or children. Activities are partly rigid or repetitive and partly constructive, even without adult support. With adult structuring, able to use dolls and people, make puppets talk, and engage in brief sequences of symbolic play (e.g., the boy doll won't eat, mommy doll gets mad, knocks the boy doll down).

Level 5 Objects used functionally. May be extraordinarily competent and knowledgeable in activities involving their circumscribed areas of interest (e.g., board games, computers, electronic games, or high-level word and number tasks). May engage in these intellectual activities with pleasure and may even appear to use them as a form of play. Activities are partly rigid or repetitive and partly constructive, even without adult support. Use dolls as people, make puppets talk, use an object as if it were a different object (e.g., block as phone receiver), act out simple sequences, and, with adult help, engage in simple role-taking games.

Reproduced from Allen (1988), with permission.

its etiology is attested to by the power of these later subtyping schema. Indeed, Fein and associates (1986) have argued that the social deficit is primary because of

(1) the dissociability of social and cognitive impairments both within and across developmentally disabled populations, (2) the special difficulty autistic children may have with social or affective stimuli, and (3) the rarity of social isolation even in severely neurologically damaged children, and its resistance to modification in autistic children. In addition, other specific cognitive deficits suggested to be central to autism (4) can be found in at least as severe a form in sociable retarded children, (5) are theoretically inadequate to explain autistic aloofness, (6) cannot be found in all autistic children, and (7) may be the very cognitive abilities which rest most heavily on social functioning.

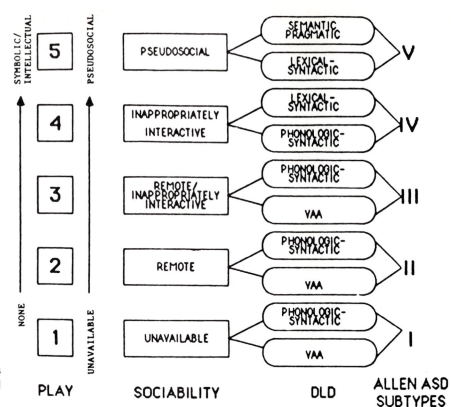

Figure 21-4. Possible relations among play skills, social skills, and language skills.

Language

Abnormal language is clearly a hallmark of autism. The eventual outcome of the disorder as a whole can often be predicted solely on the basis of language skill development. Language by 5 years is the best predictor of overall outcome (DeMyer et al., 1974). Several of the specific DLDs are discernible in preschool autistic children: verbal auditory agnosia, semantic-pragmatic deficit syndrome, lexical-syntactic deficit syndrome, and phonologic-syntactic deficit syndrome; see (Table 21-1).

Because of the prominence of the language deficits in autism, left hemisphere dysfunction has been suggested as the underlying neurologic cause. A number of neuropsychologic and electrophysiologic studies have documented a higher than normal incidence of right hemisphere specialization for language processing (Dawson et al., 1982, 1983, 1986; Prior and Bradshaw, 1979), presumably indicating left hemisphere dysfunction. Left-handers and ambidexters are found in increased numbers among autistics (Hauser et al., 1975; Golden, 1987; Soper et al., 1986).

Even if the language and gesture deficits were ac-

cepted as the critical feature in autism, Fein and colleagues (1984) argue against a left hemisphere dysfunction interpretation, in the main because aspects of language behavior like prosody and pragmatics, which are considered right hemisphere dominated (Nass and Gazzaniga, 1987), are also strikingly abnormal in the autistic child. Furthermore, although some excel on visuospatial tasks (Dawson et al., 1983), by no means all autistic children evidence spared perceptual abilities, indicative of right hemisphere intactness.

Diagnosis and Workup

The demonstration of the neurologic basis of autism has been approached from several different clinical vantages. Although a wide range of neurologic disorders have been reported to manifest an autistic phenotype (Table 21-5), none provides specific information about etiology. The decision to screen for any of these disorders depends on the complete clinical picture. The frequency of fragile X syndrome among autistic males is 7.7% and the frequency of autism among fragile X males is estimated at 12.3%

FEATURE TABLE 21-2. AUTISTIC SPECTRUM DISORDERS

Discriminating Features	Consistent Features	Variable Feature
1. Sociability deficit	1. Play impairment	1. Mental retardation
2. Language deficit	2. Stereotyped behavior	

TABLE 21-5. NEUROLOGIC CAUSES OF AUTISM

Prenatal	Metabolic
Midtrimester bleeding	Phenylketonuria
Toxemia	Histidinemia
Rubella	Lipidosis
Toxoplasmosis	Addison's disease
Lues	Hyperuricosuria
Cytomegalovirus	Hurler's syndrome
Perinatal	Hyperthyroidism
Anoxia	Celiac disease
Trauma	Adrenoleukodystrophy
Hyperbilirubinemia	Lead ingestion
Respiratory distress syndrome	Chromosomal
Hypoglycemia	Trisomy 21
Congenital	XYY syndrome
Microcephaly	XXX syndrome
Möbius's syndrome	Fragile X syndrome
Tuberous sclerosis	Acquired
Hydrocephalus	Infantile spasms
Dandy-Walker syndrome	Vascular occlusion
Cornelia de Lange syndrome	Meningitis
Oculocutaneous albinism	Herpes encephalitis
	Encephalitis

Reproduced from Golden (1987), with permission.

(Opitz, 1986). Screening of any autistic male (or, for that matter, female; Opitz, 1986) is warranted in view of the genetic implications for other family members and the possibility of prenatal diagnosis. A long, thin face and prominent ears are characteristic. Macroorchidism may not be present until after puberty.

Seizure frequency ranges from 11% (Jacobson and Janick, 1983) to 23% (Deykin et al., 1979) to 42% (Schain and Yannet, 1960). The first year of life and adolescence are common onset times (Rutter et al., 1971). All seizure types have been reported. Although there appears to be no clear predilection for temporal lobe epilepsy, which would be of theoretical interest, partial complex seizures may be more frequent than previously estimated. Furthermore, treatment of these seizures may have a positive effect on function (Nass and Petrucha, 1990; Payton and Minshew, 1987). An EEG should be obtained if there is any indication of seizures.

The neuroanatomic basis of autism is not known. Damasio and colleagues (Vilensky et al., 1981; A. R. Damasio and Maurer, 1978), extrapolating from the phenomenology of autism to adult neuropathology, suggest that the disorder results from dysfunction in a system of bilateral neural structures that includes the ring of the mesolimbic cortex located in the mesial frontal and temporal lobes, the neostriatum, and the anterior and medial nuclear groups of the thalamus. These structures are singled out as the target region of the dopaminergic mesencephalic neurons, autism presumably being the result of a neuromediator imbalance. Kinesiologic analyses revealing similarities in gait between autistic patients and those with Parkinson's disease support the view that basal

ganglia dysfunction is present in autism. The heterogeneity of the disorder is accounted for by differing degrees of involvement of the different structures in different patients. Dysfunction of the brainstem has been suggested by a number of studies documenting abnormal brainstem evoked responses, as well as by studies documenting abnormal vestibular responsiveness (Ornitz, 1987).

Although routine neuroimaging is not generally informative, research neuroimaging studies have provided some information about the basis of autism. Hauser and associates (1975) first reported dilatation of the left temporal horn based on pneumoencephalograms in 15 of 18 patients with at least some autistic features. Although the majority of patients who have been imaged by computed tomography (CT) and MRI have normal studies, focal or diffuse brain damage is reported. H. Damasio and colleagues (1980) and Rosenbloom and associates (1984) reported ventricular dilatation in a small proportion of their patients. In the 45-patient series of M. Campbell and associates (1987) and in Gillberg and Svendsen's (1983) series of 27 patients, about 25% had increased ventricular size. Evaluating 10 relatively high-functioning autistics using ^{1}H MRI, Minshew and colleagues (1986) found ventricular dilatation and atrophy only in the autistics functioning in the 70 to 85 IQ range and not in those functioning above 85. Cerebral asymmetries have also been assessed in the autistic patient. Hier and associates (1979) found a reversed parietal occipital asymmetry pattern in 57% of 116 autistic patients (in contrast to the approximately 20% with this pattern that would be anticipated among normal right-handers). This study can be criticized, however, for not controlling for sex and handedness. Others have not confirmed the high frequency of reversed asymmetry (Tsai and Stewart, 1982; Prior et al., 1984; H. Damasio et al., 1980).

Although previous studies (Williams et al., 1981; Creak, 1963; Darby, 1976; Purpura, 1979) found no relevant gross abnormalities at biopsy or postmortem of 10 patients with autism, Bauman and Kemper (1985, 1986) recently reported important cytoarchitectonic abnormalities: reduced neuronal size and increased cell packing density in hippocampal complex and amygdala. Bilateral and symmetric loss of Purkinje and granular neurons was seen in the neocerebellum and confirmed by Ritvo and colleagues (1986) in four more autistics. Both CT and MRI studies showing proportionately smaller cerebella with relatively large fourth ventricles corroborate these pathologic findings (Bauman et al., 1985; Gaffney et al., 1987; Courchesne et al., 1987).

Metabolic studies using the xenon inhalation technique revealed overall depressed regional cerebral blood flow and an abnormal resting landscape with the usual hyperfrontal flow apparent only on the left (Sherman et al., 1984). PET resting state studies of 10 high-functioning autistics using 2-deoxyglucose revealed hypermetabolism, 13% to 21% greater than that of controls, throughout the brain (Duara et al., 1984). Horwitz and associates

---

Pearls and Perils: Autistic Spectrum Disorders

1. Social deficits, rather than language deficits, may be key to defining the autistic spectrum disorders.
2. If there is no language by age 5 to 6 years, language development is unlikely and the probable outcome is poor.
3. Some children with autism may have subtle seizures and may benefit from anticonvulsants. If in any doubt, obtain an EEG.
4. Fragile X syndrome is the most common known cause of autism. Obtain chromosomes to make a prenatal diagnosis on future siblings.
5. Look for signs of parkinsonism in autistic children as a reflection of dopaminergic dysfunction.
6. The child with autism mistakenly thought to have ADD will get worse on stimulants.

(1988) reported functionally impaired interactions between frontal/parietal regions and neostriatum and thalamus, regions that subserve directed attention, in 14 adult autistic males.

Treatment

Behavioral response and the lack thereof to pharmacologic manipulation of dopaminergic and serotoninergic neurotransmitter systems have been used as arguments as to the possible neurochemic basis of autism. Lithium, tricyclic antidepressants, LSD, L-dopa, and amphetamines have all been tried with little success. The poor response to amphetamine, which actually led to worsened psychosis and stereotypies, is of clinical import, because on occasion in short-term assessment the high-functioning autistic child may appear hyperactive. Stimulants would not, however, be the treatment of choice. By contrast, dopamine blockers—particularly haldol and prolixin and less so chlorpromazine and thioridizine—appear to decrease behavioral symptoms and increase learning. These studies thus suggest that decreasing dopaminergic activity improves function in autism, a finding in direct contrast to the hypodopaminergic hypothesis put forward by A. R. Damasio and Maurer (1978). Overall the combination of behavioral modification with medical therapy produces the best results (M. Campbell et al., 1987).

In 1982, Geller and colleagues using a 2-week placebo/drug/placebo design, reported that fenflurazine, an agent that depletes central nervous system serotonin, improved the social responsiveness and IQ of three autistic males. Coincident with and continuing for several weeks after the withdrawal of the drug was a decrease

in blood serotonin level. Fenflurazine trials have now been reported in more than 100 autistic patients, with mixed success. With a sample size of 81 and using a placebo/drug/placebo design, Ritvo and associates (1986) reported that in about 25% of patients unequivocal improvement occurred, and in about 50% equivocal improvement occurred, with resultant decreased hyperactivity and stereotypies, and improved social awareness and communication. Autistic patients with higher initial IQs and lower baseline serotonin levels showed the most improvement. With a dose of 1.5 mg/kg per day, blood serotonin levels fell about 50%, regardless of initial level. By contrast, M. Campbell and colleagues (1987) reported the best success with lower-IQ subjects. August and associates (1984) reported no relationshp between response and baseline serotonin level. Thus, fenflurazine shows some promise, but one must be cautious about overestimating its efficacy.

ANNOTATED BIBLIOGRAPHY

Kanner L: Autistic disturbances of affective contact. *Nerv Child* 2:217–250, 1943.
Cohen DA, Donnellan AM, Paul R (eds): *Handbook of Autism and Pervasive Developmental Disorders.* New York, John Wiley & Sons, 1987.
  The first citation is the classic reference and the second a general review.
Fein D, Humes M, Kaplan E, Lucci D, Waterhouse L: The question of left hemisphere dysfunction in autism. *Psychol Bull* 95:258–281, 1984.
Fein D, Pennington B, Markowitz P, Braverman M, Waterhouse L: Toward a neuropsychological model of infantile autism: Are the social deficits primary? *J Am Acad Child Psychiatr* 25:198–212, 1986.
  These are excellent reviews of the neuropsychologic basis of autism.
Bauman M, Kemper TL: Histoanatomic observations of the brain in early infantile autism. *Neurology* 35:866–874, 1985.
  This is the currently definitive neuropathologic study.
Campbell M, Anderson LT, Greene WH, Deutch SI: Psychopharmacology, in Cohen DJ, Donnellan AM, Paul R (eds): *Handbook of Autism and Pervasive Developmental Disorders.* New York, John Wiley & Sons, 1987.
  This is a good review of the treatment of autism.
Gaffney GR, Tsai LY, Kuperman S, Minchin S: Cerebellar structure in autism. *Am J Dis Child* 141:1330–1332, 1987.
  This is a review of neuroimaging in autism.
Golden G: Neurologic basis of autism, in Cohen DJ, Donnellan AM, Paul R (eds): *Handbook of Autism and Pervasive Developmental Disorders.* New York, John Wiley & Sons, 1987.
  This chapter specifically addresses the neurologic abnormalities documented in autism.
Opitz JM: *X-Linked Mental Retardation 2.* New York, Alan R. Liss, 1986.
  This is a review of the fragile X syndrome.

VISUOMOTOR AND SPATIAL DYSFUNCTION

General Discussion

Although the literature on visuomotor and spatial disabilities in the school-age child is extensive (see Chapter 22), little information is available about the preschooler. However, the importance of visuomotor skills to academic achievement is attested to by the predictive power of visuomotor tasks like the Bender Gestalt Test (Koppitz, 1963). Administered in kindergarten, it predicted academic achievement in reading and math through the sixth grade. Nichols and Chen (1981), analyzing the data from the National Collaborative Perinatal Project, documented that a low score on a block sort task (which required the child to match by color, size, and shape) at age 4 years increased the risk of two of the three minimal brain dysfunction syndromes identified in the project, hyperactivity and neurologic soft signs, at age 7 years. All three minimal brain dysfunction syndromes (learning disabilities being the third) were less frequent in high-scoring sorters. Children who could not copy a circle at age 4 years (about 5% of those studied) were at increased risk for hyperactivity and neurologic soft sign syndromes at age 7 years. Those who could not copy a cross (about 30%) were at increased risk for the learning disability and neurologic soft signs syndromes. Only about 10% of the 4-year-olds were able to copy a square (mostly girls). These children were at decreased risk for all the minimal brain dysfunction syndromes. The 25% of the cohort failing the age-appropriate Porteus maze were at increased risk for all three minimal brain dysfunction syndromes.

Right hemisphere dysfunction as the etiology of visuospatial deficits in the preschooler is suggested by the documentation of such deficits in congenitally right brain–damaged preschoolers. Stiles-Davis and associates (1985) demonstrated a manipulospatial deficit, as evidenced by difficulties in creating spatial arrays during toy play, among right brain–damaged preschoolers. Failure to represent the environment properly is evident in the drawings of children with congenital right brain injury, as contrasted to their left brain–damaged counterparts and normal controls (Figure 21–5). Such findings support the view that the right hemisphere is innately specialized to mediate spatial functions (Nass and Gazzaniga, 1987).

Treatment

Successful perceptual training programs for preschoolers identified as showing perceptual delays have been reported (Lahey, 1976; Slater, 1971; Sabatino, 1974), although long-term follow-up studies are still outstanding.

ANNOTATED BIBLIOGRAPHY

Koppitz E: *The Bender Gestalt Test for Young Children.* London, Grune & Stratton, 1963.
This book reviews the use of the Bender Gestalt Test at all ages.

ATTENTION DEFICIT HYPERACTIVITY DISORDER

General Discussion

A large literature exists on attention deficit hyperactivity disorder (ADHD) in school-age children (see Chapter 22), but relatively few studies have addressed attentional problems in children of preschool ages, despite natural history data indicating that many older children with attentional problems were described as overly active, irritable, and difficult to control from infancy and toddlerhood (S. B. Campbell, 1976; Ross and Ross, 1982). M. Levine (1987) found that behavioral problems in the toddler and preschool years were significantly more common in the school-age cohort found to have ADHD than in their matched controls. In a prospective study (Palfrey et al., 1985) of 174 children from birth to kindergarten school entry, 40% of the preschoolers were found by parents, teachers, and research examiners to have some indicator of attentional difficulty, however minor or transient. Persistent attentional problems, that is, poor concentration, behavioral disorganization, poor self-monitoring, and overactivity, were found in 5%; an addi-

Pearls and Perils: Visuomotor and Spatial Dysfunction

1. Preschoolers who are even mildly delayed in perceptual development may be quite handicapped in their school progress.
2. Early perceptual deficit is related to right hemisphere dysfunction.
3. Children who show perceptual delays are at increased risk for hyperactivity and neurologic soft sign syndromes.

FEATURE TABLE 21-3. VISUOMOTOR AND SPATIAL DYSFUNCTION

Discriminating Feature	Consistent Feature	Variable Features
1. None	1. Visuomotor and spatial perception immaturity	1. Hyperactivity 2. Neurologic soft signs

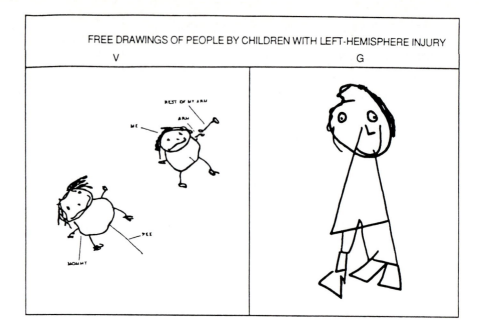

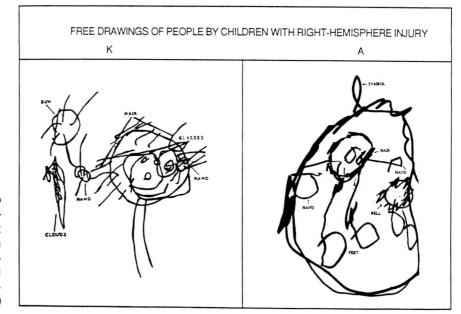

Figure 21-5. At age 5 years the two children with congenital left brain injury draw a person as a coherent whole, whereas the two children with congenital right brain damage approach the drawing in a piecemeal and inadequate fashion. *(From Stiles-Davis et al., 1985, with permission.)*

tional 8% had had significant problems, which abated before school age. Earls (1980), based on parent interviews, found hyperactivity to be a problem in 4% of 3-year-old boys and none of the girls; 8% of the boys and 4% of the girls evidenced problems with concentra-

tion. Based on teachers' reports, Kohler (1973) estimated that 2% of 4-year-old Swedish children had attentional problems.

ADHD in the preschool years largely poses management difficulties for parents and teachers. The hyperac-

FEATURE TABLE 21-4. ATTENTION DEFICIT HYPERACTIVITY DISORDER

Discriminating Feature	Consistent Features	Variable Features
1. The consistent and variable features, with no evidence of severe or profound retardation or sensory deficit	1. Difficulty with sustained attention 2. Distractibility 3. Impulsivity	1. Hyperactivity 2. Intense responsiveness to stimulation 3. Stimulus seeking

Pearls and Perils: Attention Deficit Hyperactivity Disorder

1. ADHD is a developmental disorder having its onset in infancy and toddlerhood.
2. ADHD in the preschool years poses management rather than learning difficulties.
3. The critical time to detect and intervene in ADHD is during years 3 to 4, when concerns about attention and manageability peak.
4. Complete disappearance of ADHD symptoms is rare.
5. The IQ and academic and behavioral standing of ADHD children may lag throughout childhood.

tivity component of ADHD generally tends to become less marked with age. The preschool ADHD child may show less evidence of learning delay because short bursts of attention may be sufficient for skill attainment.

Workup and Diagnosis

Consistent with the difficulty in making the diagnosis of ADHD in the preschooler, cognitive test performance on structured measures that are very useful for the older child fails to discriminate younger children with ADHD from normal children. S. B. Campbell and colleagues (1984) found no differences between groups of preschoolers (mean age 35 months) on the Matching Familiar Figures, Embedded Figures, and Draw-A-Line Slowly (Maccoby et al., 1965) tests. On the other hand, maternal ratings of behavior, using the Behar Preschool Behavior Questionnaire (Behar, 1977) and the Werry-Weiss-Peters Activity Scale (Routh et al., 1974), correlated well with free play and structured task behavioral observations to distinguish ADHD children. Rating scales appropriate for persons who have long-term contact with the child have been the most successful assessment measure used to distinguish ADHD during the early years.

ANNOTATED BIBLIOGRAPHY

Palfrey J, Levin M, Walker D, Sullivan M: The emergence of attention deficits in early childhood: A prospective study. *J Behav Dev Pediatr* 6:339–348, 1985.
Campbell SB, Breaux A, Ewing L, Szumowski E: A one year follow-up study of patient referred hyperactive preschool children. *J Am Acad Child Psychiatr* 23:243–249, 1984.
These are good general reviews.

STYLISTIC VARIATION IN TEMPERAMENT AND COGNITIVE STYLE

General Discussion

Although not formally recognized as a disorder unless found in the extreme, individual variation in temperament and cognitive style is measurable in young children and bears on their degree of success during the preschool years. Kinsbourne and Caplan (1979) suggest a continuum of temperament styles, from the impulsive style (ADHD the extreme) to the overfocused style (autism the extreme).

Signs and Symptoms

The overfocused style is characterized by prolonged deliberation and by attention in the overfocused child who is excessively persistent and slow to shift; decision making may be difficult. Overfocusers may become socially isolated and show more interest in inanimate objects than in people. This style stands in contrast to that of impulsive children, who are highly motivated for social stimulation and often intrusive in their need for social feedback. Such a continuum of attentional style can be found among the temperament categories proposed by Thomas and colleagues (1968). Carey and associates (1979) have found ADHD children aged 3 to 7 years to overlap with the difficult temperamental style, in that both share characteristics of low adaptability and negative mood. A disproportionately high number of children with the difficult temperament are referred by teachers and physicians for problems in learning and behavior. The temperament dimensions of persistence and distractibility may be useful in the early detection of impulsives and overfocusers. Nass and Koch (1987) found toddlers with right brain injury to be more difficult than their left-lesion counterparts (Figure 21–6), suggesting an organic basis for temperament differences, paralleling that found in adults with acquired pathology (Nass and Gazzaniga, 1987).

Workup and Diagnosis

Parental questionnaires, such as the Behavioral Style Questionnaire (McDevitt and Carey, 1978), are useful in discriminating temperament category in the young child.

FEATURE TABLE 21–5. STYLISTIC VARIATION IN TEMPERAMENT AND COGNITIVE STYLE

Discriminating Feature	Consistent Feature	Variable Feature
1. None	1. Inappropriate attention to stimulation	1. None

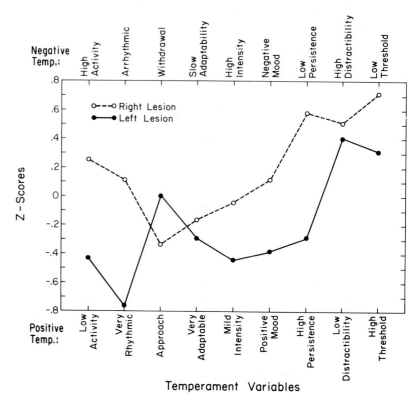

Figure 21–6. The toddler with congenital right brain injury evidences more difficult temperament characteristics than the toddler with congenital left brain damage. *(From Nass and Koch, 1987.)*

Various cognitive style dimensions have been identified (Kagan and Kogan, 1970; Santostephano, 1969). Kagan's Matching Familiar Figures Test has already been mentioned as a diagnostic tool in distinguishing ADHD children. It is also used to assess the child's position on the dimension of reflection-impulsivity. Children are relatively stable in their tendency to be either reflective (low error rate and longer response time) or impulsive (high error rate and shorter response time) (Kagan and Kogan, 1970) and performance here is predictive of other cognitive skills. Reflectives tend to do better on inductive reasoning tasks (Kagan et al., 1966) and on preschool recognition memory tests (Siegal et al., 1973).

Another well-known cognitive style dimension is field independence-dependence. The Embedded Figures Test, adapted for use with preschoolers by Coates (1972), presents a simple geometric figure followed by a complex figure within which the simple figure is embedded. The time taken to locate the figure is scored. An individual's relative positivity on the dimension appears stable (Witkin et al., 1967), but individuals also show developmental progression in their absolute performance. Differences in field independence can be detected as early as 5 years of age and are relatively stable throughout childhood even in the face of the developmental shift. Field independence has been found to correlate with analytic ability (Witkin, 1976) and drawing skills (Witkin et al., 1962) in young children. Thus, children as young as 5 years already can be reliably distinguished as showing cognitive and temperament styles that may portend sustained learning and behavioral difficulty.

Pearls and Perils: Stylistic Variation

1. Both extremes of attentional style (impulsive and overfocused) put a child at risk for learning and behavioral difficulty.
2. Cognitive style remains relatively stable throughout development.
3. The extreme of the overfocused style is the autistic child.
4. The extreme of the impulsive child is the child with ADHD.

ANNOTATED BIBLIOGRAPHY

Thomas A, Chess S, Birch HG: *Temperament and Behavior Disorders in Children.* New York, New York University Press, 1968.

This is a good introduction to the concept of temperament.
McDevitt SC, Carey WB: The measurement of temperament in 3–7 year old children. *J Child Psychol Psychiatr* 19:245–253, 1978.

This paper presents the prototype temperament questionnaire.

GLOSSARY

Functors. The small words of the language, such as prepositions and conjunctions. These are also called *closed class words* because they are limited in number.

Lexicon. The words in a language; the dictionary of word meanings.

Mean length of utterance. The number of morphemes per utterance.

Morpheme. The smallest meaningful unit in a language, occurring either in a word or as a word. A compound word like *compounding* is made up of three morphemes, *com-pounding*. Prefixes, suffixes, and inflected endings like *-ed, -s,* and *-ly* are also morphemes.

Phoneme. A distinct sound unit in a language. In English there are 46: 9 vowels and 37 consonants.

Phonology. The rules a speaker follows when combining speech sounds.

Pragmatics. The communicative intent of speech rather than its content, for example, asking a question at the right time and in the right way.

Prosody. The melody of language; the tone of voice used to ask questions, for example, or show emotion.

Semantics. The meaning of words; their definition.

Syntax. The grammar of a language; the acceptable relationship between words in a sentence.

REFERENCES

Allen DA: Autistic spectrum disorders: Clinical presentation in the preschool child. *J Child Neurol* 3:548–556, 1988.

Allen D, Mendelson L, Rapin I: Syndrome specific remediation in preschool developmental dysphasia, in French J, Harel S, Casaer P (eds): *Child Neurology and Developmental Disabilities: Selected Proceedings of the Fourth International Congress.* Baltimore, Md, Paul H Brooks, 1989.

Aram DM, Nation JE: Patterns of preschool language disorders. *J Speech Hear Res* 18:229–241, 1975.

Aram DM, Nation JE: Preschool language disorders and subsequent language and academic difficulties. *J Commun Disord* 13:159–170, 1980.

Aram DM, Nation JE: *Child Language Disorders.* St Louis, CV Mosby, 1982.

Aram DM, Ekelman BL, Nation JE: Preschoolers with language disorders: 10 years later. *J Speech Hear Res* 27:232–244, 1984.

Asperger H: Die autistischen Psychopathen im Kindesalter. *Arch Psychiatr* 17:76–137, 1944.

August GJ, Raz N, Papanicolaou AC, Baird TD, Hirsh SL, Hsu LL: Fenfluramine treatment in infantile autism. *J Nerv Men Dis* 172:604–612, 1984.

Bates E: *Language and Context: The Acquisition of Pragmatics.* New York, Academic Press, 1976.

Bates E, Marchman M: Variations in normal language development, in Plum F (ed): *Language, Communication and the Brain.* New York, Raven Press, 1988.

Bauman M, Kemper TL: Histoanatomic observations of the brain in early infantile autism. *Neurology* 35:866–874, 1985.

Bauman M, Kemper TL: Developmental cerebellar abnormalities: A consistent finding in early infantile autism. *Neurology* 36(suppl I):190, 1986.

Behar L: The preschool behavior questionnaire. *J Abnorm Child Psychol* 5:265–276, 1977.

Benson DF: *Aphasia, Alexia and Agraphia.* New York, Churchill Livingstone, 1979.

Bishop DVM: Age at onset and outcome in acquired aphasia with convulsive disorder (Landau-Kleffner syndrome). *Dev Med Child Neurol* 27:705–712, 1985.

Campbell M, Anderson LT, Greene WH, Deutch SI: Psychopharmacology, in Cohen DJ, Donnellan AM, Paul R (eds): *Handbook of Autism and Pervasive Developmental Disorders.* New York, John Wiley & Sons, 1987.

Campbell SB: Hyperactivity: Course and treatment, in Davids A (ed): *Child Personality and Psychopathology,* Vol 3. New York, John Wiley & Sons, 1976.

Campbell SB, Breaux A, Ewing L, Szumowski E: A one year follow-up study of patient referred hyperactive preschool children. *J Am Acad Child Psychiatr* 23:243–249, 1984.

Cantwell DP, Baker L: Prevalence and type of psychiatric disorders and developmental disorders in three speech and language groups. *J Commun Disord* 20:151–160, 1987.

Carey WB, McDevitt SC, Baker D: Differentiating minimal brain dysfunction and temperament. *Dev Med Child Neurol* 21:765–772, 1979.

Chapman K, Leonard LB, Rowan LE, Weiss AL: Inappropriate word extensions in the speech of young language disordered children. *J Speech Hear Disord* 48:55–62, 1983.

Coates SW: *Preschool Embedded Figures Test.* Palo Alto, Calif, Consulting Psychologists Press, 1972.

Cole AJ, Anderman F, Taylor A, et al: The Landau-Kleffner syndrome of acquired epileptic aphasia: Unusual clinical outcome, surgical experience and absence of encephalitis. *Neurology* 38:31–38, 1988.

Courchesne E, Hessellink JR, Jernigan TL, et al: Abnormal neuroanatomy in a nonretarded person with autism. *Arch Neurol* 44:335–341, 1987.

Creak M: Childhood psychosis: A review of 100 cases. *Br J Psychiatr* 109:384–389, 1963.

Curtiss S: Special grammatical abilities, in Obler L, Fein D (eds): *Neuropsychology of Special Abilities.* New York, Guilford Press, 1988.

Damasio AR, Maurer RG: A neurological model for childhood autism. *Arch Neurol* 35:777–786, 1978.

Damasio H, Maurer RG, Damasio AR, Chui HC: Computed tomographic scan findings in patients with autistic behavior. *Arch Neurol* 37:504–510, 1980.

Darby JK: Neuropathic aspects of psychosis in childhood. *J Autism Child Schizophr* 6:339–352, 1976.

Darwish H, Pearce PS: The semantic-pragmatic syndrome and corpus callosal agenesis: Prerequisites and implications. *Ann Neurol* 14:363, 1983.

Dawson G, Warrenburg S, Fuller P: Cerebral lateralization in individuals diagnosed as autistic in early childhood. *Brain and Language* 15:353–368, 1982.

Dawson G, Warrenburg S, Fuller P: Hemisphere functioning and motor imitation in autistic persons. *Brain and Cognition* 2:346–354, 1983.

Dawson G, Finlay C, Phillips S, Galpert L: Hemispheric specialization and the language abilities of autistic children. *Child Dev* 57:1440–1453, 1986.

DeMyer MK, Barton S, Alpern GD, et al: The measured intelligence of autistic children: A follow-up study. *J Autism Child Schizophr* 4:42–60, 1974.

Dennis M, Whitaker H: Language acquisition following hemidecortication. *Brain and Language* 3:404–433, 1976.

Dennis M, Hendrick EB, Hoffman HJ, Humphreys RP: The language of hydrocephalic children and adolescents. *J Clin Exp Neuropsychol* 9:593–621, 1988.

Deuel RK, Lenn NJ: Treatment of acquired epileptic aphasia. *J Pediatr* 90:959–961, 1977.

Deykin EY, McMahon PH, McMahon B: The incidence of seizures among children with autistic symptoms. *Am J Psychiatr* 136:1310–1312, 1979.

Donahue M: Linguistic and pragmatic development in learning disabled children, in Rosenberg S (ed): *Advances in Applied Psycholinguistics.* New York, Cambridge University Press, 1987.

Duara R, Rumsey J, Gady C, Kessler R, Rapoport J, Cutler N: Cerebral glucose metabolism in adult autism. *Neurology* 34:117, 1984.

Earls F: Prevalence of behavior problems in 3 year old children: A cross-national replication. *Arch Gen Psychiatr* 37:1153–1157, 1980.

Fein D, Humes M, Kaplan E, Lucci D, Waterhouse L: The question of left hemisphere dysfunction in autism. *Psychol Bull* 95:258–281, 1984.

Fein D, Waterhouse L, Lucci D, Snyder D: Cognitive subtypes in developmentally disabled children: A pilot study. *J Autism Dev Disord* 15:77–95, 1985.

Fein D, Pennington B, Markowitz P, Braverman M, Waterhouse L: Toward a neuropsychological model of infantile autism: Are the social deficits primary? *J Am Acad Child Psychiatr* 25:198–212, 1986.

Ferry P, Hall S, Hicks J: Dilapidated speech: Developmental verbal apraxia. *Dev Med Child Neurol* 17:749–756, 1975.

Filipek PA, Kennedy DN, Caviness VS, Klein S, Rapin I: In vivo magnetic resonance imaging-based volumetric brain analysis in subjects with verbal auditory agnosia. *Ann Neurol* 22:410, 1987.

Fuller P, Newcombe F, Ounsted C: Late language development in a child unable to recognize or produce speech sounds. *Arch Neurol* 40:165–168, 1983.

Gaffney GR, Tsai LY, Kuperman S, Minchin S: Cerebellar structure in autism. *Am J Dis Child* 141:1330–1332, 1987.

Garvey M, Gordon N: A follow-up study of children with disorders of speech development. *Br J Disord Commun* 8:17–28, 1973.

Geller E, Ritvo ER, Freeman BJ, Yuwiler A: Preliminary observations on the effects of fenfluramine on blood serotonin and symptoms in three autistic boys. *N Engl J Med* 307:165–169, 1982.

Geschwind N, Galaburda A: *Cerebal Laterality.* Cambridge, Mass, MIT Press, 1985.

Gillberg C, Svendsen P: Childhood psychosis and computed tomographic brain scan findings. *J Autism Dev Disord* 13:19–32, 1983.

Golden GS: Neurologic basis of autism, in Cohen, DJ, Donnellan, AM, Paul R (eds): *Handbook of Autism and Pervasive Developmental Disorders.* New York, John Wiley & Sons, 1987.

Green MCL: Speechless and backward at 3. *Br J Disord Commun* 2:134–145, 1976.

Griffiths CPS: A follow-up study of children with disorders of speech. *Br J Disord Commun* 4:46–56, 1969.

Hall KH, Tomblin JB: A follow-up study of children with articulation and language disorders. *J Speech Hear Disord* 43:227–241, 1978.

Hauser SL, DeLong GR, Rosman NP: Pneumographic findings in the infantile autism syndrome: A correlation with temporal lobe disease. *Brain* 98:667–688, 1975.

Hier DB, LeMay M, Rosenberger PB: Autism and unfavorable left-right asymmetries of the brain. *J Autism Dev Disord* 9:153–159, 1979.

Horwitz B, Rumsey J, Grady C, Rapoport S: The resting landscape in autism. *Arch Neurol* 45:749–755, 1988.

Ingram D: Speech disorders in childhood, in Lenneberg E, Lenneberg E (eds): *Foundations of Language Development.* New York, Academic Press, 1975.

Jacobson JW, Janick MP: Observed prevalence of multiple developmental disabilities. *Ment Retard* 21:87–94, 1983.

Kagan J, Kogan N: Individual variation in cognitive processes, in Musson P (ed): *Charmichael's Manual of Child Psychology,* 3rd ed. New York, John Wiley & Sons, 1970.

Kagan J, Pearson L, Welch L: Conceptual impulsivity and inductive reasonings. *Child Dev* 37:583–594, 1966.

Kanner L: Autistic disturbances of affective contact. *Nerv Child* 2:217–250, 1943.

Kertesz A: *Localization in Neuropsychology.* New York, Academic Press, 1983.

King RR, Jones C, Lasky E: In retrospect: A fifteen year follow-up report of speech and language disordered children. *Lang Speech Hear Serv Schools* 13:24–32, 1982.

Kinsbourne M, Caplan P: *Children's Learning and Attention Problems.* Boston, Little, Brown, 1979.

Kohler L: Physical examination of four year old children. *Acta Paediatr Scand* 62:181–192, 1973.

Koppitz E: *The Bender Gestalt Test for Young Children.* London, Grune & Stratton, 1963.

Lahey B: Rapid treatment of perceptual-motor problems of disadvantaged preschool children. *J Instruct Psychol* 3:38–40, 1976.

Landau WV, Kleffner FR: Syndrome of acquired aphasia with convulsive disorder in children. *Neurology* 7:523–530, 1957.

Landau W, Goldstein R, Kleffner F: Congenital aphasia: A clinico-pathologic study. *Neurology* 10:915–921, 1960.

Lassman FM, Fisch RO, Vetter DK, LaBenz ES: *Early Correlates of Speech, Language and Hearing.* Littleton, Mass, PSG Publishing, 1980.

Leonard L: What is deviant language? *J Speech Hear Disord* 37:427–446, 1979.

Leonard L: Conversational replies of children with specific language impairment. *J Speech Hear Res* 29:114–119, 1986.

Levine D, Sweet E: Localization of lesions in Broca's motor aphasia, in Kertesz (ed): *Localization in Neuropsychology.* New York, Academic Press, 1983.

Levine M: *Developmental Variation and Learning Disorders.* Cambridge, Mass, Educators Publishing Service, 1987.

Lou HC, Brandt S, Bruhn P: Progressive aphasia and epilepsy with a self-limited course, in Penny JK (ed): *Epilepsy: The Eighth International Symposium.* New York, Raven Press, 1977.

Lou HC, Hendrikson L, Bruhn P: Focal cerebral hyperfusion in children with dysphasias and/or attention deficit disorder. *Arch Neurol* 41:825–829, 1984.

Maccario M, Hefferen SJ, Keblusek SJ, Lipinsky KA: Developmental dysphasia and electroencephalographic abnormalities. *Dev Med Child Neurol* 24:141–155, 1982.

Maccoby E, Hagen JW: Effect of distortion upon central vs. incidental recall: Developmental trends. *J Exp Child Psychol* 2:280–289, 1965.

McDevitt SC, Carey WB: The measurement of temperament in 3–7 year old children. *J Child Psychol Psychiatr* 19:245–253, 1978.

McKinney W, McGreal DA: An aphasic syndrome in children. *Can Med Assoc J* 110:637–639, 1974.

Mantovani JF, Landau WM: Acquired aphasia with convulsive disorder: Course and prognosis. *Neurology* 30:524–529, 1980.

Menyuk P: Comparison of grammar of children with functionally deviant and normal speech. *J Speech Hear Res* 8:109–121, 1964.

Minshew N, Payton J, Wolf GL, Latchaw RE: ¹H NMR imaging of autistics: Implications for neurology. *Ann Neurol* 20:417, 1986.

Mohr JP: Broca's area and Broca's aphasia, in Whitaker H, Whitaker HA (eds): *Studies in Neurolinguistics*, Vol I. New York, Academic Press, 1976.

Moorehead DM, Ingram D: The development of base syntax in normal and linguistically deviant children. *J Speech Hear Res* 16:330–352, 1973.

Morley ME: *The Development and Disorders of Speech in Childhood*, 2nd ed. Baltimore, Md, Williams & Wilkins, 1965.

Nass R, Gazzaniga MS: Cerebral lateralization and specialization in the human central nervous system, in Plum F (ed): *Handbook of Physiology: The Nervous System V*. Baltimore, Md, Williams & Wilkins, 1987.

Nass R, Koch D: Differential effects of early left versus right brain damage on temperament. *Dev Neuropsychol* 3:93–99, 1987.

Nass R, Petrucha D: Pervasive developmental disorder variant of epileptic aphasia. *J Child Neurol* 5:327–328, 1989.

Nass R, Walker R: Acquired aphasia with convulsive disorder and definite pathology. Paper presented at Child Neurology Society meeting, San Antonio, 1989.

Netley C: Sex chromosome abnormalities and development of verbal and non-verbal abilities, in Ludlow C, Cooper J (eds): *Genetic Aspects of Speech and Language Disorders*. New York, Academic Press, 1983.

Nichols P, Chen T: *Minimal Brain Dysfunction*. Hillsdale, NJ, Lawrence Erlbaum, 1981.

Obler L, Fein D: *Neuropsychology of Special Abilities*. New York, Guilford Press, 1988.

Opitz JM: *X-Linked Mental Retardation 2*. New York, Alan R Liss, 1986.

Ornitz EM: Neurophysiologic studies in infantile autism, in Cohen DJ, Donnellan AM, Paul R (eds): *Handbook of Autism and Pervasive Developmental Disorders*. New York, John Wiley & Sons, 1987.

Palfrey J, Levin M, Walker D, Sullivan M: The emergence of attention deficits in early childhood: A prospective study. *J Behav Dev Pediatr* 6:339–348, 1985.

Payton J, Minshew N: Early appearance of partial complex seizures in autism. *Ann Neurol* 22:408, 1987.

Pearce PS, Darwish HZ, Gaines BH: Visual symbol and manual sign learning by children with phonologic programming deficit syndrome. *Dev Med Child Neurol* 29:743–750, 1987.

Prior MR, Bradshaw JL: Hemisphere functioning in autistic children. *Cortex* 15:73–81, 1979.

Prior MR, Tress B, Hoffman WL, Boldt D: Computed tomographic study of children with classic autism. *Arch Neurol* 41:482–484, 1984.

Purpura D: Discussion of paper by Coleman, in Katzman R (ed): *Congenital and Acquired Cognitive Disorders*. New York, Raven Press, 1979.

Rapin I: Developmental language disorders and brain dysfunction as precursors of reading disability, in Wise GA, Blaw ME, Procopis PG (eds): *Topics in Child Neurology*, Vol II. New York, Spectrum, 1982.

Rapin I, Allen D: Developmental language disorders: Nosologic considerations, in Kirk U (ed): *Neuropsychology of Language, Reading and Spelling*. New York, Academic Press, 1983.

Rapin I, Allen D: Syndromes of developmental dysphasia and adult aphasia, in Plum F (ed): *Language, Communication and Brain*. New York, Raven Press, 1988.

Rapin I, Mattis S, Rowan A, Golden G: Verbal auditory agnosia. *Dev Med Child Neurol* 19:192–207, 1977.

Ritvo E, Freeman B, Yuwiler A, et al: Fenfluramine therapy for autism: Promise and precaution. *Psychopharmacol Bull* 22:133–140, 1986.

Rosenbloom R, Campbell M, George AE, et al: High resolution CT scanning in infantile autism: A quantitative approach. *J Am Acad Child Psychiatr* 23:72–77, 1984.

Ross DM, Ross SA: *Hyperactivity: Theory, Research, and Action*. New York, John Wiley & Sons, 1982.

Routh DK, Schroeder C, O'Tuama L: Development of activity level in children. *Dev Psychol* 10:163–168, 1974.

Rubens A, Kertesz A: Localization of lesions in transcortical aphasias, in Kertez A (ed): *Localization in Neuropsychology*. New York, Academic Press, 1983.

Rutter M, Bartak L, Newman S: Autism: A central disorder of cognition and language? in Rutter M (ed): *Infantile Autism: Concepts, Characteristics and Treatment*. London, Churchill Livingstone, 1971.

Sabatino D: Home instruction utilizing teacher-moms with academic high risk preschool children. *Psychology in the Schools* 11:433–440, 1974.

Sandt-Koendermann W, Smit I, Dongen H, Hest J: A case of acquired aphasia and convulsive disorder: Some linguistic aspects of recovery and breakdown. *Brain and Language* 21:174–183, 1984.

Santostephano S: Cognitive controls and cognitive styles: An approach to diagnosing and treating cognitive disabilities in children. *Semin Psychiatr* 1:291–317, 1969.

Schain RJ, Yannet H: Infantile autism. *J Pediatr* 57:560–567, 1960.

Sherman M, Nass R, Shapiro T: Brief report: Regional cerebral blood flow in autism. *J Autism Dev Disord* 14:439–446, 1984.

Shoumaker RD, Bennett DR, Bray PF, Curliss RG: Clinical and EEG manifestations of an unusual aphasic syndrome in children. *Neurology* 24:10–16, 1974.

Siegel AW, Kirasec KC, Kilburg R: Recognition memory in reflective and impulsive preschool children. *Child Dev* 44:651–656, 1973.

Slater B: Perceptual development at the kindergarten level. *J Clin Psychol* 27:263–266, 1971.

Soper HV, Satz P, Orsini DL, Hanry RR, Zvi JC, Schulman M: Handedness patterns in autism suggest subtypes. *J Autism*

Dev Disord 16:155–167, 1986.

Stark RE, Bernstein LE, Condino R, Bender M, Tallal P, Catts H: Four year follow-up study of language impaired children. *Ann Dyslexia* 34:49–68, 1984.

Steckol KF, Leonard LB: The use of grammatical morphemes by normal and language impaired children. *J Commun Disord* 12:291–301, 1979.

Stevenson J, Richman N: The prevalence of language delay in a population of three year old children and its association with general retardation. *Dev Med Child Neurol* 18:431–441, 1976.

Stiles-Davis J, Sugarman S, Nass R: Construction of spatial and class relations in four young children with right cerebral hemisphere damage. *Brain and Cognition* 4:388–412, 1985.

Swisher LP, Pinsker E: The language characteristics of hyperverbal hydrocephalic children. *Dev Med Child Neurol* 13:746–755, 1971.

Tew B, Lawrence KM: The clinical and psychological characteristics of children with "cocktail party" syndrome. *Z Kinderchir* 28:360–367, 1979.

Thomas A, Chess S, Birch HG: *Temperament and Behavior Disorders in Children.* New York, New York University Press, 1968.

Tsai LY, Stewart MA: Handedness and EEG correlation in autistic children. *Biol Psychiatr* 17:595–598, 1982.

Vilensky, JA, Damasio AR, Maurer RG: Gait disturbances in patients with autistic behavior. *Arch Neurol* 38:646–649, 1981.

Weiner PS: The perceptual level functioning of dysphasic children. *Cortex* 5:440–457, 1972.

Weiner PS: A language delayed child at adolescence. *J Speech Hear Disord* 39:202–212, 1974.

Weiss AL, Leonard LB, Rowan LE, Chapman K: Linguistic and non-linguistic features of style in normal and language-impaired children. *J Speech Hear Disord* 48:154–164, 1983.

Williams R, Ingham RJ, Rosenthal J: A further analysis for developmental apraxia of speech in children with defective articulation. *J Speech Hear Res* 24:496–505, 1981.

Wilson B, Risucci D: A model for clinical quantitative classification. *Brain and Language* 27:281–309, 1986.

Wing L: Asperger's syndrome: A clinical account. *Psychol Med* 11:115–129, 1981.

Wing L, Attwood A: Syndromes of autism and atypical development, in Cohen DJ, Donnellan AM, Paul R (eds): *Handbook of Autism and Pervasive Developmental Disorders.* New York, John Wiley & Sons, 1987.

Wing L, Gould J: Severe impairments of social interaction and associated abnormalities in children: Epidemiology and classification. *J Autism Dev Disord* 9:11–29, 1979.

Witelson S: On hemispheric specialization and cerebral plasticity: Mark II, in Best C (ed): *Hemispheric Function and Collaboration in the Child.* Orlando, Fla, Academic Press, 1985.

Witkin HA: Psychological differentiation in cross-cultural perspective. *J Cross-Cult Psychol* 6:4–87, 1976.

Witkin HA, Dyk RB, Faterson HF, Goodenough DR, Karp SA: *Psychological Differentiation.* New York, John Wiley & Sons, 1962.

Witkin HA, Goodenough DR, Karp SA: Stability of cognitive style from childhood to young adulthood. *J Pers Soc Psychol* 7:291–300, 1967.

Wolfus B, Moscovitch M, Kinsbourne M: Subgroups of developmental language disorders. *Brain and Language* 9:152–171, 1980.

Wolpaw T, Nation JE, Aram DM: Developmental language disorders: A follow-up study. *Ill Speech Hear J* 12:14–18, 1976.

Woods BT, Carey S: Language deficits after apparent clinical recovery from childhood aphasia. *Ann Neurol* 6:405–409, 1979.

Woods B, Teuber H-L: Early onset of complementary specialization. *Trans Am Neurol Assoc* 98:113–117, 1973.

Worster-Drought C: Failure in normal speech development of neurologic origin. *Folia Phoniat* 5:130–146, 1953.

Worster-Drought C: An unusual form of acquired aphasia in children. *Dev Med Child Neurol* 13:563–571. 1971.

Disorders of Higher Cortical Function in School-Age Children

Debora L. Scheffel

Advances in the neurosciences have established clearer links between neurologic and psychologic, or cognitive, substrates of behavior, thus widening the scope of a number of disciplines, including pediatric neurology, to accommodate these developments. This in turn has fostered greater interdisciplinary cooperation and resulted in a more cohesive knowledge base to inform the treatment of children with neurologic disorders.

This chapter presents information from diverse disciplines that will be helpful to the clinical pediatric neurologist. In the discussion that follows, the term *learning disability* will be used to refer to children exhibiting developmental disorders of higher cerebral functioning, meaning that cognitive function has been disturbed as a result of an assumed neurologic dysfunction, and that the problem is one of altered process, not of a general incapacity to learn (Johnson and Myklebust, 1967).

The population of children being considered in this chapter has been variously referred to in the educational, psychologic, and medical communities by a number of terms, including *developmentally learning disabled, minimal brain dysfunction syndrome, developmental aphasia, dysgraphia, dyscalculia, dyslexia,* and *perceptually handicapped.* These terms diverge based on their relative orientation toward the etiology or behavioral manifestations of the disorder. Although children described by these terms have only fairly recently become widely recognized by the medical, psychologic, and educational disciplines, at least as early as the 1800s, physicians and educators reported cases of children who exhibited specific language difficulties or difficulties in learning to read, write, or calculate following no apparent illness or injury and in the presence of generalized intellectual competence (Morgan, 1896; Hinshelwood, 1917). Work in the early 1900s relevant to this population was aimed at relating information from the study of adults with acquired brain injuries to brain-injured mentally retarded children (Strauss and Werner, 1942) and to non-retarded children who had behavioral characteristics associated with brain damage but who had not suffered known central nervous system dysfunction (Wiederholt, 1974). Further mid–twentieth-century emphases included the translation of clinical and research findings into educational and remedial practice (e.g., Kirk, 1940; Fernald, 1943). The educational and remedial prescriptions were opportune contributions to an educational system that was increasingly coming to recognize the need to address individual differences within the classroom and receiving parental pressure to do so (Doris, 1986).

In 1963 the term *learning disability* was formally introduced to refer to children having disorders in the development of language, speech, reading, and associated communication skills needed for social interaction. Children with primarily sensory handicaps or generalized mental retardation were not to be included in the use of the term (Kirk, 1963). In that year the Association for Children with Learning Disabilities was established, and subsequent years have brought the organization and growth of learning disabilities as a discrete field of study, to which a variety of disciplines—including education, psychology, and medicine—have made and continue to make significant contributions.

Volume 42, Number 163 (August 1977) of the *Federal Register* describes a learning disability as

> a disorder in one or more of the basic psychological processes involved in understanding or in using language, spoken or written, which may manifest itself in an imperfect ability to listen, think, speak, read, write, or do math calculations. The term includes such conditions as perceptual handicaps, brain injury, minimal brain dysfunction, dyslexia, and developmental aphasia. The term does not include children who have learning problems which are primarily the result of vision, hearing, or motor handicaps, of mental retardation, of emotional disturbance, or of environmental, cultural, or economic disadvantage.

This legislative definition is primarily aimed at addressing societal needs by authorizing programs and mandating services. For research purposes, definitions more operational in character are used to select subjects. Operationalizing the definition requires specifying the magnitude of and means of arriving at a diagnosis of a disorder in one of the several categories, and establishing average intellectual competence in the presence of the disorder. Definitions for this purpose may be grouped into three categories: (1) ability-achievement discrepancy, (2) grade placement-achievement discrepancy, and (3) intelligence score scatter (Farnham-Diggory, 1986). Thus, a learning-disabled child might be identified by demonstrating a discrepancy of a given number of points (e.g., ten points or more) between IQ scores and standard scores on achievement tests, by demonstrating achievement test standard scores below a given cutoff point (e.g., below 85), or by evidencing a difference of a given number of scaled score points (e.g., fifteen points or more) on the Verbal versus Performance scales of the revised Wechsler Intelligence Scale for Children.

Numerous criticisms have been leveled at the means of defining learning-disabled children. The validity of the tests used to establish a disorder in one or more areas of cognitive functioning has been challenged (Coles, 1978). In addition, determining an appropriate cutoff score below which a child would be classified as retarded (not learning disabled), and how much discrepancy is necessary between intelligence and achievement for a child to be considered learning disabled, remain controversial issues (Siegel and Heaven, 1986).

In addition to complex identification issues affecting the composition of the population as a whole, learning-disabled children comprise a heterogeneous group. Classification research attempts to identify homogeneous subgroups within the larger population. Early studies were based on clinical inspection of psychometric data (Boder, 1973; Mattis et al., 1975), whereas multivariate statistical techniques have been used more recently to analyze psychometric data (Fisk and Rourke, 1979; Lyon, 1982). These studies differ in their use of patterns of performance or magnitude of performance differences on either academic (e.g., reading, spelling) or processing (e.g., memory, perception) tasks as the criteria to classify children (Fletcher and Morris, 1986).

Incidence statistics have changed over the past 20 years owing to increased awareness of services available to children demonstrating disorders of higher cerebral function associated with learning disabilities. The statistics are also convoluted by differing definitions used to classify children as learning disabled. In 1978 it was estimated that approximately 2% of the handicapped population were learning disabled (Farnham-Diggory, 1978). In 1981–1982, 4% of the school-age enrollment nationwide were classified as learning disabled, accounting for 38% of all children receiving special education services (U.S. Department of Education, 1983, pp. 2–4, 72). Traditionally, boys comprise the largest percentage of in-

dividuals identified as learning disabled (Johnson, 1987). Some attribute this to gender differences in hemispheric specialization (McGlone and Davidson, 1973) and to the more pervasive and debilitating effects of disorders related to linguistic functioning (more likely to be manifest in boys), in contrast to disorders in mathematics and nonverbal functioning (more likely to be manifest in girls). Whereas the elementary school emphasis on acquiring verbal skills may seem to emphasize the verbal, school-related concomitants of learning disorders, difficulty in nonacademic settings—such as exhibiting inappropriate behavior in social situations (e.g., being overly excitable or overly affectionate), poor judgment (e.g., failing to sense or respond to danger), or a tendency to get lost easily owing to difficulty understanding spatial and directional correlates—may also characterize some individuals within the population.

PATHOLOGY

Medically oriented theories of developmental learning disabilities view the associated behavioral sequelae as overt symptomatology of underlying biologic pathology. The inferred pathology is then conceptualized by different theorists as affecting, for example, perceptual systems (Frostig and Horne, 1964), perceptual-motor functioning (Kephart, 1971), neurologic organization (Delacato, 1966), or oculomotor functioning (Getman, 1981). Evidence from biologic pathology indicates that low birth weight, especially among preterm infants, represents a high risk factor for later disabilities (Johnson, 1987). Resulting problems may include those related to overall intelligence, motor development, behavioral disorders, and specific learning disabilities (Cohen, 1985). Malnutrition, especially at critical periods of growth, may result in reduced brain size and impaired intellectual development (Stoch and Smythe, 1968). Birch (1970) reports that central nervous system damage from malnutrition in the last trimester of intrauterine development or the first year of postnatal life usually has permanent effects. Furthermore, maternal drug consumption, smoking, and alcohol consumption during pregnancy have been related to later obstetric complications and hyperactive behavior in children (Ross and Ross, 1976). Persistent otitis media in childhood may also be indicated as a high risk factor (Silva et al., 1985). Relevant to endocrine gland imbalances, Gaddes (1980) notes that underproduction of thyroxin (hypothyroidism) has been associated with poor memory and depressed IQ scores, whereas overproduction (hyperthyroidism) can produce hyperactivity and difficulty with concentration and attention. Minimal hypoglycemia (low blood sugar) may be associated with word finding difficulties and depressed language competence.

Although controversial, evidence from research in vestibular functioning and hemispheric lateralization may possibly contribute to an understanding of the underlying biologic pathology seen in learning disorders. Morrison (1986) notes that dysfunctions in the vestibular system have been clinically assessed in learning-disabled children and identified by remnants of primitive reflexes, inadequate postural and equilibrium reactions, hypotonia, and dysfunctional ocular-motor reactions and control (Ayres, 1972; deQuiros, 1976). Specifically, Morrison cites evidence for a greater degree of persistence of tonic neck reflexes in pathologic groups (learning disabled and mentally retarded) than in normal groups. On procedures that evaluate balance and equilibrium reactions learning-disabled and mentally retarded groups have been found to score consistently in the pathologic range (Freides et al., 1980). Furthermore, recordings of the vestibular-ocular reflex of postrotary nystagmus have indicated deviancy in nystagmus duration as characteristic of a subsample of learning-disabled children (Ayres, 1978; Ottenbacher, 1978). Summarizing laterality studies, Obrzut et al. (1986) conclude that results from auditory, visual, and verbal-manual asymmetry techniques indicate that learning-disabled children, although demonstrating expected left hemisphere specialization for language processing, do not demonstrate left hemisphere dominance to the same degree as their normal counterparts. Interpretations of this difference in degree of lateralization include incomplete lateralization, developmental delay, and neurologic deficits. Critics of this research suggest that our understanding of specific brain-behavior relationships in these populations remains somewhat obscure.

SIGNS AND SYMPTOMS

Identifying characteristics of children exhibiting learning disabilities owing to disorders of higher cerebral function may be manifest in either school or nonschool settings. Furthermore, because these children may be described from a number of theoretic positions, symptomatology is varied. From a neuropsychologic perspective, symptomatology related to disorders of higher cerebral function issues from tasks related to anterior/posterior function, right/left hemispheric function, intersensory integration, or successive/simultaneous processing demands. Impaired functioning of brain regions or systems is evidenced by a decrement of performance in language tasks (e.g., word retrieval, auditory memory), visual-spatial functioning (e.g., visual discrimination, fine motor), or intersensory integration (recoding information from the visual to the auditory system), or inappropriate matching of successive versus simultaneous processing to task demands. Tasks that reveal disorders of planning, organization, and attention have also been used in recent years.

From a linguistic perspective, language models stressing the pervasiveness of language processing and mediation for higher cognitive functioning focus on tasks re-

flecting the child's difficulty in grasping the underlying structure of language and how it is represented, as in difficulty with rhyming, analyzing words into phonologic parts, or perceiving underlying commonalities in the semantic structure of words or connected language. Furthermore, owing to deficits in the social communicative uses of language, language characteristics affecting relationships with parents, teachers, and peers may be noted.

Cognitive psychology interprets higher cognitive functioning as reflecting capacity for general problem solving. Thus, disorders of function from this perspective are described generally by poor strategy use in problem solving. Specifically, difficulty in setting relevant goals to solve a problem, poor monitoring of performance toward a goal, inflexible task approach, poor learner awareness of task demands, and inefficient storage and retrieval of information are suggested as characteristic of disorders of cognitive functioning.

Behavioral/educational orientations report behaviors such as poor skill performance in one or more areas of reading, writing, math, or the content areas, and/or poor task completion, organization, and attention.

Other general symptomatology includes inconsistent performance on cognitive tasks (being able at times to perform adequately and at others being unable to perform at all), excessively impulsive or reflective style of response, difficulty making decisions, especially from many choices, thought perseveration, difficulty with abstract reasoning and in concept formation, slow language development, and delayed motor development. Athetoid choreiform, or rigid movements of the hands; impaired discrimination of size, right from left, and up from down; poor spatial orientation; impaired orientation in time; distorted concept of body image, impaired judgment of distance and discrimination of figure from ground; and hyperkinesis have also been noted. Aphasic-like characteristics, such as poor language comprehension or poor oral expressive language (e.g., word retrieval difficulties), reading reversals, difficulty with writing and two-dimensional representation, and social difficulties (e.g., difficulty playing in a group, overexcitability, disinhibition) may be characteristic. Hyperactivity, perceptual-motor impairments, emotional lability, general coordination deficits, disorders of attention, impulsivity, disorders of memory and thinking, specific learning disabilities (reading, arithmetic, writing, spelling), and disorders of speech and language are characteristics most often cited by referral sources (Clements, 1966, pp. 11–13).

DIAGNOSIS

Diagnostic procedures are aimed at establishing average capacity, documenting underachievement, and identifying deficits in specific underlying competencies thought to contribute to underachievement (e.g., deficient memory, poor task aproach). Because children with disorders of higher cerebral function are a heterogeneous group reflecting no single etiology or unitary characteristic, diagnostic procedures must be individualized. For example, establishing at least average intellectual potential is a necessary inclusionary criterion for this diagnostic category, yet underlying problems that may be contributing to learning difficulties may also reduce performance on intellectual measures. Thus, measures to assess intellectual potential must be selected individually so that scores that may reflect specific disabilities are not interpreted as representing generalized incapacity. Intelligence measures that sample behaviors using other than the child's processing or response areas of weakness must be selected. Furthermore, there is significant variability of measures in any given achievement area or area of processing owing to variations in task demands. A child may perform above age expectancy on one reading task and significantly below age expectancy on another, because of differences in task demands interacting with the child's strengths and weaknesses. Thus, an informed and individualized test choice is needed in each diagnostic evaluation in order to demonstrate a valid range of functioning.

In general, diagnostic procedures should include birth, medical, developmental, and psychologic/educational histories and behavioral descriptions of the problems experienced at home and at school from teachers and parents. Intact sensory functioning in vision and hearing should also be established. A battery of tests can then be chosen to assess intellectual potential (using both verbal and nonverbal measures) and areas of potential underachievement, including listening (discrimination, comprehension, memory), oral expressive language (sequencing, word retrieval, syntax, articulation, language use), reading (single words, words in context, decoding, comprehension, silent versus oral reading), writing (handwriting, spelling, syntax, discourse), mathematics (reasoning, computation), nonverbal behavior (nonverbal communication; spatial, time, left/right orientation; body image; social perception; perceptual-motor skills; visual perception and memory), and thinking/reasoning skills (Johnson, 1987). Diagnostic measures should represent a range of tasks that assess both the functioning of an integrated system (e.g., reading silently as is done in school) and performance on theoretically separable aspects of systemic functioning (e.g., the hypothesized cognitive correlates of reading, such as visual memory and auditory discrimination).

TREATMENT

Effective treatment of children with disorders of higher cerebral function is based on thorough diagnostic information yielding an understanding of the child's educational, psychologic, and social functioning; a task analysis of the skills to be taught and internalized; and ongoing modification of the approach based on dynamic evaluation of progress. Various theoretic orientations identify the skills to be taught differently. Medically oriented theories suggest that the content of instruction be skills related to the deficient underlying pathology (e.g., visual discrimination, fine motor skills, eye movements). Neuropsychologic models have proliferated in the past decade that stress the several interrelated functional systems of the brain, and suggest that instruction be aimed at reorganizing these systems so that new methods of performing target behaviors may be established. Common treatment areas include attention, developing simultaneous and successive information-processing strategies, memory, and executive functions like problem identification and monitoring. Treatment is thought to change the psychologic structure of an act and hence its cerebral organization (e.g., from slow, sequential, and discrete to smooth, rapid, and integrated performance; Luria et al., 1970; Gaddes, 1980).

Because the difficulty in specifying the relationship between the structure, chemistry, and physiology of the nervous system and principles of higher learning, some assert that the empirical approach to studying the brain results in mere tinkering with the problem of human learning, especially the language capacity (Fox, 1983). Thus, differing perspectives build heuristic models that seem to account for learning phenomena and then postulate potential areas of difficulty and their consequences. Conceptualizing disorders of higher cognitive function as language based, some feel that the difficulty is in the person's ability to grasp the underlying structure of language and how it is represented. Treatment is focused on teaching listening, speaking, reading, and writing, stressing linguistic elements such as word structure and text structure. Generally, establishing a clear mental representation of the linguisitic system and its related parts is the goal.

In contrast, cognitive models of learning suggest that problem solving is the central process in higher cerebral functioning. Reading, writing, and mathematics are seen as requiring higher-order skills, such as nonalgorithmic thinking (in which the path of action to a goal is not fully specified in advance), dealing with complexity (in which the path to a goal is not fully visible), generating multiple solutions, applying multiple criteria to problems, self-regulation, and imposing meaning and structure on apparent disorder (Resnick, 1986). Treatment is aimed not at teaching skills or content per se, but at developing self-conscious, deliberate learning strategies, such as learner awareness of task demands, an organized task completion approach, and monitoring. These strategies are taught as applied to a variety of content areas.

Finally, psychoeducational models postulate that academic deficits reflect dysfunction in the ability to perceive, remember, and integrate auditory, visual, or motor information relevant to reading, writing, and mathematics performance. Direct teaching of academic skills is the focus of treatment, with the way in which teaching is approached being informed by each child's processing strengths and weaknesses.

Generally accepted principles of treatment consistent with educational and psychologic theory (Johnson and Myklebust, 1967) include the following:

- Consider the problem in multidimensional terms.
- Maintain strengths while developing weak areas.
- Teach through intact areas of function while integrating intact with deficient areas to achieve more uniformity of performance.
- Apply no single methodology; maintain a dynamic approach based on responsivity to the child's performance.
- Address the pervasiveness of the problem as it is manifest in both the school and extraschool contexts.
- Incorporate the principles of meaningfulness (contextual realism), input before output, monitoring, simultaneity (presenting symbolic or representational stimuli simultaneous with their experiential meanings), teaching to tolerance levels, and understanding underlying concomitants of observed behaviors.

Most longitudinal follow-up studies suggest that, despite treatment intervention, problems associated with disorders of higher cerebral function persist into adulthood (Zigmond and Thornton, 1985; Miles, 1986). However, efficacy studies of early intervention suggest that early treatment can significantly affect a child's experience in school, such as by reducing the number of children assigned to special education classes and the number of children retained in school grades, and can positively affect attitudes about achievement (Lazar and Darlington, 1978). Reviewing the literature on early intervention, Reynolds and associates (1983) concluded that significant child progress gains were demonstrated in most efficacy studies from 1939 to 1982. However, studies of specific intervention variables were infrequent, owing to unavoidable nonspecific intervening variables, which precluded making definitive statements about the relationship between outcome and treatment.

DISORDERS OF ORAL LANGUAGE (DYSPHASIAS)

Of all the problems experienced by children with disorders of higher cerebral function, those with language may be the most pervasive (Wiig and Semel, 1984). It is estimated that 9 out of 10 youths classified as learning disabled exhibit accompanying language disorders (Liber-

man, et al., 1984). To acquire language normally a child must learn to hear and discriminate different phonetic sounds and to recognize the subtle auditory speech cues that occur in temporal sequence. He or she must also master the motor skills of articulation and relate surface characteristics and underlying knowledge of language to an experiential knowledge base (Gaddes, 1980). Children with normal hearing and intelligence who evidence significant impairment in understanding or using oral language have been recognized at least as early as 1825, when Gall published a treatise on the function of the brain and each of its parts (Wilson, 1965). Myklebust (1971a, b) reports a continuing interest in the subject since Gall's early publication, and the use of the term *congenital aphasia* by Broadbent in the early 1870s to describe children with impaired language function. The term *developmental dysphasia* has also been used to refer to children who exhibit either receptive or expressive impairment of language following no apparent injury or illness but due to presumed neurologic dysfunction.

The most severe dysphasic disorder is aberrant development of inner language, the ability to interpret one's own subjective experiences and communicate with one's self. This foundation for the development of receptive and expressive language occurs in the preverbal stage of cognitive development and is established from nonverbal symbolic meanings associated with experience (Johnson and Myklebust, 1967). Receptive dysphasia suggests that the child can communicate with himself or herself but has difficulty receiving linguistic information from others. Receptive dysphasia frequently occurs together with expressive language problems (i.e., expressive dysphasia), in which a child has difficulty using language fluently, accurately, and effectively for communication.

Pathology

Developmental dysphasia, associated with difficulty in developing a normal understanding and use of oral language, is thought to be due to maldevelopment of or injury to the language centers of the central nervous system pre-, peri-, or postnatally, or during the first year of life (Gaddes, 1980). Language cortical circuits in adults have been known for over 100 years. Based on neuropathologic studies with stroke patients and head injury victims, Broca, a French neurologist, identified the area in front of the left motor strip controlling muscles of the face, jaw, tongue, and speech muscles as being involved in articulation and expression of spoken speech. Wernicke, a German neurologist, identified the lateral surface of the left temporal lobe as the cortical center for understanding of oral speech.

Neuropathologic studies of dysphasic children at autopsy have been less frequently available than those of adults, and such studies have typically focused on individuals with reading deficits rather than oral language dysfunction. However, Landau et al. (1960) reported on an autopsy study of a child with developmental dysphasia. This mentally bright 6-year-old boy evidenced significantly limited understanding of spoken language. His communicative attempts consisted of jargon and gestures. After 3 years of speech/language training he developed a moderate vocabulary and learned to say simple sentences. Postmortem findings following the boy's death at age 10 showed inadequate growth of cortical layers bilaterally in the temporal lobes. The posterior portions of the parietal, temporal, and occipital lobes were reduced in size bilaterally and the medial geniculate nuclei, connecting the auditory nerves to Heschl's gyri bilaterally, were severely degenerated. It is likely that these anomalies significantly distorted the registration of language sound patterns, making understanding of oral language very difficult (Gaddes, 1980).

Roberts (1962) has reported on the case of a girl whom he followed from age 6 years until her death in adolescence. This girl incurred a high fever associated with convulsions at 15 months, which resulted in brain damage. As language developed, attempts to vocalize phonetic sounds were abnormal, resulting in severely garbled speech that only her mother could understand. She developed idiosyncratic speech with consistent meanings for herself. An electroencephalogram (EEG) revealed spike discharges over the left hemisphere mainly in the parietal lobe. Brain surgery revealed diffuse atrophy of the left hemisphere, which was surgically removed (Gaddes, 1980).

Signs and Symptoms

Developmental dysphasia includes disorders related to understanding and receiving linguistic information and to using language to communicate meaningfully. Children with difficulty at the level of reception may evidence underlying deficits in perceiving differences between speech sounds and words, remembering the sequential elements of a linguistic utterance, or integrating linguistic symbols with concepts and experiences needed to grasp the meaning of an utterance. Difficulties in receiving information orally may result in inconsistency or neglect of response to language, frustration, difficulty with attention and self-control, echolalic verbalizations, and/or inability to follow verbal directions. Difficulty with abstract concepts like *before/after, few/many,* and *all/except* is often characteristic. Because oral language is based on intentional meaning, perceiving the nuances of inferred meaning is often problematic. Understanding the significance of extralinguistic elements, such as prosody, may also be difficult.

Children with difficulty in understanding language may also have associated expressive language disorders. Diminished expressive language and syntactic poverty may be expected when receptive understanding is limited. Children may have expressive disorders related to word retrieval; sequencing sounds in words, words in sentences, or sentences in text; analyzing oral language into component parts (i.e., words into sounds or syllables or sentences into words); syntax; oral formulation and organization of ideas; and/or the auditory-motor execution of speech. Deficient performance may be observed in finding the desired word to express an idea, naming the days of the week, counting in sequence, or naming items in a common category. Sound reversals or substitutions (e.g., *binglejells/jinglebells*) and generally poor oral fluency (owing to word retrieval difficulty or difficulty planning and organizing expression) are often characteristic. Deficits in oral language development, such as sound discrimination, sequencing, and understanding of abstract linguistic concepts, often affect other language-related functions and limit academic achievement generally. Oral reading performance, reading comprehension, spelling, written expression, and arithmetic reasoning may be affected (Johnson and Myklebust, 1967; Aram and Nation, 1980; Vetter, 1982; Wiig and Semel, 1984).

Treatment

Effective treatment of developmental dysphasia must be based on differential diagnosis that distinguishes it from language impairment caused by hearing loss, mental retardation, emotional disturbance, social deprivation, or peripheral articulation problems. Once the diagnosis is established, assessment of receptive (discrimination, memory, comprehension) and expressive (retrieval, sequencing, auditory analysis/synthesis, syntax, oral formulation, and auditory-motor functioning) language functions must be undertaken in both structured (i.e., standardized tests) and unstructured (i.e., interactive classroom or home) settings (Johnson and Myklebust, 1967; Calfee and Sutter, 1982). Generally, principles for treatment of language disorders (Johnson and Myklebust, 1967) stress the importance of

- Proceeding from comprehension to expression.
- Reducing the length of language stimulation through structure; isolating parts of utterances.
- Timing presentation of language meaning units with presentation of experience.
- Proceeding from comprehension in isolation to comprehension in context.
- Selecting language taught from the child's experience.
- Proceeding from concrete meanings (unitary) to abstract meanings (multiple), beginning with real objects if needed.
- Gradually reducing the structure provided for the child to aid correct responses.

Word retrieval difficulties may be addressed by fostering self-cueing with phonologically, conceptually, or idiosyncratically related words, or with visual cues. Syntax and oral formulation problems may be addressed by activities that help the child learn the structure of language, such as sentence building, completing partial utterances, or unscrambling sentences or words in a sentence. Difficulty executing the motor patterns

FEATURE TABLE 22-1. ORAL LANGUAGE DISORDERS (DYSPHASIAS)

Discriminating Features	Consistent Features	Variable Features
1. At least average verbal or non-verbal intellectual potential 2. Significant discrepancy between intellectual potential and performance on measures of oral language functioning (where *significant* is defined by an analysis of chronologic age [CA], intellectual potential [MA], and years in school [grade age (GA)], and used to arrive at critical age and grade levels with which test scores may be compared; see example below)	1. Not a unitary disorder; heterogenous population demonstrating a variety of levels of functioning in facets of receptive and expressive language 2. Co-occur with disorders in other symbol systems such as reading, written language, and mathematics 3. Deficient functioning in any one or combination of auditory discrimination, comprehension, temporal sequencing, syntax, grammaticality, word retrieval, or formulation	1. Occur concomitant with other handicapping conditions or extrinsic influences (but are not primarily attributed to either) 2. Deficient performance in skills representing either a receptive, expressive, or global language disorder 3. Delayed language acquisition 4. Neurodevelopmental motor soft signs

Calculation of Significant Discrepancy Between Achievement and Potential

EXAMPLE: An individual 18 years, 7 months of age with an IQ of 120.

	Example	Comments	Computation
Chronologic age (CA)	= 18.6	To convert a chronologic age based on a 12-month year to a decimal in base ten: $$\frac{Months}{12} = \frac{x}{10}$$	$7/12 = x/10$ $x = 6$ $18\text{–}7 = 18.6$
Intelligence quotient (IQ)	= 120		
Mental age (MA)	= 22.3	MA = IQ score (full scale or the higher of verbal or nonverbal score) ÷ 100 × CA: $$MA = \frac{IQ}{100} \times CA$$	$\frac{120}{100} \times 18.6 = 22.3$
Grade age (GA)	= 13.4	GA = CA − 5.2 (a constant)	$18.6 - 5.2 = 13.4$
Average	= 18.1	$$\frac{CA + MA + GA}{3}$$	$\frac{18.6 + 22.3 + 13.4}{3} = 18.1$
Critical age	= 15.3	Critical age = 85% of the average (which is 1 standard deviation below the mean): Critical age = average × 0.85 Thus, age scores that fall below this critical age represent a significant discrepancy. In this example, an age score of the *Peabody Picture Vocabulary Test,* a receptive language test, of less than 15.3 would reflect a significant discrepancy between achievement and potential.	$18.1 \times 0.85 = 15.3$
Critical grade	= 10.1	Critical grade = critical age − 5.2 (a constant). Thus, a grade score falling below a critical grade of 10.1 would reflect a significant discrepancy between achievement and potential.	$15.3 - 5.2 = 10.1$

necessary for speech may be aided by fostering the child's awareness of lingual actions through imitation, using a mirror, or kinesthetic or verbal cues. In working with older school-age children, reading and writing may be used to enhance oral language (e.g., fostering organiza-tion, which may positively affect memory). These and other suggestions may be found in Johnson and Myklebust (1967), Myklebust (1971a, b), and Johnson (1985). Furthermore, working in natural communicative settings is suggested, especially with older children, as well as building in the element of awareness (i.e., explicit teaching of strategies or techniques of oral expression) so as to make the child a conscious partner in learning (Larson and McKinley, 1985).

The prognosis for children exhibiting developmental dysphasia suggests that skilled remedial teaching, begun as early as possible, is effective in sustaining the forward movement of language development throughout the school-age years in cases in which language development might have otherwise been arrested (Gaddes, 1980). However, residual language difficulties affecting communication typically persist into adolescence and adulthood (Wiig and Semel, 1984; Klecan-Aker, 1985).

DISORDERS OF WRITTEN LANGUAGE

Reading (Dyslexia)

The most commonly recognized form of developmental learning disorders is specific reading disabilities or dyslexia (Tranel et al., 1987). The term *developmental dyslexia* refers to a condition manifest by extraordinary difficulty experienced by otherwise normal children in learning to identify printed words, presumably owing to neurologic dysfunction (Vellutino, 1987). Galaburda (1985), quoting Debray-Ritzen and Debray (1979), suggests that the first reference to difficulty with the written word in two otherwise normal subjects appeared in Eugene Labiche's *La Grammaire* (1867). Thereafter, in Britain, the first medical mention of specific learning disabilities was made by James Kerr (1897), the first description of specific reading disabilities, by William Morgan (1896), and the first extensive attempt to discuss developmental reading disturbances in light of contemporary neurologic knowledge, by James Hinshelwood (1917). Since then, increasing efforts by the practitioner and research communities have been directed at this diagnostic category. Currently the estimated prevalence of reading disabilities in the United States varies from 0.5% to 15% of the school-age population (Badian, 1984).

Pathology

A total of five brains of dyslexic individuals have been studied. All have been male and have been affected by allergies or other disorders involving the immune system. Ages at autopsy have been between 12 and 30 years. Quoting the findings of Galaburda and his colleagues (1985), alterations in the brains have been of two types: (1) All cases have shown developmental anomalies in the cerebral cortex and some had alterations in subcortical structures. (2) In the four brains analyzed for asymmetry, all four showed deviation from the standard asymmetry pattern of the language regions (instead of the left temporal language region being larger, there was symmetry).

The developmental cortical alterations consist of dysplasias (disordered cellular architecture) and ectopias (presence of neural elements in places where they are normally absent). The mildest cortical dysplasia consisted of a disturbance of the normal laminar arrangement of nerve cells; the most severe dysplasia consisted of marked distortions of the cortex; certain nerve cell layers were absent, some of the layers were fused, and there was abnormal cortical folding (Galaburda, 1985, p. 27).

The ectopias consisted of collections of neurons in the first layer of the cortex (normally devoid of groups of nerve cells) or, in more severe cases, of displaced, disorganized groups of neurons. Often accompanying these cortical dysplasias and ectopias were abnormal bundles of nerve fibers and abnormal blood vessels. In all cases there was striking asymmetry of distribution anomalies, with the left hemisphere primarily affected. Lesions showed a preference for the inferior frontal gyrus (site of anterior speech zones) and for the posterior temporoparietal region (site of posterior speech zones). Furthermore, all four cases showed symmetry of the planum temporale (which normally shows asymmetry). Also the Sylvian fissures were nearly symmetric, failing to show the normal significant differences in length on the two sides.

Galaburda feels that

information from the study of cortical anomalies in other developmental disorders, from the study of fetal brains, and from experimental studies in animals, suggests that these anomalies originate in fetal life and that they cannot be a result of damage at birth or any postnatal process. All available information points to a disorder occurring during the developmental period when young neurons are migrating to their positions in the cortex (from about the sixteenth week to the twenty-fourth week of gestation) (p. 28).

The effects are most severe between 20 and 24 weeks. Galaburda concludes that these developmental lesions are accompanied by the reorganization of the architectural and connectional patterns of the hemispheres, which affect the standard pattern of asymmetry in the brain.

Geschwind and Behan (1982, 1984) examined the relationship among handedness, immune disease, and learning disorders. They found that left-handed individuals had markedly higher frequencies of immune diseases (e.g., Crohn's disease, celiac disease, thyroid disorders, ulcerative colitis, and myasthenia gravis) and of developmental learning disorders than right-handed individuals. Smith et al. (1983), studying several families in which dyslexia was prevalent, have been able to link the dyslexic trait to chromosome 15 in that most affected members of the family share a common morphologic pattern of this chromosome. The current focus of research in this area is to explore further the immunologic and hormonal influences on the development of hemispheric asymmetry and cortical anomalies.

Signs and Symptoms

Dyslexic and reading-disabled children represent a heterogeneous population and hence a varied symptomatology. Discrete subgroups within the reading-disabled population have been proposed by a number of researchers. The assumption is that dyslexia can result from a defect in any one of several independent processes, including, for example, language skills, motor-speech fluency, or visual-spatial perception (Mattis et al., 1975). These three groups do not exhaust the list of possible critical defects but illustrate the presence of differential symptomatology.

Children with underlying language disorders may exhibit faulty letter-sound associations, poor word retrieval, or deficiencies in vocabulary development. Motor-speech dysfluency may be manifest by poor use of phonic skills in word attack, dysphonetic spelling and reading errors (i.e., errors that do not resemble the sounds in the target word), and an inability to blend phonemes or reproduce graphemes. Underlying visual-perceptual disorders may be suggested by poor discrimination of visual-verbal similarities and poor storage and retrieval of visually represented letters/words. Traditionally, visual or auditory deficits have been thought to underlie contrasting symptomatology associated with reading failure. Visual deficits—such as visual discrimination difficulties, poor visual scanning, visual reversals, difficulty retaining visual sequences, and relating visually recognized word parts to the whole (e.g., *plastic/plasticity*)—have been observed to co-occur, in contrast to auditory deficits, such as difficulty distinguishing similarities and differences between sounds (as in short vowel sounds), segmenting and blending sounds in words, and relating visual symbols to their auditory counterparts (Johnson and Myklebust, 1967). In general, difficulties often cited

include slow reading rate, letter reversals (e.g., *b/d*), limited ability to use information from known words to decode others related to them, difficulty using contextual cues to aid in identification of unfamiliar words, and general difficulty with transfer, coupled wtih the need for extensive practice for achieving automaticity. Reading comprehension difficulties are typically evidenced when oral language deficits in understanding spoken vocabulary, syntax, or discourse are present. Comprehension and oral decoding deficits may or may not co-occur.

Treatment

Treatment for children with dyslexia should be based on a complete assessment of auditory and visual subprocesses and intersensory integration, and an evaluation of reading performance itself under conditions of single-word decoding, reading extended text, silent and oral reading, and considering word identification and comprehension. Sufficient oral language measures are indicated, because many impaired readers are also impaired in the language domain, and these impairments influence reading performance. Evaluation and subsequent remediation with tasks in units that most closely approximate reading as it occurs in a child's everyday experience is preferable to contrived tasks alone (Vellutino and Shub, 1982). For children who evidence deficits in auditory language functioning, treatment foci include initial emphasis on developing a sight vocabulary, working from decoding larger to smaller word components (Johnson and Myklebust, 1967), and developing comprehension, if needed, through attention to word knowledge and sentence and text structure. Fostering awareness of the structure of language by explicitly teaching the graphic (visual patterns), phonologic (auditory patterns), orthographic (word structure), semantic, and syntactic regu-

FEATURE TABLE 22-2. READING DISORDERS (DYSLEXIA)

Discriminating Features	Consistent Features	Variable Features
1. At least average verbal or nonverbal intellectual potential 2. Significant discrepancy between intellectual potential and performance on measures of reading (where *significant* is defined by an analysis of chronologic age [CA], intellectual potential [MA], and years in school [grade age (GA)], and used to arrive at critical age and grade levels with which test scores may be compared; see example in Feature Table 22–1)	1. Not a unitary disorder; heterogenous population demonstrating a variety of levels of functioning in facets of reading performance 2. Co-occur with language disorders 3. Co-occur with writing disorders 4 Deficient functioning in any one or combination of reading silently or orally, individual words or words in context, decoding or comprehension, or rate	1. Occur concomitant with other handicapping conditions or extrinsic influences (but are not primarily attributed to either) 2. Deficient performance in skills representing either disrupted visual processes (e.g., poor sight vocabulary, reversals), disrupted lexical or semantic access (e.g., poor reading comprehension), disrupted phonemic processes (e.g., poor decoding of multisyllabic words), or combinations thereof 3. 35 to 45 percent heritable 4. Neurodevelopmental motor soft signs 5. Neurologic soft signs of abnormality (asymmetries of associated movements and reflexes, choreiform movements, diffuse EEG abnormalities)

larities of language has recently been strongly advocated (Liberman, 1983).

Children whose visual functioning is deficient may have difficulty retaining the image of whole words, thus initially requiring a more phonetic approach. Teaching isolated sounds and blending them into meaningful wholes may be indicated if auditory skills are adequate. Work on improving visual memory, sequentialization, and efficient visual scanning may also be helpful (Johnson and Myklebust, 1967). Teaching more efficient learning strategies in general—such as techniques, principles, or rules needed to facilitate the acquisition, manipulation, integration, storage, or retrieval of information necessary for reading—has also been suggested (Schumaker et al., 1982). Bakker and Licht (1986), using a neuropsychologic stimulation model (versus an information processing model), have reported positive results by selective presentation of musical and visual verbal stimuli to the right and left hemispheres, respectively, to stimulate otherwise weak hemispheric processing of information that contrasting hemispheres are best suited to interpret.

In a survey of studies that have followed school or clinic groups of dyslexic children to adulthood (Herjanic and Penick, 1972), two general conclusions were reported: (1) Regarding educational and vocational status, most dyslexic students finish high school, many go on for further training, and most are employed in either skilled or unskilled jobs. (2) At least some aspects of reading disabilities persist into adulthood; even the most vocationally successful groups report or show some residual problems, such as slow reading rate and poor spelling, in adulthood (Forell and Hood, 1985). Spreen (1982) found that reading disabilities affect the occupational, social, and personal lives of impaired individuals. Most dyslexics, however, find employment and live independent lives, though those with lower intelligence (i.e., IQs below 80) have less optimistic outcomes (Rawson, 1968).

Written Language (Dysgraphia)

Lerner (1981) notes that writing is the most prevalent communicative difficulty for children labeled learning impaired. Writing requires a level of abstraction not equaled in oral language in that it is removed in time and space from its intended audience. Whereas oral speech is acquired spontaneously, the ability to communicate in writing is a result of conscious effort and explicit learning. Writing requires the intention to communicate, formulation of the message (retrieval of the auditory-language symbols and sequencing of the content), retrieval of the graphic-language symbols corresponding to the auditory-language symbols, and retrieval and execution of the graphomotor sequences necessary for writing (Gaddes, 1980).

The term *dysgraphia* has been used to refer to a partial inability to write because of a dysfunction in the brain. It is a defect that is symbolic in nature in that the individual cannot combine auditory and visual verbal information into the motor actions needed for writing (Myklebust, 1965). Dysgraphia was first recognized in adults. Orton (1937) identified developmental dysgraphia in children who were developmentally retarded in learning to write and attributed it to abnormal development of necessary areas of the brain. In addition, Sweeney and Rourke (1985) assert that distinct neurologic deficits prompt development of a variety of unsuccessful spelling patterns and strategies. Other problems evidenced in children with written language deficits may be observed in mechanics (i.e., punctuation and capitalization), syntax, and ideation. Although the formal features of writing (i.e., handwriting, spelling, punctuation) have often been emphasized over elements such as ideation, organization of ideas, and creativity of expression, research findings suggest that 90% or more of learning-disabled individuals have significant deficits in written expressive language across the range of subskills comprising this area of functioning (Blalock, 1981; Gregg, 1983).

Pathology

Most lesion studies of individuals with writing disorders have been conducted with adults. Luria's work (1966) with adults suggests that the occipito-temporal-parietal areas bilaterally, and the left manual sensorimotor strips, are all intimately involved in written language. Areas responsible for creating and planning the message may be more diffusely represented, but the auditory-visual-motor areas seem largely responsible for the mechanical production (Gaddes, 1980).

Gaddes (1980) reports a number of case studies of children sustaining traumatic brain injury and their effect on written language. Cerebellar ataxia is a disorder of neuromuscular coordination resulting from disturbances in the cerebellum that may affect any motor activity, including legibility of writing and speed of production when it affects the hands. This condition does not cause paralysis but an inability to coordinate motor movements in a normal manner (Myklebust, 1965). EEG dysrhythmia activity over the manual area of the dominant left motor strip has been reported in the case of a 6-year-old boy evidencing significantly disturbed writing and manual skills (Gaddes, 1980). In this case, the boy's dysgraphia was caused by apraxia, difficulty in relating the mental images of words and the motor system for writing. Apraxia is thought to be a symptom of injury to the sensorimotor elaboration areas of the cortex such that there is a deficiency in remembering the motor sequences for writing (Myklebust, 1965). Gaddes (1980), citing Luria (1973), reports that, if a dysgraphic child's visual-motor integration is so defective as to preclude copying, a brain lesion most likely exists bilaterally in the parietal-occipital lobes, or unilaterally in the same area of the language-dominant hemisphere.

Morton and Kershner (1987) report that cases of acquired and developmental disabilities in reading and spelling indicate that accessing the visual-spatial features and gestalt of word configurations (i.e., recognizing that a word "looks right") may be a right hemisphere function (though some oppose this view; see Sweeney and Rourke, 1985), whereas the left hemisphere may be specialized for generating phonologic codes and for applying sound-to-sound correspondence rules (Aaron, 1982; Hynd and Hynd, 1984). Gaddes (1980) asserts further that dysfunction in the left motor or premotor area of the brain may result in sequencing problems in spelling (in addition to awkward or slow handwriting); minimal dysfunction in the posterior parts of the brain may result in poor letter and word recognition; temporal lobe dysfunction in the language-dominant hemisphere may result in poor phonetic discrimination and associated aphasic symptomatology; whereas diffuse damage is likely to impair the cross-modal integration relating these several cortical areas. Behaviorally, this may translate into poor handwriting, defective spelling, or inferior linguistic expression.

Signs and Symptoms

There are three main disorders associated with written expression (Johnson and Myklebust, 1967; Gaddes, 1980; Chalfant and Scheffelin, 1969). These include disorders of visual-motor integration, perceptual/memory deficits, and formulation and syntax. Deficits in visual-motor integration are indicated when the child can speak and read but cannot recall and execute the motor patterns necessary to transduce from the visual system to the motor system. The child may have difficulty with a number of learned motor activities, such as tying shoes, opening containers, or gross motor activities (e.g., bicycle riding), in addition to writing problems. The chief identifying characteristic of this disorder in writing is an inability to copy.

Perceptual deficits (in either the auditory or the visual system) result in errors in spelling related to visual discrimination (e.g., writing letters/words visually similar to the target letter/word) or auditory perception (e.g., misarticulation and misspelling, writing letters/words that sound like the target letter/word). Difficulty with revisualization or reauditorization is manifest by adequate recognition of letters or words but inability to recall the visual image of a letter or word, or to recall the sounds of the letters from hearing the spoken word. Children with revisualization deficits can copy because their difficulty is not in executing the motor patterns of writing but in invoking images of the visual symbols. Reading errors related to deficits in visual discrimination, sequencing, or memory will be evidenced in spelling errors of similar origin (e.g., *trial/trail*); auditory misperception of words will similarly be evident in spelling, as in miswriting words or omission of syllables (Johnson and Myklebust, 1967). Significant auditory deficits coupled with adequate visual functioning typically result in phonetically inaccurate spelling errors on nonautomatized words that may be impossible for the reader to decipher (e.g., *alogads/alligator*). In contrast, a child with good auditory skills but poor visual memory may spell words incorrectly but phonetically accurate, and thus comprehensible to the reader (e.g., *vare/very*) (Boder, 1973).

Finally, deficiency in formulation and syntax may be evidenced by children who have underlying oral language comprehension or expressive language deficits. Characteristics of a child's oral syntax (e.g., simplicity or inaccuracy of expression) may be manifest in written expression, and comprehension deficits such as limitations in word meaning may be reflected in concrete ideation in writing and limited content. Dysnomia in oral language may be reflected in written language by inability to recall desired words.

Treatment

Treatment of children with dysfunction in the use of written language is based on an assessment of the subskills

FEATURE TABLE 22-3. WRITING DISORDERS (DYSGRAPHIA)

Discriminating Features	Consistent Features	Variable Features
1. At least average verbal or nonverbal intellectual potential 2. Significant discrepancy between intellectual potential and performance on measures of writing (where *significant* is defined by an analysis of chronologic age [CA], intellectual potential [MA], and years in school [grade age (GA)], and used to arrive at critical age and grade levels with which test scores may be compared; see example in Feature Table 22–1)	1. Not a unitary disorder; heterogenous population demonstrating a variety of levels of functioning in facets of writing performance 2. Co-occur with reading and language disorders 3. Deficient functioning in any one or combination of motor control or planning affecting legibility, spelling, syntax/grammaticality, ideation, or formulation	1. Occur concomitant with other handicapping conditions or extrinsic influences (but are not primarily attributed to either) 2. Deficient performance in skills representing either disrupted visual-motor, auditory-verbal (e.g., syntax or dysphonetic spelling errors), visual-verbal (e.g., over-phoneticized spellings, capitalization omissions), or combined processing deficits

involved in writing and written language itself. Auditory, visual, and motor processes, and spelling, punctuation, capitalization, syntax, and ideation must be evaluated. Analysis of several samples of discourse with varying degrees of structure is also helpful. Instruction-for-writing deficits owing to execution of motor patterns may be addressed by demonstrating motor movements accompanied by verbal instructions. Observation of writing movements, not still models, appears to be most effective (Furner, 1983), along with fostering self-verbalization to cue memory. Directional cues (e.g., arrows) and stencils or templates may also be helpful (Johnson and Myklebust, 1967). Developing the underlying auditory skills of phonetically inaccurate spellers by phonetic analysis and synthesis of words into letter chunks and individual letters is indicated. Intensive visual analysis by increasing the visual salience of visual-spatial features of word configurations may correct visually based spelling errors. Formulation and syntax difficulties may be helped by using oral language to teach monitoring of errors, doing structured written exercises for punctuation and syntactic patterns, and using oral language based on experience to foster ideation. Strategy training has also been advocated (Deshler et al., 1981), such as in organizational techniques, error monitoring, and self-reinforcement.

Clinical observation suggests that some of the problems reported in children impaired in written language persist into adulthood (Vogel, 1985). Spelling difficulties often persist even if reading problems are largely ameliorated (Rutter and Yule, 1973). In mechanics, punctuation is particularly problematic for learning-disabled adults (Herbert and Czerniejewski, 1976). Blalock (1981) reports that knowledge of the rules of punctuation and capitalization continues to be severely limited for some learning-impaired adults, whereas others have difficulty monitoring their written work.

Other approaches employ the use of word processors and tape recorders as compensatory devices.

DISORDERS OF MATHEMATICAL FUNCTION (DYSCALCULIAS)

Mathematics is a symbolic language that expresses relationships of quantity, space, form, distance, order, and time (Johnson and Myklebust, 1967). Initially the child assimilates and integrates nonverbal experience, on which an understanding of mathematic relationships is based, and then learns to express these relationships symbolically. Successful performance relates to developing a concept of number (abstract mental concepts having meaning in terms of quantity); a concept of relative value (e.g., size, distance) related to a system of spatial coordinates; and an understanding of and the ability to use the language of mathematics, as in numerical operations (e.g., +, −) and sequencing (e.g., the sequence of steps needed to solve a long-division problem, or the meaning

of sequence in the number sentence *five divided by four* versus *four divided by five*).

Some make a distinction between arithmetic and mathematics, the former being a branch of mathematics dealing with real numbers and their computation, and the latter, the broader term for the abstract science of space and numbers dealing with spatial configurations and the interrelations and abstractions of numeration (Chalfant and Scheffelin, 1969). McCloskey and associates (1985) point out the difference between reading and writing numbers, and calculation of numbers. Some classify the ability to read numbers (numerals) as part of the dyslexic syndrome while reserving the term *dyscalculia* for defective ability to perform calculation (Hermann, 1959).

Comparatively little attention has been devoted to children with disorders in mathematic reasoning and performance, as contrasted with reading disorders (Pellegrino and Goldman, 1987). However, Kosc (1981) estimates that 6% of the school-age population with normal intelligence is dyscalculic. Other incidence statistics are widely varied. McLeod and Crump (1978) suggest that only 10% of learning-disabled students have severe deficits in mathematics, but over half of the population may require supplementary instruction in mathematics, especially at intermediate and secondary school levels (McLeod and Armstrong, 1982).

Pathology

Disorders of calculation were first observed in adults. "Henschen (1919) observed that difficulties in identifying and naming printed or written figures or numbers could occur without disorders of calculation, and that number blindness could occur without any accompanying blindness for words. He described this condition and named it *acalculia*" (Chalfant and Scheffelin, 1969, p. 122). In postmortem studies, Henschen found acalculia to be present with accompanying lesions in the occipital, frontal, parietal, and temporal areas. On the basis of his findings, he concluded that the integrity of several areas of the cortex is likely necessary for calculation and that there was a separate system responsible for use of language (Chalfant and Scheffelin, 1969). Gerstmann (1927) found dyscalculia to co-occur with other characteristics (i.e., finger agnosia, right-left disorientation, agraphia), constituting a syndrome. Based on autopsy studies with adults, he associated the syndrome with organic damage to the parieto-occipital region in the dominant hemisphere corresponding to the angular gyrus and the second occipital convolution (Chalfant and Scheffelin, 1969). However, subsequent research (Heimberger et al., 1957) has failed to support the conclusion that the brain damage responsible for Gerstmann's syndrome is limited to a prescribed area. Luria (1966) suggests that lesions in the left infero-parietal or parieto-occipital area cause disintegration of visual-spatial synthesis, resulting in alexia for numbers and consequent difficulty with calculation; lesions of the left temporal region result in difficulty calculating aloud or relying on speech processes for solving arithmetic problems; lesions of the frontal lobes affect the regulatory role of the verbal system necessary for planning a problem-solving approach; and lesions in the occipital area affect visual retention and the visualization necessary for manipulating numbers.

Developmental dyscalculia and disorders of mathematic functioning are less well defined than the acquired condition. However, the limited number of cases that have come to postmortem suggest that the difficulty is related to abnormal development or underdevelopment of the parietal, temporal, and occipital cortexes bilaterally, and of the intercerebral mechanisms with hearing and language (Gaddes, 1980). Tranel and colleagues (1987) studied a group of developmentally dyscalculic patients, ages 14 years to middle adulthood, who demonstrated a constellation of symptomatology, including chronic emotional and social maladjustment; defective nonverbal, visuo-spatial cognitive functioning; and academic failure in arithmetic not accompanied by failure in reading and spelling. Paralinguistic skills were deficient but verbal functioning was intact. Of the 11 subjects, two showed left hemispheric neurologic deficits, including asymmetric posturing of the left arm and hand during complex gait, left pronator drift, and facial asymmetry. All but one of the other patients reported a significant history of physical clumsiness and awkwardness. Computed tomographic scans were normal in all patients; however, five EEGs revealed diffuse, mild abnormalities.

Grunau and Low (1987), examining the neurophysiologic correlates of mathematics performance in 41 adolescents, ages 12 to 15 years, reported that "changes from resting values in theta activity (measured during a perceptual task) at both right- and left-hemisphere locations, left-hemisphere theta activity during a verbal task, and right-hemisphere alpha activity during a visual-perceptual task made significant contributions to iden-

tification of adolescents' arithmetic calculation skills." This would suggest that calculation operations are not lateralized, consistent with findings of other research (Strang and Rourke, 1985). Giannitrapani (1982) performed factor analyses on EEG power density scores recorded during a verbal task and a mental arithmetic task and also found none of the factors related to silent arithmetic to reflect strong asymmetrics. Apparently tasks such as computation require spatial visualization in interaction with sequential reasoning and depend on left and right hemisphere cooperation (Grunau and Low, 1987).

Signs and Symptoms

Dysfunction in the understanding or use of mathematics may be associated either with language problems or visual-spatial abilities, or with disorders in logical and quantitative thinking (Kosc, 1981). Oral language deficits may be seen in difficulty understanding the words used to describe operations or word meaning in story problems. Reauditorization problems, as in difficulty recalling the auditory equivalents of numerical symbols, affect oral problem solving and oral number fact drills. Strang and Rourke (1985) have found that the majority of children who experience difficulties in arithmetic calculation do so because of deficiencies in one or more linguistic abilities. Visual-spatial disturbances may be manifest as difficulty aligning numbers in computation or conceptualizing mathematic values related to relative size or distance, while visual-perceptual problems may be evidenced in misreading operational signs (e.g., $=$, $+$), numbers (e.g., 9/6), or inattention to the significance of sequence (e.g., 574/547). Difficulty with nonverbal symbolic representation and quantitative thinking may be suggested by inability to estimate calculation outcomes, count meaningfully (i.e., establish one-to-one correspondence), grasp the meaning of process signs, or interpret graphs or maps. Furthermore, graphomotor

FEATURE TABLE 22-4. DISORDERS OF MATHEMATICAL FUNCTIONING (DYSCALCULIA)

Discriminating Features	Consistent Features	Variable Features
1. At least average verbal or non-verbal intellectual potential 2. Significant discrepancy between intellectual potential and performance on measures of mathematics achievement (where *significant* is defined by an analysis of chronologic age [CA], intellectual potential [MA], and years in school [grade age (GA)], and used to arrive at critical age and grade levels with which test scores may be compared; see example in Feature Table 22-1)	1. Not a unitary disorder; heterogenous population demonstrating a variety of levels of functioning in facets of mathematics performance 2. Deficient functioning in any one or combination of performing written/oral mathematic calculations, or understanding/application of mathematic concepts	1. Occur concomitant with other handicapping conditions or extrinsic influences (but are not primarily attributed to either) 2. Deficient performance in skills representing either a language-based disorder (e.g., poor comprehension of instructional vocabulary), disrupted visual-nonverbal processing (e.g., inaccurate reading of operational signs), or a combination thereof 3. Associated wtih slow eye-hand coordination, poor tactile form recognition, finger-agnosia, cognitive inflexibility, gross motor incoordination, and/or poor socio-emotional adjustment, if nonlanguage based

production of the symbols of mathematics is affected by dysgraphia, in which the child may be unable to retrieve and execute the motor patterns necessary to write numbers (Johnson and Myklebust, 1967). Deficient performance may also be seen in problem-solving procedures (such as in remembering and following a sequence of steps), monitoring performance, shifting set (as when two operations are required to solve a problem), and general impulsivity in problem solving strategies (Moses, 1984; Pellegrino and Goldman, 1987).

Strang and Rourke (1985) suggest evidence for a nonverbal perceptual organizational output deficit (NPOOD) syndrome represented by difficulty with mechanical arithmetic coupled with poor socioemotional adjustment, gross motor incoordination, and difficulty with all types of written work. This is consistent with clinical observations that poor mathematic performance may co-occur with poor spatial and left-right orientation (e.g., as in the tendency to get lost easily), physical clumsiness or awkwardness, and low social maturity (Johnson and Myklebust, 1967).

Treatment

Effective treatment of disorders of mathematic functioning is based on comprehensive assessment of performance in arithmetic calculation and word problem solving, and the underlying functions contributing to adequate performance in both. These include language abilities (comprehension, reauditorization, auditory sequencing, reading), graphomotor skills, visual-spatial organization, revisualization, visual sequencing, and nonverbal concepts of form, shape, distance, time, and quantity (Johnson and Myklebust, 1967). Kosc (1981) stresses the importance of determining if the disturbance in mathematic abilities is isolated or combined with disturbances in other symbolic-communicative functions, and of differentiating among verbal, spatial, reasoning, and other forms of dyscalculia. He also suggests examining the strategies and compensatory techniques the child uses, and the effect of outside assistance during problem solving. Strang and Rourke (1985) suggest that mechanical arithmetic be made as much a verbal task as possible, using oral and written cues initially to represent the visual aspects of the operation. This technique is the most effective for children who have strong auditory and language skills. Children with accompanying language disorders may need direct instruction in the language of mathematics (e.g., *less than, greater than*).

Suggestions to aid in the visual/conceptual aspects of mathematic problem solving include using graph paper to help align the numbers for calculation, color coding portions of the problem to cue the proper sequence of steps, using concrete physical aids (e.g., cuisinaire rods, number lines) to represent mathematic concepts (e.g., conservation of quantity regardless of varying the size of the units comprising it), and relating the mathematic operation to everyday living. Visual presentations may be helpful for those who have difficulty remembering or visualizing figures and numerical/spatial relationships (Johnson and Mykelbust, 1967). Cognitive strategies training has been used successfully with children with mathematic deficits (Montague and Bos, 1986) in teaching children how to structure problems, do stepwise analysis of solution procedures, and monitor performance. In general the focus must be on logic and rational thought using memory (as in memorization of math facts) and other subskills to serve this end.

Results of intervention studies suggest that children with disorders reflected in mathematic performance respond positively to systematic, direct instruction, including cumulative and distributed practice of math facts, direct instruction in math vocabulary, and in the procedures and monitoring of problem solving (Johnson, 1987). However, there is evidence to suggest that disorders in mathematic functioning in children persist into adolescence and adulthood. Johnson and Blalock (1982) found that many adults in a clinical sample of 93 individuals had difficulty with one or more aspects of mathematics and arithmetic. Although most understood the basic operations, their general independence and social maturity was limited by difficulty in computation and mathematic reasoning.

DISORDERS OF NONVERBAL FUNCTION

Over twenty years ago, Johnson and Myklebust (1967) discussed the presence of nonverbal learning disorders in children. They described a group of children having a constellation of problems, including defective body image, inability to learn gross motor patterns, poor sense of orientation in time and space, social imperception, and distractibility. They also found problems of social perception to occur frequently in association with disorders of arithmetic. These children were thought to be characterized by an inability to acquire the significance of many of the nonverbal aspects of daily experience owing to right hemisphere dysfunction. Since Johnson and Myklebust (1967) first delineated nonverbal learning disorders, there has been comparatively little interest in this area (Badian, 1986), even though nonverbal disorders, especially associated with social imperception, can be among the most debilitating.

Pathology

Spatial disorientation in adults—difficulty in right-left discrimination and in perceiving one's own body in space—has been attributed to damage to the occipital cortex and to cortical lesions in the infero-parietal and parietal-occipital areas (Luria, 1966). A number of studies also suggest that frontal lobe damage interferes with the ability to actively search, scan, or examine objects visually (Chalfant and Scheffelin, 1969), an effect possibly related to social imperception and spatial disorientation.

Findings related to the underlying pathology of neuropsychologic functions associated with nonverbal learning disorders in children are limited. Gaddes (1980) reported on the case of a boy diagnosed as having developmental right hemisphere dysfunction characterized by significant difficulty with spatial imaging and directionality. An EEG carried out at age 13 years showed a minimal dysrhythmia in the right occipital, parietal, and motor strip areas. More recently, Rourke (1987) and his colleagues have been investigating children who present with nonverbal learning disorders. Rourke reports bilateral tactile-perceptual deficits, usually more marked on the left side of the body, and bilateral psychomotor coordination deficiencies, similarly more marked on the left side of the body, in this population. Badian (1986), studying subjects ages 7 to 14 years, examined a number of her low-nonverbal-functioning subjects through brain electrical activity mapping (BEAM) (Duffy and McAnulty, 1985). At age 9 years, the BEAMs of the three subjects examined revealed abnormal brain activity bilaterally or in the right hemisphere, including the right temporal lobe. Rourke and associates (1983) have reported three case studies of children with right hemisphere dysfunction or documented damage. They describe the test results of these cases as suggestive of moderate chronic dysfunction of the temporo-parietal and possibly adjacent frontal regions of the right hemisphere (Badian, 1986).

Signs and Symptoms

Children with nonverbal disorders of learning may remain undiagnosed by their schools or are often referred for diagnostic evaluation at older ages than children with language-based problems. Difficulties commonly precipitating diagnosis include problems in arithmetic, reading comprehension, and general organizational skills, affecting, for example, written language, study habits, and task completion (Badian, 1986). Difficulties may be noted in nonachievement areas of functioning, such as engaging in pretend behavior; understanding the significance and implications of gestures, facial expressions, and body language in general; understanding humor; and understanding the relevance of time, space, size, or direction. Social immaturity, deficient social perception, disturbances in body image and self-perception, poor perception of visual nonverbal stimuli (e.g., pictures), and difficulty with nonverbal motor learning (e.g., cutting with scissors, skipping), are also characteristic. These deficits are due to a fundamental distortion of the child's perception of experience itself, not chiefly to the ability to use symbols to represent experience (Johnson and Myklebust, 1967).

Treatment

As in other areas of functioning, effective treatment is based on an assessment of a child's perception of nonverbal experience as related to orientation in space, time, left-right orientation, body image, social perception, and perceptual-motor skills. Teaching aimed at improving attention to significant aspects of nonverbal experience, and associating meaning therewith, is the focus (Johnson and Myklebust, 1967). Children who have difficulty organizing their environment visually and spatially may be helped by being taught to use verbalization, visual reference points, and a systematic way to scan their environment visually. Acquiring concepts of left-right orientation begins with teaching the child orientation to his own body's left and right sides, then left-right orientation with reference to others and then to objects. Using a mirror to develop body image and tactile stimulation, as in having the child close his or her eyes and identify on which side he or she has been touched, may be effective. Improving the child's sense of social nonverbal meanings, such as the use of gesture, may be encouraged by using pictures, films, or role-playing situations to teach the use and meaning of visual movement patterns. Verbalizing the social significance of the actions of others may also help to improve a child's awareness of social nuances. The meaning of facial expressions is an impor-

FEATURE TABLE 22–5. DISORDERS OF NONVERBAL FUNCTIONING

Discriminating Features	Consistent Features	Variable Features
1. At least average verbal or nonverbal intellectual potential 2. Significant discrepancy between intellectual potential and performance on measures of nonverbal functioning (where *significant* is defined by an analysis of chronologic age [CA], intellectual potential [MA], and years in school [grade age (GA)], and used to arrive at critical age and grade levels with which test scores may be compared; see example in Feature Table 22–1)	1. Not a unitary disorder; heterogenous population demonstrating a variety of levels of functioning on nonverbal tasks 2. Co-occur with relative proficiency in rote verbal capacities necessary for aspects of reading and spelling performance	1. Occur concomitant with other handicapping conditions or extrinsic influences (but are not primarily attributed to either) 2. Deficits in tactile perception, psychomotor coordination, and visual-spatial and organizational functioning 3. Deficits in aspects of higher language functioning (i.e., understanding humor, figurative language, and/or pragmatics) 4. Deficits in social perception, judgment, and/or interaction skills

tant area to address; this may be done by associating pictures of emotive experiences with facial expressions that might match them. Having a child practice facial expressions using a mirror may also be helpful. Children having difficulty with nonverbal motor learning, such as learning to ride a bicycle, need to learn ways of relating motor patterns they see to their own motor system. Helping a child form a kinesthetic image of the move-

ment, teaching him or her to verbally guide his actions, using a mirror, and breaking motor patterns into component parts may be helpful. These and other suggestions are elaborated by Johnson and Myklebust (1967). In general, the focus of treatment is on life skills by teaching a child to structure and understand nonverbal experience and to develop social facility and independence.

Follow-up studies conducted with children having disorders of nonverbal functioning suggest that these children are often dependent on adults for a longer period of time than normal children (Ozols and Rourke, 1985). Strang and Rourke (1985) studied eight adults with nonverbal disorders (NPOOD syndrome) and found that none held a job commensurate with his or her academic qualifications, and all exhibited emotional and social difficulties and poor adjustment in adult life. Because nonverbal disorders of learning often remain undiagnosed in childhood or are diagnosed later than other disorders (Badian, 1986), perhaps greater awareness of this area of difficulty will result in greater emphasis on developing early, effective intervention, thus attenuating the effect of these disorders in adulthood.

Pearls and Perils: Disorders of Higher Cerebral Function

1. Though there is evidence for a neurologic pathology underlying disorders of higher cerebral function in children, the evidence is incomplete and remains subject to multiple interpretations. Thus, when communicating this kind of information to parents or others, it must be ethically stated as such.
2. Testing instruments used to identify intellectual potential and levels or patterns of achievement or processing performance are imprecise. The way in which the child achieved the score is far more significant than the score itself. Thus, care in interpretation of raw test data is indicated.
3. Cultural and stylistic differences must be considered when interpreting the test or school performance of children who represent minority populations. Changing the context of performance may significantly alter the way in which the child responds and hence the conclusions drawn from that performance.
4. It is important to gain an understanding of the child as he or she functions in a structured school or testing context as well as in out-of-school, everyday settings of his or her choice. Understanding the role of context as it interacts with higher cognitive functioning is essential.
5. It is important to note that tests, such as those of memory or perception, are related to performance behaviors of interest (e.g., reading) by theoretical assumptions. The ways in which they relate are assumed on the basis of theories, which may change dramatically over time. Thus, the professional must be aware of the way in which these connections are represented, especially to nonprofessionals who might not be aware of the theoretical, not factual, basis of stated conclusions.
6. Effective treatment must be based on a range of activities wherein the adult and the child vary the distribution of control and mediation guiding task completion. If treatment is unitary and based on repeated, uniform, prestructured remedial sessions, generalization and transfer of learning are compromised.

CONCLUSION

This chapter has been organized into discrete sections discussing disorders of oral language, written language, mathematical functioning, and nonverbal functioning. Within each section, treatment suggestions have been given. The Pearls and Perils represent general suggestions that may be helpful in understanding and evaluating children evidencing disorders of higher cerebral function and in recommending treatment.

ANNOTATED BIBLIOGRAPHY

Ceci S (ed): *Handbook of Cognitive, Social and Neuropsychological Aspects of Learning Disabilities.* Hillsdale, NJ, Lawrence Erlbaum, 1986.

This volume is an eclectic collection of chapters on learning disorders in children, addressing controversial definitional issues, micro- and macro-level analyses of cognitive functioning (e.g., memory versus comprehension), psychosocial aspects of learning disorders, and neuropsychologic concomitants of learning disorders. The volume is noteworthy in its interdisciplinary treatment of learning disorders.

Cole M, Griffin P: A socio-historical approach to remediation. *Newsl Lab Compar Hum Cogn* 5(4):69–74, 1986.

This article represents an interesting discussion of treatment, emphasizing the role of language and context in mediating higher psychologic functioning. A way of understanding the relationship between subprocesses/components and the larger functional system of which they are a part, is discussed from a sociohistorical perspective.

Johnson D, Myklebust H: *Learning Disabilities: Educational Principles and Practices.* New York, Grune & Stratton, 1967.

A classic in the field of learning disabilities, this volume contains a series of informative chapters on the characteristics and treatment of childhood disorders of higher cognitive functioning. Chapters are organized according to areas of dysfunction and there is an explicit attempt to relate underlying deficits in processing to behavioral manifestations in reading, arithmetic, and other areas of underachievement.

Kirk U (ed): *Neuropsychology of Language, Reading, and Spelling.* New York, Academic Press, 1983.

This volume is a collection of chapters addressing issues related to neurodevelopmental factors in childhood cognitive disorders, peripheral mechanisms, and central mechanisms; there is also a series of discussions on developmental disorders in language, reading, and spelling from a neuropsychologic perspective.

Obrzut J, Hynd G (eds): *Child Neuropsychology,* Vol I: *Theory and Research.* New York, Harcourt, Brace, Jovanovich, 1986.

Obrzut J, Hynd G (eds): *Child Neuropsychology,* Vol II: *Clinical Practice.* New York, Harcourt, Brace, Jovanovich, 1986.

This extensive two-volume set presents current theory and research on important neurodevelopmental issues in Volume I, and a series of chapters on specific childhood neuropsychologic disorders, neuropsychologic evaluation of these disorders, and intervention and treatment in Volume II.

Rourke BP, Fisk JL, Strang JD: *The Neuropsychological Assessment of Children: A Treatment-Oriented Approach.* New York, Guilford Press, 1986.

This volume presents a coherent treatment-oriented framework for evaluating and discussing assessment issues and provides detailed case studies that illustrate this framework, as well as major assessment and intervention issues in childhood neuropsychology. The strength of the text is in its use of illustrative case studies and attention to treatment issues, which are often neglected in favor of assessment issues.

REFERENCES

Aaron P: The neuropsychology of developmental dyslexia, in Malatesha R, Aaron P (eds): *Reading Disorders.* Toronto, John Wiley & Sons, 1982.

Aram D, Nation J: Preschool language disorders and subsequent academic difficulties. *J Commun Dis* 13:159–170, 1980.

Ayres AJ: *Sensory Integration and Learning Disorders.* Los Angeles, Western Psychological Services, 1972.

Ayres AJ: Learning disabilities and the vestibular system. *J Learn Disabil* 11:30–41, 1978.

Badian NA: Reading disabilities in an epidemiological context: Incidence and environmental correlates. *Annu Rev Learn Disabil* 2:4–11, 1984.

Badian N: Nonverbal disorders of learning: The reverse of dyslexia? *Ann Dyslexia* 36:253–269, 1986.

Bakker D, Licht R: Learning to read: Changing horses in midstream, in Pavlidis GT, Fisher DF (eds): *Dyslexia: Its Neuropsychology and Treatment.* New York, John Wiley & Sons, 1986.

Birch HG: Nutritional factors in mental retardation. Paper presented at the Fifth Annual Neuropsychology Workshop, University of Victoria, Victoria, BC, Canada, 1970.

Blalock J: Persistent problems and concerns of young adults with learning disabilities, in Cruickshank W, Silvers A (eds): *Bridges to Tomorrow: The Best of ACLD,* Vol II. Syracuse, NY, Syracuse University Press, 1981.

Boder E: Developmental dyslexia: A diagnostic approach based on three atypical reading-spelling patterns. *Dev Med Child Neurol* 15:663–667, 1973.

Calfee R, Sutter L: Oral languagement assessment through formal discussion. *Top Lang Disord* 2(4):45–55, 1982.

Chalfant JC, Scheffelin MA: *Central Processing Dysfunctions in Children: A Review of Research.* NINDS Monograph No 9. Bethesda, Md, US Department of Health, Education, and Welfare, 1969.

Clements SD: *Minimal Brain Dysfunction in Children: Classification of Symptoms of Learning Disabled Children.* NINDS Monograph No 3. Bethesda, Md, US Department of Health, Education, and Welfare, 1966.

Cohen S: Low birthweight, in Brown CC (ed): *Childhood Learning Disabilities and Prenatal Risk: An Interdisciplinary Data Review for Health Care Professionals and Parents.* Skillman, NJ, Johnson & Johnson, 1985.

Coles G: The learning-disabilities test battery: Empirical and social issues. *Harv Educ Rev* 48(3):313–340, 1978.

Debray-Ritzen P, Debray FJ: *Comment Dépister une Dyslexie Chez un Petit Ecolier.* Paris, Fernand Nathan, 1979.

Delacato CH: *Neurological Organization and Reading.* Springfield, Ill, Charles C Thomas, 1966.

deQuiros J: Diagnosis of vestibular disorders in the learning disabled. *J Learn Disabil* 9:50–57, 1976.

Deshler DD, Alley GR, Warner MM, Schumaker JB: Instructional practices for promoting skill acquisition and generalization in severely learning disabled adolescents. *Learn Disabil Q* 4:415–421, 1981.

Doris J: Learning disabilities, in Ceci S (ed): *Handbook of Cognitive, Social, and Neuropsychological Aspects of Learning Disabilities.* Hillsdale, NJ, Lawrence Erlbaum, 1986.

Duffy FH, McAnulty GB: Brain electrical activity mapping (BEAM): The search for a physiological signature of dyslexia, in Duffy FH, Geschwind N (eds): *Dyslexia: A Neuroscientific Approach to Clinical Evaluation.* Boston, Little, Brown, 1985.

Farnham-Diggory S: Commentary: Time, now, for a little serious complexity, in Ceci S (ed): *Handbook of Cognitive, Social, and Neuropsychological Aspects of Learning Disabilities.* Hillsdale, NJ, Lawrence Erlbaum, 1986.

Farnham-Diggory S: *Learning Disabilities: A Psychological Perspective.* Cambridge, Mass, Harvard University Press, 1978.

Fernald GM: *Remedial Techniques in Basic School Subjects.* New York, McGraw-Hill, 1943.

Fisk JL, Rourke BP: Identification of subtypes of learning disabled children at three age levels. A neuropsychological, multivariate approach. *J Clin Neuropsychol* 1:289–310, 1979.

Fletcher JM, Morris R: Classification of disabled learners: Beyond exclusionary definitions, in Ceci S (ed): *Handbook of Cognitive, Social, and Neuropsychological Aspects of Learning Disabilities.* Hillsdale, NJ, Lawrence Erlbaum, 1986.

Forell E, Hood J: A longitudinal study of two groups of children with early reading problems. *Ann Dyslexia* 35:97–116, 1985.

Fox J: Debate on learning theory is shifting. *Science* 222:1219–1222, 1983.

Freides D, Barbat J, van Kampen-Horowitz L, et al: Blind evaluation of body reflexes and motor skills in learning disability. *J Autism Dev Disord* 10:159–171, 1980.

Frostig ML, Horne D: *The Frostig Program for the Develop-ment of Visual Perception.* Chicago, Follett, 1964.

Furner B: Developing handwriting ability: A perceptual learn-ing process. *Top Learn Learn Disabil* 3(3):41–54, 1983.

Gaddes WH: *Learning Disabilities and Brain Function: A Neuropsychological Approach.* New York, Springer-Verlag, 1980.

Galaburda A: Developmental dyslexia: A review of biological interactions. *Ann Dyslexia* 35:21–33, 1985.

Gerstmann J: Fingeragnosie und isolierte Agraphie: Ein neues Syndrome. *Z Neurol Psychiatr* 108:152–177, 1927.

Geschwind N, Behan P: Left-handedness: Association with im-mune disease, migraine and developmental learning disorder. *Proc Nat Acad Sci USA* 79:5097, 1982.

Geschwind N, Behan P: Laterality, hormones and immunity, in Geschwind N, Galaburda AM (eds): *Cerebral Dominance: The Biological Foundation.* Cambridge, Mass: Harvard University Press, 1984.

Getman GN: Vision: Its role and integrations in learning processes. *J Learn Disabil* 14:577–580, 1981.

Giannitrapani D: Localization of language and arithmetic func-tions via EEG factor analysis. *Psychol Psychiatr Behav* 7:39–55, 1982.

Gregg KN: College learning disabled writers: Error patterns and instructional alternatives. *J Learn Disabil* 16:334–338, 1983.

Grunau R, Low M: Cognitive and task-related EEG correlates of arithmetic performance in adolescents. *J Clin Exp Neuro-psychol* 9(5):563–574, 1987.

Heimberger R, De Meyer W, Reitan R: Neurological Signifi-cance of Gerstmann's Syndrome. Paper read at American Academy of Neurology, 1957.

Henschen SEZ: Über Sprach, Musik, und Rechenmechanismen und ihre Lokalisationen in Grosshirn. *Z Ges Neurol Psychiatr* 52:273–298, 1919.

Herbert MA, Czerniejewski C: Language and learning therapy in a community college. *Bull Orton Soc* 26:96–106, 1976.

Herjanic BM, Penick ED: Adult outcome of disabled child readers. *J Spec Educ* 6:397–410, 1972.

Hermann K: *Reading Disability.* Springfield, Ill, Charles C Thomas, 1959.

Hinshelwood J: *Congenital Word-Blindness.* Chicago, Medical Book Company, 1917.

Hynd G, Hynd C: Dyxlexia: Neuroanatomical/neurolinguistic perspectives. *Read Res Q* 19:482–498, 1984.

Johnson D: Using reading and writing to improve oral language skills. *Top Lang Disord* 5(3):55–69, 1985.

Johnson DJ: Review of Research on Specific Reading, Writing, and Mathematics Disorders. Unpublished manuscript, 1987.

Johnson DJ, Myklebust H: *Learning Disabilities: Educational Principles and Practices.* New York, Grune & Stratton, 1967.

Johnson DJ, Blalock J: Problems of mathematics in children with language disorders, in Lass N, McReynolds L, Northern J, Yoder D (eds): *Speech, Language and Hearing,* Vol 2. Philadelphia, WB Saunders, 1982.

Kephart NC: *The Slow Learner in the Classroom,* 2nd ed Columbus, Ohio, Charles E Merrill, 1971.

Kerr, J: School hygiene, in its mental, moral and physical aspects. Howard Medical Prize Essay. *J R Stat Soc* 60:613, 1897.

Kirk SA: Behavioral diagnosis and remediation of learning disabilities, in *Proceedings of the Annual Meeting of the Con-ference on Exploration into the Problems of the Perceptual-ly Handicapped Child,* Vol 1, 1963.

Kirk SA: *Teaching Reading to Slow Learning Children.* New York, Houghton Mifflin, 1940.

Klecan-Aker J: Syntactic abilities in normal and language defi-cient middle school children. *Top Lang Disord* 5(3):46–54, 1985.

Kosc L: Neuropsychological implications of diagnosis and treat-ment of mathematical learning disabilities. *Top Learn Learn Disabil* 1:19–30, 1981.

Landau WM, Goldstein R, Kleffner FR: Congenital aphasia, a clinicopathologic study. *Neurology* 10:915–921, 1960.

Larson V, McKinley N. General intervention principles with language impaired adolescents. *Top Lang Disord* 5(3):70–77, 1985.

Lazar I, Darlington RB: *Lasting Effects After Preschool.* DHEW Publication No (OHDS) 79-30178. Washington DC, Govern-ment Printing Office, 1978.

Lerner J: *Children with Learning Disabilities,* 3rd ed. Boston, Houghton Mifflin, 1981.

Liberman RG, Moore SP, Hutchinson EC: What's the Difference between Language Impaired and Learning Disabled Children? Paper presented at the meeting of the American Speech-Language-Hearing Association, San Francisco, November 1984.

Liberman I: A language-oriented view of reading and its disabilities, in Myklebust HR (ed): *Progress in Learning Disabilities,* Vol 5. New York, Grune & Stratton, 1983.

Luria AR: *Higher Cortical Functions in Man.* New York, Basic Books, 1966.

Luria AR: *The Working Brain.* Harmondsworth UK: Penguin Books, 1973.

Luria AR, Simernitskaya GG, Tubylevich B: The structure of psychological processes in relation to cerebral organization. *Neuropsychologia* 8:13–19, 1970.

Lyon R: Subgroups of LD readers: Clinical and empirical identi-fication, in Mykelbust HR (ed): *Progress in Learning Disabilities,* Vol 5. New York, Grune & Stratton, 1982.

McCloskey M, Caramazza A, Basili A: Cognitive mechanisms in number processing and calculation: Evidence from dyscalculia. *Brain and Cognition* 4:171–196, 1985.

McGlone J, Davidson W: The relation between cerebral speech laterality and spatial ability with special reference to sex and hand preference. *Neuropsychologia* 11:105–113, 1973.

McLeod T, Armstrong S: Learning disabilities in mathematics—Skill deficits and remedial approaches at the intermediate and secondary level. *Learn Disabil Q* 5(3):305–311, 1982.

McLeod T, Crump W: The relationship of visuo-spatial skills and verbal ability to learning disabilities in mathematics. *J Learn Disabil* 11:237–241, 1978.

Mattis S, French JH, Rapin I: Dyslexia in children and young adults: Three independent neuropsychological syndromes. *Dev Med Child Neurol* 17:150–163, 1975.

Miles T: On the persistence of dyslexic difficulties into adulthood, in Pavlidis GT, Fisher DF (eds): *Dyslexia: Its Neuropsychology and Treatment,* New York, John Wiley & Sons, 1986.

Montague M, Bos C: The effect of cognitive strategy training on verbal math problem solving performance of learning dis-abled adolescents. *J Learn Disabil* 19:26–33, 1986.

Morgan WP: A case of congenital word blindness. *Br Med J* 2:1378, 1896.

Morton LL, Kershner JR: Hemisphere asymmetries, spelling ability, and classroom seating in fourth graders. *Brain and Cognition* 6:101–111, 1987.

Morrison D: Neurobehavioral dysfunction and learning disabilities in children, in Ceci S (ed): *Handbook of Cognitive, Social and Neuropsychological Aspects of Learning Disabilities.* Hillsdale, NJ, Lawrence Erlbaum, 1986.

Moses J: Neurological analysis of calculation deficits. *Focus on Learning Problems in Mathematics* 6:1–12, 1984.

Mykelbust HR: Childhood aphasia: An evolving concept, in Travis LE (ed): *Handbook of Speech Pathology and Audiology.* New York, Appleton-Century-Crofts, 1971.

Mykelbust HR: Childhood aphasia: Identification, diagnosis, remediation, in Travis LE (ed): *Handbook of Speech Pathology and Audiology.* New York, Appleton-Century-Crofts, 1971b.

Myklebust HR: *Development and Disorders of Written Language,* Vol 1: *Picture Story Language Test.* New York, Grune & Stratton, 1965.

Obrzut J, Hynd GW, Bolick C: Lateral asymmetries in learning disabled children: A review, in Ceci S (ed): *Handbook of Cognitive, Social, and Neuropsychological Aspects of Learning Disabilities.* Hillsdale, NJ, Lawrence Erlbaum, 1986.

Orton S: *Reading, Writing, and Speech Problems in Children.* New York, WW Norton, 1937.

Ottenbacher K: Identifying vestibular processing dysfunction in learning disabled children. *Am J Occup Ther* 32:217–221, 1978.

Ozols E, Rourke B: Dimensions of social sensitivity in two types of learning disabled children, in Rourke B (ed): *Neuropsychology of Learning Disabilities: Essentials in Subtype Analysis.* New York, Guilford Press, 1985.

Pellegrino J, Goldman S: Information processing and elementary mathematics. *J Learn Disabil* 20:23–32, 1987.

Rawson M: *Developmental Language Disability: Adult Accomplishments of Dyslexic Boys.* Baltimore, Md, Johns Hopkins University Press, 1968.

Resnick L: Education and Learning to Think: A Special Report for the Commission on Behavioral and Social Sciences and Education, National Research Council, 1986.

Reynolds L, Egan R, Lerner J: Efficacy of early intervention on pre-academic deficits: A review of the literature. *Top Early Child Spec Educ* 3:3, 47–56, 1983.

Roberts, L: Childhood aphasia and handedness, in West R (ed): *Childhood Aphasia.* San Francisco, California Society for Crippled Children and Adults, 1962.

Ross DM, Ross SA: *Hyperactivity: Research, Theory, and Action.* New York, John Wiley & Sons, 1976.

Rourke B: Syndrome of nonverbal learning disabilities: The final common pathway of white-matter disease/dysfunction? *Clinical Neuropsychol* 1(3):209–234, 1987.

Rourke BP, Bakker D, Fisk JL, Strang JD: *Child Neuropsychology: An Introduction to Theory, Research, and Clinical Practice.* New York, Guilford Press, 1983.

Rutter M, Yule W: Specific reading retardation, in Mann L, Sabatino D (eds): *The First Review of Special Education.* Philadelphia, Buttonwood Farms, 1973.

Schumaker J, Deshler D, Alley G, Warner M, Denton P: Multipass: A learning strategy for improving reading comprehension. *Learn Disabil Q* 5:295–304, 1982.

Siegel L, Heaven R: Categorization of learning disabilities, in Ceci S: *Handbook of Cognitive, Social, and Neuropsychological Aspects of Learning Disabilities.* Hillsdale, NJ, Lawrence Erlbaum, 1986.

Silva P, Stewart I, Kirkland C, Simpson A: How impaired are children who experience persistent bilateral otitis media with effusion? in Duane DD, Leong CK (eds): *Understanding Learning Disabilities: International and Multidisciplinary Views.* New York, Plenum Press, 1985.

Smith SD, Kimberling WJ, Pennington BF, et al: Specific reading disability: Identification of an inherited form through linkage analysis. *Science* 219:1345, 1983.

Spreen O: Adult outcomes of reading disorders, in Malatesha R, Aaron P (eds): *Reading Disorders: Varieties and Treatments.* New York, Academic Press, 1982.

Stoch MB, Smythe PM: Undernutrition during infancy, and subsequent brain growth and intellectual development, in Scrimshaw NS, Gordon JE (eds): *Malnutrition, Learning and Behavior.* Cambridge, Mass, MIT Press, 1968.

Strang J, Rourke B: Arithmetic disability subtypes: The neuropsychological significance of specific arithmetical impairment in childhood, in Rourke B (ed): *Neuropsychology of Learning Disabilities: Essentials of Subtype Analysis.* New York, Guilford Press, 1985.

Strauss AA, Werner H: Disorders of conceptual thinking in the brain injured child. *J Nerv Ment Dis* 96:153–172, 1942.

Sweeney J, Rourke B: Spelling disability subtypes, in Rourke B (ed): *Neuropsychology of Learning Disabilities: Essentials of Subtype Analysis.* New York, Guilford Press, 1985.

Tranel D, Hall L, Olson S, Tranel N: Evidence for a right-hemisphere developmental learning disability. *Dev Neuropsychol* 3(2):113–127, 1987.

US Department of Education, Office of Special Education and Rehabilitative Services: *Fifth Annual Report to Congress on the Implementation of Public Law 94–142: The Education for All Handicapped Children Act.* Washington, DC, Government Printing Office, 1983.

Vellutino F: Dyslexia. *Scientific American* 256(3):34–41, 1987.

Vellutino F, Shub M: Assessment of disorders in formal school language: Disorders in reading. *Top Lang Disord* 2(4):13–19, 1982.

Vetter DK: Language disorders and schooling. *Top Lang Disord* 2(4):13–19, 1982.

Vogel S: Syntactic complexity in written expression of LD college writers. *Ann Dyslexia* 35:137–157, 1985.

Wiederholt JL: Historical perspectives in the education of the learning disabled, in Mann L, Sabatino D (eds): *The Second Review of Special Education.* Philadelphia, Journal of Special Education Press, 1974.

Wiig EH, Semel EM: *Language Assessment and Intervention for the Learning Disabled.* Columbus, Ohio, Charles E Merrill, 1984.

Wilson LF: Assessment of congenital aphasia, in Rappaport SR (ed): *Childhood Aphasia and Brain Damage.* Narberth, Pa: Livingston, 1965.

Zigmond N, Thornton H: Follow-up of postsecondary age learning disabled graduates and drop-outs. *Learn Disabil Res* 1(1):50–55, 1985.

Section III

Common Pediatric Neurologic Problems

An Approach to Understanding, Diagnosis, and Treatment

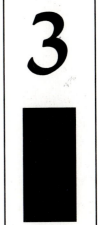

Coma
John Bodensteiner

The management of the child with persistently altered consciousness is one of the most challenging and rewarding problems in clinical medicine. The responsibility for the initial management of the comatose patient frequently falls on the primary care physician (pediatrician or family practitioner), and it is therefore helpful for that physician to have some knowledge of the basics of diagnosis and management of these problems. This chapter will

1. Define the terminology used to describe altered states of consciousness.
2. Briefly examine the mechanisms of maintenance of consciousness and conditions resulting in alteration of these mechanisms.
3. Discuss the diagnostic approach to a child in coma.
4. Touch on some of the general aspects of managing the child in coma.

TERMINOLOGY

It is important to use consistent terminology when dealing with patients with altered states of consciousness. The lack of uniformity in the way terms are used is such a problem that many have chosen to abandon the terms altogether and develop a numeric scale, such as the Glasgow Coma Scale. Although numeric scales are of value in introducing uniformity to quantification of patient responsiveness, there is still a need for terms like *obtundation, stupor,* and *coma.*

Consciousness is defined as the normal state of awareness of one's environment and one's self within that environment. A patient who is normally aware of himself and the environment is said to be *fully alert.* In this condition age-appropriate complex tasks can be performed without difficulty and the patient is oriented to person, place, time, and situation. Assuming that the patient has the means by which to communicate this awareness to the examiner (not always a valid assumption), it is relatively easy to demonstrate these responses.

If a patient is not fully oriented but is able to maintain arousal or wakefulness normally, he or she is said to be *confused.* This patient is unable to carry out complex tasks but may be able to do simple tasks. *Delirium* is an agitated form of confusion.

In the remainder of the altered states there is also a defect in the ability to maintain arousal or wakefulness. The mildest of these states is *lethargy.* The lethargic patient fails to maintain wakefulness unless receiving stimuli, such as verbal or visual input or pain. If left alone this patient will drift into a sleep-like state, but, even with arousal, he or she is unable to perform complex tasks. A patient who is only able to be aroused to a verbally responsive state by noxious stimulus and who drifts back to an unconscious state quickly when the stimulus is withdrawn is described as *obtunded.*

Stupor is a state in which the patient is unconscious at rest and will respond with semipurposeful avoidance (poorly organized withdrawal) and vocalizations only with persistent noxious stimuli. *Coma* is used to describe the mental status of a patient who is unarousable to noxious stimuli, whether they be tactile, verbal, visual, or other. Vigorous stimulation may produce decorticate (arms flexed, legs extended) or decerebrate (arms and legs extended) postures or other brainstem overflow responses. Spinal flexion responses may also occur or there may be no observable response to stimuli.

The use of less precisely defined terms such as *semicomatose* cannot be recommended because of the imprecise and variable definitions used for these terms. With each usage of these terms the definition intended must be restated.

MECHANISMS INVOLVED IN THE MAINTENANCE OF CONSCIOUSNESS

The exact mechanisms involved in maintenance of consciousness are still obscure, but it is apparent that two structures of major importance are the brainstem reticular activating system and the cerebral cortex.

The brainstem reticular activating system is a diffuse population of neurons that exists in the central core of the brainstem from the caudal aspect of the medulla up to the hypothalamus. This system contains a number of distinct nuclei and some less well-defined cell populations. In the medulla and pons the organization of the brainstem reticular activating system is somewhat more rigid, with the medial third of the system containing very large neurons called the "gigantocellular" area. The lateral aspect of the reticular formation at this level consists of smaller neurons and is more diffusely distributed.

The brainstem reticular activating system interacts with all of the major somatic and special sensory pathways of the central nervous system. There appears to be especially rich input from the spinothalamic tract into the reticular activating system. Projections from the cerebral cortex to the brainstem reticular activating system appear to modulate the activity of the system. This cerebral modulation is perhaps the mechanism that underlies the ability of the nervous system to consciously focus selectively on incoming information. There are three major ascending pathways from the brainstem reticular activating system to the more rostral regions of the central nervous system. The first of these is the pathway to the thalamic reticular nucleus, which then relays signals on to the cerebral cortex. The thalamic reticular nucleus appears to be inhibitory to the cerebral cortex and may be the physiologic site of the thalamic recruitment that is seen in the various electroencephalographic (EEG) stages of sleep. The second major ascending pathway from the brainstem reticular activating system is the relay through the limbic system, the hypothalamus, and on to the cerebral cortex. This pathway modulates vegetative drives, such as hunger, thirst, and probably sexual responses. The third major pathway is made up of those direct afferent fibers that appear to arise from pontine nuclei and pass through the dorsal tegmental bundle to the cingulum and orbital frontal and medial temporal lobes. Although only partially elucidated functionally, this tract appears to play a role in arousal and integrative cognitive mechanisms.

The cerebral cortex itself has a great influence on consciousness and conscious awareness as well as the modulation of behavior. From the pharmacologic standpoint, cholinergic and monoaminergic neurons appear to be important in the maintenance of consciousness, although many other neurotransmitter systems also have some input into this system. A simplified view would indicate that the monoamine and cholinergic fibers are the most important of the neurotransmitters.

Alterations in consciousness are generally associated with acute or subacute lesions and are not seen in chronic lesions (which are more likely to produce a dementia-like picture). In order for a subacute or acute lesion to affect consciousness, the lesion must (1) involve the brain diffusely or result in bilateral impairment of cerebral func-

tions, or (2) result in failure of the brainstem reticular activating system.

The degree of impairment of consciousness is roughly proportionate to the size of the lesion, but from a clinical standpoint this dictum is not very helpful.

DIAGNOSTIC APPROACH TO THE CHILD WITH ALTERED CONSCIOUSNESS

Determining the exact cause of the alteration of consciousness can be extremely difficult. Unfortunately, there is no single simple solution to this problem. No one laboratory test or screening procedure will sort out the multitude of possibilities and permit a hard and fast diagnosis. Despite the bewildering number of conditions that can cause altered states of consciousness, it is possible to divide them into a relatively few categories that will allow a more rational approach to the evaluation of the patient. If it is true that, in order for a lesion to cause coma, it must either produce bilateral dysfunction of the cerebral hemispheres (diffuse or multifocal injury to the hemispheres), or damage or depress the physiologic function of the reticular activating system, or both, then we can have any of the following:

1. *Supratentorial* mass lesions, which compress or displace the diencephalon and brainstem.
2. *Subtentorial destructive* or *expanding* lesions, which damage or compress the reticular activating system.
3. *Metabolic encephalopathies*, which affect the brain diffusely and depress both the cortex and the brainstem reticular activating system.

Once the general category is determined, the evaluation can be focused on the conditions most important to that category.

Faced with an acutely ill patient with a persistent alteration of consciousness, the physician may be aided in the approach by considering the following:

1. The first order of business is to determine whether the disturbance is functional or organic. (In pediatric practice psychogenic or functional alteration of consciousness is much less likely than in the adult or adolescent patient.)
2. If the disturbance is organic: Is it *focal* (the findings can be explained by a single lesion)? Is it *multifocal* (one must have more than a single lesion to account for the findings)? Or is it *diffuse* (no evidence of focal nature at all)?
3. What is the clinical course? Is the patient getting better, stable, or getting worse? The answer to these questions will allow one to prioritize the next few diagnostic and therapeutic steps.
4. Finally, what is the specific pathologic process

causing the coma? Subsequently, does medical or surgical treatment carry a greater likelihood of effectiveness?

The physician must also keep in mind that the brain must be protected as soon as possible against ongoing damage in order to prevent more serious or irreversible damage to the nervous system. This is often approached in the context of acute brain resuscitation and we will discuss the principles of emergency management in the next section of this chapter.

DIAGNOSIS AND TREATMENT

In many cases of altered consciousness a reliable history is not obtained. Lack of a history often leads one to rely too much on physical examination and laboratory clues as to etiology, severity, and the appropriate therapeutic course.

Once the vital functions have been stabilized and the patient is not in imminent danger of circulatory or respiratory collapse, the physician should proceed with prudent haste to the history and physical examination.

Whenever possible, a complete history should be obtained, usually from relatives, friends, other observers, or sometimes police. Particularly important in the history are the nature and onset of coma, the previous health of the patient, the patient's use of medications or drugs, the possibility of exposure to poisons, trauma, or a history of heart disease, seizures, or other disorders.

During the general physical examination the physician should look at the vital signs. A careful search should be made for physical evidence of trauma. Signs that might suggest such conditions as an acute or chronic medical illness, the self-administration of drugs, diabetes, or subacute bacterial endocarditis are important. The neck should be examined for nuchal rigidity unless of course the possibility of a cervical spinal fracture is considered likely.

The neurologic examination of the comatose patient has been carefully studied, and attempts have been made to quantify the various aspects of the examination. Several parameters have been shown to be helpful, particularly when examined in serial fashion (Table 23-1). It is therefore suggested that a serial recording of the responses be made so that changes in the patient's condition might be more clearly seen. The following sections discuss the neurologic features to be noted.

Verbal Responsiveness

The optimum response represents clear, oriented, intelligent speech. This is of course impossible in toddlers and younger children; therefore, appropriate speech for age is to be substituted as the normal response in those age groups. Incomprehensible speech, isolated words, or

TABLE 23-1. IMPORTANT FEATURES OF THE EXAMINATION IN COMA

Verbal responsiveness
Ocular system
    Eye opening
    Pupillary responses
    Spontaneous eye movements
Ocular reflexes
    Oculocephalic responses
    Oculovestibular responses
    Corneal responses
Respiratory pattern
Motor system
    Motor responses
    Deep tendon reflex responses
    Skeletal muscle tone

moans would be considered inadequate responses and no vocal response would, of course, be the worst possible response.

Ocular System

Eye Opening

Normally a patient will open the eyes or maintain eye opening spontaneously. A somewhat compromised patient will open the eyes to verbal stimuli. More severely compromised patients require a more noxious stimulus to produce eye opening. The comatose patient will not open the eyes even to noxious stimuli. There are some conditions in which the eyes remain open despite extensive central nervous system damage; however, these conditions will be of interest primarily to the neurologic consultant.

Pupillary Response

The presence of a pupillary response to light is normal. This test should be carried out with a very bright light and the response recorded in terms of change in pupillary size or percentage of normal response. The examiner may require a magnifying lens to identify subtle pupillary responses. The resting position of the pupil may also be important with respect to the etiology of the coma. For example, in most cases of barbiturate poisoning, the pupil is small and may be only minimally responsive, and in severe poisoning it may be completely unresponsive.

The resting position of the pupil is also important in structurally mediated coma, as there is a high incidence of abnormal findings and often the findings are of localizing value. Abnormal pupils are generally not the result of lesions involving the cerebral cortex. Damage to the ventrolateral hypothalamus produces ipsilateral pupillary constriction. Midbrain tectal damage may interrupt the pupillary light reflex while sparing the accommodation reflex, resulting in midposition unresponsive pupils that spontaneously dilate and constrict. In nuclear (tegmental) lesions the pupils show no spontaneous movement. Pontine lesions characteristically produce pinpoint pupils that are very slightly reactive. Finally, lesions in the lateral medullary or ventrolateral cervical cord may produce a homolateral Horner's syndrome.

The physician should be aware of the confounding possibilities of third-nerve paralysis, which can alter the pupillary signs and responses.

Spontaneous Eye Movements

A normally alert patient will spontaneously direct the eyes to objects of interest in the environment, whereas the compromised patient may show roving, nonfocusing, conjugate eye movement. The slightly more impaired patient may have dysconjugate eye movement. Patients with various brainstem-level dysfunctions may show miscellaneous abnormalities of movement, such as ocular bobbing or opsoclonus.

Ocular Reflexes

Oculocephalic Responses

Normal oculocephalic responses consist of the maintenance of fixation while the head is passively turned horizontally or vertically. The minimally compromised patient shows tonic deviation of the eyes to the opposite direction of head turn with subsequent correction to straight-ahead conjugate gaze. Decreased oculocephalic responses consist of less than 30° of movement of the eyes or bilateral failure of abduction of the eyes. The total absence of oculocephalic responses is the poorest level of function and results from brainstem dysfunction as low as the level of the sixth cranial nerve (the pontomedullary junction).

Oculovestibular Responses

The oculovestibular system is tested by irrigation of the external auditory canal with ice water. The head is usually raised 30° above the horizontal plane and 10 to 15 cc of ice water is instilled slowly into the external auditory canal by means of a short catheter. Care should be taken not to perforate the eardrum. A normal awake response includes rapid nystagmus toward the nonirrigated ear, often accompanied by a sensation of nausea. Patients with disturbed consciousness may show a tonic deviation of the eyes to the side of irrigation. The more severely impaired patient will show abduction of the eye on the ipsilateral side with failure of adduction of the opposite eye. A worse response would be no movement of the eyes to irrigation of the ear canal. The levels of brain function tested by calorics are the same as those tested by the oculovestibular responses; the cold water, however, is a much better stimulus to the vestibular system than head turning.

Corneal Responses

The corneal responses are tested by touching the cornea with a wisp of cotton. The entire cornea must be tested because the innervation of various portions of the cor-

nea may arise from different sources. Normal response is indicated by an attempt to close the eye as well as contralateral eye closure. The effort to close the eye is confirmed by the presence of Bell's phenomenon (upward deviation of the eye with attempted closure).

Respiratory Pattern

A number of respiratory patterns may represent abnormalities and this should be considered in the context of the possibility of metabolic acidosis or alkalosis altering the respiratory pattern. It is considered normal when the patient breathes regularly. The impaired patient may have periodic breathing, ataxic or irregular breathing, or combinations of these. The correlation between the location of the lesion and the respiratory pattern is not precise; however, the following may be seen: forebrain damage associated with Cheyne-Stokes respirations, hypothalamic upper midbrain lesions associated with central "neurogenic" hyperventilation and "neurogenic" pulmonary edema, pontine tegmentum lesions associated with pseudobulbar paralysis of voluntary control of breathing, lower pontine lesions associated with apneustic or short-cycle anoxic-hypercapnic breathing, and finally medullary lesions with ataxic or gasping respirations. The respiratory patterns are helpful only in patients who are not being mechanically ventilated.

Motor System

Motor Responses

A normal patient will follow commands with normal strength. The best score is given to that individual. If the verbal command evokes no response, the individual is tested with a noxious stimulus. A patient who makes an attempt to remove that noxious stimulus is considered to have a localizing response, particularly when the arm will cross the midline or reach above shoulder level to remove a noxious stimulus. A more primitive response is a nonlocalizing withdrawal type of response to the noxious stimulus. More primitive still is the assumption of a stereotyped posture with noxious stimulus. This may be either a decorticate or decerebrate posture, depending on the degree and level of brain dysfunction. No response is coded only when a strong noxious stimulus is applied to more than one site with no response in a patient who is free of paralyzing agents.

Deep Tendon Reflex Responses

A comatose patient may have diffusely increased deep tendon reflexes if he or she has increased intracranial pressure (ICP). Alternatively there may be depressed or absent reflexes in metabolic coma or more advanced stages of coma. Normal reflexes may be seen and are not of major significance.

Skeletal Muscle Tone

Hypertonicity is described as an increased resistance throughout the range of passive motion. Increased flex-

FEATURE TABLE 23-1. SUPRATENTORIAL MASS LESIONS

Discriminating Features	Consistent Features	Variable Features
1. Initial focal cerebral dysfunction 2. Focal slowing on EEG	1. Asymmetric motor signs 2. Lack of cranial nerve abnormalities	1. Rostral-caudal progression of signs 2. Altered mental status (late)

or or extensor muscle tone will be seen in decorticate and decerebrate rigidity, respectively, and the worst response is in an individual with flaccid or no muscle tone.

Differential Diagnosis

After having completed the history and physical examination of the patient in coma, one may have a reasonable idea of which of the major differential diagnostic categories is most likely. It is appropriate to note some of the characteristics that should by this time be pointing the physician in one of these three general directions:

1. *Supratentorial* mass lesions cause coma by compressing or displacing the diencephalon or brainstem.
   a. The initial signs are usually those of *focal* cerebral dysfunction.
   b. The signs may follow a rostral-caudal progression of cerebral dysfunction associated with increasing ICP (identified by Plum and Posner).
   c. The neurologic signs at any given time may point to the dysfunction of a particular anatomic area, such as the diencephalon, midbrain, pons, or medulla. This is again according to Plum and Posner's description of the rostral-caudal progression of brain dysfunction with a supratentorial lesion.
   d. Very importantly, the motor signs with supratentorial mass lesions may be asymmetric.
2. *Subtentorial* mass lesions causing coma compress or destroy the brainstem structures.
   a. Generally, symptoms or signs localizing neurologic abnormalities to the brainstem precede or accompany the onset of coma.
   b. In these patients there almost always is oculovestibular abnormality, and cranial nerve palsies are usually present as well.
   c. Finally, the presence of unusual respiratory patterns is common, even early on, in a coma produced by compression of the brainstem.

3. *Metabolic* problems causing coma disturb the function of both the cerebrum and the brainstem.
   a. These patients are characterized by confusion and stupor commonly preceding motor signs without the presence of focal neurologic deficits.
   b. The motor signs are most often symmetric and pupillary response is preserved until very late.
   c. Seizures and movement disorders, including myoclonus, tremor, and asterixis, are all common in the metabolic comas, usually preceding the onset of the coma.
   d. Disturbances of acid-base balance with hyper- or hypoventilation should suggest this possibility. The presence of an abnormal odor on the breath should also suggest this possibility.
   e. The EEG in metabolic coma usually consists of diffuse slowing, sometimes with high-voltage delta activity or triphasic waves. With mass lesions or supratentorial lesions, focal slowing is more commonly seen.

Subsequent Steps

If the physician engaged in the evaluation of a comatose patient is able to identify the lesion as having focal characteristics and as being either supratentorial or subtentorial, a computed tomographic and/or MR scan should be considered very strongly to confirm the presence of the suspected supratentorial or subtentorial mass lesions. If a mass lesion is identified, the pediatrician may want to stabilize the patient and call in neurologic or neurosurgical consultative help to manage the patient further. If there are no focal neurologic dysfunctions the most probable diagnosis is metabolic coma. When metabolic coma is considered, the patient usually has no evidence of focal neurologic disease, although on rare occasions metabolic coma may result in asymmetric findings. The patient frequently manifests hyperventilation or hypoventilation in metabolic coma; however, it is not unusual to see ataxic or irregular breathing patterns of other types. The individual with metabolic coma usual-

FEATURE TABLE 23-2. SUBTENTORIAL MASS LESIONS

Discriminating Features	Consistent Feature	Variable Features
1. Initial cranial nerve abnormalities *plus* 2. Contralateral long tract signs	1. Oculomotor abnormalities	1. Respiratory rate abnormalities 2. No rostral-caudal progression of signs

FEATURE TABLE 23-3. METABOLIC ENCEPHALOPATHIES

Discriminating Features	Consistent Features	Variable Features
1. Stupor precedes motor signs 2. Diffusely slow EEG	1. No focal features 2. Abnormal respiratory pattern	1. Movement abnormalities (asterixis, myoclonus) 2. Peculiar breath odor 3. Acid-base or electrolyte abnormalities

ly will have preservation (though depressed) of symmetric pupillary responses and oculovestibular and oculocephalic responses, indicating the absence of structural brainstem disease.

Once metabolic coma is suspected, the identification of the precise etiology of the coma is one of the more challenging problems in medicine. The following is a list of possible studies to be considered in a patient with metabolic coma (Table 23–2). It should be noted that, because drug ingestion is the most common cause of coma, blood and urine for toxicology studies should be obtained from all patients with coma of unknown origin. In addition, samples of venous blood should be drawn for measure-

TABLE 23-2. THE LABORATORY EVALUATION OF METABOLIC COMA

First-priority tests
Venous blood
  Glucose
  NH_3
  Electrolytes (Na, K, Cl, CO_2, Ca, PO_4)
  Osmolality
Arterial blood
  pH
  PO_2
  PCO_2
  HCO_3
  HbCO if color abnormal
Cerebrospinal fluid
  Cell count
  Gram stain
  Glucose
EKG

Second-priority tests
Venous blood
  Toxic drug screen
  Liver function tests
  Coagulation studies
  Thyroid function
  Adrenal function
  Cultures
Urine
  Toxic drug screen
  Culture
Cerebrospinal fluid
  Protein
  Culture and antigens
  Observe spun specimen

ment of serum glucose, electrolytes, NH_3, calcium, PCO_2, phosphate, urea, and creatinine, as well as serum osmolality. Arterial blood may be obtained for pH, PO_2, PCO_2, bicarbonate, and methemoglobin or carboxyhemoglobin studies (particularly if the color of the blood is unusual). Study of the cerebrospinal fluid should be considered as part of the evaluation of a coma of uncertain origin, particularly if one has ruled out or considers unlikely a focal mass lesion. In addition to these tests, an electrocardiogram (EKG) should be done to look for the possibility of cardiac effects from drugs or electrolyte imabalances. It is suggested that extra samples be obtained and saved for later analysis, including samples of venous blood for sedative or toxic drug determinations, liver function tests, coagulation studies, thyroid studies, adrenal function studies, blood cultures, or viral cultures. Urine should be saved for toxic and metabolic screens as well as culture, and cerebrospinal fluid should be saved for viral and fungal cultures to be performed if indicated.

Once the cause of the metabolic coma has been identified, attempts should be made to remove, neutralize, or reverse the effects of the metabolic derangement or the intoxication causing the problem. The specifics of this procedure depend on the nature of the offending agent or metabolic disturbance; details can be found in various sources, including publications from poison control centers, textbooks, and journal articles.

INITIAL MANAGEMENT OF THE COMATOSE PATIENT

The general principles of the early management of the comatose patient are similar regardless of the nature of the underlying problem. It is therefore appropriate to consider the emergency management of the unconscious patient. In practice the initial stabilization of the patient and the diagnostic evaluation are carried out simultaneously; however, for the sake of discussion, these aspects will be addressed separately.

The initial management, even before the diagnostic process begins, should include ascertainment of the vital signs and implementation of the "ABCs" of resuscitation. These include the assurance of the airway and establishment of oxygenation. Particular attention should be paid

Pearls and Perils: Coma

1. Discrete lesions causing coma must involve the cortex diffusely and bilaterally or the reticular activating system to produce changes in consciousness.
2. A depressed mental status with no focal features suggests a metabolic problem.
3. Diffusely increased reflexes and tone may indicate increased ICP.
4. Brainstem dysfunction with diffuse hyporeflexia is not uncommon in intoxication with depressant medications (e.g., barbiturate poisoning).
5. Be sure to smell the comatose patient's breath, as this may provide valuable clues to the nature of the coma (e.g., ethanol intoxication, diabetic ketoacidosis, hydrocarbon ingestion).
6. Retinal hemorrhage should suggest suddenly increased ICP and is not specific for any particular etiology (consider trauma, inflicted or otherwise, and intracranial hemorrhage).
7. The early focal signs in patients with discrete lesions may be overlooked unless specifically sought out by history and examination.
8. Unilateral cerebral lesions producing coma may not follow the usual rostral-caudal progression of signs because, by the time a unilateral lesion has resulted in coma, the brainstem will already have been compromised.
9. Papilledema may take several hours to develop with increased ICP.
10. The depression following a seizure may resemble diffuse metabolic coma or focal lesions (if the seizure was focal, as in Todd's paralysis). The seizure may have been unobserved or its significance unappreciated; be sure to think of this possibility when taking the history.
11. Unobserved falls may be the cause of unexplained coma; look for evidence of trauma.
12. In patients with unexplained coma, a CT scan should be performed before lumbar puncture.

to the removal of foreign materials from the airway and the use of supplemental oxygen if necessary. The physician should evaluate the respiratory excursions and the effectiveness thereof. This may require the measurement of arterial blood gases, but, as a general rule, breath sounds heard by auscultation and visual observation may provide adequate information regarding the effectiveness of respiration. The establishment of adequate respiration may or may not require the placement of an airway. If one contemplates the subsequent utilization of more energetic measures or the need for ICP management, the placement of an endotracheal tube should be considered.

The physician should also pay attention to the circulation, maintenance of blood pressure, pulse, and a regular cardiac rhythm for the delivery of oxygenated blood to the central nervous system. The maintenance of a mean arterial blood pressure of greater than 65 mm Hg will be adequate to ensure cerebral perfusion in most circumstances. Generally it is recommended that some form of continuous pressure monitoring be employed, particularly because the treatment of increased ICP may adversely affect the circulation. Fluid restriction and osmotic diuretics may contribute to hypovolemia, and barbiturates (either exogenous or therapeutically employed) may cause systemic hypotension. Measurement of the cardiac filling pressures, output, and vascular resistance may also be helpful in maintenance of adequate circulation.

After the ABCs have been attended to, three groups of problems must be considered, based on their priority for immediate treatment. The first is the administration of glucose and/or the treatment of seizures. It is commonly recommended that glucose be given in the management of coma of unknown origin. Glucose should be given because it is the primary substrate for brain metabolism and because hypoglycemia can be diagnosed only by laboratory tests; these require time to carry out and the brain may be irreversibly damaged during that interval. It is hoped that the administration of this glucose will prevent brain damage while the laboratory determinations are being performed. Although one might argue that hyperosmolar glucose in a patient with diabetic coma may worsen the disease, the risk of permanent damage in the hypoglycemic patient outweighs the temporary worsening of the encephalopathy seen in the hyperosmolar hyperglycemic patient. Therefore, I would suggest the administration of 1 g glucose/kg body weight in the form of a 50% solution to a comatose patient in whom the diagnosis is not clear.

If seizures are present, as they sometimes are in metabolic coma, one should try to stop the seizures even before the evaluation is completed because of the adverse effect on cerebral circulation and metabolism of ongoing seizures. Management strategies for seizures are discussed elsewhere.

The second priority of management is the identification and treatment of specific infections, such as encephalitis or meningitis, and the management of ICP. The management of infectious processes requires the appropriate use of antibiotics as the primary therapy. The management of increased ICP may be necessary to provide time in order to carry out or complete the diagnostic evaluation or to arrange for the appropriate specific therapy.

In general terms, the first principle in the management of increased ICP is to avoid those problems that can exacerbate the pressure elevation. Among the most frequent of these exacerbating factors are fever, seizures, awkward head position, hypoxia, and "fighting the respirator." These problems can be avoided by proper positioning, treating seizures, and ensuring adequate sedation and oxygenation of the patient.

Specific therapy for intracranial hypertension may then be considered. The choice of modalities and the order in which the modalities are to be used will vary and should be individualized for each patient. The first modality used in many patients will be hyperventilation. The patient is hyperventilated to blow off the carbon dioxide, resulting in decreased cerebral blood flow. The amount of reduction of ICP will depend on both the degree of lowering of the P_{CO_2} and the compliance of the intracranial contents. Most often maximum effect is achieved when the P_{CO_2} is maintained around 25 mm Hg. It is also important to maintain the position of the neck and head to decrease ICP and improve venous return from the head.

It is important to avoid excessive administration of fluids to a patient who is comatose; however, in some situations the use of osmotic diuretics such as mannitol with or without Lasix should be considered. In the acutely ill patient, in order to buy time for further diagnostic evaluation, mannitol should be used. The osmotic diuretics act by reducing total brain water and usually extract more water from normal brain tissue than edematous tissue. Although larger quantities of mannitol have been recommended in the past, the trend is toward smaller, more frequent doses in the neighborhood of 0.25 g/kg body weight, repeated every 4 to 6 hours as necessary. This should provide the time necessary for evaluation of the problem. The use of Lasix to enhance the effect of the mannitol has become common in the recent past. The administration of 1 mg/kg body weight of Lasix prior to mannitol administration is recommended. This has been shown to increase the duration of the effect of the mannitol on ICP as well as to increase the magnitude of the total effect. The limiting factor in osmotic treatment for increased ICP is the fact that at serum osmolalities above 330 mOsm there is little additional benefit and a greatly increased risk of vascular collapse, resulting in acute renal tubular necrosis, shock, and other problems. In those patients in whom the ICP will be an ongoing problem the management is greatly facilitated by the availability of ICP monitoring. Certainly before one considers the use of hypothermia or high-dose barbiturates in the management of ICP, some means of monitoring the pressure should be secured.

A third priority requires the identification of some less critical abnormalities—such as specific electrolyte abnormalities, greatly increased body temperature, or a specific toxin or poison—which would allow for specific treatment. Although most of the causes of unexplained coma will fall into this category, the stabilization of the patient and attention to the ABCs of management take precedence. For discussions of the specific therapies for the various etiologies of coma the reader is referred to the literature.

ANNOTATED BIBLIOGRAPHY

Plum F, Posner JB: The Diagnosis of Stupor and Coma, 3rd ed. Philadelphia, FA Davis, 1980.

This text has for years been considered the landmark publication in dealing with the diagnostic problems of stupor and coma. It contains a wealth of information regarding pathophysiology, physical examination, etiology, treatment, and prognosis of patients in coma. This book should be considered must reading for anyone dealing with comatose patients on a regular basis.

Roper AH (ed): Critical care neurology. Semin Neurol 4(4), 1984.

This issue of Seminars in Neurology contains 14 articles regarding various aspects of critical care neurology; many of these are excellent, containing information regarding theory, pathophysiology, and treatment of lesions causing coma. Also included are discussions of monitoring devices and new concepts in the field. This issue will be of use to those with more than a passing interest in neurologic problems.

Roper AH: Fundamentals of Critical Care in Neurology and Neurosurgery, Parts I and II. Neurology and Neurosurgery Update 3(11, 12). Princeton, NJ, Continuing Professional Education Center, 1982.

These two issues of the Neurology and Neurosurgery Update series contain a superb review of the basic problems in the management of critically ill neurologic patients, increased ICP, and respiratory problems in these types of patients. Roper does not discuss the diagnostic aspects of coma of unknown origin. These articles are devoted primarily to management issues.

Raphaely R, Swedlow D, Downes J, Bruce D: Management of severe pediatric head trauma. Pediatr Clin North Am 27:715–727, 1980.

Although this article discusses issues concerning only one of the causes of pediatric coma, it is nevertheless an excellent treatment and discussion of the theory as well as the practice of the management of increased ICP.

Batzdorf U: The management of cerebral edema in pediatric practice. Pediatrics 58:78–87, 1976.

This is a review of the physiology of cerebral edema and an approach to the management of the problem. Although limited in scope, this is a useful and easily read article.

Bruce DA, Schut L, Bruno LA, et al: Outcome following severe head injuries in children. J Neurosurg 48:679–688, 1978.

This article reviews the experience with 53 children and the factors related to the outcome of these head-injured patients.

Cottrell JE, Robustelli A, Post K, et al: Furosemide and mannitol induced changes in intracranial pressure and serum osmolality and electrolytes. Anesthesiology 47:28–30, 1977.

Furosemide appears to be preferable to mannitol if the desired result is diuresis. Recent data would suggest that the use of mannitol and furosemide together may be more effective than the use of either alone.

Crockard HA, Coppel DL, Morrow WFK: Evaluation of hyperventilation in treatment of head injuries. Br Med J 4:634–640, 1973.

The authors demonstrate the usefulness of blowing off carbon dioxide in the management of increased ICP.

Woodcock J, Roper AH, Kennedy SK: High dose barbiturates in non-trauma brain swelling: ICP reduction and effect on outcome. *Stroke* 13:785–787, 1982.

  The use of barbiturates to lower ICP in a variety of non-traumatic conditions is discussed. All patients had persistent elevations of ICP and only one failed to respond to intravenous barbiturates. The impression was that the survival was improved by the use of these drugs.

Shapiro HM, Marshall LF: Intracranial pressure responses to PEEP in head-injured patients. *J Trauma* 18:264–256, 1978.

  The interrelationship of positive end expiratory pressure (PEEP) and ICP is discussed and demonstrated in this study. Emphasis is placed on the need to measure the ICP directly when using PEEP in head-injured patients.

Malik AB: Mechanisms of neurogenic pulmonary edema. *Circ Res* 57:1–18, 1985.

Robertson GL, Aycinena P, Zerbe RL: Neurogenic disorders of osmoregulation. *Am J Med* 72:339–353, 1982.

  These two articles discuss two common complications of many of the lesions that cause coma in children, namely inappropriate antidiuretic hormone secretion and neurogenic pulmonary edema. Neither are entirely within the scope of this chapter but both are conditions the pediatric physician should know about.

Brain Resuscitation Clinical Trial I Study Group: Randomized clinical study of thiopental loading in comatose survivors of cardiac arrest. *N Engl J Med* 314:397–403, 1986.

  This study shows that (1) a randomized controlled trial is often necessary to prove the effectiveness of a new therapy and (2) thiopental may be effective for the control of ICP, but it does not prove useful as a prophylaxis for anoxic cerebral damage.

Teasdale G, Jennett B: Assessment of coma and impaired consciousness. A practical scale. *Lancet* 2:81–84, 1974.

  This article describes the so-called Glasgow Coma Scale, which is one of the most frequently used objective lists of clinical features that may be helpful in the determination of severity of injury and therefore outcome.

Levy DE, Caronna JJ, Singer B, et al: Predicting outcome from hypoxic-ischemic coma. *JAMA* 253:1420–1426, 1985.

  This article describes the outcome in 210 patients with hypoxic-ischemic coma and delineates the features that are important in identifying prognosis. The patients were not children; however, the principles remain valid.

Headaches
Peter B. Rosenberger

Headache is one of the most common sources of human discomfort, afflicting in some form between 40% and 70% of the population, depending on the conditions of the survey. When one considers also that it is one of the most common presenting symptoms of disease of the central nervous system, it is not surprising that headache is such an important part of the "bread and butter" of child neurology. It is thus not a subject to which the practitioner of our specialty needs introduction. It is hoped that this chapter will instead provide a guide to a more systematic clinical approach to this frequently encountered, usually routine, sometimes frustrating, and occasionally frightening malady.

WHAT HURTS IN THE HEAD?

All headache syndromes have in common that they involve one or more of the structures of the head and neck. It is thus reasonable to begin a discussion of the complaint with a consideration of the physical events involved. This question may be addressed from two viewpoints—physiologic and anatomic.

The pain receptor is probably the simplest in all of sensory physiology. It appears to consist of little more than the bare dendritic nerve ending—the simplest expression of the basic physiologic property of *irritability*, for which nervous tissue is so highly specialized. Any one of a number of external events, it appears, may bring about the change in membrane permeability required to shift the ionic balance, and thus the electrical charge, across the membrane, a shift which, if given sufficient impetus to spread along the membrane surface, will in turn give rise to the action potential that allows nervous transmission. Precipitating external events include physical pressure, chemical irritation, rapid changes in temperature, and perhaps light energy.

Anatomically speaking, pain-sensitive structures account for less than half of the total mass of the head and neck. Working from the outside in, they include first the skin, subcutaneous tissue, and muscles and tendons of the scalp and neck. The bone of the cranium is not pain sensitive, but the periosteum is exquisitely so. Underneath the skull, the fibrous tissues of the pachy- and leptomeninges comprise one of the two important pain-sensitive structures. The other is the blood vessels. Brain tissue itself is not pain sensitive, with two exceptions: the extracerebral fibers of the fifth, seventh, ninth, tenth, and eleventh cranial nerves, and the gray matter of certain somatosensory segments of the thalamus.

HEADACHE SYNDROMES

Many classifications of headache syndromes are available in the current literature. Those of most relevance to the child practitioner appear in the review of Rothner (1979) and the monographs of Friedman and Harms (1967) and Barlow (1984). Of historical importance is the review of Bille (1962), chiefly for its revelation of the high prevalence of clinically significant headache syndromes in children.

Most reviews attempt a basic distinction between "primary" headaches, those whose only clinical relevance is the discomfort itself, and "secondary" headaches, those that are symptomatic of other intracranial disease. The distinction is of limited physiologic validity, because all head pain is presumably symptomatic of some pathophysiologic process. Furthermore, in practice it is often arbitrary and imprecise, as for example in the separation of migraine from vascular headaches with specific etiologies. However, it is of considerable practical value to the clinician, who when faced with a "primary" headache syndrome will concentrate on relief of pain, but who with "symptomatic" headaches must treat the underlying cause as well, for reasons not necessarily limited to pain relief. One of the most important functions of the neurologic consultation for a child with headaches is to make this distinction as quickly and accurately as possible.

Primary ("Benign") Headache Syndromes

Primary headaches constitute the vast majority of headache syndromes in office practice. Previous classifications have differed only slightly from one another. Most make a distinction between tension and migraine. There is often disagreement about where to classify headaches related to depression. Barlow (1984) prefers the term *psychogenic* for both tension and depressive headaches. Our feeling is that the term *depression* connotes an additional mechanism not found in the large majority of tension headaches. Separation of the two also avoids the semantic difficulties some neurologists have with the term *psychogenic*.

Tension Headaches

Most observers agree that the headaches of simple nervous tension involve primarily structures outside the cranial cavity, namely muscles and tendons of the scalp and neck. The mechanism is assumed to be simple traction on pain sensors during prolonged muscular contraction. The time of onset is nearly always later in the day, or at least seldom first thing in the morning, sometimes with a "crescendo" pattern. The mode of onset is usually gradual, seldom sharply paroxysmal. The location is bifrontal, bi-occipital, or bitemporal, in that order of frequency in our experience; always bilateral; and more or less symmetric. The type of pain is usually steady rather than throbbing, and simple tension headaches are usually less severe, rarely driving the patient to tears or anguished complaint. Associated symptoms might include fatigue, stressful circumstances, or overt emotional distress. Relief by rest or relaxation is common, although the headache does not usually drive the patient to seek sleep or withdraw from the scene. The tension headache rarely outlasts a good night's sleep. Relief by simple analgesics accounts in large measure for the enormous popularity of these medications.

Migraine

Although migraine has been known in children for at least a half century, its prevalence was not appreciated until the classic studies of Vahlquist (1955) and Bille (1962), showing it to occur in between 3% and 5% of normal schoolchildren, depending on age. The term derives from a French version of "hemicrania," which Rothner (1979) attributes to Galen, in the first century A.D. The contemporary pediatric neurologist recognizes migraine as a syn-

---

Pearls and Perils: Migraine

1. "Sick headaches" are migraine until proven otherwise.
2. Migraine is a "great imitator" of a variety of other nervous system diseases.
3. Arteriovenous malformations may present with typical migraine headaches.
4. Headache and vomiting, most commonly due to migraine, are also cardinal signs of elevated intracranial pressure.

---

drome of remarkably protean manifestations, only one of which is headache.

Beginning with the classic studies of Graham, Wolff, and co-workers in the 1930s, a number of lines of evidence have suggested that the mechanism of migraine is spasm or constriction of cerebral arteries, causing focal neurologic deficit through focal cerebral ischemia, followed by reflex dilatation, causing the pain, usually from extracerebral branches of the same vessels. Observations by Lauritzen and associates (1983) would seem further to confirm this hypothesis. Direct observations of changes in vessel diameter during the attack remain ancedotal, but the widely recognized (although fortunately rarely occurring) complication of permanent vascular occlusion following migraine attacks is also consistent with the vascular hypothesis.

The clinical features of migraine are extremely variable. An important initial distinction is between the headache itself and other symptoms usually deriving from vascular spasm. It is customary to refer to the headache and certain immediately associated symptoms as "common migraine," and to the more full-blown neurologic syndrome as "classic migraine" (or sometimes as "complicated migraine," if the other symptoms are especially prominent). Onset may be at any time of day, including first thing in the morning; migraine rarely awakens the patient at night. Mode of onset is classically precipitous, more typically subacute. Duration is usually a few hours, but may be up to several days off and on. Location is classically unilateral, not necessarily on the same side for all attacks; however, a substantial minority, perhaps one third, of migraine attacks are bilateral to some degree. Supraorbital, posterior parietal, occipital, and temporal are the favored locations, more or less in that order of frequency. Severity is highly variable; the combination of symptoms in a migraine attack may be seriously debilitating, but the patient does not often scream with pain.

Associated symptoms are frequent and often helpful in the differential diagnosis. Nausea, with or without vomiting, is the most common, leading to the adage that "sick headaches are migraine until proven otherwise." Dizziness, photophobia, phonophobia, and postical sleep are frequent; the patient's insistence on lying down in a dark, quiet room is another hallmark of the syndrome.

Pearls and Perils: Tension Headaches

1. Tension headaches arise from anatomic structures outside the cranium.
2. Most people with headaches of whatever origin show some tension.

Often (though not always) the patient will report complete relief of the headache on awakening. Less frequent are symptoms of focal neurologic deficit assumed to be related to vascular spasm. Visual sensations may include dancing lights or scintillations, occasionally limited to one visual hemifield, and visual loss, which ranges from small scotomata, sometimes progressive in size over time, to complete blindness.

Oculomotor deficits may include either isolated opthalmoplegias or gaze palsies. Hermipareses, hemisensory deficits, and cortical function deficits ranging from general confusion (Gascon and Barlow, 1970) to specific aphasias may ensue. The syndrome of alternating hemiplegia in infants and children, first described by Verret and Steele (1971), is thought to be of migrainous origin.

The Relation of Migraine to Epilepsy. It has been recognized for some time that epileptic patients have an increased prevalence of migraine, and that electroencephalographic (EEG) abnormalities occur with greater than chance frequency in migraine sufferers (Ziegler and Wong, 1976). Milner (1958) and Basser (1969), recalling the phenomenon of spreading depression first described by Leao (1944a,b), suggested that this relation has a physiologic basis. Further studies by Whitehouse and colleagues (1967) and others suggested that the EEG finding of "14/6 per second positive spikes" might underlie not only migraine but a spectrum of paroxysmal disorders in children, including cyclic vomiting, abdominal pain, and possibly behavioral disturbances. Demonstrations by Lombroso et al. (1966) of a high prevalence of the 14/6 EEG pattern in nonsymptomatic populations suggested that the waveform might be a normal variant, and the notion that migraine might be an epileptic phenomenon is currently out of fashion. However, studies by DeLong and co-workers (1987) have shown a significant association between the 14/6 finding and aggressive behavior, suggesting that the prep school setting of Lombroso's studies might not represent an entirely "normal" population. In addition, our records include several EEG tracings showing the 14/6 waveform immediately followed by high-voltage slow and sometimes sharp waves. Our feeling is that the book is not yet shut on the 14/6 wave.

Depression

The prevalence of depression, including major depressive disease, among children has only relatively recently been recognized. Headache is one of the most common complaints. The mechanism of depressive headache is poorly understood, but probably has to do with the effect of mood on the perception of pain. The aggravation of minor aches and pains by a depressed mood is a common experience for all of us, and especially graphic in children. It is likely that the headache of depression begins with a tension headache, which contributes to depression and is in turn exaggerated in a sort of vicious circle.

Time of onset is frequently "every waking moment,"

Pearls and Perils: Depression

1. The depressive headache has other causes; it is only magnified by the depression.
2. Graphic description of the headache usually signifies a depressive element.
3. A depressed child with a headache may also have a brain tumor, especially in the major temporal lobe.

---

including at night. Depressed people often sleep poorly, and may complain of pain during their wakeful periods, but are probably not awakened by the headache itself. Mode of onset is usually gradual and relatively steady and unchanging during the time of complaint. Location is variable but usually symmetric, and may be circumferential or involve the vertex. The complaint is often voiced in graphic terms: "like my head is in a vise" or "like a spike through the head." Associated symptoms are those of depression, including sadness and dysphoria, suicidal thoughts, loss of psychic energy, anhedonia, social withdrawal, and vegetative dysfunction, such as insomnia, anorexia or overeating, and constipation.

Secondary or ("Symptomatic") Headache Syndromes

In the care of the child with headache, the physician's mission is twofold: diagnostic and therapeutic. The diagnostic mission in turn has two chief aims: to determine the most appropriate therapy to relieve the patient's suffering, and to uncover and treat a disease process of which the headache may be symptomatic. It is for consideration of this latter possibility that the patient is most often referred to the child neurologist.

The pathophysiologic processes of which headaches are most frequently symptomatic in children may be divided into four main categories: tumor, trauma, infection, and vascular disease. Exposure to certain toxins may also precipitate headaches.

Tumor

Tumor usually causes headache by exerting tension on meninges and/or blood vessels. This may be direct, from the tumor mass itself, or indirect, through edema or blockage of flow of cerebrospinal fluid. Disease processes involved include the solid tumors common to children (glioma, medulloblastoma, ependymoma, teratoma), and the leukemias, which most commonly infiltrate the meninges rather than the brain substance.

Time of onset is usually throughout the day. If the mechanism is raised intracranial pressure, the headache will be aggravated by the recumbent posture, and thus most severe during the night or first thing in the morning. With the exception of cluster headaches, the headache that awakens the patient in the middle of the night should always raise the suspicion of tumor. Mode of onset is classically relentlessly progressive over days to weeks, but the headache may wax and wane, being relatively less bothersome for hours to days at a time. Location may be focal, giving a clue to the location of the tumor, or generalized if intracranial hypertension is involved. One caveat regarding localization is that pain caused by stretching of the tentorium in the occipital region may be referred to the ophthalmic distribution of the trigeminal nerve. Severity is variable, but tumor headaches tend to be among the more bothersome and distressing examples of this malady.

Associated symptoms and signs may include vomiting and papilledema, the other two features of Cushing's triad. The time-honored notion that the vomiting is projectile with tumor is not reliable. There may be focal dysfunction owing to the tumor mass, or visual disturbance if papilledema compromises the blood supply to the optic nerve. The rate at which intracranial hypertension develops may determine the symptom pattern; slowly rising pressure may lead to severe papilledema in the absence of other symptoms. Systemic symptoms such as anorexia and cachexia may be further clues to a neoplastic process.

Trauma

Physical trauma to structures of the head can cause pain through a wide variety of mechanisms. Mild trauma can simply bruise the skin and subcutaneous tissue. If the periosteum is torn and stretched by hematoma, intense pain will result. Stretching and rupture of blood vessels can be caused by concussion (sudden acceleration or deceleration of the brain mass within the cranial cavity) or contusion (actual bruising of brain substance). The meninges, either the dura or the arachnoid or both, can

be stretched or ruptured by hematoma, or irritated by extravasated blood. Through mechanisms poorly understood, migraine can be precipitated or aggravated by mild head trauma (Haas and Sovner, 1969, Matthews, 1972). Finally, although again the mechanism is unclear, concussions or contusions that leave the patient otherwise entirely intact may be followed weeks or months thereafter by a poorly defined asthenic syndrome including nonspecific headaches, loss of psychic energy, and mild personality changes.

The disease process involved in every case includes at least a direct physical irritation of pain sensors. Although the severity of the trauma may vary widely, posttraumatic headaches are rare with trauma insufficient to cause at least some disturbance of consciousness. An important exception is epidural hematoma, which can result from apparently insignificant trauma, and whose acute onset is frequently heralded by severe focal headache several hours later.

Time and mode of onset will vary according to mechanism. Head pain from direct tissue injury will usually be apparent as soon as consciousness is recovered. Because any head trauma that disturbs consciousness is accompanied by some degree of amnesia, if only for the blow itself, the patient's retrospective report of headache onset may omit a period of days to weeks during which he or she was entirely conscious and complaining of pain, but for which he or she is later amnesic. With this reservation, time of onset is a valuable datum, distinguishing for example the epidural (hours to days) from the subdural (days to weeks) hematoma in most cases.

The posttraumatic headache is usually subacute to chronic, steady rather than throbbing, and of mild to moderate severity, with the above-mentioned exception of the acute epidural hematoma: Location may be quite focal to the point of trauma, except when an expanding mass of blood is involved, in which case the rules of referred pain mentioned in connection with tumor may apply. Associated symptoms may be those of focal brain dysfunction owing to traumatic injury. A rapidly expanding hematoma may cause herniation of the medial temporal lobe over the tentorium, compressing the midbrain and cerebral peduncle and paralyzing the third cranial nerve. Fractures in the base of the skull may cause leakage of cerebrospinal fluid through the nose (rhinorrhea) and also extravasation of blood into infraorbital or postauricular subcutaneous tissue or into the middle ear. Low cerebrospinal fluid pressure may also be the result of leakage from a lumbar puncture—the "post-L.P. headache" (Spielman, 1982).

Infection

Infection causes head pain through various mechanisms. The most common is direct irritation of meninges or blood vessels by the infectious agent or the inflammatory response it produces. A focus of infection, such as an intracerebral abcess, subdural empyema, or sinusitis,

Pearls and Perils: Infection

1. Both meningitis and migraine can cause photophobia, phonophobia, or both.

may of course act as an expanding mass, exerting pressure on meninges, blood vessels, or periosteum.

The disease process responsible may involve any structure or tissue type in the head. Infections probably account for headache more often than is recognized. Meningitis, vasculitis, encephalitis, and sinusitis are the principal processes, probably in that order of frequency. Viruses are by far the most common agents, but bacteria, fungi, and even spirochetes must be considered, chiefly because of their relative treatability.

Time of onset depends on underlying pathology, but for the most part shows no diurnal variation. Mode of onset may be rapid with acute infection (especially bacterial), and subacute with more indolent agents or when the mechanism of pain is pressure. Location tends to be generalized with meningitis or encephalitis, but may be focal with abscess, empyema, or sinusitis. Associated symptoms and signs may be crucial to diagnosis. They include signs of meningeal irritation or meningismus

FEATURE TABLE 24–1. HEADACHE

Type	Time of Onset	Mode of Onset	Location	Character	Associated Symptoms	Duration
Primary						
Tension	After noon	Subacute	Occipital/ bifrontal/ bitemporal	Steady	Tension/ emotional stress	Hours
Migraine	Anytime/early morning not night	Acute/ subacute	Unilateral; periorbital/ parietal/ occipital/ temporal	Throbbing/ steady	Nausea/ vomiting, dizziness, photophobia, focal neurologic deficit	Hours/ day
Depression	Anytime, including at night	Chronic; "every waking moment"	Bilateral; vertex, circumference	Boring/ gnawing/ drilling	Dysphria anhedonia, withdrawal, suicidal thoughts	Days/ weeks
Secondary						
Tumor	Anytime	Chronic; waxing/waning	Site of tumor or non-focal	Steady	Focal neurologic deficits or increased intracranial pressure	Weeks
Trauma	Anytime	Subacute/ chronic	Site of trauma or exp. mass	Steady	Focal neurologic deficit, herniation	Days/ weeks
Infection	Anytime	Acute/ subacute	Focal/nonfocal	Steady	Meningismus, photophobia, hyperacusis, systemic	Hours/ days/ weeks
Vascular	Anytime	Acute; "explosive" with subarachnoid hemorrhage	Focal/nonfocal; retro-orbital	Steady/ throbbing	Meningismus, fundal hemorrhages; focal deficit; systemic vascular	Hours/ days/ weeks
Toxic	Anytime	Dependent on toxin	Nonfocal	Steady	Vomiting, systemic; neuropathy	Hours/ days/ weeks

(back pain on straight leg raising, photophobia, hyperacusis), toxic signs of acute infection, and evidence of preexisting infection giving rise to abcess (pneumonia, otitis, congenital heart disease). Severity is highly variable, and not of much help in diagnosis.

Vascular Disease

Vascular disease (apart from migraine) causes head pain by one of two mechanisms: tension on blood vessels or meningeal irritation from bleeding. Principal disease processes responsible include arteriovenous malformation (AVM), aneurysm, and collagen-vascular disease. Of the three, AVM, although by no means a common childhood disease, is by far the most frequent. As a cause of subarachnoid hemorrhage, AVMs outnumber aneurysms by nearly 10 to 1 in children (approximately the opposite of the case with adults).

Clinical features of other vascular headaches are very similar to those of migraine; over half of AVM patients in some series have presented with migraine-like headaches. An important exception is subarachnoid hemorrhage, which produces the most acute-onset headaches known. As with adults, "explosive" headaches in children should be considered a symptom of subarachnoid hemorrhage until proven otherwise. Associated symptoms and signs may be quite helpful in diagnosis; they include meningismus and fundal hemorrhages from subarachnoid bleeding, localizing neurologic deficit from AVM, and multiple systemic signs of collagen-vascular disease.

Toxins

Toxins presumably cause headache either by direct effect on pain receptors or indirectly through elevated intracranial pressure from tissue edema. Offending agents may be divided into two large categories: endogenous and exogenous. The former include chiefly ammonia, which in children is usually produced by inborn errors of urea cycle metabolism or by severe liver disease, as in Reye's syndrome; and, less commonly, amino and organic acids in various inborn errors. The latter include tyramine and phenylethylamine (present in foods that aggravate migraine), monosodium glutamate (the offender in the "Chinese restaurant syndrome"), alcohol, heavy metals, and toxic doses of vitamin A. The bacterial toxins of the "toxic shock syndrome" should probably be included in

---

Pearls and Perils: Vascular Disease

1. Most vascular anomalies in children, even on the surface, are AVMs rather than aneurysms.
2. "Explosive" headache should be considered a symptom of subarachnoid hemorrhage until proven otherwise.
3. The early symptoms of AVM may be indistinguishable from those of migraine.

Pearls and Perils: Toxins

1. The headache of hyperammonemia owing to metabolic error may immediately follow protein ingestion.

---

this category rather than under infectious diseases, because the site of infection is remote.

Time and mode of onset of toxic headaches are usually related to toxin exposure, and may be acute, as with alcohol or tyramine, or chronic, as with heavy metals. Headaches in hyperammonemic states can be remarkably paroxysmal and related to specific high-protein meals. As the patient is sometimes both young and mentally subnormal, they may be difficult to diagnose or even to recognize as the cause of distress. Location is usually generalized and severity variable. Associated symptoms may include vomiting or other evidence of acute systemic illness. With the exception of heavy metal poisoning, focal neurologic deficit is not usually involved. Signs of elevated intracranial pressure may be present with hypervitaminosis-A.

THE HEADACHE WORKUP

In the minds of a majority of our patients, and also of more primary care physicians than we would like to admit, neurologic workup of headache is synonymous with laboratory tests, usually electrodiagnostic and/or radiologic. Pressures for defensive medicine notwithstanding, the specialist needs to bear in mind that, although such tests may satisfy the patient, they make a minimal contribution to diagnosis in the great majority of headache cases. History and physical examination are still the essential tools.

History of the Present Illness

The history is the cornerstone of neurologic diagnosis, and headaches are no exception. Although with many neurologic disorders it is better to elicit the history from the parent before the child is brought in, any child who can talk can make at least some contribution to a headache history. Our practice is in most cases to have the child in on the consultation from the start.

History of the present illness must in every case make reference to six important features of the headache. The first is *duration* of the illness (not the headache). Does the patient complain of a headache or headaches? If the latter, how long has the present series lasted, and is it the first? The usual story is that headaches have bothered the child infrequently for years, but that in recent weeks to months the frequency and/or severity has increased. Can precipitants or determinants of this increase be identified?

Concerning the acute headache that has brought the patient to attention, the clinician wants to know first about the *time of onset*. The critical distinction here is between those headaches that occur at any time of day (more likely migraine or secondary) and those that always appear after late morning (more likely tension). The problem with this distinction is that emotional upset can aggravate migraine; it is nevertheless worth asking about. Are headaches present when the patient awakens in the morning? A positive response practically rules out simple tension headaches. Are they worst in the early morning or do they ever awaken the patient at night? If so, increased intracranial pressure must be suspected, because the intracranial pressure is normally higher in the recumbent position. The converse situation (headaches aggravated by upright posture, relieved by lying down) is characteristic of the post–lumbar puncture headache, but more often accounted for by migraine. Other headaches that awaken the patient at night include cluster headaches and those secondary to depression.

The next question concerns the *mode of onset*. Here the clinician wishes to place the headache on the continuum between paroxysmal and ever-present. At one end of the spectrum is the "explosive" headache, which should always raise the suspicion of subarachnoid hemorrhage. At the other end is the depressive headache, present every waking moment of the day and night. In between, in descending order, are the sharply paroxysmal cluster headache, the widely variant but usually paroxysmal migraine episode, the subacute but recurrent tension headache, and the chronic but waxing and waning headache of tumor or other expanding mass. A crescendo increase in severity over hours usually signifies a tension headache; however, the epidural hematoma following seemingly benign head trauma can also behave in this fashion.

Next the clinician must ask about the *location* of the headache. It is helpful to ask the pediatric patient to "put one finger on where it hurts." Unilaterality versus bilaterality is the first judgment to make. Unilateral headaches will in most cases occur at least some of the time on the opposite side as well. It is an uncommon benign headache, even of the migraine variety, that always occurs in exactly the same location. Such a report should raise the suspicion of more serious focal pathology. Careful questioning will usually distinguish sinus headache from either periorbital headaches of vascular origin or tension headaches in the frontalis muscle tendons.

One should ask next about *associated symptoms*, and their temporal relation to the headache. The classic migraine attack is usually recognized; it begins with symptoms of focal neurologic deficit secondary to vasospasm, then progresses to headache, presumably the result of reflex vasodilatation, as mentioned earlier. However, the clinician soon learns that this classic presentation is seen in a small minority of migraine cases. The more usual story is of "sick headache," accompanied by nausea and dizziness, sometimes with photophobia and vomiting. A not uncommon report is that the headache "feels better" once vomiting has occurred. Nasal stuffiness and/or tearing may provide the clue to cluster headache. Sinus headache will usually be accompanied by other signs of sinus infection. Vomiting can of course occur as a result of elevated intracranial pressure; in such cases it will often be less clearly associated with episodes of headache. Symptoms of depression (sadness, social withdrawal, crying spells, thoughts or threats of suicide, anorexia, insomnia or hypersomnia, constipation) can be elicited reliably from the pediatric patient, who is less likely than the adult simply to blame the depression on the headache.

Finally, the clinician wishes to know about *response to therapy*. This is a much easier task with the pediatric patient, who as a rule has taken either no medication or small occasional doses of simple analgesics. Reliable data will seldom be available at the initial consultation, this is one of the important tasks of early management, to be discussed subsequently.

Past and Family History

A complete pediatric past history—including prenatal, perinatal, neonatal, and developmental details—is an important part of the neurologist's headache workup. One wants to rule out the entire range of developmental malformations, congenital and early childhood diseases that can cause elevated intracranial pressure, and electrolyte or metabolic imbalance. In addition the clinician wants to know how successfully the child is functioning in school and with peers at play. The clinical precept that the migraineur is a hard-driving, successful, over-worrying child probably has some truth to it. On the other hand, tension headaches may be a symptom of maladjustment and underachievement, and the depressive headache may be the cause rather than the result of these symptoms.

A positive family history of migraine or other headache is such a constant feature of the migraine syndrome as to put the diagnosis in doubt when absent. The same may be said to a lesser extent of major depressive disease. Occasionally, however, a careful chronology of the co-occurrence of child's and parent's headaches will suggest that the child's symptoms are more sympathetic than inherited. Less frequently, family history will uncover one of the heritable metabolic errors.

Physical Examination

The complaint of headache demands a general physical as well as neurologic examination. The former should include measurement of the blood pressure, auscultation of the head and neck for bruits, palpation of the abdomen, and a check for signs of meningeal irritation. The optic fundi must be well visualized in every case, especially the optic disks, for evidence of papilledema. Care should be taken to observe for pulsations of the retinal veins, which when present provide reasonable assurance of a cerebrospinal fluid pressure of less than 200 mm H₂O. Absence of the pulsations is not necessarily an abnormal finding, but disappearance of pulsations from one exam to the next can be a valuable early sign of papilledema.

The neurologic examination should aim to elicit signs of focal neurologic deficit, especially when the complaint is of focal headache. While transient focal deficit is common in migraine attacks (ophthalmaplegia, hemiparesis, and hemisensory loss being the most frequent in children), a stable localizing or lateralizing sign should raise the suspicion of more stable cerebral pathology.

Laboratory Studies

The headlong rush of technology, as well as a variety of pressures, all tend to drive the clinician toward greater dependence on laboratory studies in the workup of headache. Nevertheless, a certain amount of restraint is justified and desirable.

The *electroencephalogram* is obviously helpful when epileptic seizure is suspected, or as a measure of the physiologic effect of focal cerebral pathology. Its utility in migraine depends on one's position on the question of the relation between migraine and epilepsy, discussed earlier. Our practice is to obtain an EEG whenever the headache is frankly paroxysmal and/or focal.

The *computed tomographic (CT) scan* has revolutionized neurologic diagnosis within most of our professional lifetimes. It provides information regarding focal tissue pathology that previously was available only through a combination of painstaking clinical inference and more invasive imaging studies, such as pneumoencephalogram and arteriogram. When CT scans were more expensive and difficult to obtain, our rule in the case of headache was to reserve them for cases showing either a stable neurologic deficit or cause for suspicion of elevated intracranial pressure. More recently our threshold of decision has lowered to include focal headaches with transient functional deficit, headaches with persistent vomiting, and even nonspecific headaches that respond poorly to prophylactic treatment.

Intravenous injection of a radio-opaque contrast medium is usually necessary for optimal imaging of tissue pathology by the CT technique. There is some controversy regarding the use of contrast CT scans in migraine, the concern being the possible aggravation of vasospasm.

Principally because of the expense, magnetic resonance imaging is not performed as an initial procedure.

Angiography was once the principal imaging technique available for detection of mass lesions in the brain substance. This function has now been largely assumed by the CT scan, and these days the angiogram is largely reserved for vascular pathology. When headache is the complaint, AVM and aneurysm are the usual vascular culprits (as mentioned previously), although in children vascular occlusion (usually embolism) produces headache more frequently than in adults. There are well-docu-

mented cases of stroke immediately following angiography in migraine sufferers, justifying considerable caution in its use in this condition, particularly during an acute symptomatic episode.

Lumbar puncture for examination of the cerebrospinal fluid is a valuable tool for investigation of selected cases of headache. It is usually employed to detect infection or as an indirect measure of intracranial pressure. When employed for the latter purpose, it is nearly always performed after the CT scan, and deferred if the scan shows evidence of elevated pressure, for fear of precipitating uncal or medullary herniation. However, spinal fluid examination is sometimes judged so necessary to the workup as to justify a careful lumbar puncture, with minimal fluid removal and readily available decompression, even in cases showing other evidence of elevated pressure.

MANAGEMENT OF RECURRENT HEADACHE SYNDROMES

The acute, one-time headache, if sufficiently severe to bring the child to the neurologist, demands chiefly a diagnosis of the cause. Management is usually limited to effective short-term analgesia. It is for the recurrent headache syndrome that management becomes a critical issue, sometimes demanding the best skills and experience the physician has to offer.

First Line of Defense—Diagnostic Therapy

The patient with recurrent headaches who consults the neurologist must understand from the outset that effective management of the headaches is not going to begin with the initial consultation. We believe one of the most valuable lessons we can teach our patients is a respect for "hard data." Thus, our first recommendation for management in nearly every case is that the patient keep a written "headache diary." It should be kept over a period of several weeks, usually between 4 and 12, depending on the initially reported frequency of the complaint. We wish to know about each headache during that interval: (1) the date and time of onset; (2) location; (3) character, special features, and associated symptoms; (4) what if any medication was taken and when; and (5) how long the headache lasted.

During the period of data collection, we usually recommend as initial therapy adequate doses of simple analgesics, the first choice for children being acetaminophen. In response to the patient's frequent objection that this has "already been tried," we explain that these are in fact powerful and effective medications, available over the counter simply because they are so free of harmful side effects, but that they must be taken religiously and in adequate doses. We recommend as an initial dose a single regular-strength adult tablet (325 mg) for the child weighing 15 to 30 kg or two tablets for the child over

30 kg, taken at the very first sign of the headache, repeated every 3 hours if necessary. We ensure round-the-clock availability of adequate consultation by telephone in the event of a change or increase in symptoms, and instruct the patient to return with the headache diary at the end of the designated period. If indicated, we arrange for an EEG at the time of the return visit, giving instructions for preparation for sleep study in every case.

Longer-Term Pharmacotherapy

Simple analgesics do the job in about one in four cases in our experience. For the other three, stronger measures are called for. These may be classified as *episodic* or *prophylactic.*

Episodic therapy of simple tension headaches, when simple analgesics are not sufficient, should first be tried with preparations combining these medications with either mild sedatives or mild stimulants, depending on the nature of the complaint. With very rare exceptions, narcotics should be entirely avoided in children.

Episodic therapy of migraine is usually accomplished by ergot alkaloid preparations, either alone or in combination with caffeine. These drugs are relatively less effective in children; they tend to be more effective when premonitory symptoms of vasospasm can be clearly identified (thus allowing the medication to be given before the appearance of the headache), and are also more effective in older children and adolescents, especially females. A single tablet of Cafergot (100 mg caffeine, 2 mg ergotamine tartrate) should be given at the very first appearance of symptoms and repeated three to four times at half-hour intervals if necessary, with a maximum of 10 to 12 tablets per week. Alternatively, ergotamine tartrate (2 mg) may be given sublingually on a similar schedule. Cafergot is available as a rectal suppository, and this is an obvious advantage when vomiting is a prominent symptom. Antihistamine preparations may be of some benefit for cluster headaches, although these are best treated as migraine.

Prophylactic headache therapy is usually reserved for migraine and depressive headache. A certain minimum frequency of occurrence, usually once every 2 to 3 weeks, is required for prophylactic therapy to make sense. It has definite limitations for the younger child, who is particularly resistant to the idea of taking a medication for a symptom that is not occurring. For a given dose of a prophylactic medication, a minimum period of five to six times the baseline occurrence rate is necessary for determination of effect. It is important for future reference that any prophylactic medication tried have an adequate trial before going on to the next one.

For prophylaxis of migraine, propranolol is the current drug of first choice. It is well tolerated by children, and, except for aggravation of asthma and reduction of the heart rate, has few side effects. For the child under age 14 years, an initial dosage of 10 mg three times daily is appropriate. If this is not effective, the dose should be increased by 10 mg/day each week to a final dose of 20 mg three times daily before the drug is given up. The older adolescent may be treated as an adult, with approximately twice the above-mentioned doses. When effective, the medication may be taken safely for years, although it is prudent to recommend a trial of discontinuation after a symptom-free period of a year, especially if the dose is high.

Phenytoin was extensively used for childhood migraine before propranolol was available, especially during the years when the concept of a relation between migraine and epilepsy was popular. Its utility in current therapy depends to some extent on one's point of view on that question. Our feeling is that phenytoin is worth a try whenever the EEG is frankly paroxysmal, especially when the abnormality is focal and in a location corresponding to the symptom. It does have more side effects than propranolol, and on very rare occasions (toxic hepatitis and/or lymphadenopathy) these effects can be serious and even life threatening. Dosages are similar to those for seizure prophylaxis: up to 5 mg/kg, aiming for blood levels of 10 μg/mL or slightly higher.

Cyproheptadine, an antihistamine and antiserotonin agent sometimes used for appetite stimulation, is a relatively benign medication that can afford prophylaxis of migraine. Its side effects are usually limited to sedation. Dosages range from 2 to 4 mg two to four times daily.

Amitriptyline, a tricyclic antidepressant, has been shown to have an effect for migraine prophylaxis that may be independent of its antidepressant effect. It should be started in doses as small as 25 mg/day and increased by 25 mg/day each week to a maximum of 75 mg/day for children below pubertal age. For assessment of effect, 2 to 3 weeks are necessary even when headaches are as frequent as daily. In addition to the well-known side effects of dry mouth, blurred vision, orthostatic hypotension, and gastrointestinal upset, it can cause a difficulty with concentration that can be especially bothersome for good students, a group that includes many migraineurs.

Behavior Therapy and Relaxation Training

Emotional tension is so obvious a precipitant of headache that any effort to treat headache by reducing tension makes eminent a priori sense entirely apart from experimental demonstration of its efficacy. Some systematic approaches in recent years have shown very promising results. These are well described by Diamond and Dalessio (1982) and depend for the most part on the application of principles of operant conditioning to biofeedback, with the "reinforcing consequence" of the appropriate behavior consisting of some physiologic measure of relaxation (e.g., electromyogram of the frontalis muscle; change in pulse, blood pressure, or skin temperature). The feasibility of application of these techniques to children has been demonstrated. Behavior therapy has the obvious advantage of avoiding drugs, and at least potentially offers the patient strategies that have lifelong benefit. On the minus side, it is heavily demanding of the time of highly trained professionals, and thus will probably prove prohibitively expensive until such time as it can be highly automated.

Avoidance and Prevention

While recommendations for avoidance are not applicable to all cases of headache, they are overlooked by the clinician with surprising frequency. We have already mentioned the sensitivity of some migraine sufferers to certain foods, chiefly those containing tyramine, phenylethylamine, nitrites, or monosodium glutamate (Medina and Diamond, 1978; Swaiman and Frank, 1978). Tables of foods to be avoided are readily available (cf. Diamond and Dalessio, 1982). Briefly, they include ripened cheeses, nuts, peanut butter, chocolate, most alcoholic beverages but especially red wine, citrus fruits, processed meats, and Chinese foods.

Avoidance of extreme changes in temperature, especially of ingested foods or liquids, will protect the susceptible child from "ice cream headaches" (Raskin and Knittle, 1976). In addition, some children, especially adolescent females, experience aggravation of migraine on sudden body contact with cold water. We treated one such young lady who would complain of transient blindness on stepping into cold water at the seashore.

The role of allergy in migraine or other headaches is controversial. As is the case with hyperactive behavior, allergy and migraine are both so common that the clinician will frequently encounter children who suffer from both. The association of specific allergies with migraine, or the efficacy of allergen avoidance in headache prophylaxis, has not been demonstrated to our satisfaction in properly controlled studies.

Finally, the wisdom of avoidance of fatigue and undue stress seems self-evident. It is probably of particular benefit for the migraine sufferer, and especially relevant in today's super-competitive scholastic atmosphere.

ANNOTATED BIBLIOGRAPHY

Barlow CF: *Headaches and Migraine in Childhood.* Philadelphia, Lippincott, 1984.
  The most concise yet comprehensive review currently available. Generously embellished with case reports from the author's own experience.
Diamond S, Dalessio DJ: *The Practicing Physician's Approach to Headache.* Baltimore, Md, Williams & Wilkins, 1982.
  Current and readable, with good tables and graphs.
Diamond S (ed): Headache: Its diagnosis and management. *Headache* 19(3), 1979.

Proceedings of a symposium held December 5–6, 1978. Not entirely current, but contains several comprehensive reviews by leading authorities on individual topics.

REFERENCES

Barlow CF: *Headaches and Migraine in Childhood.* Philadelphia, JB Lippincott, 1984.
Basser LS: The relation of migraine and epilepsy. *Brain* 92: 285–300, 1969.
Bille B: Migraine in school children. *Acta Paediatr* 51(suppl)136:1–151, 1962.
DeLong GR, Rosenberger PB, Hildreth S, Silver I: The 14/6 associated clinical complex: A rejected hypothesis revisited. *J Child Neurol* 2:117–127, 1987.
Diamond S, Dalessio DJ: *The Practicing Physician's Approach to Headache.* Baltimore, Md, Williams & Wilkins, 1982.
Friedman AP, Harms E (eds): *Headaches in Children.* Springfield, Ill, Charles C Thomas, 1967.
Gascon G, Barlow CF: Juvenile migraine presenting as an acute confusional state. *Pediatrics* 45:628–635, 1970.
Haas DC, Sovner RD: Migraine attacks triggered by mild head trauma, and their relation to certain post-traumatic disorders of childhood. *J Neurol Neurosurg Psychiatr* 32:548–554, 1969.
Lauritzen M, Olsen TS, Lassen NA, Paulsen OB: Change in regional cerebral blood flow during the course of classic migraine attacks. *Ann Neurol* 13:633–641, 1983.
Leao AAP: Spreading depression of activity in the cerebral cortex. *J Neurophysiol* 7:359–390, 1944a.
Leao AAP: Pial circulation of spreading depression of activity in cerebral cortex. *J Neurophysiol* 7:391–396, 1944b.
Lombroso CT, Schwartz IH, Clark D, et al: Ctenoids in healthy youths. *Neurology* 16:1152–1158, 1966.
Matthews EB: Footballer's migraine. *Br Med J* 2:326–327, 1972.
Medina JL, Diamond S: The role of diet in migraine. *Headache* 18:31–34, 1978.
Milner PM: Note on a possible correspondence between the scotomas of migraine and spreading depression of Leao. *Electroencephalogr Clin Neurophysiol* 10:705, 1958.
Raskin NH, Knittle SC: Ice cream headache and orthostatic symptoms in patients with migraine. *Headache* 16:222–225, 1976.
Rothner AD: Headaches in children: A review. *Headache* 19:156–162, 1979.
Spielman FJ: Post-lumbar puncture headache. *Headache* 22:280–283, 1982.
Swaiman KF, Frank Y: Seizure headaches in children. *Dev Med Child Neurol* 20:580–585, 1978.
Vahlquist B: Migraine in children. *Int Arch Allergy* 7:348–355, 1955.
Verret S, Steele J: Alternating hemiplegia in childhood. *Pediatrics* 47:675–680, 1971.
Whitehouse D, Pappas JA, Escala PH, Livingston S: EEG changes in children with migraine. *N Eng J Med* 276:23–27, 1967.
Ziegler DK, Wong G: Migraine in children: Clinical and electroencephalographic study of families. A possible relation to epilepsy. *Epilepsia* 8:171–187, 1976.

Febrile Seizures

Deborah G. Hirtz
Karin B. Nelson

Since the time of Hippocrates, infants and young children have been known to be vulnerable to convulsions at the onset of acute febrile illness. Febrile seizures are the most common convulsive disorder of early childhood, occurring in approximately 2% to 5% of young children in the United States.

A febrile seizure was defined at a National Institutes of Health consensus conference (Consensus Statement, 1981) as

> an event in infancy or childhood, usually occurring between three months and five years of age, associated with fever but without evidence of intracranial infection or defined cause. Seizures with fever in children who have suffered a previous nonfebrile seizure are excluded. Febrile seizures are to be distinguished from epilepsy, which is characterized by recurrent nonfebrile seizures.

Young children may experience seizures during a febrile illness caused by such disorders as meningitis, dehydration, or toxic encephalopathy. These are not considered febrile seizures, and do not have the same prognosis, because the underlying illness may cause central nervous system damage in such cases.

Febrile seizures are often categorized into two subgroups: simple febrile seizures, which are brief and generalized, and complex febrile seizures, which are prolonged, focal, or multiple (more than one seizure in 24 hours) or followed by neurologic deficit. A family history of febrile or afebrile seizures or preexisting neurologic abnormality may accompany seizures in either of these categories (Table 25–1).

An older classification, proposed by Livingston, divided febrile seizures into "simple febrile seizures" and "epilepsy triggered by fever." The latter definition included febrile seizures that were prolonged or focal, or febrile seizures in a child with a family history of afebrile seizures. Although the features described by Livingston

do have a relationship to prognosis, these factors have been shown to have far less predictive power for later epilepsy than was indicated in his original studies (Annegers et al., 1979; van den Berg and Yerushalmy, 1969), and thus these definitions are no longer generally used.

CLINICAL PRESENTATION

Febrile seizures tend to occur early in the course of a febrile illness when the fever is rising rapidly. In some cases, the seizure is the first sign of the illness. The age of the child is usually between 3 months and 5 years. The most common seizure type is tonic-clonic. There may be an initial cry, followed by loss of consciousness and muscular rigidity (tonic phase). During the tonic phase, usually lasting less than 30 seconds, there may be apnea and incontinence. This is followed by a clonic phase consisting of repetitive, rhythmic jerking movements of the extremities or face. When movements have ceased, a period of postictal sleep or lethargy, usually brief, may follow.

Seizure types other than tonic-clonic may also occur. The seizure may consist simply of staring with stiffening or limpness, or the eyes may roll back. There may be jerking movements without prior stiffening. The movements may be focal, starting in one limb or one side of the body, and with or without generalization. The duration of the seizure is usually less than 15 minutes; in one large study less than 8% of febrile seizures were longer than 15 minutes (Nelson and Ellenberg, 1976).

Most of the febrile illnesses associated with febrile seizures are due to infections, such as tonsillitis, upper respiratory infections, or otitis media. One study isolated bacterial pathogens in 4% of cases and implicated common viral infections in 86% (Lewis et al., 1979).

In several infectious illnesses of early childhood,

TABLE 25-1. FEBRILE SEIZURES: DEFINITIONS

	Simple	Complex
Duration	< 15 minutes	May be ≥ 15 minutes
Type	Generalized	May be generalized or focal
Number during one illness	One	May be multiple
Followed by transient neurologic deficit	Never	Possible
Family history of febrile seizures	Possible	Possible
Family history of nonfebrile seizures	Possible	Possible
Preexisting neurologic abnormality	Possible	Possible

TABLE 25-2. DIAGNOSES TO BE CONSIDERED IN THE FEBRILE, CONVULSING CHILD

Bacterial or viral infection
Meningitis (bacterial, viral, granulomatous)
Encephalitis
Hypernatremic dehydration
Subdural or epidural empyema
Carotid arteritis complicating pharyngitis
Septic embolization
Reye's syndrome
Lead intoxication
Hemolytic uremic syndrome
Cortical thrombophlebitis

seizures may occur with fever, as during the prodrome of roseola infantum or shigella. With roseola infantum, the fever rises abruptly and the child may seize but looks well, and the diagnosis is not made until the appearance of a rash a few days later. Shigella gastroenteritis commonly presents with a seizure and a very high temperature, followed by passage of a green liquid stool as the lumbar puncture is being done to rule out meningitis. The pathogenesis of seizures in shigella may be related in part to a neurotoxin and not only to the occurrence of fever. One author has suggested that *Campylobacter* infections may cause a clinical picture similar to shigella (Buchta, 1983).

There are serious and potentially fatal conditions, not febrile seizures by definition, that can present as seizures with fever but which require prompt and specific treatment (Table 25-2). The possibility of bacterial meningitis should always be considered, particularly if the child is too young to exhibit typical symptoms such as meningismus. Viral meningitis or encephalitis may also present with seizures and fever, as may hypernatremic dehydration owing to gastrointestinal infection, acute toxic encephalopathy, or cerebrovascular accidents of infancy.

Children with preexisting epilepsy or brain damage may have their seizure thresholds lowered by fever. If a child has previously had one or more afebrile seizures, a seizure occurring with fever should be treated as an epileptic seizure and not as a febrile convulsion.

EPIDEMIOLOGY

In the United States, South America, and Western Europe, between 2% and 5% of all children experience convulsions with febrile illness before age 5 years (Hauser, 1981). Febrile seizures are reported to be about twice as common in certain Asian countries as in Europe and America. A study by Tsuboi (1984) found prevalence rates among 3-year old children from two locations in Japan to be 8.3% and 9.9%. The incidence of febrile seizures in Asian countries may be higher because of closer observation, with children sleeping in parents' rooms, and high housing density. However, there may be true racial or geographic differences.

In the recently reported National Birth Cohort Study from Britain (Verity et al., 1985a, b) as well as the National Institute of Neurological and Communicative Disorders and Stroke Collaborative Perinatal Project (NCPP; Nelson and Ellenberg, 1976) the first febrile seizure was complex in approximately 20% of cases; that is, it either lasted longer than 15 minutes, was multiple (two seizures or more within 24 hours), or was focal. Two thirds of the children had only a single febrile seizure, and 13% had only two episodes when observed over a 7-year period.

In about half of children with febrile convulsions, onset is in the second year of life. About 90% begin by 3 years. The average age of onset is 18 to 22 months. Febrile seizures are more common in males.

FEATURE TABLE 25-1. FEBRILE SEIZURES

Discriminating Feature	Consistent Features	Variable Features
1. Seizures in the presence of fever	1. Absence of previous afebrile seizure 2. Absence of CNS infection	1. Usually age 3 months to 5 years 2. Focal or generalized 3. May be multiple within one illness 4. Usually brief, may be prolonged 5. Family history of febrile seizures

The incidence of febrile convulsions is slightly but not statistically significantly higher in blacks than in whites. In the National Birth Cohort Study, the prevalence of a history of febrile convulsions was not related to social class. There was also no increased incidence in children with a history of allergic conditions.

A report by Sunderland and colleagues (1982) found statistically significant variations in incidence rates for febrile convulsions in relation to season and year of birth. However, others feel it is likely to be the age at time of exposure to febrile illness rather the season of birth that influences the incidence of febrile convulsions (Tsuboi and Okada, 1984).

Genetics

Febrile convulsions are more frequently found among family members of children with febrile convulsions than in the general population. In Japan (Tsuboi, 1984) as many as 17% of parents and 22% of siblings are affected, and reports from studies of Western countries have cited lower frequencies. In the NCPP, a family history of febrile seizures was identified in 7.3% of parents or prior-born siblings on prenatal questionnaires (Nelson and Ellenberg, 1978), and in the study by Verity and associates (1985a, b) a history of febrile convulsions was present in 16% of family members (including all relatives) of children with febrile convulsions. In Rochester, Minnesota, all relatives of febrile convulsions probands had a two- to three-fold increase in risk for convulsions with fever (Hauser et al., 1985).

There may be an increase in family history of afebrile seizures for children with febrile seizures, but the evidence is not as clear. Some studies have ascertained that afebrile seizure disorders are more frequent in siblings of children with febrile seizures (Metrakos and Metrakos, 1970; van den Berg, 1974). In the NCPP, a history of seizures without fever in a parent or sibling was present in 5.6% of children with febrile seizures (Nelson and Ellenberg, 1978), and it was present in 9.7% of all relatives in the British study (Verity et al., 1985a, b). Hauser and colleagues (1985) found that the relative risk for epilepsy was raised in siblings of children with febrile seizures (2.5), but was not increased in other relatives.

Younger siblings of the child with febrile convulsions have a 10% to 20% risk of having febrile convulsions. If both parents and a previous child have had febrile convulsions, the risk for another sibling may be increased to as high as one in three (Baraitser, 1983).

Although it is well accepted that familial factors, probably genetic, cause a predisposition to febrile seizures, the pattern of heredity is not known. An autosomal recessive mode of inheritance is unlikely because of the excess of affected parents and risk to siblings below 25%. A dominant mode of inheritance with reduced penetrance (Annegers et al., 1982) or a polygenetic mode (Tsuboi, 1977) are most plausible.

Recurrence

About one third of children who experience a single febrile seizure will experience a second. Of those who have a second, half will have two or more subsequent recurrences. About 9% of children with febrile seizures will have three or more. About three fourths of recurrences take place within 1 year, and 90% within 2 years.

The earlier the age at which the first febrile convulsion occurs, the greater the chance that there will be further convulsions (Table 25–3). A family history of febrile or nonfebrile convulsions, or both, also has been associated with an increased risk of recurrence. In neither the NCPP nor the British Birth Cohort Study were complex convulsions (i.e., focal, lasting longer than 15 minutes, followed by neurologic deficit, or multiple within 1 day) more often followed by recurrences. If the initial seizure was complex, the risk of a recurrence being complex was not increased. If the initial febrile seizure was brief, prolonged recurrence was very unlikely (only 1.4% in the NCPP). If the initial seizure was prolonged, prolonged recurrences were still unlikely (Nelson and Ellenberg, 1978; Verity et al., 1985a, b)

A higher number of febrile seizure recurrences does not appear to influence prognosis adversely with regard to later epilepsy or intellectual function. In two large studies, risk factors were more important than number of recurrences in predicting later epilepsy.

Epilepsy

Most population-based studies estimate that less than 5% of children with febrile seizures will go on to develop epilepsy (Ellenberg and Nelson, 1980). Other reports from selected populations of children with febrile seizures tend to cite a much higher rate of development of epilepsy than those from large population-based studies. For example, the report from the British National Child Development Study emphasizes that the differences seen depend to a large extent on sample selection: of 202 febrile seizure patients seen by general practitioners, 0.5% later had afebrile seizures. In contrast, 12% of children admitted to hospitals or referred to specialists had subsequent afebrile seizures (Ross et al., 1980).

Not all children with febrile seizures are equally at risk. Livingston (1958) believed there was a very high rate

TABLE 25–3. LIKELIHOOD OF RECURRENCE BY AGE AT FIRST FEBRILE SEIZURE

Age at First Febrile Seizure	Proportion with at Least One Recurrence
≤1 year	1/2
≤2 years	1/3
≤3 years	1/4
≤4 years	1/5

of later epilepsy in children with prolonged febrile seizures, abnormal electroencephalograms (EEGs), or focal febrile seizures, or who were over 6 years of age at first febrile fit. Later studies failed to confirm the *degree* of risk stated by Livingston for these children, but did establish that there was some degree of increased risk for later epilepsy among children with some of the risk factors mentioned by Livingston.

Nelson and Ellenberg (1976) found the following factors to be associated with increase in risk for epilepsy: suspect or abnormal neurologic development prior to the first febrile seizure, a history of afebrile seizures in a parent or sibling, and a complex first febrile seizure, that is, one that is focal, lasts over 15 minutes, or is multiple within 1 day. About 60% of the children in the NCPP had none of the above risk factors, of whom about 2% developed one or more afebrile seizures by age 7 years, a rate no different from that for children with no febrile seizures. About 34% of the children with febrile seizures had one risk factor; of these, 3% later experienced at least one afebrile seizure. An increase in the rate of later epilepsy appeared in those children with two or more risk factors: 13% of these children later had one or more afebrile seizures (Figure 25–1).

Neurologic abnormality occurring in the child before any seizure tends to be an important factor increasing the risk for epilepsy (Addy, 1986). In the NCPP, prolonged convulsions were followed by epilepsy in 1.4% of children with no prior neurologic abnormality and in 9% of children who were neurologically abnormal (Nelson and Ellenberg, 1978). Similarly, the risk of epilepsy after a first complex convulsion was 10% in a neurologically abnormal child but was not significantly increased in normal children (1.7% versus 1.1%) (Nelson and Ellenberg, 1976).

In general, the number of febrile seizure recurrences does not appear to be a factor in the later risk of epilepsy.

Half of the children who develop epilepsy after febrile seizures have the first afebrile seizure after a single febrile seizure. Almost half of the children who go on to develop epilepsy after febrile seizures do not have any of the identified risk factors. Abnormalities seen on EEG either acutely or in follow-up do not predict which children will develop epilepsy.

Variable types of afebrile seizures may occur following febrile seizures. Of the 34 children with febrile seizures in the NCPP who developed epilepsy, later seizure types included generalized motor, minor motor, partial motor, and clinically typical or atypical absence (Nelson and Ellenberg, 1976). In a series reported by Hirata and colleagues (1985), 20 children developed afebrile seizures out of 280 cases with febrile seizures. Among these 20, the distribution of seizure types was similar to that found in the NCPP. Sofijanov and associates (1983) compared a group of epileptic children with a history of febrile convulsions to a group of children without such a history and also found that all types of epilepsy were seen in patients with febrile convulsions.

Partial Complex Seizures

Some authors have suggested that febrile seizures, particularly if they are prolonged, may predispose to later complex partial seizures (temporal lobe or psychomotor epilepsy) (Falconer, 1971; Rasmussen, 1979). However, the early reports were from retrospective, uncontrolled series that did not exclude patients who may have had acute central nervous system (CNS) infections.

The bulk of the recent evidence supporting this hypothesis comes from experimental studies in rats. Evidence from recent clinical studies is more controversial. In several large studies, when epilepsy develops following febrile seizures, the proportion of complex partial seizures is no higher than in the general population

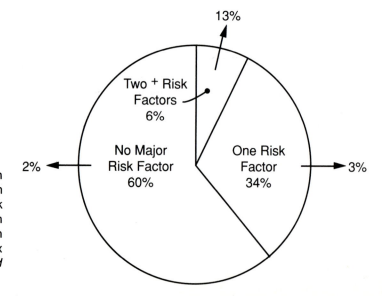

Figure 25–1. Afebrile seizures by age 7 years in children with febrile seizures, based on results from the NCPP on the outcomes of 1706 children. The risk factors evaluated were history of afebrile seizures in the immediate family, suspect or abnormal status in the child prior to first febrile seizure, and complex first febrile seizure. *(Reproduced from Nelson and Ellenberg, 1981, with permission.)*

of epileptics. Others report increased frequency of complex partial seizures in children with prolonged or focal febrile seizures. Schmidt and colleagues (1985) studied 155 patients with complex partial seizures, and concluded that there may be an association between febrile convulsions with complicating features and complex partial seizures. Epidemiologic studies from the Rochester, Minnesota, population (Hauser, 1981) have also shown that children with febrile seizures with focal features, repeated episodes, and long duration were at increased risk for later partial seizures.

Despite these data, it is unlikely that one or a few brief febrile seizures will damage selected vulnerable neurons and lead to later complex partial seizures. Children who have febrile convulsions are at slightly increased risk of complex partial seizures as well as other types of epilepsy compared to the general population. However, only a very small percentage of children with febrile seizures develop complex partial seizures, and a causal relationship has not been proven. According to Leviton and Cowan (1981), three theories may account for the association. The febrile seizures could cause the increase in risk for complex partial seizures; the febrile seizure could be the first manifestation of a seizure disorder; or separate but associated risk factors could exist for both disorders.

NEUROLOGIC OUTCOME

Children who have febrile seizures generally have normal intelligence. The British National Birth Cohort Study confirmed the lack of any significant impact of febrile seizures on later intellectual ability. Children in this study with a history of febrile convulsions did not differ from their peers in behavior, height, head circumference, or performance on simple intellectual tests. Children with simple as compared to complex febrile convulsions also did not differ in outcome. Children with febrile seizures did have an increased rate of hearing and speech problems (which may have been secondary to a higher rate of ear infections), and more frequently reported sleep disturbances (Verity et al., 1985a, b). However, this observation was of uncertain significance.

Two other large prospective studies agree that children with febrile seizures are normally intelligent. In the NCPP, in a sibling study, there was no effect on IQ or academic performance at age 7 years in children who were neurologically normal prior to the first febrile seizure and who did not develop afebrile seizures (Ellenberg and Nelson, 1978). In the National Child Development Study in Great Britain (Ross et al., 1980), children with febrile convulsions did as well as the remainder of the population in school performance at 7 and 11 years. With regard to motor handicap following febrile seizures, two large prospective series have not found any apparent

association with febrile seizures (Nelson and Ellenberg, 1978; Verity et al., 1985a, b).

There are some reports of a significant incidence of mental retardation in febrile seizure patients, but children with prior abnormalities and acute CNS infection at the time of the seizure were not excluded from these studies (Aicardi and Chevrie, 1976). Smith and Wallace (1982) have reported that children who have many recurrences tend to have a fall in developmental quotient; however, initial groups were not comparable with regard to expectation for intellectual outcome.

In summary, there is no evidence that febrile seizures cause a decrease in intellectual capacity.

MANAGEMENT

Acute Management

In most cases, a child with a febrile seizure is not brought to medical attention until after the seizure has ended. But an actively convulsing febrile child may present to an emergency room or doctor's office. In that case, the airway must be kept clear, proper oxygenation maintained, intravenous access established, and medication administered to stop the convulsion. Diazepam (0.2 to 0.3 mg/kg given at a maximum rate of 1 mg/min intravenously) is usually the first drug used and may be repeated up to a total dose of no more than 5 mg. Phenobarbital (10 mg/kg intravenously) may be used, or rectal diazepam in a dose of 0.5 mg/kg if an intravenous line cannot be readily established. It is important to be alert for, and prepared to deal with, respiratory depression, particularly if other anticonvulsant drugs have been previously administered.

When the child is seen following a febrile convulsion and is no longer convulsing, the most important task is to identify whether there is an underlying illness that may require treatment. After taking steps to control the fever, the physician should carefully examine the child and take the history. This should include a complete review of the patient's history and developmental progress, and a family history of febrile and afebrile seizures. If this was not the first episode, details of previous seizures should be noted. Particular attention in the physical examination should be paid to the level of consciousness, the presence of meningismus or a tense or bulging fontanelle, measurement of head circumference, and muscle strength, tone, and symmetry.

Lumbar Puncture

The most urgent diagnostic decision is whether or not a lumbar puncture (LP) should be done to rule out meningitis. In the younger child, classic meningeal signs may not be present and the index of suspicion should be very high; this is especially true for infants under 1 year of age. Various guidelines have been suggested based on age or the number of previous febrile convulsions (Wolf, 1978; Ouelette, 1977). Clearly, cerebrospinal fluid must be obtained if there is clinical suspicion of meningitis (such as prolonged lethargy), regardless of the child's age, number of prior febrile seizures, or family history, or the presence of another source of infection. Many authors recommend routine LP if the child is either less than 2 years or less than 18 months old because specific signs such as a stiff neck or bulging fontanelle may be absent. There is general agreement that an LP should be performed in all children under 1 year of age.

Joffe et al. (1983) reviewed the records of 241 children ages 6 months to 6 years who were seen for a first episode of seizure and fever in order to identify factors that could serve as guidelines in selection of patients warranting an LP. They found five items on the history and physical examination that identified all of the 13 children with meningitis and would have spared 62% of those without meningitis from LP. The findings were the following: a physician visit within 48 hours before the seizure, the occurrence of convulsions on arrival at the emergency room, a focal seizure, and suspicious findings on physical or neurologic examination (e.g., rash or petechiae, cyanosis, hypotension, respiratory distress, stiff neck, increased tone, lack of responsiveness, or tense fontanelle). However, use of these criteria is only recommended if a careful history and physical examination have been performed and if close follow-up for children not receiving LP is available.

A British physician (Clarke, 1985) cautions that there may be some circumstances under which an LP may be hazardous if carried out during or immediately after a seizure. Bacterial meningitis may be associated with raised intracranial pressure. Focal neurologic signs or coma may be present in a child with a febrile seizure and meningitis, and may indicate elevated intracranial pressure. In this situation LP may be hazardous. He suggests that in such cases it may be safer to give mannitol before the LP, or even to treat bacterial meningitis with antibiotics while deferring the LP. Clearly, should increased intracranial pressure be suspected clinically, the decision to perform LP must be made by an experienced physician, who will weigh the risk in delaying a diagnosis of meningitis against the risk of lumbar puncture.

Laboratory Studies

The search for a cause for the fever should begin with a careful examination. There is no routine laboratory evaluation in cases of febrile seizure (Table 25-4). In patients without an obvious source for the fever, blood cultures as well as urine culture, complete blood count, and chest x ray may be indicated. Occult bacteriemia, especially pneumococcal, has been reported as a possible important cause of febrile convulsions, which may often be overlooked (McIntyre et al., 1983). Other common

TABLE 25-4. EVALUATION AFTER FEBRILE CONVULSIONS

1. Workup of fever:
   History
   Physical examination
   Blood culture
   Throat culture
   Chest x ray   } As clinically indicated
   Urinalysis
   Urine culture
   Complete blood count
   Lumbar puncture
2. As clinically indicated: measurement of:
   Electrolytes
   Blood urea nitrogen
   Calcium
   Phosphorus
   Glucose
   Toxins
3. If there are focal abnormalities, a history of trauma, or a specific neurologic deficit present following the seizure:
   CT scan or MRI
   EEG

causes of fever may be more obvious, such as tonsillitis, otitis media, or upper respiratory viruses.

The recent trend is toward reducing the number of diagnostic tests performed in children presenting with febrile seizures, because physicians are under pressure to reduce unnecessary expenditures and because the yield from these tests, routinely used, is negligible. Electrolytes, blood glucose, blood urea nitrogen, calcium, and phosphorus should be evaluated when there is a specific indication, such as the presence of vomiting, diarrhea, or a history consistent with possible hypoglycemia. Skull x rays should be ordered only when there is a history of trauma, and a computed tomographic (CT) scan is indicated only if there is a history of significant head trauma or progressive neurologic changes, or neurologic abnormalities present after the seizure is over. In some situations of prolonged or focal seizures, a CT scan may be considered, but it still should not be routine.

The EEG has not been proven to be helpful in the evaluation of febrile seizures, although it is often ordered. Although studies describe increases in abnormalities in the EEG in febrile seizure patients, it has not been shown to be predictive of either febrile seizure recurrence or later epilepsy. An EEG done within 1 week of a febrile seizure will often be abnormal, most frequently because of occipital slowing. The incidence of paroxysmal abnormalities increases with age, and they may be found in 40% or more of children with febrile seizures followed for several years. Alvarez and associates (1983) have noted the presence of hypnagogic paroxysmal spike wave activity in almost a quarter of children with febrile convulsions, an incidence significantly higher than that in a control population. However, the children who had this abnormality could not be distinguished clinically from those who did not.

Although there may be a higher incidence of EEG abnormalities in children with febrile seizures, the EEG has not been shown to be helpful in predicting recurrences or the risk for later epilepsy. It may sometimes play a role in the management of children with focal febrile seizures, particularly if the seizures are followed by focal neurologic abnormalities, to identify underlying structural pathology.

Hospitalization

Hospitalization is usually unnecessary after a febrile seizure. The decision to hospitalize a child with a febrile seizure depends largely on the specific clinical situation and the family. Whenever possible, children presenting with a febrile seizure should be kept in an emergency room holding area for up to several hours and then reevaluated. The majority of children will have improved after a short time. If they are alert and the etiology of the fever is clear, they can be sent home, provided that follow-up care can be assured. It is advisable to schedule a follow-up appointment within a few days for reevaluation and education of the parents. If the child's clinical condition is still unstable, or if there is any question concerning the etiology of the seizure or the possibility of meningitis, the child should be admitted. If follow-up contact with the family is uncertain, or if the parents seem unreliable or unable to cope, hospitalization may be advisable.

In a survey of pediatricians published in 1975 (Asnes et al., 1975), nearly one quarter routinely hospitalized a child with a first febrile seizure, and 62% occasionally hospitalized these patients. A multispecialty survey (Hirtz et al., 1986) found that about one fifth of neurologists, pediatricians, and child neurologists frequently or routinely hospitalize children with febrile seizures. Frequent or routine hospitalization was more commonly practiced if the child had medical complications or after prolonged seizures. The current trend is away from hospitalization when possible, for reasons that include pressure to avoid unnecessary costs, increased awareness of the favorable outlook for these patients, and wish to avoid exposure of other hospitalized children to the viral illnesses commonly present in youngsters with febrile seizures.

One study was designed to determine if it was possible to predict which children with febrile seizures would have a second seizure during the same febrile illness (Green and MacFaul, 1985). Of 199 children with febrile seizures, 32 (16%) experienced more than one seizure in the same illness, 13 occurring before hospital admission and 19 after admission. All of these seizures occurred within 24 hours of admission. No factors were found predictive of which seizures would be "multiple," that is, recurring during the same illness.

Parental Counseling

The parents of a child with a first febrile convulsion are likely to be extremely upset and in a state of panic. When a seizure is first witnessed, parents often think the child is dead or dying (Hansen, 1984). They may pick up and shake the child, bang him or her on the back, try to insert fingers or an object between the teeth, or desperately attempt mouth-to-mouth resuscitation. These actions may actually endanger a convulsing child.

After the parents have had an opportunity to calm down and are assured that their child is alive, they need instructions on management of possible recurrences, which may occur either during the same illness or later on. Information and counseling are needed after the acute event and also later, when parents have had a chance to formulate questions. Information and instructions in a written format are helpful. The following points need to be stressed:

1. Although the seizure may have been quite frightening to witness, the child will not have suffered brain damage as a result of the fit, and the likelihood of future epilepsy is very small.
2. There is a risk of another convulsion when the child has another febrile illness, as well as a small risk of another convulsion within 24 hours.
3. If a febrile seizure recurs, parents must be told to stay calm, to place the child on his or her side or stomach with face downwards on a protected surface, and not to force anything between the teeth. It is very important that parents observe the child, note any focal features (especially at onset), and time the duration of the seizure. If the seizure lasts longer than 10 minutes, then the child should be brought to the nearest medical facility by car or ambulance.

It is reasonable to avoid high fevers when possible in a child who has experienced a febrile seizure, so parents should be instructed in temperature taking and fever management. Parents should be cautioned against overwrapping their children, which will exacerbate fever. Instructions on measurement of fever, dosage and timing of antipyretics, and sponging should be given, in writing, if appropriate. The exact temperature required to induce a febrile seizure is not known, but is generally thought to be 38°C or greater. Because the rate of rise of the fever may be as important as its height, there will be circumstances under which parents are unaware of a rapidly rising fever until a seizure recurs. Thus it must be stressed to them that, although treating their child's fevers is appropriate, they should not hold themselves responsible if seizures recur.

The parents may ask questions and should be counseled on the prognosis for their child. It should be stressed that, in general, children with febrile seizures do very well. Physicians can feel comfortable in reassuring parents that children do not die because of febrile convulsions; in large cohort studies no deaths were reported. Earlier studies reporting deaths among hospitalized children with febrile seizures included cases of severe preexisting handicap and meningitis. Factors affecting recurrence rate and risk of epilepsy should be discussed, as well as the reasons influencing the physician's decision to initiate or withhold anticonvulsant therapy. If medication is prescribed, a full discussion of the goals, risks, benefits, and side effects is needed.

Questions regarding the advisability of continuation of routine childhood immunizations may arise, because most routine immunizations are scheduled at the age of susceptibility to febrile seizures. In the NCPP, seizures following childhood immunizations had the characteristics and benign outcome of febrile seizures (Hirtz et al., 1983). Other recent studies have noted an increase in febrile but not afebrile seizures following diphtheria-pertussis-tetanus immunization (Walker et al., 1988; Griffin et al., 1990). In each child, the advantages of the protection offered by the vaccine must be weighed against the possible complications of immunization, and the advisability of immunization with pertussis should be reevaluated at each subsequent medical visit. The risks and benefits of immunization should be discussed fully with parents and a record made of the discussion, whatever the conclusion. If immunizations are given, prompt administration of antipyretics for fever and close observation are warranted for 48 hours following diphtheria-pertussis-tetanus immunization and during the seventh through tenth days after measles immunization.

Long-Term Management

Although antipyretics such as aspirin and acetaminophen do reduce fever, they cannot be relied on to prevent febrile seizures. Often, a febrile seizure may be the first sign that the child is feverish and antipyretics cannot be administered early enough in the course of a febrile illness to prevent an initial rapid rise of fever. Nevertheless, it is important to make certain parents are aware of proper dosage and administration of antipyretics and of sponging techniques, and that they try to reduce their child's fever when possible. Treatment of the primary illness causing the fever should be instituted as soon as possible, when there is a treatment, for example in cases of otitis media.

There is no convincing evidence to date that treating children with febrile seizures with anticonvulsant therapy can prevent the development of epilepsy, and there are case reports from Japan of adequately treated children who went on to develop epilepsy (Hirata, 1985). An extremely large randomized and controlled trial would be necessary to determine if treatment reduces the risk of afebrile seizures; such a trial may never be undertaken.

The intermittent use of phenobarbital at the time of febrile illness has been tried by some physicians with the intent of preventing febrile seizure recurrences. This therapy is not effective. An acute dose does not achieve a therapeutic blood level unless the dose is so large as to be dangerous, because the half-life of phenobarbital is 24 to 100 hours and it takes at least five half-lives to achieve a steady-state blood level. The tendency to use intermittent phenobarbital prophylaxis appears to be declining. A 1975 questionnaire revealed that intermittent therapy was commonly used by pediatricians (Asnes et al., 1975). A more recent survey (Hirtz et al., 1986) revealed that 14% of pediatricians frequently or routinely prescribed intermittent therapy for febrile seizures, but that the practice was directly related to the age of the physician and was much less frequent among younger physicians.

A number of series have reported that continuous daily treatment with phenobarbital or valproate decreases the risk of recurrent febrile seizures (Lee and Melchior, 1981; Mamelle et al., 1984; Wolf et al., 1977). Most of these studies have dealt with children with a first uncomplicated febrile seizure. Not all reports have confirmed the efficacy of the treatment. Newton (1988) has questioned whether many of the studies with positive results were methodologically appropriate. Pooled analysis of British trials of treatment with phenobarbital or valproate, including both published and previously unpublished trials (Newton, 1988), did not show significant reduction in recurrent seizures with either agent. Two new randomized trials (McKinlay, 1989; Farwell et al., 1990),

---

Pearls and Perils: Febrile Seizures

1. Most children with febrile seizures do extremely well. The closer the clinical picture is to the typical case, the more assured is a good prognosis.
2. The earlier the age at which the first febrile convulsion occurs, the more likely are recurrences.
3. There is no increase in risk of intellectual deficit owing to the occurrence of febrile seizures.
4. The number of febrile seizure recurrences does not directly relate to the risk of later epilepsy.
5. Intermittent phenobarbital at the time of fever only is not effective in preventing recurrences.
6. Diagnostic laboratory tests should never be routine, but should be justified by the specific clinical setting.
7. The risk for later epilepsy after febrile seizures is relatively increased but still low when:
   a. There is neurologic or developmental abnormality before any seizures.
   b. There is a history of seizures without fever in a parent or sibling.
   c. The first febrile seizure is focal, is multiple, or lasts longer than 15 minutes.

which examined selected populations of children with febrile seizures at increased risk of subsequent seizures and analyzed according to intention to treat, do not demonstrate efficacy for phenobarbital, nor (in the former) valproate, for the chronic treatment of febrile seizures.

For some time there has been concern that barbiturates may pose a risk to cognitive and behavioral function in children. In a recent randomized clinical trial designed to address this question, mean IQ was 7 points lower in children with early, complex, or repeated febrile seizures who were randomly assigned to treatment for 2 years with phenobarbital, as compared with children given a placebo (Farwell et al., 1990). There was no difference in occurrence of subsequent seizures between the group assigned to phenobarbital and the group assigned to the placebo. Thus evidence based on samples of children selected for characteristics that make them candidates for consideration of long-term medical therapy after febrile seizures suggests that phenobarbital may adversely affect cognitive function and may offer no countervailing benefit in reducing the risk of later seizures.

There are a few effective alternatives to phenobarbital, but none to date that are problem-free. Sodium valproate has been found to be effective in the prevention of febrile seizure recurrences (Lee and Melchior, 1981; Mamelle et al., 1984). The dose of valproate recommended is 20 to 35 mg/kg per day. The incidence of side effects was very low in these studies. However, rare but life-threatening complications of pancreatitis and acute liver failure have been reported with sodium valproate, and it is appropriate to exercise caution in considering its use in a relatively benign disorder such as febrile convulsions. Less serious complications include weight gain, gastrointestinal dysfunction, and hair loss.

Alternative modes of therapy to phenobarbital and valproate for prevention of febrile seizure recurrence are limited. Carbamazepine does not prevent febrile seizure recurrences (Antony and Hawke, 1983) and phenytoin is also ineffective (Melchior et al., 1971).

In countries outside the United States, intermittent oral and rectal diazepam has been successfully used for febrile seizure prophylaxis. Both routes provide therapeutic anticonvulsant levels within minutes. When rectal administration of diazepam at the onset of illness was compared to daily phenobarbital, febrile seizure recurrences were less frequent with diazepam, even though in a few cases parents did not recognize illness was present until the seizure occurred (Thorn, 1981). Diazepam administered rectally was given every 12 hours for fever (38.5°C) and was effective in preventing recurrences. However, some mild transient sedation was seen in one third of the children (Knudsen, 1985). Others have successfully used diazepam orally at the onset of fever (Minagawa et al., 1985; Dianese, 1979). Another successful strategy has been home treatment with rectal diazepam once a seizure begins, a regimen designed to prevent prolonged convulsions. At present in this country, rectal or oral diazepam at the time of illness has not been widely used because of the concern over the possibility of sedation of a sick child, and further study in a controlled clinical trial is appropriate. However, the prescription of rectal diazepam may be useful in selected cases for certain qualified parents to administer at home for the prevention of lengthy recurrent convulsions.

CONCLUSION

Although febrile seizures may be frightening to witness, the child who has one or several will usually do quite well. Only a small number of children will later develop epilepsy, and unless exceedingly lengthy the seizures do not appear to cause brain damage or result in later intellectual or motor handicaps.

Parental reassurance and counseling form the cornerstone of management of the child with febrile seizures. Treatment has not been shown to prevent the development of epilepsy. Few children need be placed on treatment to prevent recurrences. These would predominantly be children whose clinical picture is quite atypical, such as the child who has experienced focal paralysis following a febrile seizure. Potential risks of anticonvulsant therapy must be weighed against benefits. Further investigations of new therapies are needed before we can be assured that they are both safe and efficacious. Fortunately, the great majority of children with febrile seizures will have a good outcome whatever management strategy their physician chooses.

ANNOTATED BIBLIOGRAPHY

Addy DP: Nosology of febrile convulsions. *Arch Dis Child* 61:318–320, 1986.

A discussion of factors that have an impact on the prognosis of the child with febrile seizures. The evidence resulting from the major studies is very well presented and summarized, and logical conclusions are drawn. Where questions remain, they are well defined.

Hirtz DG, Nelson KB: The natural history of febrile seizures. *Annu Rev Med* 34:453–471, 1983.

This is a previously published review by the current authors with more emphasis on results of published studies on febrile seizures.

Verity CM, Butler NR, Golding J: Febrile convulsions in a national cohort followed up from birth. I. Prevalence and recurrence in the first five years of life. *Br Med J* 290:1307–1310, 1985.

Verity CM, Butler NR, Golding J: Febrile convulsions in a national cohort followed up from birth. II. Medical history and intellectual ability at 5 years of age. *Br Med J* 290:1311–1314, 1985.

This study gives the results of follow-up of about 16,000 neonatal survivors born in 1 week in Britain in 1970. Children with febrile convulsions were compared to their peers at 5 years. This study is in good agreement with the results of the previous large American studies, but unfortunately also repeats some of their weaknesses, such as lack of reporting of treatment.

Farwell JR, Lee YJ, Hirtz DG, Sulzbacher SI, Ellenberg JH, Nelson KB: Phenobarbital for febrile seizures: Effects on intelligence and seizure recurrence. *N Engl J Med* 322:364–369, 1990.

This article reports the results of a randomized, double-blind, placebo-controlled study to investigate the side effects of phenobarbital for prevention of febrile seizures. An adverse effect on intellectual function was seen.

REFERENCES

Addy DP: Nosology of febrile convulsions. *Arch Dis Child* 61:318–320, 1986.

Aicardi J, Chevrie JJ: Febrile convulsions, neurological sequelae, and mental retardation, in Brazier MAB, Coceani F (eds): *Brain Dysfunction in Infantile Febrile Convulsions.* New York, Raven Press, 1976, p 247–257.

Alvarez N, Lombroso CT, Medina C, Cantton B: Paroxysmal spike and wave activity in drowsiness in young children: Its relationship to febrile convulsions. *Electroencephalogr Clin Neurophysiol* 56:406–413, 1983.

Annegers JP, Hauser WA, Elveback LR, Kurland LT: The risk of epilepsy following febrile convulsions. *Neurology* 29:297–303, 1979.

Annegers JF, Hauser WA, Anderson VE, Kurland LT: The risk of seizure disorders among relatives of patients with childhood onset epilepsy. *Neurology* 32:174–179, 1982.

Antony JH, Hawke SHB: Phenobarbital compared with carbamazepine in prevention of recurrent febrile convulsions. *Am J Dis Child* 137:842–895, 1983.

Asnes RS, Novick LF, Nealis J, Nguyen M: The first febrile seizure: A study of current pediatric practice. *J Pediatr* 87:485–488, 1975.

Baraitser M: Relevance of a family history of seizures. *Arch Dis Child* 58:404–405, 1983.

Buchta RM: Campylobacter enteritis associated with convulsions. *Am J Dis Child* 137:919, 1983.

Clarke MA: Convulsions and lumbar puncture. *Dev Med Child Neurol* 27:541–542, 1985.

Consensus Statement on Febrile Seizures, in Nelson KB, Ellenberg JH (eds): *Febrile Seizures.* New York, Raven Press, 1981, p 301.

Dianese G: Prophylactic diazepam in febrile convulsions. *Arch Dis Child* 54:244–245, 1979.

Ellenberg JH, Nelson KB: Febrile seizures and later intellectual performance. *Arch Neurol* 35:17–21, 1978.

Ellenberg JH, Nelson KB: Sample selection and the natural history of disease—Studies of febrile seizures. *JAMA* 243:1337–1340, 1980.

Ellenberg JH, Nelson KB: Long-term clinical trials on the use of prophylaxis for prevention of recurrences of febrile seizures and epilepsy, in Nelson KB, Ellenberg JH (eds): *Febrile Seizures.* New York, Raven Press, 1981, p 267–278.

Falconer MA: Genetic and related etiological factors in temporal lobe epilepsy. *Epilepsia* 12:13–31, 1971.

Farwell JR, Lee YJ, Hirtz DG, Sulzbacher SI, Ellenberg JH, Nelson KB: Phenobarbital for febrile seizures: Effects on intelligence and seizure recurrence. *N Engl J Med* 322:364–369, 1990.

Green AL, MacFaul RV: Duration of admission for febrile convulsions? *Arch Dis Child* 60:1182–1184, 1985.

Griffin MR, Ray WA, Mortimer EA, Fenichel GM, Schaffner W: Risk of seizures and encephalopathy after immunization with the diphtheria-tetanus-pertussis vaccine. *JAMA* 263:1641–1645, 1990.

Hansen A, Abitbol V, Ibsen KK, et al: Conditions for children and their parents in hospitals. III. Parents' reactions in connection with admission of the child with the diagnosis of the first febrile seizure. *Ugeskr Laeg* 196:689–691, 1984.

Hauser WA: The natural history of febrile seizures, in Nelson KB, Ellenbrg JH (eds): *Febrile Seizures.* New York, Raven Press, 1981, p 5–17.

Hauser WA, Annegers JF, Anderson VE, Kurland LT: The risk of seizure disorders among relatives of children with febrile convulsions. *Neurology* 35:1268–1273, 1985.

Hirata Y, Mizuno Y, Nakano M, Sohmiya K: Epilepsy following febrile convulsions. *Brain Dev* 7:1–75, 1985.

Hirtz DG, Nelson KB, Ellenberg JH: Seizures following childhood immunizations. *J Pediatr* 102:14–18, 1983.

Hirtz DG, Lee YJ, Ellenberg JH, Nelson KB: Survey on the management of febrile seizures. *Am J Dis Child* 140:909–914, 1986.

Joffe A, McCormick M, De Angeles C: Which children with febrile seizures need lumbar puncture? *Am J Dis Child* 137:1153–1156, 1983.

Knudsen FU: Recurrence risk after first febrile seizure and effect of short term diazepam prophylaxis. *Arch Dis Child* 60:1045–1049, 1985.

Lee K, Melchior JC: Sodium valproate versus phenobarbital in the prophylactic treatment of febrile convulsions in childhood. *Eur J Pediatr* 137:151–153, 1981.

Leviton A, Cowan LD: Do febrile seizures increase the risk of complex partial seizures? An epidemiologic assessment, in Nelson KB, Ellenberg JH (eds): *Febrile Seizures.* New York, Raven Press, 1981, p 65–74.

Lewis HM, Parry JV, Parry RP, et al: Role of viruses in febrile convulsions. *Arch Dis Child* 54:869–876, 1979.

Livingston S: Convulsive disorders in infants and children. *Adv Pediatr* 10:1113–1119, 1958.

McIntyre P, Kennedy R, Harris F: Occult pneumococcal bacteraemia and febrile convulsions. *Br Med J* 286:203–206, 1983.

McKinlay I, Newton R: Intention to treat febrile convulsions with rectal diazepam, valproate, or phenobarbitone. *Dev Med Child Neurol* 31:617–625, 1989.

Mamelle N, Mamelle JC, Plasse JD, Revol M, Gilly R: Prevention of recurrent febrile convulsions—A randomized therapeutic assay: Sodium valproate, phenobarbital and placebo. *Neuropediatrics* 15:37–42, 1984.

Melchior JD, Buchthal F, Lennox-Buchthal M: The ineffectiveness of diphenylhydantoin in preventing febrile convulsions in the age of greatest risk, under three years. *Epilepsia* 12:55–62, 1971.

Metrakos JD, Metrakos K: Genetic factors in epilepsy. *Mod Probl Pharmacopsychiatr* 4:71–86, 1970.

Minagawa K, Mizuno S, Shirai H, Miura H: A pharmacokinetic study on the effectiveness of intermittent oral diazepam in the prevention of recurrent febrile convulsions. *No To Hat-tatsu* 17:162–167, 1985.

Nelson KB, Ellenberg JH: Predictors of epilepsy in children who have experienced febrile seizures. *N Engl J Med* 295:1029–1033, 1976.

Nelson KB, Ellenberg JH: Prognosis in children with febrile seizures. *Pediatrics* 61:720–727, 1978.

Newton RW: Randomized controlled trials of phenobarbitone and valproate in febrile convulsions. *Arch Dis Child* 63:1189–1191, 1988.

Ouelette EM: Managing febrile seizures. *Drug Ther* 2:37–39, 1977.

Rasmussen T: Relative significance of isolated infantile convulsions as a primary cause of focal epilepsy. *Epilepsia* 20:395–401, 1979.

Ross EM, Peckham CS, West P, Butler NR: Epilepsy in childhood: Findings from the National Child Development Study. *Br Med J* 1:207–210, 1980.

Schmidt D, Tasi JJ, Janz D: Febrile seizures in patients with complex partial seizures. *Acta Neurol Scand* 72:68–71, 1985.

Smith JA, Wallace ST: Febrile convulsions: Intellectual progress in relation to anticonvulsant therapy and to recurrence of fits. *Arch Dis Child* 57:104–107, 1982.

Sofijanov N, Sadikario A, Dukovski M, Kuturec M: Febrile convulsions and later development of epilepsy. *Am J Dis Child* 137:123–126, 1983.

Sunderland R, Carpenter RC, Gardner A: Are all born equal? Incidence of febrile convulsions by season of birth. *Br Med J* 284:624–626, 1982.

Thorn I: Prevention of recurrent febrile seizures: Intermittent prophylaxis with diazepam compared with continuous treatment with phenobarbital, in Nelson KB, Ellenberg JH (eds): *Febrile Seizures*. New York, Raven Press, 1981, p 119–126.

Tsuboi T: Genetic aspects of febrile convulsions. *Hum Genet* 38:169–173, 1977.

Tsuboi T: Epidemiology of febrile and afebrile convulsions in children in Japan. *Neurology* 34:175–181, 1984.

Tsuboi T, Okada S: Seasonal variation of febrile convulsions in Japan. *Acta Neurol Scand* 69:285–292, 1984.

van den Berg BJ, Yerushalmy J: Studies on convulsive disorders in young children. I. Incidence of febrile and nonfebrile convulsions by age and other factors. *Pediatr Res* 3:298–304, 1969.

van den Berg BJ: Studies on convulsive disorders in young children. IV. Incidence of convulsions among siblings. *Dev Med Child Neurol* 16:457–464, 1974.

Verity CM, Butler NR, Golding J: Febrile convulsons in a national cohort followed up from birth. I. Prevalence and recurrence in the first five years of life. *Br Med J* 290:1307–1310, 1985a.

Verity CM, Butler NR, Golding J: Febrile convulsions in a national cohort followed up from birth. II. Medical history and intellectual ability at 5 years of age. *Br Med J* 290:1311–1315, 1985b.

Walker AM, Jick H, Perera DR, Knauss TA, Thompson RS: Neurologic events following diphtheria-tetanus-pertussis immunization. *Pediatrics* 81:345–349, 1988.

Wolf SM: Laboratory evaluation of the child with a febrile convulsion. *Pediatrics* 62:1074–1076, 1978.

Wolf SM, Carr A, Davis DC, et al: The value of phenobarbital in the child who has had a single febrile seizure: A controlled, prospective study. *Pediatrics* 59:378–385, 1977.

The Hyperactive Child

Mary B. McMurray
Russell A. Barkley

The problem of the "hyperactive child" is a common one, the incidence being variously reported from as low as 0.5% to as high as 20% of the school-age population (Ross and Ross, 1982). This latter figure would suggest that the problem is almost a variation of normal. More commonly a figure of 2% to 4% is quoted (*Diagnostic and Statistical Manual of Mental Disorders*, 1987 [DSM-III-R]). The physician who treats children will encounter the condition with some frequency and is often the first professional to whom parents will turn for help.

The syndrome of attentional difficulties, impulsive behavior, distractibility, and overactivity has been known for many years. There have been numerous attempts at definition and the establishment of nomenclature (Barkley, 1981). Among the names that have been applied are Strauss's syndrome, minimal brain dysfunction, minimal brain damage, and hyperkinesis. Most recently these have been replaced by attention deficit disorder (ADD; *Diagnositc and Statistical Manual of Mental Disorders*, 1980 [DSM-III]), which focuses on the primary problem of difficulty in sustaining attention to task. DSM-III divided children with ADD into those with or without hyperactivity, depending on whether or not they showed overt increased motor activity. The validity of this distinction is now under question (Carlson, 1986). DSM-III-R combines the two as attention deficit hyperactivity disorder (ADHD) and gives the following diagnostic criteria:

A. 1. often fidgets with hands or feet or squirms in seat (in adolescents may be limited to subjective feelings of restlessness)
   2. has difficulty remaining seated when required to do so
   3. is easily distracted by extraneous stimuli
   4. has difficulty awaiting turn in games or group situations
   5. often blurts out answers to questions before they have been completed
   6. has difficulty following through on instructions from others (not due to oppositional behavior or failure of comprehension), e.g., fails to finish chores
   7. has difficulty sustaining attention in tasks or play activities
   8. often shifts from one uncompleted activity to another
   9. has difficulty playing quietly
   10. often talks excessively
   11. often interrupts or intrudes on others, e.g., butts into other children's games
   12. often does not seem to listen to what is being said to him or her
   13. often loses things necessary for tasks or activities at school or at home (e.g., toys, pencils, books, assignments)
   14. often engages in physically dangerous activities without considering possible consequences (not for the purpose of thrill-seeking), e.g., runs into street without looking

   Note: The above items are listed in descending order of discriminating power based on data from a national field trial of the DSM-III-R criteria for Disruptive Behavior Disorders.

B. Onset before the age of seven.

C. Does not meet the criteria for a Pervasive Developmental Disorder.

Despite the prevalence of the hyperactive syndrome and its description in the medical literature since at least the turn of the century (Still, 1902), its existence as a clinical entity has continually been questioned. There are those on the one hand who feel that the term has been used as a wastebasket diagnosis for children who present with a variety of socially unacceptable behaviors. The term has been used to excuse or explain the conduct of children who are aggressive, disruptive, or poorly disciplined. At the same time, numerous professionals who have worked with and studied hyperactive children recognize a cluster of symptoms that will lead them to make the diagnosis and also recognize a commonality of associated symptoms and response to treatment (Barkley, 1982). It seems therefore that, if strict criteria are used when referring to the symptom complex ADHD, it may be a valid and useful term.

The variation in incidence of the syndrome depends to a great extent on whom one asks (Lambert et al., 1978). Like beauty, "hyperactivity" is often in the eye of the beholder and depends on the standards and expectations of the individual who is judging a child or group of children as well as the circumstances under which the assessment is being made. Classroom teachers may rank up to 50% of their pupils as being overactive and disruptive (Trites et al., 1979), whereas parents may tolerate a much higher level of motor activity (especially if they have no other children to use as a comparison or if they have a large household in which the general level of activity is high). Pediatricians are often at a loss to detect an abnormality in a child's behavior during a routine office visit, despite reports from parents and teachers that their patience and sanity are being challenged on a daily basis (Sleator and Ullman, 1981). On the other hand, a physician surveying the devastation of an examining room after such a visit may be the first to suggest that the child's activity level falls outside the bounds of normal.

There is universal agreement that more boys than girls are diagnosed as being "ADHD," with the most common ratio quoted being 5:1 among clinic-referred children (Ross and Ross, 1982). In the general population, though, it is estimated at 2.5:1 (DMS-III-R). The reason for this differential is not clear, but it may be partly due to a multifatorial genetic component and may be linked to other developmental and cognitive problems for which males are more at risk than females. Females may compensate earlier, and to some extent the disparity may also be due, in part, to factors associated with probability of referral (i.e., because boys are more aggressive and aggression often leads to referral, more boys than girls will be referred for ADHD given its high correlation with aggression).

SIGNS AND SYMPTOMS

The primary symptom that distinguishes ADHD children from others is an inability to attend to a task for an expected period of time (Douglas, 1983). For some children this occurs in almost all situations, including high-interest activities. Others demonstrate a lack of sustained attention only when they are doing things that are difficult or uninteresting or require a high level of concentration (Zentall, 1985). This can be viewed as an exaggeration of the normal response to having to study or work on a project that demands focused attention. This difficulty will obviously have a major impact in the classroom when it limits the amount of information learned (or retained) and may lead to negative interactions with the teacher (Whalen et al., 1980). These in turn can produce a lowering of self-esteem and poor self-image.

Concomitant with the short attention span there is distractibility. This inability to inhibit responses to environmental stimuli unrelated to the task leads the child to address his attention constantly to sights, sounds, and movements within his range of vision and hearing. In the classroom, a teacher who finds that the child is unable to remember what has been said or that his paper is unfinished may label the child as lazy or unmotivated. At home, the parent who finds the child diverted from a requested task will be understandably upset and probably will interpret the behavior as frank disobedience. Nevertheless, there is great controversy among researchers as to whether ADHD children are truly more distractible or whether this response simply represents the rapid extinction of sustained attention (Barkley, 1988).

Another common symptom in the ADHD child is impulsivity, causing the child to show poor self-monitoring (Douglas, 1983). Teachers will report that this is a youngster who when asked a question will blurt out the first thing that comes into his head. Papers may be done quickly but inaccurately. These children speak out inappropriately in class and have trouble waiting their turn. On the playground, the child may get into frequent fights because he does not consider the consquences of his actions.

Excessive motor activity is frequently the symptom that prompts the parents to seek help in managing their youngsters (Porrino et al., 1983). Sometimes a mother will report in retrospect that this was a baby who was overactive in the womb, but more commonly the excessive activity is first noticed when the baby reaches toddlerhood. Often the early motor milestones are achieved early and the toddler's waking hours are spent in a whirlwind of motion. Much of the energy may be expended in repetitive purposeless activity. At this age ADHD children may get themselves into dangerous situations

FEATURE TABLE 26-1. ATTENTION DEFICIT HYPERACTIVITY DISORDER

Discriminating Feature	Consistent Features	Variable Features
1. Difficulty in sustaining attention to task	1. Distractibility 2. Impulsivity 3. Hyperactivity	1. Positive response to stimulants 2. Specific learning disability 3. Poor social skills 4. Neurodevelopmental immaturity 5. Conduct disorder

through lack of forethought or insight. Their caretakers, therefore, are constantly engaged in preserving the safety of the child and their property. However, it should be noted that up to 30% of ADHD children show little if any difficulties with increased motor activity (Carlson, 1986).

In the preschool years there is often more opportunity to compare a child's activity level with that of peers. Nursery school teachers will point out that the hyperactive child cannot stay with a task for the same amount of time as the others and so seldom finishes a project (Campbell et al., 1978). He cannot sit still for circle time or snack and demands a lot of staff attention. His mother may be called to pick him up early from a birthday party or play session because his behavior is too disruptive to the other children.

It is in grammar school, however, that the child's activity level tends to be most troublesome. It is often in the first few years of school that the problem first comes to light. The high level of activity, which may have been passed off as "just normal boy behavior" or as something that he would outgrow, now becomes a real impediment to his ability to learn in the classroom and often earns negative attention from his teacher and classmates. The hours spent in the classroom are the time when a child's behavior is most expected to conform to that of others of the same age, and walking around in the classroom, disturbing other children, or dropping books and pencils is poorly tolerated. At home this is the youngster who has trouble sitting through mealtimes with the rest of the family and who while watching a TV program may be in and out of the room constantly or bouncing a ball while watching the screen (Tarver-Behring et al., 1985).

As the child enters the second decade, he often is more able to control the more overt motor actions, such as running around inside the house or getting out of his seat in class, but he still may be noted to move around and change position frequently when sitting, shuffle his feet often, and fidget with any object within his reach (Weiss and Hechtman, 1986).

The overactive behavior frequently includes verbal activity (Barkley et al., 1983). The children are frequently referred to as being "motor mouths" who talk constantly and are liable to skip from one subject to another in a free-flowing stream of conversation. They often fail to contain their verbalizations or vocal noises in situations in which quiet is expected, such as in church, a movie theater, and the classroom, or in conversations between adults.

This symptom of saying inappropriate things at inappropriate times is part of the overall difficulty with social skills that most hyperactive children display (Pelham and Bender, 1982). The majority of children seem to acquire, by a combination of instinct and learning, the ability to interact in a suitable manner with a variety of people. When 4-year-olds are put together in a nursery school class, they generally know how to start a game or make a friend, and will address a teacher in a different manner than they would another child. ADHD children, on the other hand, often lack this ability. The problem is not uncommonly compounded by language difficulties, and so they fail to pick up from their companions' verbal or body language responses the fact that their behavior does not fit the situation (Cunningham and Siegel, 1987). In grammar school, the social isolation is often compounded by active teasing. Friendships formed tend to be transient. Social ineptitude can last throughout life, although by the time of middle to late adolescence it may be less problematic, because personality differences are better tolerated as one gets older and it is acceptable to have only a few friendships, perhaps centered around particular interests rather than being a part of a large group. Mutual experiences may lead ADHD children to seek each other out as companions.

There is a wide area of overlap between attention deficit and other learning disabilities. As many as 30% to 40% of hyperactive children are found to be failing academically (Safer and Allen, 1976). Some of this overlap is specious. Children with attention difficulties may do poorly in academic areas because they fail to assimilate information and finish work. Conversely, children with specific learning disabilities are liable to be fidgety and distractible in class because they do not understand much of what is going on and are frustrated by their inability to perform tasks mastered relatively easily by classmates. Nevertheless, there remains a large group in whom both conditions coexist. Specific learning disabilities must not be overlooked or treatment may be only partially effective at best.

Although the early motor milestones may be reached quickly, ADHD children are often poorly coordinated (Hartsough and Lambert, 1985). Both gross and fine motor skills may be immature when compared with the average for age, making such children clumsy in the gym and on the playing field and leading to poor handwriting. Some will achieve success in sports by dint of fearlessness and strength.

Approximately 75% of parents of hyperactive children complain about discipline problems (Barkley, 1981). These range from noncompliance through defiance to aggressive and destructive behavior. The differentiation between conduct disorder and hyperactivity may be a difficult one and has been a factor in the wide variation in reported incidence of ADHD. In particular, British writers tend to classify children who have aggressive, acting-out behavior under the diagnosis of conduct disorder, whereas their United States colleagues would consider that a proportion of such children had a primary attentional deficit (Taylor, 1986). Certainly many patients fit the criteria for both diagnoses, again raising the question of whether the overlap reflects common genetic or environmental etiologic influences.

It is readily understandable that children who are inattentive and distractible and who may have several of the symptoms described earlier very frequently come to suffer from poor self-esteem by late childhood. Many have no area of their lives in which they feel successful. In the family they suffer the criticism of their parents and the resentment of their siblings, who feel that they are being deprived of parental attention and may be embarrassed by their brother's or sister's behavior. At school, they are under pressure because of poor academic performance and discipline problems as well as difficulties with peers. And there can be little satisfaction from after-school sports for youngsters whose coordination is poor and who have trouble following the course of a game. Children who are constantly being told they are no good will sooner or later come to believe it and some will progress to overt depression (Barkley, 1981).

Anxiety is another emotional problem that can complicate the attention deficit. Such anxiety is more often seen in those ADHD children who are not hyperactive (Carlson, 1986). There is sometimes a cyclic progression of failure, which creates anxiety, which further interferes with performance.

WORKUP AND DIAGNOSIS

Attempts to identify neurochemical differences in ADHD children that would make a laboratory diagnosis possible have thus far brought no definitive results. The diagnosis remains a clinical one (Shaywitz et al., 1983). Meticulous history taking and observation are essential. The time to listen to the parents' story and the child's feelings and to explain the nature of the problem is probably the most important thing a physician can offer to a family. The evaluation process in itself can, in this way, be therapeutic.

Although perinatal hypoxia or central nervous system infection or trauma can be significant etiologic factors (Streissguth et al., 1984), a direct relationship is usually difficult to establish. Rather the review of the past medical history may serve to educate parents about what did not cause their child's handicap and to allay feelings of guilt that they may have been harboring. A chronic or recurrent illness affects many aspects of a young person's life and some will experience behavioral or emotional problems as a result. Medical conditions that can have a direct effect on a child's behavior or learning ability include lead intoxication, seizure disorders, cranial irradiation for leukemia or other malignancy, intracranial space-occupying lesions, and hyperthyroidism or hypothyroidism. If the child is using medications chronically or intermittently, especially theophylline preparations, anticonvulsants, and antihistamine-decongestant preparations, one should ask the parents if they notice a change in the child's behavior when taking them.

When asking about accidents that the child has sustained it is useful to know not only of major trauma but also whether this is a child who has sustained more than his share of cuts, bumps, and scrapes. The hyperactive child's lack of judgment, impulsivity, and poor coordination often earn him preferred customer status at the local emergency room. Accidental ingestions are also a common historic finding and may occur later than the toddler stage, which is the most common age for such incidents in the general population. Given the higher risk of ADHD children for physical abuse, questioning of such accidents must be thorough yet diplomatic.

The developmental pattern varies just as widely for hyperactive children as for those who do not have this handicap, but as one interviews large numbers of their parents certain trends do emerge. Many will be described as good babies who slept well and fed easily, but retrospective information suggests that more ADHD children than normal started out in life as colicky, difficult-to-schedule infants (Chamberlin, 1977). However, there are no good prospective studies to confirm this. While early motor milestones are often passed at an earlier than average age, later accomplishments like riding a bicycle or dribbling a soccer ball may take longer for the hyperactive child to master. Language milestones, on the other hand, may be delayed compared to the average from early on, especially in ADHD girls. Although the older child may talk a great deal, language may be immature and it is useful to ask if speech and langue therapy has ever been received or recommended. The developmental history should include the times of mastering self-help and independence skills, to determine how the child is functioning in his world. As the child's development is being reviewed, parents can be asked when they first thought that their child seemed different from the norm. Some will claim that they knew from birth that he was going to be difficult. Others will say that when the child started to become independently mobile they noticed that he was much more active than expected. Or it may have been at the time when they expected to be able to sit down with the child to play interactively or teach him that they found that he did not have the attention span necessary for this. Still others will have felt that their child's behavior was perfectly normal until they had a report from a nursery school or grade school teacher that he could not concentrate. Once it has been pointed out that a problem exists parents may acknowledge that in retrospect the child has always been very busy. The presence of other children in the home for comparison will obviously have a bearing on when parents notice a deviation from the expected norm and seek help.

In a large number of cases (40%) a complete family history will reveal other members who either have been diagnosed as having attention deficit (Biederman et al., 1986) and hyperactivity or, without ever having been identified or treated, have been noticed to have similar traits to the patient. Gentle probing may be required to discover educational difficulties in the parents themselves, who may be embarrassed to bring these up spontaneously, but specific questions about how far each parent progressed in school and whether they repeated grades or received extra help will produce a surprising number of positive responses. Frequently one will hear that a grandmother has stated that the parent was "just like" the patient when he or she was growing up. Medical conditions occurring on either side of the family should be recorded, in particular any neurologic problems such as seizures or tics. Similarly mental retardation and developmental problems are important to know about. Physicians are sometimes diffident about asking about the occurrence of mental health problems, such as depression, alcoholism, other substance dependencies, or sociopathy in family members, but if this is done sensitively in the context of completing a family medical history, it will seldom cause offense and can provide significant information (Biederman et al., 1987). Parents may in fact be relieved to bring up the subject if they have been worried that their child may end up with a similar condition.

The child's educational history, starting with any preschool experience and continuing through the years of formal education, should be elicited, noting particularly any grades that have been repeated, testing done by the schools in the past, and whether extra services have been provided. Have there been moves involving different school systems? It is also useful to know whether the family is pleased with the services the school is providing and if they have a good relationship and maintain good communication with the school personnel.

Some detailed accounting of behavioral problems should include when and in what situations the offenses occur. It is also useful to record how parents and other supervisors react to the behaviors and what subsequent interactions take place as a result of those reactions (Barkley, 1981). What discipline methods are used in the home currently and were used in the past, and what formalized help have parents sought and obtained for managing the problems?

The examination of the child should include a complete physical examination, a formal neurologic examination, and an extended neurodevelopmental assessment.

In the course of the physical examination, height, weight, and head circumference should be measured and plotted on standardized graphs. Hearing and vision should be screened and blood pressure measured. Although it is unlikely that medical conditions that would significantly affect child's functioning would not have come to attention previously, any findings on the examination suggestive of hypothyroidism or hyperthyroidism, lead intoxication, anemia, or other chronic illness obviously need to be pursued further.

On the formal neurologic examination one looks for subtle signs of previous central nervous system insult or of a progressive neurologic condition. Abnormalities of muscle tone or a difference in strength, tone, or deep tendon reflex response between the two sides may have gone unnoticed previously. Similarly nystagmus, ataxia, tremor, decreased visual field, or fundal abnormalities should be noted and investigated.

The extended neurodevelopmental examination provides a system for looking at the progression of higher neurologic function in the areas of motor coordination, visual-perceptual skills, language skills, and cognitive function through the school-age years. Test items have been developed in an attempt to find a clinical window that would allow one to identify more specifically areas of functional deficit. This part of the examination also allows the examiner to observe the child over a period of time and engaged in a variety of tasks, and this is often its most useful function. Many parents have been frustrated to find that their child demonstrated none of the behaviors that they have complained of during the course of a 10-minute standard physical examination (Sleator and Ullman, 1981). If the physician then declares the child to be normal and in no need of treatment, the parent will be forced to look elsewhere for help and support.

There are several standardized neurodevelopmental test batteries. The PEEX (Levine and Rappaport, 1983) and PEERAMID (Levine, 1985), devised by Dr. Melvin Levine, are among the more comprehensive, and several shorter versions have been devised for office screening. Many clinicians choose a few test items in the various areas so that they become familiar with their administration and age norms and are able to judge where a particular child falls on the continuum. The areas of development assessed should include gross and fine motor coordination, with recording of any motor impersistence, synkinesia, or motor overflow movements. The efficiency of eye tracking and rapid alternating movements should be observed as well as the ability to identify right and left body parts both on self and on a person standing opposite.

When one sits the child down at a table with paper and pencil, fidgety and distractible behavior may become more apparent (Barkley et al., 1988). Useful activities for this part of the examination are handwriting, which allows the physician to observe pencil grasp and facility of execution as well as the finished product, and form copying, which will assess the child's visual-perceptual skills. A few math problems at the child's current level of function will demonstrate how he approaches school work, and in all these tasks one will have an opportunity to see how he organizes his work on the page, whether he monitors and self-corrects, whether his approach to the task is impulsive, and how well he is able to maintain his attention on the work.

Whether the physician wishes to include one of the standardized reading tests and/or screening of receptive and expressive language abilities will depend on what other testing has been performed or is planned by other professionals, either in school or elsewhere, as well as on the interest of the individual clinician and the time available. Other sources of information to aid the diagnostic process can include behavior checklists (Barkley, 1987a), reports of previous assessments, and authorized telephone communication with school personnel and with others who are evaluating or treating the patient.

A number of specific tests have been devised to provide objective measures of a subject's vigilance and impulsivity. Those most commonly employed include the Kagan Matching Familiar Figures Test, the Gordon Diagnostic System, and the Swanson-Kinsbourne Paired Associates Learning Test (Barkley, 1988). For the most part, these tests will be used in clinics specializing in ADHD and for research purposes, because they require time and trained personnel for administration.

Laboratory tests are seldom helpful in making the diagnosis of attention deficit. As a rule they should be undertaken only if there is a clinical indication by the history and physical exam. An electroencephalogram should be performed when there is suspicion of a seizure disorder, including absence spells. To order one on every child who presents with hyperactive symptoms will result in a number of readings in the "slightly abnormal" category and put one in the dilemma of having to interpret these results to the families. Other tests that can be helpful in specific cases include a complete blood count, measurements of lead level and blood glucose, and thyroid studies.

TREATMENT

As decribed previously, the child with ADHD presents with problems in several areas of functioning. In formulating a treatment plan, all of these must be considered. The initial explanation and discussion of the disorder can in itself be very helpful. A child who has been putting forth his best effort to obey directions, finish his work, and remember facts but is constantly chastised for being lazy and disobedient can be very relieved to know that someone believes that he is trying and understands his difficulties. He needs to hear too that he is not "dumb" or "retarded," as his classmates may have said or as he himself may have concluded. For the parent, too—who may have been told on one hand that there is nothing wrong with the child or that he will grow out of it, or on the other hand that the fault lies with the parent for poor child-rearing practices and lack of adequate disciplinary measures—a description of the syndrome can help dispel years of guilt and frustration. At the same time one needs to convey the message that freedom from blame does not relieve the child or his parents from the responsibility of dealing with the problem.

Psychotherapy in one or several forms is usually indicated. It may be in the context of individual counseling for the child to help him deal with his handicap and improve his self-image. A group of children can benefit from sharing their experiences and learning that there are others with similar problems, or a group may be formed to work on social skills training. Parents can almost always benefit from behavior modification training to help them deal with the undesirable behaviors that are occurring in their child and to train them to identify and reinforce the desirable traits (Barkley, 1987b). This too can be done in group sessions to allow for the exchange of ideas, but some parents who have particular situations to work on or who prefer privacy will need individual therapy. In either case it is importnat that both parents be involved if both have contact with the child. If there are others who regularly have responsibility for caring for the child, they may be involved in the training also so that he can experience consistency from the adults in his life.

Family counseling is another form of therapy that can be used when there are interactional issues deserving attention. This can also be a format for siblings to express their feelings about living with such a difficult brother or sister and about getting less than an equal share of parental attention. Some parents are too overwhelmed by their own personal or marital problems and need to work in individual or couples counseling before they can be available to deal with their child's difficulties.

The school program must be adjusted to meet the special needs of the ADHD child (Barkley, 1981). Specific learning disabilties must be identified so that appropriate remediation may be instituted. Because of his distractibility, the child will work best under close supervision of an adult; this can be facilitated in a number of ways, ranging from moving his desk nearer the teacher's to small group or individual tutoring. A few children will require a separate classroom designed either for children who have special academic requirements or for those whose behavioral difficulties preclude them from the regular classroom. The physical environment should also be considered. The open classroom with several projects going on at one time provides too much stimulation. A quiet room without a lot of visual distractions is preferred and a partition that blocks out the sights and sounds of the general classroom activities can be used some of the time.

The same considerations apply to homework time. A quiet place should be provided and the monitoring of an adult helps to keep the child on task. However, as a general rule, parents should not be expected to provide supplementary teaching and there should be a limit set on the amount of unfinished work that is to be completed at home. For the most part, school issues should be confined to school hours and the time spent at home should be for social and family activities.

The mainstay of treatment for many ADHD children is stimulant medication (Cantwell and Carlson, 1978), but it must be made clear to patients and parents at the outset that this is never the sole solution to the problem. Nor should response to stimulant medication be used as a diagnostic tool (Donnelly and Rappaport, 1985).

Pearls and Perils: The Hyperactive Child

1. It is critical that clinicians maintain an extensive file of potential referral agencies to whom families of ADHD children can be directed for additional, nonmedical services. Knowing where to refer for child management training, parent counseling, special educational tutoring, social skills training, marital counseling, substance abuse detoxification, and therapy for parental depression is indispensable in dealing with these multiproblem families.

2. Be sure to base the diagnosis on multiple sources of information (e.g., teachers) rather than relying exclusively on office behavior or parental reports. However, because each source of information has its limitations, combining sources often corrects for the problems with each.

3. There is no set age at which stimulant medication for treatment of ADHD should be stopped. It should be continued into adulthood if still effective.

4. The concept of a drug/placebo evaluation is acceptable to most people regardless of their preconceived ideas about the use of stimulant medication.

5. Avoid the diagnosis in children under 2 years of age. It is best to require that the child have had behavioral problems for at least 12 months before becoming confident in a diagnosis of ADHD. When in doubt, express the diagnosis as "Probably ADHD" or "At Risk for Later ADHD" and wait 6 to 12 months to avoid excessive diagnosis of what at times is a transient behavioral problem.

6. Watch for and query parents about parental psychopathology, such as depression, anxiety disorders, substance abuse, or marital discord. Where present, they can result in exaggerated reports of child misconduct. These factors are also strongly related to poor response to parent training programs as well as poor monitoring and usage of medication in the home. Where they are present, referral for their treatment first, before or simultaneous with undertaking extensive child treatment, may be warranted.

7. Be attuned to the possibilities of child physical or emotional abuse. The symptoms of ADHD often prove stressful to even the best caregivers. Where caregivers are already compromised by parental psychiatric disorders, economic hardship, or marital disharmony, clinicians should become more vigilant for indications of abuse.

8. Take extra caution to question parents about the child's history of tic disorders, Gilles de la Tourette's syndrome, or excessive anxiety, as these may contraindicate stimulant medication therapy. High anxiety levels in children are the single best predictors of *adverse* reactions to stimulants. Even where anxiety is not at issue, a personal or family history of tics or Tourette syndrome may increase the risk of tic reactions to stimulant medication.

9. While titrating medication, always obtain information directly from the child's school teacher on the effects of medication in the classroom. Do not rely exclusively on parents for these reports as theirs is second-hand information. Question teachers (and parents!) about the *range* of side effects rather than simply the most common. Agitation, depression, severe insomnia, weight loss, and emotional irritability should all be pursued, among others. For parents, this should be done monthly when the prescription is renewed.

10. Not all children who are overactive have an innate attentional problem. Anxiety, depression, or specific learning disability can be the underlying cause of the behavior.

11. Medication may slow a child down sufficiently that he or she no longer poses an overt behavioral problem. Take care that other emotional and educational needs are not overlooked.

Stimulants have been used to treat ADHD children since 1937, when Bradley noted the improvement in behavior and classroom performance of a group of these children in a residential school who were treated with amphetamines. Twenty years later methylphenidate (Ritalin) became available and the use of the stimulants increased rapidly. Since that time there has been considerable controversy, much of it in the popular media, about the extent to which stimulants are used. It is estimated that between 2% and 3.6% of the school-age population is currently receiving stimulants, that is, about 50% of those who have been diagnosed as having ADHD (Safer and Krager, 1988). This would indicate that usage is not excessive, although certainly there are instances of inappropriate prescribing.

The three stimulant medications most commonly prescribed at this time are methylphenidate (Ritalin), dextroamphetamine (Dexedrine), and pemoline (Cylert). Most studies indicate that 70% to 80% of ADHD children have a positive response to stimulants (Barkley, 1977). Contrary to the original assumption that they produced a paradoxic effect of sedation, their action should still be considered to be stimulant in nature in that these drugs alert the parts of the brain that will allow the child to concentrate on his work and to block out the extraneous stimuli that cause him to be distracted from the task at hand (Donnelly and Rappaport, 1985).

Methylphenidate is the drug preferred by most clinicians for medical treatment of attention deficit. Because it has been on the market for over 30 years, there is a large body of cumulative experience involving children who have taken the drug over periods varying from a few weeks to several years. The evidence suggests that, when prescribed after appropriate evaluation and monitored carefully, it is a safe drug with a reassuring lack of long-term side effects. Because children do not experience the euphoria that adults get from the drug, addiction does not occur. Methylphenidate is a piperidine derivative and is chemically related to the amphetamines. Its mode of action appears to be release and perhaps reuptake of stored catecholamines. The usual dosage ranges from 0.3 to 1.0 mg/kg per day, but a few patients will require up to 2.0 mg/kg to achieve optimal response. The dosage must be tailored to the individual child rather than prescribed on a rote basis.

The effects of Ritalin are usually apparent about 30 minutes after ingestion and last for 4 to 6 hours. This will generally mean giving two doses, one with breakfast and one with lunch, for the child to function well during the school day. Some will benefit from a third dose in the late afternoon to get them through homework time and after-school social activities, but this needs to be balanced against possible loss of appetite at dinner and wakefulness at bedtime. A sustained-release form of Ritalin with an 8- to 12-hour action time became available in 1984. This has not proven as effective in clinical practice as had been hoped, especially for younger children, but may be worth trying in the child over 10 years old, for whom receiving medication in school tends to be more problematic (Pelham et al., 1987).

The most common side effects encountered by children taking Ritalin include anorexia, insomnia, abdominal pain, headache, and increases in heart rate and blood pressure (Barkley, 1977). A decrease in growth velocity may occur that does not appear to be entirely due to appetite suppression. There is evidence that catch-up growth will take place after about 2 years if the drug is continued. A few children will encounter dysphoria and this is an indication for stopping the drug or reducing the dosage. Stimulants should be used cautiously in patients with seizure disorder, with close monitoring for increase in seizure activity, and, since the metabolism of anticonvulsants can be affected, levels should be checked more frequently after starting methylphenidate. A more serious although rare side effect is precipitation of motor tics, which may persist after the drug is discontinued (Barkley, 1987c). The development of tics is an indication to stop the pills immediately, and a strong family history of Gilles de la Tourette syndrome or tics is a contraindication for prescribing methylphenidate. The drug is also not recommended for children with symptomatic heart disease. Methylphenidate has not been approved for use in chil-

dren under 6 years of age; it is usually not effective in the preschool years but may be helpful in the same child in grade school.

Dextroamphetamine (Dexedrine) is thought to stimulate release of newly synthesized catecholamines and has a clinical action similar to that of Ritalin. The therapeutic action lasts about 4 to 6 hours for the tablets and 8 to 10 hours for the long-acting spansules, but Dexedrine has a longer half-life than Ritalin. Dosage for ADHD children is in the range of 0.15 to 0.5 mg/kg per dose. Dexedrine will sometimes be effective in children who have not had a satisfactory response to Ritalin, especially those in the younger age groups. The amphetamines have a considerable reputation for abuse and addiction, so prescribing should be carefully monitored.

Pemoline (Cylert) has been available since the early 1970s. It is a central nervous system stimulant chemically unrelated to the amphetamines and methylphenidate, but its pharmacologic action is similar. It has a half-life of 12 hours and its once-a-day regimen avoids administration in school. There is a lag time of several days before Cylert reaches its maximum effect and in some cases this may extend to 3 to 4 weeks. The recommended starting dosage is 37.5 mg/day, increasing by 18.75 mg/week until the maximum effect is obtained. Tablets are available in 18.75, 37.5, and 75 mg dosages. An occasional side effect is elevation of the liver enzymes, which should therefore be checked regularly. The enzyme dysfunction is generally reversed when the drug is stopped.

Whereas a majority of children with ADHD will benefit from treatment with stimulant medication, it has been shown that approximately 30% will also report an initial positive response to placebo (Barkley, 1977). In order to determine true responses and to reduce inappropriate prescribing, an initial test period using a double-blind drug/placebo procedure may be instituted (Barkley et al., 1988). This can be quite simple, using an on-off technique over a 2-, 4-, or 6-week period, with information about the child's behavior and side effects being reported directly from the parents and teacher or by means of a short behavioral checklist. A more elaborate process can include different dosage regimens, detailed questionnaires to record teachers' and parents' impressions of various aspects of the child's behavior, and specific testing performed in the office while the child is on each dose. In this way one can determine not only whether the drug is effective but also what the optimal dosage is for the particular patient. The performance of any type of drug/placebo trial requires the help of a pharmacist to prepare look-alike capsules with the appropriate contents and to retain the sequence code until the trial is completed.

When prescribing stimulants for a child with ADHD, a number of factors must be considered. Whether the patient should take the medication only on school days or 7 days a week and during vacation time depends on whether the benefit is mainly in improved classroom performance or also includes better social skills and behavior at home. How long the medication is given for is determined by how long the child may require it and the length of time it remains effective. At least once a year it should be discontinued for a period of about 2 weeks at a time when things are stable and the teacher can provide feedback. The time to stop it permanently is when the child does just as well without it as with it. Although for many patients this point will be reached in the midteen years, there is wide individual variation, with some patients being able to stop the drug in elementary school while others will continue to derive benefit from it into the third and fourth decades of life. The prescribing physician must take responsibility for monitoring the patient with respect to growth velocity, heart rate, and blood pressure, as well as the clinical effectiveness and any side effects of the drug. Office visits every 3 months seem prudent for such monitoring. Adjustments in dosage and regimen should be made as deemed appropriate.

Other medications that may be helpful in patients for whom the stimulants are either ineffective or contraindicated include the tricyclic antidepressants (imipramine, desipramine) (Puig-Antich et al., 1985; Pliska, 1987), which appear to be particularly helpful for anxious or depressed ADHD children. The major tranquilizers (thioridazine, haloperidol), and the minor tranquilizers (diazepam, oxazepam) may help in rare instances when aggression or anxiety is a significant symptom.

When a problem affects as many children as are diagnosed with ADHD, parents search far and wide for treatments and cures. It is not surprising, therefore, that a number of controversial treatment methods have been proposed. Because their proponents are generally more available and willing to promote their theories in the popular media than are busy clinicians or legitimate researchers, they tend to enjoy considerable publicity. Commonly, these therapies involve dietary manipulation, either by elimination of certain substances or by supplementation with vitamins and minerals. Most popular among these has been the Feingold or Kaiser-Permanente diet, which excludes artificial additives and preservatives as well as naturally occurring salicylates. The 80% success rate initially claimed by Dr. Feingold could not be reproduced on carefully controlled double-blind crossover trials (Conners, 1980). Rather, such methods indicate that about 5% of hyperactive children show some improvement. Similarly, controlled experiments failed to show a difference in children's behavior associated with increased intake of sugar (Milich et al., 1986). Certainly many of us might be healthier for a reduced intake of food additives and sugar, but we should not expect to be more compliant as a result. Also, in its strictest form, the Feingold diet forbids some of the fruits and vegetables that children usually like and the suggested substitutes may not be as acceptable to the young palate, so that overall nutrition could be impaired. Parents who wish to try these methods should be apprised of the scientific evidence available and of the fact that a perceived change in the child's behavior may be the result of a placebo ef-

fect and increased parent-child interaction around the issue of diet. Other fads with no proven efficacy have included sensory integration training, visual tracking exercises, allergen therapy, and chiropractic manipulations.

PROGNOSIS

The outlook for children diagnosed with ADHD has to be guarded (Weiss and Hechtman, 1986). Although a positive response to medication can bring about a dramatic change in a student's ability to attend and produce work in the classroom and parents will report a "day and night" difference in the child's social interactions and compliance, follow-up studies on the whole give a rather pessimistic view. To date there is no evidence that treatment can improve long-term academic achievement. When followed into adolescence and young adulthood, ADHD children as a group have a higher incidence of juvenile delinquency, criminal activity, alcoholism, and other substance dependency than the general population. They also do worse than average when it come to educational attainment, employment records, and career achievement, although there has been at least one study that showed that they tend to be viewed more positively by their employers than they had been by their teachers (Weiss et al., 1978). Outcome in these children is not so much related to degree of ADHD as to the coexistence and severity of conduct problems, intelligence, marital discord, and parent psychopathology.

Despite this rather negative prognosis in groups, one should be as optimistic as possible when evaluating, advising, and following the individual patient and family. With appropriate medical treatment, counseling, and school programming, up to 60% of ADHD children can be expected to grow into satisfactorily functioning adults. The same basic temperamental characteristics will usually persist but can take on a more positive aspect with maturity. Thus overactivity can translate into increased energy and productivity and impulsivity can become creativity. It can be pointed out that, once the school years are over, an individual has a much wider choice of how to spend the working portion of the day, and someone with ADHD will probably elect to have a job that involves variation of activities and does not require him to sit at a desk for hours at a time. Thus the ADHD child has the potential to be more successful and accepted as an adult than as a child. The task of the professionals working with him is to help him reach that point on as smooth a course as possible.

ANNOTATED BIBLIOGRAPHY

Barkley RA: *Hyperactive Children: A Handbook For Diagnosis and Treatment.* New York: Guilford Press, 1981.
    Provides a comprehensive description of the syndrome of

hyperactivity and a very practical detailed account of methods used for intervention and treatment. It is a very useful book for the practitioner who is evaluating and treating ADHD children.

Taylor EA (ed): *The Overactive Child.* Philadelphia, JB Lippincott, 1986.

This volume, part of the Clinics in Developmental Medicine series, gives a very nice overview of the literature on ADHD and exposes the reader to a number of different points of view.

Wender P: *The Hyperactive Child, Adolescent and Adult.* New York, Oxford University Press, 1987.

An excellent review that can be used by parents and teachers.

Weiss G, Hechtman L: *Hyperactive Children Grown Up.* New York, Guilford Press, 1986.

The best summary of the literature presently available on follow-up of ADHD.

Ingersoll B: *Your Hyperactive Child.* Philadelphia, WB Saunders, 1988.

A superb review for parents.

REFERENCES

Barkley RA: A review of stimulant drug research with hyperactive children. *J Child Psychol Psychiatr* 18:137–165, 1977.

Barkley RA: *Hyperactive Children: A Handbook for Diagnosis and Treatment.* New York, Guilford Press, 1981.

Barkley RA: Specific guidelines for defining hyperactivity in children (attention deficit disorder with hyperactivity), in Lahey B, Kazdin A (eds): *Advances in Clinical Child Psychology,* Vol 5. New York, Plenum Press, 1982, p 137–180.

Barkley, RA: Child behavior rating scales and checklists, in Rutter M, Tuma H, Lann I (eds): *Assessment and Diagnosis in Child Psychopathology.* New York, Guilford Press, 1987a, p 113–155.

Barkley RA: *Defiant Children: A Clinician's Manual for Parent Training.* New York, Guilford Press, 1987b.

Barkley RA: Tic disorders and Tourette's syndrome, in Mash E, Terdal L (eds): *Behavioral Assessment of Childhood Disorders,* 2nd ed. New York, Guilford Press, 1987c, p 552–585.

Barkley RA: Attention deficit-hyperactivity disorder, in Mash E, Terdal L (eds): *Behavioral Assessment of Childhood Disorders,* 2nd ed. New York, Guilford Press, 1988, p 69–104.

Barkley RA, Cunningham C, Karlsson J: The speech of children and their mothers: Comparison with normal children and stimulant drug effects. *J Learn Disabil* 16:105–110, 1983.

Barkley RA, Fischer M, Newby R, Breen M: Development of a multi-method clinical protocol for assessing stimulant drug responses in ADHD children. *J Clin Child Psychol* 17:14–24, 1988.

Biederman J, Munir K, Knee D et al: A family study of patients with attention deficit disorder and normal controls. *J Psychiatr Res* 20:263–274, 1986.

Biederman J, Munir K, Knee D, et al: High rate of affective disorders in probands with attention deficit disorders and in their relatives: A controlled family study. *Am J Psychiatr* 144:330–333, 1987.

Bradley W: The behavior of children receiving benzedrine. *Am J Psychiatr* 94:577–585, 1937.

Campbell SB, Schleifer M, Weiss G: Continuities in maternal reports and child behaviors over time in hyperactive and comparison groups. *J Abnorm Child Psychol* 6:33–45, 1978.

Cantwell D, Carlson G: Stimulants, in Werry J (ed): *Pediatric Psychopharmacology.* New York: Brunner/Mazel, 1978, p 171–207.

Carlson C: Attention deficit disorder without hyperactivity: A Review of Preliminary Experimental Evidence, in Lahey B, Kazdin A (eds): *Advances in Clinical Child Psychology,* Vol 9. New York, Plenum Press, 1986, p 153–176.

Chamberlin RW: Can we identify a group of children at age two who are at risk for the development of behavioral or emotional problems in kindergarten or first grade? *Pediatrics* 59 (suppl):971–981, 1977.

Conners CK: *Food Additives and Hyperactive Children.* New York, Plenum Press, 1980.

Cunningham CE, Siegel LS: Peer interactions of normal and attention-deficit disordered boys during free-play, cooperative task, and simulated classroom situations. *J Abnorm Child Psychol* 15:247–268, 1987.

Diagnostic and Statistical Manual of Mental Disorders, 3rd ed. Washington, DC, American Psychiatric Association, 1980.

Diagnostic and Statistical Manual of Mental Disorders, 3rd ed rev. Washington, DC, American Psychiatric Association, 1987.

Donnelly MK, Rappaport JL: Attention deficit disorders, in Weiner JM (ed): *Diagnosis and Psychopharmacology of Childhood and Adolescent Disorders.* New York, John Wiley & Sons, 1985, p 178–198.

Douglas VI: Attention and cognitive problems, in Rutter M (ed): *Developmental Neuropsychiatry.* New York, Guilford Press, 1983, p 280–329.

Hartsough CS, Lambert NM: Medical factors in hyperactive children and normal children: Prenatal, developmental, and health history findings. *Am J Orthopsychiatr* 55:190–201, 1985.

Lambert NM, Sandocal J, Sassone D: Prevalence of hyperactivity in elementary school children as a function of social system definers. *Am J Orthopsychiatr* 48:446–463, 1978.

Levine MD: *Pediatric Examination of Educational Readiness at Middle Childhood.* Cambridge, Mass, Educators Publishing Service, 1985.

Levine MD, Rappaport L: *Pediatric Early Elementary Examination.* Cambridge, Mass, Educators Publishing Service, 1983.

Milich R, Wolraich M, Lindgren S: Sugar and hyperactivity: A critical review of empirical findings. *Clin Psychol Rev* 6:493–513, 1986.

Pelham WE, Bender ME: Peer relationships in hyperactive children: Description and treatment, in Gadow K, Bialer E (eds): *Advances in Learning and Behavioral Disabilities,* Vol 1. Greenwich, Conn, JAI Press, 1982, p 365–436.

Pelham WE, Sturges J, Hoza J, et al: Sustained release and standard methylphenidate effects on cognitive and social behavior in children with attention deficit disorder. *Pediatrics* 80:491–501, 1987.

Pliska SR: Tricyclic antidepressants in the treatment of children with attention deficit disorder. *J Am Acad Child Adolesc Psychiatr* 26:127–132, 1987.

Porrino LJ, Rapoport JL, Behar D, Sceery W, Ismond DR, Bunney WE: A naturalistic assessment of the motor activity of hyperactive boys. *Arch Gen Psychiatr* 40:681–687, 1983.

Puig-Antich J, Ryan N, Rabinovich H: Affective disorders in childhood and adolescence, in Weiner JM (ed): *Diagnosis and*

Psychopharmacology of Childhood and Adolescent Disorders. New York, John Wiley & Sons, 1985, p 151–177.

Ross DM, Ross SA: *Hyperactivity: Current Issues, Research, and Theory,* 2nd ed. New York, John Wiley & Sons, 1982.

Safer DJ, Allen R: *Hyperactive Children.* Baltimore, Md, University Park Press, 1976.

Safer DJ, Krager JM: A survey of medication treatment for hyperactive/inattentive students. *JAMA* 260:2256–2258, 1988.

Shaywitz B, Shaywitz S, Cohen D: Monoaminergic mechanisms in hyperactivity, in Rutter M (ed): *Developmental Neuropsychiatry.* New York, Guilford Press, 1983, p 330–347.

Sleator EK, Ullman RK: Can the physician diagnose hyperactivity in the office? *Pediatrics* 67:13–17, 1981.

Still GF: Some abnormal psychical conditions in children. *Lancet* 1:1008–1012, 1077–1082, 1163–1168, 1902.

Streissguth AP, Martin DC, Barr HM, Sandman BM, Kirchner GL, Darby BL: Intrauterine alcohol and nicotine exposure: Attention and reaction time in 4-year-old children. *Dev Psychol* 20:533–541, 1984.

Tarver-Behring S, Barkley R, Karlsson J: The mother-child interactions of hyperactive boys and their normal siblings. *Am J Orthopsychiatr* 55:202–209, 1985.

Taylor EA: Childhood hyperactivity. *Br J Psychiatr* 149:562–573, 1986.

Trites RL, Dugas F, Lynch G, Ferguson B: Incidence of hyperactivity. *J Pediatr Psychol* 4:179–188, 1979.

Weiss G, Hechtman L: *Hyperactive Children Grown Up.* New York, Guilford Press, 1986.

Weiss G, Hechtman L, Perlman T: Hyperactives as young adults: School, employer, and self-rating scales obtained during ten-year follow-up evaluation. *Am J Orthopsychiatr* 48:438–445, 1978.

Whalen CK, Henker B, Dotemoto S: Methylphenidate and hyperactivity: Effects on teacher behaviors. *Science* 208:1280–1282, 1980.

Zentall SS: A context for hyperactivity, in Gadow KD (ed): *Advances in Learning and Behavioral Disabilities,* Vol 4. Greenwich, Conn, JAI Press, 1985, p 273–343.

Sleep Disorders

Ronald B. David

Clinically, sleep disorders in children span the severity continuum from mildly irritating to life threatening. In clinical practice sleep disorders are extremely common and at times quite frustrating to treat.

NORMAL SLEEP

Although the sleep of infants and children differs from that of adults, both have in common periods of arousal and periods of inhibition. These periods are characterized by electroencephalographic (EEG) stages during normal adult sleep. Dement and Kleitman (1957) described four stages of EEG activity during normal adult sleep. Stage 1 shows low-voltage fast activity; stage 2 is characterized by the presence of sleep spindles and K complexes with low-voltage background activity. Stages 3 and 4 show varying degrees of slow, high-voltage activity referred to as slow wave sleep. In stage 1, there may occur binocularly synchronous eye movements, decreased muscle tone, and accelerated irregular respiratory and heart rates. This stage is referred to as rapid eye movement (REM) sleep. Non–rapid eye movement (NREM) sleep occurs during stages 1 through 4 of sleep and is characterized by the persistence of muscle tone and slowed regular cardiac and respiratory rates. REM and NREM states are two discrete states of neurophysiologic activity. REM sleep is a period of high activity while NREM sleep is a more basal and regular state. The two stages alternate and together they constitute a sleep cycle. A typical adult sleep cycle begins with NREM sleep and descends through stages 1 to 4. Stages 3 and 2 then progress to a period of REM sleep, and the cycle is repeated. Generally up to six cycles occur throughout the night. REM sleep is associated with dreaming, although there is also mental activity during stages 1 and 2 of NREM sleep. Sleep cycles are generally approximately 90 minutes in duration and the deepest stages of sleep occur early in the cycle.

Significant differences occur between the sleep of adults and that of infants or children. Infant sleep is characterized by three distinct stages: (1) active REM sleep, (2) quiet sleep; and (3) indeterminate sleep. Active REM sleep and quiet sleep may be the infant equivalents of adult REM and NREM sleep. The adult and infant stages are similar in that they are active and basal in character, but the infant stages lack the orderly structure of those of adults. Indeterminate sleep is seen in premature infants of 34 weeks' gestation as well as in newborns 3 months of age. In the term infant, active REM sleep occurs 45% to 50% of the time, indeterminate sleep occurs 10% to 15% of the time, and quiet sleep occurs 35% to 45% of the time. The proportion of quiet sleep increases with age. Active REM declines until later childhood, when normal adult patterns are established.

The amount of sleep obtained during a 24-hour cycle gradually decreases from an average of 12 to 16 hours for infants under 6 months of age to an average of 10 to 12 hours for 5-year-old children. The decrease is due to shortening and eventual abandonment of daytime naps, although this pattern is variable.

The duration of a sleep cycle (active REM/quiet sleep) varies with age. For example, term infants have a periodicity of 45 to 50 minutes, whereas older children and adults have a periodicity of 90 to 100 minutes. Infants under 34 weeks' conceptual age do not demonstrate cycling. Other immature infants show shorter cycles. Adults generally enter sleep with an initial NREM period, followed by proportionally greater REM as the night proceeds. Newborns enter sleep initially through active REM sleep and cycle regularly, with uniform distribution of active REM sleep throughout the night. In adults, sleep and wakefulness generally follow day and night. This pattern of sleep and wakefulness is established in infants by 3 months of age, although cycling may occur earlier. The initial, relatively brief transitions from wakefulness to sleep in the very young infant gradually merge into a more typical diurnal pattern by 8 months of age. This pattern is still generally interrupted, however, by two brief naps. The process of developing the more mature pattern of sleep and wakefulness is referred to as "settling." Moore and Ucko (1957) found that 70% of infants, age 3 months, slept from midnight to 5:00 AM and that this proportion increased to 83% by 6 months and to 90% by 9 months. While 10% to 30% of infants may have problems sleeping through the night, this pattern is still normal. Infants spend more relative and actual time in REM sleep over a 24-hour period than do adults. Adults spend only 20% of their night's sleep in REM sleep.

It should be emphasized that there is a great deal of variability in what are considered to be "norms." If an infant or child's sleep pattern is neither problematic nor symptomatic, then it should be considered within normal limits for that child.

SLEEP DISORDERS

Guilleminault (1987) and Anders and Weinstein (1972) have classified the disorders of sleep in infancy and childhood. Based on their approach we may group these into (1) hypersomnias, those disorders in which sleep is excessive; (2) insomnias, those conditions in which sleep is abnormally short, and (3) dyssomnias, those disorders in which sleep is disturbed by episodic events. A fourth category includes conditions produced secondarily, including fever, endocrine disorders, metabolic disorders, seizure disorders, and those disorders that are of a psychogenic origin. The fourth category will not be reviewed here.

Hypersomnias

Hypersomnias include two major conditions that produce primary excessive daytime sleepiness (EDS). The first is narcolepsy, and the second is obstructive sleep apnea syndrome.

Narcolepsy

Although a pattern of EDS with narcolepsy may be evident before 11 years of age, the typical age of onset for narcolepsy is between 15 and 25 years of age. Cataplexy is defined by episodic inability to perform voluntary movements associated with a sudden loss of body tone. Hypnagogic hallucinations consist of vivid visual or auditory images occurring at the onset of sleep, which are typically frightening. Sleep paralysis is the sudden awareness while falling asleep that the individual can neither cry out nor move. Yoss and Daly (1957) suggest that this narcoleptic tetrad occurs only about 10% of the time and that a genetic factor is present, as indicated by a higher than predicted familial incidence of the disorder. Sleep attacks are associated with cataplexy about 75% of the time and with sleep paralysis and hypnagogic hallucinations 20% to 30% of the time.

The cataplectic attacks vary in severity from a state of absolute immobility to limited involvement of muscle groups such as the jaw or neck. Cataplectic attacks are considered pathognomonic of narcolepsy and may precede the development of EDS by several years.

Cataplexy, however, generally develops with EDS. Cataplexy is not observed before 12 years of age.

Hypnagogic hallucinations are not uncommon in normal individuals. However, they rarely occur successively. Such hallucinations are frightening experiences and children may fail to report them even though prompted. The hallucinations are usually shadows without form, colored or uncolored. Such hypnagogic hallucinations are frequently associated with sleep paralysis. In the face of such hallucinations, the child may find himself or herself unable to move, and may scream or simply fall asleep. The only recollection may be of an unusual event at onset of sleep or of a nightmare.

Narcoleptic children generally exhibit a prolonged initial REM sleep both with EDS and during the night, and frequently present with cataplexy, sleep paralysis, and hypnagogic hallucinations. It has been suggested by Dement and associates (1966) that the definition of narcolepsy be limited to those hypersomnias characterized by attacks of REM sleep. It is therefore thought that the recording of REM sleep at sleep's onset is suggestive of narcolepsy in any child with EDS. The diagnosis is confirmed by a history of cataplexy.

In the non-Oriental population, 99% of individuals with narcolepsy are HLA-DR2 positive. This antigen is also present in approximately 30% of the otherwise asymptomatic population. Therefore, in a symptomatic patient, its absence virtually excludes the diagnosis of narcolepsy.

Treatment of narcolepsy consists initially of informing the child and parents of the nature of the condition. Other caregivers, including the child's teachers, should also be informed. An explanation of the symptoms of cataplexy, hypnagogic hallucinations, or sleep paralysis should also be given to both parents and child. Medication generally prescribed for children includes methylphenidate and amphetamines. Imiprimine or chlorimiprimine are effective agents for sleep paralysis, cataplexy, and hypnagogic hallucinations.

Obstructive Sleep Apnea Syndrome

The review of obstructive sleep apnea by Guilleminault and colleagues (1981) divides this condition into two modes of presentation: breathing irregularity secondary to a medical condition, and the "primary" obstructive sleep apnea syndrome. The precipitating medical conditions include facial dysmorphisms, such as Pierre Robin and Treacher Collins syndromes and Crouzon's disease. The syndrome is also associated with neuromuscular disorders, including myotonic dystrophy, cerebral palsy, and Chiari malformations, as well as with more general medical problems, including Prader-Willi syndrome. Common presenting complaints in both groups are hyperactivity and antisocial behavior. Clinical presentations include failure to thrive, abnormal weight for age, acute cardiac or cardiorespiratory failure, hyperactivity, and frequent upper airway infections. Continuous heavy snoring is reported in all cases, as well as disruptive nocturnal sleep, sleepwalking, nightmares, and enuresis. Polygraphic analysis of sleep shows a complete disappearance of stage 3 NREM sleep in 86% of cases. There is less of a decrease in REM sleep.

Therapeutic recommendations are based on the severity of the obstructive apnea syndrome as documented by polygraphic data as well as on the syndrome's effects on daytime social and intellectual function. Also considered are structural problems identified on lateral x rays of the neck undertaken to investigate soft tissue enlargement, computed tomograms of the neck, and maxillofacial, orthodontic, and otolaryngologic conditions. Recommendations are divided into medical and surgical. Medical measures include modification of diet and prescription of steroids, protriptyline, and acetazolamide. Surgical approaches include tonsillectomy and/or adenoidectomy. Reconstructive facial surgery and orthodontic treatment are recommended when there is severe evidence of sleep-related oxygen desaturation. Tracheostomy could be considered, but is only performed when other approaches have proven to be ineffective.

Insomnias

Insomnias in infants occur as a deviance from normal night settling that is problematic or symptomatic. Dreyfus-Brisac and Monod (1965) have reported a complete lack of sleep cycling in infants with evidence of severe neurologic insult. Unusual frequent and irregular sleep stage shifts occur in children with lesser degrees of neurologic involvement. Infants of diabetic mothers, toxemic mothers, and addicted mothers all demonstrate abnormaliites in quiet sleep organization and/or the maturation of various EEG waveforms. Abnormalities of active REM sleep have been reported in chromosomal disorders, autism, and mental retardation. These infants are at high risk for insomnia.

Infantile Colic
Infantile colic is generally agreed to be a self-limiting condition occurring during the first 3 months of life. Infants usually experience flatulence and discomfort. The condition usually disappears by the fourth month and, although it may give rise to parental anxiety and tension, there is nothing to suggest that it is caused by parental behavior. Milk consumption may alleviate or exacerbate the condition. Antispasmodics may have some or no effect. A trial-and-error approach to treatment is generally advocated for this problem. The family's well-being should not be minimized. During the second half of the first year, changes in routine are frequently reported to be the cause for infant awakening. These changes may include illnesses and injury, or even a new sleeping place. By this age, parental anxiety and fear frequently compound the situation. It should be remembered that a 2 to 4-week course of chloral hydrate is frequently more effective than programs that are more time consuming

or alter basic family dynamics, particularly when it can be demonstrated that the sleep problem is accelerating.

Preschool to Early School Years
Lozoff and colleagues (1985), based on their own findings, indicated that 20% to 30% of children experience a bedtime or night awakening difficulty during the first 4 years of life. Sleep disturbance appears to occur in children whose mothers' attention has been withdrawn as a consequence of family illness or accident, unaccustomed separation, or maternal depression. Sleeping in the parents' bed, it was presumed, occurred as a reaction to sleep problems. From a speculative standpoint, the security that sleeping with the parents affords could be viewed as an attempt to compensate for feelings of separation and insecurity. However, the experience of many clinicians suggests that this habit, once routinized, becomes difficult to break, even though the separation fear may have long since vanished. A diary of the child's sleep-wake patterns can be crucial in determining the child's needs for a stable pattern when compared with those of normal children. If daytime naps are excessively long, then shortening naps may be helpful in decreasing nocturnal wakefulness. On the other hand, it has been observed that many mothers cherish their child's daytime nap for the freedom it affords, even though the nap may be indirectly responsible for nighttime wakefulness. The development of a more normal sleep pattern should be recommended. Chloral hydrate or another hypnotic may be helpful in establishing a more desirable sleep-wake pattern for parent and child. Once again, the effect of this problem on the child and family's overall well-being cannot be overemphasized.

It is rare in children 3 to 7 years of age not to find some sleep-related difficulty. The most prevalent may be difficulty falling asleep but not awakening, nightmares, or fear of ghosts. Objects in a darkened room assume surrealistic significance for a child. To relieve the anxiety associated with going to sleep, presleep rituals are often developed, and the bedtime hour can take on the characteristics of a parent-child power struggle. Appropriate counselling in this regard is needed.

Middle Childhood
Insomnia appears to be less of a problem in the middle childhood years. Morrison and associates (1985) suggest three causes of insomnia: psychologic, behavioral, and physical. Psychologic causes include anxiety and depression; depression is highly correlated with early awakening and the inability to return to sleep, whereas anxiety is associated with difficulty falling asleep. Behavioral causes include irregular bedtime and rising hours, long daytime naps, and excessive consumption of caffeine-containing foods or drinks. Physical causes are associated with allergies, asthma, or the side effects of prescribed as well as illicit drugs.

FEATURE TABLE 27-1. APNEA OF PREMATURITY

Discriminating Features	Consistent Features	Variable Features
1. Prematurity 2. Predominance of mixed apnea pattern 3. Exclusion of other causes of apnea (e.g., pneumothorax, sepsis)	1. Age of onset: birth to 2 weeks 2. Mixed apnea type 3. Variable-frequency, severe apneic episodes with risk of sudden death 4. Good response to theophyllin therapy	1. Central or obstructive apnea pattern 2. Predisposing GE reflex 3. Predisposing upper respiratory infection 4. Failure to thrive 5. Therapeutic response to stimulation

Adolescence

Up to 50% of adolescents have chronic insomnia or occasional poor sleep. Three parameters define the chronic condition: (1) 45 minutes or more are required to fall asleep on three or more successive nights a week; (2) one or more awakenings followed by at least 30 minutes of wakefulness occur on three or more nights a week; and (3) three or more awakenings occur on three or more nights a week. The treatment of adolescent insomnia should focus on alleviation of the cause. Symptomatic treatment approaches can best be developed as a consequence of an overall sleep evaluation, which is best achieved in a sleep laboratory. The evaluation should be supplemented by an accurate sleep diary recording the approximate bedtime, the number of sleep interruptions, and the time of arousal. Relaxation techniques can be a helpful form of treatment. Because prescribed and unprescribed drugs can frequently be at the root of insomnia, the use of hypnotics is discouraged. Estimates suggest, however, that up to 50% of insomniacs sooner or later use over-the-counter or prescribed hypnotics.

Dyssomnias and Sleep Apnea

Of the episodic dyssomnias, sleep apnea in infants represents a major diagnostic and therapeutic problem, owing principally to the life-threatening nature of these episodes. A number of syndromes can produce apnea during both sleep and waking states, and only those conditions producing apnea principally during sleep will be considered. It should be noted that normal infants have apneic episodes during sleep, with many parents remarking that "my baby stops breathing, but seems to start back on his or her own after a while." The medical literature contains many reviews of apnea. Causes include apnea of prematurity, congenital central hypoventilation syndrome in the newborn, and apneas of infancy.

Apnea of Prematurity

More than 80% of infants with birth weights of under 1000 g will have one or more apneic episodes. Gestationally older infants have fewer apneas. Spells may occur one per week or several per hour. The frequency generally decreases at 2 to 3 weeks of age and the spells cease by a postconceptual age of 40 weeks. Apnea of prematurity appears to be linked to immature neural mechanisms, although the systems that are affected are unclear. It has been suggested that in up to half of the cases these episodes begin with one or more inspiratory efforts without air flow occurring. This effort at inspiration is followed by cessation of all respiratory effort. Most episodes of obstructive breathing occur at the end of the spell.

FEATURE TABLE 27-2. CONGENITAL CENTRAL HYPOVENTILATION SYNDROME

Discriminating Features	Consistent Features	Variable Features
1. Shallow respiratory effort during quiet sleep 2. Elevated $PaCO_2$ and reduced PaO_2 3. Decreased respiratory effort when breathing 5% carbon dioxide 4. Exclusion of lung or cardiac disease 5. Exclusion of respiratory muscle weakness and deformities of chest wall or diaphragm	1. Onset: birth to 1 week 2. Central apnea 3. Frequent apneas 4. Failure to thrive 5. Severe apneic episode 6. Risk of sudden death	1. Triggered by upper respiratory infection 2. Severe cyanosis and respiratory acidosis at birth 3. Swallowing and feeding difficulties 4. Cyanosis during feedings rather than sleep 5. Recurrent aspiration pneumonia 6. Generalized hypotonia 7. Stridor

FEATURE TABLE 27–3. APNEA OF INFANCY

Discriminating Features	Consistent Features	Variable Features
1. By exclusion, sepsis 2. Obstructive apnea 3. Apnea, seizures 4. GE reflux	1. Age of onset: 1 week to 1 year 2. Infrequent apneic episodes of greater than 15 to 20 seconds 3. Tracings of respirations showing periodic breathing 4. Short apneas with or without clinical cyanosis 5. Bradycardia during apnea	1. Family history of apnea of infancy 2. Associated upper respiratory infection

On pneumography, the spells show evidence of obstruction as well as central apnea or a "mixed apnea" picture. The obstructed site most often is the pharynx. During most of the spells, the infant makes one or more swallowing efforts. These may coincide with the apneas, although not necessarily. Bradycardia (less than 100 beats per minute) occurs 5 to 10 seconds after the onset of apnea, with cyanosis appearing within 20 seconds. In the absence of spontaneous recovery, gentle stimulation of the infant produces a resumption of ventilation.

Predisposing factors may include neck positioning, hiccups and feeding, infections, anemia, enterocolitis, and cardiopulmonary conditions. Each condition can either cause or exacerbate the condition.

The treatment of apnea of prematurity includes theophylline with a loading dose of 6 mg/kg and maintenance doses of 2 mg/kg every 8 hours. Theophylline levels should be monitored. Generally the lowest level required to maintain the infant free of apnea is recommended. This reduces the risk of potential side effects. Positive pressure airway ventilation may prevent spells in the hospital. Electronic monitoring of respiration at home may be required at the time of discharge, with appropriate parent education.

The long-term prognosis for apnea of prematurity is good, although subsequent neurologic abnormalities have been reported in a higher proportion of these patients, as opposed to other preterm infants.

Congenital Central Hypoventilation Syndrome

Congenital central hypoventilation syndrome (CCHS) is an unusual condition affecting the autonomic control of respiration. Episodic apnea occurs primarily during sleep. Originally described by Mellins and colleagues (1970), this condition is occasionally referred to as Ondine's curse. CCHS is most severe in quiet sleep. Hypoventilation is associated with reduced tidal volume, although in some infants a reduction of respiratory frequency is more prominent. In addition to slow, shallow breathing patterns, episodes of episodic central apnea also occur in quiet sleep and contribute to respiratory insufficiency. Such episodes may be associated with obstructive apnea.

Infants with this condition generally show symptoms at birth or shortly thereafter. Hypoxic seizures may herald the onset of the condition, although the EEG is normal. Life support systems may be needed, as sudden death may occur during sleep. Furthermore, there may be difficulties with swallowing and feeding. These infants may have cyanosis during feeding, rather than during sleep, associated with recurrent aspiration. Cor pulmonale and pulmonary hypertension may ensue and are secondary to chronic decreased ventilation and/or pneumonia. These infants are particularly susceptible to respiratory tract infections and respiratory failure.

Hypoventilation, in the absence of other conditions, is associated with shallow slow respiratory efforts dur-

FEATURE TABLE 27–4. OBSTRUCTIVE APNEA OF INFANCY

Discriminating Features	Consistent Features	Variable Features
1. Intubation or simple airway relieves obstruction while auscultating air flow at neck 2. Cineradiographic evidence of obstruction site	1. Facial or airway deformities from birth 2. Obstructive apnea type, frequent apneic episodes during sleep 3. Positive response to airway pressure or intubation 4. Snoring 5. Polysomnographic evidence of obstructed air flow	1. Mixed apnea type triggered by posture 2. Concurrent or frequent upper respiratory infection 3. Failure to thrive 4. Severe apneic episodes 5. Cor pulmonale

FEATURE TABLE 27–5. FEEDING-ASSOCIATED AND GASTROESOPHAGEAL REFLUX–INDUCED APNEAS OF INFANCY

Discriminating Features	Consistent Features	Variable Features
Feeding-Associated Apnea of Infancy		
1. Cyanosis and apnea early in feeding	1. Occurs during early feeding 2. Cyanosis transient	1. Central mixed or obstructive apnea type 2. Bradycardia
Gastroesophageal Reflux-Induced Apnea of Infancy		
1. pH probe evidence of gastroesophageal reflux	1. Occurs shortly after feeding during sleep or wakefulness 2. May frequently complicate other apneas	1. Vomitus in mouth 2. Radiographic evidence of GE reflux on barium swallow in distal esophagus

ing quiet sleep with elevated $PaCO_2$ and reduced PaO_2. Pneumography may show obstructive as well as central respiratory pauses, but not of sufficient degree to suggest obstructive apnea. If the upper airway obstruction is relieved by intubation and the evidence of hypoventilation persists, then CCHS should be considered. Increased respiratory effort and response to breathing 5% carbon dioxide in air or oxygen is present in obstructive apnea, but absent in CCHS.

Management of CCHS is difficult. All cases have required long-term assisted ventilation during sleep. Tracheostomy with positive pressure or volume ventilation during sleep has been used. Some patients have received the assistance of electrical diaphragmatic pacing. Children who are on ventilators at home require careful supervision. The longest reported survival is 4 years, with most children dying within the first year of life. This condition is generally considered a permanent one, although there are occasional reports of patients who no longer require mechanical ventilation.

Apnea of Infancy

Apnea of infancy (AOI) occurs in term neonates and post-neonatal infants. It is either idiopathic or secondary to a specific cause. The idiopathic variety has been referred to as aborted or near-miss sudden infant death syndrome (SIDS). Affected infants are usually under 1 year of age. Although most episodes occur while the infant is asleep, some episodes may occur during wakefulness or feedings.

In some infants there may be an associated upper respiratory infection. A number of the etiologic agents have been identified in these infants, and include obstructive apnea of infancy (OAOI), gastroesophageal (GE) reflux, and apneic seizures. The manifestations are generally cyanosis or pallor, opisthotonos, or loss of response to stimuli if apnea is prolonged. Such manifestations may also me associated with gasping respiration.

Pneumography and polysomnography have identified alterations in the respiratory pattern of these infants. These include apnea during sleep (apnea defined as respiration absent for more than 15 to 20 seconds). Periodic breathing (brief periods of apnea in chains of at least three) is frequently seen, but its significance is controversial. These infants may show evidence on polysomnography of central obstructive or mixed apnea, which attests to the heterogeneity within this idiopathic variety. Some infants in this category are later found to demonstrate obstructive sleep apnea as well as pallid breath-holding spells. Up to 60% of infants who have had this event will have a repeat episode. The natural history of this condition is of course unknown, but the fact that up to 25% of these infants may die of SIDS attests to the link between this interrupted form of AOI and SIDS.

The laboratory evaluation for AOI should include a complete blood count with differential; measurement of serum electrolytes, urea, and blood gases; electrocardiogram, EEG; chest x ray; and pneumogram.

The management strategy of choice for these infants

FEATURE TABLE 27–6. APNEIC SEIZURES

Discriminating Features	Consistent Features	Variable Features
1. Simultaneous EEG and respiratory monitoring 2. Response to anticonvulsants with EEG patterns consistent with clinical seizures	1. Apnea sole symptom 2. Bradycardia late in episode compared with other apneas	1. Cyanosis may or may not be present 2. Associated meningitis or metabolic cause of seizures

FEATURE TABLE 27-7. SLEEP MYOCLONIC MOVEMENTS

Discriminating Features	Consistent Features	Variable Features
1. Diagnosis of exclusion in otherwise normal neonates 2. Occurring during sleep and associated with normal EEG	1. Confined to neonates 2. Associated with arousal 3. Normal EEG 4. Normal neurologic examination and history 5. Distal myoclonus	1. None

is home apnea monitoring. Parents should be instructed in the use of home monitors, their function and malfunctions, as well as in cardiopulmonary resuscitation.

Obstructive Apnea of Infancy

OAOI is of unknown etiology and has been described in the previous section. Obstructive apnea is of course not uncommon in infants under 6 months of age, although obviously the presenting symptom is apnea rather than hypersomnia. In the very young infant facial defects such as mandibular hypoplasia or choanal atresia or stenosis cause airway narrowing. Snoring is almost universal in infants with this form of sleep apnea. The snoring often has a stridorous quality and can be confused with laryngeal stridor. There may also be an increase of motor activity during sleep or unusual sleeping postures.

The physical examination of these infants should include observation during sleep to note the presence of snoring as well as respiratory effort. The infant's neck may also be slightly flexed to induce or promote obstruction, with observation of respiratory effort. The subsequent placement of a nasal pharyngeal airway with repetition of this manuever should eliminate the obstruction and serve as a useful diagnostic procedure. Other diagnostic considerations and treatment implications have been previously noted.

Feeding-Associated Apnea of Infancy

Burnard (1973) suggested that 50% of normal healthy full-term infants show evidence of apnea as manifested by cyanosis during their first feeding.

Others have demonstrated consistent evidence of mild hypoxia during the initiation of the feeding process.

This alone or in combination with other forms of AOI can produce or exacerbate symptoms.

AOI associated with GE reflux was described by Menon and colleagues (1985). They identified a 17-fold increase in risk of prolonged apnea after the brief period immediately following regurgitation episodes. GE reflux occurs both during wakefulness and during REM sleep. It is generally preceded by a startled facial expression, body rigidity, and coughing. A barium swallow is used widely for diagnosis. However, false positives as well as false negatives limit its usefulness, and the use of the pH probe represents a more sensitive way of establishing a diagnosis of GE reflux. The relationship between GE reflux and AOI is controversial.

A variety of treatment techniques have been used, including thickening feedings, adjusting the amount and time of feedings, and employing a variety of postprandial positions, principally use of an infant seat. Drugs to speed gastric emptying or those increasing lower esophageal tone have also been used.

Apneic Seizures

Apnea associated with epilepsy is a well-known clinical phenomenon. The association of apnea with AOI represents a differential diagnostic consideration. The only manifestation of a seizure in some infants may be apnea.

Coulter (1984) suggests that apnea is variable, lasting from several seconds to more than a minute with or without cyanosis. It is suggested that bradycardia occurs later than in other forms of apnea. Because the interictal EEG may be normal, combined EEG and respiratory monitoring during the spells is necessary to make the diagnosis. If seizures are suspected, an empiric trial of anticonvulsant treatment may be helpful diagnostically and therapeutically.

FEATURE TABLE 27-8. MOVEMENTS OF REM SLEEP

Discriminating Features	Consistent Features	Variable Feature
1. Occur only during REM sleep 2. Recollection of dream sequence	1. None	1. Brought on by fearful or anxious experiences, recent or past

FEATURE TABLE 27-9. NIGHTMARES

Discriminating Features	Consistent Features	Variable Features
1. Fearful dreams 2. Recollection of details of the dreams 3. Occur during REM sleep	1. None	1. None

Other Dyssomnias

Sleep Myoclonic Movements. Sleep myoclonic movements are regarded as brief, involuntary, repetitive, arrhythmic, stereotyped movements that are either focal or generalized. They never last more than 5 seconds and may be only half a second in duration. Such movements differ from shuddering or tremulousness, which have a rhythmic quality. In infants studied by Coulter and Allen (1982), these movements occurred during the early stages of sleep and involved distal parts of the upper extremities. The movements are principally evidenced by rapid flexion of the fingers, wrists, and elbows. Ankle dorsiflexion was also present. These movements differ from the single asymmetric proximal myoclonus seen in adults. Benign sleep myoclonus should be differentiated from myoclonic seizures and benign infantile myoclonus as described by Lombroso and Fejerman (1977), benign familial neonatal seizures as described by Pettit and Fenichel (1980), and the myoclonic jerks of opsoclonus-myoclonus. All may further be confused with auditory reflex myoclonus, the hyperacusis observed in the lipidoses, and the benign sleep myoclonus of neonates. Hypnagogic myoclonus as described by Oswald (1959) consists of single asymmetric proximal myoclonic movements seen on falling asleep. These occur only on falling asleep and are differentiated from benign myoclonic jerks in that the latter occur during sleep arousal states.

In describing REM sleep, investigators have noted active periods of body movement associated with rapid eye movements under closed lids. This type of movement may be confused with myoclonus or clonic seizures. The movements are asymmetric, arrhythmic, and confined to REM sleep. They are therefore associated with rapid eye movement phenomena.

Nightmares. Nightmares are extremely common. These occur during REM sleep. The child is generally awakened by a bad dream and, for a short period after the dream, can recount the experiences of the dream sequence.

Night Terrors (Pavor Nocturnus). In night terrors the child will suddenly sit up in bed and scream. He or she may appear to be focusing on a distant object and is dyspneic, often diaphoretic, and obviously anxious. There is tachycardia and vocalization; the child may be inconsolable for 10 to 20 minutes or even longer. There is generally amnesia for the event. Gastaut and Broughton (1965) recorded seven nocturnal sequences. In all cases, the attack occurred during sudden arousal from stage 4 NREM sleep. These children, unlike normal children, had a relative tachycardia during slow wave sleep and increased cardiac rates during the arousal episodes. The child cannot be wrested from the event; he or she is unaware of the surroundings. Dilatation of the pupils and sweating occur.

Diazepam (5 to 20 mg/day) is the agent of choice in severe cases.

Somniloquy (Sleep Talking). Somniloquy is generally considered to be a phenomenon of the first decade of life. Reimao and Lefevre (1980) suggested that it occurred throughout the childhood years, with half of the children

FEATURE TABLE 27-10. NIGHT TERRORS

Discriminating Features	Consistent Features	Variable Features
1. Amnesia for the episode 2. Occur on arousal from stage 4 NREM sleep on polysomnogram	1. Extreme autonomic activity 2. Tachycardia 3. Dyspnea 4. Diaphoresis 5. Vocalizations 6. Distress and/or anxiety 7. Glassy-eyed staring 8. Inconsolable 9. Amnesia for the event	1. Duration of the attack 2. Degree of inconsolability 3. Fragmentary immediate memory of dream

FEATURE TABLE 27–11. SOMNILOQUY

Discriminating Feature	Consistent Features	Variable Feature
1. Talking associated with sleep arousal state(s) during NREM sleep	1. Usually sounds or short phrases 2. Often relate to recent experiences	1. Associated with somnabulism

in a sample of over 2000 reporting it at least once a year, but less than 10% reporting it every day. It varies between a few scarcely intelligible sounds to full phrases. Rechtschaffen and associates found that the subject matter related often to the immediate preceding experience. It is a myth that sleep talkers reveal their innermost secrets. For the most part, their ramblings are incomprehensible. Sleep talking is associated with emergent sleep stage transitions during NREM sleep.

Somnambulism (Sleep Walking). It has been estimated that up to 15% of all children have sleep walked at least once, and 1% to 6% have shown persistent sleep walking up to four times a week. Characteristically there is body movement, with the child sitting up in bed. The eyes are open, although glassy. Movements are stilted and efforts to communicate with the child are met with garbled speech or single-syllable answers. The duration of the walk may be up to 30 minutes. Preceding the episode, the EEG shows evidence of high-voltage, slow-wave bursts. The majority of incidences occur 1 to 3 hours following sleep onset; they are associated with the transition from stage 3 or 4 NREM sleep to lighter stages, frequently prior to the first REM.

Sleep walking may need to be curbed to protect the sleep walker. Management may include the installation of simple door locks, and sleep walking also responds to treatment with diazepam (5 to 20 mg/day).

Nocturnal Enuresis (Bed Wetting). Bed wetting past the age of four is probably the most common dyssomnic disorder of children; 17% of children between 3 and 15 years of age may show the disorder. Broughton (1968) defined enuresis as occurring generally between the first and third hours after sleep onset, as the child is making

the transition from NREM stage 3 or 4 to the first REM period. This state is associated with tachycardia, tachypnea, decreased skin resistance, and penile erection. Urination usually occurs within 4 minutes after the onset of the episode, in a moment of relatively quiet sleep. Immediately following the episode, children are difficult to awaken. They report that they have not been dreaming and there is amnesia for the episode. Studies suggest that enuretics have higher bladder pressure during stage 4 NREM sleep than do controls, associated with more frequent spontaneous bladder contractions.

Imiprimine is presently the drug of choice in the management of enuresis, owing either to its anticholinergic properties or its stimulant effect on sleep stage patterns. Conditioning therapies using alarms as well as manipulation of liquid intake are also reported to be effective. Recently desmopressin acetate (antidiuretic hormone) nasal spray has been used. It is effective, though expensive to use regularly. It is often used for overnight stays away from home in children refractory to other treatments.

Bruxism. Tooth grinding may occur in up to 50% of children, although it is a prominent habit in fewer than 10%. The cause of bruxism is unknown; it is quite common in the neurologically impaired, but occurs more often in normal children. Bruxism during the day, in contrast to nocturnal bruxism, is believed to occur more as a consequence of psychologic factors. Protective mouth guards or tooth caps may be helpful for control of nocturnal bruxism.

Rocking or Bed Rocking. Children frequently will rock themselves to sleep. This condition appears to occur in neurologically impaired children to a greater extent than

FEATURE TABLE 27–12. SOMNAMBULISM

Discriminating Features	Consistent Features	Variable Features
1. Presence of high-voltage, slow-frequency delta bursts preceding event on EEG (polysomnogram) 2. Arousal from stage 3 or 4 NREM sleep preceding movement	1. Body movement 2. Glassy-eyed appearance, simple movements 3. Difficult to arouse 4. Amnesic for episode 5. Normal EEG	1. Duration of walk 2. Associated somniloquy

FEATURE TABLE 27–13. ENURESIS

Discriminating Features	Consistent Features	Variable Features
1. Enuresis in the absence of urinary tract anomalies 2. Enuresis unassociated with either diabetes mellitus or diabetes insipidus 3. Enuresis occurring during the shift from the deeper stages of NREM sleep to REM sleep on polysomnography	1. Tachycardia, tachypnea 2. Penile erection 3. Decreased skin resistance prior to onset of enuresis 4. Unresponsive during episode 5. Amnesia for episode	1. Frequency of enuretic episodes 2. Age of spontaneous cessation

in other populations. The etiology of this condition is unknown and the condition is generally self-limiting, although it may persist into adolescence or adult life. Occasionally children who engage in severe head banging need to be fitted with protective helmets and to have their beds padded.

Pearls and Perils: Sleep Disorders

1. It is often difficult for children to report hypnagogic hallucinations. The only clue to their existence may be a child's fight against sleepiness.
2. Sleep paralysis and hypnagogic hallucinations are not uncommon in normal children.
3. Parents are often reassured by comparing benign nocturnal movements to the sleep movements frequently witnessed in domestic pets.
4. There is no clear consensus with respect to home apnea monitoring for prematures, term neonates, or older infants who have experienced apnea. The decision ultimately rests with the clinical judgment of the physician. Parental anxiety is an indication for home monitoring.
5. There is likewise no clear consensus with respect to when to discontinue home apnea monitoring. The decision is again based on the clinical judgment of the physician. Parental anxiety is an indication for continued home monitoring.
6. Long-term hypnotic medication should not be given to children except in rare and closely supervised situations.
7. As distressing as night terrors are for parents, they are seldom or completely recalled by the child.
8. Sleep-walking (somnambulism) can be a dangerous event. Although some reactivity is preserved, judgment and a normal sense of danger are impaired.

ANNOTATED BIBLIOGRAPHY

Anders TF, Weinstein P: Sleep and its disorders in infants and children: Review. *Pediatrics* 50:312–324, 1972.
> This is a succinct, but not recent, review of sleep disorders in children.

Guilleminault C: *Sleep and Its Disorders in Children.* Raven Press, 1987.
> This is an extremely complete review of sleep disorders in children.

Thach BT, Bradley T: Sleep apnea in infancy and childhood, *Med Clin North Am* 69:1289–1315, 1985.
> This recent, though not current, reference provides the reader with a general background and overview of sleep apnea disorders in infants and children. It contains 148 references and is well written and readable.

BIBLIOGRAPHY

Anders TF, Guilleminault C: Pathophysiology of sleep disorders in pediatrics. I. Sleep disorders in infancy. *Adv Pediatr* 22:137–150, 1976a.

Anders TF, Guilleminault C: Pathophysiology of sleep disorders in pediatrics. II. Sleep disorders in children. *Adv Pediatr* 22:151–174, 1976b.

Anders TF, Weinstein P: Sleep and its disorders in children: Review. *Pediatrics* 50:312–324, 1972.

Aserinsky E, Kleitman N: Motility cycle in sleeping infants as manifested by ocular and gross body activity. *J Appl Physiol* 8:11–18, 1955.

Broughton RJ: Sleep disorders: Disorders of arousal? *Science* 159:1070–1078, 1968.

Burnard FD: Apnea and cyanosis during feeding in the neonate. *Proc* 8th Singapore/Malaysia *Cong Med* 8:220–222, 1973.

Coulter DL: Partial seizures with apnea and bradycardia. *Arch Neurol* 41:173–174, 1984.

Coulter DL, Allen RJ: Benign neonatal sleep myoclonus. *Arch Neurol* 39:191–192, 1982.

Dement W, Kleitman N: Cyclic variation in EEG during sleep and the relationship to eye movement, body motility and dreaming. *Electroencephalogr Clin Neurol* 9:673–690, 1957.

Dement W, Techtschaffen A, Guleuitch G: A polygraphic study of the narcoleptic sleep attack. *Neurology* 16:18–33, 1966.

Dreyfus-Brisac C, Monod N: Sleep of the premature in full-term neonates—A polygraphic study. *Proc R Soc Med* 58:6–7, 1965.

Gastaut H, Broughton RJ: Clinical and polygraphic study of episodic phenomena during sleep, in Wortis J (ed): *Recent Advances in Biological Psychiatry,* Vol 7. New York, Plenum Press, 1965, p 197–221.

Guilleminault C: *Sleep and Its Disorders in Children.* Raven Press, 1987.

Guilleminault C, Anders TF: The pathophysiology of sleep disorders in pediatrics, part two. *Adv Pediatr* 22:151–174, 1976.

Guilleminault C, Korobkin R, Winkle R: Review of 50 children with obstructive sleep apnea syndrome. *Lung* 159:275–287, 1981.

Lombroso CT, Fejerman N: Benign myoclonus of early infancy. *Ann Neurol* 1:138–143, 1977.

Lozoff B, Wolf AW, Davis NS: Sleep problems seen in pediatric practice. *Pediatrics* 75:477–483, 1985.

Mellins RB, Balfourhn H, Turino GM, Winters RW: Failure of automatic control of ventilation (Ondine's curse) reported of an infant born with this syndrome in review of literature. *Medicine* 49:487–504, 1970.

Menon A, Schefft G, Thach BT: Apnea associated with regurgitation in infants. *J Pediatr* 106:625–629, 1985.

Moore T, Ucko C: Night wakening in early infancy. *Arch Dis Child* 32:333–342, 1957.

Morrison JR, Kujawae E Jr, Storey BA: Causes and treatment of insomnia among adolescents, *Gen School Health* 55:148–150, 1985.

Oswald I: Sudden body jerks on falling asleep. *Brain* 82:92–103, 1959.

Pettit RE, Fenichel GM: Benign familial neonatal seizures. *Arch Neurol* 37:45–48, 1980.

Price VA, Coates TJ, Thoresen CE, Grinstead OA: Prevalence and correlates of poor sleep among adolescents. *Am J Dis Child* 132:583–586, 1978.

Rechtschaffen A, Goodenou D, Shapiro A: Patterns of sleep talking. *Arch Gen Psychiatr* 7:418, 1962.

Reimao RN, Lefevre AB: Prevalence of sleep talking in childhood. *Brain Dev* 2:353–357, 1980.

Yoss RE, Daly D: Criteria for the diagnosis of narcoleptic syndrome. *Proc Staff Meet Mayo Clin* 32:320–328, 1957.

Index of Annotated Literature

Index